TAYLOR'S MANUAL
OF FAMILY MEDICINE

T0200025

TAYLOR'S MANUAL OF FAMILY MEDICINE

Fourth Edition

Editors

Paul M. Paulman, MD, FAAFP

Professor/Predoctoral Director
Assistant Dean for Clinical Skills and Quality
Department of Family Medicine
University of Nebraska Medical Center
Omaha, Nebraska

Audrey A. Paulman, MD, MM, FAAFP

Clinical Professor
Department of Family Medicine
University of Nebraska Medical Center
Omaha, Nebraska

Kimberly J. Jarzynka, MD, FAAFP

Associate Professor/Residency Program Director
Department of Family Medicine
University of Nebraska Medical Center
Omaha, Nebraska

Nathan P. Falk, MD, CAQSM, FAAFP

Department of Family Medicine
University of Nebraska Medical Center
Omaha, Nebraska

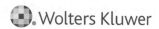
. Wolters Kluwer

Philadelphia · Baltimore · New York · London
Buenos Aires · Hong Kong · Sydney · Tokyo

Executive Editor: Rebecca Gaertner
Senior Product Development Editor: Kristina Oberle
Production Project Manager: David Orzechowski
Marketing Manager: Stephanie Kindlick
Design Coordinator: Teresa Mallon
Senior Manufacturing Coordinator: Beth Welsh
Prepress Vendor: S4Carlisle Publishing Services

4th edition

9 8 7 6 5 4 3 2 1

Printed in China

Library of Congress Cataloging-in-Publication Data
Taylor's manual of family medicine / editors, Paul M. Paulman, Audrey A. Paulman, Kimberly J. Jarzynka, Nathan P. Falk. — Fourth edition.
    p.; cm.
Manual of family medicine
Includes bibliographical references and index.
ISBN 978-1-4963-0068-3 (alk. paper)
    I. Paulman, Paul M., 1953-, editor. II. Paulman, Audrey A., editor. III. Jarzynka, Kimberly, editor.
IV. Falk, Nathan P., editor. V. Title: Manual of family medicine.
    [DNLM: 1. Family Practice—methods—Handbooks. WB 39]
    RC55
    616—dc23

                                                                            2015001706

The editors of **Taylor's Manual of Family Medicine** would like to dedicate this book to our section editors and chapter authors who worked diligently to create a book that will be useful to those who provide primary care for their patients.

Section Editors

Elisabeth L. Backer, MD
Associate Professor
Department of Family Medicine
University of Nebraska Medical Center
Omaha, Nebraska

Jonathan Bassett, MD
Faculty Physician
Eglin Family Medicine Residency
Eglin Air Force Base
Valparaiso, Florida

Christopher W. Bunt, MD, FAAFP
Assistant Professor
Department of Family Medicine
Uniformed Services University of the Health Sciences
Bethesda, Maryland

Timothy J. Coker, MD, FAAFP
Associate Program Director
Ehrling Bergquist Family Medicine Residency
Offutt Air Force Base
Omaha, Nebraska

Courtney Ann Dawley, DO
Faculty Family and Sports Medicine
Travis Family Medicine Residency
Travis Air Force Base
Fairfield, California

Gretchen M. Dickson, MD, MBA
Program Director and Assistant Professor
University of Kansas School of Medicine—Wichita
Family Medicine Residency at Wesley Medical Center
Wichita, Kansas

Ashley J. Falk, MD
Assistant Professor
Department of Family Medicine
University of Nebraska Medical Center
Omaha, Nebraska

Toby D. Free, MD
Assistant Professor
Department of Family Medicine
University of Nebraska Medical Center
Omaha, Nebraska

Kathryn K. Garner, MD
USAF National Capital Region Family Medicine
Residency Staff
Fort Belvoir Community Hospital Simulation Center
Medical Director
Fort Belvoir Community Hospital
Fort Belvoir, Virginia

David Harnisch Sr., MD, FAAFP, FACOG
Associate Professor
Department of Family Medicine
University of Nebraska Medical Center
Omaha, Nebraska

William Henry Hay, MD
Clinical Associate Professor
Department of Family Medicine
University of Nebraska Medical Center
Omaha, Nebraska

Douglas J. Inciarte, MD
Assistant Professor of Family Medicine
Medical Director Oakview Family Medicine
Department of Family Medicine
University of Nebraska Medical Center
Omaha, Nebraska

Rick Kellerman, MD
Professor/Chair
Department of Family and Community Medicine
University of Kansas School of Medicine—Wichita
Wichita, Kansas

Jessica B. Koran-Scholl, PhD
Associate Professor, Director of Behavioral Health
Department of Family Medicine
University of Nebraska Medical Center
Omaha, Nebraska

Shou Ling Leong, MD, FAAFP
Associate Vice-Chair for Education and Predoctoral
Director Professor of Family and Community
Medicine
Penn State College of Medicine
Hershey, Pennsylvania

Michael A. Malone, MD
Assistant Professor Department of Family and
Community Medicine
Penn State College of Medicine
Hershey, Pennsylvania

Jim Medder, MD, MPH
Associate Professor
Department of Family Medicine
University of Nebraska Medical Center
Omaha, Nebraska

Scott E. Moser, MD, FAAFP
Professor, Vice Chair for Education
Department of Family and Community Medicine
University of Kansas School of Medicine—Wichita
Wichita, Kansas

Shawn P. Murdock, MD
Adjunct Assistant Professor
Department of Family Medicine
University of Nebraska Medical Center
Rural Training Track Residency Program
Midlands Family Medicine
North Platte, Nebraska

Laeth Nasir, MBBS
Professor and Chairman
Department of Family Medicine
Creighton University
Omaha, Nebraska

Jason M. Patera, MD
Assistant Professor
Department of Family Medicine
University of Nebraska Medical Center
Omaha, Nebraska

Amber M. Tyler, MD, EMDM
Assistant Professor
Department of Family Medicine
Univesity of Nebraska Medical Center
Omaha, Nebraska

Contributors

Alan M. Adelman, MD, MS
Professor Vice Chair for Research and Academic Affairs
Department of Family and Community Medicine
Penn State College of Medicine
Hershey, Pennsylvania

William A. Alto, MD, MPH
Swedish Cherry Hill Family Medicine Faculty Site Director
Seattle Indian Health Board
Seattle, Washington

Matthew R. Anderson, MD, MS
Assistant Professor
Department of Family & Social Medicine
Montefiore Medical Center/Albert Einstein College of Medicine
Bronx, New York

Ferdinando Andrade, MD
Resident Physician
Department of Family Medicine
University of Nebraska Medical Center
Omaha, Nebraska

Hina Anjum, MD
House Officer III
Department of Family Medicine
University of Nebraska Medical Center
Omaha, Nebraska

Syed M. Atif, MD
Penn State Hershey Family Medicine Residency Program
Penn State Milton S. Hershey Medical Center
Hershey, Pennsylvania

Elisabeth L. Backer, MD
Associate Professor
Department of Family Medicine
University of Nebraska Medical Center
Omaha, Nebraska

Justin M. Bailey, MD, FAAFP
Associate Professor of Clinical Medicine
Department of Family Medicine
University of Washington School of Medicine
Boise, Idaho

Matthew G. Balderston, MD
Resident Physician
Department of Family Medicine
Eglin Air Force Base
Valparaiso, Florida

Sarah M. Balloga, MD
51st Medical Group
Osan Air Base
Republic of Korea

Denise Barnard, MD, FACC
Clinical Professor of Medicine
Division of Cardiovascular Medicine
Advanced Heart Failure Treatment Program UCSD Health Sciences/Sulpizio Cardiovascular Center
University of California, San Diego School of Medicine
La Jolla, California

Matthew Barnes, MD
Assistant Professor
Uniformed Services University
United States Air Force
Bethesda, Maryland

Jonathan Bassett, MD
Faculty Physician
Eglin Family Medicine Residency
Eglin Air Force Base
Valparaiso, Florida

Dennis J. Baumgardner, MD
Clinical Adjunct Professor of Family Medicine
University of Wisconsin School of Medicine and Public Health
Director of Research
Aurora UW Medical Group
Associate Director
Center for Urban Population Health
Milwaukee, Wisconsin

Keely J. Beam, Ed. S
Iowa Area Education Association
Red Oak, Iowa

Jared D. Beck, DO
Family Medicine House Officer
Department of Family Medicine
University of Nebraska Medical Medical Center
Omaha, Nebraska

Marvin Moe Bell, MD, MPH
Clinical Professor
Family and Community Medicine
University of Arizona College of Medicine
Phoenix, Arizona

Jennifer L. Bepko, MD
Faculty
David Grant Family Practice Residency Program
David Grant Medical Center
Travis Air Force Base
Fairfield, California

Kevin J. Berg, MD, FAAFP
Teaching Physician Department of Family Medicine
Family Medicine Residency at Hackensack
UMC Mountainside
Verona, New Jersey

Danish E. Bhatti, MD
Assistant Professor
Department of Neurological Sciencese
University of Nebraska Medical Center
Omaha, Nebraska

Michelle Anne Bholat, MD, MPH
Professor/Executive Vice Chair of Family Medicine
David Geffen School of Medicine at UCLA
Los Angeles, California

Paul A. Botros, MD
PGY II Family and Community Medicine
Penn State Milton S. Hershey Medical Center
Palmyra, Pennsylvania

Rachel Bramson, MD
Associate Professor
Department of Family and Community Medicine
Texas A&M Health Science Center College of
*   Medicine*
Bryan, Texas

Kevin P. Brazill, DO
Resident Physician
The University of Cincinnati/The Christ Hospital
*   Family Medicine & Psychiatry Residency Program*
Cincinnati, Ohio

Daniel E. Brewer, MD
Professor
Department of Family Medicine
University of Tennessee
Knoxville, Tennessee

Dawn Brink-Cymerman, MD
Family Medicine Residency Faculty
St. Joseph's Hospital
Assistant Professor of Medicine
Department of Family Medicine
SUNY Upstate
Syracuse, New York

Gabriel Briscoe, MD
Resident
David Grant Family Practice Residency Program
David Grant Medical Center
Travis Air Force Base
Fairfield, California

Brandon D. Brown, MD
Chief Resident
Family Medicine
Medical University of South Carolina
Charleston, South Carolina

Michael L. Brown, MD
Assistant Professor
Department of Psychiatry
Texas A&M University System Health Science Center
College of Medicine
College Station, Texas

Christopher W. Bunt, MD, FAAFP
Assistant Professor
Department of Family Medicine
Uniformed Services
University of the Health Sciences
Bethesda, Maryland

Bruce M. Bushwick, MD
Chair, Department of Family Medicine
York Hospital, WellSpan Health
Clinical Assistant Professor of Family and Community
*   Medicine*
Pennsylvania State University
Hershey, Pennsylvania

Dustin C. Carpenter, MD
Community Hospital—Fairfax
Mound City Family Medicine
Mound City, Kansas

Marc D. Carrigan, MD
Clinical Assistant Professor
Associate Director Family Medicine Residency
University of Illinois College of Medicine
Peoria, Illinois

Stephanie T. Carter-Henry, MD, MS
Assistant Professor/Education Director
University of Massachusetts Medical School
UMass Memorial Health Care/Hahnemann
*   Family Health Center*
Worcester, Massachusetts

Jacintha S. Cauffield, PharmD, BCPS
Associate Professor of Pharmacy Practice
Lloyd L. Gregory School of Pharmacy
Palm Beach Atlantic University
West Palm Beach, Florida

Jennifer G. Chang, Maj, USAF, MC
Faculty Physician
Ehrling Bergquist Family Medicine Residency
Offutt Air Force Base
Omaha, Nebraska

Linda F. Chang, PharmD, MPH, BCPS
Assistant Dean of Medical Education and Evaluation
Clinical Associate Professor
Department of Medical Education and Evaluation
University of Illinois College of Medicine at Rockford
Rockford, Illinois

Jason Chao, MD
Professor
Department of Family Medicine and Community
*   Health*
Case Western Reserve University
Cleveland, Ohio

Ayesha F. Chaudry, MD
Family Medicine Resident
University of Nebraska Medical Center
Omaha, Nebraska

Anthony M. Cheng, MD
Resident Physician
Department of Family Medicine
Oregon Health & Science University
Portland, Oregon

S. Lindsey Clarke, MD, FAAFP
MUSC AHEC Professor (Greenwood/Family
Medicine)
Self Regional Healthcare
Family Medicine Residency Program
Greenwood, South Carolina

Deborah S. Clements, MD, FAAFP
Nancy and Warren Furey Professor of Community
Medicine
Chair of the Department of Family and Community
Medicine
Northwestern University Feinberg School of Medicine
Chicago, Illinois

Charles W. Coffey, MD, MBA, MPH
Resident Physician
Department of Internal Medicine and Pediatrics
University of Kansas School of Medicine—Wichita
Wichita, Kansas

Timothy J. Coker, MD, FAAFP
Associate Program Director
Ehrling Bergquist Family Medicine Residency
Offutt Air Force Base
Omaha, Nebraska

Brian R. Coleman, MD
Associate Professor
Department of Family Medicine
University of Oklahoma Health Sciences Center
Oklahoma City, Oklahoma

Douglas R. Collins, MD, CTropMed
Adjunct Assistant Professor
Department of Family and Community Medicine
University of Cincinnati
Cincinnati, Ohio

Amy E. Curry, MD
Clinical Assistant Professor
Department of Family and Community Medicine
Associate Director
University of Kansas School of Medicine—Wichita
Family Medince Resdidency Program at Via Christi
Wichita, Kansas

Mel P. Daly, MD
Geriatrician
Gilchrist Greater Living
Geriatric Medicine
Associate Professor of Medicine
Johns Hopkins University, School of Medicine
Baltimore, Maryland

Robert Daro, MD
House Officer
Deparment of Family Medicine
Rural Training Track, University of Nebraska of
Medical Center
Omaha, Nebraska

Marilyn S. Darr, MD, PharmD
Associate Residency Program Director
Clinic Operations
Family Medicine of SW Washington
PeaceHealth Medical group
Vancouver, Washington

Courtney Ann Dawley, DO
Faculty Family and Sports Medicine
Travis Family Medicine Residency
Travis Air Force Base
Fairfield, California

Elizabeth K. Dayton, DO
House Officer III
Department of Family Medicine
University of Nebraska Medical Center
Omaha, Nebraska

Alexei DeCastro, MD
Assistant Professor
CAQ Sports Medicine
Director, MUSC/Trident Family Medicine
Residency Program
MUSC Department of Family Medicine
Medical University of South Carolina
Charleston, South Carolina

Natasha N. Desai, MD
Fellow, Department of Orthopedics
Children's Hospital of Philadelphia and Hospital at
University of Pennsylvania
Philadelphia, Pennsylvania

Urmi A. Desai, MD
Assistant Professor of Medicine
Center for Family and Community Medicine
Columbia University Medical Center
New York, New York

Gretchen M. Dickson, MD, MBA
Program Director and Assistant Professor
University of Kansas School of Medicine—Wichita
Family Medicine Residency at Wesley Medical Center
Wichita, Kansas

Lisa Grill Dodson, MD
Campus Dean
Medical College of Wisconsin—Central Wisconsin
Campus
Wausau, Wisconsin

Philip T. Dooley, MD
Assistant Professor of Family Medicine
Uniformed Services University of the Health Sciences
Eglin Family Medicine Residency
Eglin Air Force Base
Valparaiso, Florida

Patrick T. Dowling, MD, MPH
Professor and Chair
Department of Family Medicine
David Geffen School of Medicine at UCLA
Los Angeles, California

Nancy C. Elder, MD, MSPH
Professor/Director of Research
Department of Family and Community Medicine
University of Cincinnati
Cincinnati, Ohio

Paul Evans, DO, FAAFP, FACOFP
Vice President and Dean
Professor of Family Medicine
Marian University College of Osteopathic Medicine
Indianapolis, Indiana

F. Samuel Faber, MD
Associate Professor
Department of Family and Community Medicine
Penn State Milton S. Hershey Medical Center
Hershey, Pennsylvania

Ashley J. Falk, MD
Assistant Professor
Department of Family Medicine
University of Nebraska Medical Center
Omaha, Nebraska

Nathan P. Falk, MD, CAQSM, FAAFP
Department of Family Medicine
University of Nebraska Medical Center
Omaha, Nebraska

Pierre Fayad, MD, FAHA, FAAN
Professor Residency Program Director
Director, Nebraska Stroke Center
Department of Neurological Sciences
University of Nebraska Medical Center
Omaha, Nebraska

J. Americo M. Fernandes Filho, MD
Associate Professor of Neurology
Department of Neurological Sciences
University of Nebraska Medical Center
Chief, Neurology Section
VA Nebraska-Western Iowa Health Care System
Omaha, Nebraska

Kathryn Helena Filutowski, MD
Department of Family Medicine
University of Nebraska Medical Center
Omaha, Nebraska

Jonathon M. Firnhaber, MD
Associate Professor/Residency Director
Department of Family Medicine
East Carolina University
Greenville, North Carolina

Carey Christiansen Ford, MD
Staff Physician
Urgent Care Center of Richmond Hill
Richmond Hill, Georgia

Peter H. Forman, MD, FAAFP
Assistant Clinical Professor
Department of Family and Community Medicine
Albany Medical Center
Albany, New York

Ryan Frank, MD
Co-Chief Resident, HO III
Department of Family Medicine
University of Nebraska Medical Center
Omaha, Nebraska

Toby D. Free, MD
Assistant Professor
Department of Family Medicine
University of Nebraska Medical Center
Omaha, Nebraska

Jessica-Renee Gamboa, MD
Family Medicine Resident
Department of Family Medicine
David Grant Medical Center
Travis Air Force Base
Fairfield, California

Kathryn K. Garner, MD, USAF
Medical Director
National Capital Region Family Medicine Residency
  Staff
Fort Belvoir Community Hospital Simulation Center
Fort Belvoir Community Hospital
Fort Belvoir, Virginia

Louis Paul Gianutsos, MD, MPH
Program Director
Swedish Family Medicine Residency Cherry Hill
Clinical Associate Professor of Family Medicine
University of Washington
Seattle, Washington

Stephanie A. Gill, MD, MPH
Assistant Professor
Department of Family and Community Medicine
Penn State Milton S. Hershey Medical Center
Hershey, Pennsylvania

John R. Gimpel, DO, MEd
President and CEO
National Board of Osteopathic Medical Examiners
Conshohocken, Pennsylvania

Jeremy Golding, MD
Professor of Family Medicine and OB-GYN
University of Massachusetts Medical School
UMass Memorial Health Care/Hahnemann Family
  Health Center
Worcester, Massachusetts

Kristen H. Goodell, MD
Director for Innovation in Medical Education
Center for Primary Care
Harvard Medical School
Boston, Massachusetts

Mark Duane Goodman, MD
Professor of Family Medicine
Creighton University School of Medicine
Omaha, Nebraska

Mark D. Goodwin, MD, FAAFP
Associate Professor
Department of Family Medicine
University of Nebraska Medical Center
Omaha, Nebraska

Joseph W. Gravel Jr., MD
Professor
Department of Family Medicine & Community Health
University of Massachusetts Medical School
Program Director
Lawrence Family Medicine Residency
Lawrence, Massachusetts

Kevin L. Gray, MD
Eglin AFB Family Medicine Residency
Eglin Air Force Base
Valparaiso, Florida

Richard E. Gray, Capt, USAF, MC
Doctor of Osteopathic Medicine
Family Medicine Faculty
Offutt Air Force Base
University of Nebraska Medical Center Family
  Medicine Residency
Omaha, Nebraska

Samuel N. Grief, MD, FCFP
Associate Professor
Department of Family Medicine
University of Illinois at Chicago
Chicago, Illinois

James E. Hannigan, MD
Oncology
Adventist La Grange Memorial Hospital
La Grange, Illinois

Jimmy H. Hara, MD, FAAFP
Professor and Associate Dean
Charles Drew University College of Medicine
Professor of Clinical Family Medicine
David Geffen School of Medicine at UCLA
Los Angeles, California

David Harnisch Sr., MD, FAAFP, FACOG
Associate Professor
Department of Family Medicine
University of Nebraska Medical Center
Omaha, Nebraska

Wendell M. Harry, MD
Assistant Clinical Professor
UCSF Natividad Family Medicine Residency
  Program
Salinas, California

Fred E. Heidrich, MD, MPH
Clinical Professor of Family Medicine
University of Washington School of Medicine
Family Physician
Group Health Permanente
Seattle, Washington

James J. Helmer Jr., MD, FAAFP
Family, Geriatric, and Hospice & Palliative Medicine
Professor
Department of Family Medicine
UCLA Ventura Family Medicine Residency Program
Ventura, California

Chantell R. Hemsley, MD
Family Medicine Resident Physician
David Grant Medical Center
Travis Air Force Base
Fairfield, California

Michael J. Henehan, DO
Adjunct Clinical Professor
Division of General Medical Disciplines
Stanford University School of Medicine
Stanford, California

Charles E. Henley, DO, MS, MPH, FAAFP, FACOEP
Associate Dean for Clinical Affairs
Marian College of Osteopathic Medicine
Indianapolis, Indiana

Nadine S. Hewamudalige, MD
PGY II Family and Community Medicine
Penn State Milton S. Hershey Medical Center
Palmyra, Pennsylvania

Amy White Hockenbrock, MS, MD
Family Medicine/Sports Medicine Fellow
Department of Family Medicine
O'Connor Hospital of San Jose
Family Medicine Associates of San Jose
San Jose, California

Stephen Horras, MD
Resident
David Grant Family Practice Residency Program
David Grant Medical Center
Travis Air Force Base
Fairfield, California

Alexandria D. Howard, MD
Senior Instructor
Department of Family Medicine & Community
Health
University Hospitals Case Medical Center
Case Western Reserve University School of Medicine
Cleveland, Ohio

Thomas M. Howard, MD
Program Director
Sports Medicine Fellowship
VCU-Fairfax Family Practice
Fairfax, Virginia

Yaowen Eliot Hu, MD
Herndon Family Medicine
Fairfax Family Practice Sports Medicine Fellowship
Team Physician
George Mason University
Fairfax, Virginia

William J. Hueston, MD
Professor of Family Medicine
Senior Associate Dean for Academic Affairs
Medical College of Wisconsin
Milwaukee, Wisconsin

Scott W. Hughes, MD, FAAFP
Associate Professor
Family Medicine Residency
Offutt Air Force Base
Omaha, Nebraska

Daniel G. Hunter-Smith, MD
Program Director
Adventist La Grange Memorial Hospital Family
Medicine Residency
La Grange, Illinois

Douglas J. Inciarte, MD
Assistant Professor of Family Medicine
Medical Director Oakview Family Medicine
Department of Family Medicine
University of Nebraska Medical Center
Omaha, Nebraska

Sumaira Iqbal, MD
Family Medicine Resident PGY3
Department of Family Medicine
Mount Sinai Hospital
Chicago, Illinois

Lena Jafilan, MD
Resident Physician
Department of Family Medicine
Penn State Milton S. Hershey Medical Center
Hershey, Pennsylvania

Charis James, MD, MPH
Resident Physician
Department of Family and Community Medicine
Penn State Milton S. Hershey Medical Center
Hershey, Pennsylvania

James W. Jarvis, MD, FAAFP
Associate Clinical Professor
Director of Family Medicine Residency Program
Chief of Family Medicine Service
Eastern Maine Medical Center
Bangor, Maine

Kimberly J. Jarzynka, MD, FAAFP
Associate Professor/Residency Program Director
Department of Family Medicine
University of Nebraska Medical Center
Omaha, Nebraska

Julie Jeter, MD
Assistant Professor/Clinical Director
Department of Family Medicine
University of Tennessee, Graduate School of
Medicine
Knoxville, Tennessee

Lisa M. Johnson, MD
Assistant Professor
Department of Family Medicine and Rural Health
Florida State University College of Medicine
Tallahassee, Florida

Emily J. Jones, MD
Family Medicine Associates
North Platte, Nebraska

Jeffrey G. Jones, MD, MPH, DTMH
Medical Director
St. Francis TravelWell
Indianapolis, Indiana

Brian N. Julich, MD
Flight Surgeon
United States Air Force Medical Corps
Department of Flight Medicine
Seymour-Johnson Air Force Base
Goldsboro, North Carolina

Brian P. Jundt, MD
House Officer
Department of Family Medicine
University of Nebraska Medical Center
Omaha, Nebraska

Dena M. Jundt, MD
House Officer
Department of Family Medicine
University of Nebraska Medical Center
Omaha, Nebraska

Rahul Kapur, MD
Associate Professor
Family Medicine and Sports Medicine
Department of Family Medicine and Community
Health and Penn Sports Medicine Center
University of Pennsylvania
Philadelphia, Pennsylvania

Daphne J. Karel, MD, FAAFP
AHEC Associate Professor of Family Medicine
Self Regional Family Medicine Residency Program
Greenwood, South Carolina

Neha Kaushik, MD
Penn State College of Medicine
Hershey, Pennsylvania

Rick Kellerman, MD
Professor/Chair
Department of Family and Community Medicine
University of Kansas School of Medicine—Wichita
Wichita, Kansas

Zackary J. Kent, MD
Faculty Physician
Family Medicine Residency
Offutt Air Force Base
Omaha, Nebraska

Sara Shelton Kerley, MD
Major
United States Air Force Medical Corps
Joint Base
Charleston, South Carolina

Birgit Khandalavala, MD
Assistant Professor
Department of Family Medicine
University of Nebraska Medical Center
Omaha, Nebraska

Michael R. King, MD, MPH, FAAFP
Associate Professor
Residency Program Director
Department of Family & Community Medicine
University of Kentucky College of Medicine
Lexington, Kentucky

Mitchell S. King, MD
Clinical Professor
Department of Family and Community Medicine
University of Illinois College of Medicine
Rockford, Illinois

Jeffrey T. Kirchner, DO, FAAFP, AAHIVS
Associate Director
Family Medicine Residency
Lancaster General Hospital
Lancaster, Pennsylvania

Jessica B. Koran-Scholl, PhD
Associate Professor
Director of Behavioral Health
Department of Family Medicine
University of Nebraska Medical Center
Omaha, Nebraska

Kelly Gray Koren, MD
Family Physician
Department of Family Medicine
Fort Belvoir Community Hospital
Fort Belvoir, Virginia

Mindy J. Lacey, MD
Assistant Professor
Department of Family Medicine
University of Nebraska Medical Center
Omaha, Nebraska

Amy E. Lacroix, MD
Associate Professor
Director of Adolescent Medicine
Department of Pediatric Medicine
University of Nebraska Medical Center
Omaha, Nebraska

Valerie B. Laing, MD
Laing Dermatology & Skin Cancer Center
Knightdale, North Carolina

Lars C. Larsen, MD
Professor
Department of Family Medicine
The Brody School of Medicine at East Carolina
  University
Greenville, North Carolina

Kim Edward LeBlanc, MD, PhD, CAQSM, FAAFP, FACSM
Executive Director
Clinical Skills Evaluation Collaboration
Philadelphia, Pennsylvania

Douglas Lewis, MD
Associate Director
University of Kanas School of Medicine—Wichita
Family Medicine Residency at Via Christi
  Medical Center
Assistant Clinical Professor
University of Kanas School of Medicine—Wichita
Department of Family and Community Medicine
Wichita, Kansas

Janet C. Lindemann, MD, MBA
Dean of Medical Student Education
Professor of Family Medicine
University of South Dakota
Sanford School of Medicine
Sioux Falls, South Dakota

Nicholas Longstreet, MD
Resident
David Grant Family Practice Residency Program
David Grant Medical Center
Travis Air Force Base
Fairfield, California

Paul E. Lyons, MD
Professor and Chair
Family Medicine
Senior Associate Dean for Education
University of California, Riverside School of Medicine
Riverside, California

Megan C. Madsen, DO, PGY-3
Chief Resident
Department of Family Medicine
Abington Memorial Hospital
Philadelphia, Pennsylvania

Russell G. Maier, MD
Residency Director
Central Washington Family Medicine
Yakima, Washington
Clinical Professor
Department of Family Medicine
University of Washington School of Medicine
Seattle, Washington

Stella C. Major, MBBS, FRCGP
Associate Professor of Clinical Medicine
Director of Clinical Skills Center & Medicine,
*   Patient and Society II Course*
Weill Cornell Medical College in Qatar
Doha, Qatar
Honorary Senior Lecturer
Department of Primary Care and Social Medicine
Imperial College London
London, England

Robert Mallin, MD
Dean of Medical Education
College of Medicine
American University of Antigua
Coolidge, Antigua West Indies

Michael A. Malone, MD
Assistant Professor
Department of Family and Community Medicine
Penn State College of Medicine
Hershey, Pennsylvania

Laura C. Mayans, MD
Assistant Professor
Department of Family and Community Medicine
University of Kansas School of Medicine—Wichita
Wichita, Kansas

Stephanie Eve Owen McCullough, MD
Faculty Physician
Family Medicine Residency of Idaho
Boise, Idaho

Glenn D. Miller, MD
Clinical Professor of Family Medicine
Department of Family and Community Medicine
University of Illinois College of Medicine at Peoria
Peoria, Illinois

Hilary B. Miller, MD
Department of Family Medicine
University of Nebraska Medical Center
Omaha, Nebraska

Nasser Mohamed, MD
Family Medicine/Primary Care Sports Medicine
University of Connecticut
Farmington, Connecticut

Svetlana Moore, MD
Family Medicine Physician
Family Medicine, Sutter North Medical Group
Yuba City, California

Najib I. Murr, MD
Assistant Professor
Associate Residency Director
Department of Neurological Sciences
University of Nebraska Medical Center
Omaha, Nebraska

Arwa Nasir, MBBS, MSc, MPH
Division Chief of General Pediatrics
Associate Professor of Pediatrics
Department of Pediatrics
University of Nebraska Medical Center
Omaha, Nebraska

Laeth Nasir, MBBS
Professor and Chairman
Department of Family Medicine
Creighton University
Omaha Nebraska

Munima Nasir, MD
Assistant Professor
Department of Family & Community Medicine
Penn State Hershey Medical Center
Hershey, Pennsylvania

Carole V. Nistler, MD
Chair
Department of Family Medicine
Olmsted Medical Center
Rochester, Minnesota

Parminder Nizran, MD
Penn State Hershey Family Medicine Residency
*   Program*
Penn State Milton S. Hershey Medical Center
Hershey, Pennsylvania

Christine O'Dea, MD
Assistant Professor
Director of Global Health Education
The Christ Hospital/University of Cincinnati Family
*   Medicine Residency*
Cincinnati, Ohio

Michael L. O'Dell, MSHA, MD
Professor Chair
Department of Community and
*   Family Medicine*
Faculty
Department of Biomedical and Health Informatics
University of Missouri at Kansas City
Kansas City, Missouri

Michael Ryan Odom, MD
Family Medicine
David Grant Medical Center
Travis Air Force Base
Fairfield, California

Cynthia G. Olsen, MD, CMD
Professor
Department of Family Medicine
Boonshoft School of Medicine
Wright State University
Dayton, Ohio

Josephine K. Olsen, DO
Resident
Eglin Family Medicine Residency
United States Air Force
Ft. Walton Beach, Florida

John J. Olshefski, MD, PGY-3
Family Medicine Residency Clinic
Eglin Air Force Base
Valparaiso, Florida

Alisha E. O'Malley, MD, PGY-2
Department of Family Medicine
University of Nebraska Medical Center
Omaha, Nebraska

Matthew O'Neill, MD
Dayton, Ohio

Cayce Onks, DO, MS
Assistant Professor
Departments of Family & Communinty Medicine
and Orthopedics & Rehabilitation
Penn State Milton S. Hershey Medical Center
Hershey, Pennsylvania

Eugene Orientale Jr., MD
Professor/Program Director
Department of Family Medicine
University of Connecticut Health Center
Farmington, Connecticut

Sean M. Oser, MD, MPH
Assistant Professor
Department of Family & Community Medicine
Penn State College of Medicine
Hershey, Pennsylvania

Tamara K. Oser, MD
Assistant Professor
Department of Family & Community Medicine
Penn State College of Medicine
Hershey, Pennsylvania

Susan M. Ott, MD
Professor of Medicine
Department of Medicine
University of Washington Seattle
Seattle, Washington

Kalpana P. Padala, MD, MS
Geriatrician/Research
Geriatrics Research Education and Clinical Center
(GRECC)
Central Arkansas Veterans Healthcare System
(CAVHS)
Assistant Professor
Department of Geriatrics
University of Arkansas for Medical Sciences
Little Rock, Arkansas

Prasad R. Padala, MD, MS, FACHE
Associate Director, Clinical
Geriatric Research Education and Clinical Center
(GRECC)
Associate Professor of Psychiatry and Geriatrics
North Little Rock, Arkansas

Heather L. Paladine, MD
Assistant Professor of Medicine
Columbia University Medical Center
Center for Family and Community Medicine
New York, New York

Jenny Papazian, MD
Fellow in Cardiovascular Medicine
University of California
San Diego School of Medicine
La Jolla, California

Jennifer Parker, MD, FAAP, FACP
Associate Professor, Program Director
Internal Medicine-Pediatrics
University of Nebraska Medical Center
Omaha, Nebraska

Sarah Parrott, DO
Assistant Professor
Department of Primary Care
College of Osteopathic Medicine
Kansas City University of Medicine and Biosciences
Kansas City, Missouri

Jason M. Patera, MD
Assistant Professor
Department of Family Medicine
University of Nebraska Medical Center
Omaha, Nebraska

Eric M. Pauli, MD
Assistant Professor, Director of Endoscopic Surgery
Department of Surgery
Penn State Hershey Medical Center
Hershey, Pennsylvania

Audrey A. Paulman, MD, MM, FAAFP
Clinical Professor
Department of Family Medicine
University of Nebraska Medical Center
Omaha, Nebraska

Paul M. Paulman, MD, FAAFP
Professor/Predoctoral Director
Assistant Dean for Clinical Skills and Quality
Department of Family Medicine
University of Nebraska Medical Center
Omaha, Nebraska

Rebecca L. Peebles, DO, Capt, USAF, MC
Family Medicine Resident
David Grant Medical Center
Travis Air Force Base, California

Oscar O. Perez Jr., DO, FAAFP
Assistant Clinical Professor
Associate Residency Director
Department of Family and Community Medicine
University of Kentucky College of Medicine
Lexington, Kentucky

Ryan C. Petering, MD
Assistant Professor
Medical Director Sports Medicine
Department of Family Medicine and Orthopedics
Oregon Health & Science University
Portland, Oregon

Elizabeth S. Pietralczyk, MD
Assistant Director
Maternity Care Services
Eglin Air Force Base Family Medicine Residency
Eglin Air Force Base
Valparaiso, Florida

Richard W. Pretorius, MD, MPH
Vice Chair for Medical Student Education
Department of Family Medicine
State University of New York at Buffalo
Buffalo, New York

Bridgette Pudwill, MD
Family Medicine Resident
HOIII University of Nebraska Medical Center
Omaha, Nebraska

George G.A. Pujalte, MD, FACSM
Chief, Sports Medicine
Divisions of Primary Care, and Orthopedics
Mayo Clinic Health System
Waycross, Georgia

Martin A. Quan, MD
Professor of Clinical Family Medicine
Vice Chair for Academic Affairs
Department of Family Medicine
David Geffen School of Medicine at UCLA
Los Angeles, California

Kalyanakrishnan Ramakrishnan, MD
Professor, Department of Family and Preventive
  Medicine
University of Oklahoma Health Sciences Center
Oklahoma City, Oklahoma

Shri Lalitha Rayavarapu, MD
House Officer III
Department of Family Medicine
University of Nebraska Medical Center
Omaha, Nebraska

Joshua J. Raymond, MD, MPH
Assistant Professor
Geriatric Fellowship Director
Department of Family and Community Medicine
Robert Wood Johnson Medical School
Rutgers University
CentraState Family Medicine Residency
Freehold, New Jersey

Colton R. Redding, DO
Resident Physician
Department of Family Medicine
University of Connecticut
Farmington, Connecticut

David Richard, MD, FAAFP
Associate Professor/Clerkship
Director/Medical Director, PA Program
Department of Family and Community Medicine
Penn State College of Medicine
Hershey, Pennsylvania

James P. Richardson, MD, MPH
Chief
Geriatric and Palliative Medicine
St. Agnes Hospital
Clinical Professor of Family Medicine
University of Maryland School of Medicine
Baltimore, Maryland

Mari A. Ricker, MD
Associate Professor
Department of Family and Community Medicine
University of Arizona College of Medicine
Tucson, Arizona

Angela M. Riegel, DO
Faculty Physician
Offutt Family Medicine Residency
Offutt Air Force Base
Omaha, Nebraska

Lyrad K. Riley, MD, FAAFP
Director of Maternity Care Services
Eglin Family Medicine Residency
Eglin Air Force Base
Valparaiso, Florida

Timothy D. Riley, MD
Assistant Professor
Department of Family and Community Medicine
Penn State Milton S. Hershey Medical Center
Hershey, Pennsylvania

Cynthia Rizk, MD
Department of Family & Community Medicine
Penn State Milton S. Hershey Medical Center
Hershey, Pennsylvania

Tessa Rohrberg, MD
Resident Physician
University of Kansas School of Medicine
Wichita Family Medicine Residency Program at
Wesley Medical Center
Wichita, Kansas

Irina Rozin, BSc, MSc
University of Nebraska
Medical Center College of Medicine
Omaha, Nebraska

Payam Sazegar, MD
Clinical Assistant Professor
Department of Family and Community Medicine
University of California—San Francisco
San Francisco, California

Matthew C. Schaffer, MD
Director of Curriculum Development
UPMC St. Margaret Family Medicine Residency
Pittsburgh, Pennsylvania

Ted C. Schaffer, MD
Program Director UPMC St. Margaret
Family Medicine Residency
Pittsburgh, Pennsylvania

L. Peter Schwiebert, MD
Professor
Department of Family and Preventive Medicine
University of Oklahoma Health Sciences Center
Oklahoma City, Oklahoma

Jarrett K. Sell, MD
Assistant Professor
Department of Family and Community Medicine
Penn State Milton S. Hershey Medical Center
Hershey, Pennsylvania

Sanjeev K. Sharma, MD
Associate Professor
Department of Family Medicine
Creighton University School of Medicine
Omaha, Nebraska

John P. Sheehan, MD, FACE
Associate Clinical Professor of Medicine
Case Western Reserve University
Medical Director
North Coast Institute of Diabetes and Endocrinology,
Inc.
Cleveland, Ohio

Ahad Shiraz, MD
Family Medicine Resident-PGY2
Department of Family and Community Medicine
Penn State Milton S. Hershey Medical Center
Hershey, Pennsylvania

Avery L. Sides, MD
Family Medicine Physician
Fall River Health Services
Hot Springs, South Dakota

Manel Silva, MD, MPH
Director of HIV Services
Lutheran Family Health Center
Brooklyn, New York

Sabrina L. Silver, DO
Captain, USAF, MC Family Medicine Residency,
HO III
University of Nebraska Medical Center
Omaha, Nebraska

Kevin C. Sisk, DO
Chief Resident
Department of Family Medicine
University of Nebraska Medical Center
Omaha, Nebraska

Neil S. Skolnik, MD
Professor of Family and Community Medicine
Temple University School of Medicine
Associate Director
Family Medicine Residency Program
Abington Memorial Hospital
Jenkintown, Pennsylvania

Dawn M. Sloan, MD
Staff Family Physician
Kimbrough Ambulatory Care Center
Fort Meade, Maryland

Beth-Erin S. Smith, MD, MPH
Adjunct Assistant Professor
Department of Family Medicine
University of Cincinnati College of Medicine
Cincinnati, Ohio

Charles Kent Smith, MD
Professor of Family Medicine
Senior Associate Dean for Students
Case Western Reserve University School of Medicine
Cleveland, Ohio

John L. Smith, MD
Associate Professor
Department of Family Medicine
University of Nebraska Medical Center
Omaha, Nebraska

Jitendrakumar D. Sodvadiya, MD
Department of Family Medicine
University of Nebraska Medical Center
Omaha, Nebraska

David K. Solondz, MD
Family Medicine & Acupuncture
Providence Medical Group—Cascade
Affiliate Instructor
Oregon Health & Science University
Portland, Oregon

Rhonda A. Sparks, MD
Clinical Professor
Department of Family Medicine
Medical Director
Clinical Skills Education and Testing Center
University of Oklahoma College of Medicine
Oklahoma City, Oklahoma

Anthony J. Strickland, MD
House Officer
Department of Family Medicine
University of Nebraska Medical Center
Omaha, Nebraska

Denise K.C. Sur, MD
Vice Chair for Education
Clinical Professor
Residency Director
Department of Family Medicine
David Geffen School of Medicine at UCLA
Los Angeles, California

Joshua J. Sypal, MD
House Officer
Department of Family Medicine
University of Nebraska Medical Center
Omaha, Nebraska

Abraham R. Taylor, MD
Assistant Professor
Department of Family and Community Medicine
Penn State Milton S. Hershey Medical Center
Hershey, Pennsylvania

Nathan J. Timmer, MD
Family Medicine Physician
Avera Medical Group
Mitchell, South Dakota

William L. Toffler, MD
Professor/Director of Medical Student Education
Department of Family Medicine
Oregon Health & Science University
Portland, Oregon

Diego R. Torres-Russotto, MD
Associate Professor, Department of Neurological
Sciences
Director, UNMC Movement Disorders Program
Medical Director, TNMC Movement Disorders
Center
Director, Movement Disorders Fellowship Program
Director, Neurology Clinical Clerkship
University of Nebraska Medical Center
Omaha, Nebraska

Marc Tunzi, MD, MA
Assistant Director
Family Medicine Residency
Natividad Medical Center
Salinas, California
Clinical Professor
Department of Family and Community Medicine
University of California
San Francisco, California

Amber M. Tyler, MD, EMDM
Assistant Professor
Department of Family Medicine
Univesity of Nebraska Medical Center
Omaha, Nebraska

Margaret M. Ulchaker, MSN, RN, CDE, CNP, NP-C, BC-ADM
Clinical Instructor
School of Nursing
Case Western Reserve University
Endocrine Nurse Practitioner
North Coast Institute of Diabetes and
Endocrinology, Inc.
Cleveland, Ohio

Daniel J. Van Durme, MD, MPH
Professor and Chair
Department of Family Medicine and Rural Health
Florida State University College of Medicine
Tallahassee, Florida

Chelsey Villaneuva, MD
Resident
David Grant Family Practice Residency Program
David Grant Medical Center
Travis Air Force Base
Fairfield, California

Abdul Waheed, MD
Assistant Professor
Department of Family & Community Medicine
Penn State College of Medicine
Penn State Milton S. Hershey Medical Center
Hershey, Pennsylvania

Anne D. Walling, MB, ChB
Professor Associate Dean for Faculty Affairs and
Professional Development
Department of Family and Community Medicine
University of Kansas School of Medicine
Wichita, Kansas

Anne Walsh, PA-C, MMSc, DFAAPA
Instructor of Clinical Family Medicine
Keck School of Medicine
University of Southern California
Los Angeles, California

Kristen Hood Watson, MD
Assistant Professor
Family Medicine Co-Clerkship
Director Department of Family Medicine
Medical University of South Carolina
Charleston, South Carolina

Rebecca Wester, MD
Associate Professor
Department of Family Medicine/Geriatrics
University of Nebraska Medical Center
Omaha, Nebraska

Katrina N. Wherry, MD
Staff Physician
Family Medicine
Family Health Clinic
Joint Base Elmendorf Richardson
Anchorage, Alaska

Sean P. Wherry, MD
Staff Physician
Family Medicine
Family Health Clinic
Joint Base Elmendorf Richardson
Anchorage, Alaska

Brett Wilhoit, MD
Family Medicine Resident
MUSC/Trident Family Medicine Residency Program
MUSC Department of Family Medicine
Medical University of South Carolina
Charleston, South Carolina

Pamela M. Williams, MD
Associate Professor/Program Director
David Grant USAF Medical Center
Family Medicine Residency
Travis Air Force Base
Fairfield, California

Jennifer Wipperman, MD, MPH
Assistant Professor
Department of Family and Community Medicine
Associate Director
University of Kansas School of Medicine
Wichita Family Medicine Residency Program
at Via Christi
Wichita, Kansas

Lei Yu, BM
College of Medicine, Class of 2016
University of Nebraska Medical Center
Omaha, Nebraska

Kent Jian Zhao, MD
Faculty Physician
Clarkson Family Medicine Residency Program
Nebraska Medicine
Omaha, Nebraska

Jay Zimmermann, MD
Assistant Professor
Department of Family and Community Medicine
Penn State Milton S. Hershey Medical Center
Hershey, Pennsylvania

Preface

Taylor's Manual of Family Medicine, Fourth Edition, is designed for the busy practitioner. The manual is a point-of-care reference and is intended to provide timely answers for the most commonly encountered clinical problems in family medicine and primary care.

The editors, authors, and production staff involved with the manual have made every effort to continue the practical style and format first used by Dr. Robert Taylor in the second edition of the manual.

Where appropriate, new chapters have been added, some chapters have been removed, or their content assigned to other pertinent chapters. All chapters in this edition have been updated with the latest clinical information and evidence, including electronic resources.

The content of the manual emphasizes ambulatory care, with references as appropriate for hospital, extended care facility, or home care.

Providers of primary care will also find the content and outline of the manual useful in preparation for certification or recertification examinations.

The hundreds of authors and section editors contributing to this work have done a great job bringing practical, easy-to-understand, clinically useful information to their chapters.

The production staff at Wolters Kluwer have been outstanding partners in this project. The editors offer special thanks to Kristina Oberle, who continues to provide any support necessary to complete this book. We thank you, Kristina.

We hope you find this edition of *Taylor's Manual of Family Medicine* useful and that it is the book you reach for when you have a clinical question in your busy practice.

Paul M. Paulman, MD

Contents

CHAPTER 1

Disease Prevention and Health Promotion

Section Editor: Jim Medder

Health Maintenance Overview

Paul E. Lyons

Family physicians and other primary care providers should follow evidence-based guidelines and customize interventions based on the patient's personal profile or risk assessment (e.g., age, gender, family history, and other indicators of high-risk status).[1] They should also use efficient office systems to monitor and track the effectiveness of preventive interventions and to ensure compliance with recommendations. This chapter focuses on how to do it.

CAUSES OF DEATH

Childhood is the age of unintentional injuries, cancer, and congenital disease, and adolescence the age of unintentional injuries, suicide, and homicide; however, adulthood represents the age of acquired illness. Environment, genetics, health behaviors, and advancing age contribute to a population that will increasingly manifest significant medical conditions. Even for adults a uniform approach is not entirely possible; for those aged 25 to 44, the most common cause of mortality is injuries (including unintentional injuries, homicide, and suicide), followed next by cancer, and then by heart disease. The younger age group represents a generally healthy group of patients with a relatively low risk for the most common chronic diseases, and thus will have considerably fewer screening tests, but because most injuries are preventable, counseling is more important for this age group.

For those older adults aged 45 to 64, cancer is the primary cause of death, followed next by heart disease, and then by unintentional injuries. Deaths in adults aged 65 and older resemble those for the overall population (see Table 1.1-1).[2] As the population ages, however, it seems apparent that those over the age of 65 are not a homogeneous group either. Recognize that the "young elderly" do not always fit the stereotypical profile of a geriatric patient and that the "older elderly" may have additional concerns that do not always apply to their younger peers.

Patients should be viewed as a continuum rather than a series of distinct groups. The age groups are useful for organizational purposes, but must always be interpreted in the context of an individual patient and his or her personal medical story. The specific medical issues of each age group are influenced by the medical conditions of the previous age group and will, in turn, affect the health of patients as they age into the next age group. For this reason, comprehensive care of any given patient requires knowledge of current medical concerns as well as those that have gone before and those that will come, and will require a willingness to help patients to help themselves achieve longer, healthier lives.

HEALTH CARE MAINTENANCE

Primary care physicians often see patients who present for a health maintenance visit, sometimes referred to by patients as a "checkup" or "physical." Health maintenance is an integral component of the care and treatment of patients and one of the most important aspects of responsible health care by family physicians. Counseling and patient education activities, directed at asymptomatic healthy individuals, are as highly valued as the diagnosis and treatment of illnesses.[1]

Table 1.1-1	Causes of Death (2011)		
Rank	**Cause of death**	**Number**	**%**
	All causes	2,512,873	100
1	Diseases of heart	596,339	24
2	Malignant neoplasms	575,313	23
3	Chronic lower respiratory diseases	143,382	6
4	Cerebrovascular diseases	128,931	5
5	Accidents (unintentional injuries)	122,777	5
6	Alzheimer disease	84,691	3
7	Diabetes mellitus	73,282	3
8	Influenza and pneumonia	53,667	2
9	Nephritis and nephrotic syndrome	45,731	2
10	Intentional self-harm (suicide)	38,285	2
11	Septicemia	35,539	1
12	Chronic liver disease and cirrhosis	33,539	1
13	Essential hypertension/renal disease	27,477	1
14	Parkinson disease	23,107	1
15	Pneumonitis, aspiration	18,090	1
	All other causes (residual)	512,723	20

The leading causes of death and disability among adults are largely related to personal health and lifestyle behaviors or the actual causes of death (see Table 1.1-2), and may therefore be preventable through routine health maintenance interventions in the form of counseling, screening, immunizations, and preventive medications.[3] These interventions are best delivered longitudinally as an integral component of the provider–patient contact—whatever the chief complaint—rather than as periodic, annual, or comprehensive physical examinations. As many provider–patient encounters occur only during times of illness or injury, the family physician must be prepared to be "opportunistic" and address health maintenance as a clinical issue whenever "teachable moments" arise, keeping in mind that, ultimately, patients must feel empowered to be responsible for their own health status. A few general guidelines will assist this process:

- **Form a therapeutic alliance with the patient.** All meaningful change will come from the patient. It is the role of the physician to provide the necessary tools for all patients to be as healthy as possible. It is not the physician's role to make the patient change.
- **Listen fully, look carefully, test sparingly.** The history will provide the overwhelming majority of the necessary information. The physical examination will add small but important additional pieces of information. Screening tests have an important but limited role in adult care and should be ordered with careful consideration of their role in patient management.

Table 1.1-2	Actual Causes of Death in Adults (2000)		
Rank	**Cause of death**	**Number**	**%**
1	Tobacco	435,000	18
2–3	Diet/activity patterns	400,000	17
4	Alcohol	85,000	4
5	Microbial agents	75,000	3
6	Toxic agents	55,000	2
7	Motor vehicles	43,000	2
8	Firearms	29,000	1
9	Sexual behavior	20,000	1
10	Illicit use of drugs	17,000	1
	Total	1,159,000	48

- **Counsel patiently.** Behavior change is incremental and slow. Do not assume that the absence of change means the patient did not hear what you said. Repetition, understanding, encouragement, and patience will provide the best results. The family physician's adult patients are assumed to be motivated to protect and improve their health status and capable of being responsible for the maintenance of their health. Adults are motivated by economic issues related to work and family care responsibilities as well as the need for independence and security for their future as retirees.

RISK ASSESSMENT: HISTORY AND PHYSICAL EXAM

The history will help direct the physical examination, screening tests, immunizations, preventive medications, and patient counseling/education. A systematic approach to patients will allow for a structured, thorough, and focused visit that meets the current and future needs of your patients. Each of these visits will begin with the history. This history may be relatively comprehensive if the patient is new or may represent a review and/or update of important interval developments. The past history, social history, and family history are particularly important in the risk assessment.

Besides identifying chronic diseases and medications, including preventive meds, the past history can include a health maintenance section that lists previous screening tests and immunizations. The social history includes important health behaviors, such as physical activity, dietary habits, substance use, etc., but it may also contribute to a broader understanding of the patient (e.g., hobbies, education, family status) and yield information with potentially important implications for the health of the patient (e.g., high-risk occupations, incarceration, travel to endemic disease areas, exercise and diet patterns).

A review of medical conditions that occur in the patient's family allows the physician to develop a broader understanding of health concerns that may arise in the future for the patient. A general family history should encompass three generations: up one generation (parents), down one generation (children, if any), and the index generation (siblings, if any). Basic information in the family history includes age, whether the person is alive or dead, and important medical conditions for each person. For persons who are dead, the age and cause of death should be noted as well as any additional medical conditions that may have been present.

Screening Tests

Screening to detect the presence of asymptomatic disease is an important component of health maintenance and can often be accomplished at any patient visit. Frame[4] developed criteria to consider when selecting a disease and test to use for screening:

- The condition must have a significant effect on the quality and quantity of life.
- Acceptable methods of treatment must be available.
- The condition must have an asymptomatic period during which detection and treatment significantly reduce morbidity and mortality.
- Treatment in the asymptomatic phase must yield a therapeutic result superior to that obtained by delaying treatment until symptoms appear.
- Tests that are acceptable to patients must be available at a reasonable cost to detect the condition in the asymptomatic period.
- The incidence of the condition must be sufficient to justify the cost of screening.
- Test sensitivity, specificity, and positive predictive value are important factors in the selection and evaluation of screening tests. Poor sensitivity or specificity can lead to a high rate of false-positive and false-negative results, both of which carry potentially serious consequences for patients.

Follow-Up of Screened Patients is an Important Adult Health Maintenance Strategy

The single most important factor predicting whether cancer screening is obtained in the office setting may be the incorporation of a routine health maintenance visit in the practice regimen.[5] Screening results must be evaluated and incorporated into the patient record as this information is necessary to identify individuals for needed follow-up testing. Accuracy in testing and reporting of results is an important consideration. Laboratories used to analyze screening tests must adhere to national standards. Potential screening costs and morbidity may become issues for patients in the event of follow-up testing and treatment.

Immunizations[6]

Vaccination against infectious diseases is an important and cost-effective component of health maintenance. Many children and adults have not received the vaccines and toxoids that are indicated to protect them against potentially life-threatening diseases. Office procedures to improve compliance with immunization schedules are recommended and consistent with general office-based strategies to incorporate preventive services.

- Have office staff routinely assess patient's immunization status, making sure that appropriately complete checklists are being used.
- Generate reminders automatically.
- Send reminder postcards.
- Establish standing orders in outpatient and inpatient settings that allow nurses to administer routine immunizations (e.g., annual influenza vaccine).
- Provide patients with materials on vaccine-preventable diseases.
- Provide medical record audit feedback to clinicians on their patients' panel immunization rates.

Preventive Medications

This important component of adult health maintenance, often underutilized, involves the use of medications or supplements prospectively to prevent potential future diseases. Indications (benefits), risks of use and nonuse, dosage, precautions, and possible side effects of preventive medications are basic issues for the family physician in helping patients decide whether or not to adopt a specific intervention as a health maintenance strategy.

Counseling and Patient Education

Adult health maintenance programs should promote lifestyle change by explaining the links between risk factors and health status. Risk factor assessment and counseling with adult patients should help them acquire information, motivation, and skills to adopt and maintain healthy behaviors. Recommended counseling strategies include the following:

- Develop/utilize a therapeutic alliance.
- Counsel all patients.
- Ensure that patients understand the relationship between behavior and health.
- Jointly assess barriers to change.
- Gain patient commitment to change.
- Involve patients in selecting risk factors to change.
- Be creative, flexible, and practical, and use a combination of strategies.
- Design a behavior modification plan.
- Monitor progress through follow-up contact.
- Involve office staff (team approach).

EFFECTIVE PHYSICIAN AND OFFICE-BASED STRATEGIES

The following strategies have been shown to enhance the quality and quantity of health maintenance interventions.[7]

- **Involve the office staff.** A team approach to the delivery of preventive services is highly effective. Nursing and other members of office or clinic staff are often able to communicate with patients very effectively. Examples of specific staff functions include reviewing records to prompt clinicians and patients regarding preventive care, updating patient care flow sheets or computerized records, issuing reminders to patients and clinicians, following up on test results, and helping patients gain access to community resources. All immunizations and many screening activities can be successfully provided by nurses or allied health professionals. The team approach resolves the major barrier physicians face in implementing preventive care and recommendations: lack of time.[8]
- **Incorporate routine documentation tools into your practice.** Use chart-based or electronic medical record (EMR) systems, and include reminder postcards/emails for patients to alert them to the need for specific prevention interventions. Also use patient flow sheets for preventive care (e.g., smoker, due for Td or mammogram), wall charts and posters that inform patients that health maintenance is a practice priority, and prevention prescription pads to allow the clinician to write brief risk-reduction behavioral prescriptions for patients.
- **Facilitate patient adherence.** Make available patient education materials and information regarding community resources to help patients. Patient-held mini-records or direct patient access to their EMR promote increased responsibility among patients for their own health maintenance activities.[9] Patient education materials should also be appropriately directed in terms of the patient's literacy level and other pertinent factors (e.g., older than 60 years, requiring large print, etc.).
- **Establish health maintenance guidelines (standards and objectives) for the practice, and evaluate achievement through audits and continuous quality improvement approaches.** Practice systems to foster adult health maintenance activities can be most effectively evaluated through periodic

reviews of charts or EMRs and specifying other indicators of quality. To obtain or maintain National Commission on Quality Assurance (NCQA) accreditation, health care organizations are now required to conduct such audits, which usually include such indicators as immunization history and various cancer screening tests.

- **Develop minicounseling topics.** Ten preventive topics, 3 to 10 minutes in duration and updated as necessary, can maximize the impact of "teachable moments." The list may include exercise, smoking cessation, stress reduction, injury prevention, discipline and parenting skills, and family health promotion.
- **Reminder or prompting systems.** Generate adherence reminders, either manually or by computer, as a systemized approach to tracking patients in need of routine preventive care.[10]

REFERENCES

1. U.S. Preventive Services Task Force. http://www.uspreventiveservicestaskforce.org/recommendations.htm. Accessed June 5, 2014.
2. Hoyert DL, Xu J. Deaths: leading causes for 2012. *Natl Vital Stat Rep* 62(6):9–10.
3. Mokdad AH, Marks JS, Stroup DF, et al. Actual causes of death in the United States, 2000. *JAMA* 2004;291(10):1238–1245.
4. Frame PS. Health maintenance in clinical practice: strategies and barriers. *Am Fam Physician* 1992;45(3):1192–1200.
5. Ruffin MT, Gorenflo DQ, Woodman B. Predictors of screening for breast, cervical, colorectal, and prostatic cancer among community-based primary care practices. *J Am Board Fam Pract* 2000;13:1–10.
6. Immunization Schedules. Centers for Disease Control and Prevention. http://www.cdc.gov/vaccines/schedules/index.html. Accessed June 2, 2014.
7. Yano EM, Fink A, Hirsch SH, et al. Helping practices reach primary care goals. Lessons from the literature. *Arch Intern Med* 1995;155(11):1146–1156.
8. Strange KC, Fedirko T, Zyzanski SJ, et al. How do family physicians prioritize delivery of multiple preventive services? *J Fam Pract* 1994;38(3):231–237.
9. Krist AH, Woolf SH, Rothemich SF, et al. Interactive preventive health record to enhance delivery of recommended care: a randomized trial. *Ann Fam Med* 2012;10(4):312–319.
10. Frame PS. Computerized health maintenance tracking systems: a clinician's guide to necessary and optional features. A report from the American Cancer Society Advisory Group on Preventive Health Care Reminder Systems. *J Am Board Fam Pract* 1995;8(3):221–229.

Health Maintenance for Infants and Children

Mindy J. Lacey

Health maintenance visits provide the physician with an excellent opportunity to practice preventive medicine and establish an ongoing relationship with the child and his or her family. At each visit, the child should be evaluated for early disease processes, development, and behavioral problems. In addition, the appropriate screening tests, immunizations, anticipatory guidance, and counseling must be provided. A good resource is the book *Bright Futures: Guidelines for Health Supervision of Infants, Children, and Adolescents* from the American Academy of Pediatrics (AAP) and other resources available online at their web site. This chapter covers children from birth to 10 years.[1]

HISTORY AND PHYSICAL EXAMINATION
History

The initial history should address birth history, family history, social history, living environment, allergies, medications, and a complete medical history (including injuries, dietary history, growth, development, and behavioral problems). With each visit the history should be reviewed and updated for any changes.

Physical Examination

The physical examination should be complete with particular attention to those aspects appropriate for the child's age.

Developmental Assessment

The child's developmental level should be assessed at each visit. The Denver Developmental Screening Test is a widely used assessment tool. Table 1.2-1 includes a listing of some developmental highlights that can be used for a rapid and informal developmental screening. Some questionnaires, such as "Ages and Stages Questionnaires," can be purchased and may be used to help evaluate communication, gross motor, fine motor, problem-solving, and personal–social skills of children at different ages.[2]

SCREENING

Table 1.2-2 presents a summary of the screening recommendations outlined below. A listing and schedule of all AAP Recommendations for Preventive Pediatric Health Care is available at the

Table 1.2-1	Developmental Milestones[a]
Age	**Developmental milestones**
2 wk	Lifts head prone
	Follows to midline
	Responds to noise
2 mo	Smiles responsively
	Follows past midline
	Lifts head 45 degrees
4 mo	Grasps rattle
	Rolls over one way
	Laughs
	Squeals
6 mo	Sits briefly without support
	Reaches for objects
	Smiles spontaneously
9 mo	Transfers object from one hand to another
	Stands holding on
	Plays peek-a-boo
	Feeds self a cracker
1 yr	Stands momentarily
	Walks holding on to furniture
	Says mama, dada (now specific)
	Thumb–finger grasp
15 mo	Stands alone
	Walks alone
	Drinks from a cup
	Says three words other than mama, dada
18 mo	Mimics household chores (sweeping)
	Makes tower of two or three cubes
	Indicates wants
2 yr	Points to body parts
	Scribbles
	Handles a spoon well
	Says two-word sentences
	Kicks a ball

[a]These milestones should have been attained by 75% to 90% of children by the age indicated.

Table 1.2-2	Childhood Screening Recommendations

Condition	Recommendation
Congenital diseases	Newborn screening
Growth	Length, weight, and head circumference first 2 yr; BMI percentile starting at age 2 yr
Hypertension	Blood pressure starting at age 3 yr
Hearing	Newborn hearing screen; subjective assessment at all visits
Vision	Red reflex and corneal light reflex during first week of life and at 6 mo; cover–uncover test during first year; and visual acuity starting at 3 yr
Anemia	Age 9–12 mo with hemoglobin/hematocrit
Autism	Surveillance at each visit; ASD screen at age 18 and 24 mo
Tuberculosis	Screening questions; TB skin test if high-risk
Lead	Screening questions 6 mo–6 yr; blood lead test if high-risk
Lipid disorders	Screen all children aged 9–11 yr (and 18–21 yr) and high-risk children over 3 yr with lipid profile

Bright Futures link: http://www.aap.org/en-us/professional-resources/practice-support/Periodicity/Periodicity%20Schedule_FINAL.pdf.

- **Newborn screening.** Every state has its own regulations, and, as such, clinicians should be familiar with their own state's guidelines. Most states screen for at least phenylketonuria (PKU), congenital hypothyroidism, galactosemia, and sickle cell disease. Infants screened for PKU earlier than 24 hours after birth should be screened again before the second week of life. Other commonly screened diseases include congenital adrenal hyperplasia, maple syrup urine disease, homocysteinurea, biotinidase deficiency, and cystic fibrosis.[3] Primary care physicians must be aware that the expanded newborn screen can have up to 3% false-positive results, which can lead to increased parental stress, additional testing, and cost.[4]
- **Growth.** Measuring growth and following its progression over time can help identify significant childhood conditions. Length, weight, and head circumference should be measured at birth, at 2 to 4 weeks, and at 2, 4, 6, 9, 12, 15, 18, and 24 months of age. BMI percentiles should be plotted and calculated annually for all patients aged 2 years and older.[5,6] BMI percentiles between 85 and 95 are classified as overweight, while obesity is in the 95th percentile or greater. Some disease-specific growth charts are available, for example, premature infants and Down syndrome. The United States Preventive Services Task Force[7] (USPSTF) recommends that clinicians screen children aged 6 years and older for obesity and offer or refer them to comprehensive, intensive behavioral interventions to promote improvement in weight status.
- **Blood pressure.** Blood pressure should be measured beginning at 3 years of age during routine office visits. Hypertension in children is defined as persistent blood pressure elevation at or above the 95th percentile based on gender, age, and height tables, while prehypertension is between the 90th and 95th percentiles.[8]
- **Hearing.** All states require universal newborn hearing screening, with both the USPSTF and the AAP supporting that recommendation. The AAP also recommends follow-up periodic hearing screening, including audiometry and subjective assessments of hearing, including checking for a response to noise produced outside an infant's field of vision, noting an absence of babbling at 6 months of age, assessing speech development, and inquiring about parental concerns. These should be performed repeatedly, especially during the first year of life.[1,7]
- **Vision.** All children should be screened for a red reflex (looking for malignancy of the retina) and a symmetrical corneal light reflex (looking for esotropia) during the first week of life and again at 6 months of age. In the first year of life, children should also be screened with the cover–uncover test. At age 3 years, a photo screen is recommended by some groups. The AAP recommends picture tests, such as LH test or Allen cards, at age 3 to 4 years old. AAP also states that children over 4 years old can be screened with Snellen letters, Snellen numbers, and Tumbling E charts.[9]
- **Anemia.** All children should be screened for anemia using either hemoglobin or hematocrit testing at approximately 9 to 12 months of age. Preterm infants and low-birth-weight infants who are fed

with low-iron formulas should be screened by 6 months of age. Children with the following risk factors should have a repeat screening for anemia 6 months after their initial screen: preterm or low-birth-weight infants, breastfed infants who do not receive iron-supplemented foods after 6 months of age, children who consume more than 24 ounces of cow's milk a day after age 12 months, and infants in low-income families.[1]

- **Autism.** AAP recommends surveillance for autism spectrum disorder (ASD) at each visit and routine autism screening at 18 and 24 months. Surveillance factors include a sibling with autism; parental concern, inconsistent hearing, unusual responsiveness; other caregiver concern; and clinician concern. Various ASD screening tools are available.[1]
- **Tuberculosis.** Annual tuberculosis (TB) testing is recommended for children in high-risk populations. High-risk questionnaire with a yes to any of these questions necessitates screening with a tuberculin skin test.[10]
  - Does your child have regular contact with adults who are at high risk for tuberculosis (such as homeless or incarcerated persons, persons with HIV, persons who use illicit drugs)?
  - Has your child had contact with someone infected with tuberculosis?
  - Is your child infected with HIV or other immunosuppressive disorders?
  - Was any household member, including your child, born in an area where TB is common (i.e., Africa, Asia, Latin America, Caribbean)? Or has anyone in your family traveled to one of these areas?
- **Lead.** All children aged 6 months to 6 years should be assessed for risk of lead exposure using a structured questionnaire (see questions below).[1] Any child for whom an answer to any of the questions is yes should be considered high risk and have whole-blood lead level testing. Those with blood levels less than 10 µg per dL should be retested once a year until age 6. Some groups advocate screening all children at 12 months of age. Recommended questions for assessing lead exposure risk (one yes or I don't know is considered positive):
  - Does your child live in or regularly visit a house that was built before 1950 and has peeling or chipping paint?
  - Does your child live in or regularly visit a house built before 1978 with recent, ongoing, or planned renovation or remodeling?
  - Does your child have a brother or sister, housemate, or playmate being followed or treated for lead poisoning (blood lead levels greater than 15 µg per dL)?
  - Does your child live with an adult whose job or hobby involves exposure to lead? (Examples include stained glass work, furniture refinishing, and ceramics.)
  - Does your child live near an active lead smelter, battery recycling plant, or other industry likely to release lead?
- **Lipid disorders.** In 2011, an expert panel sponsored by the United States National Heart, Lung, and Blood Institute (NHLBI) revised the guidelines that were initially developed by the AAP and the National Cholesterol Education Program (NCEP). In these guidelines, universal screening is recommended for children aged 9 to 11 years (and again for adolescents between ages 18 and 21 years), while children at high risk for cardiovascular disease should be screened as early as age 3 years. A high-risk child is one who has a family history of premature cardiovascular disease diagnosed at <55 years old for males (father or brothers) or <65 years for females (mother or sisters), a parent who has a serum cholesterol >240 mg per dL, or the child has risk factors, such as obesity, hypertension, diabetes, cigarette smoking, or moderate or high-risk conditions. The recommended screening is with either nonfasting non-HDL lipid profiles or fasting lipid profiles.[11]
- **Genetics.** Tracing the illnesses suffered by parents, grandparents, and other blood relatives can help the primary care physician predict the disorders to which a child may be at risk and take action to keep the patient and the patient's family healthy. Family history (preferably a three-generation genogram) is the single most important genetic tool.

IMMUNIZATIONS

The Advisory Committee on Immunization Practices (ACIP), the Committee on Infectious Diseases of the American Academy of Pediatrics, and representatives from the American Academy of Family Physicians have worked together to develop the recommended childhood immunization schedule. Recommendations are updated annually and can be found at http://www.cdc.gov/vaccines. The following information is based on 2014 recommendations.[12]

- **Hepatitis B.** All children should be immunized against hepatitis B at birth, 1 to 2, and 6 to 18 months of life. Infants born to mothers positive for hepatitis B surface antigen (HBsAg) should receive hepatitis B vaccine and hepatitis B immune globulin within 12 hours of delivery. Infants born to mothers with unknown HBsAg status should receive hepatitis B vaccine, and mother's blood should be drawn; if positive for HBsAg, then immune globulin should be administered to the infant within 1 week of delivery. All older children and adolescents at high risk for hepatitis B infections should receive a complete series of immunizations.

- **Rotavirus.** This vaccine is available as a live attenuated rotavirus and is given as a liquid by mouth at 2, 4, and 6 months of age. The maximum age for the final dose is 8 months.
- **Diphtheria, tetanus, and pertussis.** All children should be immunized against diphtheria, tetanus, and pertussis (DTaP) at 2, 4, 6, and 15 to 18 months of age (the fourth vaccine can be given any time between 12 and 18 months, provided at least 6 months have passed since the third vaccination). This vaccine contains an acellular pertussis preparation that has fewer side effects than whole-cell pertussis preparations. If a child younger than 7 years has a contraindication to pertussis vaccine, DT should be used.
- *Haemophilus influenzae* **type B.** All children should be immunized against *H. influenzae* type B (Hib) at 2, 4, 6, and 12 to 15 months.
- **Pneumococcal disease.** All children should be immunized with the 13-valent pneumococcal conjugate vaccine (PCV13) at 2, 4, 6, and 12 to 15 months. Children aged 2 years and older who are at increased risk for *Streptococcus pneumoniae* infections (e.g., those with sickle cell disease, cochlear implants, HIV infection, and other immunocompromised or chronic medical conditions) who did not receive PCV13 should be vaccinated according to the high-risk schedule with PCV13 and PPSV23.
- **Poliovirus.** All children should be immunized against polio with the inactivated poliovirus vaccine (IPV) at 2 months, 4 months, 6 to 18 months, and 4 to 6 years of age. To eliminate the risk for vaccine-associated paralytic poliomyelitis, use of an all-IPV schedule is now recommended.
- **Influenza vaccine.** Influenza vaccine is recommended annually for all children aged 6 months and older, especially those with the following risk factors: asthma, cardiac disease, sickle cell disease, HIV, diabetes, and children who are household members of health care workers. Children receiving the inactivated influenza vaccine (IIV) should be given an age-appropriate dose (0.25 mL if aged 6 to 35 months and 0.5 mL if $\geq$3 years). Children $\leq$8 years old who are receiving the vaccination for the first time should receive two doses. Healthy children >2 years old can receive the live attenuated influenza vaccine (LAIV).
- **Measles, mumps, and rubella.** All children should be immunized against measles–mumps–rubella (MMR) at 12 to 15 months and 4 to 6 years of age. For infants aged 6 to 11 months, administer one dose prior to any international travel, and for infants aged 12 months and older, administer two doses prior to departure, with the second dose 4 weeks after the first. MMR is a live attenuated viral vaccine.
- **Varicella.** All children who have no history of varicella infection should be given the varicella zoster vaccine (VZV) at 12 to 18 months of age. It is a live attenuated viral vaccine.
- **Hepatitis A.** All children should be immunized against hepatitis A, with the first dose at 12 months of age and the second dose 6 to 18 months after the first dose.
- **Contraindications to vaccines in general include:** Prior anaphylactic reaction to vaccine or any vaccine component (i.e., egg protein for influenza vaccine), and moderate or severe acute illness. Do not postpone vaccinations for mild illness, which become missed opportunities.[13]

ANTICIPATORY GUIDANCE AND COUNSELING

Providing anticipatory guidance and health education surrounding issues likely to be encountered at specific ages is a cornerstone of the pediatric health maintenance visit. Clinicians should be familiar with common parental questions and be prepared to provide counseling and advice about child development, child behavior, discipline, nutrition, and safety.

- **Dental and oral health.** Dental and oral health counseling should be provided routinely, with referral for a dental visit occurring at 2 to 3 years of age. Parents should be instructed to wipe their infants' gums and teeth with a moist washcloth after each feeding. Once multiple teeth have appeared, parents should brush their infants' teeth daily using a pea-sized amount of toothpaste. To prevent tooth decay, infants should not be permitted to fall asleep with a bottle containing anything other than water. Infants should be encouraged to begin using a cup instead of a bottle at age 1 year. Fluoride supplementation should be administered according to the following guidelines:
  - Infants who are exclusively breastfed and those who live in an area without adequately fluoridated water should receive fluoride supplementation beginning at age 6 months and continuing until approximately age 16 years.
  - Children who live in an area where the local water supply contains less than 0.3 parts per million (ppm) of fluoride should receive 0.25 mg fluoride daily until age 3 years, 0.5 mg fluoride daily from 3 to 6 years, and 1.0 mg daily from 6 to 16 years.

- Children who live in an area where the local water supply contains 0.3 to 0.6 ppm of fluoride require no supplementation until age 3. From age 3 to 6 years, they should receive 0.25 mg fluoride daily, and from age 6 to 16 years, they should receive 0.5 mg daily.
- No fluoride supplementation is required for children living in areas with more than 0.6 ppm of fluoride in the local water supply.[1]
- **Safety.** Age-specific safety counseling should be provided routinely. Among the safety issues to be addressed are the following:
- Sudden infant death syndrome: A sleeping infant should be positioned on his or her back and should not sleep prone.
- Car seats/booster seats: The AAP recommends that infants should be rear facing until 2 years old. Children should transition from a rear-facing seat and use a forward-facing seat with a harness until they reach the maximum weight or height for that seat. The next step is a booster seat, which will make sure the vehicle's lap-and-shoulder belt fits properly. The shoulder belt should lie across the middle of the chest and shoulder, not near the neck or face. The lap belt should fit low and snug on the hips and upper thighs, not across the belly. Most children will need a booster seat until they have reached 4 feet 9 inches tall and are between 8 and 12 years old.[14]
- Use stair and window gates to prevent falls.
- Keep objects that can cause suffocation and choking away from small children.
- Avoid scald burns by reducing the water temperature of hot water heaters to below 120°F.
- Keep medicines and other dangerous substances locked up and in child-resistant containers.
- Always ensure that children wear safety helmets when riding bicycles.
- Smoke alarms should be installed and maintained in the home.
- If a firearm is kept in the home, it should be stored unloaded and locked away, separately from ammunition.

REFERENCES

1. Bright Futures. American Academy of Pediatrics. http://brightfutures.aap.org/. Accessed June 2, 2014.
2. Ages & Stages Questionnaire. Brookes Publishing Company. http://agesandstages.com/. Accessed June 2, 2014.
3. Newborn Screening Information. National Newborn Screening & Global Resource Center. http://genes-r-us.uthscsa.edu/. Accessed June 2, 2014.
4. McCandless S. A primer on expanded newborn screening by tandem mass spectrometry. *Primary Care Clin Office Pract* 2004;3:583–604.
5. Barlow SE; Expert Committee. Expert Committee recommendations regarding the prevention, assessment, and treatment of child and adolescent overweight and obesity: summary report. *Pediatrics* 2007;120(4):S164–S192.
6. Krebs NF, Jacobson MS; American Academy of Pediatrics Committee on Nutrition. Prevention of pediatric overweight and obesity. *Pediatrics* 2003;112(2):424–430.
7. U.S. Preventive Services Task Force. http://www.uspreventiveservicestaskforce.org/Page/Name/recommendations. Accessed January 30, 2015.
8. Spagnolo A, Giussani M, Ambruzzi AM, et al. Focus on prevention, diagnosis and treatment of hypertension in children and adolescents. *Ital J Pediatr* 2013;39:20. doi:10.1186/1824-7288-39-20.
9. Committee on Practice and Ambulatory Medicine, Section on Ophthalmology. American Association of Certified Orthoptists, American Association for Pediatric Ophthalmology and Strabismus, American Academy of Ophthalmology. Eye examination in infants, children, and young adults by pediatricians. *Pediatrics* 2003;111(4, pt 1):902–907.
10. Potter B, Rindfleisch K, Kraus CK. Management of active tuberculosis. *Am Fam Physician* 2005;72(11):2225–2232. http://www.aafp.org/afp/20051201/2225.html. Accessed April 28, 2014.
11. Expert Panel on Integrated Guidelines for Cardiovascular Health and Risk Reduction in Children and Adolescents; National Heart, Lung, and Blood Institute. Expert panel on integrated guidelines for cardiovascular health and risk reduction in children and adolescents: summary report. *Pediatrics* 2011;128(5):S213.
12. Immunization schedules. Centers for Disease Control and Prevention. Retrieved from http://www.cdc.gov/vaccines/schedules/index.html. Accessed June 2, 2014.
13. Chart of contraindications and precautions to commonly used vaccines. Centers for Disease Control and Prevention. Retrieved from http://www.cdc.gov/vaccines/recs/vac-admin/contraindications-vacc.htm. Accessed June 2, 2014.
14. AAP updates recommendation on care seats. American Academy of Pediatrics. http://www.aap.org/en-us/about-the-aap/aap-press-room/pages/AAP-Updates-Recommendation-on-Car-Seats.aspx. Accessed June 2, 2014.

Health Maintenance for Adolescents

Avery L. Sides

The adolescent health care visit is one of the best opportunities to impart preventive medicine, as most adolescents are healthy, and should be conducted yearly as the choices made during adolescence will result in consequences that may persist into adulthood.[1] Three of four adolescents engage in risky behavior, with over 70% of adolescent deaths related to motor vehicle crashes, unintentional injuries, homicide, and suicide.[2-4]

This chapter will cover four elements of the adolescent health care visit; the history and physical, screening, immunizations, and counseling. Special emphasis is placed on screening, as this is the optimal time to diagnose and treat adolescents to promote health. Bright Futures is a national health promotion and disease prevention initiative from the American Academy of Pediatrics (AAP) that addresses children's health needs in the context of family and community and is the basis for most recommendations in this chapter; their web site has many useful downloadable tools and resources.[1] Table 1.3-1 summarizes preventive services discussed in this chapter for those aged 11 to 21 years.

HISTORY AND PHYSICAL EXAMINATION

The history portion of the adolescent exam differs slightly as adolescence is the time to begin allowing the child to take part in their care. It is important to outline the appointment for both the youth and the parent. Interviewing the parent to cover concerns followed by having the parent, friend, and/or partner leave the room to cover other aspects of the history without others present is crucial to proper risk assessment. Many youth may not divulge information in the presence of others. It is important to discuss confidentiality with the patient, so that he or she is assured that what they say will remain confidential.

While discussing sexuality or sexual practices, it is important to normalize this for the patient as well. Providers that appear uncomfortable with this discussion will promote discomfort with the patient. While interacting with the adolescent, providers should display respect for the youth, avoid assumptions, ask specific questions, avoid medical jargon, and listen to responses without interruption. Fostering the provider–patient relationship during adolescence will create a trusting relationship as the patient ages, enhancing health care for the patient.[5]

The health care maintenance visit during adolescence should focus on determining risks, such as obesity, high blood pressure, substance use, cardiovascular disease, and sexually transmitted disease. The exam should be complete with attention paid to signs of abuse or self-inflicted trauma. Laboratory testing or imaging should be based on the individual's risk assessment, history, and physical exam.[6]

SCREENING

- **Obesity and eating disorders.** Adolescents should be questioned about body image and behaviors that may suggest an eating disorder. Excessive weight loss or gain may be a sign of anxiety or depression. Adolescents should be screened for obesity yearly. Obesity is defined as BMI greater than the 95th percentile for age and sex, and overweight is defined as BMI between the 85th and 95th percentiles, while underweight is BMI less than 5% for age and sex.[7] Obese adolescents should be referred to counseling and behavioral interventions to promote improved weight status.[7]
- **Hypertension.** The goals for screening adolescents for hypertension are to identify primary versus secondary hypertension in order to potentially reverse the causes of secondary hypertension, identify those who need antihypertensive treatment, and identify comorbid risk factors in those found to have prehypertension or hypertension.[1,6]

  The 2004 National High Blood Pressure Education Program Working Group definitions are used to classify blood pressure measurements in the United States. Blood pressure percentiles are based upon gender, age, and height. The systolic and diastolic pressures are considered equal, with the higher value determining the blood pressure category.

  Systolic and diastolic blood pressures both below the 90th percentile are considered normal. Prehypertension is defined as systolic and/or diastolic pressures above the 90th percentile but below

Table 1.3-1   Health Care Maintenance for Adolescents Aged 11 to 21 Years

Condition	Recommendation
Screening	
Obesity/eating disorders	BMI, screening questions
Hypertension	Blood pressure
Substance use	Screening questions
Depression/suicide	Screening questions
Abuse (physical, sexual, emotional)	Screening questions
Learning/school problems	Screening questions
Sexual behaviors	Screening questions; STI testing as indicated
HIV	Screen one time ages 15–65 yr with HIV test
Hearing	Screening questions about difficulty understanding and hearing; audiometry if positive
Vision	Once during each age stage (11–14, 15–17, and 18–21) with Snellen chart
Tuberculosis	Screening questions for risk factors; TST if positive
Lipid disorders	Screen everyone between the ages of 9–11 and ages 18–21 and high-risk adolescents ages 12–17 with lipid profile
Anemia	Screening questions about eating habits/menses; hemoglobin/hematocrit if positive
Immunizations	
Influenza	Annually
Tetanus–diphtheria–pertussis	Tdap ages 11–12
Human Papillomavirus	Ages 11–12 (three-dose series)
Meningococcus	Ages 11–12; booster ages 16–18
Catch-up and high-risk conditions	Assess at each visit
Counseling	
Dietary habits, obesity, eating disorders, regular exercise, strengthening exercises, screen time, tobacco, alcohol, drug use, sexual behaviors, contraception, injuries (helmets & seat belts), hearing loss, bullying/online activities, skin protection, and dental health	Periodically

the 95th percentile or exceeding 120/80. If either the systolic and/or the diastolic pressure is over the 95th percentile, the patient is considered hypertensive. Hypertension is further delineated into stage I (mild) or stage II (severe). Stage I is defined as systolic and/or diastolic pressures between the 95th percentile and 5 mmHg above the 99th percentile. Stage II is defined as systolic and/or diastolic pressures 5 mmHg above the 99th percentile.[8]

Secondary hypertension is more likely in adolescents that are prepubertal, those with stage II hypertension, or those with diastolic and/or nocturnal hypertension, which can be detected with ambulatory blood pressure monitoring. On the other hand, those more likely to have primary hypertension are postpubertal, have mild or stage I hypertension, are overweight, or have a significant family history of hypertension.[8] Most adolescents, especially those likely to have secondary hypertension, may need to be referred to a specialist with experience in childhood hypertension or a pediatric nephrologist.

- **Substance use.** Adolescent youth should be asked about tobacco, drinking, or illicit drug use. If there is a positive response to questions regarding adolescent drug use, screening tools, such as the CRAFFT questionnaire found in Bright Futures documents, should be used for further evaluation.[1]
- **Depression.** Adolescence is a critical period for the development of depressive disorders; however, depression can be seen even in younger children. Depression occurs in 2.8% of children younger than 13 and in 5.6% of adolescents aged 13 to 18.[6] The AAP recommends asking each youth directly

about depression and suicide. There are a few tools that can be used by primary care physicians to screen for depression, including PHQ-2/PHQ-9, the Beck Depression Inventory, Reynolds Adolescent Depression Screen, and Mood and Feelings Questionnaire. The depression tools listed are a good start for screening, but results should be interpreted along with other information, such as that from parents or guardian.

- **Suicide.** Suicide is the third leading cause of death in children and adolescents. Suicidal ideation can occur in the prepubertal ages, although attempts and completions are rare.[2] Increasing attempts and completion rates occur with increasing age. Female youth are more likely to have suicidal ideations, a specific plan, as well as attempts; however, males are more likely to complete suicide. Risk factors for suicidal behavior in children include psychiatric disorders, previous attempts, family history of mood disorders or suicidal behavior, history of physical or sexual abuse, and exposure to violence. Other questions to ask include potentiating factors, such as access to means, alcohol or drug use, exposure to suicide, social stress or isolation, as well as emotional or cognitive factors. Although potentiating factors do not contribute to suicide directly, they interact with risk factors, leading to more risky behaviors.[9–11]

- **Physical, sexual, emotional abuse.** Abuse is prevalent in the United States, with violence as a major cause of death and disability for American children. Victims and witnesses to abuse have both physical and psychiatric sequelae.[12]

    Although school remains one of the safest places for youth, it is clear that violence is everywhere.[11] Primary prevention is key for providers seeing youth in their practice, and they should screen for violence and other risk factors during all wellness exams.[13] Risk factors for violence or violence-related injuries include previous history of fighting or violence-related injury, access to firearms, alcohol and drug use, gang involvement, and exposure to domestic violence, child abuse, media violence, and violent discipline. If a youth discloses abuse during the encounter, ensure safety for the youth and report all cases of child abuse.[4,11]

    Screening for violence includes both a family assessment and an environmental assessment. Youth should be asked about family function, stress or coping mechanisms, and support systems. Environmental assessment includes screening for access to weapons, namely guns. Youth should be asked about school performance, as abrupt decline may be a sign of bullying, depression, abuse, or family stresses.[4,11,14]

- **Learning or school problems.** Learning disorders are not uncommon among children. Risk factors for developmental disorders include poverty, male sex, presence of smoke, being adopted, and having a two-parent stepfamily or other family structure. Adolescent youth should be asked about difficulties at school, including academic performance and interactions with peers, with further evaluation for diagnosis and treatment for those at risk.

- **Sexual behavior.** Middle adolescence (ages 14 to 17) is characterized by increasing sexual interests. The average age of coitus initiation in America is 16. As adolescents age, there are higher rates of sexual activity as well as higher rates of sexually transmitted disease acquisition. Nearly half of new sexually transmitted infections are diagnosed in individuals between the ages of 15 and 25.

    To counsel youth effectively, it is important to discuss their sexual orientation (physical and/or emotional attraction to the same and/or opposite gender) and gender identity (person's private sense or subjective experience of their own gender, generally described as one's private sense of being a man or a woman). It is important not to assume individuals are heterosexual; as many as 10% of adolescent females and 6% of adolescent males report sexual encounters with the same sex.[15] Knowing gender identity and sexual orientation will allow the provider to appropriately counsel the individual about safe sexual practices and refer individuals who are struggling with their gender identity and sexual orientation to resources for support.

    The AAP stated, in a published statement in 2004, that as the social norm is to be heterosexual, lesbian, gay, bisexual, transgender, or questioning (LGBTQ) teens may feel "abnormal." Providers should also be aware of how reactions to "coming out" will affect LGBTQ youth, especially negative parental reactions. Without proper support and guidance, LGBTQ youth have increased risk of personal violence, mental health issues, substance abuse issues, and risky sexual behaviors. Providers should help all youth sort through feelings and behaviors, helping them remain healthy and promote positive expressions of their sexuality.[9,10,16–18]

    All youth should be asked specific questions regarding their sexual behavior and be assessed for risks of sexually transmitted infections. Youth may answer "no" to the question of current sexual activity, as they may not perceive oral, anal, or current vaginal intercourse as "being sexually active."[19] It is important to ask about the most recent activity, recent partners, total number of partners, condom use, and contraception use for themselves or their partner.

One should differentiate condom use as sexually transmitted infection prevention from its use as a birth control method to increase compliance for youth using another form of birth control.[20] When asking about birth control, it is important to ask about difficulty with continuation, concerns, and side effects as half of the unintended pregnancies in this age group are due to issues with adherence with birth control.[20] It is also important to ask when a patient may want to conceive.[21] Discussing these aspects of sexuality will promote discussion and patient autonomy.

Youth that are sexually active should be screened for sexually transmitted infections, including chlamydia and gonorrhea, as well as HIV and syphilis per the Bright Futures recommendations. The United States Preventive Services Task Force (USPSTF) recommends one-time universal HIV screening in the 15- to 65-year-old age group.[6] One should also consider screening for trichomoniasis as well as hepatitis. Infections with chlamydia, trichomoniasis, and HPV make up 90% of infections in the adolescent age group.[22–24] The USPSTF recommendations for Pap smear testing now recommend delaying Pap smears until the age of 21.[6]

- **Hearing.** Adolescents should be questioned about difficulty understanding and hearing in a variety of environments at each annual visit. If a patient indicates a positive response, the patient should be referred for audiometry and appropriate follow-up.[1]
- **Vision.** Bright Futures recommends a vision test once in early (ages 11 to 14), once in middle (ages 15 to 17), and once in late (ages 18 to 21) adolescence. In years that the individual does not require vision testing, the adolescent should be asked questions regarding vision difficulties.[1]
- **Tuberculosis.** Screening for tuberculosis is indicated only in children at risk for latent tuberculosis infection or progression of a latent infection. In the absence of risk factors, testing is not indicated. There is no indication for routine testing in children entering daycare, school, or attending camps.[25] The AAP advises risk assessment for tuberculosis at the first visit to establish care and annually.[1] Risk factors for tuberculosis include living in an endemic region, another person in the household with a positive tuberculin skin test, and reactivation due to immunosuppressive condition or medications.[25]

  Tuberculin skin test (TST) is recommended for screening. Those tested should undergo a thorough history and physical for signs of disseminated disease. Testing early after an exposure may result in a false negative TST or interferon-γ release assay. If initial testing is negative, repeat testing is indicated at 8 to 12 weeks after exposure to the infected individual.[25]

  Immigrants should be tested 8 to 12 weeks after immigration, although if high risk, immediate testing may be indicated. Immigrants may have a false negative and should be retested between in 3 to 6 months. A positive test in these individuals is considered a TST over 10 mm.[26]

  Those who have received the Bacille Calmette–Guerin (BCG) vaccination may have a positive TST. The interferon-γ release assay may be used to distinguish between latent tuberculosis, in which the assay will be positive, and BCG vaccination, in which the test will be negative.[26]
- **Hyperlipidemia.** Bright Futures currently recommends universal screening of LDL, HDL, and triglycerides during the late adolescent (ages 18 to 21) exam.[1] NHLBI recommends universal screening in early adolescence (ages 9 to 11) and again in late adolescence (18 to 21), with selective screening between the ages of 3 to 8 and 12 to 17 for those at high risk based on positive family history or presence of high-risk conditions.[27] The USPSTF does not recommend universal pediatric screening.[6] Nonfasting non–HDL-C is the recommended laboratory test, but Bright Futures recommends a full fasting lipid profile.[1,27]

  Risk factors for dyslipidemia include significant smoke exposure, premature family history of coronary artery disease, parental history of dyslipidemia or total cholesterol over 240, obesity, or childhood hypertension. Certain pediatric diseases or conditions are associated with atherosclerosis and should be assessed as well, including diabetes type 1 and 2, chronic kidney disease, cardiac transplant recipients, Kawasaki disease, chronic inflammatory diseases, cancer survivors, as well as being homozygous or heterozygous for familial hypercholesterolemia.[1,27]
- **Anemia.** Adolescents should be screened for risk of anemia by asking about their eating habits, including vegan and vegetarian patterns, as well as menstruation patterns to assess those at risk.[1]

IMMUNIZATIONS[28]

Adolescents should have their immunizations reviewed at every wellness exam and as necessary. Students that are beginning college or youth in a detention facility should be reviewed carefully. At age 11 to 12 years (or later for catch-up), they should receive:

- Annual influenza vaccine (all ages)
- Tetanus, diphtheria, acellular pertussis (Tdap)
- Human papillomavirus vaccine (three-dose series)
- Meningococcal vaccine with booster at age 16 to 18

The following are recommended if not previously given (catch-up):

- Hepatitis B
- Inactivated poliovirus
- Measles, mumps, and rubella
- Varicella
- Hepatitis A

The following should be provided for specific high-risk populations:

- Pneumococcus (PCV13/PPSV23)
- Hepatitis A

ANTICIPATORY GUIDANCE (COUNSELING) FOR ADOLESCENTS

Bright Futures recommends that the following be discussed at wellness exams. Providers may not have enough time to discuss each point at every exam, so the topics may be covered over the course of multiple wellness exams. It is also important to discuss the needs of the changing adolescent with parents at least once during early, middle, and late adolescence. Topics for discussion include:

- Healthy dietary habits with discussion about healthy weight, obesity, eating disorders, and appropriate weight loss behaviors[7];
- Participating in regular exercise, including 60 minutes of exercise most days of the week, strengthening exercises, and limiting screen time to 2 hours daily[27];
- Abstinence from tobacco, alcohol, and other illicit substances, including anabolic steroids;
- Responsible sexual behaviors, including abstinence or proper protection and contraception[29–31];
- Use of bicycle and motorcycle helmets as well as car seat belts;
- Hearing loss prevention; wearing hearing protection regularly[6];
- Discussion on bullying and how to deal with bullying[32];
- Refraining from online behaviors that may have negative consequences, including online relationships with strangers, sharing personal information online, or engaging in "sexting"[33,34];
- Using UV protection.
    The USPSTF recommends counseling children, adolescents, and young adults aged 10 to 24 years who have fair skin to minimize their exposure to ultraviolet radiation.[35] Individuals at increased risk of melanoma and individuals highly exposed to sunlight should apply a broad-spectrum sunscreen with an SPF of 15 or higher daily and thoroughly before going out. Because of inconsistent application, the American Academy of Dermatology recommends the use of a sunscreen with an **SPF of at least 30** during sun exposure.[35]
- Routine dental care, including daily brushing/flossing and periodic dental visits.

CONCLUSION

The adolescent health care maintenance visit is an opportunity for evaluation of risks but also the adolescent's strengths.[36] This chapter covered history and physical examination of the adolescent, screening, immunizations, and anticipatory guidance for the adolescent. The goal during the exam is to promote a healthy lifestyle and healthy choices.[37]

REFERENCES

1. Bright Futures. American Academy of Pediatrics. http://brightfutures.aap.org/. Accessed March 2, 2014.
2. National Center for Chronic Disease Prevention and Health Promotion (CDC). Healthy youth. Publications and links. 2006. http://www.cdc.gov/HealthyYouth/publications/index.htm. Accessed March 2, 2014.
3. Eaton DK, Kann L, Kinchen S, et al. Youth risk behavior surveillance—United States, 2011. *MMWR Surveill Summ* 2012;61(4):1–162.
4. Henry-Reid LM, O'Connor KG, Klein JD, et al. Current pediatrician practices in identifying high-risk behaviors of adolescents. *Pediatrics* 2010;125(4):e741–e747.
5. Tylee A, Haller DM, Graham T, et al. Youth-friendly primary-care services: how are we doing and what more needs to be done? *Lancet* 2007;369:1565–1573.
6. Child and Adolescent Guidelines. United States Preventive Task Force. http://www.uspreventiveservices taskforce.org/tfchildcat.htm. Accessed March 4, 2014.
7. Barton M; for U.S. Preventive Services Task Force. Screening for obesity in children and adolescents: U.S. Preventive Services Task Force recommendation statement. *Pediatrics* 2010;125(2):e396–e418.
8. Luma G, Spiotta R. Hypertension in children and adolescents. *Am Fam Physician* 2006;73(9):1558–1568.
9. Hatzenbuehler ML. The social environment and suicide attempts in lesbian, gay, and bisexual youth. *Pediatrics* 2011;127(5):896–903.

10. Eisenberg ME, Resnick MD. Suicidality among gay, lesbian and bisexual youth: the role of protective factors. *J Adolesc Health* 2006;39(5):662–668.

11. Turner CF, Ku L, Rogers SM, et al. Adolescent sexual behavior, drug use, and violence: increased reporting with computer survey technology. *Science* 1998;280:867–873.

12. Family Planning. Healthy People 2020. http://healthypeople.gov/2020/topicsobjectives2020/overview .aspx?topicid=13. Accessed March 1, 2014.

13. Miller E, Decker MR, Raj A, et al. Intimate partner violence and health care-seeking patterns among female users of urban adolescent clinics. *Matern Child Health J* 2010;14(4):910–917.

14. Strasburger VC, Jordan AB, Donnerstein E. Health effects of media on children and adolescents. *Pediatrics* 2010;125(4):756–767.

15. Pathela P, Schillinger JA. Sexual behaviors and sexual violence: adolescents with opposite-, same-, or both-sex partners. *Pediatrics* 2010;126(5):879–886.

16. Committee on Adolescence. Office-based care for lesbian, gay, bisexual, transgender, and questioning youth. *Pediatrics* 2013;132(1):198–203.

17. McCabe J, Brewster KL, Tillman KH. Patterns and correlates of same-sex sexual activity among U.S. teenagers and young adults. *Perspect Sex Reprod Health* 2011;43(3):142–150.

18. The health of lesbian, gay, bisexual, and transgender people: building a foundation for better understanding. Committee on Lesbian, Gay, Bisexual, and Transgender Health Issues and Research Gaps and Opportunities, Board on the Health of Select Populations, Institute of Medicine of the National Academies. http://www.iom.edu/Reports/2011/The-Health-of-Lesbian-Gay-Bisexual-and-Transgender-People .aspx. Accessed June 20, 2014.

19. Bleakley A, Hennessy M, Fishbein M, et al. How sources of sexual information relate to adolescents' beliefs about sex. *Am J Health Behav* 2009;33(1):37–48.

20. Frost JJ, Darroch JE. Factors associated with contraceptive choice and inconsistent method use, United States, 2004. *Perspect Sex Reprod Health* 2008;40(2):94–104.

21. National Campaign to Prevent Teen and Unplanned Pregnancy. Sex and tech: results from a survey of teens and young adults. 2008. http://thenationalcampaign.org/resource/sex-and-tech. Accessed June 20, 2014.

22. Weinstock H, Berman S, Cates W Jr. Sexually transmitted diseases among American youth: incidence and prevalence estimates, 2000. *Perspect Sex Reprod Health* 2004;36(1):6–10.

23. Forhan SE, Gottlieb SL, Sternberg MR, et al. Prevalence of sexually transmitted infections among female adolescents aged 14 to 19 in the United States. *Pediatrics* 2009;124(6):1505–1512.

24. Kann L, Olsen EO, McManus T, et al. Sexual identity, sex of sexual contacts, and health-risk behaviors among students in grades 9–12—youth risk behavior surveillance, selected sites, United States, 2001–2009. *MMWR Surveill Summ* 2011;60(7):1–133.

25. Perez-Velez CM. Pediatric tuberculosis: new guidelines and recommendations. *Pediatrics* 2012;24(3):319–328.

26. Cruz AT, Starke JR. Treatment of tuberculosis in children. Expert review article. *Infect Ther* 2008;6(6):939–957.

27. Expert Panel on Integrated Guidelines for Cardiovascular Health and Risk Reduction in Children and Adolescents; National Heart, Lung, and Blood Institute. Expert panel on integrated guidelines for cardiovascular health and risk reduction in children and adolescents: summary report. *Pediatrics* 2011;128(5):S213–S256.

28. Immunization schedules. Centers for Disease Control and Prevention. http://www.cdc.gov/vaccines/ schedules/index.html. Accessed June 2, 2014.

29. Sexually Transmitted Diseases. Healthy People 2020. http://healthypeople.gov/2020/topicsobjectives 2020/overview.aspx?topicid=37. Accessed March 1, 2014.

30. Ogle S, Glasier A, Riley SC. Communication between parents and their children about sexual health. *Contraception* 2008;77(4):283–288.

31. Chandra A, Mosher WD, Copen C, et al. Sexual behavior, sexual attraction, and sexual identity in the United States: data from the 2006–2008 National Survey of Family Growth. *Natl Health Stat Report* 2011;(36):1–36.

32. Rideout VJ, Foehr UG, Roberts DF. *Generation M2: media in the lives of 8- to 18-year-olds*. Menlo Park, CA: Kaiser Family Foundation; 2010.

33. Braun-Courville DK, Rojas M. Exposure to sexually explicit web sites and adolescent sexual attitudes and behaviors. *J Adolesc Health* 2009;45(2):156–162.

34. Council on Communications and Media, American Academy of Pediatrics. Policy statement—sexuality, contraception, and the media. *Pediatrics* 2010;126(3):576–582.

35. de Maleissye MF, Beauchet A, Saiag P, et al. Sunscreen use and melanocytic nevi in children: a systematic review. *Pediatr Dermatol* 2013;30(1):51–59.

36. Adolescent Health Updated Editorial Board. Use a strengths-based approach to adolescent preventive care. *AAP News* 2009;30:13.

37. Adolescent friendly health services: an agenda for change. The World Health Organization 2004. www .who.int/child_adolescent_health/documents/fch_cah_02_14/en/index.html. Accessed March 4, 2014.

1.4 Health Maintenance for the Adult Patient

Paul E. Lyons

The recommendations in this chapter are primarily based on the findings of the U.S. Preventive Services Task Force (USPSTF)[1] and the Commission on Health of the Public and Science (CHPS) of the American Academy of Family Physicians (AAFP).[2] Recommendations listed in Table 1.4-1 summarize preventive services for adults aged 19 to 64 years.

SCREENING

- **Obesity.** All adults should be screened for obesity at each visit by measuring weight and height and calculating BMI. A BMI of 30 or greater is defined as obese, while BMI between 25 and 30 is

TABLE 1.4-1	Health Care Maintenance for Adults Aged 19 to 64 Years
Condition	**Screening recommendation**
Obesity	BMI at each visit
Hypertension	BP every 1–2 yr
Tobacco use	Screening questions
Alcohol misuse	Screening questions
Depression	Screening questions
Intimate partner violence	Women of childbearing age
Chlamydia	Sexually active women aged 24 and younger
Hepatitis C	One time if born between 1945 and 1965
HIV	One time for ages 15–65 yr
Lipid disorder	Fasting lipid profile for men aged 35 and older every 5 yr
Cervical cancer	Women aged 21–65 with Pap smear every 3 yr or at ages 30–65 every 5 yr with cytology and HPV testing
Breast cancer	Women aged 50–74 with mammogram every 2 yr; screening before age 50 should be individualized
Colorectal cancer	Ages 50–75; colonoscopy every 10 yr or FOBT annually
Immunizations	
Influenza	Annually
Tetanus–diphtheria–pertussis	Td every 10 yr; substitute one time with Tdap
Varicella	Without prior immunity or exposure; two doses
Human papillomavirus	Women aged 19–26; men aged 19–21; three doses
Zoster	One time at age 60 or older
Measles–mumps–rubella	Born after 1956 and lack immunity; one or two doses
High-risk conditions	Assess at each visit
Preventive Medications	
Cardiovascular disease	Assess 10-yr risk of CVD every 4–6 yr for ages 40–75 to determine preventive benefit of statin therapy
Cardiovascular disease	Aspirin for men aged 45–79 and women aged 55–79 when potential benefit outweighs potential harm
Neural tube defects	Folate (0.4 mg) for women planning or capable of pregnancy
Counseling	
Nutrition, physical activity, smoking, alcohol and drugs, sexual behavior, HIV exposure, family planning, injuries, skin cancer, and dental health	Periodically

identified as overweight. Obese patients should be referred to intensive, multicomponent behavioral interventions.

- **Hypertension.** Blood pressure readings should be obtained at every office visit and at least once every 2 years.
- **Tobacco use.** The USPSTF recommends that all adults be asked about tobacco use and provided counseling as appropriate, including parents with children in the home.
- **Alcohol misuse.** All adults should be periodically screened for alcohol misuse, and those involved in risky drinking should be counseled appropriately. Several screening tools are available, including the AUDIT-C (see Chapter 5.3).
- **Depression.** Screening for depression is recommended when staff-assisted depression care supports (staff other than the primary care physician) are available in the office to assure accurate diagnosis, effective treatment, and follow-up. PHQ-2 (Patient Health Questionnaire-2) is a useful screening tool that when positive should be followed by the PHQ-9 for more definitive diagnosis (see Chapter 5.2).[3]
- **Intimate partner violence.** All women of childbearing age should be screened for domestic violence and provided with or referred to appropriate intervention services.
- **Chlamydia.** All sexually active women aged 24 and younger should be screened for Chlamydia, while older women at high risk should also be screened. The evidence is insufficient to make a recommendation for screening men.
- **Hepatitis C.** In addition to screening high-risk individuals, everyone born between 1945 and 1965 should be screened once. This age group may have been exposed prior to screening the blood supply, which began in 1992, and may benefit from treatment if detected at an early stage.
- **HIV.** All adults up to age 65 should be screened once. High-risk individuals should be screened at any age and more frequently. Some 20% to 25% of individuals with HIV are not aware of their status.
- **Lipid disorders.** The USPSTF recommends screening all men regardless of risk starting at age 35, and women at high risk at age 45; men and women should be screened earlier if high risk. Although the appropriate frequency of screenings has not been established, given the prevalence of cardiovascular disease in this age group, screening should occur at least every 5 years. Also, given the importance of lipid subfractions in therapeutic decisions, a fasting lipid profile should be obtained. Abnormal results should be followed up by a second confirmatory test, and secondary causes of dyslipidemia should be ruled out. All patients, but especially those at high risk, should be counseled about intake of dietary saturated fat and other measures to reduce cardiovascular disease (CVD). Other risk factors for CVD, including smoking, diabetes, and hypertension, should be identified and addressed (see Chapter 17.4). (See "Statin therapy for cardiovascular disease prevention" below.)
- **Cervical cancer screening.** Recommendations include:
  - Routine cytology (Pap smear) age 21 to 65 every 3 years or for women at age 30 to 65 cytology plus human papillomavirus testing every 5 years;
  - No routine screening prior to age 21;
  - No routine screening after age 65 for women with adequate screening history and no high-risk screening factors;
  - No routine screening for women who have had a hysterectomy with no history of high-grade cervical neoplasia or cancer;
  - No HPV screening in women younger than 30 (see Chapter 13.4).
- **Breast cancer.** Screening for breast cancer is a dynamic and evolving area in medicine. The USPSTF is currently developing a draft research plan to review current recommendations. The 2009 USPSTF recommendations included several statements:
  - A recommendation for biennial screening from 50 to 74;
  - Screening prior to age 50 should be individualized;
  - Insufficient evidence exists on which to base a recommendation for screening after age 74;
  - Insufficient evidence to recommend for or against the benefits of clinical breast exam above those of mammogram;
  - Recommendation against teaching breast self-examination (see Chapter 13.8).
- **Colorectal cancer (CRC).** This is another important cause of cancer-related death in the United States (see Chapter 11.11). CRC screening for those at average risk should begin at age 50 and continue until age 75. The task force recommends against routine screening for those 76 to 85 years old, but recognizes that individual patients may warrant screening in this age group. The task force recommends against screening for any patients older than 85. Screening should be directed to high-risk adults before age 50. It is important to elicit family history to determine risk status, which should

include history of colon cancer or adenomas and sporadic polyps in first-degree relatives, all now considered to be important predictors.

Three screening modalities are routinely recommended: Colonoscopy, fecal occult blood tests (FOBTs), and a combination of FOBT and sigmoidoscopy. Annual FOBT remains the most cost-effective screening tool; if the test result is positive, follow-up examination with colonoscopy should be undertaken. FOBT every 3 years with flexible sigmoidoscopy every 5 years is a second option, while colonoscopy every 10 years is widely recommended. With a history of colon polyps, people should receive more frequent colonoscopic screening.

- **Prostate cancer.** Prostate-specific antigen (PSA) for prostate cancer is not recommended by the USPSTF. The benefits of PSA screening remain controversial, whereas the risks resulting from screening are quantifiable and substantial. Clinicians should discuss the pros and cons of PSA screening with patients so they can make an informed personal decision about screening. If PSA tests are obtained, age-specific reference ranges should be used to eliminate unnecessary biopsies in patients older than 60 years with elevations due to the normal aging process. Digital rectal examination is not recommended as a screen for prostate cancer (see Chapter 12.6).
- **Skin cancer.** The USPSTF states that there is insufficient evidence to determine the risks and benefits of routine whole body screening by primary care clinicians or patient skin self-examination for the detection of cutaneous melanoma, basal cell cancer, or squamous cell cancer. Patients with a history of skin cancer should consider having a complete skin exam annually.
- **Lung cancer.** Annual screening for lung cancer with low-dose computed tomography (LDCT) in adults aged 55 to 80 years who have a 30 pack-year smoking history and currently smoke or have quit within the past 15 years is recommended by the USPSTF. However, the American Academy of Family Physicians believes that there is insufficient evidence for this recommendation.

IMMUNIZATIONS[4]

- **Influenza:** Annually for all adults unless specifically contraindicated.
- **Tetanus, diphtheria, pertussis:** Td booster every 10 years; substitute one time with Tdap.
- **Varicella:** Consider for healthy persons without a history of chickenpox or prior immunization (consider serologic titer option). Two doses are recommended.
- **Human papillomavirus:** All women aged 19 to 26, all men aged 19 to 21, and men at high risk aged 22 to 26, if not previously vaccinated. Three doses are recommended.
- **Zoster:** A single dose recommended for all adults aged 60 or older (regardless of previous history of zoster).
- **Measles–mumps–rubella:** If born after 1956 and lacking evidence of immunity to measles.
- **High-risk groups:** The following immunizations are recommended if another risk factor (other than age) is present:
  - Pneumoccoccal (PCV13/PPSV23)
  - Meningococcus
  - Hepatitis A
  - Hepatitis B
  - *Haemophilus influenzae* type B (Hib).

PREVENTIVE MEDICATIONS

- **Statin therapy for cardiovascular disease (CVD) prevention.** The 2013 American College of Cardiology/American Heart Association guidelines recommend calculation of 10-year risk of cardiovascular disease every 4 to 6 years for those aged 40 to 75 years who are not already on cholesterol-lowering drug therapy, do not have cardiovascular disease or diabetes mellitus, and have LDL-C ≤190. Statin therapy is recommended for those with estimated ≥7.5% 10-year risk (risk calculators are available at the American Heart Association website).[5]
- **Aspirin therapy.** Longitudinal trials indicate a benefit for women as well as men from daily or every-other-day use of aspirin after age 40 to prevent vascular disease, especially if the patient is at high risk or has a family history of coronary artery disease and no risk of stroke or bleeding. The USPSTF currently recommends the use of aspirin for all men aged 45 to 79 and women 55 to 79 when the risk of GI hemorrhage is outweighed by cardiovascular benefit. The task force found insufficient evidence to recommend for or against use after age 80, and recommends against use prior to 45 for men or 55 for women.
- **Folate.** Women planning or capable of pregnancy should take 0.4 mg folate supplement daily.

COUNSELING AND PATIENT EDUCATION

- **Diet.** The USPSTF currently finds that there is insufficient evidence to recommend diet or exercise counseling in patients without underlying disease. Selective counseling may be appropriate. Nutritional assessment of intake of fat—saturated fats, polyunsaturated fatty acids (PUFAs), monounsaturated fatty acids (MUFAs)—cholesterol, complex carbohydrates, fiber, sodium, iron (women), and calcium (women) should be initiated. Specific recommendations include the following: Eat a variety of foods; maintain a healthy weight; choose a diet low in saturated fat and cholesterol; choose a diet with plenty of vegetables, fruits, and grain products; use complex carbohydrates in moderation, and limit intake of simple carbohydrates; use salt and sodium in moderation; and, if alcoholic beverages are used, use them in moderation.

  Calcium is especially important for women beginning in their teen decade to reduce the risk of osteoporosis and bone fracture. Average daily intake should be 1,000 to 1,200 mg. The USPSTF finds insufficient evidence to assess risks and benefits of calcium supplementation greater than 1,000 mg per day. The adverse effect of carbonated drinks with phosphorus on calcium and bone growth should also be discussed. Vitamin (especially antioxidants) and mineral supplementation should also be discussed with patients. Scientific evidence to date suggests that improving diet is more effective than supplementation alone.

- **Exercise.** Patients should be given at least a brief exercise prescription, including selection of an exercise program to provide a source of regular physical activity tailored to their health status and lifestyle. Regular exercise at moderate intensity (150 minutes per week) or vigorous intensity (75 minutes per week) plus muscle strengthening activities at least twice a week can improve strength, flexibility, and cardiovascular fitness. Weight-bearing exercise is especially important for perimenopausal and postmenopausal women to avoid or decrease bone loss and osteoporosis.

- **Substance use.** Include advice on cessation of tobacco use, limiting of alcohol consumption, health effects of other drugs, and not driving or doing other dangerous activities while under the influence of intoxicants (see Chapter 5.7).

  Smoking is the leading cause of preventable death in the United States. Studies have shown that multiple intervention strategies (one-to-one counseling, self-help materials, referral to community or online programs, prescription of nicotine substitutes, and use of bupropion or varenicline) are most effective.[6] The basics of smoking cessation counseling should include the following:
  - Providing a smoke-free environment,
  - Designating an office smoking cessation coordinator,
  - Asking patients at every opportunity whether they smoke, and assessing their readiness to stop if they do smoke,
  - Adding tobacco use to problem list in medical record If the patient smokes as a way of cueing office staff for ongoing interventions,
  - Providing multiple interventions to assist the smoker to stop, and
  - Following up to support patients who are motivated to stop.

- **Sexual practices.** Clinicians should take a complete sexual history, including sexual orientation/gender identity. Counseling efforts should focus on prevention of sexually transmitted diseases, including human immunodeficiency virus (HIV), and prevention of unwanted pregnancy. Sexually active adults should be advised that the most effective strategy to prevent infection is to abstain or maintain a mutually monogamous sexual relationship with an uninfected partner. "Safe-sex" recommendations, including partner selection and condom use, should also be provided (see Chapter 19.4). Women of childbearing age need to be advised of the dangers of HIV and other sexually transmitted infections during pregnancy. Empathy and confidentiality are important aspects of this counseling.

  Contraceptive options should be discussed with sexually active adults of childbearing age who do not desire pregnancy, including information on efficacy limitations and proper use of available contraception techniques (see Chapter 14.1).

- **Injury prevention.** Minimum counseling efforts in this area include use of safety belts in motor vehicles and helmets on motorcycles and bicycles, wearing other protective equipment during sports activities, prevention of violent behavior, safe use and storage of firearms, use of smoke and carbon monoxide detectors, and not smoking near bedding or upholstery.

  Intentional injuries include suicide and violence, and patients should be questioned regarding their risk with directed interventions when indicators are present. Injury to women as a result of intimate partner violence is one of the nation's most widespread and least reported health problems.

  Unintentional injuries include motor vehicle–related injuries and environmental and household injuries. Advise patients never to drive while under the influence. To avoid other types of injuries, patients should be advised against alcohol, tobacco, or psychoactive drug use when participating in potentially dangerous activities; advised to check their smoke detectors regularly; and counseled to child-proof their homes as indicated and to remove hazards to prevent falls among elderly household members.

- **Skin cancer.** The USPSTF recommends counseling young adults up to 24 years who have fair skin to minimize their exposure to ultraviolet radiation. Chronic overexposure to sunlight is responsible for 95% of all basal cell carcinomas. Individuals should be encouraged to use a sunscreen with a protection factor of at least 15.
- **Dental health.** Good personal oral hygiene, daily brushing and flossing, use of fluoride, and avoidance of sugary foods can control plaque and gingivitis. Individuals with current or a history of tobacco use or heavy alcohol use are at risk for oral–pharyngeal cancers and should be advised to get thorough checkups periodically. Individuals engaged in sports potentially leading to dental trauma should be encouraged to use mouth guards.
- **Preconception counseling.** Counseling and risk assessment can reduce the risk of congenital malformations and low birth weight, markedly improving outcomes by reducing infant morbidity and mortality. In addition to emphasizing general health promotion (taking folate supplement; achieving healthy weight; abstinence from alcohol, drugs, and tobacco products; and lowering risk of sexually transmitted disease), control of chronic diseases and recognition of their medications for teratogenic effects should be discussed (e.g., hypertension, diabetes, seizures, hyperthryoidism, acne, asthma).

  Evaluations of a couple considering conception can also include determining their emotional readiness to have children, the availability of sufficient financial resources, the risk of occupational or environmental toxin exposure for either person, and the need for genetic counseling and possible genetic diagnostic interventions. Counseling to reduce exposure to infections (rubella, cytomegalovirus, hepatitis B, toxoplasmosis, tuberculosis, herpes simplex virus, chlamydia, gonorrhea, syphilis, human papillomavirus) and updating immunization status are very important (e.g., hepatitis B, influenza, MMR, Td/Tdap, varicella).[7]

REFERENCES

1. U.S. Preventive Services Task Force. http://www.uspreventiveservicestaskforce.org/Page/Name/recommendations. Accessed January 30, 2015.
2. Commission on Health of the Public and Science, The American Academy of Family Physicians. http://www.aafp.org/patient-care/clinical-recommendations/cps.html. Accessed June 1, 2014.
3. Maurer DM, Darnall CR. Screening for depression. *Am Fam Physician* 2012;85(2):139–144.
4. Immunization schedules. Centers for Disease Control and Prevention. http://www.cdc.gov/vaccines/schedules/index.html. Accessed June 2, 2014.
5. Stone NJ, Robinson J, Lichtenstein AH, et al. 2013 ACC/AHA Guideline on the treatment of blood cholesterol to reduce atherosclerotic cardiovascular risk in adults: a report of the American College of Cardiology/American Heart Association Task Force on Practice Guidelines. http://circ.ahajournals.org/content/early/2013/11/11/01.cir.0000437738.63853.7a.full.pdf. Accessed March 29, 2014.
6. Larzelere MM, Williams DE. Promoting smoking cessation. *Am Fam Physician* 2012;85(6):591–598.
7. Farahi N, Zolotor A. Recommendations for preconception counseling and care. *Am Fam Physician* 2013;88(8):499–506.

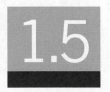

1.5 Health Maintenance for Older Adults

James P. Richardson

The proportion of the population that is elderly continues to grow. Because of the large influx of "baby boomers" that began in 2010, this demographic group will increase in size dramatically, guaranteeing that geriatric medicine will be a large part of every family physician's practice. Today's 65-year-old will live for an average of 19 years more. Thus, health promotion is not an activity that patients "outgrow."

Many health promotion activities recommended in the past have not been supported by evidence of their effectiveness. Additionally, physicians cannot simply extrapolate recommendations for younger age groups because older adults often suffer from multiple comorbidities and reduced function.[1] Physicians are often confused by the plethora of recommendations from government agencies, professional groups, and experts. A good source for the practitioner is the web site of the U.S. Preventive Services Task Force (USPSTF)[2]: www.USPreventiveServicesTaskForce.org. The task force concisely reviews the evidence for more than 100 health promotion activities, ranking recommendations by the strength of the evidence. The USPSTF now evaluates prevention topics on a continuing basis, and the task force's web site should be monitored for future recommendations and revisions.

The following recommendations are largely consistent with the USPSTF guidelines but also include those of other organizations, such as the American Cancer Society,[3] and the author's own. These recommendations primarily apply to asymptomatic people without risk factors. See Table 1.5-1 for a summary of recommendations for those aged 65 and older.

TABLE 1.5-1 Health Care Maintenance for Adults Aged 65 Years and Older

Condition	Recommendation
Primary Prevention/Immunizations	
Influenza	Annually
Pneumonia (PCV13 and PPSV23)	See text
Tetanus–diphtheria–pertussis	Td every 10 yr; substitute one time with Tdap
Zoster (shingles)	Once at age 60 or older
Primary Prevention/Counseling	
Prevention of sexually transmitted diseases	Periodically counsel to avoid high-risk sexual behaviors; screen as indicated
Injury prevention	Periodically counsel
Smoking cessation	Periodically counsel
Routine dental care	Recommend daily brushing/flossing and periodic visits to the dentist
Primary Prevention/Preventive Medications	
Cardiovascular disease	Assess 10-yr risk of cardiovascular disease every 4–6 yr to determine preventive benefit of statin therapy
Cardiovascular disease	Aspirin for men aged 45–79 and women aged 55–79 when potential benefit outweighs potential harm
Secondary Prevention/Cancer Screening	
Breast cancer	Women aged 50–74 with CBE/mammogram every 2 yr; under age 50 individualize screening
Cervical cancer	Women with cervices who have had adequate Pap smear screening may stop at age 65
Colorectal cancer	Ages 50–75; colonoscopy every 10 yr or FOBT annually
Secondary Prevention/Miscellaneous Screening	
Weight/height	At each visit
Hypertension	Blood pressure annually
Alcohol use	Periodically screen
Depression	Periodically screen
Osteoporosis	DXA scan women at age 65 or older
Abdominal aortic aneurysm	Men aged 65–75 who have ever smoked should have one-time screening
Tuberculosis	Screen on admission to nursing homes or assisted living facilities
Hepatitis C	Screen once if born between 1945 and 1965
Geriatric Assessment	
Vision	Periodically screen with Snellen chart
Hearing	Periodically screen with history/whisper test
Polypharmacy	Periodically review medications
Cognitive impairment	Periodically screen
Advanced directives and power-of-attorney	Periodically assess if present

INCORPORATING HEALTH MAINTENANCE INTO PRACTICE

Older patients are less likely than younger ones to request health promotion activities and are less tolerant of long appointments. A useful approach, therefore, is to attempt to include some elements of health maintenance activities with every visit. For example, a visit for hypertension follow-up in the fall is an opportune time to inquire about influenza, pneumococcal, and tetanus–diphtheria (Td) immunizations. Medicare includes a "Welcome to Medicare" visit for enrollees within the first 6 months of coverage and has recently added yearly wellness visits to encourage discussion of health promotion between patients and their doctors. Under the Affordable Care Act, patients no longer have co-pays for many of these services.[4]

Many studies show that physicians believe they recommend health maintenance to their patients more often than can actually be demonstrated. Reminder systems and aids have been found effective in increasing provision of preventive services, and the most effective are those that remove the physician from the decision loop. In other words, physicians can provide health promotion activities by involving their nurses and other staff or by using questionnaires to initiate discussions of health promotion, as encouraged in the Patient Centered Medical Home model.[5] Office protocols and prompts from electronic medical record systems also are effective (e.g., immunizations, making a return appointment for cervical cancer screening). For a more detailed discussion of implementation strategies, see Chapter 1.1.

As with all health care for older adults, health promotion activities should be individualized and take into account functional status, quality-of-life concerns, and patient preferences. Shared decision making is paramount.

PRIMARY PREVENTION

- **Definition.** Interventions that are primary types of prevention seek to prevent a given disease from ever beginning. A good example is immunizations to prevent infectious diseases.[6]
- **Immunizations.** Prevention of infectious diseases with immunizations is often neglected by patients and providers. Together, influenza and pneumonia are the eighth leading cause of deaths in elderly individuals in 2011.
  - **Influenza.** Influenza vaccine should be administered in October or November in the United States to all elderly persons who consent and are not allergic to eggs. The vaccine is effective in reducing the incidence of influenza and pneumonia, hospitalizations for these diseases, and may reduce the risk of cardiovascular disease.[7]
  - **Pneumococcal vaccine.** The Centers for Disease Control and Prevention's Advisory Committee on Immunization Practices (ACIP) now recommends the 13-valent vaccine (Prevnar) to all 65-year-old individuals. For those who have not been vaccinated, the ACIP recommends that unvaccinated elders receive a dose of Prevnar 13, followed by a dose of the 23-valent pneumococcal vaccine six to twelve months after the dose of the 13-valent vaccine. Those who have been previously vaccinated with the 23-valent vaccine should be given 13-valent vaccine no sooner than one year later. Immunocompromised individuals may be revaccinated with the 23-valent vaccine after five years, but routine revaccination is not recommended.
  - **Tetanus–diphtheria and pertussis.** While rare overall, tetanus is more common in older adults because of failure to maintain immunity with vaccinations. Immunity to tetanus and diphtheria can be maintained by giving Td boosters every 10 years to patients who have had the primary series of three immunizations over 6 months. Additionally, because pertussis has become more prevalent, persons aged 65 years and older should be vaccinated with a single dose of Tdap if they have not already received a dose. Administration of tetanus immune globulin is necessary to elderly people with tetanus-prone (i.e., "dirty") wounds who have never completed a primary series.
  - **Herpes zoster.** A vaccine to reduce the incidence of shingles, or herpes zoster, is recommended for all adults aged 60 and older who have no contraindications.
- **Prevention of sexually transmitted disease.** As with younger age groups, sexually active older adults should be counseled to avoid high-risk sexual behavior and to use condoms with new partners.
- **Injury prevention.** Injuries are a frequent cause of death in elderly individuals.
  - Elderly patients should be counseled regarding the dangers of falls and the benefits of exercise. Avoidable causes of falls include extrinsic factors, such as environmental hazards, which include poor lighting and throw rugs, and intrinsic factors, such as visual deficits, medications, and debilitation. Ensuring vitamin D sufficiency also reduces the risk of falls. Physicians should counsel older adults to gradually increase their exercise capacity by walking, gardening, or doing household chores. In addition to reduced fall risk, benefits of physical activity demonstrated in population studies include lower incidence of cardiovascular disease, dementia, osteoporosis, and improved mood.

- Everyone should be counseled to wear safety belts (and bicycle or motorcycle helmets if applicable), to maintain working smoke detectors and carbon monoxide detectors, to store firearms safely, and to keep hot water temperatures below 120°F.
- Although screening of all older drivers is not advocated, all providers should know the local laws governing driving restrictions if they become aware that a patient is no longer a safe driver. Many hospitals offer testing by occupational therapists that may help with this determination.
- **Smoking cessation.** Benefits accrue to those who stop smoking at any age. Patients' smoking history should be obtained, and smokers should be encouraged to quit. Counseling patients to stop smoking is an effective intervention.
- **Routine dental care.** Daily brushing, flossing, and periodic visits to the dentist remain important in the elderly population.

Preventive Medications

- **Statin therapy for cardiovascular disease (CVD) prevention.** In 2013, the American College of Cardiology and the American Heart Association released new guidelines on the treatment of blood cholesterol to reduce the risk of CVD. In addition to a healthy lifestyle, primary prevention with statin therapy is recommended up to age 75 years for those with a 10-year risk of CVD ≥7.5%. Calculation of risk is recommended every 4 to 6 years for those not currently on statins, who do not have CVD or diabetes, and who have LDL-C ≤190 (risk calculators are available at the American Heart Association website). The decision must therefore be individualized, based on the senior's quality of life, life expectancy, other risk factors, cost, and patient preference.[8,9]
- **Aspirin.** Although the value of aspirin is well established for secondary prevention of stroke and myocardial infarction, its role in primary prevention is less clear (for further discussion, see Chapter 1.4). The task force recommends that physicians discuss the use of aspirin with patients at high risk for CVD, although it also found that aspirin use increases the risk of gastrointestinal bleeding, and, to a smaller extent, the risk of hemorrhagic stroke, particularly in older adults. Recently, aspirin at a dose of 100 mg every other day has been demonstrated to reduce the risk of ischemic stroke, myocardial infarction, and major cardiovascular events in women older than 65.[10] Aspirin also may reduce the risk of colorectal cancer. The optimal dose of aspirin for prophylaxis is not known.
- **Multivitamins.** Vitamin supplementation does not prevent CVD or cancer and is not recommended by the task force.

SECONDARY PREVENTION

- **Definition.** Interventions that seek to detect disease before individuals become symptomatic are secondary preventive measures. Examples include blood pressure measurement to detect hypertension and prevent CVD, and cervical smears to detect cervical cancer.

Cancer Screening

- **Breast cancer.** Almost half of all breast cancers in women occur in those aged 65 years and older. The USPSTF guidelines for breast cancer screening are currently being updated at the time of publication. Beginning at age 40 years, the American Cancer Society recommends yearly clinical breast examination and mammography as long as a woman is in good health. Mammography screening in older women remains controversial because studies of mammography have included few women older than 75 years, and there is no evidence that mammography is effective after this age. Mammography combined with clinical breast examination has been proved to reduce mortality from breast cancer in women aged 50 through 69 years. The USPSTF guidelines do not recommend breast cancer screening after age 75 because of insufficient evidence. Nevertheless, because the aging breast has an increased proportion of fat, which makes it easier to examine radiologically (and therefore mammography has a higher positive predictive value in elderly individuals), clinical breast examination and mammography performed every 2 years can be recommended to women older than 70 with a life expectancy of at least 10 years. Women at increased risk for breast cancer and with low risk of adverse effects, such as thromboembolism, may benefit from treatment with risk-reducing medications, such as raloxifene or tamoxifen. As with other preventive measures, shared decision making remains paramount.
- **Cervical cancer.** A significant proportion of elderly women have never had cervical (Pap) smears, and these women with cervices who are or have been sexually active should have smears every 3 years.

Screening more frequently confers little additional benefit. Women who have had three or more technically satisfactory negative smears and are not at high risk can stop undergoing screening after age 65 (see Chapter 13.4).

- **Colorectal cancer.** Rectal examination is not a useful screen in the asymptomatic patient. Annual fecal occult blood testing (FOBT), sigmoidoscopy every 5 years with FOBT every 3 years, and colonoscopy every 10 years are all recommended protocols for colon cancer screening. There is insufficient evidence to recommend one test over the other. Because of the length of time between adenoma development and cancer, the task force recommends against routine screening between the ages of 76 and 85 and recommends against screening those older than 85 years.
- **Lung cancer.** The USPSTF recommends annual screening for lung cancer with low-dose computed tomography (LDCT) in adults aged 55 to 80 years who have a 30 pack-year smoking history and currently smoke or have quit within the past 15 years. The task force recommends that screening be discontinued once a person has not smoked for 15 years or develops a health problem that substantially limits life expectancy or the ability or willingness to have curative lung surgery. However, the American Academy of Family Physicians believes that there is insufficient evidence for this recommendation.
- **Prostate cancer.** A digital rectal examination for prostate cancer has a very low yield. The prostate-specific antigen (PSA) test is elevated in older men, not only in those with prostate cancer, but also in men with benign prostatic hypertrophy as well. Men older than 65 to 70 years most likely will die of a comorbid condition other than prostate cancer. Therefore, with the possible exception of patients who request testing and have been informed of its risks and drawbacks, PSA screening is not recommended for elderly men.
- **Skin.** A yearly examination of all skin for patients with significant sunlight exposure or with a history of skin cancer is recommended. The task force found the evidence insufficient to recommend routine screening in the general population.

Screening for Other Conditions/Diseases

- **Weight/height.** Assess for underweight/overweight/obesity, and monitor for changes that may indicate underlying disease or nutritional issues.
- **Hypertension.** Blood pressure should be measured at least yearly.
- **Alcohol use.** As alcoholism develops in some older people late in life due at least in part to slower metabolism, screening with the Cut down, Annoyed, Guilty, and Eye opener (CAGE) questions or AUDIT-C (see Chapter 5.3) is recommended.
- **Depression.** Depression is common in elderly individuals. Screening for depression is recommended by the USPSTF when staff-assisted depression care supports (staff other than the primary care physician) are available in the office to assure accurate diagnosis, effective treatment, and follow-up.[2] Many simple depression-screening instruments (e.g., Geriatric Depression Scale) are available.[11]
- **Osteoporosis.** Screening for osteoporosis in women by dual-energy x-ray absorptiometry (DXA) is recommended at age 65 or older. Younger women should be screened if their fracture risk is equal to or greater than that of a 65-year-old white female who has no additional risk factors.
- **Abdominal aortic aneurysm.** Men between the ages of 65 and 75 who are current or former smokers should have at least one ultrasound of the abdominal aorta.
- **Tuberculosis.** Routine purified protein derivative (PPD) testing is not necessary for community-dwelling elderly individuals who are not HIV-positive, but should be administered on admission to nursing homes or assisted living facilities. Two-stage testing (repeating the PPD 1 to 2 weeks after the first in those with an initial negative result) is necessary because of the booster phenomenon.
- **Hepatitis C.** Everyone born between 1945 and 1965 should be screened once in addition to screening high-risk individuals. This age group may have been exposed prior to routine screening of the blood supply, which began in 1992, and may benefit from treatment if detected at an early stage.
- **Hypothyroidism.** Routine screening is not recommended, but clinicians should have a low threshold for ordering thyroid function tests, for example, serum thyroid-stimulating hormone level (TSH and free T_4), because of its subtle presentation in this age cohort.
- **Glaucoma.** Routine screening by primary care physicians is not recommended. High-risk populations (blacks older than 40, whites older than 65, and those with a positive family history, diabetes, or severe myopia) may be referred to eye specialists for screening. The optimal interval for screening is not known.

GERIATRIC ASSESSMENT

Although not as strongly supported by evidence as the above recommendations, most experts recommend some or all of the following activities for elderly individuals.[11]

- **Special senses.** Visual and hearing losses contribute to functional decline and cognitive impairment. Vision may be tested with the Snellen chart, and hearing loss may be screened by history or a whisper test.
- **Polypharmacy.** Simplifying drug regimens improves compliance, reduces the incidence of adverse drug reactions, and saves money. Common offending drugs are those whose indications were never clear or the indications for which have disappeared (e.g., digoxin). Anticholinergic drugs (e.g., antispasmodics, antihistamines) and sedatives are particularly problematic for older adults.
- **Cognitive impairment.** Dementia is common in elderly individuals. The Folstein Mini-Mental State Examination is specific but not very sensitive for dementia, especially in well-educated or intelligent older adults.[12] Many experts prefer the Montreal Cognitive Assessment (MoCA) as a more accurate test.[13]
- **Advance directives and power-of-attorney.** Although all elderly individuals should be encouraged to record their desires in formal advance directive instruments, simply recording the patient's desires in the medical record is often very helpful to other providers and family members should the patient become unable to make his or her own decisions (see Chapter 22.5). More importantly, older adults should be encouraged to grant a power-of-attorney to someone to make decisions for them, should they become unable to communicate or lose decision-making capacity.

REFERENCES

1. Richardson JP. Considerations for health promotion and disease prevention in older adults. *Medscape* 2006. http://www.medscape.com/viewarticle/531942. Accessed March 31, 2014.
2. U.S. Preventive Services Task Force. http://www.uspreventiveservicestaskforce.org/Page/Name/ recommendations. Accessed January 30, 2015.
3. American Cancer Society. http://www.cancer.org/index. Accessed June 18, 2014.
4. Centers for Medicare and Medicaid. Your guide to Medicare's Preventive Services. https://www .medicare.gov/Pubs/pdf/10110.pdf. Accessed March 29, 2014.
5. Agency for Healthcare Research and Quality. Patient Centered Medical Home Research Center. http:// pcmh.ahrq.gov. Accessed March 29, 2014.
6. Immunization Schedules. Centers for Disease Control and Prevention. http://www.cdc.gov/vaccines/ schedules/index.html. Accessed June 2, 2014.
7. Warren-Gash C, Hayward AC, Hemingway H, et al. Influenza infection and risk of acute myocardial infarction in England and Wales: a CALIBER self-controlled case series. *J Infect Dis* 2012;206:1652–1659.
8. Stone NJ, Robinson JG, Lichtenstein AH, et al. Treatment of blood cholesterol to reduce atherosclerotic cardiovascular disease risk in adults: synopsis of the 2013 American College of Cardiology/American Heart Association cholesterol guidelines. *Ann Intern Med* 2014:339–343.
9. American Heart Association. http://my.americanheart.org/professional/StatementsGuidelines/Prevention Guidelines/Prevention-Guidelines_UCM_457698_SubHomePage.jsp. Accessed March 29, 2014.
10. Ridker PM, Cook NR, Lee I-M, et al. A randomized trial of low-dose aspirin in the primary prevention of cardiovascular disease in women. *N Engl J Med* 2005;352:1293–1304.
11. Gallo JJ, Bogner HR, Fulmer T, et al., eds. *Handbook of geriatric assessment.* 4th ed. Gaithersburg, MD: Aspen Publishers; 2006.
12. Folstein MF, Folstein SE, McHugh PR. Mini-mental state: a practical method for grading the cognitive state of patients for the clinician. *J Psychiatr Res* 1975;12:189–198.
13. Roalf DR, Moberg PJ, Xie SX, et al. Comparative accuracies of two common screening instruments for classification of Alzheimer's disease, mild cognitive impairment, and healthy aging. *Alzheimers Dement* 2013;9:529–537.

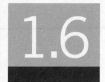

Health Care for the International Traveler

Douglas P. Collins, Christine O'Dea, Kevin P. Brazill,
Beth-Erin S. Smith, Nancy C. Elder

GENERAL PRINCIPLES[1]

More Americans than ever are traveling to developing countries. Accidents are the leading cause of mortality, while traveler's diarrhea is the leading cause of morbidity. Other serious infectious diseases are also a threat to travelers and can be decreased through pretravel consultation.

APPROACH TO THE PATIENT[1]

- **History** should include information about previous travel (including problems encountered), current itinerary (destinations, length of visit, type of accommodations, planned activities), and personal history (age, chronic diseases or problems, disabilities, habits, occupation, avocations). In addition, an up-to-date medication list, including over-the-counter and herbal preparations, should be obtained, and an immunization history taken.
- **Physical examination** for young healthy patients needs nothing additional to that performed for healthcare maintenance. Patients with chronic illness will need special attention to maximize their current health prior to departure.

INTERVENTIONS AND RECOMMENDATIONS
Traveler's Diarrhea (TD)[2–5]

- **Epidemiology**
  - By far the most common illness seen in international travelers.
  - 20% to 60% of travelers to high-risk countries will experience TD.
  - Symptoms last 4 days without treatment, 1/5 are bedridden for 1 day, 1/3 forced to alter activities.
- **Definition**
  - Three or more unformed stools in 24 hours and at least one of the following: fever, nausea, vomiting, abdominal cramps, tenesmus, bloody stools. In children, defined as a twofold increase in number of stools.
  - Dysentery is defined as diarrhea with fever and bloody, mucoid stools.
- **Etiology**
  - 50% to 80% bacterial etiology. *Escherichia coli (especially Enterotoxigenic/ETEC and Enteroaggregative/EAEC species)* is the number one overall cause. Primarily *E. coli* in Latin America, Caribbean, and Africa. In South and Southeast Asia, *Campylobacter, Salmonella,* and *Shigella* are relatively more important.
  - Protozoa (such as *Giardia, Entamoeba,* and *Cryptosporidium*) are less common; suspect if symptoms last more than 2 weeks.
  - Viruses (especially *Rotavirus* and *Norovirus*) are most common viral causes; Norovirus has become increasingly important, particularly in cruise ship settings.
- **Transmission**
  - Contaminated food and water with fecal material is the primary route of transmission, including salads, unpeeled fruits, poorly cooked meats, unpasteurized dairy, and tap water. Food from street vendors is especially risky. Person-to-person spread is rare.
  - Freezing does not kill; thus, ice can be contaminated; even liquor with high alcohol content does not sterilize contaminated ice.
- **Risk factors**
  - Include: low-budget and adventure travel; living in a high-risk region (missionaries, Peace Corps workers); immunodeficiency; extremes of age; prior gastric surgery; lower GI acidity (proton pump inhibitor and H_2 blocker use). Recent studies show a genetic susceptibility to TD; therefore, previous history of TD is also a risk factor.

- **Complications**
  - 5% to 10% will develop Irritable Bowel Syndrome (Post-Infectious IBS)
- **Behavioral counseling for prevention**
  - "Boil it, cook it, peel it, or forget it." Bottled water safest. Water that has been boiled 1 minute is considered safe to drink. Travelers should avoid swimming in unclean waters. All foods need to be heated >65°C (not just warmed). Advise carrying alcohol hand-gel (>60% alcohol) for portable hand washing before meals.
  - There is little evidence that behavioral counseling lowers risk of TD.
- **Chemoprophylaxis for prevention**
  - Consider for those who are at high risk (Inflammatory bowel disease, history of TD, immunodeficiency, chronically ill/insulin-dependent diabetes, leukemia, reduced gastric acidity) or in whom diarrhea during trip cannot be afforded (athletes, high-profile speakers, politicians). Do not use for longer than 2 to 3 weeks. Consider geography when selecting an antibiotic.
  - Antibiotic options include: Ciprofloxacin 250 to 500 mg daily from day of arrival until 2 days after return, no longer than 3 weeks (90% protective with side effects of skin rash, vaginal candidiasis, mild phototoxicity, gastrointestinal sensitivity, and rarely anaphylaxis. Not for children or in pregnancy); Rifaximin 200 to 550 mg daily.
  - Bismuth subsalicylate. Less effective than antibiotics (65% protective), and QID dosing limits utility. Not for patients on anticoagulation, other salicylates. Can interfere with doxycycline absorption. Stools and tongue temporarily discolored black. Avoid in children <3 years old.
  - Probiotics. Protection up to 47% with *Lactobacillus* GG (Culturelle) in one study; other studies show limited or no benefit, and optimal dosing is unknown.
- **Treatment**
  - **Antimicrobials.** Consider geography/resistance patterns, and types of travel when prescribing.
    - ○ Drug of choice for empiric self-treatment is ciprofloxacin 500 mg twice daily or 750 mg once daily, may repeat on days 2 and 3 as needed. However, increasing rates of resistance are a concern, especially in *Campylobacter* in Southeast Asia. Avoid in children and pregnancy. Alternative quinolones such as levofloxacin may also be used. Zithromax is recommended for children with TD at 5 to 10 mg per kg once and is the drug of choice in pregnancy. It is also recommended in places with high rates of quinolone-resistance. Adult dosing is 1 g once or 500 mg for up to 3 days.
    - ○ Rifaximin useful for nondysenteric TD in patients 12 and over, 200 mg TID for 3 days, especially where *E. coli* predominant as cause, such as Central America.
- **Antidiarrheals**
  - ○ Loperamide 4 mg at initial loose stool and then 2 mg after each loose stool up to 16 mg per day. Avoid in children less than 2 years old.
  - ○ Limited clinical evidence suggests antimotility medications should not be used in cases of dysentery, but are likely safe when used with an antibiotic.
  - ○ Rehydration is the most important treatment. Oral rehydration solution (ORS) options should be reviewed with travelers at high risk.

Malaria[5-8]

- **Epidemiology.** There are 200 to 300 million cases and 1 million deaths from malaria each year. 3.3 billion people in 97 countries live in areas at risk in Central and South America, Africa, the Middle East, South and Southeast Asia, and Oceania. Approximately 1,500 cases are diagnosed in the United States annually, mostly in travelers, and the prevalence is increasing.
- **Cause.** Five species of the *Plasmodium* protozoa *(P. malariae, P. vivax, P. falciparum, P. ovale, and P. knowlesi)* are now recognized to cause human infection. They are passed from infected female anopheles mosquitoes to humans, usually during dusk-to-dawn feeding, and cause disease. *P. falciparum* is life-threatening and the species of major concern.
- **Clinical presentation.** Malaria can present in a variety of ways, but flulike symptoms (fever, chills, muscle aches, headache) predominate. Severe *P. falciparum* may cause coma (cerebral malaria), liver, and kidney failure; *P. vivax* and *P. ovale* may remain dormant in the liver for years, reappearing months to years later.
- **Behavioral counseling.** The *ABCD* approach is recommended to guide travelers: Awareness, Bite avoidance, Chemoprophylaxis, and early Diagnosis of febrile illness. Prevent mosquito bites by avoiding being outdoors at dusk and dawn; wearing light-colored, full-length clothing, socks, and closed shoes; using insect repellent with sufficient concentrations of diethyltoluamide (DEET) (20% to 30% concentration advised: 4% is effective for 90 minutes, 23% is effective for approximately 5 hours, and concentrations above 30% are no more effective; DEET, even at high concentrations, is considered

safe for children over 2 months old and for pregnant women) or Picaridin 20% (comparable to 35% DEET in efficacy); using mosquito nets and clothing treated with permethrin; sleeping indoors or under a mosquito net. Educate patients about malarial symptoms and the need for urgent medical evaluation and treatment. The importance of insect bite avoidance to prevent other diseases, such as Dengue Fever, Japanese Encephalitis, and Yellow Fever, should be emphasized.

- **Medications**
  - **Prophylaxis**
    - ○ Resistance is constantly changing. Chloroquine resistance is common; mefloquine resistance exists. Check up-to-date recommendations at websites such as www.cdc.gov/travel.
    - ○ Chloroquine (Aralen) is for adults, children, and pregnant women. Side effects are rare and minor (nausea, headache, dizziness). Adult dose is one 500-mg tablet (8.3 mg per kg salt for children) per week, starting 2 weeks prior to travel and continuing 4 weeks after leaving malaria area.
    - ○ Mefloquine (Lariam) is for adults and children over 9 kg only. Significant side effects, especially in those with seizure disorder, psychiatric history, or cardiac conduct abnormalities, include neuropsychiatric disturbances. Adult dose is one 250-mg tablet (5-mg per kg salt for children, taken with food due to bitter taste) per week, starting 2 weeks prior to travel and continuing 4 weeks after leaving malaria area. Preferred medication for pregnant patient if chloroquine resistance.
    - ○ Doxycycline (Vibramycin) is for adults and children over age 8 only. Side effects include photosensitivity and vaginitis. Adult dose is one 100-mg tablet (2 mg per kg for children) per day, starting 2 days prior to travel and continuing 4 weeks after leaving malaria area.
    - ○ Atovaquone/proguanil (A/P) (Malarone) is for adults and children over 11 kg only. Side effects are relatively less common and include abdominal pain, nausea, headache, and oral ulcers. Adult dose is one A/P 250-/100-mg tablet with food daily (pediatric tablet is A/P 62.5/25 mg; number of tablets depends on weight), starting 2 days prior to travel and continuing 7 days after leaving malaria area. Higher cost of A/P is often a concern for patients.
    - ○ Primaquine may be indicated for non-G6PD deficient patients traveling to *P. vivax* only regions.
  - **Presumptive self-treatment**
    - ○ Consider for travelers unable to access medical care within 24 hours. Atovaquone/proguanil (Malarone) four tablets as a single dose daily for 3 days or Artemether/lumefantrine (CoArtem) are options. Travelers should avoid self-treating with the medication they have been taking for prophylaxis.
  - **Treatment**
    - ○ Treatment depends on region where malaria was acquired, the species of Plasmodium, and the severity of disease.
    - ○ Guidelines should always be checked. Details can be found at www.cdc.gov/malaria. A 24-hour CDC Malaria Hotline is also available. The World Health Organization's international guidelines can be found at www.who.int/malaria.
    - ○ Medications for treatment usually involve combination therapy and may include the medications above and/or quinine sulfate for uncomplicated malaria; IV quinidine gluconate or artesunate for severe malaria; clindamycin may be used instead of doxycycline when the latter is contraindicated. Quinine and quinidine can cause cinchonism (characterized by tinnitus, hearing loss, and headache) and cardiac toxicity.

Vaccine-Preventable Infectious Diseases[1,5,9]

- **Tetanus, diphtheria, and pertussis**
  - Still highly endemic in the developing world.
  - Immunization
    - ○ DTaP series for younger children
    - ○ Tdap booster advised for those 11 to 18 years old who have completed their childhood vaccinations, ≥19 years old who have never received at least one previous dose of an acellular pertussis–containing vaccine, and in pregnant women.
    - ○ Td recommended booster every 10 years for adults; 5 years if prolonged trip planned with limited access to care and moderate or high risk of injury.
- **Influenza**
  - Highly endemic across the world. The season in the northern hemisphere may extend from October through May; in the southern hemisphere it is April through November. However, in tropical areas, influenza can occur year round.
    - ○ Due to antigenic drift, vaccine is changed each year to cover the most common strains circulating. The new vaccines are usually available each September and include coverage of two influenza A strains, including H1N1, and one (if trivalent) or two (if quadrivalent) influenza B strains.

- ○ Influenza vaccine contraindicated in those allergic to eggs. High-risk travelers may consider carrying an antiviral drug like oseltamavir.
- ○ Travelers ≥6 months of age without contraindications should be vaccinated using the intramuscular or intradermal vaccination. Live intranasal vaccine is approved for healthy individuals aged 2 to 49.
- **Measles**
  - Highly contagious; transmission rate is approximately 90% to those who are unvaccinated. High incidence of complications resulting after the acute phase. Can cause birth defects in those who are pregnant.
  - Immunization
    - ○ Indicated for all travelers ≥ 12 months of age born in 1957 or later without history of two doses of live vaccine at any point in life or titers indicating immunity. Contraindicated in the immunosuppressed or pregnant. A single dose of MMR should be given for traveling infants 6 to 11 months of age; a two-dose series should still be given beginning at 12 months.
    - ○ The live virus vaccine (mumps–measles–rubella, MMR) is generally well tolerated, but side effects can include fever and/or rash 7 to 12 days after vaccination.
- **Polio**
  - Incidence has been reduced by approximately 99% overall, but outbreaks still occur in the developing world. Outbreak information is available at the CDC website.
  - Immunization
    - ○ All travelers should have at least three doses. Those traveling to higher-risk areas should also have a one-time adult booster dose. Live attenuated oral vaccine not to be used in immunosuppressed, pregnancy.
- **Hepatitis B**
  - Endemic in areas of Asia and Africa with infections in approximately 15% of population. Vaccination series recommended for those travelers at high risk: adventure travelers, dental or healthcare workers, medical/dental tourists, or those who may have a new sexual partner during the stay.
  - Immunization
    - ○ Three-dose series (0, 1 to 2, and 4 to 6 months).
    - ○ An accelerated three-dose schedule is available (given on days 0, 7, and 14), but requires fourth dose at 12 months for lifelong immunity.
- **Hepatitis A**
  - Most frequent vaccine-preventable travel-related illness. Risk is 20 per 100,000 rural travelers per month in some countries. Now a routine childhood immunization in the United States and indicated for most travelers to the developing world. No vaccination is needed if natural immunity has occurred from previous infection.
  - Immunization
    - ○ Two-dose series with second dose at least 6 months after the first. First dose provides 95% immunity at 4 weeks; second dose provides long-term immunity.
    - ○ A combination hepatitis A/B vaccine is also available.
    - ○ For adults >40 years with immunosuppression or certain chronic diseases who will be traveling to an endemic area in <2 weeks, immune globulin is additionally recommended.
- **Typhoid fever**
  - Bacterial infection spread fecal–oral route, person to person, through contaminated food or water. Infection results in high fevers, abdominal pain, and frequently diarrhea. Especially high risk for pregnant travelers. Immunization recommended for most travel to the developing world or any travel that will include adventurous dietary habits, prolonged stays, or predominantly rural itineraries. Even after vaccination, it is possible to be infected after eating food that has a high level of bacteria.
  - Immunizations: Two vaccines exist:
    - ○ Oral Typhoid TY21a vaccine (Vivotif Berna): Efficacy of 50% to 90% for this live attenuated strain of *Salmonella typhi*. Duration of immunity is 5 to 6 years. Four doses taken on days 0, 2, 4, and 6. Pills must be kept refrigerated, and not taken within 24 hours of mefloquine or antibiotics. Approved for ages ≥6 years, but should not be given to the immunocompromised.
    - ○ Injectable capsular polysaccharide vaccine (Typhim Vi): Efficacy of 60% to 80%. Duration of immunity is 2 to 3 years. Well tolerated and low side effects. Safe for children aged 2 years and older and for those with immunodeficiencies.

- **Yellow fever**
  - Mosquito-spread viral illness found in South America and sub-Saharan Africa. Mosquito precautions (see Malaria) are essential.
  - Immunization
    - Live virus vaccine with efficacy >95%.
    - Proof of immunization (International Certificate of Vaccination) at approved site can be required for travel to or from endemic countries. Single dose becomes effective in 10 days, and protection lasts at least 10 years.
    - Up to 5% of persons can experience flulike symptoms 5 to 14 days after immunization, and rarely (approximately 1 in 100,000) neurologic/encephalitis or visceral organ disease can occur. It is important to discuss the risks and benefits of this vaccine with patients. Not for patients with egg allergies, younger than 6 months (it is preferable to wait to ≥9 months), or in pregnant or immunosuppressed patients.
- **Meningococcal meningitis**
  - Epidemics common in sub-Saharan Africa "Meningitis Belt," particularly December to June, but uncommon in travelers from the United States. Travelers to endemic areas of the world should be offered vaccination. Legally required for pilgrims making the Hajj or Umrah pilgrimage to Mecca, Saudi Arabia.
  - Immunization
    - Vaccines protect against serogroups A, C, Y, and W-135, but not B.
    - Meningococcal polysaccharide-protein conjugate vaccine (MCV4) available as *Menactra* (For persons 2 to 55 years of age, one-dose series, and for children 9 to 23 months, two-dose series) or *Menveo* (For persons 2 to 55 years of age). Increased effectiveness compared with MPSV4, see below, low risk of side effects, and may be used in pregnancy and immunosuppression.
    - Meningococcal polysaccharide vaccine (MPSV4, *Menomune*): For children aged ≥2 years, or acceptable alternative for older age groups; similar side effect profile to MCV4.
- **Cholera**
  - Epidemics of diarrhea in developing world. The best treatment is rehydration, and the best prophylaxis is hand washing and food/water precautions.
  - Immunization: Dukoral, Shanchol, and ORC-Vax are vaccines not licensed in the United States and not recommended by the CDC for pretravel vaccination except for travelers to high-risk situations (refugee camps, outbreak settings, healthcare providers in endemic areas).
- **Rabies**
  - Endemic in most of the developed world. All animal bites or exposures in the developing world should be followed by vigorous washing and medical attention.
  - Vaccine not indicated for most travelers but can be considered in high-risk persons (those with potential occupational exposure, children traveling to higher-risk areas) or those who will be staying, especially >1 month, in remote areas with limited access to evacuation.
  - Postexposure treatment includes immediate immune globulin, a multiple-dose series of active vaccine if no pre-exposure vaccination, and 2 additional active vaccines if already vaccinated pre-exposure.
  - Immunization
    - Inactivated viral preparation
    - Three-dose series on days 0, 7, 21, or 28
    - Chloroquine and mefloquine should not be taken until completion of vaccination series.
- **Japanese encephalitis**
  - Transmitted by mosquitoes. Endemic or epidemic in some Asian countries, India, and parts of Australia. Low risk for short-term travelers and those staying in urban areas. Prevention of mosquito bites is critical for prevention (see Malaria).
  - Immunization
    - Inactivated vero cell culture (Ixiaro) is the only vaccine available in the United States.
    - Recommended for those who will be traveling in an endemic area for ≥1 month or ≤1 month if planning nonurban outdoor activities during transmission season.
    - Given subcutaneously on days 0 and 28
    - Approved for travelers 2 months of age or older. Safety not yet studied in pregnant women, and therefore deferring is advised unless risk of infection outweighs theoretical risk of vaccination.
    - Local symptoms occur in around 10% of recipients. Contains protamine sulfate and may cause hypersensitivity.

INJURIES AND ACCIDENTS[1]

Definition and Epidemiology

- Injuries are among the leading causes of death and disability in the world, and they are the leading cause of preventable deaths in travelers. Traveling U.S. Citizens are 10 times more likely to die abroad as a result of a catastrophic injury than as a result of acquiring an infectious disease. Most deaths and injuries are a result of motor vehicle accidents.
- In young adult travelers, death rates due to injury are increased by a factor of 2 to 3, and most of these deaths are traffic or swimming related. While men are more likely to be injured as a result of accidents, women are more likely to fall victim to violence or sexual assaults.
- Unintentional injuries include road traffic accidents, falls, fires, poisoning, and drowning, as well as injuries incurred during extreme sporting events, and recreational drug and alcohol use.
- Injuries are the primary reason U.S. Citizens are carried back to the United States by medical evacuation each year, and in many countries, trauma services including safe blood transfusion are not readily available for lifesaving emergent care.

Behavioral Counseling

- Travelers should be counseled on avoiding situations when traffic accidents frequently occur: at dusk, in poor weather conditions, at crossroads, while speeding, when traffic rules are unclear, and while passing other drivers.
- Seat belts should be required as a condition of vehicle rental (as well as airbags if available), and those traveling with small children should bring appropriate car seats.
- Drivers should never engage in mobile phone activity (talking, texting, other) while operating an automobile, bicycle, or motorcycle.
- Motorcycles, scooters, open trucks, and small, unscheduled aircraft should be avoided. For those using two-wheeled vehicles, including bicycles, helmets of sufficient quality should be worn at all times by drivers and riders.
- Travelers should ensure that companies specializing in extreme or recreational sports are credentialed and provide proper supervision and safety equipment.
- Travelers should select lodging that includes smoke detectors, sprinklers, and locks on the doors. Rooms adjacent to stairwells or dark passageways should be avoided. In addition, it is recommended that travelers stay no higher than the sixth floor in hotels since fire ladders generally do not extend beyond six stories.
- Violence is also a threat to travelers abroad, particularly to poorer regions. Homicide is the second leading cause of death behind accidents for Americans overseas. Travelers should avoid wearing expensive clothing, guard belongings, travel in pairs, travel during the day, and vary daily routines and routes.
- Evacuation plans should be thought through in advance in cases of instability or medical emergency. Health and evacuation insurance is an option for travelers if their destinations include countries where there may not be access to good medical care.

SEXUALLY TRANSMITTED INFECTIONS[1,10]

Definition and Epidemiology

- Casual sexual encounters (including vaginal, anal, and oral–genital contact) and sexual promiscuity during travel play a major role in the transmission of sexually transmitted infections (STIs). An estimated 448 million people worldwide have some form of an STI.
- Abstinence or mutual monogamy is the most reliable way to avoid acquisition and transmission of STIs. Correct and consistent use of a latex (or polyurethane if latex allergy) condom can reduce the risk of STI transmission. If used with a latex condom, lubricants should be water-based, not petroleum-based.
- Many STIs, including HIV, have high prevalence even in the most remote travel destinations, particularly in sub-Saharan Africa, Southeast Asia, Eastern Europe, and northern countries in South America.
- Some STIs are more prevalent in developing countries (e.g., chancroid, lymphogranuloma venereum, and granuloma inguinale), and increased rates of infectious syphilis and quinolone-resistant gonorrhea have recently been reported among men who have sex with men. Vaccines against hepatitis A and B are highly recommended for men who have sex with men.

Behavioral Counseling

- Travelers should be counseled to avoid sexual interactions with groups of efficient STI transmitters (commercial sex workers, IV drug users) in endemic areas.

- Meeting sexual partners online with plans to meet in person is a particularly dangerous activity and should be avoided.
- Any traveler who may have been exposed to an STI or who develops a vaginal or urethral discharge, an unexplained rash or genital lesion, throat lesions, or genital or pelvic pain should seek medical care immediately.
- Screening for asymptomatic infection should be encouraged among travelers who have had casual sexual activity since infection can often occur without overt symptoms.

Medications

- Knowledge of the clinical presentation, frequency of infection, and antimicrobial resistance patterns (e.g., quinolone-resistant *Neisseria gonorrhoeae*) is important in the management of STIs that occur in travelers to specific destinations.
- Treatment should be directed toward a specific pathogen for most STIs where reliable testing is available. Empiric treatment can be used in situations where laboratory testing is not available. A typical regimen in the United States for chlamydia, gonorrhea, and trichomoniasis includes ceftriaxone 250 mg IM once, azithromycin 1 g orally once, and metronidazole 2 g orally once.

ALTITUDE ILLNESS[5,11-13]
Definition and Epidemiology

- A number of acute syndromes occur at high altitude. Some may occur at altitudes as low as 2,500 m, and all are more likely with increasing altitude and increased rate of ascent.
- Acute mountain sickness (AMS) is defined as the presence of headache in an unacclimatized person who has recently arrived at an altitude above 2,500 m (8,000 feet) plus the presence of one or more of the following: gastrointestinal symptoms (anorexia, nausea, vomiting), insomnia, dizziness, and fatigue or weakness. Physical exam findings can include edema and crackles on lung auscultation. The symptoms typically develop within 6 to 10 hours after ascent, but can occur as early as 1 hour or as late as 96 hours.
- High altitude cerebral edema (HACE) is a clinical diagnosis, defined as the onset of ataxia and/or altered consciousness in someone with AMS, usually occurring within 48 to 72 hours upon arrival at a given altitude (often above 3,000 m). Symptoms may include headache, confusion, loss of coordination, decreased mental status, or coma. Physical exam findings my include papilledema and loss of cerebellar control.
- High altitude pulmonary edema (HAPE) accounts for the majority of deaths due to high altitude disease and usually begins 24 to 96 hours after arriving at altitude. Diagnosis of HAPE requires two of the following symptoms: chest tightness, dyspnea at rest, weakness or cough; and two of the following physical exam findings: increased heart rate or respiratory rate, and wheezing/rales or cyanosis. Production of frothy, rusty sputum may also be present.
- Risk factors include a history of high altitude illness, rapid rate of ascent, residence at an altitude below 900 m, physical exertion, obesity, age less than 50 years, and certain preexisting cardiopulmonary conditions.

Behavioral Counseling

- Altitude illness can be prevented or modified by paying attention to the speed, height, and duration of ascent. Ascending to an altitude of greater than 2,700 m immediately is not recommended.
- "Staging" is the process of remaining at an intermediate altitude for a few days before attempting the ultimate altitude. It is recommended that the patient ascend no more than 300 m per day if the altitude is greater than 2,400 m. The most important factor in ascent is thought to be the altitude at which the patient is located during each sleeping period.
- If symptoms of AMS occur, further ascent should be delayed until symptoms resolve. If symptoms worsen, last more than 24 to 48 hours, or if symptoms of HAPE or HACE occur, then descent should begin immediately.
- Adequate hydration can help decrease symptoms, as can good physical conditioning (but even athletes in excellent condition can experience altitude illness).

Medications

- Acetazolamide can help prevent or mitigate the symptoms of AMS. For prophylaxis of moderate- to high-risk patients, the dose is 125 mg twice daily (or 500 mg daily with slow-release formulation) started the day before the ascent. The dose can be increased to 250 mg orally twice a day if the patient develops AMS during the ascent. The prophylaxis should be continued for the first 2 days at high altitude. When treating symptoms, the dose is 250 mg twice a day until symptoms resolve.

- Dexamethasone can be administered in doses of 2 mg every 6 hours or 4 mg every 12 hours. If a patient will not be able to acclimate and will be doing intense physical activity, the dose can be increased to 4 mg every 12 hours. Total time of therapy with steroids should not be longer than 10 days. Additionally, combining acetazolamide and dexamethasone may have additive benefits in cases where there is a rapid progression of symptoms, particularly if descent will be delayed.
- Oxygen therapy can help alleviate many of the symptoms of AMS in the acute setting, and can be lifesaving in HAPE and HACE.
- Theophylline has been shown to have some efficacy in preventing or reducing the severity of AMS in several small studies.
- Nifedipine can be used to prevent HAPE in people with a previous history. The usual dose is 30 mg twice daily one day prior to ascent and then three times daily once climbers reach 3,400 m. Nifedipine 10 mg initially and then 20 to 30 mg every 12 hours can be used for the acute treatment of HAPE while descent is being arranged.
- Portable hyperbaric chambers, which are becoming common equipment on mountaineering expeditions, may be a useful and lifesaving temporizing measure while descent is arranged in HACE and HAPE.

ADDITIONAL CONSIDERATIONS[5,14]

- **Jet lag**, the disturbance of biorhythms resulting from a rapid time zone change in travel, is common, and typically more severe after eastward travel. Increased sunlight exposure, daytime caffeine, short naps, and remaining well hydrated may be helpful. Melatonin or a short-acting sleeping medication such as zolpidem may be helpful to some travelers.
- Travelers are at increased risk of prolonged immobilization and related **venous thromboembolism** (VTE), particularly during cramped air travel. Certain risk factors (history of VTE, obesity, malignancy, pregnancy, and advanced age) increase the risk. Lower extremity exercises during travel (such as frequent walking and calf pumping), increased hydration, compression stockings, and, for high-risk patients, prophylactic doses of low-molecular-weight heparin are considerations to reduce risk.
- **Motion sickness** is a common occurrence for travelers, particularly by sea or air. Food and drink containing ginger may reduce nausea. Medications that may be helpful in appropriate patients include scopolamine patch, promethazine, dimenhydrinate, or meclizine. Anticholinergic medication side effects (such as increased falls in elderly) are a concern.
- **Sun protection** advice, including use of sunscreen (SPF of at least 30) and protective clothing (including wide-brimmed hat), should be given to travelers to sunny climates (especially to higher altitudes or closer to the equator).
- Prior to travel, maximize the health status of those with chronic health problems, such as diabetes, asthma, heart disease, arthritis, etc. Cardiovascular disease is the most common cause of death for Americans traveling abroad.
- Educate travelers using life-sustaining medications (asthma inhalers, antianginal medications, etc.) to bring twice as much as needed for the trip, in two separate containers in two separate locations (one always carried by the patient).
- Provide travelers with a medication list with generic names and doses, and include over-the-counter and herbal remedies. Travelers should also have copies of important medical records, including electrocardiograms, lists of diagnoses, and details on implantable devices (pacemakers, valves, defibrillators, etc.).
- Consider the fetal impact of immunizations and prophylactic medications in pregnant women, and advise women about their own immunocompromised state. Adjust itineraries to avoid areas where teratogenic medications would be necessary for malaria prophylaxis. Discourage women with high-risk pregnancies from any international travel.
- Immigrants visiting friends and relatives ("VFRs") account for a disproportionately high volume of international travel. They are at increased risk of travel-related illness, as they have longer stays and spend time in high-risk areas. In addition, they rarely receive pretravel care, and often take inappropriate or no prophylaxis for malaria or other conditions. Physicians need to proactively query their immigrant patients about plans to visit friends and relatives abroad, and offer appropriate, culturally sensitive care.

REFERENCES

1. CDC Health Information for International Travel 2014. Centers for Disease Control and Prevention. www.cdc.gov/travel/yellowbook/2014. Accessed March 21, 2014.
2. de la Cabada Bauche J, DuPont HL. New developments in traveler's diarrhea. *Gastroenterol Hepatol* 2011;7(2):88–95.
3. Kollaritsch H, Paulke-Korinek M, Wiedermann, U. Traveler's diarrhea. *Infect Dis Clin North Am* 2012;26(3):691–706.
4. Xavier RJ, Thomas HJ. Gastrointestinal diseases. In: Magill AJ, Ryan ET, Hill D, et al., eds. *Hunter's tropical medicine and emerging infectious diseases*. 9th ed. Philadelphia, PA: Elsevier Saunders; 2013:18–27.
5. Advice for travelers, Treatment Guidelines from the Medical Letter. *Med Lett* 2012;(10):45–56.
6. World Malaria Report 2013. World Health Organization. http://www.who.int/malaria/publications/world_malaria_report_2013/en/. Accessed March 21, 2014.
7. Taylor T, Agbenyega T. Malaria. In: Magill AJ, Ryan ET, Hill D, et al., eds. *Hunter's tropical medicine and emerging infectious diseases*. 9th ed. Philadelphia, PA: Elsevier Saunders; 2013:696–717.
8. Johnson BA, Kalra MG. Prevention of malaria in travelers. *Am Fam Physician* 2012;85(10):973–977.
9. Jong E. Immunizations for travelers. In: Jong EC, Sanford C, eds. *The travel and tropical medicine manual*. 4th ed. Philadelphia, PA: Elsevier Saunders; 2008:50–75.
10. Workowski KA, Berman S; Centers for Disease Control and Prevention (CDC). Sexually transmitted diseases treatment guidelines, 2010. *MMWR* 2010;59(RR-12). http://www.cdc.gov/STD/treatment/2010/STD-Treatment-2010-RR5912.pdf. Accessed March 21, 2014.
11. Litch JA, Bishop RA. Altitude illness. In: Jong EC, Sanford C, eds. *The travel and tropical medicine manual*. 4th ed. Philadelphia, PA: Elsevier Saunders; 2008:152–162.
12. Fiore DC, Hall S, Shoja P. Altitude illness: risk factors, prevention, presentation and treatment. *Am Fam Physician* 2010;82(9):1103–1110.
13. Luks AM, McIntosh SE, Grissom CK, et al. Wilderness Medical Society consensus guidelines for the prevention and treatment of acute altitude illness. *Wilderness Environ Med* 2010;21(2):146–155.
14. Bazemore AW, Huntington M. The pretravel consultation. *Am Fam Physician* 2009;80(6):583–590.

CHAPTER 2

Common Presenting Problems

Section Editor: Gretchen M. Dickson

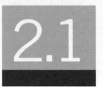

Weight Loss

Samuel N. Grief

Involuntary or unintentional weight loss is a common complaint in primary care offices.[1,2] Involuntary weight loss is associated with more adverse health outcomes.[3] Gastrointestinal and psychiatric disorders are usually the most prevalent causes of unintentional weight loss.[2–4] Although malignancy is a leading cause of weight loss, extensive and costly workups for occult cancers are rarely beneficial.[1,5,6] Evaluation of weight loss is not a simple task, given the extensive potential list of causes (Table 2.1-1). In more than one study, 10% to 36% of weight loss remains undiagnosed.[1,2,4] Yet basic principles of taking a comprehensive history, performing a pertinent and focused physical examination, and ordering appropriate laboratory testing will quickly uncover most causes of weight loss in the outpatient setting.

DIAGNOSTIC APPROACH

Weight loss is a challenging problem, often surrounded by fears on the part of both patient and physician of an occult malignancy. The key to the diagnosis of involuntary weight loss is a careful and complete history and age-appropriate physical examination. The approach begins broadly and then quickly focuses on specifics derived from the initial evaluation.

Quantify Loss

A loss of 5% or more from the baseline body weight (not ideal body weight) over 6 months is significant.[2,4,7,8] Some authorities now suggest that a minimum of 10% weight loss over the same period warrants action.[1,9] Unintentional weight loss may be a result of loss of fat, muscle atrophy, fluid loss, or a combination of these.[9]

Serial measurements are the best method of verifying weight loss, but other considerations include family report and changes in clothing or belt size. For infants and young children, slowing or cessation of growth are red flags to initiate a diagnostic evaluation.

TABLE 2.1-1	Major Causes of Weight Loss

Decreased intake
Malignancy, congestive heart failure, medications, dementia, depression, grief, electrolyte disturbances, poor dentition or taste, gastric or esophageal disease, electrolyte disorders, alcoholism, financial hardship, social isolation, HIV and AIDS
Increased nutrient loss
Profuse vomiting or diarrhea, diabetes mellitus
Increased metabolic demand
Fever, malignancy, tuberculosis, hyperthyroidism, chronic infection, drug abuse (cocaine, stimulants)
Impaired absorption
Cholestasis, infection (parasitic, other), medications, pancreatic insufficiency, diabetic or HIV enteropathy, inflammatory bowel disease, celiac sprue, surgery

TABLE 2.1-2	Weight Loss MD: A Mnemonic for Common Causes of Unintentional Weight Loss in Adults[31]
W	Wasting disease (e.g., cancer, AIDS)
E	Eating problems or disorders (anorexia nervosa, inability to feed self)
I	Income deprivation, Infectious (e.g., HIV, TB)
G	Gastrointestinal problems (e.g., inflammatory bowel disease, parasitic infestation, chronic diarrhea, gastroparesis, celiac disease)
H	Hyperthyroidism, hyperparathyroidism, hypoadrenalism
T	Toxic substances (e.g., alcohol, laxatives, lead, illicit drugs)
L	Low-calorie diet (e.g., commercial weight loss programs, self-imposed diets)
O	Oral problems (e.g., sores, ulcers, caries, poor dentition or dentures)
S	Swallowing disorders (e.g., amyotrophic lateral sclerosis, Parkinson disease, progressive supranuclear palsy)
S	Social problems (e.g., isolation, neglect, stress)
M	Medication side effects or metabolic conditions (e.g., diabetes, thyroid disease)[11]
D	Depression or other psychiatric disorders (e.g., schizophrenia, obsessive–compulsive disorder)

AIDS: Acquired Immune Deficiency Syndrome
HIV: Human Immunodeficiency Virus
TB: Tuberculosis

- **Categories of weight loss.** The causes of weight loss can be divided into four major categories: decreased intake; increased nutrient loss; increased metabolic demand; and impaired absorption (Table 2.1-1). A novel way of approaching typical causes of weight loss is by using the mnemonic device "Weight Loss MD" (Table 2.1-2). Since gastrointestinal (GI) causes are frequently implicated in weight loss, it may be suitable to divide causes of weight loss into GI and non-GI causes.[3] Involuntary weight loss exceeding 20% of usual, baseline weight is often associated with severe protein-energy malnutrition, nutritional deficiencies, and multiorgan dysfunction.[10]

Special Considerations

A tailored approach in elderly people includes greater emphasis on social and environmental factors.[4,8,11,12] Unintentional weight loss in elderly people is often associated with increased morbidity and mortality.[4,8,12–14] The approach in human immunodeficiency virus (HIV) and acquired immune deficiency syndrome (AIDS) is more comprehensive, and special attention is given to disease-specific infections, nutritional changes, psychosocial issues, and neoplasia.[15–17] In the pediatric population, failure to thrive is still the most appropriate term for improper growth among infants and young children.[18] Anorexia nervosa and other psychiatric or behavioral disorders are the most common causes of weight loss in older children.[19]

Other populations at high risk for unintentional weight loss are those suffering major burns and trauma and those with spinal cord injury, as well as patients in outpatient rehabilitation and in nursing homes due to comorbid factors such as aging and disability.[20,21]

History

- **Initial data.** Begin with open-ended, general questioning followed by a complete review of systems. How do you feel about your weight? This open-ended question provides an opportunity for patients to disclose any concerns about their weight loss and help uncover undiagnosed eating disorders. More specific questions include: Is the loss intentional? Are you dieting, taking diuretics or laxatives, or suffering from any eating disorders? A yes to any of these questions would be classified as voluntary weight loss. It is valuable to quantify the patient's average daily or weekly intake of food and drink and total calories. Food frequency questionnaires are useful tools for the above and are best administered by registered dietitians.[22] The frequency of meals, appetite changes, and difficulty with food preparation can also be elicited. Quantify tobacco, alcohol, and drug usage as these substances often replace food intake and increase the risk of nutritional deficiencies and subsequent weight loss. Focused and relevant past medical, surgical, psychiatric, and family histories will often provide clues to the underlying cause of weight loss. Ask about past bariatric or gastric bypass surgeries, previous or current mood disorders, and any history of endocrinopathies. Inquire about exercise habits—excessive exercise or forms of physical activity may hint at underlying body dysmorphic disorders.[23] Medications (especially anorexiants) and herbal or vitamin supplements may also factor into weight considerations, and a detailed list of all pharmaceuticals should be obtained.[2,8,13] Social factors, including stress, isolation, and the cost and effort required to prepare and consume food, can have a major impact on weight.[13,24]

- **Specific historical data.** The patient's symptoms and complaints should direct the clinician to greater detail. Focus your history using the mnemonic device Weight Loss MD (Table 2.1-2). Ask all patients about constitutional symptoms to evaluate their general state of health: Any nausea or vomiting? Change in bowel habits? Fever? How is their appetite? Energy level?

Physical Examination

The importance of a complete physical exam in evaluating unexplained weight loss has been confirmed.[6] In the pediatric population, physical findings are helpful in distinguishing causes of involuntary weight loss.[25] First, quantify loss by serial weight measurements whenever possible. Measurement of vital signs, including body mass index, temperature, blood pressure, respiratory and heart rates, is always important. A more focused examination based on clues from the history is often appropriate. Physical findings such as a goiter, clubbing, hepatosplenomegaly, and/or generalized lymphadenopathy may also be relevant findings.[25]

Testing

- **Basic laboratories.** Debate continues regarding the most useful and cost-effective laboratory testing for involuntary weight loss. A simple and structured approach is best.[1–4,8] The first line of testing should include complete blood count, thyrotropin (thyroid-stimulating hormone; TSH) assay, urinalysis, and fecal occult blood testing. A comprehensive chemistry panel including serum glucose, transaminases, blood urea nitrogen, creatinine, and electrolytes (calcium, magnesium, phosphorus, sodium, and potassium) is essential. A chest radiograph is often included in the initial battery of tests.[1]
- **Comprehensive analysis.** Careful observation and follow-up are superior management strategies to undirected diagnostic testing.[1–4,8] An initial basic evaluation can often provide reassurance regarding lack of an ominous cause to the involuntary weight loss.[6] When indicated, targeted ultrasounds, upper gastrointestinal radiographs, endoscopy, and colonoscopy are the most useful second-line tests.[1] National Cancer Institute or U.S. Preventive Services Task Force age-specific screening guidelines should be evaluated and up-to-date for the patient. These can be accessed on the internet at http://www.ahrq.gov/clinic/uspstfix.htm.

    Computed tomography and other expensive investigations are seldom beneficial in the absence of a specific indication.[1,2,8] Tumor markers are third-line tests and may not be as helpful as previously thought in uncovering the cause of involuntary weight loss.[14]

Differential Diagnosis

The integration of history, examination, and laboratory data will usually reveal the cause of involuntary weight loss. Cancer, including gastrointestinal malignancies, accounts for 24% of cases, whereas lung cancer represents 5% of cases. Gastrointestinal diseases account for another 25% to 31%.[7] Using a cancer scoring system to stratify older patients into risk categories for cancer due to unexplained, unintentional weight loss has not proven to be of value in identifying an underlying cause.[5] If the initial steps in the evaluation are not conclusive, the best approach is careful observation. Follow-up examinations and testing should be done monthly for 6 months. If a physical cause exists, it will almost always be found within this period of time.[1,4] If an organic cause is present, this simple approach will expose it more than 75% of the time.[1,2] If an organic cause is not identified within the first 6 months, it is unlikely that one will be found.[4] However, these undifferentiated patients typically do well, and assuming they do not have continued and progressive weight loss, they have an excellent overall prognosis.[5] Malignancy is a significant cause of weight loss; however, a truly occult malignancy is rare, and an exhaustive search for one is neither cost-effective nor supported by the literature.[1–6]

TREATMENT

Nonpharmacologic and pharmacologic treatments are usually comingled in the treatment plan for unintentional weight loss.

- **Nonpharmacologic treatment.** Involving ancillary health care providers, such as dietitians, social workers, home health care nurses, and immediate or extended family members, is beneficial.[1,4] Increasing physical activity in patients with low energy may stimulate appetite and result in modest weight gain.[1,4] Nutritional supplements are a common modality in treating weight loss and often work best when used in conjunction with other treatment options.[13,26] Counseling patients to consume nutritional supplements in between, rather than instead of meals, is the best approach[13,26] A broad-spectrum vitamin and mineral supplement should be considered in all patients with unintentional weight loss.[13,26]

- **Pharmacologic treatment.** Several medications have been used in attempts to stave off continued weight loss and establish weight gain. Megestrol acetate is indicated for unexplained, significant weight loss in patients with AIDS.[27] Recent literature has shown megestrol is also effective in weight gain among the cachectic, geriatric patients.[28] Dronabinol is indicated for weight loss in patients with AIDS and in patients with cancer undergoing chemotherapy.[29] Other appetite stimulants or weight-gain–inducing medications include cyproheptadine, ghrelin, growth hormone, vitamin supplements, antidepressants, antipsychotics, and other mood-stabilizing drugs.[11,28,30] Treatment with any medication should involve close monitoring for side effects and initially be for a short period (<3 months); further treatment depends on response and condition of the patient.[26]

REFERENCES

1. Evans AT, Gupta R. Approach to the patient with weight loss. http://www.uptodate.com/contents/approach-to-the-patient-with-weight-loss?detectedLanguage=en&source=search_result&search=unexplained+weight+loss&selectedTitle=1%7E150&provider=noProvider. Accessed November 4, 2013.
2. McMinn J, Steel C, Bowman A. Investigation and management of unintentional weight loss in older adults. *BMJ* 2011;342:d1732.
3. Proctor DD. Approach to the patient with gastrointestinal disease. In: Goldman L, Ausiello D, eds. *Cecil medicine*. 23rd ed. St. Louis, MO: Saunders; 2008:840–841.
4. Alibhai SMH, Greenwood C, Payette H. An approach to the management of unintentional weight loss in elderly people. *CMAJ* 2005;172(6):773–780.
5. Chen SP, Peng LN, Lin MH, et al. Evaluating probability of cancer among older people with unexplained, unintentional weight loss. *Arch Gerontol Geriatr* 2010;50 (Suppl 1):S27–S29. doi: 10.1016/S0167-4943(10)70008-X.
6. Metalidis C, Knockaert DC, Bobbaers H, et al. Involuntary weight loss. Does a negative baseline evaluation provide adequate reassurance? [published online ahead of print November 26, 2007]. *Eur J Intern Med* 2008;19(5):345–349. doi: 10.1016/j.ejim.2007.09.019.
7. Sahyoun NR, Serdula MK, Galuska DA, et al. The epidemiology of recent involuntary weight loss in the United States population. *J Nutr Health Aging* 2004;8(6):510.
8. Huffman GB. Evaluating and treating unintentional weight loss in the elderly. *Am Fam Physician* 2002;15;65(4):640–650.
9. National Cancer Institute (November 2011). "Nutrition in cancer care (PDQ)". *Physician Data Query*. National Cancer Institute.
10. Bistrian BR. Nutritional assessment. In: Goldman L, Schafer AI, eds. *Cecil medicine*. 24th ed. Philadelphia, PA: Saunders Elsevier; 2011:chap 221.
11. Zanni G, Involuntary Weight Loss - An Ignored Vital Sign in Seniors. *Pharmacy Times*, January 15, 2010. http://www.pharmacytimes.com/publications/issue/2010/January2010/FeatureFocusWeightLoss-0110. Accessed November 5, 2013.
12. Gazewood JD, Mehr DR. Diagnosis and management of weight loss in the elderly. *J Fam Pract* 1998;47:19–25.
13. Stajkovic S, Aitken EM, Holroyd-Leduc J. Unintentional weight loss in older adults. *CMAJ* 2011;183(4):443–449.
14. Wu JM, Lin MH, Peng LN, et al. Evaluating diagnostic strategy of older patients with unexplained unintentional body weight loss: a hospital-based study [published online ahead of print November 10, 2010]. *Arch Gerontol Geriatr* 2011;53(1):e51–e54. doi: 10.1016/j.archger.2010.10.016.
15. Carter M, Hughson G. Unintentional weight loss. In: *NAM, Aids map*. http://www.aidsmap.com/Unintentional-weight-loss/page/1044802/. Published June 14, 2012.
16. Siddiqui J, Phillips AL, Freedland ES, et al. Prevalence and cost of HIV-associated weight loss in a managed care population. *Curr Med Res Opin* 2009;25(5):1307–1317.
17. Tang AM, Jacobson DL, et al. Increasing risk of 5% or greater unintentional weight loss in a cohort of HIV-infected patients, 1995–2003. *JAIDS* 2005;40(1):70–76.
18. Olsen EM. Failure to thrive: still a problem of definition. *Clin Pediatr* 2006;45:1–6.
19. Behrman RE, Kliegman RM, Schor N, et al. *Nelson textbook of pediatrics*. Chap 26. 19th ed. Amsterdam: Elsevier; 2011.
20. Demling RH, DeSanti L. Involuntary weight loss and protein-energy malnutrition: diagnosis and treatment. *Medscape* 2001. http://www.medscape.org/viewarticle/416589_2. Accessed November 5, 2013.
21. Salva A, Coll-Planas L, Bruce S, et al. Nutritional assessment of residents in long-term care facilities (LTCFs): recommendations of the task force on nutrition and ageing of the IAGG European region and the IANA. *J Nutr Health Aging* 2009;13(6):475–483.
22. Liu L, Wang PP, Roebothan B, et al. Assessing the validity of a self-administered food-frequency questionnaire (FFQ) in the adult population of Newfoundland and Labrador, Canada. *Nutr J* 2013;12:49.
23. van der Meer J, van Rood YR, van der Wee NJ, et al. Prevalence, demographic and clinical characteristics of body dysmorphic disorder among psychiatric outpatients with mood, anxiety or somatoform disorders [published online ahead of print October 27, 2011]. *Nord J Psychiatry*. 2012;66(4):232–238. doi: 10.3109/08039488.2011.623315.

24. Sorbye LW, Schroll M, Finne Soveri H, et al. Unintended weight loss in the elderly living at home: the aged in Home Care Project (AdHOC). *J Nutr Health Aging* 2008;12(1):10–16
25. Caglar D. Evaluation of weight loss in infants over six months of age, children, and adolescents. Accessed April 9, 2013. http://www.uptodate.com/contents/evaluation-of-weight-loss-in-infants-over-six-months-of-age-children-and-adolescents.
26. Smith KL, Greenwood C, Payette H, et al. An approach to the nonpharmacologic and pharmacologic management of unintentional weight loss among older adults. *Geriatrics & Aging* 2007;10(2):91–98.
27. Medline Plus. AHFS* Consumer Medication Information. The American Society of Health-System Pharmacists, Inc. U.S. National Library of Medicine, U.S. Department of Health and Human Services National Institutes of Health. http://www.nlm.nih.gov/medlineplus/druginfo/meds/a682003.html.
28. Yaxley A, Miller MD, Fraser RJ, et al. Pharmacological interventions for geriatric cachexia: a narrative review of the literature. *J Nutr Health Aging* 2012;16(2):148–154.
29. Medline Plus. AHFS* Consumer Medication Information. The American Society of Health-System Pharmacists, Inc. U.S. National Library of Medicine, U.S. Department of Health and Human Services National Institutes of Health. http://www.nlm.nih.gov/medlineplus/druginfo/meds/a607054.html
30. Berkowitz RI, Fabricatore AN. Obesity, psychiatric status and psychiatric medications. *Psychiatr Clin North Am* 2005;28(1):39–54.
31. Grief, SN. Weight loss. In: Paulman P, Paulman A, Harrison J, eds. *Taylor's Manual of Family Medicine*. 3rd ed. Philadelphia, PA: Lippincott Williams & Wilkins; 2008:47–50.

2.2 Fatigue

Janet C. Lindemann

GENERAL PRINCIPLES
Definition
Fatigue is defined as a subjective state of lack of energy, exhaustion, or tiredness with a decreased capacity for physical or mental work, and persists despite sufficient rest.

Epidemiology
One of the most common complaints in the general population, fatigue is the chief complaint in nearly 10% of patients presenting to a primary care physician and is reported as a symptom in over 20% of all patient encounters. Women complain of fatigue approximately twice as often as men. A medical or psychiatric cause is identified in about two-thirds of cases of fatigue.[1] The prognosis of idiopathic fatigue is surprisingly poor with half of patients still fatigued 6 months later.

Classification
Fatigue may be classified as acute fatigue, prolonged fatigue, chronic fatigue, and chronic fatigue syndrome. Acute fatigue is short-lived and generally attributable to physical exertion or an acute illness. Prolonged fatigue is defined as persistent fatigue lasting 1 month or longer, while chronic fatigue is defined as similar symptoms lasting 6 months or more.

Chronic fatigue syndrome is specifically defined by the Centers for Disease Control and Prevention as clinically evaluated, unexplained, persistent, or relapsing fatigue lasting 6 months or more with four or more of the following associated symptoms: impaired memory or concentration, sore throat, tender cervical or axillary lymph nodes, muscle pain, pain in several joints, new headaches, unrefreshing sleep, or malaise after exertion.[2] The impairment in functioning and psychological distress is more severe in chronic fatigue syndrome than idiopathic chronic fatigue, and the prognosis is worse. Less than 10% of patients with chronic fatigue have chronic fatigue syndrome.

DIAGNOSIS
History
The clinical evaluation of fatigue is rooted in a thorough medical and psychosocial history. Allowing the patient to speak uninterrupted for the first several minutes in the interview often provides important clues. Key aspects of history include onset and nature of the fatigue, medical and psychiatric

histories, family and social histories, medications and substance use, dietary and exercise habits, life events, and family relationships. A mental status examination and screening for depression should be considered if warranted by presenting symptoms.

Physical Examination

The physical examination, though often unrevealing, should include thyroid gland assessment; full cardiopulmonary examination to detect evidence of CHF, valvular disease, or chronic lung disease; full neurologic examination, including muscle strength, bulk, and tone; and examination of the lymphatic system to assess for lymphadenopathy.

Laboratory and Imaging

Laboratory testing for the diagnosis of fatigue does not often yield answers. Studies show that only about 15% of patients in primary care settings have an organic cause for their fatigue and that laboratory results rarely affect management. The following recommendations for the laboratory investigation of fatigue are adapted from guidelines developed by Dutch, Canadian, and Australian general practice groups[3]:

- Consider monitoring for a month after initial presentation, while initiating conservative management.
- If proceeding with laboratory evaluation, it should include complete blood count, electrolytes, glucose, liver and kidney function tests, thyroid function tests, and urinalysis.
- Clues from the history and examination may indicate the need for erythrocyte sedimentation rate, monospot, antinuclear antigen testing, or chest radiography.

Differential Diagnosis

The mnemonic, **DEAD TIRED** (Table 2.2-1), illustrates the common causes of fatigue. Depression, environment or lifestyle issues, anxiety and anemia are among the most common causes of fatigue. Diabetes and other endocrine disorders, including thyroid disease, should be considered as well as an undiscovered tumor. Many infections, especially those of viral origin, cause fatigue, as well as insomnia and sleep disorders such as obstructive sleep apnea. Rheumatologic disorders, such as rheumatoid arthritis, systemic lupus eythematosus, and fibromyalgia, are often accompanied by fatigue. Endocarditis, while rare, is a must-not-miss diagnosis, as are other cardiac conditions such as coronary artery disease. Finally, drugs, either prescription or of personal use or abuse, should be considered. The following medications may cause fatigue[4]:

- Antihistamines
- Benzodiazepines
- β Blockers
- Blood pressure medications
- Diuretics
- Glucocorticoids
- Narcotic pain medications
- Nonsteroidal anti-inflammatory drugs (NSAIDs)
- Selective serotonin reuptake inhibitors
- Sleeping medications
- Tricyclic antidepressants

A pearl that is sometimes useful is that fatigue from organic disease is relieved by sleep and decreased activity, while fatigue from anxiety or depression may improve with exercise and is often not relieved by rest.[5]

TABLE 2.2-1	Common Causes of Fatigue: DEAD TIRED		
D	Depression	T	Thyroid, Tumors
E	Environment/lifestyle	I	Infection, Insomnia
A	Anxiety, Anemia	R	Rheumatologic
D	Diabetes/endocrine	E	Endocarditis/cardiovascular
		D	Drugs (medications or substance abuse)

From Lindeman J. Fatigue. In: Bope ET, Kellerman RD, eds. *Conn's current therapy, 2014*. Philadelphia, PA: Saunders Elsevier; 2013:12.

TREATMENT

Behavioral

Early and active management of fatigue may prevent its progression to chronicity. When an underlying cause can be identified, this should be treated. When no disease is identified, a broader biopsychosocial strategy is necessary. This begins with acknowledgement and reassurance, along with education about the common causes and natural course of fatigue. Cognitive behavioral therapy is a brief pragmatic psychotherapeutic approach that incorporates graded increases in activity while paying attention to the patient's beliefs and concerns. Identifying unhelpful beliefs, such as *this is all due to a virus*, and suggesting alternative approaches that reproduce positive outcomes can be helpful. Graded exercise therapy may also be of benefit.

Medications

If there is evidence of depression, a trial of an antidepressant is appropriate. Randomized trials have shown cognitive behavioral therapy to be equally as effective as medication for mild to moderate depression.

Referrals

Specialty referrals may be appropriate in the following situations:

- Children with chronic fatigue.
- Suspicion of severe psychiatric illness.
- Suspicion of occult malignancy.
- Evidence of significant sleep disorder.

REFERENCES

1. Rosenthal TC, Majeroni BA, Pretorius R, et al. Fatigue: an overview. *Am Fam Physician* 2008;78(10):1173–1179.
2. Centers for Disease Control and Prevention. Chronic fatigue syndrome. Atlanta, GA. http://www.cdc .gov/cfs/general/index.html. Accessed March 3, 2014.
3. Harrison M. Pathology testing in the tired patient: a rational approach. *Aust Fam Physician* 2008;37(11):908–910.
4. O'Connell TX. Fatigue. In: O'Connell TX, Dor K, eds. *Instant work-ups: a clinical guide to obstetric and gynecologic care.* 1st ed. Philadelphia, PA: Saunders; 2009:76–82.
5. Ponka D, Kirlew M. Top 10 differential diagnoses in family medicine: fatigue. *Can Fam Physician* 2007;53:892.

2.3 Dizziness

Jennifer Wipperman

Dizziness is a common, often frustrating, complaint encountered by family physicians. The differential diagnosis for dizziness is extensive, and frequently patients have multiple contributing etiologies. While most causes of dizziness are benign, a few may be life-threatening. However, with a thorough history and physical exam, most patients can be effectively diagnosed and serious causes ruled out.

DEFINITION

Dizziness is a general term that should be classified into four subtypes:

- *Presyncope.* A feeling of lightheadedness; patients note that they feel like they are "about to pass out."
- *Vertigo.* A false sense of motion of the self or the environment, most often described as a spinning sensation, but also as a tilting or swaying motion. Causes include benign paroxysmal positional vertigo (BPPV), vestibular neuritis, migraine, and cerebrovascular attacks.
- *Disequilibrium.* A sense of imbalance, most often noted while walking.
- *Nonspecific dizziness.* A vague sense of dizziness that patients struggle to describe.

The most common type of dizziness seen in general practice is vertigo; however, the distribution of causes varies with age.[1] The elderly are more likely to have multiple etiologies, and more likely to have a serious cause such as stroke.[2] Younger patients are more likely to present with benign causes such as vasovagal presyncope or psychiatric conditions.

DIAGNOSIS

The diagnosis of the disorder(s) causing a patient's dizziness is made clinically. Further testing with labs or imaging is mainly for diagnostic confirmation and for ruling out other causes.

History

An accurate, unbiased history is essential to forming the correct diagnosis. Patients should be asked to describe their dizziness in an open-ended manner, without leading questions. Historical clues help define the problem, which include:

- *Triggers.* Vertigo that is triggered by head position changes, such as rolling over in bed or looking up to a shelf, is characteristic of BPPV. Lightheadedness upon standing is indicative of orthostasis. While standing can trigger both BPPV and orthostasis, orthostasis will not be triggered by head position changes alone. Recent head trauma may be associated with BPPV. A need to hold on to an object or countertop to maintain balance is often seen with disequilibrium.
- *Timing.* The acute onset of constant, severe vertigo may be seen in vestibular neuritis/acute labrynthitis or stroke. Episodic vertigo lasting less than a minute is usually BPPV. Vertigo lasting minutes to hours is more likely Meniere disease or TIA, while vertigo associated with migraine often lasts hours to days. Presyncope is always episodic, while nonspecific dizziness is more constant in nature.
- *Associated symptoms.* Migraine symptoms that accompany vertigo are indicative of vestibular migraine. Ear symptoms such as tinnitus and hearing loss may be seen in Meniere disease or acute labrynthitis. Presyncope is often accompanied by sweating, nausea, and blurry vision. Neurologic symptoms are concerning for central causes such as stroke or intracranial mass. Symptoms of chest pain, palpitations, and dyspnea imply cardiac causes, but may be seen in psychiatric dizziness as well.
- *Past medical history.* A prior history of diabetes, hypertension, stroke, or coronary artery disease is associated with cardiovascular causes of dizziness. Long-standing, poorly controlled diabetes mellitus predisposes to autonomic and peripheral neuropathy. Patients with vestibular migraine usually have a prior history of migraine.
- *Family history.* Many etiologies have a familial preponderance such as migraine, BPPV, stroke, and Meniere disease.
- *Medications.* Anticonvulsants and antidepressants are often associated with nonspecific dizziness. Overtreatment of hypertension may lead to orthostasis.

Physical Exam

A thorough physical exam is the second essential step to diagnosis. Specific exam findings include:

- *Eye and ear.* Cerumen impaction, otitis media, vesicles on the tympanic membrane (herpes zoster oticus), hearing or visual changes, nystagmus
- *Cardiovascular.* Orthostatic blood pressure, carotid bruit, heart murmur, arrhythmia, signs of peripheral vascular disease
- *Neurologic.* Focal findings, such as sensory changes, abnormal Rhomberg, abnormal gait
- *Specialized physical exam tests* may help diagnose the cause of dizziness. If BPPV is suspected, the Dix–Hallpike maneuver is diagnostic for posterior canal BPPV, and the supine roll maneuver for lateral canal BPPV. To perform the Dix–Hallpike (DH), the patient sits with legs extended on the exam table. The patient looks up and to the side at a 45-degree angle. The examiner quickly lowers the patient to a lying position with head hanging off the exam table in the same 45-degree angle. The examiner observes the patient's eyes, and if a typical nystagmus and vertigo occur (latency of 5 to 20 seconds, crescendo–decrescendo pattern, torsional up-beating nystagmus, and lasts less than 60 seconds), then it is a positive test for the affected ear on the side tested. The test should be repeated on the opposite side, as BPPV can be bilateral. If the DH is normal, then the supine roll maneuver should be performed. The patient lies on his back, head facing up. The examiner quickly moves the patient's head 90 degrees to the side, and waits for horizontal nystagmus and vertigo. As with the DH, the supine roll test should be repeated on the other side.

The head-thrust and visual fixation tests are useful for differentiating between stroke and vestibular neuritis. For the head-thrust test, the examiner moves the patient's head quickly 10 degrees to the left and right, observing for a saccade. If a saccade is present, this is indicative of a peripheral lesion causing vertigo, such as vestibular neuritis. If there is no saccade, then a central cause, like stroke or intracranial mass, is suspected. The visual fixation test is helpful in patients who have spontaneous nystagmus. Nystagmus that stops by visually focusing on an object in the room indicates a peripheral lesion. Central causes of vertigo will exhibit a nystagmus that cannot be suppressed with visual fixation.

Having a patient hyperventilate may help confirm a suspicion of nonspecific, psychogenic dizziness. In this case, hyperventilation will cause a dizziness that approximates the patient's symptoms.

Labs and Imaging

Additional evaluation with labs and imaging is generally not necessary. However, if stroke or an intracranial mass is suspected, an MRI of the brain is the imaging of choice because it best visualizes the posterior fossa. Vascular studies such as carotid doppler or MRA of intracranial vessels may be helpful in suspected cerebrovascular accident (CVA). Audiograms are helpful for confirming Meniere disease or if there is a concern for hearing loss. In cases of suspected arrhythmia, an EKG or Holter monitoring may be indicated. Vestibular function testing is helpful in cases of vertigo where the diagnosis is unclear.

TREATMENT

Dizziness is a symptom, not a disease. Therefore, to treat dizziness, the underlying problem should be targeted. Symptomatic medications, such as meclizine, antihistamines or benzodiazepines, should be used sparingly since they can worsen vertigo. Patients with vertigo often improve because the brain adapts and compensates for the initial deficit. However, vestibular suppressant medications can block central compensation and lead to chronic dizziness. These medications often increase fall risk in elderly patients as well, and thus are best avoided.

Elderly patients usually have multifactorial, chronic dizziness that is better managed than cured. All contributing factors should be elicited and treated, and function preserved. It is essential to ensure proper hearing and vision. Gait may be aided with assistant devices. Physical therapy is particularly useful for the elderly, including vestibular rehabilitation, which has been shown to decrease risk of falls. BPPV should be treated with a specific form of physical therapy called the *Epley maneuver*, or canalith repositioning procedure.

Vestibular rehabilitation is a useful treatment for multiple causes of vertigo, including vestibular neuritis, BPPV, and Meniere disease. It hastens recovery and improves balance, gait, and vision by increasing central compensation for vestibular dysfunction. Exercises consist of balance and gait training, as well as coordination of head and eye movements.

REFERENCES

1. Kroenke K, Lucas CA, Rosenberg ML, et al. Causes of persistent dizziness. A prospective study of 100 patients in ambulatory care. *Ann Intern Med* 1992;117(11):898–904.
2. Newman-Toker DE, Hsieh YH, Camargo CA Jr, et al. Spectrum of dizziness visits to US emergency departments: cross-sectional analysis from a nationally representative sample. *Mayo Clin Proc* 2008;83(7):765–775.

2.4 Cough

Stephanie Eve Owen McCullough, Justin M. Bailey

GENERAL PRINCIPLES
Definition

According to the most recent CDC data from 2010, cough was the most frequent principal reason for ambulatory care visits, comprising over 30 million visits annually.[1] For the purposes of diagnosis and treatment, cough can be easily categorized as acute (<3 weeks' duration), subacute (3 to 8 weeks' duration), or chronic (>8 weeks' duration).

DIAGNOSIS

Acute Cough

Most acute cough is of viral etiology and presents as an upper respiratory tract infection (URTI), viral rhinosinusitis, or acute bronchitis. Other causes of acute cough include exacerbation of preexisting conditions, such as asthma, bronchiectasis, or chronic obstructive pulmonary disease (COPD); occupational or environmental irritants; or serious conditions such as pneumonia, pulmonary embolus, congestive heart failure, or lung cancer.[2]

There are no specifically recommended tests for URTI. In patients with findings consistent with acute bronchitis, a chest x-ray may be warranted to exclude acute pneumonia if the physical exam demonstrates heart rate >100 beats per minute, respiratory rate >24 breaths per minute, oral temperature >38°C, or abnormalities on chest exam (especially in the presence of preexisting pulmonary disease, cardiac disease, or diabetes).[3] Specific instances in which further diagnostic testing might be considered include:

- influenza or RSV testing if there have been suspected exposures
- pertussis testing in high-risk patients (e.g., infants, immunosuppressed, chronically ill) with suspected exposures
- chest radiography if oxygen saturation is <90%
- D dimer and, if appropriate, chest computerized tomography (CT) if there are symptoms consistent with or risk factors for pulmonary embolus (known coagulopathy or personal venous thromboembolism, family history of venous thromboembolism, recent surgery or immobilization, pregnancy or estrogen use)

Note that, in the setting of an URTI, abnormalities seen on sinus films or CT scans are often due to congestion from the infection and not diagnostic of a bacterial sinus infection.[3]

Subacute Cough

The differential for subacute and chronic cough often overlap. However, **postinfectious** cough is the most common cause of subacute cough.[4] It is believed to be secondary to mucus hypersecretion and impaired clearance, but other superimposed factors, including upper airway cough syndrome and asthma, may contribute as well. Thus, if the cough has no relationship to a recent URTI or LRTI, it is reasonable to proceed with evaluation for chronic cough, as discussed below.

One should maintain a high index of suspicion for pertussis, especially if the cough is biphasic, associated with posttussive emesis, occurs in severe paroxysms, or has the characteristic inspiratory whooping sound. Laboratory confirmation can be performed via nasopharyngeal swabs for PCR, or for culture (if within 2 weeks of onset of symptoms).[5]

In a patient with known COPD or bronchiectasis, an acute exacerbation could persist into the subacute period. In these more complicated patients, consider chest x-ray or spirometry based on symptoms (e.g., wheezing, tachycardia, hemoptysis) and physical examination findings.

Chronic Cough

To assist in narrowing the differential for a patient with chronic cough, the clinician might proceed by first stopping any angiotension-converting enzyme (ACE) inhibitors, encouraging smoking cessation, and confirming a normal chest x-ray. Note that the ACE inhibitor–induced cough can present from hours to months after initiation of the medication. Similarly, resolution is generally within 1 to 4 weeks of discontinuation, with literature reports of cough lingering as long as 3 months after the medication was stopped.[6] In patients with a normal chest x-ray, not on an ACE inhibitor medication, the following etiologies can be considered:

- **Upper airway cough syndrome (UACS) (i.e., postnasal drip, sinusitis, rhinitis).** Patients with this syndrome may need to frequently clear the throat and often have nasal congestion and/or hoarseness. There may be a history of allergic or nonallergic rhinitis or sinusitis symptoms. However, there is no definitive symptom or physical finding that defines this entity. Patients may even be asymptomatic. The diagnosis is usually established by response to treatment (see below). If the patient suspected of UACS does not respond to treatment, sinus imaging may be indicated, with the understanding that positive predictive value is poor.[7]
- **Asthma.** It should be recognized that typical symptoms of asthma may not be present in patients with cough-variant asthma. When considering asthma, first do spirometry. If that is normal but the diagnosis of cough-variant asthma is still expected, definitive testing in the form of a methacholine challenge test may be explored. If this test is not easily available, empiric treatment for asthma may be tried (see below).

- **Nonasthmatic eosinophilic bronchitis (NAEB).** This entity is characterized by a chronic cough, no reversible airway obstruction, a negative methacholine challenge test, and a high eosinophil count in induced sputum. Patients often have an occupational or environmental allergy that triggers the cough.[8]
- **Gastroesophageal reflux disease (GERD).** In the nonsmoker with a normal chest x-ray, who is not taking an ACE inhibitor and has not responded to empirical treatments for UACS or asthma, reflux-related cough may be considered. Patients with cough-generating GERD do not always have typical reflux symptoms. It is important to recognize that esophageal reflux may be present in patients with other concurrent causes of chronic cough; thus, a temporal association with symptoms is important. The GERD evaluation can be costly. Additionally, endoscopy and barium esophagoscopy are not useful for establishing a temporal relationship, and esophageal pH monitoring is not useful for detecting the nonacid reflux that can cause cough. Thus, more invasive diagnostic evaluation may be preceded by a medication trial, as discussed below.[7,9,10]
- **Obstructive sleep apnea (OSA).** While the aforementioned etiologies ought to be addressed prior to relating a patient's chronic cough to OSA, there have been several literature reports of higher prevalence of chronic cough in patients with OSA diagnoses, and of improved cough symptoms after CPAP treatment in patients with OSA. It has been theorized that OSA-associated GERD, UACS, and airway inflammation may be contributing mechanisms. Thus, this diagnosis ought to be considered, and completion of the Epworth Sleepiness Scale and/or polysomnography may be considered in a patient with refractory chronic cough.[11–13]
- **Tuberculosis.** Although a less common etiology than those discussed above, consider tuberculosis infection in patients who are from areas with high prevalence or with risk factors (e.g., immunosuppressed or institutionalized).
- **Rare causes.** Sarcoidosis, congestive heart failure, pulmonary fibrosis, lung tumors, arterial venous malformations, retrotracheal masses, tracheal diverticula, trachealbronchialmalacia, chronic tonsillar enlargement, external auditory pressure (cerumen impaction, foreign body in external ear canal), and premature ventricular contractions have all been associated with chronic cough.
- **Unexplained cough.** If the patient continues to have cough after the above workup and/or empiric treatments for UACS and silent GERD, referral to a pulmonary or ENT specialist is reasonable. A diagnosis of habit or psychogenic cough should be made only after an extensive evaluation of other causes has been done.

TREATMENT

Empirical treatment of cough is a reasonable approach given that a few common etiologies are responsible for a great majority of cases. It has been demonstrated in the literature that the majority of chronic cough patients can be managed via primary care without intensive investigations or other referrals.[10]

Acute Cough

- **Common cold.** First-generation antihistamines (such as brompheniramine or chlorpheniramine) combined with a decongestant (pseudoephedrine) are the recommended treatment as per the 2006 ACCP guidelines. However, in a 2012 Cochrane Review of over-the-counter (OTC) medications for the treatment of acute cough in adults and children, studies assessing the efficacy of antihistamines, decongestants, antitussives, and expectorants produced conflicting results.[14] The efficacy of newer nonsedating antihistamines and other OTC products has not been clearly demonstrated.[3] In addition, it is difficult to determine when it is preferable to suppress cough rather than promote expectoration.[2] In those unable to take an antihistamine/decongestant, intranasal ipratropium or tiotropium may be considered if there are prominent rhinitis symptoms. Short-term use of narcotic antitussives or dextromethorphan may be considered for cough suppression. If the patient is wheezing, inhaled beta-agonists may be useful.[2] Use of honey for cough treatment has been studied in children, and based on a 2012 Cochrane review, honey may be slightly better than diphenhydramine in reducing cough frequency and did not differ significantly from dextromethorphan.[15] Other OTC expectorants, cough syrups, drops, or antibiotics are not usually recommended.

Subacute Cough

- **Postinfectious cough.** If the cough interferes with the patient's quality of life, an inhaled anticholinergic (such as ipratropium) may be helpful. If the cough persists, inhaled corticosteroids may be trialed. In some algorithms, a first-generation antihistamine with decongestant is utilized for 3 weeks when postnasal drip is thought to be contributing.[14] If the patient has severe paroxysms, a 1-week course of oral prednisone may be considered, though evidence is limited.[3] At this time, montelukast does not appear to be effective treatment for postinfectious cough.[17,18] Additionally, long-acting beta-agonists, antihistamines, and corticosteroids have no evidence demonstrating effectiveness in pertussis infection. The effectiveness of antibiotic therapy decreases over time and is not recommended if a cough secondary to pertussis has been present more than 3 weeks. A macrolide is recommended as antibiotic treatment of choice when appropriate. Patients suspected of having acute pertussis should be isolated for 5 days from the start of treatment, and vaccination with either Tdap is crucial for controlling pertussis infection rates.[3]

- **Acute exacerbation of chronic bronchitis.** Note that this course of illness may extend from acute to chronic in nature. A short course (1 to 2 weeks) of appropriate antibiotic therapy (such as doxycycline, TMP-SMX, amoxicillin/clavulante, or macrolide) may be utilized if infection is suspected. Use maximum doses of bronchodilators (e.g., short-acting beta agonist or anticholinergic). For severe exacerbations or for those with significant underlying disease, a short course of oral corticosteroids may be necessary. A recent Cochrane review suggests that mucolytics may produce a small reduction in acute exacerbations, but appear to have little effect on quality of life.[19]

Chronic cough

Guidelines from the American College of Chest Physicians recommend empiric treatment trials addressing the following diagnoses in the order that follows, progressing to the next after treatment of the former has been ineffective.

- **Upper airway cough syndrome.** Intranasal corticosteroids are often effective initial therapy and can be combined with first-generation antihistamines with decongestants. Consider imaging if the above are ineffective, to exclude chronic sinusitis.[3,7,20]
- **Cough-variant asthma.** Recommended treatment is with inhaled corticosteroids and bronchodilators for 8 weeks. If the cough is refractory, ensure adequate inhaler technique and compliance, and consider adding an oral leukotriene receptor agonist. If that is not effective, a one-to-two-week course of oral corticosteroids may be necessary.[3,7]
- **Nonasthmatic eosinophilic bronchitis.** First, the patient should be directed to avoid any suspected allergen or sensitizer. Inhaled corticosteroids, as for asthma, are the key anti-inflammatory therapy, and it may be reasonable to initiate treatment without induced sputum if the other diagnostic criteria are met.[8]
- **GERD cough.** Once to twice daily proton pump inhibitors for 2 months should be trialed. Recommended lifestyle changes should include tobacco cessation, less than 45 grams of fat in 24 hours, and avoidance of coffee, tea, soda, chocolate, mints, citrus, tomatoes, and alcohol. Additionally, weight loss and elevation of the head of the bed should be initiated. Prokinetic agents (such as metoclopramide) should be reserved for those with definitive diagnosis.[3,9,10]

It is important for the family physician to recognize the pathophysiological upregulation of the cough reflex that promotes cough hypersensitivity. There are multiple theories regarding the etiologies of this cough hypersensitivity, including a neuropathic disorder of the afferent pathways. Abnormal sensations (e.g., throat tickling or itching, choking sensation, throat clearing, hoarseness, dysphonia, dysphagia) often accompany chronic cough and may support the sensory neuropathy theory. Mechanisms of upper airway neuropathy may include GERD (repeated acid exposures), vitamin deficiencies, diabetes, and inflammation (e.g., asthma, recent viral illness) to name a few. There is literature support for use of amitriptyline and gabapentin in patients with chronic cough, especially if the efforts discussed above are not producing sufficient therapeutic result.[21]

SUMMARY

For patients with a chronic cough (>8 weeks' duration) who are nonsmokers, are not taking ACE inhibitors, and have a normal chest film, the diagnosis is likely upper airway cough syndrome (UACS, formerly called postnasal drip), asthma, or GERD.

The patient suspected of having UACS should be treated empirically with intranasal corticosteroids, potentially with a first-generation antihistamine/decongestant combination.

The patient suspected of having cough-variant asthma should have spirometry and, if suggestive, be treated with a standard antiasthma regimen of inhaled corticosteroids and bronchodilators. If spirometry is not supportive of asthma, consider empiric treatment with inhaled corticosteroids for possible eosinophilic bronchitis.

The patient with otherwise unexplained chronic cough may have reflux disease and should be treated with lifestyle modifications and acid suppression therapy. In patients with chronic cough, recognize the potential contribution of cough hypersensitivity, and consider treatment with amitriptyline or gabapentin. For patients with chronic cough in whom the etiology is not clear, a series of empiric therapies may be tried with referrals and additional evaluation utilized as needed.

REFERENCES

1. National Ambulatory Medical Care Survey, 2010. Centers for Disease Control. http://www.cdc.gov/nchs/data/ahcd/namcs_summary/2010_namcs_web_tables.pdf. Accessed February 24, 2014.
2. Dicpinigaitis PV, Colice GL, Goolsby MJ, et al. Acute cough: a diagnostic and therapeutic challenge. *Cough* 2009;5:11.
3. Irwin RS, Baumann MH, Bolser DC, et al. Diagnosis and management of cough. Executive summary: ACCP evidence-based clinical practice guidelines. *Chest* 2006;129:1S–23S.
4. Kwon N, Oh M, Min T, et al. Causes and clinical features of subacute cough. *Chest* 2006;129:1142–1147.
5. Madison JM, Irwin RS. Cough: a worldwide problem. *Otolaryngol Clin North Am* 2010;43(1):1–13.
6. Dicpinigaitis PV. Angiotensin-converting enzyme inhibitor-induced cough: ACCP evidence based clinical practice guidelines. *Chest* 2006;129(1S):169S–173S.
7. Birring S. Controversies in the evaluation and management of chronic cough. *Am J Respir Crit Care Med* 2011;183:708–715.
8. Cornere M. Chronic cough: a respiratory viewpoint. *Curr Opin Otolaryngol Head Neck Surg.* 2013; 21:530–534.
9. Gawron AJ, Kahrilas PJ, Pandolfino JE. Chronic cough: a gastroenterology perspective. *Curr Opin Otolaryngol Head Neck Surg* 2013;21:523–529.
10. Ojoo JC, Everett CF, Mulrennan SA, et al. Management of patients with chronic cough using a clinical protocol: a prospective observational study. *Cough* 2013;9(2):1.
11. Sundar KM, Daly SE, Willis AM. A longitudinal study of CPAP therapy for patients with chronic cough and obstructive sleep apnea. *Cough* 2013;9(19).
12. Wang T, Lo Y, Liu W, et al. Chronic cough and obstructive sleep apnea in a sleep laboratory-based pulmonary practice. *Cough* 2013;9(24).
13. Faruqi S, Fahim A, Morice A. Chronic cough and obstructive sleep apnoea: reflux-associated cough hypersensitivity? *Eur Resp J* 2012;40(4):1049–1050.
14. Smith SM, Schroeder K, Fahey T. Over the counter medications for acute cough in children and adults in ambulatory settings [Review]). *Cochrane Database Syst Rev* 2012;15(8).
15. Oduwole O, Meremikwu MM, Oyo-Ita A, et al. Honey for acute cough for children. *Cochran Database Syst Rev* 2012; 3.
16. Kwon N, Oh M, Min T, et al. Causes and clinical features of subacute cough. *Cough* 2006;129:1142–1147.
17. Wang K, Birring SS, Taylor K, et al. Montelukast for postinfectious cough in adults: a double-blind randomised placebo-controlled trial. *Lancet Respir Med* 2014;3:35–43.
18. Grant CC. Postinfectious cough and pertussis in primary care. *Lancet Respir Med* 2014;2–3.
19. Poole P, Black PN, Cates CJ. Mucolytic agents for chronic bronchitis or chronic obstructive pulmonary disease. *Cochran Database Syst Rev* 2012;8:CD001287.
20. Athanasiadis T, Allen JE. Chronic cough: an otorhinolaryngology perspective. 2013;21:517–522.
21. Chung KF, McGarvey L, Mazzone SB. Chronic cough as a neuropathic disorder. *Lancet Respir Med* 2013;1(5):414–422.

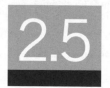

2.5 Chest Pain

Douglas Lewis

GENERAL PRINCIPLES

Definition

Chest pain accounts for 1% of all primary care visits and 6 million emergency department visits annually.[1] Arising from multiple body systems, the difficulty of accurate diagnosis increases because chest pain can be a disease process where patients appear well while actually having a life-threatening condition.[2] Missed diagnoses can be minimized by following a systematic diagnostic approach based on risk factor analysis, observation, electrocardiography (ECG), and serial biomarkers.[4] A useful strategy may be consideration of potential causes following an anatomical trail progressing from the heart outward: cardiac muscle, pericardium, chest vasculature, mediastinum, lung tissue, lung airspace, bronchial tree, trachea, lung pleura, esophagus, diaphragm, stomach, gall bladder, ribs, skeletal muscle, skin, and brain (psychiatric). Such an approach focuses the clinician on the primary etiology to be excluded, cardiac, and may also facilitate education of patients and families on potential causes.

DIAGNOSIS

Clinical Presentation

A commonly accepted adverse event rate for Emergency Department and primary care physician outcomes is <1% adverse events at 30 days following a negative assessment.[5] To achieve such a target rate, a clinician must first rule out life-threatening etiologies.[4] An initial rapid assessment of vital signs, patient appearance, and pain characteristics may be sufficient for a physician to determine suspicion of life-threatening etiologies and arrange transport to an appropriate Emergency Department.[6] When the situation is nonemergent, a careful history and physical examination with particular attention to risk factors for cardiac etiologies assists in prioritization. Immediate assessment in the Emergency Department has been recommended for patients with the following: chest pain, pressure, tightness, or heaviness that radiates to the neck, jaw, shoulders, back, or arms and/or associated with weakness, dizziness, lightheadedness, or loss of consciousness.[7]

History

Critical historical elements include a detailed description of the pain, noting the conditions of onset, timing, severity, alleviating/aggravating features, recurrence, and other associated symptoms such as diaphoresis or shortness of breath. Chest pain that is not typical of myocardial ischemia includes pleuritic pain, pain isolated to the middle or low abdomen, pain localized with the tip of one finger, pain reproduced with movement or palpation of chest wall and/or arms, pain that persists for many hours, pain lasting for only a few seconds, or pain that radiates to the lower extremities.[8] Careful attention should be given to risk factors for cardiovascular disease as aids to diagnostic accuracy: male gender, high-stress environment, hypertension, diabetes, hyperlipidemia, smoking, personal history of coronary artery disease (CAD), family history of CAD, obesity, and substance abuse. However, as the classic risk factors have not been demonstrated to be independent predictors of a myocardial infarction, clinical decisions based on their absence may underestimate true risk.[8] The diagnostic complexity makes validated prediction rules attractive, but the American Heart Association has not considered any as reliable enough to support discharge from the Emergency Department and instead advises that low-risk patients be admitted to a chest pain unit for cardiac stress testing.[9] A prediction rule has been developed wherein patients under the age of 40 without risk factors may be safely discharged from the Emergency Department if the initial cardiac troponin level is less than the 99th percentile reference limit; however, it has yet to be fully validated.[10]

Differential Diagnosis

Emergent (Immediately Life Threatening):
- **Acute coronary syndrome (ACS):** This term is applied to those in whom there exists evidence of myocardial ischemia or infarction and/or unstable angina.[11] ACS patients may present with symptoms of chest heaviness, pressure, or squeezing in the substernal or anterior chest that may radiate to the upper back, neck, jaw, shoulder, or arm. Accompanying symptoms may include shortness of breath, nausea, diaphoresis, hypotension, and/or lightheadedness. Pain is generally of gradual onset with increasing intensity during exertion. Unstable angina can be defined as angina at rest or any chest pain that has significantly changed from previous baseline.[12] Pain relief after administration of sublingual nitroglycerin or a "GI cocktail" is not a reliable indicator of ischemic versus nonischemic etiology.[13]
- **Pericardial tamponade:** Tamponade occurs when fluid collects between the pericardium and the heart and can be of varying degrees of severity. Pain is only associated with acute pericarditis from infection as the proximal pleura sees involvement. Malignancy and uremia result in a painless effusion. It is classically positional, increasing with supine positioning and somewhat relieved in the sitting position, especially when leaning forward.[6]
- **Pulmonary embolism (PE):** Many presentations of pain are possible, including painless dyspnea. However, pain may also worsen with deep inspiration. A high index of suspicion is essential as the reported 1:1,000 annual incidence likely underrepresents the true incidence.[6]
- **Tension pneumothorax:** Often, a sudden, ipsilateral sharp stabbing pain over the chest wall is described with a tension pneumothorax. A tension pneumothorax is a clinical, rather than

radiographic, diagnosis made with a classic history of trauma or sports participation. Tracheal deviation to the contralateral side may be seen on exam.

- **Aortic dissection:** Three per 100,000 patients per year presenting to the Emergency Department with chest pain have an aortic dissection.[6] Pain is described as abrupt in onset, tearing or ripping in nature, and located in the center of the chest with radiation to the back. It does not change with position. The location of pain is generally associated with the portion and the extent of the aorta involved.
- **Mediastinitis:** Most often, mediastinitis results from esophageal compromise. The pain is generally of a burning nature and tends to be in the epigastric region as well as in the chest.[6]

NonEmergent (Not Immediately Life Threatening):

- **Stable angina:** Chest discomfort may be similar in character to that of ACS but occurs only with exertion that pushes the myocardium beyond its available oxygen supply. It recurs often at relatively predictable points and resolves with decreasing myocardial oxygen demand.[14]
- **Spontaneous pneumothorax:** In contrast to tension pneumothorax, a spontaneous pneumothorax often occurs at rest without an inciting event. Pain is on the ipsilateral side.
- **Pneumonia:** Pain from an infectious, consolidating process in the lung airspace that occurs with pneumonia is located around the site of infection and may have a pleuritic component. Pain is particularly pleuritic in nature when the infiltrate is peripheral. Diaphragmatic irritation may cause shoulder pain on the ipsilateral side.
- **Tracheo-bronchitis:** Tracheo-bronchitis presents as a burning or aching after prolonged coughing typically accompanying or following a respiratory tract infection.[6]
- **Pleural pain:** Pleural pain can be either sharp and knifelike or dull and aching and is typically felt superficially in the chest wall. Pleural pain is associated with deep breathing, coughing, and positional changes and is generally a sign of an inflammatory process or reaction.
- **Esophagitis and gastroesophageal reflux (GERD):** Reflux causes a deep burning pain that may be indistinguishable from a myocardial infarction or angina. It is often felt in the epigastrium or substernally. The onset of pain is gradual but with a chronic course. Specific foods, alcohol, and nonsteroidal anti-inflammatory drugs (NSAIDS) are common triggers.[6]
- **Gastric or duodenal ulcer:** Gastric ulcers generally cause pain with eating, whereas duodenal ulcers hurt when one is hungry ("hunger ulcer"). The pain is a deep burning or a dull ache felt in the epigastrium but can be substernal. Milk, histamine blockers, or antacids may relieve pain.
- **Cholecystitis:** Gall bladder pain is often preceded by a meal of high fat content. It is cramp-like and/or burning and is generally felt in the right upper quadrant, epigastrium, or even the back.
- **Musculoskeletal:** Pain due to musculoskeletal disease is generally sharp, well localized, and reproducible with motion or palpation on examination.
- **Herpes zoster (shingles):** The pain from shingles may precede the onset of the skin eruption for hours to days. It may be described as burning, hypersensitive, or even numbness, and may be experienced as radiating. The distribution of the pain is dermatomal.
- **Less common etiologies:** Sarcoidosis, sickle cell crisis, Tietze Syndrome (atraumatic chest wall inflammatory pain),[15] and vasculitis are less likely causes of chest pain. A psychosomatic diagnosis should in general be made only after adequate investigation to rule out a more serious cause.

Physical Examination

The physical exam may assist in diagnosis, although some analyses demonstrate that the traditional history and physical exam are unhelpful in determination of a cardiac cause.[16]

- **Vital signs:** Tachycardia is often associated with acute coronary syndrome, pulmonary emboli, pneumothorax, cardiac tamponade, and aortic dissection, but can also be present with simple anxiety. Bradycardia may be associated with acute coronary syndrome. Hypotension is generally suggestive of an emergent etiology, yet young females may be relatively hypotensive in their normal state. Blood pressure differences between arms suggest aortic dissection.
- **Inspection:** Cyanosis indicates hypoxemia or low cardiac output, which can accompany all emergent causes. Diaphoresis, nausea, and emesis are often associated with acute coronary syndrome, but are not especially specific. The use of accessory muscles most often points to a pulmonary etiology. Tracheal deviation suggests tension pneumothorax on the contralateral side.
- **Auscultation:** Absent breath sounds are consistent with a pneumothorax. Pulmonary friction rubs indicate pleural inflammation and possible infection or infarction. Pericardial friction rubs suggest pericardial inflammation from infection, infiltration, or infarction. Cardiac murmurs and/or gallops, especially if new in onset, can suggest papillary muscle dysfunction from myocardial injury.

- **Palpation:** Pain on palpation of the chest wall is suggestive of musculoskeletal disease. Hyperesthesia with or without a rash suggests herpes zoster. Localized tenderness in the right upper quadrant is suggestive of a biliary, hepatic, or even pancreatic process. Midepigastric tenderness suggests duodenal or gastric ulceration but may also be present in biliary disease. Calf pain may indicate a deep vein thrombosis (DVT) and prompt investigation for pulmonary emboli.

Laboratory and Imaging Electrocardiogram

A completely normal 12-lead ECG does not rule out myocardial ischemia. However, it is a noninvasive and inexpensive test. Both the American Heart Association and the American College of Cardiology recommend that an ECG be completed and interpreted within 10 minutes of a patient with chest pain arriving in the Emergency Department.[14] The initial ECG is often not diagnostic in patients with acute coronary syndrome but may demonstrate changes when repeated at 10-minute intervals if the patient remains symptomatic and there is a high clinical suspicion. A normal ECG has been demonstrated to have a negative predictive value of 80% to 90% without regard to whether or not there was chest pain at the time it was obtained.[17] Comparison with a prior baseline ECG is advisable as it improves diagnostic accuracy when identifying the two major patterns of acute myocardial infarction.

- **ST elevation myocardial infarction (STEMI):** New 1 mm of ST-segment elevation at the J point in two anatomically contiguous leads other than V2–V3 is indicative of a STEMI. If elevation is noted in V2–V3, there must be 2 mm of elevation in men >40 years of age, 2.5 mm of elevation in men <40 years of age, and 1.5 mm of elevation in women. New LBBB is considered a STEMI equivalent. Most STEMI's will evolve into evidence of a Q-wave infarction.[18]
- **Non–ST-elevation MI (non-STEMI):** New horizontal or downward sloping ST-segment depression in two anatomically contiguous leads and/or new T-wave inversion in two anatomically contiguous leads suggests a NSTEMI. Diagnosis of this type of myocardial infarction is confirmed by detection of cardiac biomarkers.[19]

  Q-waves are suggestive of prior myocardial infarction. Signs of right ventricular strain such as right axis deviation, right bundle branch block, and T-wave inversion in V1–V4 can occur with pulmonary emboli. Diffuse ST-segment elevation with PR depression may be suggestive of pericarditis. Left bundle branch block can interfere with accurate ECG interpretation but when new, can indicate myocardial damage.[6]

Cardiac Biomarkers

Cardiac biomarkers are essential in the diagnosis of myocardial infarction. Cardiac troponins are very specific, and an advanced troponin-I assay demonstrates elevation within 3 hours, peaks at 12 hours, and remains elevated for up to 10 days following a myocardial infarction. Lacking specificity, the half-life of CK-MB in the circulation is shorter, making it useful in estimating the timing of infarction. CK-MB is generally twice normal at 6 hours and peaks at 24 hours. Even if the initial biomarkers demonstrate no abnormality, a single set is not sufficient to rule out myocardial injury. Serial sets of biomarkers at 6 to 8 hour intervals are necessary to demonstrate no myocardial damage. In addition, a complete metabolic profile can give an indication of liver or biliary function, and a complete blood count can indicate the inflammation of infectious etiologies or anemia suggestive of aortic dissection. In a patient that has a low-test probability for pulmonary emboli, a sensitive D-dimer is useful in ruling out the diagnosis and when normal in a low probability patient, eliminates the need for further diagnostic testing.[19]

Imaging/Ancillary Testing

- **Chest x-ray** may assist in determining the etiology of chest pain. Readily demonstrable causes include pneumonia, spontaneous pneumothorax, pleural effusion, enlarged cardiac size (possibly from pericardial tamponade), pulmonary edema (from congestive heart failure due to myocardial injury and dysfunction), and esophageal rupture. Most patients with acute coronary syndrome have a normal chest x-ray.[9]
- **Cardiac echocardiography (ECHO)** is invaluable in the evaluation of patients suspected of having acute coronary syndrome as regional wall motion abnormalities can be detected within seconds of arterial occlusion and before ECG changes appear.[2] It also readily demonstrates the effusion of pericarditis and can be useful in the detection of a pulmonary embolus significant enough to cause a dilated right ventricle.[9] The addition of stress via treadmill or pharmaceuticals increases the ability to detect inducible ischemia.[6]
- **Exercise Treadmill Test (ETT):** Traditional Bruce protocol or modified Bruce protocol treadmill exercise stress testing is appropriate for patients who have the ability to and lack contraindications to

exercise. Patients who achieve more than 10 metabolic equivalents (METS) with negative findings on ECG are at very low risk of ischemia.[2] It is acceptable in carefully selected, low-risk patients to have ETT completed as an outpatient procedure.[2]

- **Nuclear imaging:** Thallium-201 and technetium-99 sestamibi accumulate in myocardial tissue in correlation with myocardial blood flow. Subsequently, areas of ischemia are demonstrated by reduced radioactive counts. Stress testing can be added via either treadmill or pharmaceuticals to increase the accuracy of determining risk of ischemia ranging from those of low risk to high risk.[2]
- **Coronary angiography** has been considered the gold standard for the diagnosis and interventional treatment of CAD. Angiography is reserved for:
  - Patients with active infarction for reperfusion access to perform angioplasty and/or stenting to limit myocardial damage;
  - Patients with markedly positive noninvasive tests indicating CAD;
  - Patients at high risk for CAD in whom empiric therapy has failed;
  - Patients with unstable angina or persistent angina;
  - Patients with contraindications to noninvasive testing options.

TREATMENT

A patient with acute ST-segment elevation is a candidate for immediate reperfusion therapy. Percutaneous coronary intervention (PCI) is preferred to fibrinolysis as outcomes are better, complications are less, and it has the highest survival benefit in high-risk patients. However, these advantages are realized only at PCI-capable high-volume hospitals. Stenting with bare metal stents decreases the rates of restenosis compared with balloon angioplasty, but no mortality benefit has yet been demonstrated. When PCI cannot be administered within 120 minutes of first medical contact, fibrinolysis is recommended. Fibrinolysis should be done within 12 hours of symptom onset.[18]

In patients with a non-STEMI or with unstable angina, reperfusion therapy has no demonstrated benefit. For both NSTEMI and unstable angina, anti-ischemic therapies are the mainstay of treatment, including aspirin upon arrival to the hospital, bed rest, oxygen supplementation, sublingual and/or intravenous nitroglycerin (NTG), morphine sulfate if NTG has not relieved pain symptoms, beta-blockers, and angiotensin converting enzyme inhibitors. Medications initiated during the acute hospitalization should be continued upon discharge. An early invasive strategy with coronary angiography is acceptable for patients who are unstable, who are affected with refractory angina, or who are at elevated risk for cardiac events.[20]

REFERENCES

1. Hsiao CJ, Cherry DK, Beatty PC, et al. National ambulatory medical care survey: 2007 summary. *Natl Health Stat Report* 2010;(27):1–32.
2. Kontos MC, Diercks DB, Kirk JD. Emergency department and office-based evaluation of patients with chest pain. *Mayo Clin Proc* 2010;85(3):284–299.
3. Physician Insurers Association of America. *Acute myocardial infarction study*. Rockville, MD: Physician Insurers Association of America; 1996:1.
4. Parsonage WA, Cullen L, Younger JF. The approach to patients with possible cardiac chest pain. *Med J Aus* 2013;199(1):1–5.
5. Than M, Herbert M, Flaws D, et al. What is an acceptable risk of major adverse cardiac event in chest pain patients soon after discharge from the emergency department? A clinical survey. *Int J Cardiol* 2013;166:752–754.
6. Sabatine MS, Cannon CP. Approach to the patient with chest pain. In: Bonow RO, Mann DL, Zipes DP, et al, eds. *Braunwald's heart disease: a textbook of cardiovascular medicine*. Philadelphia, PA: Elsevier Saunders; 2011:1076–1086.
7. National Heart Attack Program Coordinating Committee, 60 Minutes to Treatment Working Group. Emergency department; rapid identification and treatment of patients with acute myocardial infarction. *Ann Emerg Med* 1994;23:311–329.
8. Anderson JL, Adams CD, Antman EM, et al. ACC/AHA 2007 guidelines for the management of patients with unstable angina/non ST-elevation myocardial infarction: A report of the American College of Cardiology/American Heart Association Task Force on Practice Guidelines: Developed in collaboration with the American College of Emergency Physicians, the Society for Cardiovascular Angiography and Interventions, and the Society of Thoracic Surgeons: Endorsed by the American Association of Cardiovascular and Pulmonary Rehabilitation and the Society for Academic Emergency Medicine. *J Am Coll Cardiol* 2007;50(7):e1–e157.
9. Amsterdam EA, Kirk JD, Bluemke DA, et al. Testing of low-risk patients presenting to the emergency department with chest pain; a scientific statement from the American Heart Association. *Circulation* 2010;122:1756–1776.

10. Hess EP, Brison RJ, Perry JJ, et al. Development of a clinical prediction rule for 30-day cardiac events in emergency department patients with chest pain and possible acute coronary syndrome. *Ann Emerg Med* 2012;59(2):115–125e1.
11. McGonachy JR. Oza RS. Outpatient diagnosis of acute chest pain in adults. *Am Fam Physician* 2013;87(3):177–182.
12. Braunwald E. Unstable angina. A classification. *Circulation* 1989:80(2):410–414.
13. Grailey, K, Glasziou, PP. Diagnostic accuracy of nitroglycerine as a 'test of treatment' for cardiac chest pain; a systematic review. *Emerg Med J* 2012;29:173–176.
14. Wright RS, Anderson JL, Adams CD, et al. 2011 ACCF?AHA focused update of the guidelines for the management of patients with unstable angina/non-ST elevation myocardial infarction (updating the 2007 guideline): a report of the American College of Cardiology Foundation/American Heart Association Task Force on Practice Guidelines. *Circulation* 2011;123(18):2022–2060.
15. Grodin L, Farina G. Tietze's syndrome in the emergency department: a rare etiology of atraumatic chest pain. *Case Rep Clin Med* 2013;2(3):208–210.
16. Bruyninckx R, Aertgeerts B, Bruyninckx P, et al. Signs and symptoms in diagnosing acute myocardial infarction and acute coronary syndrome: a diagnostic meta-analysis. *Br J Gen Pract* 2008;58(547):105–111.
17. Turnipseed SD, Trythall WS, Diercks DB, et al. Frequency of acute coronary syndrome in patients with normal electrocardiogram performed during presence or absence of chest pain. *Acad Emerg Med* 2009;16:495–499.
18. Kushner FG, Ascheim DD, Casey DE, et al. 2013 ACCF/AHA Guideline for the Management of ST-Elevation Myocardial Infarction: A Report of the American College of Cardiology Foundation/American Heart Association Task Force on Practice Guidelines. *JACC* 2013;61(4):e78–e140.
19. van Belle A, Buller HR, Huisman MV, et al. Effectiveness of managing suspected pulmonary embolism using an algorithm combining clinical probability, D-dimer testing, and computed tomography. *JAMA* 2006;295(2):172–179.
20. Anderson JL, Adams CD, Antman EM, et al. 2012 ACCF/AHA Focused Update Incorporated Into the ACCF/AHA 2007 Guidelines for the Management of Patients With Unstable Angina/Non-ST-Elevation Myocardial Infarction: A Report of the American College of Cardiology Foundation/American Heart Association Task Force on Practice Guidelines. *Circulation* 2013;127:e1–e187.

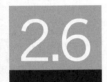

2.6 Abdominal Pain

Laura C. Mayans

GENERAL PRINCIPLES

Abdominal pain is one of the top 10 complaints seen in outpatient offices and is the chief complaint in 5% to 10% of emergency room visits. Etiologies of abdominal pain can range from minor conditions to life-threatening emergencies, and a specific diagnosis is not found in up to 30% of patients, despite broad testing and evaluation. Often the first priority is to determine whether the pain is acute or chronic in nature. Sudden or severe abdominal pain more often requires emergent evaluation and intervention. A careful history and physical exam are needed to identify acute emergencies and direct further diagnostic efforts.

DIAGNOSIS

History

A thorough and accurate history is an important component in the evaluation of abdominal pain and serves to direct any subsequent workup. Initial onset, timing and frequency of pain, quality of the pain, and location of pain all help to determine the underlying etiology and help guide judicious use of ancillary tests. Knowing the onset of pain helps to categorize the condition as acute, subacute, or chronic. The quality of the pain, such as sharp, burning, dull, focal, or radiating can aid in classifying the pain as peritoneal or visceral. Often peritoneal pain is worsened with movement while visceral pain often causes the patient to continually move in an effort to find a comfortable position. The location of the pain helps to narrow possible etiologies anatomically, though it is not advisable to completely eliminate a possible cause based solely on location. Referred pain is common and can result from serious underlying conditions. Frequency and timing are useful in evaluating pain of gradual onset or pain that is recurrent. Patients should also be asked about associated signs and symptoms, such as nausea, vomiting, fever, diarrhea, constipation, or anorexia as well as aggravating or relieving factors. Past medical history can be significant if this pain has occurred before. A history of previous abdominal surgeries increases the likelihood of bowel obstruction from adhesions or hernia. Medication and social history are important as the use of certain over-the-counter medications, alcohol, and tobacco are risk factors for conditions such as gastritis and ulcers.

Physical Examination

A thorough physical exam includes inspection, auscultation, percussion, and palpation. Inspection should be done first, looking for distension, discoloration, or scars. It should be done upright and then the patient should be placed supine, with the knees slightly bent, for additional inspection and for the remainder of the abdominal exam. Auscultation should be performed next. Attention to frequency and quality of bowel sounds and presence of bruits is important. Abnormal bowel sounds can be a sign of partial or complete obstruction or ileus. It is recommended to perform some light palpation with the stethoscope during auscultation as there is often less guarding and embellishment at this point in the exam. Percussion and palpation occur last. Abnormal internal organ size can often be appreciated, and pain can be better localized. It is important to assess pain with palpation as well as rebound tenderness and guarding. When present, rebound tenderness and guarding are more suggestive of peritoneal irritation and acute and urgent underlying etiologies such as appendicitis, ruptured ectopic pregnancy, perforated viscus, or bacterial peritonitis. Rectal and pelvic exams should always be considered when evaluating abdominal pain.

Diagnostic Studies

Most patients presenting with acute or chronic abdominal pain should undergo basic laboratory studies including a complete blood count and basic metabolic panel. In many situations, a urinalysis can also be helpful. Women of childbearing age, regardless of contraceptive status, should receive a pregnancy test. Other labs should be ordered on the basis of location, quality, and pattern of pain. Right upper quadrant (RUQ) pain is often evaluated with liver function studies, liver enzymes, alkaline phosphatase, and bilirubin. Hepatitis panels can also be considered. For more centrally located or epigastric pain, a lipase to evaluate for pancreatitis is indicated. If the pain is associated with diarrhea, often stool studies are needed and include ova and parasites, culture for organisms such as *Salmonella*, *Shigella*, or *Campylobacter*, and *Clostridium difficile* toxin assays. If inflammatory bowel disease is suspected, an erythrocyte sedimentation rate (ESR) and/or c-reactive protein (CRP) are indicated. Elderly individuals with hypothyroidism can present with vague abdominal pain, and so thyroid stimulating hormone (TSH) could be considered in this population. An electrocardiogram (ECG) should also be considered in people with high risk for cardiac disease.

Imaging studies used in the evaluation of abdominal pain include plain film x-rays, ultrasound, and CT scan. Plain film x-rays can show dilated bowel loops suggestive of obstruction, some masses, free air indicating organ perforation, and some stones. Ultrasound is particularly useful in the setting of RUQ pain to evaluate the liver and biliary system. Still, CT scan is often the imaging modality of choice in both acute and chronic abdominal pain. Many acute and chronic conditions can be easily and reliably identified on CT scan, including appendicitis, renal calculi, diverticulitis, abdominal aortic aneurysms, pancreatic lesions, bowel obstruction, and more. Endoscopy is also increasingly used in the evaluation of both upper and lower abdominal pain and allows collection of tissue biopsies for the diagnosis of conditions such as *Helicobacter pylori* infection, inflammatory bowel disease, and cancer.

ACUTE ABDOMINAL PAIN AND THE ACUTE ABDOMEN

Acute abdominal pain is generally defined as severe pain of sudden onset and short duration in a previously healthy person.[1] An acute abdomen refers to an underlying etiology that needs emergent intervention that is often, but not always, surgical.[2] The American College of Emergency Physicians (ACEP) issued a consensus statement regarding recommendations for the management of acute abdominal pain, and several important guidelines come from this clinical policy. First, they advise against limiting the differential diagnosis based solely on the location of pain. They also stress that there is insufficient evidence to use the presence or absence of fever to distinguish surgical causes from medical causes, particularly in the elderly. Patients at high risk for atypical presentations of acute abdominal pain, such as the elderly, diabetics, or people with cardiac risk factors, should be identified early, and an ECG should be considered. When the underlying cause of abdominal pain is unclear, serial abdominal examinations and ancillary testing are often needed. Finally, narcotics should not be withheld for fear of obscuring a diagnosis. Incremental doses of IV narcotics ease pain but do not appear to eliminate tenderness to palpation.[3] Recent randomized trials have shown that morphine administration neither obscures the correct diagnosis nor delays appropriate treatment.[4] Signs and symptoms of an acute abdomen include pain that is of sudden onset or pain that is progressively worsening, fever, rebound tenderness, rigidity, elevated WBCs, hematemesis or rectal bleeding, and hemodynamic instability. The following are conditions that frequently present acutely:

- **Acute appendicitis.** Appendicitis typically presents with progressively worsening pain that begins periumbilically and later localizes to McBurney's point in the right lower quadrant (RLQ). It is often associated with anorexia, nausea, low grade fever, and elevated WBCs with a left shift. Rebound and guarding are often present, and the typical patient attempts to remain very still in order to avoid worsening the pain. Although not required, CT scan of the abdomen is often performed to confirm the diagnosis prior to emergent surgery.
- **Mesenteric lymphadenitis.** Mesenteric lymphadenitis is inflammation of the mesenteric lymph nodes, often due to a viral infection. It very closely mimics acute appendicitis and can lead to unnecessary abdominal surgeries. Accurate differentiation of the two is still very difficult, but often a CT scan is diagnostic. While it is an acute process, mesenteric lymphadenitis is not life-threatening. It is a self-limited disease that will resolve without any intervention.[5]
- **Perforation.** A perforation can occur in the gall bladder, pancreas, stomach, bowel, or bladder. However, perforations from gastric or duodenal ulcers and from diverticulitis are most common. Leakage of the contents of the viscus organ into the abdominal cavity causes peritoneal irritation and manifests as sudden and severe pain. Signs and symptoms of an acute abdomen are also present, such as rebound, guarding, rigidity, elevated WBC count, and possibly hemodynamic instability. Immediate surgery is indicated, and if delayed, the abdominal cavity can become infected, leading to peritonitis. Perforations also lead to free air between the liver and the diaphragm, easily seen on upright abdominal x-rays.
- **Complete intestinal obstruction.** Both the small and the large bowel can become obstructed. Common causes include strangulated hernias, volvulus, tumors, adhesions, inflammatory bowel disease, or even fecal impaction. Complete obstruction is a surgical emergency, while partial obstruction can often be managed medically. Common presenting symptoms are severe pain, often generalized or umbilical, vomiting, absence of flatus and inability to pass feces (can be variable depending on location of obstruction), and progressive abdominal distension. Auscultation often reveals high-pitched, "tinkling" bowel sounds. Abdominal films often show intestinal air–fluid levels, though this can be seen in both complete obstruction and ileus.
- **Mesenteric vascular occlusion.** Mesenteric vasculature can become occluded by either a thrombosis or an embolism. Most often affected is the superior mesenteric artery. This leads to infarction and subsequent gangrene of the intestinal segment. In thrombotic arterial occlusion, often a history of abdominal angina or intermittent cramping precedes the occlusion. An embolic etiology is often seen in patients with underlying heart arrhythmias, particularly atrial fibrillation. No matter what the cause of the obstruction, prompt surgical intervention is required to preserve bowel function and life. Symptoms can be insidious and may occur for up to 3 to 4 days before the patient seeks treatment. They include anorexia, bloody diarrhea, and steady and progressively worsening crampy abdominal pain that is often out of proportion to the findings on exam. Fever, leukocytosis, and hemodynamic instability are very late findings. CT angiography is often necessary to confirm the diagnosis.
- **Ruptured abdominal aortic aneurysm.** A ruptured AAA is a life-threatening emergency that necessitates immediate surgical intervention. Symptoms include sudden abdominal or flank pain, abdominal rigidity, anxiety, nausea and vomiting as well as hemodynamic instability that can progress to shock. A pulsatile abdominal mass is common, though it should be noted that after rupture, the aneurysm may no longer pulsate. Abdominal ultrasound or CT can be used to definitively diagnose a ruptured AAA.
- **Ectopic pregnancy.** This diagnosis should be explored in any woman of reproductive age with abdominal pain. Most ectopic pregnancies will rupture by the eighth week, though depending on the exact location of implantation, it could be later. Pain will often gradually increase over hours to

days preceding rupture and is often located in the hypogastric or iliac regions. Menstrual history, physical exam, urine pregnancy test as well as quantitative hCG, and pelvic ultrasound are used for diagnosis. A prior history of tubal ligation does not negate ectopic pregnancy as a possible diagnosis, and a full evaluation should still be completed.

SUBACUTE AND CHRONIC ABDOMINAL PAIN

Longer-lasting pain is classified as subacute or chronic abdominal pain. Subacute pain is classified as lasting days to weeks. Chronic pain is generally defined as lasting a month or more. The range of severity of such problems is large, from self-limited etiologies to evolving, potentially more serious etiologies. Common examples are discussed below.

- **Gastritis.** Also called dyspepsia, gastritis is inflammation of the lining of the stomach. It accounts for almost 5% of visits to primary care physicians.[6] It is characterized by episodic aching or burning pain in the epigastric region, often after eating, lasting up to several hours. It can be associated with ulcerative disease and bleeding, in which case a fecal occult blood test is often positive. A common cause that can lead to ulcers if left untreated is *H. pylori* infection. *H. pylori* testing should be strongly considered, and upper endoscopy may be warranted in older patients or in patients with persistent symptoms despite treatment.
- **Diverticulitis.** Diverticulitis is the infection and/or inflammation of a colonic diverticulum and is associated with fever, anorexia, abdominal pain, and abnormal bowel movements. Pain is most often in the left lower quadrant (LLQ) and leukocytosis is often present. It can occur in young adults, but is more common in the middle-aged and older. It can be diagnosed clinically, and if symptoms are mild, antibiotics can be given in the outpatient setting. If the patient is more severely ill, abdominal CT is warranted to look for complications such as abscesses or perforation, and the patient may need to be admitted for inpatient treatment and monitoring.
- **Cholelithiasis.** Stones in the gall bladder (cholelithiasis) or in the common bile duct (choledocholithiasis) cause RUQ pain, usually following fatty meals, owing to transient obstruction by the stones. Pain can be severe and debilitating and is often associated with nausea. If complete obstruction occurs, acute infection and inflammation of the gall bladder ensues (cholecystitis). In this case, pain is more severe, longer lasting, and often associated with fever and leukocytosis. In all cases, surgery is required for cure, though it does not have to be performed urgently.
- **Pancreatitis.** Pancreatitis can present as acute, subacute, or chronic abdominal pain and is most often associated with gall stones or alcohol ingestion. Pain is usually gnawing, in the epigastric, umbilical, or RUQ regions, and often radiates to the back. It is frequently associated with nausea and vomiting. Most cases are mild with rapid recovery and no lasting effects. However, severe pancreatitis can be life-threatening. Workup includes a lipase level, which is more sensitive than amylase but does not correspond to severity of disease, and often abdominal CT to rule out the presence of pancreatic pseudocysts.
- **Irritable bowel syndrome.** It is estimated that symptoms consistent with IBS are present in up to 20% of adults.[7] Most, however, never seek a physician's care. The exact etiology is still unknown, but symptoms include abdominal pain and cramping, constipation or diarrhea or both, mucus in the stools, and it is often associated with anxiety or depression. Physical exam is usually nonspecific, and diagnosis is made clinically. Workup usually involves tests to rule out other similar organic diseases, and treatment is symptomatic.
- **Inflammatory bowel disease.** Inflammatory bowel disease includes Crohn's Disease and Ulcerative Colitis. Incidence is bimodal and typically occurs between the ages of 15 and 25 and 55 and 65 years of age. Ulcerative colitis is confined to the colon, while Crohn's can affect the entire digestive tract. In both cases, symptoms often include recurrent flares of abdominal pain that can be severe; diarrhea, often bloody; anorexia; and anemia. Diagnosis is made via tissue biopsy performed during colonoscopy.
- **Special female considerations.** Pain from female pelvic organs also manifests as abdominal pain. Specific etiologies to be aware of in females with abdominal pain are ovarian cysts or torsion, endometriosis, pelvic inflammatory disease, and pregnancy-related concerns, such as ectopic pregnancy discussed above. Often abdominal pain in females requires a pelvic exam and pregnancy test in those of reproductive age.
- **Other causes.** Possible etiologies of abdominal pain are vast, and other less common etiologies to be aware of include nephrolithiasis, acute or chronic hepatitis, porphyria, Henoch–Shonlein Purpura, food sensitivities, and drug ingestions.

REFERENCES

1. Greenberger NJ, Blumber, RS, Burakoff R, eds. *Current diagnosis and treatment gastroenterology, hepatology, and endoscopy.* 2nd ed. New York, NY: McGraw-Hill; 2012.
2. Silen W. *Cope's early diagnosis of the acute abdomen.* 22nd ed. New York, NY: Oxford University Press; 2010.
3. American College of Emergency Physicians. Clinical policy: critical issues for the initial evaluation and management of patients presenting with a chief complaint of nontraumatic acute abdominal pain. *Ann Emerg Med* 2000;36:406–415.
4. Aghamohammadi D, Gholipouri C, Hosseinzadeh H, et al. An evaluation of the effect of morphine on abdominal pain and peritoneal irritation sign in patients with acute surgical abdomen. *J Cardiovasc Thorac Res* 2012;4(2):45–48
5. Toorenvliet B, Vellenkoop A, Bakker R, et al. Clinical differentiation between acute appendicitis and acute mesenteric lymphadenitis in children. *Eur J Pediatr Surg* 2011;21:120–123.
6. Heidelbaugh JJ. Abdominal pain. In: Paulman PM, Harrison J, Paulman A, et al, eds. *Signs and symptoms in family medicine, a literature-based approach.* Philadelphia, PA: Mosby; 2012:1–25.
7. Barter CM, Dunne L. Abdominal pain. In: South-Paul JE, Matheny SC, Lewis EL, eds. *Current diagnosis and treatment family medicine.* 3rd ed. New York, NY: McGraw-Hill; 2011:319–336.

2.7

Jaundice

Glenn D. Miller, Marc D. Carrigan

GENERAL PRINCIPLES

Definition

Jaundice is a yellowish discoloration of the skin, sclerae, and mucous membranes caused by an accumulation of bilirubin. Other causes of yellowish pigmentation, unrelated to hyperbilirubinemia, are excessive ingestion of foods rich in carotene (carrots) or lycopene (tomatoes) or certain drugs (quinacrine or busulfan).

Pathophysiology

Jaundice is not clinically evident until serum bilirubin levels exceed 3.0 mg per dL.[1] Bile metabolism may be altered at four major points: overproduction (hemolysis), failure of uptake or excretion by the hepatocyte (transport defect), failure of conjugation (hepatocellular), or obstruction (extra- or intrahepatic).

DIAGNOSIS

Clinical Presentation

Signs and symptoms vary with the underlying etiology. Patients may be asymptomatic or have specific clinical manifestations that will help differentiate the cause.

History

Nonspecific symptoms of liver disease include anorexia, nausea, vomiting, weight loss, fatigue, and malaise. Generalized pruritus is often associated with cholestasis while fever and chills are associated with biliary obstruction and cholangitis. Chronic weight loss, especially preceding the jaundice, suggests malignancy.

Drug, alcohol or toxin exposure may precipitate jaundice. Agents known to cause jaundice are acetaminophen, certain antibiotics, chemotherapeutic agents, psychotropic medications, cholesterol-lowering agents, anticonvulsants, sex hormones, nonsteroidal anti-inflammatory drugs, inhalation anesthetics, thiazide diuretics, oral hypoglycemics, certain antihypertensives, certain antiarrhythmics, salicylates, cimetidine, warfarin, colchicine, allopurinol, penicillamine, gold, sulfa derivatives, and solvents.

Blood transfusions, intravenous drug use, sexual contact, travel to endemic areas, ingestion of contaminated foods, and contact with jaundiced persons are associated with viral hepatitis.

History of gallstones, biliary surgery, previous episodes of jaundice or inflammatory bowel disease, acholic stools, sudden-onset jaundice, and right upper quadrant pain suggest extrahepatic cholestasis.

Family history of jaundice suggests an inherited defect in conjugation or bilirubin transport, hemolytic disorder, Wilson disease, α_1-antitrypsin deficiency, hemochromatosis, or benign idiopathic cholestasis.

Abdominal pain suggests hepatic inflammation or congestion, obstruction, abscess, or tumor. Colicky right upper quadrant pain is more often associated with common bile duct obstruction.

Physical Examination

Palmar erythema, spider angiomas, gynecomastia, testicular atrophy, or ascites suggests chronic liver disease or cirrhosis. Other findings that suggest a diagnosis include Kayser–Fleischer rings (Wilson disease), xanthelasma (chronic cholestatic liver disease, especially primary biliary cirrhosis), and large liver nodules (metastatic disease). Additionally, signs of congestive heart failure suggest that passive congestion of the liver may be responsible for jaundice symptoms. A physician should note that hepatosplenomegaly, abdominal tenderness, mass lesions, and cachexia are suggestive of inflammatory or neoplastic disease. In particular, a Courvoisier gallbladder (a nontender, palpable gallbladder) is a sign of pancreatic cancer.

Laboratory Studies

Initial laboratory tests should include aminotransferases —aspartate aminotransferase (AST) and alanine aminotransferase (ALT)—total and direct bilirubin, and alkaline phosphatase.

A prothrombin time and albumin should be obtained if severe liver dysfunction is suspected.

Specific tests include viral hepatitis serology, antimitochondrial antibody (primary biliary cirrhosis), iron studies (hemochromatosis), ceruloplasmin and urine copper levels (Wilson disease), and antinuclear and smooth muscle antibodies (autoimmune hepatitis). Gamma-glutamyl transpeptidase (GGTP), leucine aminopeptidase, and 5'-nucleotidase are used to confirm hepatic origin of alkaline phosphatase. **Liver biopsy may be necessary to completely determine the etiology.**

Imaging

If imaging is necessary for diagnosis, right upper quadrant ultrasound is the first study that should be performed as it is inexpensive, rapid, noninvasive, and does not expose the patient to radiation or contrast media. Ultrasound accurately identifies stones within the gallbladder and biliary system, differentiates intra- from extrahepatic obstruction, and can identify larger (>1 cm) intra- and extrahepatic masses within the liver and surrounding area.[2]

Computed tomographic (CT) scan has higher resolution than ultrasound and can detect smaller lesions (>5 mm), but is more costly and exposes the patient to ionizing radiation and sometimes contrast media.

Magnetic resonance cholangiopancreatography (MRCP) provides images of the biliary tree without contrast media. It can differentiate intra- from extrahepatic obstruction, visualize choledocholithiasis, and differentiate pancreatitis from pancreatic cancer.[3]

Endoscopic retrograde cholangiopancreatography (ERCP) allows direct visualization of the biliary tree by passing a camera into the bile ducts and injecting contrast media. It is primarily used as a therapeutic procedure that allows for extraction of common bile duct and pancreatic duct stones, biliary stent placement, sphincterotomy, and tissue sampling.[4]

Percutaneous transhepatic cholangiography is similar to ERCP but requires passing a needle through the liver parenchyma into a peripheral bile duct to inject contrast media.

Differential Diagnosis

The differential diagnosis can be classified as disorders of bilirubin metabolism, liver disease, and bile duct obstruction.[5] Evaluating the clinical presentation and pattern of initial laboratory tests delineates specific causes of jaundice.

Normal aminotransferases, alkaline phosphatase, and albumin suggest hemolysis or a defect of bilirubin conjugation or transport. Elevated unconjugated (indirect) bilirubin (>80% to 85% of total) is seen with hemolysis or hereditary conjugating defects. An initial laboratory workup including a complete blood count, peripheral blood smear, reticulocyte count, and lactate dehydrogenase (LDH) is helpful in these patients. If a high reticulocyte count, decreased hemoglobin, or abnormal red cell forms are noted, hemolysis should be suspected. Additional laboratory findings of hemolysis include the presence of plasma-free hemoglobin, low haptoglobin, and the presence of hemoglobinuria.[6]

If laboratory results are not consistent with hemolysis, suspect a defect in conjugation, especially if the total bilirubin is less than 6 mg per dL and conjugated bilirubin is normal.

Gilbert syndrome is the most common conjugating defect affecting 7% of the population. In Gilbert syndrome, bilirubin is usually less than 3 mg per dL[7] but increases with fever, fasting, or stress, and patients are asymptomatic and have normal liver histology.

Crigler–Najjar syndrome is rare. In Type I, bilirubin levels rise to 45 mg per dL, and death occurs in infancy. In Type II, bilirubin values may reach 25 mg per dL, but it is uncommon for severe sequelae to occur.[7]

Elevated conjugated (direct) bilirubin (>50% of total) suggests a congenital defect in conjugated bilirubin transport. These conditions appear in childhood or adolescence with bilirubin levels up to 20 mg per dL, but cause no clinical sequelae. They follow an autosomal recessive inheritance pattern. Patients with Rotor syndrome demonstrate visualization of the gallbladder on oral cholecystogram (OCG). In Dubin–Johnson syndrome, the gallbladder is not seen on OCG; black cetrilobular pigment is found on liver biopsy.[7]

Predominant elevation of aminotransferases suggests hepatocellular injury. Acute or chronic viral hepatitis can be diagnosed by viral hepatitis serology. Alcoholic hepatitis clinically resembles viral or toxic hepatitis, but AST is usually greater than ALT (a reversal of the usual ratio); diagnosis is based on a history of heavy alcohol intake, absence of other causes of hepatitis, and liver biopsy. Wilson disease is confirmed by low ceruloplasmin levels and Kayser–Fleischer rings or by liver biopsy. Hemochromatosis is suspected in patients with a history of hepatomegaly, idiopathic cardiomyopathy, skin pigmentation, loss of libido, diabetes mellitus, or arthritis; elevated transferrin saturation and ferritin levels suggest the diagnosis, which is confirmed by genetic testing or liver biopsy. α_1-Antitrypsin deficiency is associated with obstructive pulmonary disease and cirrhosis, and is confirmed by decreased α_1-antitrypsin levels.

Congestive and ischemic diseases including right-sided congestive heart failure, constrictive pericarditis, Budd–Chiari syndrome (hepatic vein or inferior vena cava obstruction), portal vein thrombosis, veno-occlusive disease, and hypotension are causes of jaundice and hepatocellular injury. Fatty liver disease should be considered in obese or alcoholic patients.

Liver diseases in pregnancy that cause hepatocellular injury are severe preeclampsia, HELLP syndrome, and acute fatty liver of pregnancy. Drug-induced hepatitis can be confirmed by drug levels (e.g., acetaminophen), agent-specific patterns of hepatotoxicity, and, occasionally, liver biopsy. Autoimmune hepatitis is suspected when antinuclear antibodies, smooth muscle antibodies, or antimitochondrial antibodies are present; liver biopsy is helpful.

Predominant elevation of alkaline phosphatase suggests cholestasis. Aminotransferases may also be elevated. 5′-nucleotidase and GGTP are usually elevated; if not, consider a bone source.

If extrahepatic cholestasis is suspected based on history and physical examination, possible causes include choledocholithiasis, malignancies (pancreatic, bile duct, lymphoma, metastases), biliary stricture, sclerosing cholangitis, chronic pancreatitis, biliary atresia, and other rare conditions (Asian cholangiohepatitis, ascariasis, hemobilia). Extrahepatic biliary obstruction requires prompt removal of the obstruction. To image the biliary tree, ultrasound is usually preferred owing to lower cost, better detection of gallbladder stones, and avoidance of radiation exposure. CT gives better visualization of the pancreas and should be chosen if pancreatic pathology is suspected. Because ultrasound or CT scan can fail to detect up to 40% of intraductal stones, perform ERCP or percutaneous transhepatic cholangiography if suspicion is high.

If intrahepatic cholestasis is suspected on the basis of history and physical examination, specific laboratory tests directed at suspected pathology should be ordered. Consider ultrasound to rule out extrahepatic obstruction. Acute and chronic hepatitis (viral, alcohol, and drug-induced) can be diagnosed by viral hepatitis serology, verification of toxin exposure, and specific toxin levels.

Cirrhosis is most commonly caused by long-term alcohol use and viral infections, especially hepatitis C. Rarer causes include genetic and metabolic diseases (Wilson disease, hemochromatosis, and α_1-antitrypsin deficiency) and autoimmune diseases (primary biliary cirrhosis, primary sclerosing cholangitis, and lupoid hepatitis). Liver biopsy may be helpful if the diagnosis or cause is unclear.

Chronic cholestatic syndromes include primary biliary cirrhosis and primary sclerosing cholangitis. Primary biliary cirrhosis is usually seen in middle-aged women; antimitochondrial antibodies are elevated in more than 90% of patients; liver biopsy confirms the diagnosis.

Primary sclerosing cholangitis may be seen as an isolated finding or in association with inflammatory bowel disease, other fibrosclerosing syndromes, or AIDS; diagnosis is confirmed by ERCP or magnetic resonance cholangiogram.

Benign recurrent intrahepatic cholestasis is diagnosed by recurrent episodes, family history, and absence of obstruction on cholangiography. Cholestasis of pregnancy is usually seen in the third trimester and often recurs in subsequent pregnancies or in association with estrogen use. It is diagnosed by elevated serum bile acids. Cholestasis can also be seen with sepsis, parenteral nutrition, postoperative state, or neoplasm.

Neonatal Jaundice

Evaluation of the newborn with jaundice is influenced by the level of bilirubin elevation relative to the infant's age, blood group incompatibility, gestational age at birth, neonatal infection, and breast-feeding status. Clinical jaundice <24 hours of age, blood group incompatibility, prematurity, and exclusive breast-feeding are risk factors for severe hyperbilirubinemia. Initial testing for significant jaundice includes total and direct bilirubin, CBC, reticulocyte count, examination of the peripheral blood smear, blood typing (mother and baby), and Coombs test.

If unconjugated bilirubin is elevated, consider physiologic jaundice as a diagnosis. Physiologic jaundice has an onset between days 2 and 4 of life, total bilirubin <15 mg per dL and has a predominantly unconjugated bilirubin pattern (direct <1.5 mg per dL). Such jaundice occurs in 50% of newborns and usually resolves in 1 week in term infants and 2 weeks in preterm infants. If significant hemolysis is noted, consider Rh and ABO incompatibility, spherocytosis, enzyme deficiency, and hemoglobinopathy in the differential diagnosis. Breast milk jaundice occurs between days 4 and 7 of life, and peaks during the third week of life. This jaundice also causes elevated unconjugated bilirubin and resolves between 3 and 10 weeks of age. Polycythemia and cephalohematoma may also contribute to jaundice in the newborn.

If conjugated bilirubin is elevated, consider causes such as biliary atresia, sepsis, hepatitis, TORCH (toxoplasmosis, syphilis, rubella, cytomegalovirus, and herpes virus), and galactosemia. Biliary atresia should be ruled out in any newborn with direct bilirubin >2 as it needs to be treated as soon as possible to prevent permanent damage to the liver.

REFERENCES

1. Pratt DS, Kaplan MM. Jaundice. In: Longo DL, Fauci AS, Kasper DL, et al, eds. *Harrison's principles of internal medicine.* 18 ed. New York, NY: McGraw-Hill; 2012. http://accessmedicine.mhmedical.com/content.aspx?bookid=331&Sectionid=40726762. Accessed February 20, 2014.
2. Rogoveanu I, Gheonea DI, Saftoiu A, et al. The role of imaging methods in identifying the causes of extrahepatic cholestasis. *J Gastrointestin Liver Dis* 2006;15(3):265–271.
3. Adamek HE, Albert J, Breer H, et al. Pancreatic cancer detection with magnetic resonance cholangiopancreatography and endoscopic retrograde cholangiopancreatography: a prospective controlled study. *Lancet* 2000;356(9225):190–193.
4. Adler DG, Baron TH, Davila RE, et al. ASGE guideline: the role of ERCP in diseases of the biliary tract and the pancreas. *Gastrointest Endosc* 2005;62:1–8.
5. Lidofsky SD. Jaundice. In: Feldman M, Friedman LS, Brandt LJ, eds. *Sleisenger and Fordtran's gastrointestinal and liver disease.* 9th ed. Philadelphia, PA: Saunders; 2010:323–335. http://www.mdconsult.com/das/book/pdf/436471517-3/978-1-4160-6189-2/4-u1.0-B978-1-4160-6189-2..00020-2..DOCPDF.pdf?isbn=978-1-4160-6189-2&eid=4-u1.0-B978-1-4160-6189-2..00020-2..DOCPDF. Accessed January 29, 2014.
6. Bunn HR. Approach to the anemias. In: Goldman L, Schafer AI, eds. *Goldman's cecil medicine.* 24th ed. New York, NY: Elsevier Saunders; 2012:1038–1039. http://www.mdconsult.com/das/book/pdf/435065669-3/978-1-4377-1604-7/4-u1.0-B978-1-4377-1604-7..00161-5..DOCPDF.pdf?isbn=978-1-4377-1604-7&eid=4-u1.0-B978-1-4377-1604-7..00161-5..DOCPDF. Accessed January 14, 2014.
7. Berk P, Korenblat K. Approach to the patient with jaundice or abnormal liver tests. In: Goldman L, Schafer AI, eds. *Goldman's cecil medicine.* 24th ed. New York, NY: Elsevier Saunders; 2012:956–966. http://www.mdconsult.com/das/book/pdf/436471517-3/978-1-4377-1604-7/4-u1.0-B978-1-4377-1604-7..00149-4..DOCPDF.pdf?isbn=978-1-4377-1604-7&eid=4-u1.0-B978-1-4377-1604-7..00149-4..DOCPDF. Accessed January 29, 2014.

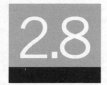

Edema

Gretchen M. Dickson, Charles W. Coffey

GENERAL PRINCIPLES

Definition

Edema is swelling in the body caused by a disruption of homeostasis that results in an abnormal collection of fluid in tissue. Edema is typically not a disease process in and of itself; rather, it is the manifestation of another disease process; that is, edema is a symptom, not a disease.

Pathophysiology

The normal forces that keep the body free of edema are the interplay between[1] hydrostatic pressure[2], oncotic pressure, and[3] vessel permeability. They are expressed mathematically by the Starling Equation:

$$Jv = Kf([Pc - Pi] - \sigma[\pi c - \pi i])$$

where Jv is the net fluid movement between compartments, $[Pc - Pi] - \sigma[\pi c - \pi i]$ is the driving force, Pc is the capillary hydrostatic pressure, Pi is the interstitial hydrostatic pressure, πc is the capillary oncotic pressure, πi is the interstitial oncotic pressure, Kf is the filtration coefficient, and σ is the reflection coefficient.

As demonstrated in the equation, net hydrostatic and oncotic pressure depend on the pressures in the capillary and interstium, while permeability is not dependent on any other forces. If any of these forces are disrupted or overwhelmed by a disease state or outside force, edema can result.

TABLE 2.8-1	Common Causes of Edema	
Cardiovascular	**Lymphatic**	**Pulmonary**
• Congestive Heart Failure	• Lymphedema	• Cor pulmonale
• Myocardial Infarction	• Postsurgical trauma	• Pulmonary contusion
Endocrine	**Nutrition**	**Venous**
• Hypothyroidism	• Protein calorie malnutrition	• Deep vein thrombosis
• Diabetes mellitus, uncontrolled	• Protein losing enteropathy	• Venous insufficiency
		• Compression secondary to mass effect
Renal	**Gastrointestinal**	**Other**
• Chronic kidney disease	• Ulcerative colitis	• Trauma
• Acute kidney injury	• Pseudomembranous colitis	• Burns
• Nephrotic syndrome	• Celiac sprue	• Acute or chronic
• Nephritic syndrome	• Hepatorenal syndrome	inflammation
	• Cirrhosis	
	• Hemochromatosis	
Medications		
• Calcium channel blockers (dihydropyridine>nondihydropyridine)		
• Hydralazine		
• Minoxidil		
• Glucocorticoids		
• Insulin		
• Estrogen		
• Testosterone		
• Aromatase inhibitors		
• Nonsteroidal anti-inflammatories		

Hydrostatic pressure is the outward pressure exerted on the walls of blood vessels and lymphatics by the fluid inside those vessels. Increases in hydrostatic pressure, when $Pc > Pi$, can result from venous obstruction, expanded plasma volume, and arteriolar vasodilation.

Venous obstruction occurs when there is a downstream obstruction in blood or lymphatic flow. As long as upstream flow continues, hydrostatic pressure in the vessel will increase, eventually resulting in extravasation of fluid. An example of obstruction is venous return from the legs of a pregnant woman. The venous blood returning to the right atrium from the lower extremities has to overcome a greater pressure due to partial obstruction from the fetal pressure on the inferior vena cava resulting in lower extremity edema.

Plasma volume expansion is often the result of sodium imbalance in the body. As sodium concentration increases in the plasma, so too does fluid by the process of diffusion. Increasing the amount of fluid in a closed system results in increased hydrostatic pressure and consequent extravasation of free fluid into the surrounding tissue. Common causes of expanded plasma volume include heart failure, nephritic syndrome, and hepatic cirrhosis.

Edema associated with arteriolar vasodilation is a common side effect of certain classes of antihypertensive medications, most notably dihydropyridine calcium antagonists. These antihypertensive medications act at the level of the arteriole to lower systemic vascular resistance by decreasing the contractility of vascular smooth muscle. This relaxation of smooth muscle results in increased "pooling" of blood and resultant extravasation of free fluid.

Oncotic pressure is the inward pressure that plasma proteins exert on surrounding fluid. Albumin makes up the largest constituent of oncotic pressure, accounting for ~80% of plasma protein. As such, anything that lowers albumin concentration in the plasma, when $\pi i > \pi c$, can result in edema.

For example, in the presence of liver disease or malnutrition, albumin synthesis is relatively low and hypoalbuminemia results. Hypoalbuminemia results in decreased capillary oncotic pressure and extravasation of fluid. Similarly, albumin can be lost via the kidneys or GI tract. Disease states such as nephrotic syndrome and protein losing enteropathies result in an efflux of protein from the vascular space, subsequently driving capillary oncotic pressure down and resulting in edema.

Vascular permeability in the body is generally a static force, represented in the Starling equation by Kf, whereas hydrostatic and oncotic pressure are variable forces. While vascular permeability is not dependent upon another force for equilibrium, it can be altered by a myriad of insults that decrease the integrity of the vessel, including infection, trauma, burns, and autoimmune insults.

Etiology

A diverse spectrum of disease states, from insignificant to life-threatening, can lead to Starling disturbance. As a result, edema can be thought of as a spectrum of conditions from benign to life-threatening, depending on the underlying etiology. As a result, elucidating the cause of edema is fundamental for a physician. Table 2.8-1 highlights common causes of edema by organ system.

DIAGNOSIS

History

"If a diagnosis cannot be gleaned from a history, go back and take the history again." This adage is especially true when working to understand the etiology of edema. Edema can be a manifestation of innumerable disease states, many of which can be life-threatening. A thorough history must be obtained in order to fully elucidate the etiology of edema as important clues can be ascertained from each component of the history. Important historical considerations include the onset, location, and duration of edema. A description of the severity of edema and any inciting or ameliorating events is also important. Past medical history of congestive heart failure, Crohn's disease, or COPD may lead a physician to a diagnosis as might a surgical history of lymphatic disruption or gastric bypass. A thorough review of medications and review of systems is also critical to elucidating the cause of edema.

Physical Examination

A thorough physical examination should be performed to help a physician narrow the broad differential diagnosis associated with edema. A physician might especially note a new murmur, friction rubs, rhythm disturbance, or distant heart sounds on the cardiac examination, or crackles, rhonchi, or decreased breath sounds on pulmonary examination. Likewise, an abdominal examination may reveal ascites, organomegaly, or a fluid wave, while the neurologic examination may expose confusion, lethargy, or generalized weakness.

Characteristics about the edema itself that are important to note include the distribution and symmetry of the swelling. In particular, a physician should note whether edema is dependent or nondependent. If edema is observed to be nonpitting, it is more likely to be the result of myxedema or moderate to severe lymphedema. Also, tenderness associated with edema and overlying skin discolorations or lesions should be identified. Tenderness may suggest infection or increased pressure on normal tissues, while skin lesions can reveal a nidus of infection or signs consistent with venous insufficiency.

Differential Diagnosis

The differential diagnosis for edema is vast, and testing should be focused on determining the underlying etiology.

TREATMENT

Treatment should always be directed at management of underlying conditions. Empiric treatment may mask disease severity without correcting the imbalance in Starling forces, and therefore lead to missing a potentially serious underlying disease.

Behavioral

In cases of dependent edema, elevation of the affected limbs above the level of the hips may temporarily reduce symptoms. Compression apparel can be a useful adjunct when treating dependent edema. Compression apparel, most commonly stockings, increases pressure in the lower extremities and/or abdomen to help increase venous return to the heart and minimize pooling. Compression garments should have graduated pressures, with highest pressure at the ankles and lowest at the top of the garment. Improperly fitting compression garments can be harmful.

Medications

Diuretics are the foundation for correction of peripheral edema, as they are relatively safe and well tolerated by patients. Diuretics target the most common causes of edema, increased relative hydrostatic pressure. By reducing intravascular pressure and volume through diuresis, excess interstitial fluid can diffuse back into the vascular system, thereby alleviating the edema. The goal of diuretic therapy is to bring the Starling forces back into equilibrium, but excess diuresis can result in intravascular volume depletion and dehydration.

With congestive heart failure or renal disease, correction of peripheral edema occurs rapidly because the body's full capillary system can be employed to reabsorb the excess interstitial fluid. Loop diuretics are first-line treatment in patients with congestive heart failure. In cirrhosis, however, aldosterone receptor antagonists such as spironolactone are first-line, because these patients often develop secondary hyperaldosteronism. Rapid diuresis must be avoided in patients with ascites because only the peritoneal capillaries are available to draw off interstitial fluid and the maximal threshold is quickly surpassed. Periodic paracenteses are sometimes used to avoid high diuretic doses, although the fluid drawn off is eventually replaced. In cases where edema is not caused by changes in hydrostatic pressure (changes in vascular permeability, decreased capillary oncotic pressures, lymphedema) diuretics have little effect and can be harmful.

Patient Education

Patients are often the first to notice edema, and are often concerned about its cosmetic consequences. Offering reassurance and focusing discussion on the underlying disease can greatly allay the patient's concerns.

REFERENCES

1. Messerli FH. Vasodilatory edema: a common side effect of antihypertensive therapy. *Curr Cardiol Rep* 2002;4(6):479–482.
2. Guyton A, Hall J. Chapter 16: the microcirculation and the lymphatic system. In: Gruliow R. *Textbook of medical physiology*. 11th ed. Philadelphia, PA: Elsevier; 2006:187–188.
3. Lee YT, Sung JJ. Protein-losing enteropathy. *Gastrointest Endosc* 2004;60(5):801–802.
4. Vincent JL. Relevance of albumin in modern critical care medicine. *Best Pract Res Clin Anaesthesiol* 2009;23(2):183–191.

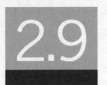

Pelvic Pain

Tessa Rohrberg, Gretchen M. Dickson

GENERAL PRINCIPLES

Pelvic pain is defined as pain in the lower abdomen or pelvic region and can be acute or chronic in nature. The true bony pelvis is that cavity bordered anteriorly by the pubic symphysis and superior rami, laterally by the ischium and ilium, and posteriorly by the sacrum and coccyx. This area contains the bladder, distal ureters, colon, rectum, pelvic neurovascular structures, and pelvic muscles. In women, it also contains the uterus, ovaries, and fallopian tubes, while in men it includes the prostate gland. Pelvic pain is much more common in women than in men, and so this chapter focuses on female pelvic pain (see Special Considerations for a brief discussion of pelvic pain in men). Pelvic pain is a very common complaint in family medicine and can originate from a variety of causes. The pathophysiology and management of pelvic pain depends on the nature of the underlying cause. Pelvic pain is most commonly classified by acute and chronic diagnoses and can be further classified by defining location, comparing age groups, or by reviewing urgent to nonurgent etiologies.

DIAGNOSIS (ACUTE)

Acute pelvic pain is often described as pain in the lower abdomen or pelvis lasting less than 3 months.[1] Occasionally, the underlying pelvic pathology may lead to upper quadrant or generalized abdominal pain, with or without peritoneal signs. The differential diagnosis of acute pelvic pain is best separated into locations and age groups. A differential diagnosis of pelvic pain is listed in Table 2.9-1. The clinical presentation of acute pelvic pain varies according to the etiology. The patient complaining of pain may be mildly symptomatic to acutely ill and toxic appearing. It is important to identify urgent etiologies, such as ectopic pregnancy, ruptured ovarian cyst, ovarian torsion, appendicitis, and pelvic inflammatory disease (PID).[1]

History

As with any pain complaint, the history should begin with attempting to elucidate the PQRSTs of the pain: palliative and provocative factors, the quality of the pain, the region of the pain and if there is any radiation of the pain, the severity of the pain, and the timing and duration of the pain. Second, the interviewer should ask about the presence of any associated symptoms. An organ system approach is helpful in narrowing the differential diagnosis and in choosing the proper diagnostic testing. This is done by querying the patient on symptoms related to systems existing in the pelvic region, including the skin (rash, blisters, paresthesias), musculoskeletal (history of strain or trauma), genitourinary (vaginal discharge, dyspareunia, vaginal bleeding, urinary frequency or urgency, dysuria, hematuria), and gastrointestinal (nausea, vomiting, anorexia, hematochezia, constipation, diarrhea) systems.

In women with pelvic pain, it is especially important to include an obstetrical, menstrual, and sexual history, asking about the last menstrual period, gravida/para status, past and current sexual partners, method of contraception, and history of sexually transmitted infections (STIs). It is helpful to know as well whether or not the patient has ever had any past abdominal or pelvic surgeries, especially appendectomy, hysterectomy, or oophorectomy.

Eliciting the patient's own explanatory model for the symptoms is often extremely helpful, as it may reveal pertinent information (past history of similar pain, past medical evaluations) or important worries the patient may have ("I'm worried that I may have ovarian cancer"). A social history is important to further investigate potential substance abuse or history of domestic violence.

Physical Examination

The physical examination should begin with review of the patient's vital signs, especially noting heart rate, blood pressure, and temperature. This should be followed by a general assessment of how ill the patient appears: for example, is the patient visibly uncomfortable (grimacing, grasping stomach, rocking back and forth).

Exam should then proceed to include the abdomen, beginning with inspection looking for any skin lesions (rash or bruises) or any obvious distension or deformity. Auscultation follows to assess

TABLE 2.9-1	Differential Diagnosis of Pelvic Pain

Acute
- Gastrointestinal
  - Appendicitis
  - Gastroenteritis
  - Interstitial lymphadenitis
  - Intestinal obstruction
  - Diverticulitis
  - Hernia
- Genitourinary
  - Pelvic inflammatory disease
  - Ovarian torsion
  - Vaginitis
  - Imperforate hymen
  - Urinary tract infection
  - Pyelonephritis
  - Urethritis

- Pregnancy
  - Ectopic pregnancy
  - Corpus luteum hematoma
  - Placental abruption
  - Miscarriage
  - Round ligament pain
  - Postpartum ovarian venous thrombosis
- Vascular
  - Aneurysm
  - Mesenteric venous thrombosis
- Skin
  - Trauma
  - Herpes zoster

Both Acute and Chronic
- Musculoskeletal
  - Trauma
  - Inflammatory arthritis
  - Piriformis syndrome
- Gastrointestinal
  - Irritable bowel syndrome
- Vascular
  - Ischemic colitis

- Genitourinary
  - Sexually transmitted infections
  - Ovarian cyst
  - Prostatitis
  - Nephrolithiasis
- Psychologic
  - Domestic violence
  - Sexual abuse

Chronic
- Musculoskeletal
  - Fibromyalgia
  - Myofascial pain
  - Peripartum pelvic pain syndrome
- Gastrointestinal
  - Constipation
  - Celiac disease
  - Colon cancer
  - Inflammatory bowel disease
- Psychologic
  - Mood disorder
  - Somatization disorder
  - Abdominal migraine
  - Vaginismus

- Genitourinary
  - Ovarian tumor
  - Primary dysmenorrhea
  - Fibroid uterus
  - Mittelschmerz
  - Endometriosis
  - Adenomyosis
  - Adhesions
  - Malignancy
  - Interstitial cystitis

for presence or absence of normal bowel sounds. Palpation should uncover any tender areas as well as assess for peritoneal signs, including rigidity, guarding, and rebound tenderness.

A pelvic exam is indicated and should begin with inspection of the external genitalia and urethral orifice, looking especially for any skin lesions or discharge that might indicate an underlying infectious process, for signs of trauma, or for any anatomic abnormality. The speculum exam is then performed to allow direct visual inspection of the vaginal mucosa and the cervix, looking for signs of infection and also for any dilation of the cervix, or blood, or tissue in the cervical os that could indicate an inevitable or threatened miscarriage. It may also be used to view anatomical abnormalities, such as an imperforate hymen or transverse vaginal septum. Samples can be obtained for STI screening and potentially for Pap smear testing (if the patient is in need of this screening). Following visualization with the speculum, the bimanual exam is completed to assess the cervix for cervical motion tenderness (also a peritoneal sign) and to assess for any uterine or adnexal masses or tenderness. The rectovaginal exam may be indicated on the basis of clinical suspicion (to rule out gastrointestinal bleed or fecal impaction, to assess for possible retrocecal appendix, etc.). Additional examination should be guided by the history and specific clinical situation.

Laboratory Studies

The most common testing ordered in the female patient with acute pelvic pain includes a urinalysis (UA) and pregnancy testing. Additional testing may include cervical cultures for *Neisseria gonorrhea* and *Chlamydia*, a vaginal wet prep and KOH slide, or a complete blood count (CBC). White blood cells, hematuria, and positive nitrite or leukocyte esterase on the UA can suggest a diagnosis of urinary tract infection, while hematuria alone could indicate an underlying renal stone. The pregnancy test is required for any woman of childbearing age. An initial positive urine or blood test may need to be followed by a more specific serum quantitative test, which measures an exact amount of the human chorionic gonadotropin (HCG) hormone (this can be helpful in dating a pregnancy and in correlating with ultrasound findings).

The vaginal wet prep can be diagnostic for bacterial vaginosis (if clue cells are seen) or *Trichomonas* vaginitis (if the flagellated trichomonads are seen). If the KOH slide is positive for yeast or fungal elements, then the diagnosis of *Candida* vaginitis is made. When diagnosing an STI, it is important to remember to screen for additional infections, as the risk is higher for a second when diagnosed with one.

A high white count on the CBC may indicate an underlying infectious process. Anemia, if present and especially if associated with tachycardia or hypotension, could indicate a more serious process, such as a ruptured ectopic pregnancy or ovarian cyst. Further lab testing may include fecal occult blood test, urine culture or stool studies, or Rh blood typing (if pregnant).[1]

Imaging

Although imaging is often not necessary in the evaluation of acute pelvic pain, there are situations where it will be helpful. If the patient is acutely ill and a reasonable diagnosis cannot be made on the basis of the history, physical, and laboratory tests, then imaging may be needed to better define the problem. It is important to use imaging to assist in making the most accurate diagnosis while using the least amount of radiation.[1]

Ultrasonography is the modality of choice and is readily available at most hospitals, and even in some private offices.[1] A pelvic ultrasound utilizing the transabdominal and transvaginal approaches can often identify many sources of pelvic pain, including an ectopic pregnancy, ovarian pathology (hemorrhagic cysts and torsion), uterine fibroids, PID, and many cases of acute appendicitis. Renal ultrasound can also be helpful in ruling out structural renal pathology and dilation of the ureters (hydronephrosis), which may result from an obstructing kidney stone.

When ultrasound imaging is inconclusive, computed tomography (CT) imaging may be considered. It can be used to assess for signs of acute appendicitis and diverticulitis. Noncontrast spiral CT scan of the renal system has largely replaced intravenous pyelogram (IVP) testing to evaluate for the presence of nephrolithiasis. Some subtle changes may show up on the CT scan in cases of PID as well.

Magnetic resonance imaging (MRI) can also be used in the setting of acute pelvic pain and may be an alternative to the ionizing radiation used in CT imaging; however, MRI is not always readily available and is more expensive.

Surgical Diagnostic Procedures

In acute cases, surgical intervention for diagnosis (most often using laparoscopy) is generally reserved for those patients who are severely ill, where a diagnosis has not yet been made, or for patients who are failing to respond to treatment.

TREATMENT (ACUTE)

Specific treatments for a variety of common causes of acute pelvic pain are outlined below. Pain control will be an important feature for all patients with acute pelvic pain. For many diagnoses, conservative treatment with ice or heat and rest, combined with over-the-counter acetaminophen or nonsteroidal anti-inflammatory drugs, is sufficient. However, some patients may require narcotics to control their pain. Dietary modification may be useful in certain situations. Behavioral therapy is generally supportive as in some cases reassurance is all that is needed.

Medications

Many of the conditions that can cause acute pelvic pain are infectious and treatable with the correct antibiotic agent. Antibiotic selection may change depending on outpatient versus inpatient management, failure to respond to first-line treatment, or in special populations such as pregnancy.

Although the exact causative agent is often not identified in cases of PID, it is often caused by *Chlamydia* or *N. gonorrhea,* so empiric antibiotic coverage must be effective against both of these agents. Commonly, the combination of intramuscular ceftriaxone in one 250-mg dose plus oral doxycycline 100 mg twice daily for 14 days with or without oral metronidazole 500 mg twice daily for 14 days.[2] Vaginitis is treated according to the causative agent: *Trichonomas* is treated with metronidazole 2 grams in a single dose or 500 mg twice daily for 7 days, *Candida* infections are treated with topical (terconazole, clotrimazole, tioconazole, and nystatin) or oral (fluconazole) antifungals, and bacterial vaginosis is also treated with metronidazole, vaginally or orally, with clindamycin vaginally as the alternative.[3] For urinary tract infection, there are many antibiotics that may be effective. These include the first-line agents of trimethoprim-sulfa, fluoroquinolones, macrodantin, and cephalexin.

Shingles can be ameliorated with the appropriate antiviral agent (acyclovir, valacyclovir, or famciclovir), especially if started early in the course.

Diverticulitis is usually managed with broad-spectrum antibiotic coverage to include Gram-negative and anaerobic bacteria, usually trimethoprim/sulfamethoxazole DS or a fluoroquinolone plus metronidazole.[4] Most gastroenteritis is viral in origin and requires only symptomatic care, though a bacterial pathogen may be more likely if the patient also has fevers, bloody diarrhea, and significant abdominal cramping.

Surgery

Surgery is the treatment of choice for acute appendicitis, ovarian torsion, and symptomatic hernias. Surgery is often indicated as well for bowel obstruction and for ectopic pregnancy (although in some instances ectopic pregnancy can also be managed medically) and may be indicated in diverticulitis or in cases of kidney stone (especially when there is concomitant obstruction).

Nonoperative

Many conditions may benefit from alternative therapies. Specifically, uterine artery embolization is now available in most communities and has provided an important nonsurgical alternative to hysterectomy or myomectomy for the treatment of uterine fibroids.

Referrals

Family physicians should refer for procedures that are beyond their scope of care and help to coordinate the plan of care. For pelvic pain with peritoneal findings, consultation with surgery (obstetrical, gynecologic, or general) is usually indicated.

Monitoring

Patients with acute pelvic pain should be monitored to ensure response to treatment. Depending on the diagnosis, patients may need to be admitted (acute abdomen) or reexamined within 48 to 72 hours. Additionally, patients should be monitored until complete resolution of symptoms, as complications may arise and also as some acute pelvic pain may become chronic pelvic pain.

Patient Education

Patient education should be provided to all patients to help them understand the etiology, treatment, and prognosis for their pelvic pain. Patients should also be educated to look for warning signs of disease progression. Follow-up should be encouraged when symptoms do not respond to therapy.

Complications

The potential complications from acute pelvic pain are wide-ranging. In most instances, the pain resolves, and there are no long-term problems. However, many complications, including progression to chronic pain, are possible. PID can lead to chronic pain, infertility, and an increased incidence of ectopic pregnancies. Because of the increased risk of complications, hospitalization for patients with PID is indicated if the patient is pregnant, has severe illness, is unable to tolerate oral medication, has a tubo-ovarian abscess, or if there is failure to improve after 3 days on initial therapy.[2] Ectopic pregnancy can cause fallopian tube rupture, which can potentially lead to fatal blood loss. Fibroids (leiomyomata) of the uterus can lead to severe pain and anemia and may necessitate hysterectomy. Kidney stones, especially if recurrent or associated with obstruction, have the potential to lead to chronic kidney disease. Given the range of potential complications and the seriousness of many of the possible diagnoses, it is important for the health care provider to be careful and thorough in managing patients presenting with acute pelvic pain.

DIAGNOSIS (CHRONIC)

Chronic pelvic pain can be defined as noncyclic pain lasting six months or more.[5] The clinical presentation of chronic pelvic pain may be quite similar to that for acute, and many acute etiologies can progress to chronic pelvic pain. Often, the pain is severe enough to cause functional disability, though a cause is not always identified. A differential diagnosis is listed in Table 2.9-1.

History

With chronic pelvic pain, the history should be expanded to focus more in depth on the psychosocial situation of the patient as chronic pelvic pain may indicate a history of physical or sexual abuse. Furthermore, the physician should explore the impact of the pain on the patient's life at work, home, or school. Keeping a symptom calendar (sometimes referred to as pain diary) may be helpful in uncovering hidden patterns or associations.[6] It is also important to ask about pain in relation to hormonal or nonhormonal patterns (endometriosis versus irritable bowel syndrome, respectively).[5] The clinician should inquire about family history significant for systemic disease or cancer. Unexplained weight loss, hematochezia, perimenopausal irregular bleeding, postmenopausal vaginal bleeding, or postcoital bleeding may indicate malignancy.

Physical Examination, Laboratory Studies, Imaging

The workup including physical examination, laboratory, and imaging studies should include the same items listed under acute pelvic pain. The examiner should pay special attention for masses, including vaginal, uterine, or rectal. Age-appropriate cancer screening may also be indicated.

Surgical Diagnostic Procedures

Diagnostic laparoscopy may be indicated in the workup of chronic pelvic when no obvious cause can be found on the initial workup. Cystoscopy may also be needed to further evaluate the bladder and urinary tract.

TREATMENT (CHRONIC)

Treatment should be directed at the underlying cause of pain. As an etiology is not always identified, a multidisciplinary approach should be used, targeting dietary, social, environmental, and psychosocial aspects. This may include exercise, nutritional supplements, or contemporary therapies such as yoga, massage, or acupuncture.[5]

Medications

Medications for infectious etiologies are discussed above. For noninfectious gynecologic diagnoses, there are often hormonal therapies that may be effective. The pain associated with endometriosis or adenomyosis can often be controlled by nonsteroidal anti-inflammatory drugs and cyclo-oxygenase-2-specific inhibitors. Combined oral contraceptives or progestins may also be used. If unsuccessful, gonadotropin-releasing hormone analogues may be helpful.[7] These same medications are also often helpful in treating the pain from primary dysmenorrhea.[8,9]

Medications are also the mainstay of therapy in the treatment of inflammatory bowel disease and, along with lifestyle modification, may be helpful in treating irritable bowel syndrome. The most commonly used medications for inflammatory bowel disease are anti-inflammatories (like 5-acetyl-salicylic acid compounds, such as sulfasalazine or mesalamine, and corticosteroids, such as prednisone and hydrocortisone) and immunosuppressant medications (like azathioprine, cyclosporine, and newer agents such as infliximab). In treating irritable bowel syndrome, it may be helpful to differentiate between constipation-predominant and diarrhea-predominant syndromes.

Selective serotonin reuptake inhibitors may be useful in treating coexisting depression. Trigger-point injections of the abdominal wall may also be beneficial for myofascial pain.[5]

Referrals

If a gastrointestinal source is suspected, referral to a gastroenterologist for consideration of colonoscopy may be indicated. Additionally, when initial management fails to lead to significant improvement, additional surgical, urological, or gynecologic consultation may be required. When there is a significant psychosocial component, referral to a mental health specialist should be included. Finally, if a history of abuse is uncovered, the physician should make the patient aware of available legal and social supports in the community.

Monitoring

Patients with chronic pelvic pain desire personalized care and often need reassurance. This is best done over several visits with appropriate referrals, as above.[5]

SPECIAL CONSIDERATIONS (PELVIC PAIN IN MEN)

The differential diagnosis of pelvic pain in men includes the skin, musculoskeletal, gastrointestinal, urologic, and vascular possibilities listed in Table 2.9-1. For men, however, the prostate and scrotal contents must also be considered. Prostatitis, which can be acute or chronic, is a common cause of pelvic pain in men as is referred pain from the scrotum.

Epididymitis, testicular torsion, torsion of the appendix testis, and varicocele can all cause pain that is referred to the pelvis. Of these, epididymitis is usually infectious and is treated with appropriate antibiotics (in younger men less than 35 years old, this is usually the same medication as used to treat PID in women, whereas for older men, fluoroquinolones are usually first-line agents). Testicular torsion is a surgical emergency, while torsion of the appendix testis (which only sometimes will have the classic "blue dot" sign) is almost always a benign, self-limited condition requiring only short-term analgesics. A varicocele is essentially a varicose vein in the scrotum and when symptomatic, or when there are concerns about fertility, urologic referral is indicated.

A patient with acute bacterial prostatitis is generally ill-appearing and often febrile. The patient will complain of pain, which may be anywhere from the lower back to the lower abdomen and pelvis. There will often be signs of urinary hesitancy or weakness of stream, and at times the patient may be unable to void altogether. Physical exam of an acutely infected prostate will reveal it to be enlarged, tender, and often boggy. The physician should avoid prostatic massage and vigorous prostate exam in this setting as there is concern this may increase bacteremia. The mainstay of treatment for acute bacterial prostatitis is antibiotic therapy targeting primarily Gram-negative pathogens using trimethoprim-sulfa or fluoroquinolones. However, in men younger than 35, there is again a higher likelihood of *N. gonorrhea* and *Chlamydia* infections, so therapy should cover these agents as well. Therapy should continue for a minimum of 2 weeks, though many experts advocate treating for a full 4-week course. Chronic bacterial prostatitis should be treated with similar antibiotics, though should have an extended 6- to 12-week course.

Some men may also suffer from chronic prostatitis/chronic pelvic pain syndrome, which is a poorly understood, noninfectious inflammation of the prostate. A variety of therapies have been tried, including trials of antibiotics, alpha blockers and nonsteroidal anti-inflammatory medications.[10] Urologic consultation may be helpful for these patients.

REFERENCES

1. Kruszka PS, Kruszka SJ. Evaluation of acute pelvic pain in women. *Am Fam Physician* 2010;82(2):141–147.
2. Gradison M. Pelvic inflammatory disease. *Am Fam Physician* 2012;85(8):791–796.
3. Hainer BL, Gibson MV. Vaginitis: diagnosis and treatment. *Am Fam Physician* 2011;83(7):807–815.
4. Wilkins T, Embry K, George R. Diagnosis and management of acute diverticulitis. *Am Fam Physician* 2013;87(9):612–620.
5. Ortiz DD. Chronic pelvic pain in women. *Am Fam Physician* 2008;77(11):1535–1542,1544.
6. Williams R, Hern T. Pelvic pain. *Hosp Physician* 2002;6:1–12.
7. Schrager S, Falleroni J, Edgoose J. Evaluation and treatment of endometriosis. *Am Fam Physician* 2013;87(2):107–113.
8. Osayande AS, Mehulic S. Diagnosis and initial management of dysmenorrhea. *Am Fam Physician* 2014;89(5):341–346.
9. Nasir L, Bope ET. Management of pelvic pain from dysmenorrhea or endometriosis. *J Am Board Fam Pract* 2004;17:S43–S47.
10. Sharp VJ, Takacs EB, Powell CR. Prostatitis: diagnosis and treatment. *Am Fam Physician* 2010;82(4):397–406.

2.10 Back Pain
Natasha N. Desai, Rahul Kapur

Back pain is common, though the etiology is often obscure. Once a serious medical or surgical problem has been eliminated, the management is usually straightforward.

Definition

Low back pain (LBP) refers to pain in the general lumbosacral levels of the back, and cervical pain refers to posterior neck pain from the lower occiput to the superior part of the scapula. The source of the back pain can often be nonspecific and can include the spine, paraspinal muscles, ligaments, facet joints, intervertebral disks, and the surrounding structures. Acute pain is defined as pain lasting less than 12 weeks, while chronic pain is pain lasting more than 12 weeks.

Epidemiology

Most people will likely experience acute low back or neck pain at some point in their lives. LBP affects at least 80% of people in their lifetime and is the 5th most common complaint for all physician visits. The highest incidence occurs in the third decade of life and the highest prevalence in the 6th decade of life.[1] Approximately 66% of people will have an episode of neck pain in their life.[2] The high prevalence leads to a multibillion-dollar cost from disability and work absenteeism.

LOW BACK PAIN
Diagnosis

Clinical Presentation

Patients can present either with insidious or abrupt onset of LBP. Most people will have self-limited LBP and will not seek medical care. Approximately 90% of all patients have nonspecific LBP. Potential causes of nonspecific LBP include musculoligamentous injuries, disk herniation with nerve impingement, sacroiliac (SI) joint derangements, degenerative changes of the bone, disk, or facet joint, spinal stenosis, spondylolisthesis, or scoliosis. It is important to distinguish these musculoskeletal causes from underlying systemic diseases. First, a clinician must rule out acute cord compression requiring surgical intervention as well as serious, nonorthopedic problems. Then, interventions can focus on symptom improvement with less focus on defining a specific lesion.

History

In diagnosing the cause of LBP, history is critical and should focus on ruling out serious conditions, particularly in patients older than 50 years. It is important to ask about the "red flags" of back pain to rule out a potentially serious condition, including trauma, cancer, unexplained weight loss or fever, failure of pain relief with bed rest, saddle anesthesia, bladder or bowel dysfunction, or a history that would indicate a risk of infection or increased risk of fracture.[3–5] It is important to note that one should not simply rely on a checklist of red flags alone. A recent study found that up to 80% of patients can have a red flag and not have a serious problem.[5]

After ensuring that a serious condition is the unlikely cause of back pain, questions should focus on characterizing the pain. A physician should inquire about the onset, frequency, and pattern of pain. For example, disk problems tend to occur suddenly, whereas other mechanical pain often comes on gradually. Information about the duration of the pain and previous episodes of back pain, as well as identification of precipitating situations at work or during exercise can be helpful. Pain below the knee, paresthesias, and weakness of the lower leg are consistent with nerve root compression, usually due to a disk protrusion or herniation. Patients with unilateral low back and buttock pain that gets worse with standing in one position may be suffering from an SI joint derangement. A history in older patients of exacerbation of pain with walking that is relieved by leaning forward is suggestive of neural claudication due to spinal stenosis.

It is also important to determine what risk factors the patient has to developing chronic back pain, also known as the "yellow flags" or psychosocial prognostic factors of back pain. Assess current functional limitations, employment factors such as job satisfaction and days missed, and the psychosocial situation when planning a course of treatment.[1,6]

Physical Examination

Many clues to the cause and severity of back pain can be ascertained as soon as the physician enters the room. For instance, the patient's posture and demeanor can provide a sense of the severity of pain. During the physical examination, the patient's posture and alignment, hip heights and signs of spinal deviation should be noted. Additionally, the spinous processes should be palpated to assess tenderness, while the paraspinal muscles should be examined for tenderness and spasm. Range-of-motion testing may reveal asymmetry or provocation of pain that can help to identify disk pathology.

The walk test is performed by the examiner's positioning his or her thumbs over the patient's posterior superior iliac spines while the patient is standing and then watching to see whether the thumbs move symmetrically when the patient's hips are flexed. Asymmetry of movement often indicates an SI problem. Straight leg raising and extension of the knee while sitting (flip test) are tests for dural impingement usually from a disk; these tests are considered positive when sciatic type pain is produced in the leg as the leg is extended. Pain on the contralateral side is a strongly positive test result.

Every back examination should include a neurologic examination that includes gait, muscle testing, sensory examination, and testing of deep tendon reflexes. Focus the exam on the L4 to S1 distribution, because 95% of lumbar disk herniations occur at L4 to L5 or L5 to S1.[5,7]

Laboratory and Radiographic Studies

In the evaluation of nontraumatic LBP, radiologic studies are not usually helpful during the first 4 weeks of the onset of back pain unless there are signs of an underlying serious condition. Magnetic resonance imaging (MRI) and computed tomography (CT) can be misleading because of their high false-positive rate. Back imaging has been shown to increase cost and exposure to radiation without improving outcomes.[8] Even after 4 weeks, these tests should be reserved for patients for whom surgery or epidural injection is contemplated.[8] Radiography is often used as the initial imaging but has low sensitivity and specificity. MRI is the preferred imaging modality, and CT is used when MRI is contraindicated.[5,7,8] Laboratory tests are not indicated for the first 4 weeks unless there is a fever or other sign of systemic illness.

Treatment

Patient Education

Patient education and managing expectations is a very important aspect of a successful outcome. Ninety percent of patients recover within 4 weeks regardless of the method of treatment.[4] Contemporary management of acute LBP, as expressed in the practice guidelines put forth jointly by the American College of Physicians (ACP) and American Pain Society (APS),[7] moves beyond exclusively addressing pain control to emphasizing improved activity tolerance and an early return to work. Informing patients of the likely favorable outcome, reducing worry, and managing expectations can improve outcome[5] and keep the patient from developing a disability mindset. Taking the time to discuss specific exercises, self-care strategies, and prevention by improving general fitness is also important.

Activity Level

Bed rest should be avoided except in extreme cases, and even then patients should be put on bed rest for only 1 or 2 days.[4] Usual activities should be resumed as soon as possible. However, all lifting and bending should be avoided temporarily, using pain as a guide for tolerable activity. Exercise is beneficial for treatment of subacute and chronic LBP. One study found that there was no difference between individual or group classes, but that supervision of back exercises in general led to better outcomes.[9]

Medication

Medication guidelines emphasize the use of the least amount of medication for the shortest period of time that is effective. One well-designed study has shown that patients treated with fewer pain medications and less bed rest than other therapy have lower costs and equal functional improvement after 1 month and 12 months.[10] Nonsteroidal anti-inflammatory drugs (NSAIDs) and acetaminophen should be used as first-line agents. NSAIDs provide better analgesia but have a greater side-effect profile. Muscle relaxants including benzodiazepines are frequently used and are beneficial, but are no more effective than NSAIDs, and no study has shown use of both NSAIDs and muscle relaxants to be better than either one alone.[7,11] Opioids are second- or third-line agents to be used for short periods, given lack of evidence and abuse potential. The ACP and APS guidelines suggest that opioids taken for longer than 2 weeks, oral steroids, and colchicine should be avoided altogether.

Physical Therapy

Physical therapy should be considered if pain persists longer than 2 weeks. No standard protocol exists. The Mckensie method, spinal stabilization exercises, and home exercises may be beneficial.[4] Spinal traction, biofeedback, and physical modalities (e.g., braces, corsets) do not have good supporting research for their efficacy. Recently, heat packs have been shown to give some benefit, especially when paired with exercise.

Injections

Epidural injections can be helpful in patients with acute radicular pain.[4] Trigger point injections and facet joint injections are also used but have not been thoroughly investigated.

Surgery

Cord compression and cauda equina syndrome require immediate surgery; otherwise, only 5% to 10% of symptomatic disk herniations require surgery. In fact, sciatica due to a herniated disk can resolve spontaneously in 9 to 12 months. Consider referral if a patient has persistent and severe sciatica and clinical evidence of nerve root compromise after 1 month of conservative care.

Alternative Medicine

Spinal manipulation by physical therapists, physicians, or chiropractors can be helpful during the first month of symptoms. There is no evidence that it is superior to other methods. It can also be used for the SI joint problems that are common in pregnancy. Other therapies proposed with conflicting evidence are yoga, Pilates, Tai Chi, acupuncture, and massage.[7]

Behavioral

A poor social situation can alter a patient's reaction to pain, especially if there is job dissatisfaction. Other factors, such as pending litigation, can complicate or prolong the treatment. Assessment by a psychiatrist or other mental health professional may be helpful if the psychologic issues are complex.

Recurrences of LBP are common, no matter what the treatment. It is important to recognize patients at risk for chronicity such as those with psychosocial risk factors such as depression or job dissatisfaction. LBP lasting longer than 12 weeks is considered chronic and carries with it a worse prognosis. The longer the pain lasts, the less the likelihood of recovery. The goal of treatment should be to improve functional capacity despite the pain. Passive modality treatments should be avoided. Medications are minimized, and alternative medications are being investigated, as mentioned above. An active exercise and reconditioning program with experienced therapists, intensive interdisciplinary rehabilitation, cognitive–behavioral therapy, or progressive relaxation can be helpful.[7] Ongoing psychosocial support is also crucial. Ligament injections are advocated by some physicians. Surgery should be avoided unless there is a proven source of pain. The alternative therapies mentioned above are available to these patients; unfortunately, few have been studied scientifically. Most do not cause harm and may be worth trying for selected patients.

CERVICAL PAIN

Diagnosis

History

As in LBP, the primary focus of the history is to rule out a serious underlying cause. A history of trauma, particularly a motor vehicle accident, should be obtained. Determining acuity and duration of pain is key. Pain that radiates down the arm and is accompanied by paresthesia in the C4 and C5 distribution indicates nerve compression, often caused by disk protrusion. Patients may describe awakening with a painful, deviated neck if they develop acute torticollis. The red and yellow flags of LBP may be similarly helpful in determining the seriousness of cervical pain.[2]

Physical Examination

A physical examination should include assessment of posture, symmetry, and range-of-motion testing. Range-of-motion testing should include side flexion, rotation, forward flexion, and extension. A complete neurologic examination of both upper extremities should be performed, including motor, sensory, and reflex testing.

Laboratory and Radiographic Studies

Unless there is a reason to suspect a systemic illness causing the pain or there is a history of trauma, no radiographs or other radiologic studies are necessary on initial evaluation.

Management

When needed, immobilization with a soft or hard cervical collar should be limited to just a few days. The patient should start gentle range-of-motion exercises immediately. If the pain persists for more than 1 week, the patient should be referred for physical therapy. Medications should be limited to mild analgesics, acetaminophen and NSAIDs, as in LBP. A muscle relaxant can be added only if there is no response to the analgesic alone, although there is little evidence to support this practice. Surgery is reserved for fractures or radiculopathy with disabling pain.

REFERENCES

1. Patrick N, Emanski E, Knaub MA. Acute and chronic low back pain. *Med Clin N Am* 2014;98:777–789.
2. Teichtahl AJ, McColl G. An approach to neck pain for the family physician. *Aust Fam Physician* 2013;42(11):774–778.
3. Downie A, Williams, CM, Henschke, et al. Red flags to screen for malignancy and fracture in patients with low back pain: systematic review. *BMJ* 2013;347:f7095.
4. Becker JA, Stumbo JR. Back pain in adults. *Prim Care Clin Office Pract* 2013;40:271–288.
5. Casazza BA. Diagnosis and treatment of acute low back pain. *Am Fam Physician* 2012;85(4):343–350.
6. Nicholas MD, Linton SJ, Watson PJ, et al. Early identification and management of psychological risk factors ("yellow flags") in patients with low back pain: a reappraisal. *Phys Ther* 2001;95(5):737–753.
7. Chou R, Qaseem A, Snow V, et al; Clinical efficacy assessment Subcommittee of the American College of Physicians; American College of Physicians; American Pain Society Low Back Pain Guidelines Panel. Diagnosis and treatment of low back pain: a joint clinical practice guideline from the American College of Physicians and the American Pain Society. *Ann Intern Med* 2007;147(7):478–91.
8. Chou R, Deyo RA, Jarvik JG. Appropriate use of lumbar imaging for evaluation of low back pain. *Radiol Clin N Am* 2012;50:569–585.
9. Henchoz Y, So AK. Exercise and nonspecific low back pain: a literature review. *Joint Bone Spine* 2008;75:532–539.
10. Von Korff M, Barlow W, Cherkin D, et al. Effects of practice style in managing back pain. *Ann Intern Med* 1994;121:187.
11. Miller SM. Low back pain: pharmacologic management. *Prim Care Clin Office Pract* 2012;39:499–510.

CHAPTER 3

Emergency Problems in Ambulatory Care

Section Editor: William Henry Hay

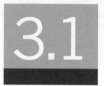

Anaphylaxis

Mark D. Goodwin

DEFINITION

Anaphylaxis has no universally accepted definition, but is generally described as an acute, potentially fatal, multiorgan system reaction mediated by sudden systemic release of mast cells and basophil mediators. Anaphylactoid and pseudoanaphylaxis have been replaced with immunologic (IgE and IgG and immune complex complement–mediated) and nonimmunologic anaphylaxis (sudden mast cell and basophil degranulation in the absence of immunoglobulins).[1,2,3,4]

EPIDEMIOLOGY

True incidence of anaphylaxis is unknown due to underdiagnosis, underreporting, and continued lack of consensus of the definition. Lifetime risk of anaphylaxis is 1% to 3% per individual, with 1% mortality rate. Incidence in the United States is 49.9/100,000 person-years. Atopy is present in only 37% to 53% of anaphylaxis, and is more important for reactions to foods, latex, and radiocontrast, but less for reactions to medications or insect stings.[1]

PATHOPHYSIOLOGY

Most anaphylaxis is IgE-mediated. Following previous sensitization, antibodies to an allergen attach to mast cells and basophils, resulting in activation and degranulation. Immunologic or not, histamine, heparin, tryptase, kallikrein, platelet-activating factor, bradykinin, tumor necrosis factor, nitrous oxide, and several types of interleukins are released and contribute to the proinflammatory cascade. Mediators induce smooth muscle spasm in the respiratory and gastrointestinal tracts, vasodilation, increased vascular permeability, and stimulation of sensory nerve endings.[5,6,7] Airway edema, increased mucous secretion, and bronchial smooth muscle tone contribute to respiratory symptoms. Decreased vascular tone and capillary leakage shift up to 35% to 50% of the vascular volume to the extravascular space within 10 minutes.[3]

ETIOLOGY

Etiology includes any agent activating mast cells or basophils. Common causes include the following:[1–8,5,6,3,9]

1. **Venoms:** Honeybees, bumblebees, wasps, yellow jackets, fire ants, etc. Up to 3% of adults and 1% of children who have been stung are anaphylactic. First reactions can be fatal.
2. **Medications:** Hormones, vitamins, corticosteroids, nonsteroidal anti-inflammatory drugs, opiates, and antibiotics (1 in 5,000 exposures to parenteral penicillin or cephalosporin causes anaphylaxis).
3. **Foods:** 30% of fatal cases of anaphylaxis most commonly with peanuts, tree nuts, fish, shellfish, cow's milk, soy, and egg.
4. **Foreign proteins:** Pertussis, typhoid vaccines, horse serum (antivenin), seminal plasma globulins (human, horse, rodent), and antitoxins.

5. **Latex:** Health care settings have successfully eliminated most latex; anaphylaxis occurs after exposure to latex gloves, condoms, balloons, padded play pits, infant pacifiers, and bottle nipples.
6. **Radiocontrast material (RCM):** With conventional high-osmolality RCM, adverse reactions, which occur independent of RCM dose or concentration, occur 5% to 8%, with life-threatening reactions seen in less than 0.1%. Use of lower-osmolality RCM reduces the risk of reactions by one-fifth. Risk factors include previous RCM reaction (16% to 44%), atopy, asthma, and cardiovascular disease. There is no evidence that inorganic iodine is present in seafood or topical iodine–containing solutions are related to RCM adverse events. Reactions can occur during hysterosalpingograms, myelograms, and retrograde pyelograms and are clinically identical to IgE-mediated reactions but do not appear to involve any immunologic mechanism. Pretreatment protocols (oral glucocortico-steroids, H1 and H2 antihistamines, ephedrine) combined with lower osmolarity agents reduce risk to approximately 1%.
7. **Idiopathic:** 33% of cases in the United States.

DIAGNOSIS

Clinical diagnosis is based on probability and pattern recognition. The presence of one of three criteria listed below predicts anaphylaxis 95% of the time.

1. Acute onset of illness (minutes to hours) with involvement of skin, mucosal tissue, or both (i.e., generalized hives; pruritus/flushing; swollen lips, tongue, uvula), and one of the following:
   a. Respiratory compromise (i.e., dyspnea, wheeze-bronchospasm, stridor, reduced peak expiratory flow, hypoxemia)
   b. Reduced blood pressure or associated symptoms of end-organ dysfunction (i.e., hypotonia [collapse], syncope, incontinence)
2. Two or more of below occurring rapidly (minutes to hours) after exposure to likely allergen:
   a. Involvement of skin, mucosal tissue, or both (i.e., generalized hives; pruritus or flushing; swollen lips, tongue, or uvula)
   b. Respiratory compromise (i.e., dyspnea, wheeze-bronchospasm, stridor, reduced peak expiratory flow, hypoxemia)
   c. Reduced blood pressure or associated symptoms (i.e., hypotonia [collapse], syncope, incontinence)
   d. Persistent gastrointestinal symptoms (i.e., abdominal cramps, vomiting)
3. Reduced blood pressure that occurs rapidly (minutes to hours) after exposure to known allergen. In adults, it is systolic blood pressure of <90 mmHg or a >30% decrease from baseline. In infants and children, definition of low systolic blood pressure is age-specific. [1,4]

CLINICAL PRESENTATION

Signs and symptoms usually develop within 5 to 30 minutes of exposure to offending allergen, but may develop within seconds or not for several hours depending upon the route of exposure. Symptoms usually resolve within minutes to hours of treatment, but reactions rarely last up to 72 hours despite treatment. Up to 20% of patients experience biphasic reaction (second acute anaphylactic reaction occurring after first response without further allergen exposure), most occurring within 8 but rarely up to 72 hours after initial reaction.[1,8,3] Signs and symptoms of anaphylaxis are based upon the organ system involved.[1–8,5,6,3,9]

1. **Skin (90% of episodes):** Pruritis, flushing, urticaria, angioedema, erythema, maculopapular/mobilliform rash, and pilor erecti.
2. **Eyes:** Conjunctival injection, lacrimation, periorbital edema, and pruritis.
3. **Respiratory tract (70% of episodes):** Pruritis of lips, tongue, palate; sneezing, rhinorrhea, nasal congestion, metallic taste, cough, wheeze, tachypnea, dyspnea, accessory muscle use, hoarse-ness, choking sensation/tightness in the throat, laryngeal/oropharyngeal edema, stridor, cyanosis, respiratory arrest.
4. **Cardiovascular (45% of episodes):** Chest pain, tachycardia, conduction disturbances, arrhyth-mias, myocardial ischemia/infarction, hypotension, bradycardia, and cardiac arrest.
5. **Gastrointestinal (45% of episodes):** Abdominal pain/cramping, nausea, vomiting, and diarrhea.
6. **Neurologic (15% of episodes):** Dizziness, syncope, seizure, and sense of impending doom.
7. **Other:** Low back pain, uterine contractions, and generalized weakness.

DIFFERENTIAL DIAGNOSIS

Any condition resulting in sudden collapse (i.e., acute myocardial ischemia, pulmonary embolism, foreign body aspiration, acute poisoning, hypoglycemia, seizure) can be confused with anaphylaxis. Other conditions resembling anaphylaxis include:

1. **Sudden syncope:** Vasovagal (most common). Urticaria and dyspnea absent with normal (or elevated) blood pressure, tachycardia, cool and pale skin. Bradycardia may occur in late/protracted anaphylaxis; arrhythmia, cerebrovascular accident, drug overdose.
2. **Shock:** Hemorrhage, hypovolemia, sepsis, and cardiogenic shock.
3. **Respiratory distress:** Status asthmaticus, chronic obstructive pulmonary disease exacerbation, epiglottitis, pulmonary edema, and vocal cord dysfunction.
4. **Angioedema:** Hereditary angioedema and angiotensin-converting inhibitor side effect.
5. **Skin symptoms:** Systemic mastocytosis, serum sickness, scromboid toxin, medication side effects (red man syndrome, oral hypoglycemics with alcohol), peri-/postmenopausal hot flushes, pheochromocytoma, carcinoid syndrome, and urticarial vasculitis.
6. **Psychiatric symptoms:** Anxiety attack, globus hystericus, hyperventilation, Munchausen stridor, Munchausen by proxy, factitious anaphylaxis, and malingering.

HISTORY

Details of onset and severity of symptoms, associated risk factors, potential exposures, previous anaphylaxis, allergies, asthma, or atopy help determine whether a reaction was anaphylactic. [1]

PHYSICAL EXAMINATION

Appearance and vital signs vary by severity of episode and organ system(s) affected. Patients are commonly restless and anxious, and may manifest any of the following.

1. **Respiratory:** Angioedema of tongue and lips; tachypnea; stridor, severe air hunger; loss of voice, hoarseness, and/or dysphonia; wheezing.
2. **Cardiovascular:** Tachycardia, hypotension; cardiovascular collapse and shock.
3. **Neurologic:** Altered mentation; depressed level of consciousness, agitation/combative.
4. **Dermatologic:** Urticaria, angioedema; generalized erythema (or flushing).
5. **Gastrointestinal:** Vomiting, diarrhea, and abdominal distention.[1,8,5,6,3,9]

MONITORING

Vital signs are assessed frequently. Continuous cardiac monitoring is done in severe reactions; in patients with cardiovascular disease, chest pain, hypotension or shock, concurrent β-blocker use, and arrhythmias; and after IV epinephrine or other vasopressors. Continuous pulse oximetry is used for respiratory symptoms and central venous pressure monitoring for hypotension or shock.

LABORATORY STUDIES

Value of confirmatory blood testing is limited. Serum histamine levels must be obtained within 15 to 60 minutes of symptom onset and require special handling (histamine breaks down with any movement). Tryptase levels increase 15 to 30 minutes after onset of symptoms and peak in 1 to 3 hours. Levels sampled on presentation, at peak, and 24 hours after presentation to assess for return to baseline. Neither test is specific.[1,5,3] Other tests may be indicated based upon the clinical situation (not to diagnose anaphylaxis).

1. Arterial blood gas if significant respiratory symptoms are present.
2. CBC, electrolytes in prolonged treatment, comorbid conditions or hospitalization.
3. Allergy testing: Skin testing, radioallergosorbent test, and serum antibody testing are more helpful after episode of anaphylaxis to identify allergen to promote future avoidance.

IMAGING

Not routinely necessary. Chest x-ray or CT may be indicated for localized physical findings, poor response of bronchospasm to treatment, or uncertain diagnosis (i.e., foreign body, PE, infiltrate, etc.).[1,2]

TREATMENT

The treatment of immunologic and nonimmunologic anaphylaxis is identical. Immediate therapy is ABC (airway, breathing, and circulation). Epinephrine is the mainstay therapy for anaphylaxis. Postponement is associated with fatal anaphylaxis. If reaction is due to insect sting, remove remaining stinger/venom sac by scraping it off. Do not pinch/squeeze the venom sac (will inject additional venom). Discontinue exposure to trigger, if relevant (i.e., discontinue intravenous medication or biological agent).[1,8,5,6,3,9]

MEDICATIONS FOR IMMEDIATE CARE

Treatment in order of importance: epinephrine, oxygen, intravenous fluids, nebulized therapy, vasopressors, antihistamines, corticosteroids, and other agents.

Epinephrine

Epinephrine is used for moderate-to-severe reactions with respiratory distress, stridor, significant gastrointestinal symptoms, laryngeal edema, hypotension, syncope, dysrhythmia, and rapidly progressing reaction. If there is any doubt, it is generally better to administer epinephrine.

Adult: 0.3 to 0.5 mL of 1:1000 IM is delivered into anterolateral thigh (<u>NOT</u> subcutaneous) q 5 to 15 minutes. Pediatric: 0.01 mL per kg q 5 to 15 minutes to maximum of 0.3 mL per dose. Patients should not suddenly sit or stand after receiving epinephrine injection. This can lead to the empty inferior vena cava/empty ventricle syndrome and sudden death. Up to 20% of patients require second dose for ongoing symptoms or biphasic anaphylaxis. In older patients or patients with known coronary artery disease, the best current evidence shows benefits far outweigh any risk.

Oxygen

Oxygen is used in respiratory distress, hypoxia, prolonged reactions, patients with preexisting hypoxemia, myocardial dysfunction, and those receiving inhaled β-agonists or requiring multiple doses of epinephrine. Use high-flow (6 to 8 L per min) delivery systems depending upon degree of distress or hypoxia. Consider in any patient. Oximetry guides oxygen treatment.

Intravenous fluids

Intravenous fluids are used for persistent hypotension despite epinephrine. Hypotension is due to dramatic shifts in intravascular volume. Even in the presence of upper airway obstruction, placing a patient in the recumbent position with lower extremities raised is preferred over elevating the head of the patient's bed, as the vascular collapse during anaphylaxis can be devastating. Saline stays in intravascular space longer than dextrose and contains no lactate, which may exacerbate metabolic acidosis. Give IV fluids aggressively, especially if the patient is taking a β-adrenergic blocker. Adults: 1 to 2 L bolus normal saline or colloid via two large-bore IV catheters (5 to 10 mL per kg in the first 5 minutes up to 65 L); Pediatric: 20 mL per kg bolus, continue as necessary (up to 30 mL per kg in the first hour).

Antihistamines

Antihistamines are NOT drugs of choice in initial anaphylaxis treatment. There is no direct outcome data regarding effectiveness of any antihistamine (H1 or H2). Alone or in combination, these agents are second-line to epinephrine. They do not treat upper or lower airway obstruction, hypotension, shock or the underlying cause of the allergic reaction. They do decrease urticaria and itching that persist after epinephrine. After oral administration, onset of action is 1 to 3 hours (too long in acute anaphylaxis). IV administration shortens time to onset of action but can cause hypotension. First-generation, potentially sedating H1 antihistamines have a poor benefit/risk ratio as they can (especially in children) adversely affect mentation, which can impair self-recognition of symptoms and complicate interpretation of CNS symptoms and signs. Data involving second-generation antihistamines are lacking but suggest they may be as efficacious as first-generation agents. However, they have the same drawback of a slow onset of action as they are all administered orally and are therefore not useful in anaphylaxis. H2 blockers may effect cardiac, gastrointestinal, and dermal signs and symptoms, but evidence of efficacy H2 blocker antihistamines is particularly sparse.

H1 blockers

Diphenhydramine: Adult: 1 to 2 mg per kg or 25 to 50 mg IV over 10 to 15 minutes, IM or PO with mild reactions q 4 to 6 hours; Pediatric: 1.25 mg per kg q 4 to 6 hours. Chlorpheniramine: Adult: 2 mg 4 tablets PO; Pediatric: age <6 years 1 tablet PO, age 6 to 12 years 2 tablets PO. Hydroxyzine: Adult: 25 mg PO; Pediatric: age <6 years 50 mg PO qd divided tid–qid, age >6 years 50 to 100 mg PO qd divided tid–qid.

H2 blockers

Ranitidine: Adult: 50 mg; Pediatric: 12.5 to 50 mg (1 mg per kg) IM or diluted to total volume of 20 mL D5W IV over 5 minutes.

Bronchodilators

Use inhaled β_2-agonist in bronchospasm, constant dry cough, and respiratory distress, especially when bronchospasm does not respond to epinephrine. Adult: Albuterol 0.5%: 0.5 to 1 mL in 2.5 mL saline nebulized q 15 minutes or continuous; Pediatric: age <2 years: 0.03 mL per kg, age >2 years: 0.5 to 1.0 mL per kg.

Corticosteroids

Corticosteroids are not drugs of choice in initial anaphylaxis treatment. Use to theoretically decrease the incidence and severity of protracted, delayed, or biphasic reactions, but evidence of effectiveness is lacking and the onset of action is slow (at least 6 hours).

Methylprednisolone: Adult: 40 to 250 mg IV or IM q 6 hours; Pediatric: 1 to 2 mg per kg IV or IM q 6 hours.

Prednisone: 1 to 2 mg per kg PO q 8 hours; continue for 6 to 24 hours for mild to moderate attacks and for 24 to 48 hours for severe attacks.

MEDICATIONS FOR REFRACTORY SYMPTOMS

If anaphylaxis is not responding to above, including repeated doses, IM epinephrine, IV epinephrine, vasopressors, and glucagon may be considered.

Epinephrine

Adult/adolescents: infusion 1 mg (1 mL) 1:1000 epinephrine in 250 mL of D5W (4.0 mg per mL) at a rate of 1 mg per min, titrated to desired hemodynamic response, to maximum 10.0 mg per min. Pediatric: 0.01 mg per kg (0.1 mL per kg 1:10,000 solution 10 mg per min; maximum dose, 0.3 mg). Potential for lethal arrhythmias, epinephrine should be administered IV only in patients profoundly hypotensive or in cardio/respiratory arrest, who failed to respond to IV volume replacement and several IM doses of epinephrine. Continuous hemodynamic monitoring is recommended but do not withhold if monitoring is not available.

Glucagon

Glucagon is used for patients with concurrent oral or ophthalmic β-adrenergic blocker use. Airway protection is important to prevent aspiration in severely drowsy or obtunded patients. Adult: 1 mg IV or IM q 1 minutes up to 5 mg or 1 mg IV bolus followed by continuous infusion of 1 to 5 mg IV per hour. Pediatric: 0.03 to 0.1 mg per kg up to 1 mg per dose repeat q 15 to 20 minutes.

Vasopressors

Alleviate hypotension when all previous measures fail. Dopamine is the vasopressor of choice (400 mg in 500 mL of 5% dextrose), at 2 to 20 mg/kg/min titrated to systolic blood pressure.

IMMEDIATE POST-ANAPHYLAXIS TREATMENT

Observation after anaphylaxis is individualized and based on comorbid conditions, distance from treatment facilities, patient's (or parent's) ability to recognize recurrence of sign and symptoms, ability to self-administer epinephrine using autoinjector, incomplete response to treatment, recurrent reactions, secondary complications, extremes of age, and inadequate social support. There are no reliable predictors of subsequent biphasic reactions. For most patients, 4 to 6 hours of observation is probably adequate, but most recommend a minimum of 24 hours for many moderate and all severe reactions. Patients should continue the oral antihistamines and prednisone for 2 to 3 days and should be educated that symptoms may recur for up to 72 hours and should use the epinephrine autoinjector and seek care immediately should reaction recur. Follow up with primary care provider in 1 to 3 days.

REFERRALS

Guidelines strongly recommended consultation with allergist/immunologist following anaphylaxis to assist in identification of causative agent, clarification of diagnosis, provision of patient education, education on management of recurrent reactions, and consideration for allergy testing and desensitization if indicated.[1,8,5]

RISK MANAGEMENT

Action plan is an important component of follow-up. Avoidance is primary and should be individualized, taking into consideration the factors such as age, activity, occupation, hobbies, residence, and access to medical care. Even when the allergen is known, avoidance is not always successful. Patients should be instructed in self-management, which includes awareness of signs of symptoms, proper use of autoinjector, and follow-up.

PATIENT EDUCATION

Emphasizing hidden allergens (i.e., food label reading), cross-reactivity between allergens and drugs, and unforeseen risks during medical procedures (latex or RCM sensitivity) is the most important prevention strategy. Patients should avoid β-blockers, ACE inhibitors, angiotensin II receptor blockers, monoamine oxidase inhibitors, and some tricyclic antidepressants to avoid treatment medication interactions, which can either exacerbate anaphylactic reactions or blunt treatment measures. Epinephrine is available as (a) Ana-kit two 0.3-mL epinephrine doses, four 2-mg chlorpheniramine tablets, (b) EpiPen 0.3 mL per dose, EpiPen Jr. 0.15 mL per dose, or (c) Twinject 0.15 mL or 0.3 mL per dose. Strongly consider wearing medical alert identification tags. Medical facilities and physicians should be aware of and implement one of the approved pretreatment protocols for radiocontrast sensitivity.

REFERENCES

1. Arnold J, Williams PM. Anaphylaxis: recognition and management. *Am Fam Physician* 2011;84(10):1111–1118.
2. Oswalt ML, Kemp SF. Anaphylaxis: office management and prevention. *Immunol Allergy Clin North Am* 2007;27(2):177–191,vi.
3. Mustafa SS. Anaphylaxis. Medscape Review. 2014.
4. Sampson HA. Second symposium on the definition and management of anaphylaxis: summary report—Second National Institute of Allergy and Infectious Disease/Food Allergy and Anaphylaxis Network symposium. *J Allergy Clin Immunol* 2006;117(2):391–397.
5. Simons FE. Anaphylaxis. *J Allergy Clin Immunol* 2010;126(4):885.
6. Brown SG, Mullins RJ, Gold MS. Anaphylaxis: diagnosis and management. *Med J Aust* 2006;185(5):283–289.
7. Simons FE, Ardusso LR, Dimov V. World Allergy Organization Anaphylaxis Guidelines: 2013 update of the evidence base. *Int Arch Allergy Immunol* 2013;162:193–204.
8. Lieberman P. The diagnosis and management of anaphylaxis practice parameter: 2010 update [Practice parameter]. *J Allergy Clin Immunol* 2010;126(3):477.
9. Simons FE, Ardusso LR, Bilò MB, et al. 2012 Update: World Allergy Organization Guidelines for the assessment and management of anaphylaxis. *Curr Opin Allergy Clin Immunol* 2012;12:389–399.
10. NICE (National Institute for Health and Clinical Excellence). Anaphylaxis: Assessment to confirm an anaphylactic episode and the decision to refer after emergency treatment for a suspected anaphylactic episode, NICE (National Institute for Health and Clinical Excellence) clinical guideline 134, published December 2011.

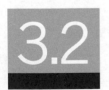

3.2 Bronchospasm
Kristen Hood Watson

GENERAL PRINCIPLES

Definition

Contraction of the bronchial smooth muscles causing narrowing and obstruction of the bronchial lumen, resulting in restricted airflow.[1]

Etiology

Asthma exacerbation, chronic obstructive pulmonary disease (COPD) exacerbation, anaphylaxis, viral or bacterial infection (pneumonia, bronchitis, bronchiolitis, sinusitis), heart failure, aspiration, allergen exposure, irritant exposure (air pollutants, smoke, organic particles, chemicals, etc.), medication exposure (NSAIDs/Aspirin, β-adrenergic receptor blockers), rhinitis, foreign body aspiration, acid reflux, exercise, stress, weather changes (cold air), envenomation, perinatal factors (preterm delivery, maternal smoking), anatomic abnormalities (laryngomalacia, bronchopulmonary dysplasia), cystic fibrosis, and obstructive sleep apnea.[2–5]

DIAGNOSIS
Clinical Presentation

- Dependent upon severity and duration of bronchospasm
- Shortness of breath, cough, difficulty speaking, wheezing (may or may not be present), tachypnea, prolonged expiration, diaphoresis, accessory muscle use, anxiety, agitation, cyanosis, mental status changes, respiratory, or cardiac arrest[3,6]
- Pediatric patients may also present with weak cry, difficulty feeding, grunting, and nasal flaring[3,5]

History

- Duration and severity of symptoms
- Precipitating factors, for example, exercise, exposure to irritants, recent illness
- Relieving factors/response to treatment
- Smoking/substance abuse history
- Current medication, compliance, and last use
- Drug or other allergies
- Prior hospitalizations and emergency department visits for bronchospasm, especially in the last year
- Prior episodes of respiratory failure, intensive care unit admission, intubation, or mechanical ventilation
- Other potentially complicating illnesses:
  - Chronic pulmonary or cardiac disease
  - Diabetes, peptic ulcer disease, hypertension, psychosis, and depression (all may be aggravated by systemic corticosteroids)[2,3]

Physical Examination

- Findings depend on severity and duration of symptoms (Table 3.2-1)
- **Other signs:** diaphoresis, central cyanosis, nasal flaring, and decreased capillary refill
- **Look for signs of complicating condition:** peripheral edema, stridor, subcutaneous emphysema, unequal breath sounds, fever, unilateral leg edema, or tenderness[2–5,7]

TABLE 3.2-1	Classifying Severity of Bronchospasm			
	Mild	**Moderate**	**Severe**	**Imminent respiratory arrest**
Talks in	Sentences	Phrases	Words	Words or unable
Alertness	May be agitated	Usually agitated	Usually agitated	Drowsy or confused
Accessory muscle use, retractions	Usually not	Common	Usually	Paradoxical movement
Wheeze	Moderate, often only end expiratory	Loud, throughout exhalation	Usually loud, throughout inhalation and exhalation	Absent wheeze
Respiratory rate	Increased	Increased	Often >30/min	Often >30/min
Heart rate	<100 bpm	100–120 bpm	>120 bpm	Bradycardia
Pulsus paradoxus	Absent <10 mmHg	May be present 10–25 mmHg	Often <25 mmHg adult, 20–40 mmHg child	Absence suggests respiratory muscle fatigue
PEFR (% predicted or personal best)	>70%	40%–69% or response lasts <2 h	<40%	<25%
SaO$_2$ (room air)	>95%	90%–95%	<95%	

Adapted from Busse WN. National Asthma Education and Prevention Program: Expert panel report III: Guidelines for the diagnosis and management of asthma. Bethesda, MD: National Heart, Lung, and Blood Institute, 2007. (NIH publication no. 07-4051.)

Monitoring
- **Pulse oximetry**
  - SaO_2 90% or less in adults or 92% or less in children indicates severe airflow obstruction
  - Oxygenation may decrease with β-agonist inhalant therapy due to increases in v/q mismatch[5]
- **Spirometry/peak expiratory flow rate (PEFR)**
  - Serial measurements document response to therapy
  - Normal values differ with size and age
  - FEV1 preferred over peak expiratory flow (PEF) if available because a low PEF cannot differentiate between obstructive versus restrictive disorders versus poor effort[6]
- **Electrocardiography/telemetry**
  - *Not* routinely obtained
  - **Indication:** Severely symptomatic, age 50, coexistent heart disease or COPD
  - **Possible findings:** sinus tachycardia, right heart strain, and supraventricular tachycardia (SVT) (consider theophylline toxicity); arrhythmias other than SVT are rare[3,6]

Laboratory Studies
- **Complete blood count** with fever, purulent sputum, or other signs of infection[2,3]
  - Leukocytosis is common with asthma exacerbations, significant stress, corticosteroid or catecholamine use
- **Arterial blood gas (ABG)** with severe distress, PEF 25% predicted or less, or SaO_2 <90% after initial treatment[3,5]
  - $PaCO_2$
    - Initially **decreased** due to increased respiratory drive and hyperventilation.
    - **Normal** indicates severe airflow obstruction, respiratory muscle fatigue, and increased risk of respiratory failure.
    - **Elevated** (>42 mmHg) indicates inadequate ventilation and impending respiratory failure.[3]
- **Serum electrolytes** with coexisting cardiovascular disease, diuretic or chronic steroid use[3,5,6]
  - Low potassium, magnesium, and/or phosphate may be secondary to frequent β_2-agonist or steroid use[3,5,6]
- **Theophylline level** with current treatment[5,6]
- **Tests for viral or bacterial infections** per clinical suspicion

Imaging
- **Chest x-ray (CXR)**
  - *Not* routinely recommended
  - **Indications (suspected complicating cardiopulmonary process):** fever, leukocytosis, elevated procalcitonin, unexplained chest pain, asymmetric breath sounds, hypoxemia, subcutaneous emphysema, peripheral edema, and high-risk comorbidities (intravenous drug use, immunosuppression, granulomatous disease, recent seizures, cancer, chest surgery, and congestive heart failure)[3,5,6]

Differential Diagnosis
- Extrathoracic upper airway obstruction
  - Anaphylaxis, postnasal drip syndrome, vocal cord abnormalities or dysfunction, hypertrophied tonsils, epiglottitis, laryngeal edema, laryngostenosis, laryngocele, postextubation granulomas, retropharyngeal abscess, peritonsillar abscess, mobile supraglottic soft tissue, obesity, tumors, Wegener granulomatosis, cricoarytenoid arteritis, abnormal arytenoid movement, relapsing polychondritis, and klebsiella rhinoscleroma[2,4–6]
- Intrathoracic upper airway obstruction
  - Tracheal stenosis, foreign body aspiration, airway tumors, intrathoracic goiter, tracheobronchomegaly, acquired tracheomalacia, herpetic tracheobronchitis, and right-sided aortic arch[2,4–6]
- Lower airway obstruction
  - Asthma, COPD, emphysema, pulmonary edema, aspiration, pulmonary embolism, pneumonia, bronchiolitis, bronchitis, gastroesophageal reflux disease, cystic fibrosis, carcinoid syndrome, bronchiectasis, lymphangitic carcinomatosis, parasitic infections, α_1-antitrypsin deficiency, and sarcoidosis[2,4–6]
- Other
  - Panic disorder, hyperventilation syndrome, conversion disorder, and myasthenia gravis[2,6]

TREATMENT
Medications

- **Oxygen:** Maintain PO_2 >90% to 92% and >95% with pregnancy and coexistent heart disease[3]
- **Short-acting $\beta\chi_2$-agonist (albuterol)**
  - **Nebulized**
    - **Intermittent:** Adult 2.5 to 5 mg or pediatric 0.15 mg per kg (minimum 2.5 mg) q 20 to 30 minutes × 3 doses, then q 1 to 4 hour prn
    - **Continuous:** If severely ill or PEFR <200, adults 10 to 15 mg per hour or pediatric 0.5 mg/kg/h
  - **Metered-dose inhaler (MDI) with spacer/holding chamber** (four to eight puffs is equivalent to one nebulized treatment)
    - Four to eight puffs q 20 to 30 minutes × 3, then q 1 to 4 hour prn
  - **Parenteral:** If seriously ill with no improvement after two to three inhaled treatments; No proven benefit compared to inhaled
    - **Epinephrine:** 1:1000 (1 mg per mL) adult 0.3 to 0.5 mg sq or pediatric 0.01 mg per kg (up to 0.3 0.5 mg per kg) sq q 20 minutes × 3 doses
    - **Terbutaline** (1 mg per mL) adult 0.25 mg or pediatric 0.01 mg per kg sq q 20 minutes × 3 doses, then q 2 to 6 hour prn[3]
- **Anticholinergics:** Add to albuterol if severe bronchospasm or slow response to initial β_2-agonist therapy. It is recommended for initial use in the emergency room as it may decrease hospital admission rates, but it is not recommended for hospital use[3,6]
  - **Ipratropium bromide (Atrovent)**
    - **Nebulized:** Adult 0.5 mg or pediatric 0.25 to 0.5 mg q 20 to 30 minutes × 3 doses, then q 2 to 4 hour prn
    - **MDI:** Adult eight puffs or pediatric four to eight puffs q 30 minutes × 3 doses, then q 2 to 4 hour prn[3]
- **Corticosteroids:** Start as soon as insufficient improvement with β-agonist is identified (<10% improvement in PEFR after first dose β-agonist, PEFR <70% after initial hour of treatment); start immediately in all patients currently taking oral corticosteroids; start early in pediatric population[3,5]
  - **Parenteral**
    - **Methylprednisolone (Solu-Medrol, Depo-Medrol)** adult 40 to 80 mg per day IV in 1 to 2 divided doses or pediatric 1 to 2 mg/kg/day IV in 1 to 2 divided doses (max 60 mg)[3]
  - **Oral:** In the absence of vomiting, efficacy is comparable to IV[3]
    - **Prednisone:** adult 40 to 80 mg per day in 1 to 2 divided doses or pediatric 1 to 2 mg/kg/day in 1 to 2 divided doses (max 60 mg) (until PEF reaches 70% predicted)[1,3]
    - **Inhaled.** Start at discharge, do not wait until after tapering oral steroid (causes confusion and medication noncompliance)
- **Methylxanthines:** Not recommended owing to the increased risk of toxicity, without added benefit[3,5]; may consider in refractory cases; check level with current treatment
  - **Theophylline (Aminophylline):** Adult 5 mg per kg over 20 minutes followed by continuous infusion of 0.5 to 0.7 mg/kg/hour or pediatric (≥2 years old) 5 mg per kg IV over 20 minutes followed by continuous infusion of 1 mg/kg/hour
- **Magnesium sulfate:** Use is controversial, results of published trials are mixed[5]; may consider in refractory cases; 2 g IV over 30 minutes or pediatric 25 to 75 mg per kg IV up to 2 g over 10 to 20 minutes[5]
  - **Leukotriene receptor antagonist:** *Not* recommended as use in acute setting is unclear; small studies indicate improvement in PEFR when given with acute bronchospasm,[5,6] may consider in refractory cases
    - **Montelukast:** Adolescent and adult 10 mg PO, pediatric 2 to 5 years old 4 mg, 6 to 14 years old 5 mg
- **Antibiotics:** *Not* recommended without signs of complicating bacterial infection (sinusitis, bronchitis, or pneumonia)[3,6]
- **Heliox:** Mixture of helium and oxygen; may improve oxygenation in refractory cases, but not proven consistently effective[5]; may consider in refractory cases
- **IV fluids:** Only to treat dehydration; young children and infants may become dehydrated owing to tachypnea and decreased oral intake[3,5]
- **Sedatives:** *Not* recommended owing to respiratory suppression unless intubated[3]
- **Mucolytics:** *Not* recommended; may worsen cough or bronchospasm[3]

Nonoperative
Endotracheal Intubation and Mechanical Ventilation
- **Indications:**
  - **Absolute:** apnea, coma

- **Other:** Altered mental status, inability to speak, increasing or decreasing pulsus paradoxus, respiratory or cardiac arrest, diaphoresis in the recumbent position, acute barotrauma, severe lactic acidosis (especially in infants), silent chest despite respiratory effort, retractions, worsening fatigue, refractory hypoxemia (PaO_2 <60 mmHg on max O_2), increasing $PaCO_2$ (50 mmHg and rising >5 mmHg per hour)[6]; see Table 3.2-1 above for findings associated with imminent respiratory arrest.
- **Risks:** Laryngeal damage, high pressures causing hypotension (auto-PEEP), barotrauma, pneumothorax, pneumomediastinum
- **Guidelines:**
  - Do not delay intubation once it is deemed necessary
  - Consult with or comanagement by physician expert in ventilatory management
  - Best done semi-electively, before the crisis of respiratory arrest
  - Perform in a controlled setting (intensive care unit or emergency room) by experienced physician
  - Maintain or replace intravascular volume to prevent hypotension caused by PPV
  - Permissive hypercapnia or controlled hypoventilation (adequate oxygenation and ventilation while minimizing high airway pressure and barotrauma)
    - Highest FiO_2 as necessary to maintain oxygenation
    - Accept hypercapnia
    - Treat respiratory acidosis with IV sodium bicarbonate
    - Adjust tidal volume, rate, and I:E ratio to minimize airway pressures
    - Continue other therapy[3]

Referrals/Consultation

- Severe, refractory, or life-threatening symptoms with intensive care unit transfer or intubation with mechanical ventilation
- Recurrent emergency department visits or hospitalizations for bronchospasm
- Atypical signs and symptoms or difficult differential diagnosis
- Other complicating conditions
- Additional diagnostic testing indicated (allergy skin testing, rhinoscopy, pulmonary function tests [PFTs], bronchoscopy)
- Additional patient education is needed (problems with adherence or allergen avoidance)
- Confirmation of occupational or environmental exposure
- Pregnant patients with severe or recurrent symptoms
- Significant psychiatric, psychosocial, or family problems that interfere with care[3]

Risk Management

Failure to initiate steroid therapy or intubation, monitor electrolyte balance, admit a wheezing patient with normal PCO_2, treat expediently, educate patients upon discharge, and identify other diagnoses (congestive heart failure, myocarditis, multiple pulmonary embolisms, surreptitious vocal cord dysfunction, panic disorder, hyperventilation, etc.)

Patient Education

Monitoring PEFR at home with written action plan, importance of taking medication, proper medication use, proper use of inhalants and spacers, trigger avoidance, oral rinsing after inhaled corticosteroids (ICS), significance of nocturnal exacerbations, and close follow-up.[3,5,6]

Follow-Up

After treatment
- **PEFR ≥ 70% and minimal or absent symptoms:** Discharge with education and close follow-up; increase frequency of short-acting β-agonist (SABA), possibly start oral steroids, consider ICS.
- **PEFR 40% to 69% and mild-to-moderate symptoms**
  - **Consider for discharge:** Improving lung function, low risk (good self-care skills and supportive home environment) and can obtain medications; discharge with education and close follow-up; increase frequency of SABA, start oral steroids, consider ICS.
  - **Hospitalize:** New-onset or labile asthma, multiple prior hospitalizations or emergency room visits, past intensive care unit admission or intubation, using >2 SABA canisters in 1 month, severe symptoms that preclude self-care, lack of plan, patient difficulty understanding severity of symptoms, other complicating conditions, psychiatric disease, drug use, or adverse socioeconomic conditions.
- **PERF <40%:** Hospitalize[3]

Complications

Medication side effects, pneumothorax, pneumomediastinum, secondary infection, respiratory distress/arrest, death.

Special Considerations

- **Socioeconomic factors:** Inability to obtain medications or medical care can lower the threshold for admission. Consider discharging patient with medications in hand or IM steroid to avoid possible nonadherence.[6]
- **Pediatrics:** May be more difficult to determine severity of illness. Treat as aggressively as adults in appropriate dosages, give corticosteroids early, more likely to become dehydrated due to increased work of respiration.[3,5]
- **Pregnancy:** Treat as aggressively as nonpregnant women to prevent maternal and fetal hypoxia. Hypoxia and respiratory acidosis can be detrimental to both the fetus and the mother. Continuous electronic fetal monitoring is recommended when fetus is potentially viable. Obstetrical and pulmonary consultation with severe or refractory symptoms.[2,8,9]

REFERENCES

1. *Mosby's Medical Dictionary.* 8th ed. St. Louis, MO: Elsevier; 2009.
2. Morris MJ. Asthma. *emedicine* (Online serial). November 18, 2013
3. Busse WN. *National Asthma Education and Prevention Program: Expert panel report III: guidelines for the diagnosis and management of asthma.* Bethesda, MD: National Heart, Lung, and Blood Institute; 2007. (NIH publication no. 07–4051.)
4. Weiss LN. The diagnosis of wheezing in children. *Am Fam Physician* 2008;77(8):1109–1114.
5. Asthma Exacerbation in Children. *Dynamed* (Online serial). March 10, 2014.
6. Asthma Exacerbation in Adults and Adolescents. *Dynamed* (Online serial). June 7, 2013.
7. Irwin RS. Diagnosis of wheezing illnesses other than asthma in adults. *UpToDate* (Online serial). February 20, 2014; Version 10.0.
8. American College of Obstetricians and Gynecologists (ACOG). *Asthma in pregnancy.* Washington, DC: American College of Obstetricians and Gynecologists; 2008. (ACOG practice bulletin #90). Retrieved from www.guideline.gov/contents.aspx?id=12630. Accessed on March 19, 2014.
9. Busse WW, Alving B, et al. *National Asthma Education and Prevention Program: Working group report on managing asthma during pregnancy: recommendations for pharmacologic treatment.* Bethesda, MD: National Heart, Lung, and Blood Institute; 2004. (NIH publication no. 05–5236.)

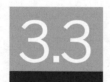

3.3 Drug Overdose

Payam Sazegar

GENERAL PRINCIPLES

- Drug overdose is the leading cause of injury-related death in the United States.[1,2]
- According to the National Safety Council (www.nsc.org), drug overdose was the leading cause of death in working-age adults in 2013.
- Rapid stabilization of any suspected overdose patient is the first priority.
- Quick determination of substances used from patient, family, friends, and ambulance staff is needed to prevent delay of therapy. The initial history often correlates poorly with the definitive diagnosis; therefore, patients should have their clothing, wallets, phones, and accessories checked for pills, prescriptions, and drug-related equipment. Further information can be obtained from toxicology screens. State prescription drug monitoring databases can also be checked when available.
- Gastric lavage, emesis, whole-bowel irrigation, activated charcoal, and use of cathartics should be considered to decrease gut absorption of toxic substances. Activated charcoal is often the preferred approach initially.
- Maintaining close contact with the US Poison Control Center (national toll-free number 1-800-222-1222) or area toxicologists will likely be needed. In some cases, patients may call this number

and be treated from home with assistance from the poison control center—if they have been asymptomatic, ingested a known nontoxic quantity of medication, and felt to be reliable.[3]
- The care team should be alert for indications of intentional overdose for self-harm or malicious intent and involve psychiatry and/or the appropriate authorities.
- Analgesics, sedatives, antipsychotics, and antidepressants are the most common drugs found in overdoses,[4] not a surprise as patients prescribed these drugs are the most likely to suffer from suicidal ideation.
- Suicide attempts, poisonings, pediatric accidental ingestion, and illicit drugs are the most commonly encountered drug overdoses. Ingestion of a toxic substance, either accidental or intentional, is the most prevalent, but has a fatality rate of <1%, with only 7% of cases requiring hospitalization.[4] Today's era of drug parties, especially among teens, is causing an increase in accidental overdoses. Experimentation with common substances and production of new illicit drugs will continue to confound clinicians. Furthermore, the number of opioid-related deaths in the United States has sharply risen over the past decade.

DIAGNOSIS

Initially assess for life-threatening complications. Treatment focuses on eliminating the drug and specific antidote and drug therapy. Look for patterns of the classic "toxidromes": sympathomimetic, anticholinergic, hallucinogenic, opioid, sedative–hypnotic, cholinergic, neuroleptic malignant syndrome, and serotonin syndromes; distinguished by physical exam, EKG changes, and unique odors. Keep in mind other causes for the patient's signs and symptoms such as infections and electrolyte disturbances.

History

Question the patient, family, friends, and the paramedics about
- Type and/or name of the drug(s)
- Time and amount of ingestion
- Any empty bottles or drug paraphernalia found at the site
- Past medical history of other significant diseases that may complicate the overdose

Physical Examination

- Vital signs (unstable vital signs demand prompt attention)
- Smell the breath for any distinctive odors; remembering other processes such as a diabetic ketoacidosis could also be occurring
- **Eyes:** pupil size and reactivity, extraocular movements, nystagmus
- **Heart:** murmurs may indicate infective endocarditis
- **Lungs:** Rales point to pneumonia or pulmonary edema
- Abdomen: liver size, peripheral stigmata of chronic liver disease
- Rectal exam can be helpful in the case of "body packers" (body packers place packages of illicit drugs in body cavities)
- **Skin:** look for sweating, a cold or clammy feeling, and needle marks
- Neurologic examination: consciousness, gag reflex, tremors, and deep tendon reflexes

Laboratory Tests and Imaging

- Bedside blood glucose: Do not delay in treating hypoglycemia
- **EKG:** QRS/QTc changes that may require urgent action
- CBC
- Electrolytes, BUN, creatinine, serum osmolality (osmolar gap may occur with alcohol ingestion)
- **Complete urinalysis:** may show rhabdomyolysis, crystals
- Chest x-ray and arterial blood gas if any respiratory impairment
- Some toxins or drug packets can be detected on radiology plain films
- Levels of suspected agents, for example, alcohol, acetaminophen, and salicylate
- Toxicology screens on the blood, urine, and gastric contents must be obtained rapidly; many substances metabolize quickly and are not detectable within a few hours of ingestion even though their affects may be longer lasting. Suspected false-negative or false-positive results will need confirmatory testing

TREATMENT
Stabilization

- In comatose or severely compromised drug overdose patients, establish an airway and ventilate the patient immediately. In lethargic or obtunded patients, check the gag reflex and, if it is not present, intubate the patient. If no blood pressure or pulse is present, begin cardiopulmonary resuscitation and also provide airway and circulatory support. Patients should be monitored for cardiac arrhythmias, and a large-diameter intravenous line should be placed. Decontamination should be considered as an additional "D" in the secondary ABCs of cardiac life support resuscitation. The preferred option is activated charcoal (1 to 2 g per kg, max 100 g), which can decrease absorption by 70% if given within 30 minutes of ingestion and by 30% if given within 30 to 60 minutes. Gastric lavage (performed with a size 36 to 40 French tube) can be helpful but only if started within 60 minutes of the drug ingestion; there is a risk of injury to the esophagus or aspiration with this procedure. Whole-bowel irrigation with bowel prep solutions such as potassium chloride (Go-Lytely) or polyethylene glycol at a rate of 1 to 2 L per hour can be used in cases of iron intoxication, lithium overdose, or a ruptured "body pack." If nasogastric administration of the solution is required, the patients must lay at a 45 degrees incline to help prevent aspiration. Airway protection and management is paramount in this procedure. It may take more than 5 hours to clear the contaminant; samples of the effluent from the rectum can be tested to ensure clearing of the drug. Serial blood tests may be required.

Medication

- During the initial treatment of drug overdose patients, empirically treat unconscious patients for possible hypoglycemia with 50 mL of 50% dextrose intravenous (IV). Administration of 100 mg of IV thiamine may help prevent an acute Wernicke syndrome in alcoholics; however, the myth that it "must" be given prior to the administration of dextrose has been debunked in the literature.[5] For potential narcotic overdoses, give naloxone (Narcan) to any patient with respiratory depression, 0.4 mg IV; if there is no response in 1 to 2 minutes, you can give 2 mg IV, and keep repeating the dose to a maximum of 10 to 20 mg IV. A helpful mnemonic to remember for the unconscious patient is "DONT" (D=Dextrose; O=Oxygen; N=Naloxone; T=Thiamine).

Referrals/Counseling

- Local poison control centers and toxicologists are good resources throughout the treatment process and especially helpful in uncommon overdoses. Psychiatrists and psychologists should be consulted in intentional overdoses after the patient has been stabilized and cleared medically. Close monitoring, usually one-on-one supervision, may be needed after the patient has regained consciousness until they are discharged or transferred. Many emergency departments and primary care centers train staff to perform the Screening, Brief Intervention, and Referral to Treatment (SBIRT).[6]

Prevention

- Physicians play a critical role in preventing prescription drug overdoses. Evaluate all patients for their overdose potential. Give low-toxicity drugs to patients with a history of depression, substance abuse, previous suicide attempts, or overdoses and to those who may be more sensitive to drugs, such as elderly, young, pregnant patients, and patients on other drugs. Female patients are more likely to overdose than male patients. Give high-risk patients smaller amounts of the drug with more frequent refills. This is especially true in patients with seizure disorders requiring barbiturates, which are up to 10 times as toxic as benzodiazepines.

SPECIFIC DRUG OVERDOSE TREATMENT
Cocaine and Amphetamines
Diagnosis

- Stimulant drug overdoses present with chest pain, cardiac arrhythmias, hypertension, stroke, paranoia, seizure, severe agitation, and asthma attacks. Hyponatremia due to excess sweating may also be present. Severe cocaine intoxication may present as bradycardia and hypotension due to cardiovascular toxicity. Death is caused by cardiac arrhythmias, status epilepticus, cerebral hemorrhage, myocardial infarction, or hyperthermia. Simultaneous alcohol use increases the production of active metabolites, causing prolonged drug toxicity.[7] Smugglers may swallow large bags of cocaine to prevent detection, a practice known as body packing. Rupture of the bags causes severe cocaine intoxication.

Treatment

- Treat hypertension with diazepam (Valium), 5 to 10 mg IV no faster than 5 mg per minute. If severe hypertension persists, start a sodium nitroprusside infusion, 0.5 to 10 mg/kg/minute. Hyperthermia needs to be aggressively treated with rapid cooling to prevent rhabdomyolysis and subsequent renal failure. Treat myocardial ischemia with nitroglycerin and aspirin. Consider using nitrates and calcium-channel blockers for the management of uncontrolled hypertension. β-Blockers should be

used with caution for cocaine-induced chest pain or myocardial ischemia, although the theoretical risk of unopposed α-adrenergic stimulation is not supported in the literature.[8] Consider thrombolytic therapy and coronary catheterization in acute myocardial infarctions.
- Treat body packers with activated charcoal (50 to 100 g in adults) and consider whole-body irrigation.
- Amphetamine psychosis, seen after "speed runs," can be managed with diazepam, 0.1 to 0.2 mg per kg IV or, in severe cases, haloperidol (Haldol), 5 to 10 mg IM or PO (but this may cause hyperthermia and a reduced seizure threshold).

Tricyclic Antidepressants
Diagnosis
- Tricyclic antidepressants (TCAs) are frequently used in suicide attempts. Patients present often with tachycardia and hypotension, and it can be lethal due to cardiac toxicity. The classic "anticholinergic toxidrome" can be present: dilated pupils ("blind as a bat"), flushing with vasodilation ("red as a beet"), elevated temperature ("hot as hades"), confusion and delirium ("mad as a hatter"), thirst and decreased salivation ("dry as a bone"). Other symptoms include decreased gastrointestinal motility and hyperreflexia. Patients presenting with arrhythmias, altered mental status, seizures, respiratory depression, or hypotension are at high risk, requiring close monitoring and hospital admission. Think of tricyclic antidepressant overdose if the patient has a QRS interval longer than 0.12 seconds with right axis deviation on the electrocardiogram. Ventricular tachycardias should be treated with IV sodium bicarbonate. Remember that many drug overdoses involve multiple drugs and some potential causes of the "anticholinergic toxidrome" include some antihistamines, antiemetics (phenothiazines), antispasmodics, and antipsychotics.

Treatment
- Because antidepressant overdoses decrease gastrointestinal motility, do gastric lavage and give activated charcoal every 4 hours. Treat cardiac toxicity and hypotension with sodium bicarbonate, 1 to 2 mEq per kg IV bolus, until the arterial pH is 7.45 to 7.55, and if this does not control arrhythmias then give lidocaine.[7] Manage seizures with benzodiazepines.
- Antidepressants such as selective serotonin-reuptake inhibitors (SSRIs) or serotonin–noradrenalin reuptake inhibitors (SNRIs) should be used in high-risk patients.
- A good suicide prevention strategy, including a crisis line to call and improved social supports, is an essential part of postdischarge care.

Ethanol and Benzodiazepines
Diagnosis
- In addition to recreational use, patients frequently use alcohol to "get the courage" to attempt suicide with other drugs. Symptoms include nystagmus, ataxia, hypoglycemia, vomiting, and coma. A blood level of 300 mg per dL causes coma in a "novice" drinker. In patients with severe coma and respiratory depression or arrest, consider the possibility of concomitant γ-hydroxybutyrate (GHB, one of the "date rape" drugs) ingestion.

Treatment
- Do a urine toxicology screen to determine whether other drugs have been ingested. Time and supportive care (which may include intubation and blood pressure support) are all that is needed for the majority of alcohol overdoses. Replenish intravascular volume depletion with good hydration and IV fluids. Benzodiazepines should be used to control agitation and systemic affects (such as seizures, hypertension and tachycardia) in alcohol withdrawal. Clonidine may also be used for autonomic symptoms. Flumazenil (Romazicon), 0.2 mg IV over 30 seconds, and repeated if needed in 1 to 2 minutes, can reverse the sedation and respiratory depressant effects in benzodiazepine overdoses, but it is rarely needed and can cause serious side effects (seizures if the patient is taking concomitant tricyclic antidepressants, and severe withdrawal effects and seizures if the patient is dependent on benzodiazepines). Temporary intubation and ventilatory support may be necessary in GHB overdoses or to prevent aspiration in sedative to hypnotic overdoses.

Opiates
Diagnosis
- Opiate overdose is an ever-increasing problem of endemic proportions in the United States. Overdose is characterized by respiratory depression, pupil constriction (which may not be seen with meperidine or diphenoxylate overdose), central nervous system depression, hypotension, and

bradycardia. In severe overdose patients, apnea and pulmonary edema may occur. If alcohol has been ingested, opiate toxicity is increased. Synthetic opioids (such as Fentanyl, Tramadol, Methadone, and Oxycodone) are often not detected in standard urine toxicology screens and require confirmatory testing.

Treatment

Naloxone should be given as soon as possible. This can be effectively delivered via the intranasal (IN) (1 to 2 mg), subcutaneous (0.4 mg), intramuscular (0.4 mg), and intravenous (0.4 mg) routes. The IN route is equally effective and also a faster and safer method of delivery,[8] so it is becoming part of the public health and harm reduction strategies to prevent deaths due to opioid overdose.[9] It can be prescribed at the same time as prescription opioids and is being dispensed by an ever-increasing number of pharmacies. In severe overdose, symptoms may recur owing to naloxone's half-life of 60 to 90 minutes, which is shorter than that of most opiates, requiring treatment of patients with repeated doses every 2 hours; daily maximum of 10 to 20 mg IV. There is no clearly established daily maximum dose for naloxone, but adverse effects have been noted with doses of 2 mg per kg.

Hallucinogens

Diagnosis

- Lysergic acid diethylamide (LSD), the most commonly abused hallucinogen, causes sympathetic stimulation with tachycardia, hallucinations, paranoia, fear, dilated pupils, sweating, and fever. Hallucinogen intoxication can be difficult to differentiate from acute schizophrenic symptoms. Patients taking hallucinogens usually have no history of mental illness, know that the symptoms are drug related, and have visual instead of auditory hallucinations. Patients who have been at a "rave" dance club commonly ingest LSD, methylene dioxymethamphetamine (ecstasy or MDMA), or methylenedioxyamphetamine (Eve or MDA).

Treatment

- Hallucinogens are rapidly absorbed into the bloodstream, and lavage and activated charcoal only increase agitation. Quiet reassurance helps patients to "come down." In severe cases, diazepam or lorazepam helps to quiet patients. MDMA can cause hyperthermia and muscle rigidity that can lead to rhabdomyolysis if untreated (cool the patient, hydrate him or her, and use benzodiazepines for rigidity).

Phencyclidine

Diagnosis

- Phencyclidine (PCP) overdose patients can be challenging to manage. Patients' behavior ranges widely, from quiet sedation to severe violence. PCP is frequently used as an adulterant in other illicit drugs, and patients may not know that they have ingested PCP. In mild intoxication, patients are lethargic, euphoric, and have hallucinations. In more severe intoxication, patients have hypertension, muscle rigidity, sweating, seizures, and coma. PCP intoxication can be suspected in any patient with nystagmus and rapidly changing behavior.

Treatment

- Because enterohepatic recirculation slows elimination, the effects of PCP last up to 24 hours. Decrease sensory input and administer activated charcoal to decrease reabsorption. Avoid the use of restraints, which can increase the risk of rhabdomyolysis. Treat violent behavior with benzodiazepines. Haloperidol may be used cautiously but it may increase muscle rigidity. Increased diuresis is advocated by some experts.[5,10]

Acetaminophen

Diagnosis

- This is based mostly on history but should be suspected in cases of elevated liver function tests in suspected drug overdose/intoxications. Acetaminophen is widely available and is frequently used for suicidal gestures. Many over-the-counter and prescription analgesics can contain acetaminophen and thus unintentional overdoses can also occur, so it is important to educate adults to not take more than 4 g per day from ALL sources. The toxic dose is approximately 150 mg per kg. A serum acetaminophen level should be drawn 4 hours after ingestion. Nomograms are available to help determine total ingested dose and whether a toxic and/or lethal dose was consumed, with "toxicity" progressing through four phases over a 2-week course.[11] Prompt recognition of the problem and instituting appropriate therapy is necessary to prevent liver failure.

Treatment
- Activated charcoal can help if given within an hour of ingestion. *N*-Acetylcysteine (NAC) is the antidote of choice for acute overdose where the serum level is in the toxic range on the nomogram. It should also be given in paracetamol and *N*-acetyl-*p*-aminophenol (APAP) overdose with elevated liver enzymes and undetectable serum APAP levels as these patients are still in the toxic phase of APAP poisoning. Intravenous NAC should be considered in severe and chronic overdose situations, especially when the AST and ALT are significantly elevated.

Referrals
- Severe acute or chronic overdose may require transfer to an intensive care unit with consultation of a liver transplant team.

Ethylene Glycol and Methanol

Diagnosis
- Both ethylene glycol and methanol are used in industrial and automotive fluids (e.g., antifreeze, brake fluid, etc.). Ingestions can be either intentional or accidental. Typical symptoms are nausea, vomiting, abdominal pain, pulmonary edema, hypotension, central nervous system depression, seizures, ataxia, and coma. Visual disturbances (blurred vision, blindness, optic disc hyperemia) are hallmarks of methanol toxicity. An anion gap metabolic acidosis with osmolar gap is present with both intoxications. Calcium oxalate crystals in the urine are suggestive of ethylene glycol intoxication.

Treatment
- Aggressive supportive care is required for both substances. Stabilization and airway management must be closely monitored. Thiamine, folate, and multivitamin supplements should be used for both. Folinic acid (1 mg per kg up to 50 mg every 4 to 6 hour for 24 hours) should be used in methanol poisoning. Ethanol can be used, either orally or intravenously, to prevent metabolism of the substances to their toxic metabolites. Maintain a blood concentration of 100 to 150 mg per dL. Fomepizole (4-methylpyrazole), an inhibitor of alcohol dehydrogenase, can be used instead, with the advantage of not exacerbating the intoxicated state. Give a loading dose of 15 mg per kg IV followed by 10 mg per kg IV bolus every 12 hours; after 48 hours, the dose is increased to 15 mg per kg IV bolus every 12 hours.[9] In either treatment, the therapy is continued until the concentration of methanol or ethylene glycol falls below 20 mg per dL. Hemodialysis can also be used in cases with significant or refractory acidosis, visual impairment, renal failure, and pulmonary edema. It is continued until the acidosis resolves.

Serotonin Syndrome

Diagnosis
- Serotonin syndrome is a potentially life-threatening condition, and early recognition is of paramount importance. It can result from intentional overdose with a single agent, drug interactions involving multiple agents, or recreational drug use. It often involves SSRIs or monoamine oxidase inhibitors, in overdoses or when they are combined with SNRIs, triptans, cocaine, amphetamines, psychedelics, dopaminergic agents, dextromethorphan, specific herbs, certain antiemetics, and some opioids. Serotonin syndrome is a clinical diagnosis involving a disturbance in three domains: autonomic instability (tachycardia, hyperthermia, elevated BP, diaphoresis, diarrhea, nausea); altered mental status (agitation, anxiety, sedation, delirium, seizures); and somatic effects (tremor, hyperreflexia, dysarthria, ataxia, myoclonic jerks, restlessness). Autonomic instability, in particular high fevers, can cause rhabdomyolysis, metabolic acidosis, renal failure, and disseminated intravascular coagulation.[12]

Treatment
- This condition requires aggressive support, including airway management, circulatory support, and seizure prophylaxis with benzodiazepines. Activated charcoal can be helpful in the setting of medication overdose. Agitation and somatic effects can be managed with benzodiazepines. Treatment with Cyproheptadine, an antiserotonergic agent, at a dose of 4 to 8 mg orally TID has been shown in case reports to reduce symptom severity.[12]
- Prevention of future events involves patient and provider education about drug interactions (including over-the-counter products) and avoidance of polypharmacy. Although symptoms typically resolve within 24 hours of discontinuation, drugs with long half-lives are known to interact for several weeks, requiring more aggressive or ongoing management.

REFERENCES

1. Warner M, Chen LH, Makuc DM, et al. *Drug poisoning deaths in the United States, 1980–2008.* NCHS data brief, no. 81. Hyattsville, MD: National Center for Health Statistics; 2011.
2. Centers for Disease Control and Prevention. Vital signs: overdoses of prescription opioid pain relievers—United States, 1999–2008. *MMWR Morb Mortal Wkly Rep* 2011;60:1487.
3. Frithsen IL, Simpson WM. Recognition and management of acute medication poisoning. *Am Fam Physician* 2010;81(3):316–323.
4. Bronstein AC, Spyker DA, Cantilena LR, et al. 2011 Annual report of the American Association of Poison Control Centers' National Poison Data System: 29th Annual Report. *Clin Toxicol (Phila)* 2012;50:911.
5. Schabelman E, Kuo E. Glucose before thiamine for Wernicke encephalopathy: a literature review. *J Emerg Med* 2012;42:488.
6. Substance Abuse & Mental Health Services Administration. Screening, Brief Intervention, and Referral to Treatment (SBIRT). http://www.samhsa.gov/prevention/SBIRT/index.aspx. Accessed April 17, 2014.
7. Mokhlesi B, Leikin JB, Murray P, et al. Adult toxicology in critical care: part II: specific poisonings. *Chest* 2003;123(3):897–922.
8. Ibrahim M, Maselli DJ, Hasan R, et al. Safety of beta-blockers in the acute management of cocaine-associated chest pain. *Am J Emerg Med* 2013;31(3):613–616.
9. Wermeling DP. A response to the opioid overdose epidemic: naloxone nasal spray. *Drug Deliv Transl Res* 2013;3(1):63–74.
10. Alapat PM, Zimmerman JL. Toxicology in the critical care unit. *Chest* 2008;133:1006–1013.
11. Rowden AK, Norvell J, Eldridge DL, et al. Acetaminophen poisoning. *Clin Lab Med* 2006;26(1):49–65.
12. Frank C. Recognition and treatment of serotonin syndrome. *Can Fam Physician* 2008;54(7):988–992.

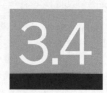

3.4 Epistaxis*

Jennifer L. Bepko, Pamela M. Williams, Stephen Horras, Nicholas Longstreet, Gabriel Briscoe, Chelsey Villaneuva

GENERAL PRINCIPLES

Definition

- Epistaxis is simply defined as **bleeding from the nose.**

Anatomy

- The vascular supply to the nose is through branches of both the internal and the external carotid arteries. Epistaxis is described as **anterior** or **posterior** based on the location of bleeding. About 90% of cases occur in the region of the **Kiesselbach plexus** along the **anterior** septum. The usual location of posterior bleeding is the posterior septum.

Epidemiology

- Epistaxis is the most common bleeding disorder of the head and neck region and is estimated to occur in about 60% of the population.[1] Only 6% to 10% will seek medical attention and account for 0.5% of emergency department visits. Epistaxis occurs in a bimodal distribution with peaks at <10 and >50 years old.[1]

Etiology

- Common causes of both anterior and posterior epistaxis are divided into **local** and **systemic** factors:
- Local:
  - Trauma/nose-picking
  - Irritants/dry nasal mucosa (oxygen administration via nasal cannula, continuous positive-airway pressure machine use)

---

*This chapter represents the views of the authors and does not represent the views of the U.S. Air Force or the Department of Defense.

- Tumors
- Medications (nasal steroids, illicit medications)
- Foreign body
- Allergic rhinitis/sinusitis
- Anatomic deformities
- Vascular malformation or telangiectasia
- Systemic:
  - Coagulopathies
  - Blood dyscrasias (hemophilia, thrombocytopenia)
  - Medications (anticoagulants/anti-inflammatories/herbals/illicit)
  - Vasculitis (Wegener granulomatosis)
  - Liver disease (cirrhosis)

DIAGNOSIS
Clinical Presentation
- Patients present with a **range of symptoms** from visible nasal bleeding to nausea, hemoptysis, and melena. **Assessment of hemodynamic stability** is a critical first step as some patients may require resuscitation prior to taking a history or performing a physical exam.

History
- In the stable patient, key historical questions include **duration** of current episode, **amount** of bleeding, **prior history** and treatment, **chronic medical conditions**, medications (prescription, recreational, nonprescription and herbal), recent illnesses, prior surgeries, known bleeding disorders, and recent trauma.

Physical Examination
- Unstable patients, such as patients with hypotension, tachycardia, or large amount of visible blood loss, should have intravenous catheters and fluids started and cardiopulmonary monitor placed prior to the physical exam. Instruments necessary for adequate visualization include nasal speculum, light source, suction, and irrigator. Determining location of bleeding is critical, and a thorough **inspection of the turbinates and septum** is mandatory.

Laboratory Studies
- Further evaluation and testing are **directed by the history and physical exam.** Patients with significant bleeding, known liver disease, and elderly, family history of bleeding disorder or patients on anticoagulation therapy should be evaluated with a complete blood count and prothrombin/partial thromboplastin time.[2] Patients with recurrent, unexplained epistaxis should be evaluated for a hereditary bleeding disorder; von Willebrand disease is the most commonly discovered bleeding disorder.

Monitoring
- The type and amount of monitoring for patient safety is **based on the resuscitation required,** extent or persistence of bleeding, and comorbid conditions. Patients may require hospital admission for ongoing monitoring and treatment.

TREATMENT
- **Behavioral**, especially in children such as no nose-picking or foreign objects in the nose.
- **Sustained compression** of the nose, with the patient **leaning forward for 5 to 20 minutes,** is the first step to control bleeding.

Medications
- For bleeding unresponsive to compression, the next step is to achieve **vasoconstriction** using either **oxymetazoline 0.05%** or **phenylephrine solution 0.5% to 1%** applied directly to the mucosa or with soaked cotton/gauze. If no response, the next step is to apply **topical anesthetic** such as **lidocaine** or **4% cocaine. Chemical cautery** may also be performed on easily visualized bleeding vessels. **Silver nitrate** sticks should be applied to the area for no more than 5 seconds to prevent destruction of healthy tissue. This procedure has limited efficacy if bleeding is profuse, and can be associated with complications such as septal perforation if applied aggressively, extensively, or on both sides of the septal wall.

Nonoperative

- For persistent anterior bleeding, the next step is **nasal packing.** This may be accomplished with Bayonet forceps and nonadherent gauze or expandable nasal tampons. There are many commercial packing materials available to ease insertion. Packing material is directed in a posterior to anterior manner, and folded in layers until the superior aspect of the cavity is filled. All packing material should be coated with **topical antibiotic** to help reduce the risk of infections such as toxin-producing Group A *Staphylococcus.* Other types of packing available include 3% bismuth tribromophenate (Xeroform), oxidized cellulose (Surgicell), and absorbable gelatin foam (Gelfoam). Packing may be left in **place for 3 to 5 days** for adequate clot formation, and moistened with normal saline frequently while in place and prior to removal.

Referrals

- All **posterior bleeding** and persistent anterior bleeding unresponsive to the above interventions should be referred for specialty care. Further options include posterior packing and/or vascular intervention (embolization and vessel ligation). Both methods have a high success rate between 75% and 100%.[3,5]

Patient Education

- Patients should be advised to return for care with any of the following: persistent bleeding, fever, hematemesis/vomiting, dizziness, dyspnea, or any concerns. Patients should also be educated on **steps to help prevent** future **occurrences:** keeping the mucosa moist with petrolatum jelly or nasal saline, avoid forceful nose blowing, no nose-picking, environmental changes (increase humidity of home/work, lower heat in sleeping areas), and avoidance of heavy lifting or straining.

Complications

- Complications include **infection** (localized or spread into surrounding tissues), **necrosis** of septum, **septal hematoma, abscess** formation, or **septal perforation.** Embolization incurs a 6% risk of complications, including cerebrovascular accident.[3]

Follow-Up

- Follow-up is based on the interventions performed. **Packing removal** should occur **3 to 5 days after placement.** Consideration should also be given to repeating any abnormal lab work and following anticoagulation status for patients on warfarin.

Special Considerations

- **Posterior bleeding:** Posterior bleeding that does not respond to anterior nasal cavity packing occurs with 9% of cases is considered an **otolaryngologic emergency,** and patients are at risk for significant complications.[5] Posterior packing requires special training, and is generally performed by an otolaryngologist. Foley bulb catheters or double balloon catheters are placed in combination with gauze packs to tamponade the posterior pharynx. Patients receiving posterior packing require hospitalization observation.

REFERENCES

1. Kucik CJ, Clenny T. Management of epistaxis. *Am Fam Physician* 2005;71:305–311.
2. Tjio E, Creagh D, Smith I. A four point questionnaire: aiding discrimination with coagulation screening in epistaxis. *Emerg Med J* 2013;30(5):428.
3. Barnes M, Spielmann P, White P. Epistaxis: a contemporary evidence based approach. *Otolaryngol Clin North Am* 2012;45:1005–1017.
4. Morgan D, Kellerman R. Epistaxis: evaluation and treatment. *Primary Care Clin Office Pract* 2014;41:63–73.
5. Spielmann R, Barnes M, White P. Controversies in the specialist management of adult epistaxis: an evidence-based review. *Clin Otolaryngol* 2012;37:382–389.

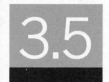

Syncope

Carole V. Nistler

GENERAL PRINCIPLES

Syncope is the transient loss of consciousness accompanied by loss of postural tone, with rapid onset and spontaneous recovery caused by a brief and abrupt cessation of global cerebral blood flow.[1] It should be distinguished from other conditions that cause altered consciousness, such as seizure, transient ischemic attack (TIA), stroke, vertigo, amnesia, concussion, migraine, hypoglycemia, drug or alcohol intoxication, or narcolepsy. These conditions either are associated with other distinctive symptoms or do not cause an abrupt loss of consciousness followed by spontaneous recovery.

Syncope is a symptom of one or more underlying causes. The most common cause of syncope is neurocardiogenic,[2] but cardiac causes, including structural heart disease and cardiac arrhythmias, are associated with up to three times the risk of death compared with other causes of syncope.[1]

The evaluation of syncope in the emergency department or other outpatient setting is directed at identifying or ruling out life-threatening causes, determining which patients require emergent hospital admission and which patients need further nonemergent evaluation.[3] Clinical decision rules, such as the San Francisco Syncope Rule, may help reinforce the decision to admit, but have not yet been shown sensitive enough to reduce the number of patients requiring admission.[4,5]

Up to 50% of patients presenting to the emergency room with syncope have no identifiable cause following their initial evaluation.[5] Similar to the evaluation of chest pain, the goal of the initial evaluation of syncope is not to determine a specific cause, but rather to stratify risk.[3]

CAUSES OF SYNCOPE

Neurocardiogenic syncope, which is also called reflex- or neurally-mediated syncope, is caused by abnormal cardiovascular reflexes that disrupt or reverse the normal compensatory autonomic response to standing or any other situation that reduces venous return to the heart.[6] Parasympathetic activity causes vasodilatation and bradycardia and overrides the normal increase in sympathetic output of the heart and blood vessels, resulting in peripheral blood pooling and right-sided heart underfilling. **Vasovagal attacks** are caused by stimuli such as emotional distress, the sight of blood, venipuncture, or prolonged standing. **Situational syncope** refers to vagal stimulation due to the Valsalva maneuver associated with coughing, sneezing, swallowing, micturition, or defecation. **Carotid sinus syncope** is caused by maneuvers that increase carotid sinus pressure such as head-turning, shaving, or wearing a tight collar. It is more common in the elderly and in men.[7]

Orthostatic syncope occurs because of a failure of the autonomic nervous system to respond appropriately to a decrease in blood pressure or to volume depletion. Causes of volume depletion include excessive sweating, vomiting or diarrhea, inadequate intake, or diuretic therapy. Autonomic dysfunction may be caused by medications, for example, β-blockers or vasodilators, chronic alcohol use, Parkinson disease, diabetes mellitus, loss of skeletal muscle tone in the elderly, and spinal cord injuries.[7]

Structural cardiac causes[2,7] include valvular heart disease, such as severe aortic or mitral stenosis, myocardial infarction or ischemia, nonischemic dilated cardiomyopathy, hypertrophic cardiomyopathy, arrhythmogenic right ventricular dysplasia/cardiomyopathy, cardiac masses such as atrial myxoma, pericardial disease, congenital anomalies of coronary arteries, and prosthetic valve dysfunction.

Cardiovascular[7] causes include pulmonary embolus, pulmonary hypertension, and acute aortic dissection.

Arrhythmogenic causes[7] of syncope may cause **bradycardia** (sinus node dysfunction, atrioventricular system disease, implanted device malfunction) or **tachycardia** (atrial fibrillation, Wolff–Parkinson–White syndrome, idiopathic ventricular tachycardia, and inherited cardiac ion channel abnormalities such as Long QT or Brugada syndrome, which predispose patients to polymorphic ventricular tachycardia). Syncope due to ventricular tachyarrhythmias is associated with increased mortality and may be an ominous sign.[2] Arrhythmogenic causes should be suspected if syncope occurs with preceding palpitations, if there are electrocardiogram (ECG) abnormalities, or if there is evidence of structural heart disease on physical exam or a family history of sudden cardiac death.[8]

Cerebrovascular disease can rarely cause syncope.[9] Vertebrobasilar artery disease is more likely to cause dizziness or drop attacks (falls without loss of consciousness) and should be associated with brain stem or focal neurologic deficits, including vertigo, dysarthria, diplopia, or ataxia. Seizures can cause loss of consciousness, and seizure-like movements can be seen following a syncopal episode due to cerebral hypoperfusion. These two conditions can be difficult to distinguish and may require both neurologic and cardiovascular evaluation.[1]

Psychogenic pseudosyncope is also called pseudoseizure because the presentation may mimic both conditions but episodes of pseudosyncope typically occur multiple times per day, which is unlikely in the case of true syncope,[7] and are associated with an underlying psychiatric disorder.

INITIAL EVALUATION

The initial evaluation of syncope should include a **history and physical examination** directed at ruling out other causes of altered consciousness not related to syncope (seizure, TIA, stroke, vertigo, migraine, alcohol intoxication, etc.) and looking for the above-listed causes of syncope. It should also include a **12-lead ECG**.[3]

The **history** should include (a) a description of the event by the patient; (b) a description of the event by any witnesses, if available; (c) any relationship of the event to emotional distress, venipuncture, immediate or prolonged standing, exercise, cough, sneeze, swallowing, micturition, defecation, head-turning, shaving, increased neck pressure, fluid loss, inadequate intake, vomiting, diarrhea, alcohol or drug use, head injury, or other trauma; (d) any preceding symptoms such as dizziness, nausea, abdominal pain, shortness of breath, diaphoresis, chest pain, heart palpitations, blurred or double vision, visual field changes, slurred speech, limb weakness, migraine-associated auras, headache, seizure-related auras, or tonic–clonic movements; and (e) any residual symptoms such as a postictal states associated with seizures, neurologic deficits associated with cerebrovascular events or fatigue, and generalized weakness following neurocardiogenic syncope.[1–3]

Medications, which may cause syncope, especially if they have been added recently, include nitrates, diuretics, vasodilators, α-adrenergic and β-blockers, antipsychotic medications, tricyclic antidepressants, antibiotics that cause QT prolongation including macrolides and quinolones, and Class 1A (e.g., procainamide, quinidine) and Class 1C (e.g. encainide, flecanide) antiarrhythmics, which have proarrhythmic properties.[2,3]

Other important elements of the history are a **past medical history** of myocardial infarction/ischemia, especially with left ventricular dysfunction, congenital heart disease, and valvular heart disease, congestive heart failure, previous cardiac arrhythmia and pacemaker or defibrillator placement. A **family history** of sudden cardiac death raises the possibility of congenital conduction abnormalities such as long QT or Brugada syndrome.[2,3]

The **physical examination** should include (a) **orthostatic blood pressure measurements** to look for evidence of orthostatic hypotension, defined as a decrease in systolic blood pressure with standing of 20 mmHg or greater[3]; (b) **differences in blood pressure or pulse between right and left arms**, which can suggest subclavian steal syndrome or aortic dissection; (c) a **cardiovascular examination** looking for carotid bruits, the murmurs of aortic stenosis, mitral stenosis or hypertrophic cardiomyopathy, signs of left ventricular dysfunction, or irregular heart rhythms. For patients suspected of carotid sinus syncope, **carotid sinus massage** can be attempted for 5 seconds in a supine patient, with cardiac monitoring and intravenous access, to detect a cardiac pause of 3 seconds or a 50-mmHg decrease in systolic blood pressure and symptoms of syncope. It should not be attempted in patients with a carotid bruit or ventricular arrhythmia, or in those who have had a myocardial infarction, TIA, or stroke within the preceding 3 months.[10]

Other relevant parts of the physical exam are (d) the **oral examination** looking for tongue-biting, which might suggest seizures; (e) the **abdominal examination** looking for evidence of gastrointestinal bleeding; and (f) the **neurologic examination** looking for focal neurologic findings.[2,3]

A **12-lead ECG** provides an assessment of cardiac rhythm, atrioventricular conduction, and previous ischemic events.[2,8] Bradycardia, prolonged PR segment, or bundle branch block may signal sick sinus syndrome or heart block. Delta waves may suggest Wolff Parkinson–White syndrome. A prolonged QT segment (QTc >450 ms) may suggest long QT syndrome. ST segment elevation in leads V1 and V2 may suggest Brugada syndrome. A previous history of ischemic heart disease or evidence of such on ECG coupled with ventricular ectopy suggests arrhythmogenic causes of syncope.

FURTHER TESTING

If the initial evaluation suggests the patient is at low risk of serious outcomes and therefore does not require hospital admission, and the initial evaluation has not revealed the cause of syncope, then the goal of further evaluation becomes identification of underlying causes of syncope in order to prevent recurrences.[2] Recurrences are associated with physical injuries and lower quality of life due to fear of dying and difficulty returning to activities such as driving or employment.[1] **Echocardiography** can identify valvular heart disease, pulmonary hypertension, right ventricular hypertrophy, hypertrophic cardiomyopathy, or anomalous coronary arteries.

Exercise testing may be indicated if the event was exercise-related.

ECG monitoring is indicated if the initial evaluation suggests any underlying cardiac cause but may also be necessary in any case of unexplained syncope because an undetected arrhythmogenic cause could be life-threatening. The type and duration of ECG monitoring depend on the frequency of symptoms. **Holter monitoring** can record 24 to 48 hours of ECG data and may be used if syncope is occurring daily. **Cardiac event monitors** depend on patient triggering to record 1 to 4 minutes of ECG data before the trigger and 30 to 60 seconds of data after the trigger. They can be used for 30 to 60 days, but their dependence on patient triggering complicates interpretation.

Implantable loop recorders (ILRs) are inserted subcutaneously and record ECG data for up to 14 months. They combine patient-activated recordings of cardiac rhythm prompted by symptoms as well as device-triggered recordings of brady- and tachy-arrhythmias. Early use of ILRs in the evaluation of syncope has led to earlier identification and treatment of arrhythmogenic causes of syncope and to reduction of recurrent episodes.[11]

Tilt-table testing has been used to confirm neurocardiogenic syncope, but its usefulness in most cases is limited. Patients with normal initial evaluations are still most likely to have neurocardiogenic syncope whether their tilt-table test is positive or not. In patients at risk for serious injury due to recurrent syncope, further investigation of arrhythmogenic causes via ECG monitoring is warranted regardless of tilt-table results.[2]

Electrophysiologic testing is of low yield without a history of or evidence of heart disease on initial evaluation. It is indicated in patients with ischemic heart disease to look for inducible ventricular tachycardia.[2]

REFERENCES

1. Rosanio S, Schwarz ER, Ware DL, et al. Syncope in adults: systematic review and proposal of a diagnostic and therapeutic algorithm. *Int J Cardiol* 2013;162(3):149–157.
2. Strickberger SA, Benson DW, Biaggioni I, et al. AHA/ACCF scientific statement on the evaluation of syncope. *Circulation* 2006;113(2):316–327.
3. Huff JS, Decker WW, Quinn JV, et al. American College of Emergency Physicians. Clnical policy: critical issues in the evaluation and management of adult patients presenting to the emergency department with syncope. *Ann Emerg Med* 2007;49:431–444.
4. Saccilotto RT, Nickel CH, Bucher HC, et al. San Francisco Syncope Rule to predict short-term serious outcomes: a systematic review. *CMAJ* 2011;183(15):E1116–E1126.
5. Kessler C, Tristano JM, De Lorenzo R. The emergency department approach to syncope: evidence-based guidelines and prediction rules. *Emerg Med Clin North Am* 2010;28(3):487–500.
6. Kapoor W. Syncope. *N Engl J Med* 2000;343:1856–1862.
7. Puppala VK, Dickinson O, Benditt DG. Syncope: classification and risk stratification. *J Cardiol* 2014;63(3):171–177.
8. Ruwald MH, Zareba W. ECG monitoring in syncope. *Prog Cardiovasc Dis* 2013;56(2):203–210.
9. Arthur W, Kaye GC. The pathophysiology of common causes of syncope. *Postgrad Med J* 2000;76:750–753.
10. Puggioni E, Guiducci V, Brignote M, et al. Results and complications of the carotid sinus massage performed according to the method of symptoms. *Am J Cardiol* 2002;89:599–601.
11. Hong P, Sulke N. Implantable diagnostic monitors in the early assessment of syncope and collapse. *Prog Cardiovasc Dis* 2013;55(4):410–417.

3.6 Cerebral Concussions

Kim Edward LeBlanc

GENERAL PRINCIPLES

Definition

As defined by the Zurich Consensus Statement in 2012:[1]

Concussion is a brain injury defined as a complex pathophysiological process affecting the brain, induced by biomechanical forces. Several common features that incorporate clinical, pathologic, and biomechanical injury constructs may be utilized in defining the nature of a concussive head injury including:

1. Concussion may be caused by a direct blow to the head, face, neck, or elsewhere on the body with an "impulsive" force transmitted to the head.
2. Concussion typically results in the rapid onset of short-lived impairment of neurological function that resolves spontaneously. However, in some cases, symptoms and signs may evolve over a number of minutes to hours.
3. Concussion may result in neuropathological changes, but the acute clinical symptoms largely reflect a functional disturbance rather than a structural injury and, as such, no abnormality is seen on standard structural neuroimaging studies.
4. Concussion results in a graded set of clinical symptoms that may or may not involve loss of consciousness. Resolution of the clinical and cognitive symptoms typically follows a sequential course. However, it is important to note that in some cases symptoms may be prolonged.

Epidemiology

Approximately 1.7 million people sustain a traumatic brain injury in the United States every year.[2] The majority of these are mild and may occur from simple falls, automobile accidents, as well as in both competitive and recreational sports.

Classification

There is no classification schema as the older grading scales have been abandoned.

DIAGNOSIS

History and Physical

Ascertain the details of the fall or sudden trauma to the head or body, usually of low velocity, resulting in onset of clinical symptoms. Symptoms may include lightheadedness, gait or balance disturbances, dizziness, headache, nausea, or feeling like in a fog.

Physical Examination

A complete neurological examination (including gait and balance testing), mental status examination, and testing of cognitive functioning should be performed and repeated as clinically indicated. You should be specifically looking for any alteration of consciousness, inability to focus, amnesia, slowed reaction time, incoordination, slurred speech, delayed responses, disorientation, and memory deficits.

Seizures may have occurred and, although frightening to bystanders, are usually benign and seldom indicative of structural intracranial pathology.[1,3]

Imaging

The Canadian CT Head Rule recommends that a head CT is required only for patients with minor head injuries (defined as witnessed loss of consciousness, definite amnesia, or witnessed disorientation in a patients with a Glasgow Coma Scale [GCS] score of 13 to 15) with one of the following:
- GCS <15 at 2 hours postinjury
- Suspected open or depressed skull fracture
- Any sign of basilar skull fracture (hemotympanum, raccoon eyes, battle's sign, CSF oto-/rhinorrhea)
- ≥2 episodes of vomiting

- Age ≥65
- Retrograde amnesia to the event ≥30 minutes or involves a "dangerous mechanism" (pedestrian struck by motor vehicle, occupant ejected from motor vehicle, or fall from >3 feet or >5 stairs.)

Neuropsychological (NP) Testing

This has been shown to have clinical value and provides significant information helpful in the management of a concussed individual, particularly adults. However, although it is a useful instrument, NP testing should not be relied upon solely to make management decisions. This would be useful particularly in patients who have a history of multiple or frequent concussions, and/or prolonged symptoms.[1,4] There are several such instruments, including ImPACT, a computerized neurocognitive assessment useful in assisting medical professionals in determining an athlete's ability to return to play (RTP). ImPACT is widely used in college and professional sports.[5]

Sport Concussion Assessment Tool—3rd Edition

The SCAT3 is a standardized tool useful in the evaluation of a concussed athlete and may be used for athletes over the age of 13 years.[6] There is also a version for those 5 to 12 years of age, the Child-SCAT3.[7]

Differential Diagnosis

Heat illness, migraine headache, muscle contraction headache, sickle-cell crisis related to exertion (particularly in hot, humid conditions or at altitude), and acute anxiety can be diagnosed.

TREATMENT
Modifiers

Certain factors may signal a more prolonged course and suggest taking a more conservative approach, including the frequency, number, and severity of previous concussions; loss of consciousness >1 minute; seizure activity; age under 18 years; high-risk sports; concussions occurring from lesser force than the previous ones (e.g., simply tapping someone's helmet in a huddle); duration of symptoms >10 days; dangerous style of play; requirement of medications; and history of recent previous concussion.

Cognitive and Physical Rest

Important in the management of concussion is allowing time for the brain to recover.[1,8] This should begin immediately following the concussive event and continue with slow return to activity over 7-day period. This includes avoiding reading, watching television, video games, and even school work. When the student returns to school, adjustments should be made, such as giving frequent breaks, reducing brightness at computer screens, allowing more quiet time, and allowing extra time to complete academic tasks. A useful reference created by the CDC may be found at http://www.cdc.gov/concussion/pdf/TBI_Returning_to_School-a.pdf.

Return to Play

Recent consensus[1] recommends a gradual RTP. Unlike in the past, a player who has suffered a concussion is never recommended to RTP on the day of the injury.

Returning to competitive or recreational sport activity requires medical clearance and full restoration of both cognitive and functional abilities. A phased return to activity can start when the patient is asymptomatic, has no academic restrictions, and has been cleared by a healthcare provider. Each phase should occur over a 24-hour period with progress to the next level if the patient remains asymptomatic: (a) no activity, (b) light aerobic exercise, (c) sport-specific exercise, (d) noncontact training drills, (e) full-contact practice and (f) RTP. If symptoms recur during any phase, the player should return to the previous asymptomatic phase and try to progress again only after a further 24-hour period of rest.

In an individual with repeated concussions, management should be similar, but a more conservative approach to return to activity is warranted.

Medications

Any medications or substances (e.g., alcohol, drugs) affecting the nervous system should be avoided. Acetaminophen and over-the-counter nonsteroidal anti-inflammatory drugs may be considered as they are fairly effective and safe.

Parental Education

The concussed individual should remain in the presence of a responsible adult for 6 to 8 hours, following the event to monitor for any signs of neurological deterioration.

In the past, sleeping was prohibited, which obviously interferes with cognitive and physical rest. However, observations should be made every few hours for signs of deterioration, such as labored breathing, increasing pulse, worsening headache, focal signs, balance problems, visual disturbance, or pupillary changes.

Prevention

Although mouth guards have been shown to prevent orofacial and dental injuries, there is no good evidence demonstrating that protective equipment, including helmets, will prevent concussions.[1] Athletes, parents, and coaches should be well informed concerning the significance of concussions and promote proper sporting techniques and avoidance of risky and/or hazardous play.

Recovery

The vast majority of those affected (80% to 90%) recover within a 7- to 10-day period of time. Children and adolescents may take longer to reach complete resolution.[1] Those symptomatic concussions falling outside of this 10-day period should be managed in a multidisciplinary fashion by clinicians with knowledge and experience in this area.

REFERENCES

1. McCrory P, Meeuwisse WH, Aubry M, et al. Consensus statement on concussion in sport: the 4th International Conference on Concussion in Sport held in Zurich, November 2012. *Br J Sports Med* 2013;47:250–258.
2. Centers for Disease Control and Prevention. Injury Prevention & Control: Traumatic Brain Injury. http://www.cdc.gov/TraumaticBrainInjury/index.html. Accessed February 24, 2014.
3. Lee ST, Lui TN. Early seizures after mild closed head injury. *J Neurosurg* 1992;76:435.
4. Echemendia R, Iverson GL, McCrea M, et al. Advances in neuropsychological assessment of sport-related concussion. *Br J Sports Med* 2013;47:294–298.
5. The Impact Test. http://www.impacttest.com. Accessed May 13, 2014.
6. Sport Concussion Assessment Tool—3rd edition. http://bjsm.bmj.com/content/47/5/259. Accessed May 13, 2014.
7. Child—Sport Concussion Assessment Tool—3rd edition. http://bjsm.bmj.com/content/47/5/263. Accessed May 13, 2014.
8. Schneider KJ, Iverson GL, Emery CA, et al. The effects of rest and treatment following sport-related concussion: a systematic review of the literature. *Br J Sports Med* 2013;47:304–307.
9. Stiell IG, Wells GA, Vandemheen K, et al. The Canadian Head CT Rule for patients with minor head injury. *Lancet* 2001;357:1391–1396.

3.7 Fractures Requiring Special Consideration

Alexei DeCastro, Brett Wilhoit

FRACTURE BASICS
Classification of Fractures

It is important to classify fractures accurately in order to properly communicate with consultants. They are described by fracture location, type, and amount of the displacement. Fracture location is usually related to anatomical landmarks or is described as involving the proximal, middle, or distal thirds of long bones. Closed (simple) fractures have no skin disruption that communicates with the bone, whereas open (compound) fractures do disrupt the skin. Complicated fractures are those with associated soft-tissue injuries. Avulsion fractures occur when a tendon or ligament pulls away from the bone with an attached fragment. Alignment refers to the relationship of the longitudinal axis to the fracture fragments. Abnormal alignment is described by degrees of angulation. Position describes the relationship of the fragments to their normal location. Displacement describes the abnormal position of the fracture fragments. Impacted fracture fragments are pushed together, whereas distracted fracture fragments are pulled apart. Direction of fracture lines is indicated by the terms *transverse, oblique, comminuted,* and *spiral.* Transverse fracture lines are perpendicular to the axis of the bone, and oblique fracture lines cross the axis of the bone at an angle. Comminuted fractures have more than two fragments. Spiral fractures result from a torsional force.

Clinical Diagnosis of Fracture

The diagnosis of fracture should be considered any time there is a history of significant acute or chronic injury to a bone, resulting in the complaint of pain. Signs of fractures include localized pain, tenderness, ecchymosis, or edema. Gross deformity, decreased function, abnormal mobility, and crepitus may also be present. Do not dismiss the possibility of a fracture because it cannot be immediately visualized on a radiograph. A careful examination for associated injuries to viscera, tendons, nerves, and blood vessels should always be included. Always suspect domestic violence if the mechanism of injury does fit the clinical presentation.

Imaging Techniques

Most fractures can be adequately visualized on plain radiographs, but some fractures require special imaging techniques. Radionuclide bone scanning is a very sensitive but nonspecific tool in the evaluation of fractures. Ultrasound is a newer tool for point-of-care testing in diagnosing fractures.[1] Computed tomography (CT) and magnetic resonance imaging (MRI) are used to evaluate suspected fractures in bones that are frequently obscured by overlying structures. CT scanning is helpful particularly in confirming fractures of the pelvic and facial bones. MRI is now considered the most sensitive modality used to diagnose occult fractures or injuries to cartilage, ligaments, and tendons.

Treatment Generalities
Stability

Stable fractures are those that maintain their position and alignment. Unstable fractures are those that tend to displace and require early immobilization. If there is any doubt about the stability of a particular fracture, it should be treated as unstable until definitive diagnosis is obtained.

Associated injuries must also be considered in the evaluation of any fracture. A detailed examination for damage to nearby viscera, nerves, blood vessels, tendons, and overlying skin must be performed. The management of traumatized viscera may take precedence over fracture management. Neurovascular injuries should be recognized early and referred for repair. Most tendon ruptures also require surgical treatment. Open fractures require special consideration because even a small skin defect that communicates with the fracture greatly increases the patient's chances of developing osteomyelitis. These wounds should generally be debrided in the operating room and the patients given prophylactic antibiotics.

Reduction is the procedure that returns displaced fracture fragments to acceptable position and alignment. What constitutes acceptable position and alignment varies with the fracture location and type, patient age, and the functional demands placed on the bone. A neurovascular examination should always be repeated after reduction.

Immobilization of fractures is initially achieved by splinting to provide pain relief and to prevent further displacement, associated injuries, and risk of fat emboli. Definitive immobilization can be achieved through internal or external fixation. Internal fixation requires a surgical procedure. External fixation is provided by splinting or casting. Choosing the correct type and length of immobilization is critical for optimal healing. Inadequate immobilization can result in displacement, delayed union, or nonunion of fracture fragments. Prolonged or improper immobilization can result in stiffness and functional impairment. Consultation should be obtained if there is doubt about the appropriate type and length of immobilization.

SKULL FRACTURES
General Principles
Definition

Fracture to any of the eight cranial bones: parietal, temporal, occipital, frontal, sphenoid, and ethmoid bones. Skull fractures are categorized by location (basilar vs. the skull convexity), pattern (linear, depressed, or comminuted), and whether they are open or closed. Complicated skull fractures are those that are open or depressed, those that involve a sinus, and those that cause intracranial air.

Diagnosis
Physical Examination

Basilar skull fractures are fractures of the base of the skull and may be manifested by a cerebrospinal otorrhea or rhinorrhea, mastoid ecchymosis (Battle sign), periorbital ecchymosis (raccoon eyes), hemotympanum, vertigo, hearing deficit, and seventh nerve palsy. Nasal discharge that is positive for glucose indicates a basilar skull fracture with cerebrospinal fluid (CSF) leak. A CSF leak can create a "ring sign" when bloody fluid is placed on a tissue or filter paper. If there is CSF mixed with the blood, it will move by capillary action further away from the center than the blood creating a halo or the "ring sign." Intracranial injury should always be suspected, and a careful assessment of the patient's neurologic status should be performed, including the use of the Glasgow Coma Scale.

Imaging

Skull radiographs should be obtained, but if they are negative and a fracture is strongly suspected, a CT scan should be obtained immediately. CT scan should also be obtained if the patient exhibits altered mental status, focal neurologic deficits, signs of a basilar skull fracture, seizures, or a palpable depression of the skull.

Treatment

Scalp lacerations may hemorrhage and should be controlled as rapidly as possible, as the rich blood supply to the scalp can result in massive blood loss. Direct pressure can be used, as well as lidocaine with epinephrine infiltrated locally. Vessels can be clamped or ligated if necessary. Open fractures should be carefully cleaned and repaired. Gentle wound exploration should be performed, with care taken not to drive bone fragments into the brain. Use of prophylactic antibiotics following an open skull fracture is controversial. In the case of a basilar skull fracture with a CSF leak, prophylactic antibiotics have not been shown to prevent meningitis and therefore are not indicated.[2] Fractures depressed beyond the thickness of the skull require operative repair. Closure of an open fracture should be undertaken only in consult with a neurosurgeon if a CT scan has not been obtained. Fractures that cross the middle meningeal artery or a major venous sinus may require neurosurgery expertise. Occipital fractures have a higher rate of subarachnoid hemorrhage, and neurosurgery should be involved. Patients with a basilar skull fractures or altered mental status should be hospitalized. Periorbital and mastoid ecchymosis are often absent initially but may develop over the course of a few hours. Most CSF leaks resolve within a week. Complications from skull fractures include intracranial injury, infections, and seizures.

MAXILLOFACIAL FRACTURES
General Principles

- **Anatomy:** Facial bones include the zygoma, maxilla, lacrimal bone, nasal bone, mandible, sphenoid, frontal, ethmoid, and palatine. Cranial nerves II, III, and VI, and branches of V course through the orbital foramina and may be compromised in orbit fractures.

Diagnosis
History and Physical Examination

Ask the patient whether he or she is having symptoms of abnormal vision, facial numbness, or abnormal alignment of the teeth. Pain on eye movement suggests injury to the orbit or globe. Inspection should evaluate facial alignment and cranial nerve VII function, which may present with unilateral facial weakness. Palpate the face looking for any tenderness or crepitus.

Imaging

Plain films or CT scan may be helpful, but should only be completed after management of head, chest, and abdominal trauma.

Treatment

- **Airway:** Always secure the airway first with maneuvers such as chin lift, jaw thrust, and oropharyngeal suctioning. With severe mandible fractures, the tongue may obstruct the airway and may need to be pulled forward. If the C-spine has been cleared, the patient with tongue obstruction from a flail mandible may need to sit upright and lean forward in order to breathe. Be careful not to get distracted from the routine trauma protocol by gross facial injuries. Avoid nasotracheal intubation as an injured cribriform plate may penetrate into the brain. Rapid sequence intubation (involving anesthesia) is risky in facial trauma because bag-valve mask may be insufficient if intubation fails, so awake intubation may be necessary. You should be prepared for cricothyroidotomy should intubation fail.
- **Nasal fractures:** In all cases involving nasal trauma, inspect the septum for a hematoma. If present, anesthetize with a topical anesthetic, incise the inferior portion of the hematoma and allow it to drain, then pack the nose with Vaseline gauze to prevent reaccumulation of blood. Nasal films are optional; however, a referral to an ear, nose, and throat (ENT) specialist is needed only if there is significant deformity or difficulty breathing through the nose requiring reduction of the nasal fracture. The best time for reduction may be within the first 3 hours immediately following injury. If not,

waiting 7 days to allow reduction of edema and swelling is preferable. If reduction is not possible within the first 7 to 10 days, then the fracture starts to heal, making reduction difficult.[3]

- **Orbital fractures:** Blowout fractures typically occur after blunt trauma to the eye or eyelids that is transferred to the weak floor of the orbit. This allows for the contents of the orbit to herniate through the floor, which may cause limitations in eye motion. Damage to the infraorbital nerve may cause anesthesia of the upper lip, nasal mucosa at the vestibule, lower eyelid, and maxillary teeth. If subcutaneous emphysema is found, suspect a sinus or facial fracture and consider starting antibiotics appropriate to sinus pathogens. Patients should avoid blowing their nose to prevent accumulation of subcutaneous air. An orbital series, which includes a Waters view, is generally no longer used; however, a CT evaluation is generally diagnostic for orbital fractures, and if positive, ENT referral should be made. Examine pupils for reactivity and whether the pupils line up in the horizontal plane. A teardrop-shaped pupil indicates a penetrated globe. Extraocular motions should be evaluated for restriction or pain. Visual acuity should be assessed using the Snellen chart, finger counting, and light perception. The swinging flashlight test may indicate optic nerve or retinal injury if the pupil initially dilates rather than constricts. If traumatic optic neuropathy is suspected, emergency ophthalmic consultation should be made in an effort to prevent blindness. Subconjunctival hemorrhage is often present with periorbital fractures. Widening of the distance between the medial canthi or pupils portends serious orbital injury.
- **Naso-ethmoidal-orbital fractures (NEO):** Suspect NEO injuries in those with trauma to the bridge of the nose or medial orbital wall. These fractures may involve lacrimal disruption and dural tears. A maxillofacial or ENT surgeon should be consulted if physical exam or CT scan suggests an NEO injury.
- **Zygomatic fractures:** Lateral subconjunctival hemorrhage often accompanies zygomatic fractures. Arch fractures are common and may be seen on arch view radiographs; these can be managed on an outpatient basis. Tripod fractures involve the infraorbital rim, diastasis of the zygomatic-frontal suture, and disruption of the zygomatic–temporal junction and are more serious. The eye may tilt when the fragment is displaced inferiorly. Tripod fractures can be seen on Waters view, and require admission for open reduction and internal fixation.
- **Mandibular fractures:** Fractures are often multiple because of the ring shape of the mandible. Malocclusion and pain on jaw movement indicate fracture. Lower lip and lower dental anesthesia occurs with mandibular fractures. Intraoral lacerations should be examined to determine whether the fracture is open or closed. Intravenous antibiotics should be started with open fractures, whereas closed fractures may be managed on an outpatient basis after consultation with an oral surgeon. If the patient has normal occlusion and a negative tongue-blade test, panoramic radiographs may be unnecessary. The tongue-blade test consists of having the patient bite down forcefully on a tongue blade. The physician then twists the tongue blade in an attempt to break the blade. Patients with an intact mandible will break the blade, whereas patients with a broken jaw will reflexively open their mouth.[4]
- **Maxillary fractures:** Fractures of the maxilla require high impact and are usually associated with multisystem trauma. Facial stability can be assessed by rocking the maxillary arch and simultaneously feeling the central face for movement with the opposite hand. Fractures of the midface may require manual reduction of the face to stem bleeding; the hard palate can be grasped at the maxillary arch and fragments realigned.

Special Circumstances

- **Penetrating facial trauma:** Gunshot wounds to the face may injure the oral cavity, and intravenous antibiotics should be given against oral flora.
- **Children:** Suspect nonaccidental trauma in cases of pediatric maxillofacial injury. Young children have a higher incidence of frontal bone injury due to its prominence, whereas adolescents have more midface fractures as their sinuses form. Cricothyroidotomy should be avoided in children younger than 12 as they are at higher risk for subglottic stenosis and tracheomalacia. Early fracture follow-up is important in all pediatric facial fractures as a child's facial skeleton heals quickly and can make delayed reduction difficult.

NECK FRACTURES

Cervical spine immobilization should always be performed when neck injury is suspected. Clinical exam of the cervical spine should involve palpation of the vertebrae and assessment of range of motion (ROM). In order to clear the C-spine, use validated clinical criteria such as the Canadian C-Spine Rule.[5] Obtain C-spine films if any the following are present: age >65 years, dangerous mechanism (fall from elevation ≥3 feet/5 stairs, axial load to head, MVC high speed [>100 km per hour], rollover, ejection, motorized recreational vehicles, bicycle struck, or collision), or parasthesia in extremities. If the patient is at low risk (simple rear-end MVC, sitting position in ED, ambulatory at any time, delayed onset of neck pain, and absence of midline C-spine tenderness), then assess clinically with ROM testing. If the patient does not fit these low risks or patient unable to rotate neck 45 degrees, then radiographs are mandatory. Views should include anteroposterior (AP), odontoid, and a lateral cervical radiograph that adequately demonstrates all seven cervical vertebra. To interpret films comfortably, remember the normal curves of the cervical spine (Figure 3.7-1): anterior and posterior vertebral body lines should form a smooth, continuous, lordotic curve, and the posterior cervical line should be a straight line connecting the bases of C1, C2, and C3. If the bases miss the line by more than 2 mm in either direction, suspect a pathologic process. Careful observation of these lines, along with the odontoid, can help the clinician rule out cervical fractures. If there is any doubt about the possibility of a significant cervical injury after viewing the cervical films, proceed with neurosurgical consultation while maintaining immobilization.

THORACOLUMBAR FRACTURES

Isolated, stable fractures that do not typically involve neurologic deficits include transverse process fractures, spinous process fractures, and pars interarticularis fractures. More serious fractures include wedge compression fractures, Chance fractures (involves the spinous process, lamina, transverse process, pedicles, and vertebral body), burst fractures, flexion distraction injuries (loss of height in the anterior portion of the vertebra with increased interspinous spaces posteriorly), and translational injuries (translation of vertebral segment on subsequent segments). Plain radiographs are generally adequate to make the diagnosis, although a CT scan may be required. Patients found to have unstable acute spine

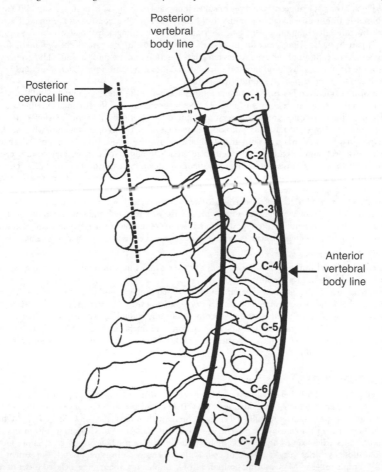

Figure 3.7-1. Normal landmarks of the cervical spine.

fractures or a fracture with a spondylolisthesis, generally require hospital admission for further evaluation, treatment, and control of pain. They will benefit from bed rest (for at least 24 hours, longer in more significant fractures), analgesics (often liberal use of narcotics is necessary to control pain), and careful and serial neurologic reassessment. In the presence of neurologic deficit, emergent neurosurgery or orthopedic consultation is necessary.

THORACIC CAGE

- **Rib fractures:** Fractures of the first or second ribs generally result from serious trauma, and attention should be directed to injury to the great vessels, cervical spine, head, and brachial plexus. Other rib fractures, if at multiple levels, may result in a flail chest. This diagnosis is made by observing paradoxical inward movement of the chest during inspiration. Underlying pulmonary contusion could cause hypoxemia as fluid moves into the injured lung secondary to acute respiratory distress syndrome. Treatment is oxygen and adequate pain control to allow adequate ventilation. If the patient cannot maintain adequate oxygenation, early ventilatory support is extremely important before the patient enters respiratory failure. A chest x-ray is necessary to confirm the injury as well as to rule out pneumothorax and hemothorax. Rib detail films are of questionable usefulness because approximately half of nondisplaced fractures cannot be seen in plain films, and treatment is the same for rib contusions and fracture. Other visceral injuries may be associated with rib trauma, and further evaluation of the liver, spleen, and kidneys may be indicated, depending on the results of the physical examination. Chest wall supports should be used cautiously, if at all, because they impair the mechanics of ventilation and the clearance of pulmonary secretions, leading to atelectasis and pneumonitis. Maintain a high suspicion for visceral injury in children because their rib cages are cartilaginous and flexible. Patients should be instructed on using a pillow for splinting and should deep-breathe and cough frequently. Healing usually takes 4 to 6 weeks.
- **Sternal fractures:** Sternal fractures can be associated with significant trauma and mortality and are commonly the result of steering wheel impact in motor vehicle collisions. Chest radiographs with lateral views of the sternum generally demonstrate the fracture. Electrocardiograms (ECG) and cardiac enzymes should be obtained serially for the first 24 hours in these patients because myocardial damage may be associated with this fracture.[6]

SHOULDER GIRDLE

- **Clavicle:** Fractures of the clavicle are grouped according to location: Group I (middle third), Group II (distal third), and Group III (proximal third). Most patients have palpable swelling and tenderness at the fracture site and generally carry the affected arm in the adducted position, resisting motion of the arm. Because these fractures may be associated with neurovascular injury, a meticulous examination should be done and documented. Routine clavicle radiographs usually demonstrate the fracture. Nondisplaced fractures can be treated with a sling or a figure-of-8 brace. Fractures of the medial third of the clavicle may be associated with intrathoracic injuries or late-onset arthritis. Clavicular fractures that involve the distal third may disrupt the coracoclavicular ligament, and there is a high risk of nonunion without operative repair. Surgical indications are complete fracture displacement, severe displacement causing tenting of the skin with the risk of puncture, neurovascular compromise, and open fractures. Distal third clavicle fractures may be managed conservatively depending on the type and the displacement.[7]

SCAPULA

Scapular fractures are relatively rare, and high energy is required to fracture this bone. Because of this type of trauma, consider coexisting injuries to the ipsilateral lung, thoracic cage, and shoulder girdle. Management of most scapular fractures includes immobilization with a sling, ice, and analgesics, with early ROM exercises. Surgical management may be necessary for significant or displaced articular fractures of the glenoid, angulated glenoid neck fractures, acromial fractures with rotator cuff tear, and displaced coracoid fractures.

HUMERUS

- **Proximal humerus:** This injury commonly occurs in elderly women who fall on an outstretched hand. A neurovascular exam should be performed with attention to sensation over the skin of the deltoid that is supplied by the axillary nerve, also called the regimental badge area. The Neer classification is used to describe proximal humerus fractures. A one-part fracture in the Neer system may have any number of fracture lines, but no major segment (greater and lesser tuberosities, anatomic neck, and surgical neck) may be significantly displaced (>1 cm separation or >45-degree angulation). Treatment of one-part fractures is immobilization, ice, analgesics, and referral. Early mobility is critical for successful treatment of proximal humeral fractures. Multipart fractures (two or more segments) should prompt emergent orthopedic consultation as they are more likely to involve neurovascular injuries, rotator cuff injury, and risk of nonunion.

- **Humeral shaft:** These fractures can occur in active young men or osteoporotic elderly women; metastatic breast cancer may present as a pathologic humerus fracture. Mid-humeral transverse fractures usually result from a direct blow. A fall on an outstretched hand may result in a spiral fracture. Neurovascular injuries are a common complication. Most closed fractures are managed nonoperatively with immobilization, ice, analgesia, and referral. Surgery may be required for pathologic fractures, fractures associated with neurovascular injuries, or very proximal or very distal humerus fractures.

ELBOW AND FOREARM FRACTURES

- **Intercondylar fractures:** These fractures are more common in adults, and any distal humerus fracture should be initially assumed to be intercondylar rather than supracondylar. A careful search should be made for a fracture line separating the condyles from each other and from the humerus. These fractures are associated with severe soft-tissue injuries. Joint reduction should be performed and the elbow immobilized, and urgent orthopedic referral made.
- **Supracondylar fractures:** These extra-articular fractures occur most commonly in children with posterior elbow dislocation. Patients with olecranon fractures have increased pain with elbow extension, whereas the pain of radial head fractures is usually aggravated by supination. Radiographs may reveal a fat-pad sign posteriorly or anteriorly. However, an anterior fat pad may be normal, whereas a posterior fat pad is always pathologic indicating an intra-articular effusion. This sign may be the only radiologic abnormality in nondisplaced radial head fractures. Suspected occult or nondisplaced radial head fractures can be treated with a posterior splint for 2 weeks followed by a sling and ROM exercises. Patients with displaced fractures of the radial head and fractures involving more than 30% of the joint surface should be referred to an orthopedist, as should those with olecranon fractures. Nondisplaced fractures are treated by casting, whereas displaced fractures require reduction and surgical fixation. Neurovascular injuries are common, as well as other complications such as nonunion, malunion, myositis ossificans, and loss of motion. Sensation and motor function should always be tested. The radial nerve provides motor function to wrist and finger extension and sensation to the dorsum of the hand. The median nerve controls wrist flexion, finger flexion, and thumb abduction, and provides sensation to the palm of the hand. The anterior interosseus nerve arises from the median nerve and has no sensory component, so specific muscles must be tested to discover injury. Testing consists of flexion at the index finger distal interphalangeal (DIP) and thumb interphalangeal joints (ask patient to make the OK sign). The ulnar nerve controls the intrinsic muscles and sensation to the ulnar side of the hand. Acute vascular injuries are possible and absence of a radial pulse is common in children, which is usually due to transient spasm. The most serious complication is Volkmann ischemic contracture, which can involve muscle and nerve necrosis and eventual severe fibrosis. Edema reduces venous outflow and arterial inflow, which induces ischemia, manifested by refusal to open the hand, pain with passive extension of the fingers and forearm tenderness. Supracondylar fractures with associated absent radial pulse should be reduced, immobilized, and emergent orthopedic referral made.
- **Olecranon fractures:** The olecranon is commonly fractured and may involve ulnar nerve injury or radial head and neck fractures. Nondisplaced fractures (<2 mm displacement) are immobilized with the elbow in 45 degrees of flexion, with orthopedic follow-up within a week. Displaced fractures are treated surgically.
- **Radial head fractures:** Radial head fractures are the most common elbow fracture and occur with a fall on an outstretched hand. A posterior fat-pad sign in a patient with an appropriate mechanism of injury is sufficient to make a diagnosis of a radial head fracture. Nondisplaced and minimally displaced fractures are treated with sling immobilization and early ROM, whereas all other fractures should be referred acutely to an orthopedist.
- **Forearm fractures:** Mid-forearm fractures are usually the result of a direct blow. Associated radioulnar joint dislocations are common. The radiographic evaluation should include views of the elbow and wrist in addition to AP and lateral views of the forearm. Fractures that involve both the radius and ulna are rarely stable and usually require surgical fixation. A long-arm cast can be used with minimally displaced or nondisplaced fractures. Open fractures can involve nerve injuries. Be alert for compartment syndrome, which may present late with signs and symptoms. Isolated nondisplaced ulnar or radial fractures can be immobilized in a long-arm cast with close follow-up; displaced fractures require open reduction and internal fixation.

- **Distal radius and ulna fractures:** Colles fracture results from falls on the outstretched hand and consists of a distal radial metaphysis fracture that is dorsally angulated and displaced. Fractures should be reduced, using finger traps while the fracture fragment is pushed distal and palmar while the patient's forearm is firmly held. Immobilization in a long-arm cast. Fractures with >20 degrees of angulation, intra-articular involvement, marked comminution, or more than 1 cm of shortening are potentially unstable and may require surgical intervention. The neurovascular examination is particularly important because of commonly associated median nerve and radial artery injuries. Smith fracture is a volar angulated fracture of the distal radius, or "reverse Colles fracture," and treatment is similar to that for Colles fracture.

WRIST FRACTURES
- **Scaphoid fracture:** Scaphoid fractures are the most common and complicated carpal fracture. They are usually caused by a fall on a hyperextended wrist. Patients have tenderness over the scaphoid in the anatomical snuffbox or with axial compression of the thumb. Another sign may be tenderness to the scaphoid tubercle, which may be more specific for scaphoid fracture. Absence of tenderness in these two areas makes fracture unlikely.[8] The radiographic evaluation should include AP, lateral, oblique, and scaphoid views. Nondisplaced scaphoid fractures frequently have negative acute radiographs. If the patient has tenderness in either of these areas but a normal x-ray, suspect occult fracture, immobilize in a short-arm thumb spica splint or cast, and reevaluate in 2 weeks. Displaced or unstable fractures should be placed in a long-arm thumb spica splint or cast. Healing of the scaphoid is hindered by its poor blood supply. Accordingly, avascular necrosis and nonunion are common complications. Patients with continued scaphoid tenderness should continue follow-up until tenderness is gone. If radiographic abnormalities are still not present, then a bone scan or MRI should be obtained.[8] Persons with confirmed fractures should be referred to an orthopedist because of the high incidence of complications.

HAND FRACTURES
- **Distal phalanx:** These can be classified as tuft, shaft, or intra-articular. Fractures at the base may be associated with flexor or extensor tendon involvement. In general, these fractures can be treated as soft-tissue injuries with protective splinting for 2 to 4 weeks. Small subungual hematomas (<25% of the nail bed area) should be drained. Larger hematomas are suggestive of a significant nail bed laceration and should be repaired for optimal cosmetic result. Extensor tendon avulsion fractures (mallet finger) require splinting for 6 weeks. Flexor tendon avulsion fractures (jersey finger) require immediate surgical referral as risk of tendon retraction is high.
- **Proximal and middle phalanx:** The physical examination should focus on ruling out the presence of rotational deformity and tendon avulsions. If the hands are held palm up and the fingers flexed, they should point toward the scaphoid. Any overlap suggests a rotational deformity. Extensor tendon avulsion fractures of the proximal interphalangeal central slip result in a boutonniere deformity, where the PIP joint is flexed and the DIP is hyperextended. Decreased active ROM accompanies tendon avulsions. Most proximal and middle phalanx fractures are stable and can be treated with buddy taping. Nondisplaced extra-articular fractures and volar plate fractures involving less than 15% of the joint surface can be splinted in flexion for 3 weeks followed by three more weeks of dynamic splinting.. Midshaft transverse fractures, spiral fractures, and intra-articular fractures often require internal fixation. Other unstable fractures can be splinted after closed reduction. Splinting should be done from the elbow to the DIP with the elbow in 20-degree extension and the metacarpophalangeal joint in 90-degree flexion.
- **Metacarpal fractures:** Metacarpal fractures are classified as head, neck, shaft, or base fractures. Metacarpal head fractures should be treated with ice, elevation, immobilization, and referral to a hand surgeon. Metacarpal neck fractures should be splinted with the wrist in 20-degree extension and the MP flexed at 90 degrees. Fracture of the fifth metacarpal neck is called a boxer's fracture and angulation of <40 degrees is acceptable. Angulation of <20 degrees is acceptable in the fourth metacarpal. In second and third metacarpal neck fractures, <15 degrees of angulation is acceptable. If the second and third metacarpal necks are significantly displaced or angulated, precise reduction and fixation is required. Nondisplaced shaft fractures can be treated with a gutter splint; otherwise, operative fixation is required. Metacarpal base fractures may be associated with carpal bone fractures; fourth and fifth metacarpal base fractures may result in paralysis of the motor branch of the ulnar nerve. Additionally, boxer's fracture have been correlated with high rates of associated psychiatric illness and possibly substance abuse.[9,10]

PELVIS AND HIP FRACTURES
- **Pelvic fractures:** Pelvic fractures should be suspected in all victims of serious or motor vehicle trauma. Fractures may occur in a single pelvic bone, the pelvic ring, or the acetabulum. Because the

pelvis is a ring, there is usually more than one fracture or ligamentous injury. Examination of the patient may reveal perineal and pelvic edema, ecchymoses, lacerations, and deformities. The pelvis should be compressed from lateral to medial and also anterior to posterior to appreciate pain or instability. The greater trochanters should be compressed and hip ROM evaluated. Rectal examination should be done, with attention to tone, bone fragments, or rectal injury. Inability to void, hematuria, or a high-riding prostate suggests urethral injury. A standard AP view of the pelvis should be obtained in all victims of serious trauma. Pelvic fractures that are unstable or that include displacement of the pelvic ring are often associated with multisystem trauma and high mortality. Significant hemorrhage is common, and the patient may present in shock. Temporary external fixation of the pelvis may be attempted with a tightly wrapped bed sheet. Single pubic or ischial ramus fractures are the most common fractures of the pelvis. Elderly fall victims often experience a single pubic or ischial ramus fracture, and these can be treated conservatively with pain control and short-term bed rest with progression to ambulation with crutches. A cushion for sitting may help relieve pain. Iliac wing fractures usually result from acute trauma, and the treatment is similar to that listed for single pubic or ischial ramus fractures. Coccyx fractures result from falls in which the individual lands in the seated position. Localized pain to palpation and pain with sitting or defecation characterize such fractures. The diagnosis can usually be confirmed by rectal examination, and radiographic results are often negative. Treatment generally involves bed rest, sitz baths, laxatives, and cushions for sitting. Acetabular fractures are common in motor vehicle accidents and occur during hip dislocations. Treatment includes reduction of the dislocation, hospital admission, and early orthopedic consultation.

- **Hip fractures:** These fractures are classified as intracapsular (femoral head and neck) or extracapsular (trochanteric, intertrochanteric, and subtrochanteric). Intracapsular fractures are at greater risk for avascular necrosis due to compromise of the femoral neck vessels. Radiographs should be obtained in all major trauma victims as well as elderly fall victims, even if the patient is ambulatory. Occult fracture should be suspected with negative films, but significant pain with weight-bearing after trauma, and MRI may be helpful. Intertrochanteric fractures cause marked external rotation and shortening of the affected limb. Morbidity and mortality are relatively high in elderly patients with hip fractures due to thromboembolic events and failure to regain normal function. Orthopedic consultation should be made emergently with intracapsular fractures, whereas extracapsular fractures should be referred urgently.

LOWER EXTREMITY

- **Distal and mid-femur fractures:** The mid-femur is a strong bone with excellent blood supply, a characteristic that predisposes patients with femoral shaft fractures to significant potential for hemorrhage. Up to 40% of isolated fractures may require transfusion, as the femur is very vascular and can result in blood loss up to 3 units.[8] The muscles surrounding the femoral shaft frequently cause a deformity and displacement of any fracture. Patients generally present with severe pain, a shortened leg, and a swollen thigh. Routine films generally demonstrate the fracture. The Ottawa Knee Rules should be utilized when deciding to obtain radiographs in the evaluation of a knee injury. If one of the following is present, knee radiographs are indicated: age >55 years, isolated patellar tenderness without other bone tenderness, tenderness of the fibular head, inability to flex to 90 degrees, or the inability to bear weight immediately after injury and in the emergency department (four steps) regardless of limping. These rules should not be used if the patient is <2 years of age, is intoxicated, has other distracting painful injuries, has decreased sensation, or whom has gross swelling that prevents proper palpation. (This applies to other Ottawa rules cited below.)

  The extremity should be immobilized, and orthopedic consultation should be urgently obtained as surgical fixation will be required. Open fractures should be irrigated and parenteral antibiotics started. Distal femoral fractures are uncommon and may be intra-articular or extra-articular. They are usually the result of direct trauma, and these patients present with pain, swelling, and deformity of the knee. Because of the close proximity of this area of the femur to the peroneal nerve (innervates space between the first and second toe) and the popliteal artery, it is essential that the neurovascular status of the leg be evaluated and documented early in the assessment of the patient. If the popliteal artery injury is suspected by decreased distal pulses, emergent angiography and vascular consult are necessary. Initial treatment would include pain control, immobilization, and emergent referral.

- **Tibia and fibula:** Tibial fractures are the most common of long-bone fractures. They may be intra-articular or extra-articular. Fractures of the tibial plateau (medial and lateral tibial condyles) are easy to miss on standard radiographic films; therefore, tibial plateau views should be obtained to clearly identify these fractures. Nondisplaced, single-plateau fractures can be immobilized and outpatient orthopedic referral made. Other plateau fractures should be referred quickly. Dislocations and fractures of the fibular head may appear innocuous, but are often a marker for more significant knee injury. Fibular fracture may even occur with an ankle sprain that tears the syndesmosis, and causes a Maisonneuve fracture. Injury to the peroneal nerve must also be suspected due to its proximity to the head of the fibula. Displaced fractures of the tibia are often associated with displaced fractures of the fibula. Orthopedic consultation is recommended for tibial and fibular fractures because of the frequently associated injuries (ligamental, meniscal, and vascular) and the frequently seen complications, which can result in chronic pain, knee dysfunction, and degenerative arthritis.

- **Patella:** Patellar fractures most commonly result from direct trauma, but a violent contraction of the quadriceps may cause an avulsion fracture. Transverse fractures are most common, followed by stellate and comminuted types. Local tenderness and swelling are the most common presenting complaints. If extensor mechanism is disrupted by a patellar fracture, the patient will be unable to extend the knee. AP, lateral, and sunrise views of the patella are usually sufficient to define most fractures. Patellar alignment is best seen with a Merchant view but is often difficult to obtain as it requires a simple device at the end of the imaging table that ensures proper knee flexion. Because bipartite and tripartite patellae are relatively common and usually bilateral, comparison views may be helpful and smooth cortical margins should be seen. A nondisplaced patellar fracture with intact extensor mechanism should be treated with a knee immobilizer, ice, elevation, and analgesics followed by long-leg casting. Aspiration of hemarthrosis may be helpful in decreasing pain. Attention must be paid to maintaining quadriceps strength with exercises to avoid atrophy. Consideration should be given to specialist referral because of the possibility of traumatic chondromalacia and avascular necrosis. In other types of patellar fractures, consultation is recommended.
- **Ankle:** The ankle joint consists of three bones (tibia, fibula, and talus) and three main ligamentous structures (lateral ligament complex, medial deltoid ligament, and the syndesmosis, which joins the tibia and fibula). The Ottawa Ankle Rules indicate that radiographs are required only if there is tenderness along the distal 6 cm of either bone or in the tip of either malleoli or if the patient is unable to bear weight for four steps either immediately or in the emergency room (accepted patients noted above in femur fractures). The standard radiographs (AP, lateral, and mortise views) are usually adequate. Special attention should be paid to the malleolar–talar space. The medial clear space (between talus and medial malleolus) should be <4 mm, and when the medial space is >4 mm, then lateral shift of talus is present, which indicates a deltoid ligament injury.

  Ankle fractures and ligamental injuries often coexist. Disruption of the ankle at only one place generally results in a stable ankle injury that can be treated by conservative means (posterior splinting, non–weight bearing, and edema control). If two or more disruptions of the ankle are present, the ankle is not stable, and treatment is immobilization and urgent referral. Unilateral avulsion fractures of the distal tip of the malleolus are often treated like second-degree sprains. If there is any doubt about optimal management, discuss the case with an orthopedic specialist because the risk for complications of ankle fractures is high.

- **Hindfoot fractures:** The hindfoot consists of the calcaneus and talus. Although standard films may demonstrate fractures in this area, a CT scan may be required for adequate visualization of injuries because occult fractures are common in this area. A posterior subtalar effusion seen on the lateral view may indicate an occult lateral process fracture. If heel or ankle pain is persistent despite conservative measures, consider an occult fracture.[11] For this reason, the clinical examination is critical in making decisions. Although full ankle motion may be present, heel pain with weight bearing after the appropriate trauma is common. Calcaneus fractures should prompt evaluation of the spine as they are usually caused by falls from a height. Compartment syndrome should be suspected in patients with calcaneal fractures. Generally, the nondisplaced fracture is treated with a well-padded posterior splint, non–weight bearing, elevation, and analgesics until swelling subsides, when a well-molded walking cast may be used. Partial weight bearing is generally needed for at least 8 weeks. Because of the high likelihood of posttraumatic arthritis and chronic pain and stiffness, patients bearing these fractures are often referred to an orthopedic specialist. If any displacement is present, prompt referral is recommended.
- **Midfoot fractures:** The midfoot consists of the navicular, cuboid, and three cuneiforms. Isolated fractures of the cuboid and cuneiforms are rare. The Ottawa Foot Rule for mid- and forefoot fractures is similar to the ankle rule, except one checks for tenderness over the navicular and the base of the fifth metatarsal.

  Additionally, an injury to the Lisfranc joint should be sought when there is a direct blow to the dorsum of the foot or an axial load is applied to the planter flexed foot. The Lisfranc joint consists of the tarsometatarsal complex and injuries here are often missed. Palpate for point tenderness over the midfoot and laxity between the first and second metatarsals in a dorsal–plantar direction. Check the alignment of the medial margin of the base of the second metatarsal with the medial margin of the intermediate cuneiform on the AP view of the foot. A fracture of the base of the second metatarsal or gap >1 mm between the bases of the first and second metatarsals on radiograph is pathognomic of a ligamentous injury. Weight bearing or stress views as well as comparison views are often needed to appreciate this injury on imaging.

Small, nondisplaced chip fractures of the navicular are usually treated with a compressive dressing for several weeks. Other nondisplaced navicular fractures can often be treated conservatively with a well-molded walking cast. Displaced navicular fractures and Lisfranc joint injuries with cuboid and cuneiform fractures should be referred for open reduction.

- **Forefoot fractures:** The metatarsals and phalanges usually result from direct crush injuries. Because of the large forces to the second and third metatarsals during the push-off phase of walking or running, this area is prone to stress fractures. Standard foot radiographic views are generally adequate to demonstrate fractures (with the exception of early stress fractures, which may require a bone scan or MRI to visualize). A secondary ossification center in the base of the fifth metatarsal may sometimes be confused with a fracture, but this area generally has smooth, bilateral sclerotic margins. Nondisplaced shaft fractures are generally treated conservatively with a walking cast or orthopedic shoe. However, the first metatarsal, if fractured, should be kept non–weight bearing. Displaced shaft fractures can be treated with closed reduction, casting, and non–weight bearing for 6 weeks. For neck fractures, open fixation is often required for displaced fractures. Fifth metatarsal fractures are the most common of the metatarsal fractures. The base of the fifth metatarsal is the most common metatarsal fracture. An avulsion fracture must be differentiated from a transverse fracture (Jones fracture) of the base. The Jones fracture (transverse fracture 15 to 31 mm distal to the proximal part of the metatarsal) can be complicated by malunion or nonunion and thus requires orthopedic referral; they require 6 weeks in a non–weight bearing cast, or surgery if there is displacement. An avulsion fracture of the tuberosity of the base can appear similar to a Jones fracture but appears as a longitudinal fracture instead. It requires only a cast shoe. Phalangeal fractures, if nondisplaced, can be treated with "buddy taping" and sometimes a cast shoe. Fractures of the first toe are not adequately immobilized by dynamic splinting, and a walking cast is usually necessary. Displaced fractures should be reduced under digital nerve block if possible; displaced fractures of the great toe may need surgical fixation.

PATHOLOGIC FRACTURES

Any fracture that results from insignificant trauma should be considered pathologic, meaning that the broken bone has preexisting disease that has resulted in a loss of structural integrity. The patient may complain of pain that existed even before the fracture, and the actual fracture site may not be especially tender. The radiograph may have an altered appearance in that the trabecular patterns of the bone near the fracture can be disrupted. The most common causes of bone disease are osteoporosis, myelomas, malignant primary bone tumors, and metastatic lesions (consider cancer of the thyroid, breast, prostate, bronchus, kidney, bladder, uterus, ovary, testicle, and adrenals). Less common—but more benign—causes include enchondromas (also called chondromas), solitary bone cysts, and giant cell tumors.

FRACTURES UNIQUE TO CHILDREN

There are several unique factors about the diagnosis and treatment of fractures in children. These include the presence of the epiphyseal plate, the tendency to suffer incomplete fractures, and the evaluation for signs of child abuse (see Chapter 20.5).

Epiphyseal plate injuries are common because this site is the weakest portion of the immature skeleton. Injuries that would result in a ligamentous strain in adults frequently fracture the epiphyseal plate in children. The physical examination reveals tenderness and edema over the epiphysis. The radiographic evaluation may be difficult, and comparison views should be considered. Epiphyseal plate fractures are most commonly classified by the Salter–Harris system (Figure 3.7-2):

- Type I: Fracture through the epiphyseal plate
- Type II: Epiphyseal plate fracture with an associated metaphyseal fragment
- Type III: Fracture through the epiphysis onto the articular surface
- Type IV: Fracture through the distal metaphysis, epiphyseal plate, and epiphysis
- Type V: Impaction of the epiphyseal plate

Types I and II are treated with casting, often after closed reduction, and enjoy a good prognosis. Types III, IV, and V have a higher risk of growth disturbance and should be referred. Type V is often diagnosed in retrospect, after a growth disturbance has occurred.

Incomplete fractures: Torus fractures occur when there is a buckling of one side of the cortex. They are usually caused by a compression force. Torus fractures occur commonly in the forearm after a fall on the outstretched hand. They are treated with a long-arm cast for 4 to 6 weeks. Greenstick fractures

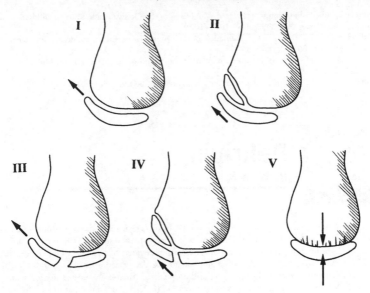

Figure 3.7-2. Salter–Harris system.

occur when a long bone is bowed, resulting in a break in only the convex side of the cortex. These are generally stable fractures that most commonly occur in the forearm. Forearm greenstick fractures with less than 15 degrees of angulation should be placed in a cast for 4 to 6 weeks. Patients whose fractures show more than 15 degrees of angulation should be referred to an orthopedist.

Physical abuse is a significant cause of early childhood fractures. Suspicion should be raised by an inconsistent or implausible explanation and by inappropriate parental behavior. The classic radiologic evidence of child abuse is multiple fractures in various stages of healing. Suspected victims should be evaluated with a skeletal survey, followed by the appropriate completion of forms and referrals to protective agencies.

REFERENCES

1. Borchers J, Best T. Common finger fractures and dislocations. *Am Fam Physician* 2012;85(8):805–810.
2. Bahk MS, Kuhn JE, Galatz LM, et al. Acromioclavicular and sternoclavicular injuries and clavicular, glenoid, and scapular fractures. *J Bone Joint Surg Am* 2009;91(10):2492–2510.
3. Weinberg ER, Tunik MG, Tsung JW. Accuracy of clinician-performed point-of-care ultrasound for the diagnosis of fractures in children and young adults [published online ahead of print May 13, 2010]. *Injury* 2010;41(8):862–868. doi:10.1016/j.injury.2010.04.020.
4. Prosser JD1, Vender JR, Solares CA. Traumatic cerebrospinal fluid leaks. *Otolaryngol Clin North Am* 2011;44(4):857–873.
5. Mondin V, Rinaldo A, Ferlito A. Management of nasal bone fractures. *Am J Otolaryngol* 2005;26(3):181–185.
6. Stiell IG, Clement CM, McKnight RD, et al. The Canadian C-spine rule versus the NEXUS low-risk criteria in patients with trauma. *N Engl J Med* 2003;349(26):2510–2518.
7. Khoriati AA, Rajakulasingam R, Shah R. Sternal fractures and their management. *J Emerg Trauma Shock* 2013;6(2):113–116.
8. Clavicular fractures in adults. In: DeLee J, Drez D, eds. *DeLee and Drez's orthopaedic sports medicine: principles and practice.* 2nd ed. Philadelphia, PA: Saunders; 2003:958–968.
9. Phillips TG, Reibach AM, Slomiany WP. Diagnosis and management of scaphoid fractures. *Am Fam Physician* 2004;70(5):879–884.
10. Lieurance R, Benjamin JB, Rappaport WD. Blood loss and transfusion in patients with isolated femur fractures. *J Orthop Trauma* 1992;6(2):175–179.
11. Alonso LL, Purcell TB. Accuracy of the tongue blade test in patients with suspected mandibular fracture. *J Emerg Med* 1995;13(3):297–304.
12. Jeanmonod RK. Punch injuries: insights into intentional closed fist injuries. *West J Emerg Med* 2011;12(1):6–10.
13. Geer SE, Williams JM. Boxer's fracture: an indicator of intentional and recurrent injury. *Am J Emerg Med* 1999;17(4):357–360.

14. Plint AC, Bulloch B, Osmond MH, et al. Validation of the Ottawa Ankle Rules in children with ankle injuries. *Acad Emerg Med* 1999;6(10):1005–1009.
15. Bulloch B, Neto G, Plint A, et al. Validation of the Ottawa Knee Rule in children: a multicenter study. *Ann Emerg Med* 2003;42(1):48–55.
16. Judd DB, Kim DH. Foot fractures frequently misdiagnosed as ankle sprains. *Am Fam Physician* 2002;66(5):785–794.
17. Eiff MP, Hatch R. *Fracture management for primary care.* 3rd ed. Elsevier; 2011.

Delirium

Rebecca Wester

Delirium is a sudden, temporary onset of confusion that causes changes in the way people think and behave. Healthcare providers often refer to delirium as "change in mental status." Delirium is regarded as reversible, which distinguishes it from dementia.[1] Healthcare providers often underappreciate delirium and its consequences. Delirium may be the only sign of an adverse drug reaction or of a significant medical illness such as pneumonia or sepsis. Older people and hospitalized patients are most at risk for delirium and are ordinarily screened with confusion assessment method (CAM). Knowing what to look for and treating the causes early can help save lives. In fact, the mortality rates for hospitalized delirious patients have been reported to be 25% to 33%, as high as the mortality rates of acute myocardial infarction or sepsis.[2]

GENERAL PRINCIPLES
Definition

The American Psychiatrics' Association's Diagnostic and statistical manual of mental disorders (DSM-5) has the following diagnostic criteria for delirium:

A. A disturbance in attention (i.e., reduced ability to direct, focus, sustain, and shift attention) and awareness (reduced orientation to the environment).
B. The disturbance develops over a short period of time (usually hours to a few days), represents a change from baseline attention and awareness, and tends to fluctuate in severity during the course of a day.
C. An additional disturbance in cognition (i.e., memory deficit, disorientation, language, visuospatial ability, or perception).

The disturbances in Criteria A and C are not better explained by another preexisting, established, or evolving neurocognitive disorder and do not occur in the context of a severely reduced level of arousal, such as coma. There is evidence from the history, physical examination, or laboratory findings that the disturbance is a direct physiological consequence of another medical condition, substance intoxication, or withdrawal (i.e., due to drug of abuse or a medication); or exposure to a toxin; or is due to multiple etiologies.[3] This means delirium always has a cause, usually multiple causes, requiring a comprehensive approach.

Epidemiology

Prevalence of delirium in the community is low (1% to 2%), but rises to 14% among >85 years of age.[3] Its prevalence in the emergency department is 10%, and rises up to 56% in older hospitalized populations.[3,4] Postoperative delirium rates are 4.5% to 6.8% for urologic cases,[2] 28% to 53% for orthopedic cases,[2] and 17% to 74% for coronary artery bypass grafting.[5] In comparison, delirium occurs in 10% to 30% of acute stroke cases[6] and 70% to 87% of intensive care unit (ICU) patients.[3] Two-thirds of the cases of delirium occur in patients with dementia.[7,8] The average duration of delirium is 1 to 2 weeks; sometimes lasting only a few hours and other times never resolving. In hospitalized patients >50 years old with delirium, 44% were found to have persistent delirium at hospital discharge, with delirium persisting in 32% at 1 month, 25% at 3 months, and 21% at 6 months following hospitalization.[9] Delirium occurs in 60% of those in postacute/long-term care facilities[3] and in up to 83% of all individuals at the end of life.[1,3] Significantly, only half of delirium cases are recognized across healthcare settings.[10] Overall, delirious hospitalized patients have longer hospital stays, are more likely to be discharged to long-term care facilities, have more loss of physical function, and have higher mortality rates.[2,3,5,6,9,11–14] Regrettably, about 40% of people who are diagnosed with delirium in the hospital are dead within a year,[8,15] independent of baseline dementia status.[7]

Classification

The American Psychiatrics' Association's Diagnostic and statistical manual of mental disorders (DSM-5) classifies delirium by:
- **Cause:** (a) substance intoxication; (b) substance withdrawal; (c) medication induced; (d) another medical condition; and (e) multiple etiologies;
- **Duration:** (a) acute (lasting few hours or days) and (b) persistent (lasting weeks to months);
- **Activity:** (a) hyperactive; (b) hypoactive; and (c) mixed level of activity.[3]

Hyperactive delirium is frequently recognized because these are the patients who are shouting and hallucinating, whereas hypoactive delirium is missed because these are the ones who seem to be the "compliant" patients. Unfortunately, patients with hypoactive delirium are more likely to die compared with those with hyperactive or mixed delirium.[15]

DIAGNOSIS

History

Determining the acuity of the "change in mental status" is the essential first step; neglecting this step or assuming baseline mental status leads to missed delirium diagnosis.[8]

The following words should trigger consideration of delirium: "not feeling right"; "weak"; "just not himself"; or "poor historian." Medications and alcohol use should be reviewed in detail. Medication errors are the easiest to miss whether it is a pharmacy error, caregiver error, patient omission (intentional or unintentionally), or medication list error.

Physical Examination

The examination should focus on whether delirium is present. The CAM is the standard screening tool for delirium.[14] This reliable and easy-to-use tool has been adapted for use across healthcare settings and translated into numerous languages.[16] The comprehensive examination, guided by the history and context, should focus on the likely cause(s) of the delirium. Focal neurologic signs are usually present if neurologic etiologies are the cause.[15]

Confusion Assessment Method

CAM is summarized in Figure 3.8-1. For delirium to be identified, both features #1 and #2 must be present plus either #3 or #4.

i. Acute onset and fluctuating course: This is a change from baseline and a change during the day. Validating history from a family member or nurse is essential. Delirium can impair sleep – awake cycles and is often worse at night (i.e., "sundowning").

ii. Inattention: This is difficulty focusing or keeping track, drifting off to sleep, or easily distracted. On rounds, this is the patient who falls asleep during an examination. You may find yourself asking the same questions over and over; or the delirious patient may end up repeating the same response. Testing inattention by asking the months of the year backwards, or serials 7's, is helpful too.

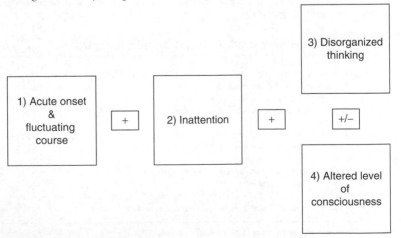

Figure 3.8-1. Confusion assessment method (CAM).

iii. **Disorganized thinking:** The patient is incoherent, rambling, irrelevant, illogical, circumstantial, or vague. The patient would be unpredictably switching from one subject to another, unclear, or with illogical flow of ideas. Any hallucinations or delusions should be ascertained.

iv. **Altered level of consciousness:** The patient is lethargic, stuporous, drowsy, or agitated. Anything other than "alert" used to describe the patient's consciousness is abnormal and considered "positive."

Laboratory and Imaging

Delirium is a clinical diagnosis. Tests investigate the cause(s) of the delirium. Order tests on the basis of history, vitals, and physical and neurologic examinations. Search for infections. A reasonable diagnostic workup would include complete blood count, electrolytes, urea, creatinine, glucose, calcium, magnesium, liver function tests, thyroid stimulating hormone, chest x-ray, urinalysis, electrocardiogram, and blood cultures. For example, order drug levels, such as digoxin if noted on their medication list; order an arterial blood gas if concerned for hypercarbia respiratory failure; order further imaging (CT chest/abdomen/pelvis) if suspicious for infection, which was not identified already. Neuroimaging studies have a low yield[8]; thus, order CT head only if there is a history of trauma, substantially impaired consciousness, new focal neurologic findings, and incomplete history, or if there is no clear alternative cause. Urine drug screen, ammonia, blood alcohol levels, and cardiac biomarkers are further diagnostic options.[8] Electroencephalography and lumbar puncture are rarely needed, unless the cause of delirium is unclear and occult seizures or meningitis are considerations.[8,15] A common pitfall is to ascribe acute changes (i.e., confusion, sepsis) to what may otherwise be normal findings in a nursing home patient. Asymptomatic bacteriuria is very common in frail seniors, found in up to 50% in the long-term care setting.[17] For example, an elderly patient who is eating and drinking poorly because of unrecognized bacterial pneumonia or an adverse drug reaction is likely to have a coexisting positive urinalysis or urine culture. Attributing the mental status change to the irrelevant positive urine test may result in failure to detect the patient's more serious underlying problem and delay of the appropriate treatment.[17]

Differential Diagnosis

Almost any medical illness, intoxication, or medication can cause delirium. It is often multifactorial, and each potential cause should be investigated. The adage "common things are common" is accurate in delirium; be vigilant not to overlook atypical presentations of common problems. For example, elderly patients are more likely to complain of weakness or dyspnea, instead of the classic chest pain symptom. It is not uncommon to hear family members of demented patients say that their loved ones are "just not themselves"; when in fact, the only symptom of their acute myocardial infarction is delirium.[2,8]

A mnemonic for the causes of delirium is given in Table 3.8-1. The most common causes include:

- *Infections* (think PUS—Pneumonia, Urinary, Skin). Subtle infections such as cholecystitis and diverticulitis should not be overlooked either.[2]
- *Medications* (Table 3.8-2). Even long-standing medications can contribute to delirium and should be evaluated.[8] The medication may be at a steady state, but the patient may have changed (i.e., lost weight or became dehydrated). Many medications have anticholinergic effects, which are thought to be additive and are often the culprits.

TABLE 3.8-1   Mnemonic for the Causes of Delirium (*DELIRIUMS*)

D—**d**rugs, **d**ehydration, **d**etox, **d**eficiencies (thiamine, niacin, B$_{12}$), **d**iscomfort (pain)

E—**e**lectrolytes (hypo-/hypernatremia, hypercalcemia), **e**motional stress, (unfamiliar) **e**nvironment, (hypertensive) **e**ncephalopathy, **e**ndocrinopathies (adrenal dysfunction)

L—**l**ungs (hypoxia or hypercarbia), **l**ow O$_2$ states (anemia, ACS, pulmonary), **l**iver (hepatic encephalopathy), **l**ack of sleep

I—**i**nfection, **i**atrogenic complications, **i**nfarction (cardiac, cerebral), **i**ctal states, **I**CU admission

R—**r**estraints (i.e., any restricted movement including Foley catheter), **r**etention (of urine or fecal impaction), **r**enal failure

I—**i**njury, **i**mpaired sensory input, **i**ntoxication (or withdrawal), **i**ntracranial bleeding

U—**U**TI, **u**nder-nutrition, **u**nder-hydration

M—**m**etabolic abnormalities (acid–base, glucose, thyroid), **m**etastasis (brain), **m**edications

S—**s**troke, **s**hock, **s**epsis, **s**urgery, **s**ubdural hematoma, **s**erotonin syndrome

---

O$_2$, oxygen; ACS, acute coronary syndrome; ICU, intensive care unit; UTI, urinary tract infection. This is not an exclusive list.

TABLE 3.8-2	Mnemonic for Medications that Cause Delirium (*ACUTE CHANGE IN MS*)

A—Antibiotics (fluoroquinolones)

C—Cardiovascular (anti-arrhythmics, digoxin, clonidine)

U—Urinary incontinence (oxybutynin, tolterodine, darifenacin, fesoterone, solifenacin, trospium)

T—Theophylline; and *all* **T**ricyclic antidepressants (TCAs) such as amitriptyline

E—*anti-***E**metics (promethazine, prochlorperazine, scopolamine, trimethobenzamide)

C—Corticosteroids

H—H2-blockers (cimetidine)

A—Anti-Parkinson (amantadine, levodopa, pramipexole, ropinirole, benztropine, trihexyphenidyl); **A**ntihistamines (hydroxyzine, diphenhydramine, loratadine); and **A**nti-spasmodic (dicyclomine, hyoscyamine, atropine products such as Lomotil)

N—NSAIDS (indomethacin)

G—Geri-psychiatric (antidepressants such as all TCAs, doxepin, paroxetine; anti-psychotics such as chlorpromazine, thioridazine, olanzapine, clozapine; sedatives such as barbiturates, benzodiazepines; mood stabilizers such as lithium, valproic acid)

E—ENT (meclizine), **E**TOH (alcohol intoxication or withdrawal)

I—Insomnia (most OTC sleep aids contain antihistamines like diphenhydramine, and herbal supplements such as valerian)

N—Narcotics (especially meperidine and pentazocine)

M—Muscle relaxants (baclofen, cyclobenzaprine, methocarbamol, carisoprodol)

S—Seizure (carbamazepine, levtiracetam, phenytoin, valproic acid[a])

[a]Most anticonvulsants are protein-bound and if the patient has poor nutrition, the amount of free (i.e., active) drug will be potentially higher than what is measured.
Abbreviations: H, histamine type 2 blockers; NSAIDS, nonsteroidal anti-inflammatory drugs; ENT, ears, nose and throat; ETOH, alcohol; OTC, over the counter.
Adapted from American Geriatrics Society. American Geriatrics Society updated Beers criteria for potentially inappropriate medications use in older adults. *J Am Geriatr Soc* 2012. All medications should be considered; this is not an exclusive list.

- *Dehydration and electrolyte abnormalities.* A third of the patients in one study arrived at the hospital dehydrated.[7]

Prevention

Primary prevention of delirium is probably the most effective treatment strategy.[4]

- The Yale Delirium Prevention Trial demonstrated the effectiveness of interventions targeting six risk factors: improving orientation and using therapeutic activities in the cognitively impaired, early mobilization, nonpharmacologic approaches to minimize the use of psychoactive drugs, interventions to prevent sleep deprivation, communication methods and adaptive equipment (i.e., eyeglasses and hearing aids) for vision and hearing impairment, and early intervention for volume depletion.[4,8] This strategy reduced delirium rates, but had no impact on delirium once it developed.[4]
- A proactive geriatric consultation reduced the incidence and severity of delirium in patients undergoing surgery for hip fracture. Goals included maintaining PO_2, hematocrit, systolic blood pressure, and correct fluid and electrolyte balance; management of pain; elimination of unnecessary medications; regulation of bowel/bladder function; adequate nutritional intake; early mobilization/rehabilitation; prevention of postoperative complications; providing appropriate environmental stimuli; and treating agitated delirium. This multicomponent strategy has a "number needed to treat (NNT)" of 5.6 cases to prevent one case of delirium. It had no impact on delirium once it started, or on patients with baseline dementia.[12]
- Haloperidol prophylaxis use in patients undergoing surgery for hip fractures did not prevent delirium. This study used low-dose haloperidol (1.5 mg per day) prophylaxis given preoperatively through postoperative day 3, and then doubled the dose if delirium occurred. It showed no difference in postoperative delirium rates, but did reduce the severity and duration of delirium episode and shorten hospital length of stay.[12]

Treatment

Once delirium develops, the emphasis switches to identification and treatment of the underlying cause(s) while maintaining safety and preventing complications.

- Correct all factors uncovered in the evaluation. Part of a comprehensive treatment strategy is to remove offending medications (Table 3.8-2).
- Provide supportive care such as nutrition, hydration, and prevent complications such as impaired mobility, pressure sores, and deep vein thrombosis.[8]
- If delirium is not resolved, reevaluate for underlying causes; follow up; and assess for possible dementia.[18]
- Behavioral nonpharmacological treatment strategies should be instituted for every patient with delirium.[8]
- Support mental stimulation. Orient patient unless reorientation causes agitation. Tolerate the patient's behavior as disagreeing may make agitation worse. Keep sentences short and simple. Explain all activities in simple terms prior to initiating activity. Use distraction to minimize agitation. Identify potential triggers and communicate findings to others. Increase sensory input by having patient wear eyeglasses and use hearing aids. Talk about current events and what is going on around the person. Have familiar objects brought from home.
- Support safety and physical activity. Promote early mobility, maintain self-care abilities, and involve physical/occupational therapy if needed. Implement scheduled toileting program.
- Modify environment to promote safety (remove hazards, bed at lowest level, etc.). Promote comfort and manage pain. Avoid restraints. Encourage family involvement and use sitters when family not available. Reassess need for invasive devices, such as IVs or foley catheters. If patient becomes agitated with a particular activity, stop that activity. Ensure that the patient is safe and approach again at a later time.
- Support healthy eating and drinking. Encourage food and drink; and provide hands-on assistance for those in need. Sometimes a simple intervention like an order: "offer food please," makes all the difference between a hungry dehydrated patient and a functional one. Ensure proper denture use and upright positioning.
- Support normal sleep–wake cycle. Promote sleep at night with a quiet room with low-level lighting. Encourage wakefulness during the day. Group medication administration and procedures (vital signs, blood draws, etc.) to allow uninterrupted sleep.[4,8]
- Support families. Provide education about delirium, its causes, and reversibility, and how to interact and family's role in restoring function. Families may have the same worries as the patient, and become frightened and disheartened instead of being hopeful and encouraging to the patient.[19]

Medications

Delirium is not the same as psychosis. There are no pharmacological agents approved by the US Food and Drug Administration (FDA) for delirium treatment. Furthermore, there is little evidence for both the

TABLE 3.8-3

Medication[a]	Suggestive dosing[8,18–20]	Comments
Haloperidol	0.25–1 mg orally every 4 h as needed	• Most widely used and studied[13,18] • QTc prolongation risk • Highly EPS, especially >3.5 mg/daily[13] • Nonsedative • Minimal anticholinergic effects • All routes available (oral/IM/IV)
Olanzapine	2.5–5 mg orally once or twice daily	• Some evidence to support its use[13,18] • Highly anticholinergic • Sedative • Weight gain • Available routes (oral/IM), not IV
Quetiapine	25–50 mg orally twice daily[b]	• Sizeable dose range • Very sedating, even at the lowest dose • Hypotension • No EPS
Risperidone	0.25–1 mg orally once or twice daily	• Dose-related EPS • >4 mg/d rarely more effective in elderly

EPS, extrapyramidal side effects; IM, intramuscular; IV, intravenous.
[a]All have black-box warning for increased mortality risk (especially strokes) in elderly dementia patients and lack FDA-approved labeling for delirium.
[b]Author recommends more conservative dosing (i.e., halved doses) in frail elderly patients.

off-label use, and the dosing of pharmacological agents for delirium treatment.[18] Haloperidol is the most used and studied pharmacologic agent for delirium treatment.[13,18] Atypical antipsychotics, compared to low-dose haloperidol (<3.5 mg per day), have been shown to be equivalent[12,13] and have no significance difference in adverse effects.[13] It is a common practice to use antipsychotics for cases involving distressed patients that are a risk to themselves or others, and when verbal/non-verbal de-escalation techniques are ineffective or inappropriate.[18] An example is a patient yanking on life-sustaining mechanical ventilation or central lines. See Table 3.8-3 for suggestive dosing. Start at the lowest clinically appropriate dose and titrate according to symptoms.[18] A cautious recommendation is to give pharmacologic treatment short term (i.e., 1 week or less).[18] Prophylactic use of either haloperidol or atypical antipsychotics to prevent delirium is not recommended, even in the ICU setting.[20] Benzodiazepines are not recommended for delirium except for alcohol or benzodiazepine withdrawal[11,18,19] as they can worsen confusion, behavioral disinhibition, and ataxia and increase falls.[21] Cholinesterase inhibitors are not effective.[12,19,22]

Referrals

Pharmacy consultants are very helpful resources. Other considerations are neurology or psychiatry consultation if the causes(s) of delirium remain elusive. Delirium is considered the great imitator among psychiatrists. Delirious patients can look psychotic, depressed, manic, anxious, or a combination of all four.

REFERENCES

1. Keeley P. Delirium at the end of life. *Am Fam Physician* 2010;81(10):1260–1261.
2. Flaherty JH. Delirium. In: Pathy MS, Sinclair AJ, Morley JE, eds. *Principles and practices of geriatrics medicine*. 4th ed. Chichester, UK: Wiley 2006:1047–1060.
3. American Psychiatric Association. *Diagnostic and statistical manual of mental disorders*. 5th ed. Washington, DC: American Psychiatric Publishing; 2013.
4. Inouye SK, Bogardus ST, Peter A, et al. A multicomponent intervention to prevent delirium in hospitalized older patients. *N Engl J Med* 1999;340(9):669–676.
5. Moller JT, Cluitmans P, Rasmussen, et al. Long-term postoperative cognitive dysfunction in the elderly ISPOCD1 study. ISPOCD investigators. International Study of Post-Operative Cognitive Dysfunction. *Lancet* 1998;351(9106):857–861.
6. Shi Q, Presutti R, Selchen D, et al. Delirium in acute stroke: a systematic review and meta-analysis. *Stroke* 2012;43:645–649.
7. Fick DM, Augustine JV, Inouye SK. Delirium superimposed on dementia: a systemic review. *J Am Geriatr Soc* 2002;50:1723–1732.
8. Inouye SK. Delirium in older persons. *N Engl J Med* 2006;354:1157–1165.
9. Cole MG, Ciampi A, Belzile E, et al. Persistent delirium in older hospital patients: a systematic review of frequency and prognosis. *Age Ageing* 2009;38(1):19–26.
10. Ryan DJ, O'Regan NA, Caoimh RO, et al. Delirium in an adult acute hospital population: predictors, prevalence and detection. *BMJ Open* 2013;3:e001772.
11. Lonergan E, Luxenberg J, Areosa S. Benzodiazepines for delirium. *Cochrane Database Syst Rev* 2009;(4): CD006379.
12. Siddiqi N, Holt R, Britton AM, et al. Interventions for preventing delirium in hospitalized patients. *Cochrane Database Syst Rev* 2007;(2):CD005563.
13. Lonergan E, Britton AM, Luxenberg J, et al. Antipsychotics for delirium. *Cochrane Database Syst Rev* 2007;(2):CD005594.
14. Inouye SK, Van Dyck CH, Alessi CA, et al. Clarifying confusion: the confusion assessment method. A new method for detection of delirium. *Ann Intern Med* 1990;113(12):941.
15. Miller M. Evaluation and management of delirium in hospitalized older patients. *Am Fam Physician* 2008;78(11):1265–1270.
16. Wei LA, Fearing MA, Sternberg EJ, et al. The confusion assessment method: a systemic review of current usage. *J Am Geriatr Soc* 2008;56(5):823.
17. American Medical Directors Association. *Urinary incontinence in the long term care setting clinical practice guideline*. Columbia, MD: AMDA; 2012.
18. National Clinical Guideline Centre. *Delirium: diagnosis, prevention and management*. Clinical Guideline 103. July, 2010. http://guidance.nice.org.uk/CG103/Guidance/pdf/English. Accessed February 26, 2014.
19. Barr J, Fraser GL, Puntillo K, et al. Clinical practice guidelines for the management of pain, agitation, and delirium in adult patients in the intensive care unit. *Crit Care Med* 2013;4(1):263–306.
20. Cook IA. *Guideline watch: practice guideline for the treatment of patients with delirium*. Arlington, VA: American Psychiatric Association; 2004.
21. American Geriatrics Society. American Geriatrics Society updated beers criteria for potentially inappropriate medications use in older adults. *J Am Geriatr Soc* 2012;60(4):616–631.
22. Overshott R, Karim S, Burns A. Cholinesterase inhibitors for delirium. *Cochrane Database Syst Rev* 2008;1:CD005317.

Problems of Infants and Children
Section Editor: Scott E. Moser

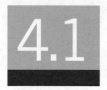

Developmental Problems in Children
Dennis J. Baumgardner

GENERAL PRINCIPLES
- Developmental problems of children include intellectual and special sensory deficits, motor dysfunction, and psychosocial disorders caused by nonprogressive central nervous system (CNS) dysfunction (behavioral problems are discussed in Chapter 4.9). Although up to 25% of children have developmental problems, diagnosis is often delayed owing to overreliance on normal variation as explanations of subtle findings, inattention to specific milestone delays when the child is otherwise normal, reliance on strictly clinical impressions or only on screening devices (failing to view each child as unique), and the physician's or parents' reluctance to discuss their fears. This problem is best approached by ongoing surveillance in the context of a continuing relationship with the family.[1–3]

DIAGNOSIS
History
- History should include open-ended questioning of the parents regarding their child's physical, cognitive, sensory, and social development, and any prior professional concern or workup. The medical history should document established developmental risk, such as known sensory deficit, chromosomal abnormality, myelomeningocele, and human immunodeficiency virus infection (which is associated with a spectrum of motor, cognitive, communication, social, and behavioral problems). For example, children with conditions such as cleft lip or palate may be otherwise unaffected or may experience physical or psychological developmental problems resulting from the cleft, and perhaps additional problems if the cleft is part of a syndrome. Sleep disorders may be a sign or sequela of developmental disorders, or (independently) negatively impact behavior, growth, cognition, or treatment plans.[4]
- Risk factor assessment builds on prenatal care assessment. Biological risk factors may be summarized as significant maternal disease, hazardous substance exposure, prematurity or obstetrical complication, congenital infection and malformation(s), and significant neonatal, infant, or childhood neurological, cardiopulmonary, infectious, somatic, or metabolic disease. Even early term infants (37 0/7 to 38 6/7 weeks) may be at risk for adverse neurodevelopmental outcomes.[5] Family history may reveal risk factors, such as familial developmental or sensory deficits, history of autism, or chromosomal abnormalities. Psychosocial risks include cognitive disability; serious emotional disturbance, substance abuse, or lack of parenting skills in caregivers; limited social or financial support; and stress, violence, or a history of abuse or neglect in the family.

Physical Examination
- Physical examination is essential for detection of risk, or workup of developmental delay.[2,3] Attention should be paid to growth abnormalities (including abnormal head circumference), signs of abuse, congenital anomalies, skin findings (e.g., neurofibromatosis, tuberous sclerosis, Sturge–Weber syndrome), eye findings (e.g., retinal pigmentation of Tay–Sachs), organomegaly (neurodegenerative disorders), postural and transition movement disorders, as well as the neurological examination. Facies may be indicative of a specific syndrome (e.g., fetal alcohol) or may lead to erroneous

conclusions. Many facially dysmorphic children have normal intelligence, whereas children deemed attractive may have any degree of cognitive impairment or autism. Red flags during history and physical examination are listed by Horridge.[2]

Developmental Surveillance

Developmental surveillance should be performed at each well-child visit by the use of milestones. This may be done "on the fly," along with immunizations, in children who are only presented for episodic care. The milestones in Table 4.1-1 were selected on the basis of objectivity, ease of parental recall or demonstration in the office, and uniformity (e.g., crawling is omitted because some children never demonstrate this prior to walking). The American Academy of Pediatrics recommends formal developmental screening at 9, 18, and 24 and/or 30 months, and autism-specific screening at the latter three time intervals.[1,6] Developmental delay is defined as actual development that is 25% (or 2 standard deviations) or more behind the expected rate, corrected for gestation, in any or all of the major streams of development (motor, speech and language, personal/social skills, and play/activities of daily living). The term global developmental delay is used when two or more streams are involved.[3]

Key points regarding milestones include the fact that development should occur in an orderly, predictable, intrinsically controlled fashion,[3] although often in spurts. A lost developmental skill, at any

Table 4.1-1	Developmental Milestones

1 mo
  Raises head when lying prone (GM)
  Retains a ring or rattle (FM)
  Gives alerting response (1 wk) (A/L/C)
  Regards face in direct line of vision (Vis, FM)
2 mo
  Raises chest when lying prone (GM)
  Social smiling (6 wk) and cooing (A/L/C)
  Follows moving object across midline (Vis, FM)
3 mo
  Up on elbows when prone (GM)
  Hands unfisted more than half of time (FM)
  Blinks to visual threat (Vis)
4 mo
  Up on hands when prone (GM)
  No head lag when pulled to sitting (GM)
  Brings hands together (FM)
  Orients to voice (A/L/C)
  Symmetrical corneal light reflexes and normal eye cover testing (Vis)
5 mo
  Sits with support (GM)
  Transfers objects (FM)
  Laughs (A/L/C)
6 mo
  Sits with minimal support (GM)
  Has unilateral reach (FM)
  Babbles (A/L/C)
7 mo
  Sits without support (GM)
  Takes pellet (crude grasp) (FM)
  Searches for dropped object (A/L/C)
8 mo
  Comes to sitting position (GM)
  Has immature pincer grasp (FM)
  Says dada/mama (inappropriate) (A/L/C)

(continued)

Table 4.1-1	Developmental Milestones *(continued)*

9 mo
  Stands holding on (GM)
  Bangs blocks together (FM)
  Plays peek-a-boo (A/L/C)
12 mo
  Walks with minimal assistance (GM)
  Has mature pincer grasp (10 mo) (FM)
  Releases voluntarily (FM)
  Says dada/mama (appropriate) and two other words (A/L/C)
  Searches for hidden object (A/L/C)
  Follows simple verbal commands (with gestures) (A/L/C)
  Drinks from cup (PS)
15 mo
  Walks alone well (GM)
  Puts in and takes out (pellets in a bottle) (FM)
  Follows simple verbal commands (without gestures) (A/L/C)
  Has three- to six-word vocabulary (A/L/C)
18 mo
  Climbs (GM)
  Stacks three or four blocks (FM)
  Knows three body parts (A/L/C)
  Imitates housework (A/L/C)
  Uses spoon (PS)
2 yr
  Runs (GM)
  Stacks four or five blocks (FM)
  Has 50-word vocabulary (A/L/C)
  Uses some two- to three-word sentences (A/L/C)
  Enjoys being read to, points to objects in book (A/L/C)
3 yr
  Walks up and down stairs, alternating feet (GM)
  Balances on one foot for 1 s (GM)
  Stacks nine blocks (FM)
  Copies a circle (FM)
  Knows own name and sex (A/L/C)
  Uses three- to four-word sentences (A/L/C)
  Dresses self except for buttons (PS)
4 yr
  Hops on one foot (GM)
  Throws a ball (GM)
  Copies a circle and a cross (FM)
  Counts to four (A/L/C)
  Recognizes three or four colors (A/L/C)
5 yr
  Walks heel-to-toe or skips (GM)
  Balances on one foot for 5–10 s (GM)
  Builds a stairway or building with blocks (FM)
  Copies a square (FM)
  Counts to 10 (A/L/C)
  Follows three commands (A/L/C)

A/L/C, auditory/linguistic/cognitive; FM, fine motor; GM, gross motor milestone; PS, personal/social; Vis, visual.

age, is a red flag. Parents and providers may focus on growth in the first 8 to 10 months, disregarding gross motor delay. Similarly, gross motor surveillance may overshadow that of fine motor development, the latter often being the earliest indicator of motor disability (hypertonia or primitive reflexes may mimic normal gross motor development in cerebral palsy). Warning flags are abnormal head size and failure to have hands unfisted at least 50% of the time by 3 months, inability to hold an object placed in the hand by 5 months, and lack of appreciation of object permanence by the end of the first year. The presence of handedness earlier than 18 months may represent an opposite-side hemiplegia. Gross motor achievement may be falsely reassuring because it does not indicate intelligence. Language development and early vocabulary are predictive of intellectual potential.

Linguistic capacity develops in sequential, critically timed phases and depends on the adequacy of stored utterances (receptive vocabulary) in infancy. A common pitfall is to ignore a language milestone delay until age 2. Articulation problems are often not identified by the parents. Specific red flags for autism spectrum disorders include no babbling or pointing by 12 months, no sharing of interest in objects with another person; no single words by 16 months, or no two-word spontaneous phrases by 24 months; any loss of language or social skills at any age; and stereotyped mannerisms, compulsive routines, and abnormal sensitivities or sensory behaviors. See Horridge[2] for other disease-specific milestones.

Further Assessment

- There is no routine laboratory workup. Normal hearing and vision should be confirmed. The results of state screening for certain inborn metabolic disorders must be known, and testing augmented if there is plateau or loss of milestone skills, vomiting and lethargy, movement or cutaneous disorders, failure to thrive, unusual body odor, or suggestive family history. Thyroid disorders should be ruled out, and complete blood count and blood chemistries are frequently obtained. Appropriate lead screening must be undertaken because relatively low-level toxicity can lead to impairment (see Chapter 1.1). Chromosomal microarray is now considered first-line testing. Children with abnormal muscle tone should be screened with creatinine phosphokinase. Chromosomal mosaicism may present subtle findings and be missed by amniocentesis. DNA testing for fragile X and specialized genetic testing is done as indicated. Learning disabilities are confirmed by neuropsychometric testing. Neuroimaging is indicated for children with focal neurologic findings, developmental regression, clinical diagnosis of cerebral palsy or stroke, abnormal head growth, craniofacial anomalies, many genetic syndromes, seizures, sensory impairments, and other unexplained findings.[2,3]

SPECIFIC SYNDROMES AND MANAGEMENT

Learning disabilities (100/1,000 children) involve "a discrepancy between a person's overall intellectual ability and actual academic performance."[7] They include specific, sometimes multiple, skill deficits in reading (dyslexia), written expression or mathematics. Etiologic factors are both genetic and neuroanatomic. Manifestations include increased effort to learn, and school distress or failure. Learning disabilities are associated with increased comorbidities, including depression, anxiety, substance abuse, and sleep and eating disorders. Sensory deficits and other disorders must be ruled out. Preschool diagnosis is often difficult, and problems may not arise until adolescence, and persist or even present in adulthood. Treatment should be individualized, in the context of the family, with the focus on educational therapy.[7]

Intellectual disability (12/1,000 children) is defined as deficits in intellectual functioning and adaptive behavior, with onset during the developmental period. Historically this would include an IQ of 70 to 75 or below (measured at age 5 or beyond), and deficits in at least 2 of the following 10 areas of adaptation: communication, self-care, home living, social skills, community use, self-direction, health and safety, functional academics, leisure, and work. These deficits may result from a variety of diseases or conditions, or no etiology may be found. Linguistic deficits contribute to the emotional and behavioral disorders that often occur.[8]

Cerebral palsy (2–3/1,000 children) is a collection of disorders that variably manifest as abnormal motion and posture caused by early nonprogressive, CNS injury (commonly during intrauterine development). It may be classified by type of motor impairment (hypertonia, hypotonia, dystonia, paresis, dyskinesia, ataxia), the area of cerebral dysfunction (pyramidal or extrapyramidal), and part of body involved. Associated impairments may include cognitive (50%), communicative, sensory perception, psychosocial, and seizures. Early neuroimaging (positive in 80%) is the most direct indication of pathogenesis, but a specific diagnosis often does not imply a specific prognosis. Treatment may include neurosurgery or orthopedic surgery or devices; PT, OT, and/or speech/nutrition therapy; medical treatment for seizures, spasticity (potentially including oral or intrathecal baclofen, or botulism toxin injections), pain, constipation, and gastroesophageal reflux and other symptoms.[9]

Autism spectrum disorder (11/1,000 children) is characterized by varying degrees of pervasive deficits of social communication and interaction, and restricted and repetitive patterns of behavior and interests. Symptoms are present in early childhood, but care may be sought at any age. There may be associated intellectual or language disabilities.[6] Exact etiology is unknown; multiple genes are involved. Up to 25% of patients manifest seizures. Early, sustained, multidisciplinary medical, educational, language, behavioral, and family therapy, and highly predictable daily routines and preparedness are treatment mainstays.[6,10] Medications targeting specific behaviors may be useful. Examples would include aripiprazole or risperidone for irritability and aggression, hyperactivity, and stereotypy, and methylphenidate for hyperactivity.[6]

Hearing impairment (6/1,000 children). Risk factors of hearing loss include family history, congenital infections, craniofacial anomalies, low birth weight, severe hyperbilirubinemia, bacterial meningitis, asphyxia, ototoxic medications, mechanical ventilation, extracorporal membrane oxygenation, and certain syndromes that may include hearing loss. Many cases will be missed by relying on risk-based screening. Universal newborn hearing screening is recommended. Prompt recognition and treatment, including early sign language instruction, can maximize language skill development and social and emotional growth.[11]

Visual impairment (25/1,000 children) is present in many of those with developmental disorders. Conversely, an increased prevalence of developmental problems is seen in the visually impaired. Careful screening (as recently reviewed[12]), prompt diagnosis, and referral to an ophthalmologist skilled in the care of children are essential.

Down syndrome (1/1,000 children), or trisomy 21, is a common cause of intellectual disability and may serve as a prototype for other chromosomal abnormalities with a wide range of medical, developmental, sensory, and emotional manifestations. Specific Down syndrome growth charts should be used along with screening for heart and visual defects, hypothyroidism, atlantoaxial instability, symptoms of celiac disease, and other associated conditions. Frequent office visits and provider education are required to anticipate and manage the various problems of children with any chromosomal abnormality or syndrome (Chapter 14.3).

Other specific chromosomal disorders such as Klinefelter syndrome (47,XXY) and trisomy X (47,XXX) may include various degrees of intellectual disabilities or behavioral problems. Other examples include microdeletions such as Williams (7q23–), Prader–Willi (15q11–13 paternal), Angelman (15q11–13 maternal), velocardiofacial-DiGeorge (22q11–), chromosomal mosaicism, and other syndromes. These and many other genetic abnormalities also frequently exhibit attention deficit hyperactivity disorder and autism spectrum phenotypes; distinctions between syndromic and non-syndromic developmental problems may be less valid.[13]

Fetal alcohol spectrum disorders (0.5/1,000 to 9/1,000 children). Fetal alcohol syndrome is diagnosed by documentation of maternal alcohol exposure and (a) 2/3 specific facial abnormalities (smooth philtrum, thin vermillion border, small palpebral fissures); (b) growth deficit; and (c) CNS abnormalities. Additional facial and hand abnormalities may be present in varying degrees. Partial syndromes are seen. CNS impairment may not be apparent in the newborn; however, lifelong consequences occur. Behavioral, learning, and adaptive difficulties are often greater than the degree of neurocognitive impairment, and may be increased by comorbid conditions and environmental exposures. Alcohol-related neurodevelopmental disorder may be present without the typical facial features. Treatment includes referral to a multidisciplinary team, and individualized interventions to stabilize the home environment and improve parent–child-school and peer interactions.[14]

Fragile X syndrome (0.25/1,000), the most common inherited cause of intellectual disability, occurs in both men and women due to a mutation that causes expansion of a CGG-trinucleotide repeat unit found on the X chromosome. In affected families, the mutation is inherited in an unstable fashion and undergoes intergenerational expansions. This syndrome can cause cognitive deficits ranging from subtle learning disabilities with a normal IQ to severe intellectual disability with social avoidance, poor adaptation, and autistic behaviors. Females and those with fewer CGG repeats may be more mildly affected. Classic findings include the triad of prominent ears, a long, narrow face, and macro-orchidism (in boys). These and other variable findings, including connective tissue dysplasias, dental and ocular abnormalities, chronic otitis media, seizures, constipation (particularly if medicated), may be subtle and less apparent in the younger child. Thus, this diagnosis should be considered in every child with delay in cognitive, adaptive, or communication milestones. DNA blood testing is diagnostic. Early intervention with appropriate therapies (medications, if needed) and family genetic counseling is beneficial.[15]

Failure to thrive (retarded physical growth) may be due to inadequate caloric intake or absorption, ineffective utilization, or excessive caloric expenditure. Causes include a variety of psychosocial, environmental, neurological, and anatomical factors and their interactions. Excellent reviews are available.[1,16] Prompt recognition and treatment are important. Prognosis is then generally favorable in full-term infants without serious underlying disorders, although long-term effects on academic performance are uncertain.

Comprehensive primary care for children with developmental delay includes a medical home with coordination and management of a team of medical and sometimes surgical and dental specialists, social workers, counselors (genetic, parental, family), habilitation or rehabilitation therapists, medical device services, and special educators. Goals must be agreed on between physician, family, therapists, and educators and written progress reports shared. Knowledge of community and social services as well as advocacy for the child and family is essential. Equally essential is prevention of exploitation, substance abuse, and incarceration in those at risk.[14]

Advice for the parents begins with frank, factual, unhurried, and compassionate discussions as soon as the diagnosis of delay is entertained.[9] Avoid speculation regarding intelligence and unnecessary pessimism. Expectations often affect outcomes: Low expectations may be a self-fulfilling prophecy. Helpful advice for rearing a child with special needs includes empowering parents,[2] setting realistic goals, having routines, avoiding hours spent finding the "perfect educational toy," and acknowledging the child's own agenda (not feeling like one has to be teaching the child every minute to "catch up"). Maximizing communication in children with language disorders and helping parents foster special gifts of their child (which often include empathy, enthusiasm, and remarkable attention to detail) should help minimize the child's frustration and consequent additional emotional, behavioral, or social disturbances. Sports activities, including Special Olympics, are often helpful for weight management, fitness, development of physical coordination, and improvement of self-esteem. Often activities involving gross motor skills are most appropriate, with attention to specific instances that increase the risk of injuries (e.g., atlantoaxial instability in Down syndrome). Consistent discipline, appropriate for the level of understanding, is important for the child, particularly in the context of his or her siblings (the child with special needs should not "get away with something" at a given developmental age if the siblings did not). Parents should avoid allowing undesirable behaviors, such as chewing on a book, because this is "progress," only to have to work very hard later to extinguish the behavior. For many older children, consider the advice of Copeland: Every child should know,(a) Where am I going? (b) What am I supposed to do when I get there? (c) How do I know if I'm doing a good job? (d) When will I be done? (e) What happens when I finish? (f) What's next?[10]

Transition to adulthood needs to be planned for. Guardianship must be established (rules vary among states). Transfers to adult-oriented specialists, therapists, jobs, recreational activities, insurance, social services, and governmental agencies must be anticipated. The family practice medical home is an excellent place of continuity for the transitioning young adult. Advocacy by the parent/guardian is important. Parents may need to consider children with rare or undefined syndromes as belonging to a broader diagnostic category in order to access support groups and needed services.

PREVENTION

• Involves optimization of preconceptual, prenatal (Chapter 14.4), and postnatal care. This includes not only avoidance of untoward exposure; early identification of toxic, metabolic, sensory, and medical disorders; and appropriate therapy and optimization of neurologic outcome; but also providing a nurturing environment. For the very premature, this should include careful application of appropriate stimuli and protected rest time. For the child in an at-risk home environment, a combination of social services, parental counseling and support groups, and an interested provider may improve outcome. Early exposure to books to encourage literacy and vocabulary building is recommended for all children. Finally, early identification of developmental delay or risk affords the best chance for affecting developmental change via a still malleable nervous system.[1,6,10,11,14] It also empowers the family to be proactive in maximizing the child's abilities, perhaps avoiding secondary emotional and physical disability.

REFERENCES

1. Grissom M, Chauhan A, Mendez R. Disorders of childhood growth and development. *FP Essent* 2013;410:11–44.
2. Horridge KA. Assessment and investigation of the child with disordered development. *Arch Dis Child Educ Pract Ed* 2011;96:9–20.
3. Silove N, Collins F, Ellaway C. Update on the investigation of children with delayed development. *J Paediatr Child Health* 2013;49:519–525.

4. Bonuck K, Grant R. Sleep problems and early developmental delay: implications for early intervention programs. *Intellect Dev Disabil* 2012;50:41–52.
5. Dong Y, Chen S, Yu J. A systematic review and meta-analysis of long-term development of early term infants. *Neonatology* 2012;102:212–221.
6. Volkmar F, Siegel M, Woodbury-Smith M, et al. Practice parameter for the assessment and treatment of children and adolescents with autism spectrum disorder. *J Am Acad Child Adolesc Psychiatry* 2014;53:237–257.
7. Rimrodt SL, Lipkin PH. Learning disabilities and school failure. *Pediatr Rev* 2011;32:315–323.
8. Tirosh E, Jaffe M. Global developmental delay and mental retardation—a pediatric perspective. *Dev Disabil Res Rev* 2011;17:85–92.
9. Aisen ML, Kerkovich D, Mast J, et al. Cerebral palsy: clinical care and neurological rehabilitation. *Lancet Neurol* 2011;10:844–852.
10. Copeland L. Help across the spectrum: a developmental pediatrician's perspective on diagnosing and treating autism spectrum disorders. *J Soc Work Disabil Rehabil* 2012;11:1–32.
11. Pimperton H, Kennedy CR. The impact of early identification of permanent childhood hearing impairment on speech and language outcomes. *Arch Dis Child* 2012;97:648–653.
12. Bell AL, Rodes ME, Kellar LC. Childhood eye examination. *Am Fam Physician* 2013;88:241–248.
13. Vorstman JAS, Ophall RA. Genetic causes of developmental disorders. *Curr Opin Neurol* 2013;26:128–136.
14. Paintner A, Williams AD, Burd L. Fetal alcohol spectrum disorders-implications for child neurology, part 2: diagnosis and management. *J Child Neurol* 2012;355–362.
15. Hersh JH, Saul RA; Committee on Genetics. Clinical report-health supervision for children with fragile X syndrome. *Pediatrics* 2011;127:994–1006.
16. Cole SZ, Lanham JS. Failure to thrive: an update. *Am Fam Physician* 2011;83:829–834.

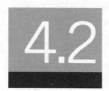

4.2 Fever in Infancy and Childhood

Peter H. Forman

GENERAL PRINCIPLES
Definition

- Fever is the elevation of body temperature to 38°C (100.4°F) or higher. Rectal temperature most accurately reflects core temperature, especially in infants. Oral or tympanic temperatures are suitable for older children but can be inaccurate.

Epidemiology

- Fever is a prominent symptom of many diseases in infants and children. Fever, as a presenting complaint, accounts for nearly one-third of pediatric outpatient visits in the United States.[1]

Pathophysiology

- Infectious agents, toxins, or mediators of inflammation stimulate monocytes, macrophages, and other cell types to release interleukin-1 (IL-1), tumor necrosis factor (TNF), IL-6, and interferons (IFNs) that act on the anterior hypothalamus (antipyretics act here). This elevates the thermoregulatory set point causing increased heat conservation and increased heat production. This process results in fever.

DIAGNOSIS
History

- Duration, height, and pattern of fever
- Constitutional: Sleepy, cranky
- Respiratory: Rhinorrhea, sore throat, otalgia, and cough
- Gastrointestinal: Vomiting and diarrhea

- Urinary: Dysuria, frequency (often absent in infants)
- Pronounced lethargy and/or irritability are red flags for serious bacterial infection (SBI)
- Noninfectious: Collagen vascular disease, malignancy, or metabolic disorder, such as hyperthyroidism; salicylate or anticholinergic poisoning; and excessive environmental temperature

Physical Examination

- Observation of the older infant or child is very helpful in determining the index of suspicion for a serious bacterial infection (SBI). A pink, alert, well-hydrated, smiling, or easily consoled infant is much less likely to have an SBI than a pale, lethargic, dehydrated, dull, or irritable child.[2]

Skin

- Petechial rash (meningococcemia)
- Maculopapular rash followed by petechial rash (Rocky Mountain spotted fever)
- Sandpaper papular rash (Strep A infection)

Head

- Bulging fontanel or nuchal rigidity (meningitis)

Eyes

- Conjunctivitis (otitis media [OM]; Kawasaki disease; measles with cough; coryza)

Ears

- Red, dull, nonmobile tympanic membranes (OM)

Nose

- Purulent rhinorrhea (sinusitis)
- Nasal flaring (pneumonia or respiratory distress)

Throat

- Stridor (laryngotracheobronchitis, i.e., croup)
- Stridor with drooling, dysphagia, or aphonia (epiglottitis)
- Petechiae on soft palate and uvula (streptococcal pharyngitis)
- Vesicles or ulcers on tongue, lips, and buccal mucosa (herpes stomatitis)
- Strawberry tongue (streptococcal pharyngitis, Kawasaki disease)

Chest

- Tachypnea, retractions, decreased breath sounds, crackles (pneumonia)
- Ronchi (bronchitis)
- Wheezing (bronchiolitis, asthma, inhaled foreign body)

Cardiac

- Murmur (subacute bacterial endocarditis, rheumatic fever; pulmonic flow murmur may be normal due to increased cardiac output from the fever itself)

Abdomen

- Local tenderness worsening with movement (appendicitis or peritonitis)

Musculoskeletal

- Refuses to bear weight or use the extremity (septic arthritis, osteomyelitis)

LABORATORY STUDIES

No test can detect every SBI in all febrile children, but the following values in infants older than 28 days deserve further investigation:

- White blood cell (WBC) count of 15,000 per μL or more or WBC count of less than 5,000 per μL
- Absolute band count of 1,500 per μL or higher
- Presence of toxic granulation or vacuolization in neutrophils

Further Investigative Studies

- *Urinalysis with culture* should be considered in male infants younger than 6 months of age, older uncircumcised male infants, and female infants younger than 2 years old when fever does not have an obvious source.

- *Blood culture* should be considered in the child younger than 36 months who is at high risk for SBI, as indicated by physical examination, fever of 39°C or higher, or WBC count of 15,000 per μL or greater.
- *Lumbar puncture* should be performed in the presence of symptoms or signs suggestive of meningitis, such as excessive irritability or lethargy, seizures, or bulging fontanel.
- *Stool smear* of bloody or mucoid diarrhea demonstrating five or more WBCs per high-power field (hpf) suggests bacterial enteritis warranting stool culture for *Salmonella*, *Shigella*, *Campylobacter*, *Yersinia*, or pathogenic *Escherichia coli*.

Imaging

- Chest radiography is indicated in the presence of pulmonary symptoms, such as tachypnea. Rales are not always heard in young children with pneumonia. If any of the following are present, there is a 33% chance of findings on chest x-ray: respiratory rate greater than 50, coryza, cough, nasal flaring, grunting, stridor, rales, rhonchi or wheezing, or WBC >20,000.
- *If none are present, there is a less than 1% chance of findings on chest x-ray.*[3]

TREATMENT

Behavioral

- Avoid fever phobia by educating parents that fever is a symptom of an underlying illness and is itself seldom dangerous.[4] The primary reason to treat fever is to make the child more comfortable.

Medications

- Fever of 38.9°C (102°F) or higher may be treated with acetaminophen, 10 to 15 mg/kg/dose q4h up to maximum of five doses per day, or ibuprofen, 5 to 10 mg/kg/dose q6–8h in children 6 months or older. The child may subsequently be sponged with lukewarm water if the temperature exceeds 40°C (104°F). The child should be encouraged to drink liquids and may be covered with a light blanket.

Special Therapy

Management of the Febrile Child at Risk for a Serious Bacterial Infection

Low-risk criteria apply to those previously healthy term infants who appear generally well (nontoxic) and have no focal bacterial infection except OM. Laboratory studies include total WBC of 5,000 to 15,000 per μL, absolute bands less than 1,500 per μL, urinalysis less than 5 WBCs per hpf or negative Gram stain result, and stool with less than 5 WBCs per hpf. These criteria do not exclude all infants with SBI but have a negative predictive value of about 98% to 99%.[5]

- **Infants younger than 28 days** should undergo a sepsis workup in the hospital and receive parenteral antibiotics pending culture results.
- **Infants 28 to 90 days old** who are toxic or at high risk should be admitted for sepsis workup and treatment. Incidence of SBI in children under 3 months old is estimated at 6% to 10%.[6] Infants who are nontoxic and at low risk may be evaluated and treated as outpatients, provided they have reliable caretakers and follow-up. Following cultures of the blood, urine, and cerebrospinal fluid (CSF), ceftriaxone (Rocephin), 50 mg per kg IM, up to 1 g maximum, should be administered. The child must be re-evaluated within 24 hours.[7]
- **Nontoxic infants aged 3 to 36 months** with a temperature less than 39°C should have fever treated symptomatically. Focal symptoms should be addressed, but the child reexamined if he or she appears worse or the fever lasts longer than 48 hours.
- **Nontoxic infants aged 3 to 36 months** with a temperature of 39°C or higher should have screening WBC count and blood culture if there is no obvious focus for infection. Incidence of SBI on children greater than 3 months is estimated at 5% to 7%.[6] Girls younger than 2 years and boys younger than 6 months (or older if uncircumcised) should have a urine culture. Chest radiography, lumbar puncture, or stool specimen should be obtained if clinically appropriate. Empirical antibiotic treatment with ceftriaxone or amoxicillin–clavulanate (Augmentin), 40 mg/kg/day of amoxicillin divided in three doses, may be considered,[7] especially if the WBC count is 15,000 per mL or greater. Oral cefixime (Suprax) 16 mg per kg on day 1 followed by 8 mg/kg/day for a total of 14 days may be used to manage urinary tract infection (UTI).[9]

Follow-Up of Infants and Children With Fever Without Source

- **Infants 28 to 90 days old** must be rechecked within 24 hours. A second dose of ceftriaxone may then be given. OM or UTI may be treated on an outpatient basis in afebrile, nontoxic, and non-bacteremia children. The afebrile well-appearing child with *Streptococcus pneumoniae* bacteremia may also be treated with oral antibiotics. Children who are still febrile, appear ill, or have a positive CSF culture result, or bacteremia other than antibiotic-sensitive *S. pneumoniae* should be admitted for sepsis workup and treatment.

- **Children 3 to 36 months old** should be rechecked in 24 to 48 hours.[8] If the child is afebrile and non-toxic, antibiotics can be discontinued after 48 hours. Oral antibiotics should be given for OM, UTIs, or antibiotic-sensitive *S. pneumoniae* bacteremia. Children who are still febrile, appear ill, or have a positive CSF culture result require further evaluation or parenteral antibiotic treatment, or both.
- **Structural evaluation of the urinary tract** should be performed on boys and young girls after their first documented UTI using bladder and renal ultrasound.

Complications

- Treatment of febrile seizures
  - Febrile seizures occur in 2% to 5% of febrile children between the ages of 6 months and 5 years. Seizures that are complex, occur upon arrival in the emergency department, or are accompanied by abnormal neurologic findings are a red flag that causes such as meningitis should be investigated. Lumbar puncture should be strongly considered in infants younger than 12 months presenting with their first febrile seizure.[10]
  - Simple seizures are generalized tonic–clonic events that last less than 15 minutes and do not recur within 24 hours.[10]
  - Complex seizures last longer than 15 minutes, demonstrate focal signs, or recur within 24 hours or in a flurry.[10]
- Ensuring adequate airway, breathing, and circulation is all that is usually required for a short febrile seizure. Intravenous lorazepam (0.05 to 0.1 mg per kg over 2 to 5 minutes) may be used for prolonged seizures or those compromising the child's cardiorespiratory status. If necessary, lorazepam may be repeated, but the clinician should be prepared to assist the child's ventilation. Rarely, intravenous phenytoin (15 to 20 mg per kg) is given slowly (1 mg/kg/minute) for persistent seizure. Rectal diazepam (0.5 mg per kg to maximum dose of 5 mg) is 80% effective in controlling febrile seizures.[11]
- Recurrent febrile seizures may occur in 50% of children younger than 12 months and 30% of children older than 12 months at the time of their first simple seizure. Recurrent seizures are also more likely if seizures were complex, multiple, or occurred in children with underlying neurologic abnormalities or a history of afebrile seizures.[12] Epilepsy may develop in 1% to 2.4% of children with simple febrile seizures (see Chapter 6.4).
- Prophylaxis of febrile seizures is rarely indicated for simple seizures but may be used for frequent or severe seizures. Phenobarbital at a blood level of 15 mg per mL is effective but causes behavioral side effects in 20% to 40% of children. Valproic acid is effective in children but can cause fatal liver failure in addition to thrombocytopenia, gastrointestinal disturbances, and pancreatitis in those younger than 3 years. Oral diazepam given at the time of fever reduces the risk of febrile seizures but can cause lethargy and ataxia that could mask a central nervous system (CNS) infection.[12]

REFERENCES

1. Finkelstien JA, Christiansen CL, Platt R. Fever in pediatric primary care: occurrence, management, and outcomes. *Pediatrics* 2000;105:260.
2. McCarthy PL. Observation scales to identify serious illness in febrile children. *Pediatrics* 1982; 70:802–809.
3. Harper M. Update on the management of the febrile infant. *Clin Pediatr Emerg Med* 2004;5(1):5–12.
4. Schmitt BD. Fever phobia. *Am J Dis Child* 1980;134:176–181.
5. Jaskiewicz JA, McCarthy CA, Richardson AC, et al; Febrile Infant Collaborative Study Group. Febrile infants at low risk for serious bacterial infection: an appraisal of the Rochester criteria and implications for management. *Pediatrics* 1994;94:390–396.
6. Rajan A, Prashant M. Evaluation of child with fever without source. *Pediatr Clin North Am* 2013;60:1049–1062.
7. Baraff LJ, Schriger DL, Bass JW, et al. Practice guideline for the management of infants and children 0 to 36 months of age with fever without source. *Pediatrics* 1993;92:1–12.
8. Bass JW, Steele RW, Wittler RR, et al. Antimicrobial treatment of occult bacteremia: a multicenter cooperative study. *Pediatr Infect Dis J* 1993;12:466–473.
9. Hoberman A, Wald ER, Hickey RW, et al. Oral versus initial intravenous therapy for urinary tract infections in young febrile children. *Pediatrics* 1999;104:79–86.

10. Provisional Committee on Quality Improvement, Subcommittee on Febrile Seizures. Practice parameter: the neurodiagnostic evaluation of the child with a first simple febrile seizure. In: *Clinical practice guidelines of the American Academy of Pediatrics.* 2nd ed. Elk Grove Village, IL: American Academy of Pediatrics; 1999:73–85.
11. Fishman MA. Febrile seizures. In: McMillan JA, ed. *Oski's pediatrics: principles and practice.* 3rd ed. Philadelphia, PA: Lippincott Williams & Wilkins; 1999:1949–1952.
12. Committee on Quality Improvement, Subcommittee on Febrile Seizures. Practice parameter: long-term treatment of the child with simple febrile seizures. In: *Clinical practice guidelines of the American Academy of Pediatrics.* 2nd ed. Elk Grove Village, IL: American Academy of Pediatrics; 1999: 105–115.

4.3 Inspiratory Stridor, Croup, and Epiglottitis

Neil S. Skolnik, Megan C. Madsen

GENERAL PRINCIPLES

Inspiratory stridor is a syndrome of upper airway obstruction characterized by a harsh sound on inspiration. Etiologic factors include croup, epiglottitis, retropharyngeal abscess, peritonsillar abscess, foreign body, extrinsic laryngeal compression (tumor, cyst, hematoma), angioedema, laryngeal webs, vascular rings, bacterial tracheitis, acquired or congenital subglottic stenosis, and laryngomalacia.

Viral croup, synonymous with laryngotracheobronchitis, is the most common form of upper airway obstruction in children aged 6 months to 6 years. It is caused by inflammation and resultant mucosal edema of the subglottic region of the larynx. Parainfluenza viruses and rhinovirus are the most frequent etiologies of croup, accounting for up to 75% of cases. A more concerning cause of inspiratory stridor is epiglottitis, a bacterial infection of the epiglottis that causes acute upper airway obstruction. Most often caused by *Haemophilus influenzae* type b infection, epiglottitis has been virtually eradicated since the introduction of routine immunization with *H. influenzae* vaccine (see Chapter 1.1).

CROUP

Clinical Presentation

The mean age of children presenting with croup is 18 months, with age ranging from 6 months to 6 years. Croup is most common in early fall and winter and is typically preceded by a couple of days of fever, coryza, and pharyngitis followed by hoarseness and a "croupy" or barking cough.

The illness is characterized by varying degrees of respiratory distress. Severe cases may progress to inspiratory stridor, flaring of the alae nasi, and suprasternal and intercostal retractions. Often parents report symptoms are worse at nighttime. Physical exam generally reveals clear lungs, but about 5% of the time there is associated wheezing. Pulse oximetry is often normal unless severe disease is present.

Diagnostic Studies

Usually no diagnostic studies are needed, and the diagnosis of croup can be made on the basis of clinical assessment. X-ray evaluation of the upper airway is often performed but does not adequately exclude a diagnosis of epiglottitis, and manipulation of the child to image the neck could cause further compromise to airway patency. Lateral neck radiography may show widening of the hypopharynx. Posteroanterior radiographs may show a narrowed subglottic region known as a steeple sign. Classic signs of croup on radiography are seen only about half the time. On laboratory evaluation, white blood cell counts are usually normal or mildly elevated but are greater than 15,000 per mm^3, approximately 20% of the time.

Treatment

The first decision in the treatment of croup is whether a child should be treated in an outpatient or inpatient setting. Indications for hospitalization include age less than 6 months, cyanosis or pallor,

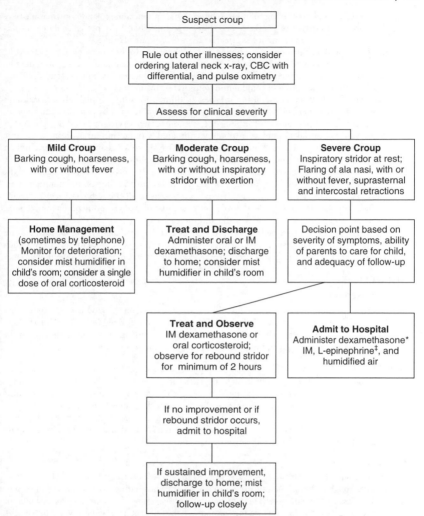

Figure 4.3-1. An algorithm for the treatment of croup. *, dosage 0.6 mg per kg; ‡, dosage L-epinephrine 1:1,000, see text for dose. (From Skolnik NS. Croup. *J Fam Pract* 1993;37:168, with permission. Copyrighted 2014. IMNG. 111815:814BN.)

stridor at rest, respiratory distress, a toxic-appearing child, and hypoxemia. A helpful algorithm for treatment is shown in Figure 4.3-1. As an initial approach to treatment, children should be kept calm during examination as agitation or crying may worsen stridor. Supplemental oxygen should be administered for patients with hypoxia or severe respiratory distress.

- **Humidified air.** Provision of humidified air, either by having the parent hold the child in his or her arms in the bathroom at home with the shower turned on to generate steam or by using a croup tent in the hospital may be reasonable; however, studies have shown little efficacy for the use of humidified air in the acute care setting.
- **Adrenal corticosteroids.** Adrenal corticosteroids should be given to all children with croup. Even in mild cases, benefits include a decrease in hospitalization and intubation rate.[1] Dexamethasone, 0.6 mg per kg IM or PO, is effective in decreasing airway obstruction, but it has a slow onset of

action and often does not take effect for up to 6 hours. Oral and intramuscular dexamethasone have equivalent efficacies. Alternatively, a single oral dose of prednisolone 1 mg per kg could be considered, but this appears to be somewhat less effective than oral dexamethasone.[2]

- **Nebulized budesonide.** Budesonide is a highly potent topical steroid that can be administered by nebulizer. It has a short onset of action and is effective in decreasing inspiratory stridor. It should be considered as an alternative for children who are unable to take oral steroids. Inhaled steroids do not show additive effects when given in conjunction with oral or IM dosing.
- L-**Epinephrine** (1:1,000) at a dose of 0.5 mL per kg diluted in 3 mL normal saline (maximum doses: <4 years 2.5 mL per dose; >4 years 5 mL per dose) administered by nebulizer can be given to acutely decrease the upper airway obstruction seen in moderate–severe croup. L-Epinephrine has been shown to have equivalent potency and safety compared with racemic epinephrine.[3] Racemic epinephrine 2.25% can be given in a dose of 0.05 mL per kg, to a maximum dose for children <10 kg of 0.25 mL and for children >10 kg of 0.5 mL. Epinephrine works through α-adrenergic effects, which lead to mucosal vasoconstriction that results in a temporary decrease in edema of the subglottic region of the larynx. Time of onset of action is less than 10 minutes, and duration of action is less than 2 hours. Treatment is very effective but transient; all children who receive racemic epinephrine must be observed for at least 3 to 4 hours because of the possibility of rebound stridor. Side effects of epinephrine include tachycardia and increased anxiety.
- **Heliox** is a gaseous mixture of oxygen and helium with a lower density than oxygen alone that reduces the resistance to airflow in narrowed upper airways. Heliox has theoretical benefit for severe cases when hypoxia is present, but more studies are necessary to determine its role in the management of croup.

EPIGLOTTITIS

Clinical Presentation

Epiglottitis tends to occur in children who are older (3 to 7 years) than the croup age group with no history of a preceding upper respiratory infection. The disease involves rapid onset of high fever, stridor, sore throat, dysphagia, and drooling. The child is often toxic in appearance and sitting up in the forward leaning position in an attempt to open the severely compromised airway.

Diagnostic Studies

Lateral neck radiography shows a swollen epiglottis, classically referred to as the "thumb sign." However, if the clinical presentation of a child suggests epiglottitis, the physician should not waste time getting a lateral neck radiograph. Visualization of the epiglottis should be performed as soon as possible in a controlled setting with facilities available for intubation and tracheotomy. Epiglottitis is confirmed by visualization of a cherry-red swollen epiglottis during intubation. Blood cultures should be obtained as the disease is often accompanied by bacteremia.

Treatment

Treatment is twofold. First, the airway must be secured to ensure adequate ventilation. This is usually accomplished through endotracheal intubation done in a controlled setting where tracheostomy can be performed if necessary. Second, intravenous antibiotics effective against *H. influenzae* type b should be started (cefuroxime, 75 mg/kg/day divided into q8h, or ceftriaxone, 100 mg/kg/day divided into q12h).

REFERENCES

1. Zoordo R, Sidani M, Murray J. Croup: an overview. *Am Fam Physician* 2011;83:9.
2. Sparrow A, Geelhoed G. Prednisolone versus dexamethasone in croup: a randomized equivalence trial. *Arch Dis Child* 2006;91(7):580–583.
3. Waisman Y, Klein BL, Boenning DA, et al. Prospective randomized double-blind study comparing l-epinephrine and racemic epinephrine aerosols in the treatment of laryngotracheitis (croup). *Pediatrics* 1992;89:302.
4. Knutson D, Aring A. Viral croup. *Am Fam Physician* 2004;69:3.
5. Skolnik NS. Croup. *J Fam Pract* 1993;37:165.
6. Scolnik D, Coates AL, Stephens D, et al. Controlled delivery of high vs low humidity vs mist therapy for croup in emergency departments. *JAMA* 2006;295:11.
7. Skolnik NS. Treatment of croup: a critical review. *Am J Dis Child* 1989;143:1045.
8. Russell K, Wiebe N, Saenz A, et al. Glucocorticoids for croup. *Cochrane Database Syst Rev* 2004;(3):CD001955.
9. Bjornson CL, Klassen TP, Williamson J, et al. A randomized trial of a single dose of oral dexamethasone for mild croup. *N Engl J Med* 2004;351;1306–1313.

10. Klassen TP, Feldman ME, Watters LK, et al. Nebulized budesonide for children with mild to moderate croup. *N Engl J Med* 1994;331:285.
11. Klassen TP. Croup. An algorithm for the treatment of croup. *Pediatr Clin North Am* 1999;46:1167.
12. Mauro RD, Poole SR, Lockhart CH. Differentiation of epiglottitis from laryngotracheitis in the child with stridor. *Am J Dis Child* 1988;142:679.
13. Johnson DW, Jacobson S, Edney PC, et al. A comparison of nebulized budesonide, intramuscular dexamethasone, and placebo for moderately severe croup. *N Engl J Med* 1998;339;498–503.
14. Tanou K, Kalampouka E, Malakasioti G, et al. Viral croup: diagnosis and a treatment algorithm. *Pediatr Pulmonol* 2014;49:421–429.

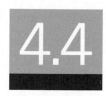

4.4 Reactive Airway Disease in Children

Dawn Brink-Cymerman

Airway hyperresponsiveness—the tendency of airways to constrict and cause obstruction due to inflammation—characterizes both asthma and wheezing respiratory illnesses in children. This collection of symptoms generally responds to medications such as bronchodilators and/or steroids. A lack of response should bring about further investigation to determine the cause. Although asthma is reactive airway disease, all reactive airway disease is not asthma.

DIAGNOSIS

History

- The most common symptoms include wheezing, shortness of breath, cough, and chest tightness. Determine whether respiratory distress has occurred previously and associated phenomena. Wheezing may be episodic as when associated with upper respiratory infections or nocturnal or seasonal.
- Associated diseases, including allergic rhinitis, eczema, or food allergies, are common.
- Aggravating factors, such as smoke, animals, exercise, upper respiratory infections, foods, and drugs, should be identified.
- A family history of allergies, eczema, or asthma is common.

Physical Examination

- Obtain vital signs, including respiratory rate, temperature, pulse, weight, and oxygen saturation.
- Observe the child's color and degree of respiratory distress and anxiety. Fatigue and cyanosis signal a severe attack, and the clinician should be prepared for respiratory failure.
- Stridor indicates an upper airway problem, such as croup or foreign body.
- Check if the wheezing is bilateral and document retractions as well as the ratio of inspiration to expiration (I/E). In children without wheezing or who have normal respirations, check for a posttussive wheeze. Lack of wheezing and presence of a normal chest examination do not exclude asthma. In fact, lack of wheezing may indicate worsening of the clinical situation as the airways become so tight, no air movement can be heard.
- Hydration status should be evaluated.
- A complete ear, nose, and throat examination should be performed with a focus on infections, nasal polyps (pathognomonic for cystic fibrosis [CF]), and signs of allergies such as allergic shiners, atopic dermatitis, or rhinorrhea.

Differential Diagnosis

The differential diagnosis of reactive airway disease is important as treatment for the various conditions is different: possibilities include the following conditions:

- **Asthma** is characterized by recurrent episodes of diffuse wheezing, dyspnea, and cough and is difficult to diagnose in children younger than 3 years but usually begins before 3 years of age. Cough without wheeze is less often a presenting symptom and should make one consider an alternative diagnosis.

- **Bronchiolitis** is characterized by the insidious onset of wheezing, tachypnea, hypoxia, and chest wall retractions associated with a 2- to 3-day history of rhinorrhea, cough, and low-grade fever in a child younger than 3 years.[1] According to evidence, bronchodilator therapy is not indicated in bronchiolitis; however, for cases caused by respiratory syncytial virus (RSV), there may be some improvement with bronchodilators, and a trial of therapy may be useful.[2]
- Other conditions may be distinguished by the wheezing pattern. A persistent wheeze present from birth may be associated with a congenital anatomic abnormality of the heart or airways. A persistent illness with wheeze may indicate **cystic fibrosis, bronchopulmonary dysplasia, laryngomalacia, agammaglobulinemia, or primary ciliary dyskinesia.**
- **Infectious causes include pneumonia, sinusitis, croup, and bronchitis. Other causes include mediastinal mass, foreign body aspiration, gastroesophageal reflux and recurrent aspiration, exposure to an irritant, and obstructive sleep apnea.**
- **Large airway obstruction** can be caused by foreign bodies, vascular rings, tracheomalacia, tumors, and laryngeal webs.

Diagnostic Tests

- **Reversibility of airway obstruction** is diagnostic of asthma and can be evaluated with a trial of epinephrine or adrenergic aerosols. If not reversible, consider a diagnosis other than asthma.
- **Complete blood count and chest radiographs** are useful when fever is present to evaluate for pneumonia. Chest x-ray is also indicated when congestive heart failure is suspected. Both tests are generally normal in reactive airway disease.
- **Pulmonary function tests** are usually reliable by age 5 to 6 years and are most useful for monitoring chronic asthma; they are not required for the diagnosis. If done to evaluate cough, provocation with methacholine might be needed.[1]
- **Sinus radiographs, pulmonary function tests, studies for reflux, and specific immunoglobulin E (IgE) antibodies or skin testing** (75% of people with asthma have environmental allergies) are indicated for patients whose asthma is resistant to the usual treatment or to evaluate for suspected inciting factors.
- **Oximetry** is useful for determining severity of respiratory compromise but is not helpful in the differential diagnosis.[3] Allergy testing can be done in children over 2 years of age, sweat chloride testing if suspicious of CF. Serum immunoglobulins and viral testing such as for RSV may be helpful also.

TREATMENT
Prevention

Warm-blooded animals should be removed from the home. Exposure to dust mites should be minimized by washing bedding and stuffed animals two times per week in water at least 130°F. Wipe off surface dust frequently using a damp cloth. Carpeting and upholstered furniture should be removed. The humidity level should be kept below 50%. Mattresses and box springs and pillows should be encased in airtight plastic covers with tape over the zipper. Regularly wash damp areas, such as shower stalls, basements, and window sills. Avoid environmental irritants. Do not allow smoking. Do not use woodstoves. Avoid strong odors or sprays. Do not clean when the patient is present. Reduce exposure to infections. Avoid daycare settings if possible, and vaccinate appropriately. If symptoms are severe or systemic and steroids are needed regularly, immunotherapy may be necessary.

Pharmacologic Therapy[4]

- **β-Adrenergic agonists** are bronchodilators effective in treating early asthmatic responses and exercise-induced asthma. They are the treatment of choice for acute episodes of bronchospasm and a rescue medication in all classes of asthma. Albuterol and levalbuterol have equal efficacy in treatment. The β-agonists are available as metered dose inhalers (MDIs), nebulizer solutions, oral preparations, and parental preparations.
- **Corticosteroids** are very potent anti-inflammatory medicines. Anti-inflammatory agents are the most important medicine in chronic recurrent asthma. They reduce inflammation, edema, and mucus secretions and restore β-adrenergic responses. There is no evidence that children will have growth reduction secondary to use of inhaled glucocorticoids over the long term. The topical agents are quickly metabolized and rarely cause systemic symptoms. Inhaled steroids are best given 10 minutes after inhaled β-agonists or are available in combined preparations. Oral doses are absorbed quickly and can be used for acute episodes.
- **Cromolyn sodium and nedocromil sodium** have few side effects. They are anti-inflammatory medicines and have no bronchodilator effect but inhibit mediator release from mast cells. The dosage is

two puffs of MDI three to four times per day or 1 unit dose via nebulizer mixed with a β-agonist. The treatment may be decreased to twice a day with adequate clinical response. They are a **nonpreferred** alternative monotherapy treatment for mild persistent asthma.

- **Theophylline** is a bronchodilator whose use has markedly decreased in recent years owing to side effects and lack of an anti-inflammatory component. It has a very narrow therapeutic window, and serum levels must be monitored frequently.
- **Anticholinergics** function as bronchodilators in most patients with asthma and enhance the effect of the β-agonists. Ipratropium bromide is poorly absorbed and has few systemic side effects. It is particularly useful in cold air–induced, irritant-induced, and emotionally induced asthma.
- **Leukotriene modifiers:** Montelukast is approved for age 2 and above, zafirlukast is approved for age 5 and above, and zileuton is approved for age 12 and above; however, these are rarely used due to the need to monitor liver functions with these medications. Leukotriene antagonists work on the inflammatory cascade in asthma, are useful in wheezing set off by allergy, and give relief of exercise-induced wheezing. They show some benefit for short-term symptom control and lower respiratory sequelae in infants with RSV.
- **Long-acting β-agonists (LABAs)** are not to be used as rescue medication or for acute bronchospasm. Salmeterol is approved for age 4 and above and formoterol is for age 5 and above with neither being first-line treatment. Studies suggest that in children an increased dose of steroids may improve airway responsiveness, by reducing inflammation, to a greater degree than the addition of an LABA.[5] According to the newest guidelines from the National Heart, Lung and Blood Institute of NIH, inhaled corticosteroids are still the preferred long-term control treatment, but a combination of LABA with corticosteroids is also an equally good treatment option.[6]
- **Influenza vaccine** is useful in preventing virus-induced episodes of asthma or reactive airway wheezing secondary to inflammation. It is now recommended for children starting at age 6 months and repeated yearly.

Management

"Step-care" management strategy of asthma, in which the number of medications and frequency of use are increased as symptoms worsen, is recommended by the National Heart, Lung and Blood Institute.[4] Treatment of comorbid conditions will benefit management. Severity is best determined when not on a long-acting controller medication, but if already on one, the ability to maintain control will be the determining factor. When determining management success or need to increase use of medication, it is important to assess patient adherence, including correct use of medication both in method and timing.

- **Mild intermittent asthma**
  - Long-term control—No daily medication needed.
  - Quick relief—Short-acting bronchodilator; inhaled β-agonists as needed.
- **Mild persistent asthma**
  - Long-term control—*Daily* anti-inflammatory: low-dose inhaled corticosteroid.
  - Cromolyn or nedocromil could be used as a second choice.
  - Quick relief—Short-acting bronchodilator; inhaled β-agonists as needed.
  - Leukotriene modifiers can be considered in this group as an alternative, but not all are responders to this medication.
- **Moderate persistent asthma**
  - Long-term control—*Daily* anti-inflammatory: inhaled corticosteroid, medium dose, *or* inhaled corticosteroid low-medium dose with long-acting bronchodilator, especially for nighttime symptoms. *If needed:* anti-inflammatory: medium–high-dose inhaled corticosteroids *and* long-acting bronchodilator, especially for nighttime symptoms.
  - Quick relief—Short-acting bronchodilator; inhaled β-agonists as needed.
- **Severe persistent asthma**
  - Long-term control—*Daily* anti-inflammatory: high-dose inhaled corticosteroid *and* long-acting bronchodilator. Oral corticosteroid tablets or syrup (2 mg/kg/day; not to exceed 60 mg/day) may be required intermittently.
  - Quick relief—Short-acting bronchodilator; inhaled β-agonists as needed.

Flowmeters

Peak flowmeters, which measure peak expiratory flow rate (PEFR), are essential to manage asthma properly but not useful in very young children due to their inability to perform the exercise properly. They also are not useful for diagnosis. The following are interpretations of flowmeter readings.

- The green zone is defined as a PEFR of 80% to 100% of personal best: No symptoms are present; the patient can engage in full activity, and no change in medication is needed.
- The yellow zone is defined as a PEFR of 50% to 80% of personal best: The patient is at increased risk for asthma attacks; treatment should be applied per the step-care management strategy (see above).
- The red zone is defined as a PEFR of less than 50%. Call the physician; *emergency care is necessary.*

Indications for Admission

Indications include continued wheezing an hour after administration of β-agonist in association with any sign of respiratory distress, persistent tachypnea, PCO greater than 40, PaO$_2$ less than 70, O$_2$ saturation less than 92%, PEFR less than 40% of predicted or personal best, or altered level of consciousness.

Indications for Consultation

Required if multiple hospital admissions, continuation of symptoms, PEFR less than 90% of predicted and never returning to baseline, and poor status following intubation, repeated use of oral corticosteroids to maintain control, additional testing that would be done only by a consultant, or treatment with immune modulators.

Resources for Patient Education

- National Asthma Education Program, DHHS, Publication No. 10-7541, 2010.
- American Lung Association, (800) 586-4872, www.lungusa.org.
- Asthma and Allergy Foundation of America, (800) 727-8462, www.aafa.org.
- Allergy and Asthma Network/Mothers of Asthmatics, Inc., (800) 878-4403, www.podi.com/health/aanma.
- National Asthma Education and Prevention Program, (301) 251-1222, www.nhlbi.nih.gov/nhlbi/nhlbi.htm.
- American Academy of Allergy, Asthma, and Immunology, (800) 822-2762, www.aaaai.org.

REFERENCES

1. Barcy TL, Graber MA. Respiratory syncytial virus infection in infants and young children. *J Fam Pract* 1997;45:473–481.
2. King VJ, Viswanathan M, Bordley WC. Pharmacologic treatment of bronchiolitis in infants and children: a systemic review. *Arch Pediatr Adolesc Med* 2004;158:127.
3. Stemple DA, Redding GJ. Management of acute asthma. *Pediatr Clin North Am* 1992;39:1311.
4. Covar RA, Spahn JD. Practical guide for the diagnosis and management of asthma. National Asthma Education Program; 2010. DHHS Publication No. 10-7541.
5. Simons FE. A comparison of beclomethasone, salmeterol, and placebo in children with asthma. Canadian Beclomethasone Dipropionate-Salmeterol Xinafoate Study Group. *N Engl J Med* 1997;337:1659.
6. National Heart, Lung and Blood Institute. Highlights of major changes in EPR-3: Full Report 2007; 2.
7. Covar RA, Spahn JD. Treating the wheezing infant. *Pediatr Clin North Am* 2003;50(3):631–654.
8. Strunk RC. Defining asthma in preschool-aged children. *Pediatrics* 2002;109:357–360.

4.5 Viral Exanthems of Children

Jeffrey T. Kirchner

GENERAL PRINCIPLES

Viral exanthems of children are common clinical problems encountered by the family physician. Numerous viral agents can produce a similar rash and other clinical symptoms, which makes the diagnosis challenging. A careful evaluation that includes age, immunization status, history of infectious diseases, exposures, medication use, prodromal period, features of the rash, fever, and the presence of pathognomonic signs is helpful in establishing a diagnosis. Laboratory testing may be available to confirm the diagnosis but often is not acutely useful due to the time delay in obtaining viral cultures or serologic antibody titers. The availability of polymerase chain reaction (PCR) and other nucleic acid–based testing has improved the ability to diagnose many infectious diseases, but these tests are expensive and often do not change management. Treatment in most cases is supportive.

MEASLES (RUBEOLA)

- **Causative agent.** Measles is caused by an RNA paramyxovirus that belongs to the genus *Morbillivirus*. Infected individuals are contagious up to 7 days after the onset of symptoms.
- **Clinical manifestations** may initially include fever, cough, conjunctivitis, and Koplik spots (an enanthem). Rash appears on the third or fourth day and begins as a purple–red maculopapular eruption along the hairline, forehead, and face. By the third day, it spreads to the feet and it fades in the order of appearance. Acute encephalitis occurs in 1 to 2 per 1,000 reported cases and may be fatal.
- **Diagnosis.** This is usually made on clinical grounds, but viral cultures of body fluids or serologic testing is confirmatory. Serology is the most common method of laboratory confirmation with detection of specific IgM in a specimen of serum diagnostic of acute infection. Acute infection can also be confirmed with a fourfold or greater increase in IgG antibody concentrations between acute and convalescent sera.[1]
- **Treatment** of uncomplicated infections is supportive. There is no specific antiviral therapy; however, vitamin A is effective and the WHO recommends administration of once-daily doses of 200,000 IU of vitamin A for 2 consecutive days to all children aged 12 months or older who have measles to reduce morbidity and mortality.[1]

RUBELLA (GERMAN MEASLES)

- **Causative agent.** Rubella is caused by a single-stranded RNA virus of the family Togaviridae. Infection is acquired via inhalation of infectious large particle aerosols, augmented by close contact with infected individuals.
- **Clinical manifestations** may include low-grade fever, postauricular adenopathy, headache, and myalgias. Rash consists of pink–red maculopapules that are discrete and do not coalesce. They appear first on the face and spread rapidly downward to the neck, arms, trunk, and lower extremities. The total duration is 3 to 4 days, with occasional brawny desquamation. Complications are rare but may include joint manifestations, thrombotic thrombocytopenic purpura, and encephalitis. Most adults are immune to rubella, but infection during pregnancy is associated with pre-term delivery and potential for congenital problems, including cardiac and neurologic disorders.
- **Diagnosis** is clinical, but this can be unreliable. Specific IgM antibody can be detected 4 days after the onset of rash and is usually detectable after primary infection for 6 to 8 weeks. Rubella infection and reinfection can be determined by a fourfold rise in rubella IgG antibody titers between acute and convalescent sera. PCR testing to detect rubella RNA is available but rarely necessary.
- **Treatment** is symptomatic and supportive. Nonimmune adults should receive a measles, mumps, and rubella (MMR) booster vaccine, especially if future pregnancy is anticipated.

ROSEOLA INFANTUM (EXANTHEM SUBITUM; SIXTH DISEASE)

- **Causative agent.** Roseola is caused by the human herpes viruses type 6 (HHV-6) and type 7 (HHV-7). Peak prevalence is 7 to 13 months and the majority of cases occur in children younger than 2 years.[3]
- **Clinical manifestations** include abrupt onset of fever, commonly 40°C to 40.6°C, which persists for 3 to 5 days with a rapid decline. Other symptoms include fussiness, rhinorrhea, and cough. Rash appears after defervescence. The lesions are pink macules or maculopapules 2 to 3 mm in diameter that blanch with pressure. They appear first on the trunk and then spread to the neck, face, and upper and lower extremities. The total duration is 1 to 2 days.
- **Diagnosis** is clinical. Serologic testing for HHV-6/7 IgM and IgG is available. Viral cultures from blood and DNA-PCR assays are available but rarely necessary.
- **Treatment** is symptomatic and supportive including the use of acetaminophen for fever.

ERYTHEMA INFECTIOSUM (FIFTH DISEASE)

- **Causative agent.** Erythema infectiosum is caused by the human parvovirus B19. Several genotypes from the family *Parvoviridae* have been identified. It is transmitted through close person-to-person contact and respiratory secretions. It is moderately contagious, with outbreaks occurring in classrooms, daycares, and families.

- **Clinical manifestations** include fever, headache, and myalgias. Rash has a sudden onset on the face, with marked erythema ("slapped cheek" appearance) with circumoral pallor. This is followed by a generalized lace-like rash on the trunk and extremities that may persist for several weeks. Heat, bathing, sunlight, or local irritation may cause a flare up of the rash. Potential complications include erythrocyte aplasia, arthropathy, and fetal hydrops.
- **Diagnosis** is clinical but may be confirmed by serologic testing for parvovirus IgM antibody. IgG antibody is present at 15 days postinfection and may be helpful for determining past infection and immune status. Detecting parvovirus B19 DNA using NAAT is now routinely performed by many laboratories but is generally indicated only for complicated cases.
- **Treatment** of uncomplicated cases is supportive. Intravenous immune globulin has been used in patients with chronic infections and immune deficiency.[4]

ENTEROVIRAL INFECTIONS

- **Causative agent or agents.** The enteroviruses consist of numerous strains of echoviruses, Coxsackie viruses, and polioviruses. Incidence of these infections is greatest in the summer and fall.
- **Clinical manifestations** are varied and include fever, gastroenteritis, respiratory disease, meningitis, and myocarditis. Rash consists of a variety of exanthems that are generalized, maculopapular, and nonpruritic but are not distinctive enough to make a specific diagnosis. Petechial lesions may be seen with type 9 echovirus and group A Coxsackie virus. Hand, foot, and mouth disease is characterized by vesicular stomatitis and cutaneous lesions of the distal extremities. Duration of the infections varies with age and viral type, lasting from a few days to 2 weeks.
- **Diagnosis** is clinical but may be difficult and often becomes one of exclusion. Although not usually necessary, laboratory diagnosis of enterovirus infections can be done by cell culture of virus, detection of enterovirus RNA with PCR testing, or by serology with acute and convalescent titers.
- **Treatment** of uncomplicated cases is symptomatic and supportive. There are currently no vaccines or specific antiviral agents for treatment of enteroviruses.

KAWASAKI DISEASE (MUCOCUTANEOUS LYMPH NODE SYNDROME)

- **Causative agent.** The etiology of Kawasaki disease (KD) remains unknown. Approximately 85% of children with KD are under the age of 5 years, with peak incidence at 18 to 24 months.[5]
- **Clinical manifestations** include fever (≥5 days), nonpurulent conjunctivitis, erythema and fissuring of the lips, induration of the hands and feet, enlarged lymph node mass (>1.5 cm), and rash. The rash is deeply erythematous and polymorphic and most commonly manifests as pruritic plaques that vary from 2 to 10 mm. They may resemble urticaria or the target lesions of erythema multiforme. Distribution is variable and may be diffuse, truncal, or limited to the extremities. It slowly fades, and desquamation may occur with resolution of clinical illness. Coronary artery (CA) aneurysms occur as sequelae of vasculitis in 15% to 25% of untreated children, and 2% to 3% die as a result of coronary vasculitis.
- **Diagnosis** is clinical and must include five of the six clinical manifestations mentioned above. Children suspected of having KD but not having all diagnostic criteria may have "incomplete" or atypical KD. They are treated the same as patients with classic KD.
- **Treatment** includes intravenous immune globulin (2 g per kg as a single dose) and aspirin (30 to 50 mg/kg/day) until afebrile for 48 hours and then decreased to 3 to 5 mg/kg/day until markers of acute inflammation (erythrocyte sedimentation rate, C-reactive protein, platelet count) normalize. Aspirin therapy can be stopped within 2 months in children with no CA abnormalities detected by echocardiography.

INFECTIOUS MONONUCLEOSIS IN CHILDREN

- **Causative agent.** Mononucleosis, usually caused by Epstein–Barr virus (EBV), occurs in children but is most commonly seen in adolescents and young adults (see Chapter 19.3).
- **Clinical manifestations** usually include fever, tonsillopharyngitis, cervical lymphadenopathy, splenomegaly, and fatigue. The rash with EBV infection occurs in 10% to 15% of patients and is generalized and maculopapular or urticarial. A rash often occurs following inappropriate prescribing of ampicillin, amoxicillin, or other antibiotics.
- **Diagnosis** is made by serologic testing for EBV antibody. Rapid tests for heterophile antibodies (Monospot) are used to screen patients for infectious mononucleosis. These tests are negative in 25% of patients during the first week of infection and in 10% during or after the second week. If clinically

necessary, a definitive diagnosis of EBV infection can be made by testing for specific IgM and IgG antibodies against viral capsid antigens, early antigens, and EBV nuclear antigen proteins.[6]
- **Treatment** is symptomatic and supportive for uncomplicated cases.

PRIMARY VARICELLA (CHICKENPOX)

- **Causative agent.** Varicella is caused by the varicella-zoster virus (VZV) and is one of the most contagious of childhood viral illnesses.
- **Clinical manifestations** include fever, headache, and malaise. Rash is characterized by the rapid evolution of macule to papule to vesicle. The vesicles, which resemble dewdrops, are 2 to 3 mm in diameter, pruritic, and rupture easily. The lesions appear in crops involving the face, extremities, and trunk. A unique feature of the rash is that the lesions in all stages may be found in the same anatomical area. They crust over by day 7 to 10.
- **Diagnosis** is clinical. Direct immunofluorescence testing can provide results in several hours. PCR also allows identification of VZV from skin lesions and other specimens. IgM serology for rapid diagnosis has not been demonstrated, and IgM indicated immunity or prior infections. Culture of VZV has a low yield and requires prolonged incubation time.
- **Treatment** is usually symptomatic and may include antipyretics and antihistamines. Oral or intravenous acyclovir may be used in complicated cases or for immunocompromised children. The live-attenuated two-series VZV vaccine is highly effective in preventing primary varicella although breakthrough cases do occur but are usually mild compared to primary infection.[7]

REFERENCES

1. Moss WJ, Griffin DE. Measles. *Lancet* 2012;379:153–164.
2. Best JM. Rubella. *Semin Fetal Neonatal Med* 2007;12(3):182–192.
3. Zero DM, Meier AS, Sleek SS. A population-based study of primary human herpesvirus 6 infection. *N Engl J Med* 2005;352:768–776.
4. Young NS, Brown KE. Parvovirus B19. *N Engl J Med* 2004;350:586–597.
5. Eleftheriou D. Management of Kawasaki disease. *Arch Dis Child* 2014;99:74–83.
6. Luzuriaga K. Infectious mononucleosis. *N Engl J Med* 2010;362:1933–2000.
7. Baxter R. Long-term effectiveness of varicella vaccine. *Pediatrics* 2013;131:1–8.

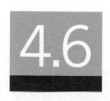

4.6 Common Musculoskeletal Problems of Children and Adolescents

John R. Gimpel

Musculoskeletal conditions in children and adolescents represent a significant percentage of visits to physicians and emergency departments, contributed to by the higher incidence of fractures, other traumatic injuries, and overuse syndromes from youth sports activities as well as from free play. Prevention in many of these issues is paramount. This chapter provides an overview of a select number of important musculoskeletal conditions, not including acute fractures.

JUVENILE IDIOPATHIC ARTHRITIS

Juvenile idiopathic arthritis (JIA) is an umbrella term for a group of common arthritic conditions that constitute the most common form of childhood arthritis and also one of the more common chronic conditions in children. As the clinical course, immunogenetic associations, and the outcomes are most often quite different from patients with adult-onset rheumatoid arthritis, the JIA classification has replaced the older Juvenile Rheumatoid Arthritis (JRA) terminology. The etiology for JIA is unknown, and the diagnosis is made by consideration of factors in the history, the physical examination, and laboratory testing. Diagnostic criteria include onset before the 16th birthday, objective arthritis (i.e., swelling, effusion, tenderness, limitation or pain with range of motion, joint warmth) in one or more joints that persists for at least 6 weeks, and exclusion of other causes of childhood arthritis. JIA can be subdivided into seven categories, each with its own unique clinical presentations, immunogenetic associations, complications, and outcomes. No specific laboratory or imaging test establishes the diagnosis of JIA. Most JIA patients do not achieve remission and require long-term treatment. Nonsteroidal anti-inflammatory drugs (NSAIDs) are most commonly used; the use of systemic corticosteroids in children should be minimized. The use of newer therapies such as methotrexate and biologic-modifying medications has contributed to improved outcomes in JIA.

SCOLIOSIS

Scoliosis is a lateral and rotational spinal curvature greater than 10 degrees and is present in 2% to 4% of adolescents at the end of their growth period. The majority of curves are due to idiopathic scoliosis and emerge in adolescence (age 10 to skeletal maturity), whereas infantile scoliosis (before age 3: less than 1% of cases) and juvenile scoliosis (age 3 to 10: 12% to 21% of cases) are much less common. Severe curves (greater than 100 degrees) are uncommon, are more likely to have an infantile or juvenile onset, and may lead to significant restrictive pulmonary disease and a shortened life expectancy. Secondary forms of scoliosis are caused by inherited disorders of connective tissue (e.g., Ehlers–Danlos syndrome, homocysteinuria, Marfan syndrome), neurologic disorders (e.g., syringomyelia, tethered cord syndrome, spinal tumors, neurofibromatosis, upper and lower motor neuron disease), and musculoskeletal conditions (e.g., herniated disc, osteogenesis imperfecta, spondylolysis, developmental dysplasia of the hip (DDH), leg length discrepancy, Klippel–Feil syndrome).

Idiopathic Adolescent Scoliosis

This is the most common spinal deformity evaluated by primary care physicians, present in 2% to 4% of the general population, and curves greater than 10 degrees are more common in females. The etiology is believed to be multifactorial, with a strong familial predisposition, thought to be a multigene dominant condition with variable phenotypic expression. The most common curve pattern is a right thoracic apex (90% of thoracic curves), followed by right thoracic–left lumbar, thoracolumbar, double thoracic, and left lumbar curves. Patients with other curve patterns or curves associated with pain or stiffness that are likely due to underlying pathology should undergo expedient evaluation.

- **Clinical presentation.** Children generally present with cosmetic concerns or are detected during routine physical examinations. Red flags for secondary causes include a left thoracic curvature, significant pain, and neurological symptoms or abnormalities on examination. Most school-based screening programs for scoliosis, commonplace in the past, have been discontinued on the basis of U.S. Preventive Services Task Force (USPSTF) recommendations and concerns for over-referral. However, physicians should remain alert for large spinal curves and other red flags when examining adolescents.
- **Physical examination.** The physical examination reveals varying asymmetries in shoulder and iliac crest height, asymmetrical scapular prominence, and a flank crease. Curves are deemed as "right" or "left" based on their convexity, and named for the location of their apex vertebrae. The Adam forward bending test is the most sensitive and should reveal a right thoracic and possibly a left lumbar prominence. The neurologic examination and gait should be normal. Height measurements with the patient sitting and standing can be repeated every 3 to 4 months to monitor the growth spurt and gauge risk of progression. A scoliometer may be useful for follow-up and reassurance for the patient and family, but can be difficult to standardize and therefore somewhat unreliable.
- **Imaging.** Patients with a scoliometer reading greater than 5 degrees or who are otherwise suspected of a significant curve can be screened with a single, standing, 36-inch posteroanterior (PA) radiograph. The vertebral levels with the greatest tilt are identified and measured by the Cobb method (the angle between intersecting lines drawn perpendicular to the top of the most tilted vertebrae above the apex and the bottom of vertebrae below the apex is the Cobb angle). Magnetic resonance imaging (MRI) should be considered in patients with onset of scoliosis before age 8, an unusual curve pattern (e.g., left thoracic), rapid curve progression (more than 1 degree per month), neurologic symptoms or deficit, or significant pain.

Risk Factors for Progression

- Spinal growth correlates with ossification of the iliac apophysis from anterolaterally to posteriomedially. Risser grades of 0 to 2 (Table 4.6-1) are associated with an increased risk, and patients closer

TABLE 4.6-1	The Risser Grading System for Spinal Maturity

Grade 0: No ossification
Grade 1: Ossification of 0%–25%
Grade 2: 26%–50%
Grade 3: 51%–75%
Grade 4: 76%–100%
Grade 5: Complete bony fusion of the apophysis

to skeletal maturity (i.e., Risser grades 3 to 4) have a somewhat lower risk of progression. Assessing the epiphyseal status on wrist radiographs can also be used.

• Girls, especially between the onset of the pubertal growth spurt (age 10 to 12) until cessation of spinal growth (Risser 4), are at the highest risk for progression of scoliosis. On average, a girl with scoliosis generally has a relatively higher risk of progression before age 12, and a relatively lower risk after age 12.5. Girls generally have a tenfold higher risk of progression than boys.

• Clinical markers of maturity, such as Tanner staging or age at menarche, are important in the evaluation. Peak curve progression occurs during Tanner stage 2 or 3. Delayed puberty and menarche are risk factors for progression. Hypoestrogen status delays maturation of osseous growth centers and allows an accentuated curve.

• Thoracic curves or curves with their apex at a higher vertebral level are at greater risk.

• Overall risk of progression: >10 degrees: 2% to 3%; >20 degrees: 0.3% to 0.5%; >30 degrees: 0.1% to 0.3%; >40 degrees, <0.1%.

Treatment

• Curvature of 0 to 10 degrees is normal.

• For curvature of 10 to 15 degrees, follow up every 6 months for clinical recheck with forward bending test and scoliometer test to check for progression.

• For curvature of 15 to 20 degrees, repeat radiographs every 3 to 4 months in a growing child with a larger curve. For smaller curves or near the end of growth, repeat radiographs in 6 to 8 months.

• For curves greater than 20 degrees, refer to an orthopedic subspecialist for consideration of close (e.g., every 6 months) follow-up, bracing, and surgical options. Bracing can be considered with curves of 25 degrees or more, and often for curves of 29 degrees and higher, particularly in patients lacking skeletal maturity. Spinal surgery with instrumentation (rod placement and bone grafting) is generally reserved for curves greater than 40 to 45 degrees in patients with growth remaining. Modern surgery is accompanied by spinal cord monitoring using somatosensory and motor-evoked potentials, minimizing complications.

SPONDYLOLYSIS AND SPONDYLOLISTHESIS

While back pain in youth in adolescents is fairly common, and there are many causes, primary care physicians should maintain a high index of suspicion for spondylolysis and spondylolisthesis in young athletes who present with back pain. Spondylolysis is a bony defect of the vertebral pars interarticularis. It is generally considered to be a stress fracture due to repetitive lumbar hyperextension and is the most common fourth and fifth lumbar vertebral levels. The pars defect may also be congenital, and is present in 5% to 6% of North Americans and more than 50% of Alaskan Native Americans or in those with a family history of spondylolysis. It is four times more common in gymnasts than in the general population, and should be considered in dancers, divers, cheerleaders, weightlifters, volleyball players, and football lineman, among other athletes, who present with back pain. Nonathletes may be genetically predisposed to pars breakdown with minimal stress, whereas athletes likely place undue stress on a normal pars. In up to one-third of athletes with back pain, spondylolysis is the cause. Spondylolisthesis is anterior displacement of the cephalad vertebral body on the caudad one, and may be related to a history of spondylolysis, where bilateral defects allow the forward slippage. Grade I spondylolisthesis is displacement of 0% to 25%; grade II, 25% to 50%; grade III, 50% to 75%; grade IV, 75% to 100%; and grade V indicates slippage greater than 100%, which means no overlap of the two vertebral bodies.

Clinical Presentation

Low back pain develops in late childhood and early adolescence and is generally mild. Those with signs of inflammatory back pain, including prolonged morning stiffness, where pain is improved by exercise, and unrelieved by rest may in fact have ankylosing spondylitis (those who are HLA B27 positive have a 20% risk; see Chapter 15.2). In contrast, with spondylolisthesis or spondylolysis, back pain is aggravated with standing and activities requiring lumbar hypertension, such as gymnastics, weightlifting, football (linemen blocking), volleyball (serving), cheerleading (tumbling), and ballet. The pain is typically relieved with rest, and is midline or slightly lateral and may be referred to the buttocks or thighs. Radicular pain is unusual except in severe subluxations (i.e., grade III slips or greater.)

Physical Examination

Patients may have a stiff-legged gait due to tight hamstrings. Excessive lumbar lordosis is often present, and there may be tenderness of the lumbar paraspinous muscles, or other evidence of somatic dysfunction (tissue texture abnormalities, asymmetry, decreased intersegmental range of motion, tenderness) at the affected level. Forward flexion does not aggravate the pain, whereas back hyperextension does. In the single-leg hyperextension ("stork" test) test, the patient stands, grasps one knee, and hyperextends the low back. Back pain on the weight-bearing side suggests an ipsilateral pars interarticularis defect.

Radiographs

The initial diagnostic workup for young athletes with back pain of 3 or more weeks duration, when indicated, should include PA, lateral, and right and left oblique radiographs of the lumbosacral spine. The most common site of involvement is between the fifth lumbar and first sacral segment. The pars interarticularis is best visualized on the oblique views, which show a lucent or sclerotic line known as the "collar of the Scottie dog." The lateral view demonstrates the amount of subluxation in spondylolisthesis. Diagnosis of early spondylolysis with plain radiographs may be difficult because the pars interarticularis may not have completely fractured; this "Scotty dog" may not be readily apparent. If radiographs are normal and suspicion remains, a bone scan or single-photon emission computed tomography (SPECT) scan is indicated. SPECT is the most sensitive test and should be done if the plain bone scan is normal. CT scans are also highly specific. MRI inadequately visualizes the pars in up to one-third of cases and should not be relied on to rule out the diagnosis, but can be beneficial to detect the entrapment and direct impingement of associated spinal nerve roots.

Treatment

- **Spondylolysis.** Any activity that causes pain should be restricted and the patient started on an antilordosis program of rehabilitation (abdominal and back flexion strengthening exercises, hamstring and hip flexor stretching). NSAID medications can be used for pain. If pain persists in spite of conservative treatment, the patient can be placed in an antilordosis corset or brace, such as a Boston overlap brace with 0 degree lordosis. The brace is worn during waking hours or up to 23 hours per day. For the first 2 to 3 weeks, the patient performs only hamstring stretches. After 2 to 3 weeks or when pain subsides, lumbosacral stretches and abdominal strengthening out of the brace is added. Sporting activity while the brace is worn can be resumed when asymptomatic. Bracing can be weaned after 4 months if the individual is pain free with full sporting activity in the brace. The brace is tapered off by decreasing wear by 1 hour per day each week. Total bracing time is generally 6 to 9 months. Patients should be followed radiographically every 4 to 6 months for possible progression to spondylolisthesis. Most patients respond to conservative management and return to full activity within 6 months of diagnosis. Patients with persistent pain should be referred.
- **Spondylolisthesis.** Patients with slippage up to 50% can be treated initially similarly to spondylolysis. Patients with slippage greater than 50% or with pain resistant to conservative treatment should be comanaged by an orthopedic or spine surgeon. Fusion surgery is reserved for patients with greater than a grade II slippage and persistent neurologic symptoms.

JUVENILE KYPHOSIS (SCHEUERMANN DISEASE)

Scheuermann disease is an idiopathic condition resulting in anterior wedging of the thoracic vertebrae and a kyphotic deformity greater than 45 degrees. It occurs in approximately 4% to 8% of the population, may be slightly more common in male adolescents than females, and affected individuals are likely genetically predisposed.

Diagnosis

Patients generally present prior to or at the onset of puberty (10 to 13 years) with a concern of a progressive "round-back" or "humpback" deformity occasionally associated with pain. Pain is generally mild and activity related, but is not activity limiting or associated with easy back fatigability. The round-back deformity is accentuated by forward bending but does not fully correct with back extension, which, along with the radiographs, helps to distinguish Scheuermann disease from postural round back. Approximately one-third of patients have associated scoliosis. Excess lumbar lordosis is common and predisposes to spondylolysis at L5 to S1. Severe kyphosis may be associated with cord compression, extradural cysts, thoracic disk herniation, or restrictive lung disease, but these manifestations are rare.

Radiographs

Complete evaluation requires full-length standing anteroposterior (AP) and lateral spine films. The lateral view shows irregularity of the involved vertebral end plates and anterior wedging of three or more contiguous vertebrae by 5 degrees or more. Kyphosis between T4 and T12 measured by the angle of Cobb is greater than 45 degrees. Only one or two vertebral bodies may be involved with thoracolumbar disease. The radiographs should also assess for associated scoliosis, lumbar hyperlordosis, and spondylolisthesis. Lateral hyperextension views are helpful in determining the flexibility of the deformity.

Treatment

- **General.** Treatment is based on the severity of deformity, presence of pain, and the patient's age. Curves of 45 to 60 degrees with no evidence of progression are treated with observation, an exercise program to correct lumbar lordosis (abdominal strengthening, increasing hip flexor, and hamstring flexibility), and thoracic spine hyperextension exercises. Recheck every 3 to 4 months.
- **Bracing** is indicated with significantly painful curves of 50 degrees or greater, progressive deformity, especially in those with an immature skeleton, or for patients with curves that are cosmetically unacceptable.[2] A modified Milwaukee brace is most commonly used in conjunction with exercises, is best if initiated before skeletal maturity, and generally requires 12 to 18 months of treatment. Comanagement with an orthopedic or spine subspecialist is warranted.
- **Surgery** is rarely indicated and reserved for those with severe deformities (generally >75 degrees) or persistent back pain unresponsive to conservative treatment.

BACK PAIN IN YOUTH: RED FLAGS FOR INFLAMMATORY CONDITIONS

Persistent back pain is generally uncommon in childhood—including the above-mentioned conditions. **Inflammatory back pain,** with onset in adolescence or preadolescence, may reflect an underlying inflammatory condition (e.g., HLA B27–associated ankylosing spondylitis or Reiter syndrome; see Chapter 15.2). Pain in these conditions is typically insidious in onset (over months), not associated with trauma or any visible abnormality described above, low back in origin, worse in the morning, associated with stiffness lasting an hour or longer, improving with exercise, and worsening after sitting.

Physical Examination

- Will sometimes reveal loss of normal lordotic curve (i.e., straightening), associated with decreased forward flexion of the lower 10 cm of the lumbosacral spine. The Schober maneuver measures 10 cm up from a line drawn between the sacroiliac "dimples" when standing fully upright and marks start and end of that distance. The child then bends forward, and the distance between the two marked spots is remeasured. The normal lumbar spine expands from the baseline 10 cm out to 15 cm (expansion of 5 cm). Loss of normal lumbar expansion can indicate an early inflammatory spondyloarthropathy.
- In addition, when hip flexion, extension, and internal and external rotation are normal—but crossing the leg, and pressing down on the knee and opposite pelvic brim (flexion, abduction, external rotation [Faber test]) causes pain in the sacroiliac joint, or the groin—there may be inflammation of the sacroiliac joint.

FLATFOOT (PES PLANUS)

Flatfoot is broadly categorized as either physiologic flexible flatfoot or pathologic flatfoot. Pathologic flatfoot in infants can be secondary to the common but benign calcaneovalgus foot or a more ominous congenital vertical talus. Older children may have a tarsal coalition, hypermobile flatfoot with tight heel cords, or neurogenic flatfoot.

Flexible Flatfoot

- **Etiology.** The normal arch is not present at birth and slowly develops around 4 to 5 years of age. Excessive laxity of the joint capsule and plantar ligaments allows the developing arch to flatten out while bearing weight. In young children, a fat pad may further obscure the arch.

- **Clinical presentation.** Children are generally asymptomatic and brought to the physician by the parents with a concern about potential problems related to the flatfoot. The child may have fatigue or aching of the foot muscles with prolonged walking or standing.
- **Physical examination.** The child's foot flattens with weight bearing but develops an arch while the child stands on tiptoe or actively dorsiflexes the great toe. Observed from behind, the calcaneus is in valgus position while the child is standing and inverts when the child stands on tiptoe. The child's ability to stand on the heels indicates adequate heel cord flexibility. The child should be able to stand both on the inner and outer borders of the feet indicating good muscular control and adequate subtalar motion.
- **Radiographs.** Radiographs are not needed unless other pathology is suspected.
- **Treatment.** Reassure parents that no treatment is necessary because there is gradual improvement with growth, generally by age 5 years. Arch supports do not generally make a difference in radiographic or clinical outcome. The occasional child who develops symptoms associated with the flatfoot (e.g., foot pain, patellofemoral pain) should be given medial longitudinal arch supports or a medial heel wedge, or both.

PATHOLOGIC FLATFOOT

Pathologic flatfoot is characterized by limited ankle motion and, frequently, foot or ankle pain. Ankle motion may be limited in dorsiflexion by a tight heel cord and in inversion and eversion by subtalar pathology.

Hypermobile Flatfoot with Tight Heel Cord

- **Etiology.** A tight heel cord combined with a flexible flatfoot forces the calcaneus into a valgus position during ambulation. This compensatory hindfoot valgus allows for more ankle dorsiflexion. The resultant abnormal foot biomechanics lead to pain.
- **Clinical presentation.** Patients complain of foot or ankle pain.
- **Diagnosis.** The patient has a flattened arch and calcaneal valgus when standing. Observation from the side shows early heel liftoff during the gait and an arch that develops as the toes dorsiflex. Subtalar motion (calcaneal inversion and eversion) is normal, but ankle dorsiflexion is limited to neutral or less.
- **Treatment.** Patients with mild symptoms can be initially treated with aggressive heel cord stretching and a medial longitudinal arch support with a medial heel wedge. Those with more severe symptoms can be treated with a short-leg walking cast, with the ankle neutral for 4 weeks followed by heel cord stretching. Surgery for heel cord lengthening and correction of heel valgus may be necessary if conservative treatment fails.

HEEL PAIN
Sever Disease

- **Calcaneal apophysitis** is common in boys between the ages of 6 and 10, especially in obese children and athletes, secondary to repetitive microtrauma or overuse of the heel and thought to be related to tensile forces from the Achilles tendon on the calcaneal apophysis. It is commonly seen in athletes playing soccer, basketball, track, and other running sports. Pain is usually on the posterior side of the calcaneus, is bilateral in 60% of patients, is more pronounced after activity, and commonly worse at the beginning of a new sports season or during a growth spurt. Tenderness can be elicited at the insertion of the Achilles tendon and on medial and lateral compression of the posterior calcaneus. Acute treatment includes temporary avoidance of high-impact activities, heel lifts or heel cups/cushions, ice massage, and NSAIDs. Once stretching is not painful, adding in calf stretching exercises, other manual therapies and orthotic devices can be helpful. Most young athletes can return to full pain-free activity within 3 to 6 weeks. In refractory cases, cast immobilization may be needed. Patients with persistent symptoms despite adequate rest and a stretching program should lead you to reconsider the possibilities of alternate diagnoses, including Achilles tendonitis, plantar fasciitis, or calcaneal stress fracture.
- **Plantar fasciitis.** Plantar heel pain that is burning, aching, and occasionally sharp and lancinating and occurs with weight bearing on arising in the morning or after prolonged sitting, often worse for the first few steps taken, is suspicious for plantar fasciitis. This is more common in adults, but can occur in overweight children and adolescents, and risk factors include pes planus, pes cavus, and sedentary lifestyle. Palpation of the medial calcaneal tubercle at the origin of the plantar fascia usually elicits tenderness, as compared with calcaneal stress fracture, where pain is elicited with medial to lateral compression of the calcaneus. Imaging is not routinely indicated initially. Treatment is similar as for

Sever disease; relative rest, consideration of orthotic devices that counteract pronation and disperse heel strike forces (e.g., arch supports, heel pads or heel cups), use of NSAID medications in select patients, ice massage and manual/myofacial treatments, and stretching exercises of heel cord and plantar fascia. Using local injections of corticosteroids via a 25-gauge needle can be helpful in resistant chronic cases; extracorporeal shock wave therapy and plantar fasciotomy are reserved for the most recalcitrant and debilitating cases that extend beyond 6 months to a year. Also remember that heel pain, stiffness in the morning, and inflammatory type back pain can be associated with inflammatory spondyloarthropathy.

BOWLEGS (TIBIA VARUS)

Varus angulation of the knee can be normal, secondary to metabolic disease, severe physiologic bowing, or osteochondrosis deformans tibiae (Blount disease).

- **Normal development.** Children are born with tibia varum, become maximally bowlegged by 6 months, and begin to straighten by 18 to 24 months. Tibia valgum or "knock-knee" develops during the second to third year and peaks by the fourth year. Development then progresses back to the normal adult alignment of slight valgus by age 7 to 8 years. **Bowlegs should be fully evaluated if they have not corrected by age 2.**
- **Metabolic etiology.** Parents should be questioned regarding diet, and the child's growth curve should be reviewed. Rickets, abnormal calcium or phosphorus metabolism, and renal disease should be considered. If a generalized disorder is suspected, screening laboratory tests should be ordered, including serum calcium, phosphorus, alkaline phosphatase, creatinine, and hematocrit.

Severe Physiologic Bowing and Blount Disease

- **Clinical presentation.** While physiologic tibia varum is a normal variation that the child will outgrow, pathologic tibia varum is referred to as Blount disease. The child typically has painless bilateral tibia varus that is of concern to the parents. Growth and development is otherwise normal. The child may experience pain along the medial side of the knee, and/or trouble walking without tripping.
- **Diagnosis.** Standing PA radiographs must be obtained while the child's feet are together or shoulder-width apart and patellae directly forward. A tibiofemoral angle of more than 20 degrees is abnormal.
- **Severe physiologic bowing.** This is characterized by medial metaphyseal beaking of the distal femur and proximal tibia, medial cortical thickening, and no pathologic changes of the proximal medial tibial epiphysis.
- **Blount disease.** This disorder is characterized by angulation under the posteromedial proximal tibial epiphysis, tibial metaphyseal irregularity, beaking of the proximal tibia, and wedging of the proximal epiphysis. It is more common in African-American children, where bowing gets worse between the ages of 2 and 4, or it can occur in overweight adolescents.

Treatment

- **Severe physiologic bowing.** Spontaneous correction generally occurs by age 7 to 8 years. Surgery may be indicated if the deformity persists past age 8.
- **Blount disease. Aggressive treatment is needed, with bracing with a hip–knee–ankle–foot orthosis or a knee–ankle–foot orthosis worn 23 hours daily. Surgical (e.g., tibial osteotomy) correction may be needed to prevent permanent damage.** Patients should be referred for consideration of surgery once the diagnosis is made or suspected.

INTOEING

General

Intoeing affects a large number of infants and children and is a major source of concern for parents, leading to consultation and questions. Understanding the primary cause of concern is helpful in counseling the parents of the child with intoeing. Knowledge of what is normal and what will self-correct with normal growth and development will prevent unnecessary treatment, identify the rare causes that need intervention, and reassure most parents that the condition will resolve over time with normal growth. The three most common causes are metatarsus adductus, internal tibial torsion, and increased femoral anteversion, and vary in proportion to the age of the child.

Rotational Profile

The parents' attention focuses on the child's feet, but the source of intoeing can be anywhere in the lower extremities. Certain definitions are needed to facilitate evaluation of the gait and the lower extremities (Figure 4.6-1).

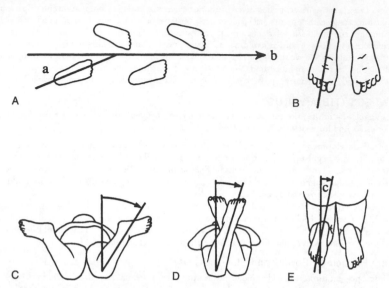

Figure 4.6-1. Rotational profile. **A:** The angle between the line of progression (b) and the foot axis is the foot progression angle (a). **B:** Foot axis. **C:** Internal (medial) femoral rotation. **D:** External (lateral) femoral rotation. **E:** Thigh–foot angle (c) is formed by the foot axis and the longitudinal axis of the femur.

- **Line of progression** is an imaginary line indicating the path of movement of the body while walking.
- **Foot axis** relates to metatarsus adductus. An imaginary line bisects the long axis of the foot from the mid-heel through the middle of the metatarsal heads.
- **Foot progression angle** is the angle of the intersection between the foot axis and the line of progression.
- **Internal and external femoral rotation** are indices of femoral version. The child lies prone with the knees flexed at 90 degrees. The pelvis is stabilized and the angle of gravity-assisted internal and external rotation of each leg is measured.
- **Thigh–foot angle** indicates tibial torsion. An imaginary line through the long axis of the foot is measured against the long axis of the femur, measured with the child in the prone position and the knees flexed at 90 degrees.

Metatarsus Adductus

- **Clinical presentation.** This is the most common cause of intoeing seen in the first year of life, either alone or combined with tibial torsion, and the most common congenital foot deformity (1 in 1,000 live births). Presentation may be unilateral or bilateral, and it is found more commonly in females, as well as more so on the left side. The most likely etiology is intrauterine positioning/crowding.
- **Physical examination.** The foot is convex laterally and concave medially, with possibly a prominence at the base of the fifth metatarsal. With the heel held in neutral position and pressure directed laterally at the first metatarsal head, a flexible deformity corrects to neutral but does not overcorrect (as do normal feet). Flexible deformities may self-correct if the lateral border of the foot is stroked. Rigid metatarsus adductus does not allow either active or passive correction of the deformity.
- **Treatment.** This condition resolves spontaneously by age 1 year in more than 90% of cases. Treatment of flexible metatarsus adductus involves having the parents passively correct the deformity with each diaper change. Referral for serial casting is necessary for rigid metatarsus (grade III) that persists beyond 6 months of age and is most effective if started early.

Internal Tibial Torsion

- **Clinical presentation.** Parents are concerned about the appearance of asymptomatic unilateral or bilateral intoeing, generally in their 1- to 2-year-old as he or she begins to walk. This is the most common cause of intoeing, being equal in males and females, but affecting the left side more so than

the right. Intrauterine positioning, sleeping in the prone position, and sitting on the feet may be the primary causes.
- **Physical examination.** The child walks with the patella facing forward and the feet pointing inward. Determine the thigh–foot angle by gazing along the axis of the lower leg with the child prone and the knee flexed (Figure 4.6-1). Be sure there is no evidence of metatarsus adductus. Normal values of the thigh–foot angle are as follows:
  - Birth: 5 degrees medial to 5 degrees lateral version
  - 12 months: up to 10 degrees lateral version
  - Adults: 10 to 20 degrees lateral version
- **Treatment.** Correction is almost always spontaneous (95% by age 8), and braces, splints, cables, and orthotics have not been shown to be effective. The condition usually corrects by age 3 to 4. The child may habitually sit with the feet turned in toward the buttocks. Although not harmful, this may slow natural correction. Getting the child his or her own chair or encouraging sitting with the legs crossed "Indian style" in front may help while the child grows. Surgical correction is reserved for patients with internal tibial torsion that persists into skeletal maturity.

Femoral Anteversion (Medial Femoral Torsion)
- **Clinical presentation.** A congenital inward twist of the femur causes turning in of the knee, leg, and foot and commonly presents between 3 and 7 years of age. This is often familial, affecting girls more than boys.
- **Physical examination.** These children walk with their patellae and feet pointing inward. The gait appears very clumsy, with frequent tripping. With the child prone and the knees bent at a right angle, the degree of internal rotation of the thighs is greater than that of external rotation. Medial rotation is normally less than 70 degrees for girls and 60 degrees for boys. Mild anteversion is 70 to 80 degrees, moderate is 80 to 90 degrees, and severe is greater than 90 degrees.
- **Treatment.** Medial femoral torsion tends to correct spontaneously with growth (80% by mid-childhood). Special braces are not necessary because it is impossible to "brace" the femur into external rotation. Rarely, patients may need surgical derotation if there is a severe torsion that persists past age 8 to 10, resulting in significant cosmetic or functional problems. Discouragement of children from sitting in the "W" position (with their lower legs outside of their thighs) may help natural correction.

COMMON HIP PROBLEMS
Developmental Dysplasia of the Hip
Formerly referred to as congenital hip dysplasia, DDH includes several conditions associated with impaired development and growth of the hip. DDH in the infant represents a spectrum from subtle hip laxity to frank dislocation. The incidence is one to two cases per 1,000 children of European descent, and is rare in patients of African descent. It is four times more common in females and three times more common in the left hip than in the right. The most significant risk factor is a positive family history; breech presentation and oligohydramnios are additional common associations. Children with untreated hip dysplasia have been shown to develop premature degenerative changes and disabling arthritic conditions in young adulthood. Newborn screening for this condition is essential for early diagnosis and treatment, and a high index of suspicion is important to avoid missed or "late" diagnosis (beyond 3 months of age) and complications. Missing the diagnosis of DDH is a common complaint in malpractice suits in pediatrics; however, the USPSTF concluded that evidence for screening is insufficient. While screening by physical examination or ultrasound leads to earlier detection, many or most cases identified as suspicious for DDH resolve spontaneously or require no intervention.

- **Physical examination.** Serial physical examination remains the primary method for diagnosing DDH in infants, particularly for high-risk infants, and should continue at well visits until the child is walking. Under optimal circumstances, the infant will be relaxed during the examination and only one hip examined at a time. Evaluation begins with observation of both lower extremities prior to the examination of each hip separately. Asymmetric skin folds or leg length inequalities are common physical findings in patient with unilateral hip dislocation.
  - **Barlow test.** With the infant supine, one hand stabilizes the pelvis and the other hand holds the hip to be examined with the thumb in the groin and the forefinger over the greater trochanter. The hip is flexed to 90 degrees, and gentle pressure is exerted posteriorly with the web space of the examiner's hand while lateral pressure is exerted with the thumb. With this maneuver, the unstable hip can be felt to dislocate from the acetabulum ("dislocatable" and "positive" test).

- **Ortolani test.** After Barlow maneuver, the hip is abducted and gently lifted. Relocation of the dislocated femoral head is palpable (and sometimes audible) in a positive Ortolani reduction test. It is important to note that "clicks" or "pops" are not diagnostic of this condition but rather indicate a palpable femoral head leaving the acetabulum. Audible high-pitched "clicks" without a sensation of instability usually have no particular significance.
- **Galeazzi sign.** This is elicited by placing the child supine with both hips and knees flexed, with a positive Galeazzi sign showing inequality of the height of the knees.
- **Older children** (greater than 3 months) may be more difficult to examine, and are less likely to exhibit a positive Ortolani test. Signs to consider include tight or limited hip abduction; apparent shortening of the femur; uneven gluteal, groin, or thigh folds; telescoping of the affected hip; positive Galeazzi sign; or a limp or waddled gait. In children who are walking, Trendelenberg symptom is a limp on the affected side and may be the first sign of a dislocated hip.
- **Imaging tests.** Ultrasonography is the study of choice in the infant but is overly sensitive as a screening tool in the first 6 weeks of life and, in general, should not be ordered until after that. Plain radiographs are useful after 4 to 6 months of age but are unreliable before 3 months of age as the femoral heads typically do not ossify until 4 to 6 months of age. Radiographs may show proximal and lateral migration of the femoral head or poor acetabular development. Because of the dependence on positioning of the hips during examinations, there are many false-positive and false-negative results.
- **Treatment.** The newborn who has a dislocated hip (positive Ortolani and irreducible) should be referred immediately to an orthopedic specialist. In the 0- to 5- or 6-month age group, treatment is generally by Pavlik harness (a brace that places the hips in flexion and abduction) for the reducible hip and traction; closed reduction or spica cast is used for the unreducible hip or older child. As a dislocatable hip (positive Barlow) may stabilize within a few weeks, use of an abduction pillow and delayed referral and reexamination in 2 weeks may be an appropriate option. Treatment is usually continued for at least 6 weeks full-time and 6 weeks part-time in younger children, or longer with older patients. Pavik harness treatment is generally 95% successful for acetabular dysplasia and subluxation, and 80% for frank dislocation. The endpoint of brace treatment is a stable hip with normal imaging studies. Avascular necrosis develops in 2.5 of 1,000 infants treated with the Pavlik harness prior to 6 months and 109 of 1,000 of those referred later. Operative treatment usually involves closed reduction under anesthesia with hip spica casting, and is generally indicated for refractory cases and children older than 6 months. Surgical release of the adductor and iliopsoas muscles may be necessary in older children who are walking, or even open reduction with femoral and/or pelvic osteotomy in children older than 2, in order to prevent or minimize premature onset of osteoarthritis.

Legg–Calvé–Perthes Disease

Also known as avascular necrosis (osteonecrosis) of the femoral head, this idiopathic disease is thought to result from a partial interruption of the blood supply to the immature femoral head. It is rare in toddlers but more common in children 4 to 8 years of age, has a male-to-female ratio of 4:1, and is bilateral 10% to 20% of the time. Risk factors include family history, low birth weight, abnormal birth presentation, higher birth order, lower socioeconomic status, and HIV.

- **Clinical presentation.** The patient usually presents with an atraumatic limp, which is painless at first and then becomes painful only after activity. Pain becomes more constant and is frequently referred to the thigh or knee. Symptoms can be variable, and this entity must be considered in any child with a limp and/or groin, thigh, or knee pain. Septic arthritis or osteomyelitis may present similarly and should be ruled out in equivocal cases.
- **Physical examination.** The child may favor the hip and be unwilling to bear weight on it for any length of time. There may be leg length discrepancy with a positive Galeazzi sign, and there is generally a decreased range of motion of the hip joint, especially abduction and internal rotation. The most sensitive physical examination maneuver for intra-articular hip pathology is the prone internal rotation test.
- **Radiographs.** The diagnosis demands a high index of clinical suspicion, as radiographs are usually normal for the first 3 to 6 weeks of the disease. Anteroposterior and frog-leg lateral radiographs may demonstrate varying degrees of fragmentation, flattening of the femoral head, and sclerosis of the proximal femur growth center with widening of the joint space. Technetium bone scanning or MRI is useful to confirm early disease.
- **Treatment.** Prompt referral to an orthopedic specialist is warranted. In younger children with early disease, treatment mainly consists of activity limitation and therapy to regain motion of the hip. The painful hip may require traction, crutches, Petrie cast, or abduction brace. Children identified and treated before 5 to 6 years of age have a lower risk of premature arthritis or permanent loss of motion. Surgical treatment is reconstructive.

Slipped Capital Femoral Epiphysis

- **Clinical presentation.** Defined as a posterior and inferior slippage of the proximal femoral epiphysis on the metaphysis (femoral neck), slipped capital femoral epiphysis (SCFE) is the major hip disorder during the adolescent growth spurt, usually presenting in 11- to 14-year-old patients and twice as often in boys as in girls. It occurs more commonly in obese children and in black or Polynesian children, and is bilateral in up to 40% of cases. The most common presentation is a chronic limp, although patients can present with acute hip pain and inability to walk, or more vague activity-related pain in the thigh, hip, groin, or knee. These symptoms warrant high suspicion and an immediate evaluation, with use of crutches or a wheelchair to make the child non–weight bearing on the way to the orthopedic referral. Most cases are stable and have a good prognosis if diagnosed early.
- **Physical examination.** The child is generally overweight (80th to 100th percentile). Range of motion is limited in hip flexion, abduction, and internal rotation, and forced internal rotation causes groin or knee pain. Obligatory external rotation of the femur with passive hip flexion is a pathognomonic sign.
- **Radiographs.** Widening of the growth plate is an early visible sign on the supine AP view, but it may be more obvious on the frog-leg lateral view as the hip slips farther posteriorly than medially. Technetium bone scanning or MRI is useful in diagnosing preslips and questionable cases.
- **Treatment.** Once identified, this merits prompt orthopedic referral for operative management. Treatment consists of avoiding any weight bearing and obtaining immediate orthopedic evaluation. *In situ* fixation with a single central screw is the most widely used surgical treatment, and it is essential to recognize this condition early to avoid the complications of hip osteonecrosis and cartilage erosion.

Transient Synovitis

This relatively common disorder (0.2% annual incidence) typically occurs in children 3 to 8 years old, and is about two times more common in boys. Sometime referred to as toxic synovitis, it is the most common cause of sudden hip pain in children, and is thought to be viral in etiology. It is an inflammation of the tissues around the hip joint, and usually presents with unilateral pain and stiffness of the hip, but is bilateral in 5% to 10% of cases, and typically symptoms have been present for less than 1 week. Fever is typically absent or low grade, and children are nontoxic in appearance. Higher fevers and systemic symptoms, while they can occur, should prompt the urgent need to rule out septic arthritis. Of patients, 30% to 50% report having had a recent upper respiratory tract infection. Children with transient synovitis appear nontoxic, and have less acute pain and range of motion restriction than those with septic arthritis. The modified roll test may help to differentiate transient synovitis from septic arthritis, where the examiner distracts the supine child by gently holding the great toe and pretending to examine the foot from different angles, while also rotating the hip. When an arc of 30 degrees or more of hip rotation is allowed without the child complaining of pain, this may more likely be transient synovitis than septic arthritis. Management is conservative, once septic arthritis has been excluded, and includes rest, NSAIDs, and return to full activity as tolerated. Radiographs, MRI, white blood count, C-reactive protein, and erythrocyte sedimentation rate can be followed by ultrasound-guided aspiration of the hip joint if necessary to exclude septic arthritis.

COMMON KNEE PROBLEMS

Osgood–Schlatter Disease

Commonly encountered in athletic children 10 to 14 years of age after a rapid growth spurt, especially in those who play jumping sports and those involved with direct pressure, such as kneeling, soccer, gymnastics, basketball, and volleyball. This disorder is an inflammatory condition and a traction apophysitis of the proximal tibial tuberosity at the insertion of the patellar tendon secondary to repetitive microtrauma.

- **Clinical presentation.** Anterior knee pain and swelling, which is bilateral in up to 30% of cases, as well as swelling and tenderness of the tibial tuberosity, are common presenting findings. Hip examination should be performed to rule out referred pain (e.g., from SCFE). Radiographs are generally not indicated unless symptoms are atypical or there are findings suggestive of osteomyelitis (e.g., warmth, erythema) or tumor. They may show anterior soft tissue swelling and fragmentation of the tibial tubercle.
- **Treatment.** Ice, NSAIDs, and occasional resting periods are recommended, but complete avoidance of sports activities is generally not necessary or recommended. Physical therapy and quadriceps stretching to improve flexibility of leg muscles can help reduce symptoms. A protective pad over the tibial tuberosity may be helpful. Osgood–Schlatter is generally a self-limited process, and the prognosis usually is excellent with conservative management.

Patellofemoral Pain Syndrome

This is a very common cause of retropatellar or peripatellar pain, particularly in adolescent female athletes. These patients typically have anterior knee pain that occurs with activity and worsens with steps or hills, and can also be triggered by prolonged sitting. It is likely due to overuse, overload, biomechanical factors, and muscular dysfunction. It is also found more commonly in patients with pes planus or pes cavus. Radiographs are appropriate in pain that persists for 4 to 6 weeks to exclude neoplasm or osteochondritis dessicans. Treatment includes ice, NSAIDs, relative rest, evaluation of footwear, manipulative treatment approaches, and quadriceps strengthening. Taping, knee sleeves, and braces are somewhat controversial, and surgical approaches are considered a last resort (e.g., lateral release if excessive lateral tracking).

BENIGN ARTHRALGIAS OF CHILDHOOD

Growing Pains

Recurrent, self-limited pains in the extremities for which the child, parents, or physicians have no definitive explanation for are often labeled as "growing pains." These are benign, and usually resolve within 1 to 2 years of onset. The pains usually begin between ages 2 and 12, and may occur in 10% to 20% of school-aged children. The etiology is unclear, but not actually caused by growth. Symptoms are bilateral and symmetrical, with usually hurt late in day or at night and usually do not interfere with daytime activities. Pain is primarily in the lower extremities, but may also occur in upper extremities, usually in conjunction with lower extremity pain. The pain is deep and bilateral in the thighs or calves. Its character is paroxysmal: quite severe at times, symptom free for days, and it may interrupt sleep. Symptoms are often relieved by massage, heat, and analgesics. Often the episodes may be associated with disruptive crying often within an hour of retiring and usually are better with parental massage. The symptoms are often accentuated by increased activity during the day, and may be related to overuse. Some have speculated that the pain originally starts with a mild increase in compartmental pressure that usually causes muscle pain more than joint pain. Physical examination in these children is normal. Often there may be significant psychological overlay. It often responds to a period of nightly ibuprofen, especially on days with pain.

Benign Hypermobility

Some patients have hypermobility of joints and yet do not have another well-characterized connective tissue disease, such as Marfan syndrome or Ehlers–Danlos syndrome. Hypermobility may be present in 10% to 15% of girls, and somewhat less in boys. These patients can often extend the elbow more than 10 degrees beyond neutral, dorsiflex the fingers at the metacarpals to 90 degrees, retroflex the knee more than 10 degrees beyond vertical into recurvatum, oppose the thumb to the forearm, and place both palms on the floor without bending the knees. Most will have a passive flat foot. Some are asymptomatic, but others have joint pains and other recurrent somatic dysfunction and have been characterized as having benign hypermobile joint syndrome. Characteristically this can be daytime pain, and may disrupt walking and prolonged activities. Small joints in the hand may hurt with writing; this responds to using large pencils or padded pen holders to increase circumference. With growth, the adolescent usually has good athletic ability, but pain after prolonged activity. There is some increase in risk of ligamentous injury that will respond to preventive, periarticular muscular strengthening (e.g., quad strengthening). Some report brief episodes of joint swelling, as well as myalgias. There may be an association with fibromyalgia in some patients, and extra-articular manifestations may include anxiety, panic attacks, mitral valve prolapse syndrome, and cognitive disorders. Further study is needed.

ACKNOWLEDGMENT

The author acknowledges contributions of Stephen R. Mitchell, Wade A. Lillegard, and John P. Fogarty for contributions to prior versions of this chapter.

REFERENCES

1. American Academy of Pediatrics. Clinical practice guideline: early detection of developmental dysplasia of the hip. *Pediatrics* 2000;105:896.
2. Screening for developmental dysplasia of the hip. Evidence synthesis no. 42. Rockville, MD: Agency for Health care Research and Quality. hppt://www.ahrq.gov/downloads/pub/prevent/pdfser/hipdyssyn.pdf. Accessed March 29, 2006.

3. Shipman SA, Helfand M, Moyer VA, et al. Screening for developmental dysplasia of the hip: a systematic literature review for the U.S. Preventive Services Task Force. *Pediatrics* 2006;117:e557–e576.

4. Frazer CH, Rappaport LA. Recurrent pains. In: Levine MD, Carey, WB, Crocker AC, eds, *Developmental behavioral pediatrics*. 3rd ed. Philadelphia, PA: WB Saunders; 1999:357.

5. Leet AI, Skaggs DL. Evaluation of the acutely limping child. *Am Fam Physician* 2000;61:4.

6. Cassas KJ, Cassettari-Wayhs A. Childhood and adolescent sports-related overuse injuries. *Am Fam Physician* 2006;73(6):1014–1022.

7. Sass P, Hassan G. Lower extremity abnormalities in children. *Am Fam Physician* 2003;68(3):461–468.

8. Screening for idiopathic scoliosis in adolescents; update of the evidence for the U.S. Preventive Services Task Force. Agency for Health care, Research and Quality. 2003. www.preventiveservices.ahrq.gov. Accessed April 16, 2006.

9. Adib N, Davies K, Grahame R, et al. Joint hypermobility syndrome in childhood. A not so benign multisystem disorder? *Rheumatology (Oxford)* 2005;44:744.

10. Osgood-Schlatter disease. In: Greene WB, ed. *Essentials of musculoskeletal care*. 2nd ed. Rosemont, IL: American Academy of Orthopedic Surgeons; 2001:719.

11. Klippel JH, et al. *Primer on the rheumatic diseases*. 13th ed. Atlanta: Arthritis Foundation; 2008.

12. Goff JD, Crawford R. Diagnosis and treatment of plantar fasciitis. *Am Fam Physician* 2011; 84(6):676–682.

13. Talley W, Goodemote P, Henry S. Managing intoeing in children. *Am Fam Physician* 2011;84(8):942–944.

14. Sawyer JR, Kapoor M. The limping child: a systemic approach to diagnosis. *Am Fam Physician* 2009;79(3):215–224.

15. Wilson JJ, Farukawa M. Evaluation of the patient with hip pain. *Am Fam Physician* 2014;89(1):27–34.

16. Atanda A, Shah SA, O'Brien K. Osteochondrosis: common causes of pain in growing bones. *Am Fam Physician* 2011;83(3):285–291.

17. Storer SK, Skaggs DL. Developmental dysplasia of the hip. *Am Fam Physician* 2006;74(8):1310–1316.

18. Reamy BV, Slakey JB. Adolescent idiopathic scoliosis: review and current concepts. *Am Fam Physician* 2001;64(1):111–117.

19. Selected Issues for the Adolescent Athlete and the Team Physician: A Consensus Statement. American College of Sports Medicine, 2008. http://www.acsm-msee.org.

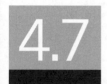

Enuresis

William L. Toffler

Enuresis, or involuntary urination, is a common problem among children. Primary enuresis describes a pattern of never having achieved bladder control. Secondary enuresis occurs in an individual who had achieved control for at least 3 months but who has subsequently lost control. Each group can be subdivided further into nocturnal (night) or diurnal (daytime) enuresis.

Primary nocturnal enuresis (PNE), sometimes simply referred to as enuresis, is the most common group, responsible for 80% of cases.[1] PNE is more prevalent in boys. Enuresis is defined as repeated, spontaneous voiding of urine during sleep in a child 5 years or older.[1] Primary diurnal enuresis in older children and secondary enuresis are much less common and may represent more serious underlying etiologies.

Delayed bladder maturation, small functional bladder capacity, diminished vasopressin release, and poor sleep arousal alone or in combination may contribute to nocturnal enuresis in a given child. Children with daytime symptoms, recurrent urinary tract infections, abnormal renal ultrasound, or known or suspected physical or neurological problems need further assessment or referral.[2]

Enuresis can be disruptive to normal family life and can generate stress between parents and child. There may be anxiety about events like sleepovers and campouts, and there are significant costs in lost time, laundry, and bedding, as well as the potential for guilt and loss of self-esteem.[2] These concerns may well offset the inherent costs of treatment. The decision to intervene depends on weighing such factors and on consideration of the degree of frustration in either the child or the parents.

DIAGNOSIS

Clinical Presentation

The presentation varies by group:
- Primary enuresis may or may not be perceived as a problem by either parent or child (or physician), whereas secondary enuresis often proves problematic regardless of age. Infectious etiologies can be accompanied by dysuria, frequency, or urgency.

Assessment

- **History.** Key questions should include periods of dryness, stress in the family, family history of enuresis (60% to 70% have a relative with enuresis[3]), bowel control (encopresis may signal stress or neurologic defect), peer interactions, and emotional changes. Never forget to ask about urinary infection symptoms (frequency, volume, stream, retention, urgency, and dysuria). Also inquire about age and results of previous efforts at bowel and bladder training, previous therapy, if any, and other health problems and medications, particularly any psychotropic or other drugs with sedative or autonomic effects. Voiding history questionnaires are useful and may be obtained from the National Kidney Foundation on the World Wide Web.[4]

    A history of snoring, mouth breathing, behavioral problems, and daytime somnolence in patients with enlarged tonsils or adenoids on examination may suggest obstructive sleep apnea. Surgical correction of airway obstruction in these patients improves or cures nocturnal enuresis and daytime wetting.[2,5]
- **Physical examination.** The physical examination is often unrevealing but helps to exclude less common anatomic or neurologic defects. Genitalia should be examined for hypospadias, fistula, or other congenital anomalies. Gait, rectal tone, perianal sensation, and anal reflex are rarely abnormal but can be screened to avoid overlooking the possibility of neurologic etiologies.
- **Laboratory studies.** Laboratory studies should be done selectively, depending on the history.
    - Urine dipstick and microscopic analysis are done to screen for infection, diabetes, and urinary tract abnormality.
    - Urine cultures may be obtained when indicated by urine microscopy. Urinalysis is a helpful screen for infection, but is usually normal.
    - Ultrasound of the kidneys, ureters, and bladder (prevoid and postvoid) may yield clues to anatomic or functional abnormalities.
    - Computed tomography urogram versus intravenous pyelogram may be necessary when greater anatomic detail is desired, or if ultrasound fails to render adequate visualization.
    - Voiding cystourethrography can be considered when an anatomic defect or physiologic dysfunction is suspected, for example, when there is a history of daytime frequency, small stream caliber, or recurrent infection.

Treatment

- **Education.** Patient and parental education are paramount when choosing a treatment plan. Helpful information may be obtained from the National Kidney Foundation.
- **Expectant management.** Enuresis spontaneously resolves in 15% of children with enuresis each year.[1] For some, the best treatment may be to monitor the child's progress. Either a parent or the child can record in a log the number of wet or dry nights per week. A review of the log at 6 months may indicate progress toward spontaneous resolution.
- **Behavioral therapy.** Evidence suggests brief positive interventions prove constructive. Other techniques include arousal training, dry bed training, hypnotherapy, and alarm systems.[1-3,6] Enuresis alarms give improvement in dry nights provided that the parents and child are motivated. It is uncertain if this leads to long-term resolution. One parent often needs to wake the child and ensure that the child rises to void. The importance of parent compliance cannot be overemphasized.
    - Advantages of the alarm system include its relatively low cost and moderate success rate 65% (range 30% to 87%).[6]
    - Disadvantages include the need for active parental participation to help wake the child (a major factor in failure), the potential inability of the alarm to awaken the child or parents, and the presence of external hardware. Relapse rates average 42% (range 4% to 55%).[6]
    - Evidence suggests equivalence among different forms of alarm, pre- and within-treatment predictors of success.[6]
- **Desmopressin.** One to two sprays of desmopressin in each nostril at bedtime has a peak effect in 2 to 3 hours and may be effective the first night. The maximum dose is 40 µg (four sprays total). In tablet form, the initial dose is 0.2 mg orally 30 to 60 minutes prior to bedtime; 0.4 mg may be more effective

and the dose may be titrated to a maximum of 0.6 mg as indicated.[2] Success occurs in approximately 60% to 70% of patients, but relapse rates can be as high as 80%.[1] Advantages include the potential for immediate results, ease of administration, and some possible long-term improvement in decreased wetting frequency even if relapse occurs. Disadvantages are desmopressin's relatively high cost and high relapse rate. Side effects, such as hyponatremia and water intoxication, are rare when the drug is used in the recommended dosages, and patients are advised to avoid excess water ingestion.[1,2]

• **Imipramine.** Less effective than desmopressin, imipramine is usually given in lower doses than those used in childhood depression, and its onset of action is rapid where its antidepressant effect is delayed. The initial dose is 10 to 25 mg at bedtime. Doses can be increased by 10 or 25 mg each 1 to 2 weeks, up to a maximum dosage of approximately 1 to 2 mg/kg/day. Although imipramine can be successful in 40% to 60% of enuretics, the evidence suggests desmopressin is better with success rates up to 70%.[1,2] Advantages include low cost, ease of administration, and, as with desmopressin, possible long-term improvement in reduction in wetting frequency after relapse. An important issue is informing parents about imipramine's potential toxicity and ensuring understanding of proper dosing. The main disadvantage of both drugs is the high relapse rate.

The synergism between behavioral and pharmaceutical treatment is questionable.[7]

• **Summary recommendation.** Success is 15% per year regardless of intervention. Some benefit is noted with brief interventions and a parental plan, the most successful of which appears to be using bladder volume alarms. Desmopressin works best for occasional nights when the child is traveling, visiting, or camping.

REFERENCES

1. Ramakrishnan K. Evaluation and treatment of enuresis. *Am Fam Physician* 2008;78(4):489–496.
2. Caldwell PJ, Deshpande AV, Von Gontard A. Management of nocturnal enuresis. *BMJ* 2013;347:f6259.
3. Akman RY. Nocturnal enuresis. *Turk Arch Ped* 2012;47:80–85.
4. https://www.kidney.org/patients/bw/pdf/voidhist.pdf
5. Firoozi F, Batniji R, Aslan AR, et al. Resolution of diurnal incontinence and nocturnal enuresis after adenotonsillectomy in children. *J Urol* 2006;175(5):1885–1888.
6. Butler RJ, Gasson SL. Enuresis alarm treatment. *Scand J Urol* 2005;39(5):349–357.
7. Gibb S, Nolan T, et al. Evidence against synergistic effect of desmopressin with conditioning and treatment of nocturnal enuresis. *J Pediatr* 2004;144(3):351–357.

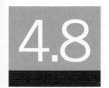

4.8 Common Poisoning in Children

Jason Chao, Alexandria D. Howard

GENERAL PRINCIPLES

The ingestion of a potentially poisonous substance is a common medical emergency in children. In 2012, nearly half of all calls to U.S. poison control centers involved children under the age of 6; three-fourths of those calls involved children 3 and younger. Ninety percent of all cases were successfully managed outside of healthcare facilities with the assistance of local poison control offices.

• The vast majority of toxic exposures in children younger than 12 are unintentional, involving household products (cosmetics and personal care products and cleaning supplies), while teenagers are most commonly the victims of intentional pharmaceutical exposure (analgesics, cough/cold preparations).

• Delayed effects of some poisons may not occur for hours to days, and chronic poisoning may occur with few overt symptoms, especially with environmental toxins. Remember to consider poisoning in the differential diagnosis of a child with serious unexplained symptoms or altered level of consciousness.

• Newly emerging sources of toxic exposure include e-cigarettes and liquid nicotine, as well as highly concentrated laundry detergent packets. In 2013, more than 10,000 exposures involving detergent packets were documented for children younger than 5.[1]

• For any potential toxic exposure, seek the advice of the local poison control center.

DIAGNOSIS

Common Toxidromes

- **Anticholinergic syndrome** (atropine, antihistamines, tricyclic antidepressants, etc.): Symptoms include mydriasis, dry skin, dry mouth, flushing, hyperthermia, urinary retention, ileus, tachycardia, hypertension, agitation, confusion, hallucinations, and seizures (see Chapter 3.3).
- **Cholinergic syndrome** (organophosphate and carbamate pesticides, certain mushrooms, etc.): Symptoms include salivation, lacrimation, bowel and bladder incontinence, emesis, abdominal cramps, miosis, bronchospasm, diaphoresis, seizures, and bradycardia. (see Chapter 21.2).
- **Sympathomimetic syndrome** (amphetamines, cocaine, etc.): Symptoms include mydriasis, sweating, fever, tachycardia, hypertension, agitation, confusion, hallucinations, seizures, nausea, vomiting, and diarrhea (see Chapter 3.3).
- **Sedative syndrome** (opiates, barbiturates, clonidine, ethanol, benzodiazepines, etc.): Symptoms include sedation from lethargy to coma, hypotension, bradycardia, respiratory depression, miosis, hypothermia, and hyporeflexia. Opiates will produce additional symptoms of miosis and decreased bowel sounds (see Chapter 3.3).

History

If possible, determine the substance(s) involved, quantity ingested, time of ingestion, any additional potential exposure and the cause of the exposure (unintentional vs. intentional). For teens or young adults, consider substance abuse and suicide attempt.

Physical Examination

Special attention should be paid to vital signs, mental status, pupil size, bowel and bladder function, mucous membranes, and skin moisture.

Laboratory Studies

- There is debate on the routine use of toxicology screens in asymptomatic children presenting soon after an exposure, given that the substance involved is usually known. Specific quantitative testing for a toxin or class of toxins can be helpful in the case of a patient who is symptomatic without a clear history of exposure or an adolescent involved in recreational drug use. Assays are available for acetaminophen, lithium, salicylate, carboxyhemoglobin, methemoglobin, theophylline, valproic acid, carbamazepine, digoxin, phenobarbital, iron, ethanol, methanol, and ethylene glycol.[2]
- Management of the clinically ill pediatric patient with potential toxic exposure should not be delayed while waiting on the results of laboratory testing. Measurement of serum electrolytes and determination of an elevated anion or osmol gap may be helpful, but a normal osmol gap cannot rule out a significant ingestion such as a toxic alcohol.
- Urine pregnancy testing should be obtained in all female patients of reproductive age.

TREATMENT

- **Stabilize the patient**
  - **Assess ABCs—airway, breathing, and circulation**. Perform a brief screening examination, including vital signs, mental status, and pupils, to identify the measures necessary in the first several minutes to prevent further deterioration of the patient. Intubate the lethargic or obtunded patient without a gag reflex.
  - Lethargic patients should be evaluated and empirically treated for hypoglycemia. Naloxone (Narcan) should be added with signs of respiratory depression and/or known opioid ingestion. Use 0.1 mg per kg, up to 2 mg IV. The dose may be doubled every 2 minutes if there is no response, not to exceed 10 mg.
- **Decontaminate skin and eyes with copious rinsing**. Eyes should be irrigated with lids open using normal saline. Care should be taken to avoid contamination of health care workers, particularly with topical agents.
- **Complete patient evaluation** is directed to clarifying the type and amount of the toxic substance as well as the timing of the exposure, evaluating the severity of its clinical effects, and searching for associated complications and trauma.
- **Supportive care** is the mainstay of therapy and should be started as soon as the patient is stabilized. Further specific treatment is based on the substance involved and the availability of an antidote.

ADJUNCT THERAPIES

- **Activated charcoal**
  - Oral activated charcoal has been shown to decrease systemic absorption of many drugs, including aspirin, acetaminophen, barbiturates, phenytoin, theophylline, and tricyclic antidepressants if administered within 60 minutes of ingestion and may be considered in the pediatric patient with ingestion of a potentially lethal dose. Give a single dose of 0.5 to 1 g per kg to a maximum of 50 g. Activated charcoal is contraindicated in patients with an unprotected airway and when its use increases the risk of aspiration.[3]
  - Multiple-dose activated charcoal, given every 2 to 4 hours, may be considered when large amounts or delayed-release drugs specifically carbamazepine, dapsone, phenobarbital, quinine, or theophylline are ingested. The use of cathartics is not recommended in children.[4]
- **Gastric lavage** has not been shown to improve clinical outcome and is associated with serious complications. The 2013 position update on gastric lavage for gastrointestinal (GI) decontamination from the American Academy of Clinical Toxicology (AACT) and the European Association of Poison Centres and Clinical Toxicologists (EAPCCT) does not support the use of gastric lavage; "gastric lavage should not be performed routinely, if at all, for the treatment of poisoned patients. In the rare situation where gastric lavage might seem appropriate, clinicians should consider treatment with activated charcoal or observation and supportive care in place of gastric lavage."[5]
- **Syrup of ipecac** remains unproven in efficacy and its use should be avoided. The American Academy of Pediatrics recommends that ipecac should no longer be a routine home treatment strategy and AACT in conjunction with EAPCCT recommend against its routine use in poisoned patients as it may delay the administration and efficacy of other more appropriate therapies.[6,7]
- **Whole-bowel irrigation** may be considered for patients presenting greater than 2 hours after the ingestion of extended-release or enteric-coated medications and/or significant amounts of iron. Polyethylene glycol solution should be administered via nasogastric tube at the following rates: 500 mL per hour (age 9 months to 5 years), 1 L per hour (age 6 to 12 years), and 1.5 to 2 L per hour (adolescents).
- **Extracorporeal hemodialysis or hemoperfusion** may be used in cases involving significant methanol, ethylene glycol or other toxic alcohol, lithium, salicylate, or theophylline ingestion.

COMMON POTENTIALLY TOXIC AGENTS

Acetaminophen

- Gastrointestinal decontamination with activated charcoal should be considered within the first hour of ingestion of a potentially toxic dose or within the first 8 hours of ingestion, if acetylcysteine cannot be administered.
- If time of ingestion is known, draw a serum level at 4 hours after ingestion; otherwise, draw the serum level on admission.
- Oral acetylcysteine (NAC) is indicated if history suggests an acute ingestion of more than 140 mg per kg or if the serum acetaminophen level falls on or above the line on a Rumack–Matthew nomogram (http://www.tylenolprofessional.com/assets/Nomogram.pdf). Treatment with NAC started within 8 hours of ingestion has been shown to effectively prevent hepatotoxicity, regardless of initial serum level. The loading dose is 140 mg per kg followed by 70 mg per kg every 4 hours for 17 doses. It may be diluted with a soft drink or juice to a 5% solution. NAC may be administered intravenously to patients with GI obstruction or inability to tolerate oral NAC.

Tricyclic Antidepressants

- Cardiac abnormalities including conduction delays (QRS >100 ms) and dysrhythmia, hypotension, and seizures may occur soon after poisoning and without warning.
- Use sodium bicarbonate infusion for ventricular tachyarrhythmia and QRS prolongation, norepinephrine for refractory hypotension and benzodiazepines for seizures. Avoid class IA and IC antidysrhythmics, which may exacerbate dysrhythmias, and flumazenil, which may precipitate seizures and cardiac arrest.

Antihistamines

- Cardiac monitoring, intravenous access, and administration of activated charcoal are indicated for potentially significant ingestion. Monitor for signs of developing anticholinergic syndrome.
- Acetaminophen and aspirin are frequently combined with antihistamine preparations, and levels for these drugs should be obtained.
- Benzodiazepines may be used for acute dystonic reactions, agitation, or seizures.

- Physostigmine (antilirium) is a specific antidote for significant anticholinergic toxicity, including tachydysrhythmias with hemodynamic compromise, refractory seizures, severe agitation, or psychosis. Use of physostigmine is contraindicated with QRS prolongation and must be given under close cardiac rhythm monitoring.

Insulin or Sulfonylureas

- Overdose of insulin or sulfonylureas, as well as ethanol, aspirin, and β-blockers, may produce hypoglycemia. Sulfonylureas may produce prolonged or recurrent hypoglycemia requiring continuous glucose infusion with glucose monitoring every 1 to 2 hours.
- All pediatric patients with symptomatic hypoglycemia should receive intravenous glucose administered as 2 to 4 mL per kg of D25 solution via slow IV push (children <12 years) or 1 to 2 mL per kg of D50 solution (children >12 years). For neonates and children with severe symptoms of hypoglycemia (convulsions, coma), give 2 mL per kg of D10 solution by slow IV push.
- Glucagon may be administered if the patient is unconscious or unable to swallow or if intravenous access cannot be obtained immediately. Give 0.5 mg intramuscularly or subcutaneously for children <20 kg or 1 mg for children >20 kg. Position the patient's head to the side to prevent aspiration from glucagon-induced emesis.
- Octreotide is recommended for serious sulfonylurea toxicity or recalcitrant hypoglycemia. Give a 1- to 2-μg per kg bolus subcutaneously or intravenously; repeat the dose every 6 hours for 2 to 3 more doses. Patients treated with octreotide should be monitored for rebound hypoglycemia for at least 24 hours after discontinuation of the therapy.

Hydrocarbons

- Ensuring an adequate airway should be the first priority in patients with hydrocarbon poisoning. All patients should receive supplement oxygen. Early intubation, mechanical ventilation, and use of positive end-expiratory pressure should be used for patients with respiratory failure. Persistent coughing, gasping, or choking is indicative of aspiration.
- Remove the patient's clothing and decontaminate skin with water followed by soap or shampoo as soon as possible after exposure as inhalation of vapors and cutaneous absorption can occur for many hours after exposure.
- Gastric decontamination is not indicated unless the hydrocarbon product is a substance known for its systemic toxicity, including camphor, halogenated hydrocarbons, aromatic hydrocarbons, and those containing metal or pesticide. Nasogastric lavage is indicated when lavage will be attempted in order to reduce the risk of vomiting and aspiration associated with a large-caliber orogastric tube.

Iron

- Volume resuscitation and supplemental oxygen are vital. Whole-bowel irrigation is indicated with ingestion of iron given the associated risk of morbidity and mortality.
- Deferoxamine (Desferal) is indicated for ingestions over 60 mg per kg of elemental iron and is given intravenously at no more than 15 mg/kg/hour for 6 hours. Continuation of therapy depends on severity of toxicity and may be necessary for up to 24 hours. Patients should be observed for recurrence of toxicity for 2 to 3 hours after discontinuation.

Lead

- Treatment for chronic lead poisoning should be in a lead-free environment. Hospitalization may be necessary if the home is not safe.
- Succimer (dimercaptosuccinic acid [DMSA]) is given orally, 10 mg per kg every 8 hours for 5 days, followed by 10 mg per kg every 12 hours for 14 days, for moderately severe lead intoxication (blood lead level [BLL] 45 to 69 μg per dL). The capsules can be mixed with juice, applesauce, or ice cream. Rebound increase in lead level is to be expected within the first week after completion of chelation therapy as lead stored in the bones redistributes to soft tissues and blood. A repeat course of DMSA may be necessary based on post-treatment BLL. Iron supplementation for iron deficiency anemia may be given concomitantly with DMSA.
- Symptomatic patients or severe lead poisoning should be admitted and treated with parenteral dimercaprol (British antilewisite, or BAL) and edetate calcium disodium (EDTA).

Salicylates

- Cases of significant salicylate toxicity may go unrecognized, given its presence in many over-the-counter products, including Bengay, oil of wintergreen, and Pepto-Bismol. Look for patients presenting with tinnitus, hyperventilation, tachycardia, and metabolic acidosis. Activated charcoal, given as a single dose, may be considered within 1 hour of ingestion.
- Treatment is directed at correction of acid–base derangements, enhancing elimination and preventing fluid deficits. Administer intravenous sodium bicarbonate as a 1- to 2-mEq per kg bolus followed by a continuous infusion, intravenous fluids to achieve urine output of 1 to 2 mL/kg/hour with a urine pH of 7.5.
- Early definitive therapy with hemodialysis is indicated for significant ingestions and critically ill patients with end-organ injury. Do not rely on the Done nomogram for predicting toxicity.[8]

Toxic Alcohols (Ethanol, Ethylene Glycol, Isopropanol, and Methanol)

- These alcohols are rapidly absorbed and toxicity may initially be attributed to ethanol intoxication. Parent alcohols are responsible for early toxicity, whereas metabolites of ethylene glycol and methanol cause end-organ damage.
- Fomepizole is a specific antidote for serious methanol or ethylene glycol ingestion. Give a 15-mg per kg loading dose, followed by 10 mg per kg every 12 hours for four doses, then 15 mg per kg every 12 hours until toxic alcohol level <20 mg per dL. If fomepizole is unavailable, an older alternative is ethanol 10% intravenous infusion titrated to a serum concentration of 100 mg per dL. Fomepizole and ethanol inhibit alcohol dehydrogenase, preventing the formation of toxic metabolites.
- Hemodialysis should be used if the patient develops metabolic acidosis or acute renal failure.

CONTINUING CARE AND PREVENTION

- Consider child neglect or abuse in poisonings under the age of 12 months. Unintentional ingestion is unusual after age 5 and poisoning is frequently due to stress, suicidal gesture or attempt, or drug-seeking behavior.
- An adequate observation period should be established after diagnosis and initial treatment. Poison prevention education is an essential component of follow-up care, and parents should be taught when and how to contact Poison Control. Involvement of social work or child protective services may be necessary, and referral source should be identified for follow-up treatment.

REFERENCES

1. American Association of Poison Control Centers. *Alerts: Laundry Detergent Packets*. Alexandria, VA: AAPCC. http://www.aapcc.org/alerts/laundry-detergent-packets. Accessed April 23, 2014.
2. McKay CA Jr. Can the laboratory help me? Toxicology laboratory testing in the possibly poisoned pediatric patient. *Clin Pediatr Emerg Med* 2005;6:116–122.
3. American Academy of Clinical Toxicology, European Association of Poisons Centres and Clinical Toxicologists. Position paper: single-dose activated charcoal. *Clin Toxicol* 2005;43:61–87.
4. American Academy of Clinical Toxicology, European Association of Poison Centres and Clinical Toxicologists. Position Statement and Practice Guidelines on the Use of Multi-Dose Activated Charcoal in the Treatment of Acute Poisoning. *Clin Toxicol* 1999;37(6):731–751.
5. American Academy of Clinical Toxicology, European Association of Poison Centres and Clinical Toxicologists. Position paper update: gastric lavage for gastrointestinal decontamination. *Clin Toxicol* 2013;51:140–146.
6. American Academy of Pediatrics Committee on Injury, Violence, and Poison Prevention. Poison treatment in the home. *Pediatrics* 2003;112:1182–1185, Reaffirmed 2007.
7. American Academy of Clinical Toxicology, European Association of Poison Centres and Clinical Toxicologists. Position paper: ipecac syrup. *Clin Toxicol* 2004;42(2):133–143.
8. Michael, JB, Sztajnkrycer, MD. Deadly pediatric poisons: nine common agents that kill at low doses. *Emerg Med Clin N Am* 2004;22:1019–1050.

4.9 Behavioral Problems of Children

Keely J. Beam

GENERAL PRINCIPLES

Appointments with the family physician (FP) provide important opportunities for screening and diagnosing behavioral problems in infants and children. FPs are often the first professionals to be consulted by parents when a behavior problem arises. Given that long-term outcomes are improved by early intervention, it is important that FPs learn to screen, diagnose, and treat behavioral problems. Due to the limited time, FPs have to spend with an individual patient; they must also know when to refer a child to a specialist for additional assessment and what community resources are available to assist both children with behavioral problems and their families.

- **Prevention of behavioral problems.** Causation of behavioral problems are numerous and may include (but are not limited to) organic/genetic factors, physical factors, prenatal factors, early trauma, developmental delays, attachment disruptions, unrealistic parental expectations, poor parenting skills, poor parental mental health, parental substance abuse, physical/sexual/emotional abuse, and neglect. FPs should be aware of these factors and the impact they have on normal development. Providing anticipatory guidance is a focus of well-child care. FPs should also be aware of services in their community that will provide assistance to families in need at no or reduced financial cost. The Individuals with Disabilities Education Act (IDEA 2004 and 2011) guarantees services to children, from birth, with issues that will or do interfere with functioning in school. Under the IDEA, public agencies have a duty to find children in need of assistance; FPs should know whom to contact, in their area, to initiate services. In cases of abuse and/or neglect, FPs should contact the appropriate authorities per their mandatory reporter requirement. Local human service departments provide many services as well as protection for children.

Assessment

Behavioral *problems* may be a function of a single setting, including the people. Behavioral *disorders* manifest themselves across settings. In order to make an appropriate diagnosis and develop an effective treatment plan, FPs should work collaboratively with parents, psychologists (school, clinical, and/or developmental), school nurses, teachers, and social workers. **Remember the R.I.O.T. outline for effective behavioral assessment:**

- **Review records.** A review of records provides FPs with insight into the evolution of the presenting problem. In addition, it will provide clues to causation, which may provide direction for treatment.
- **Interview.** Interview information, which may take the form of questionnaires or behavioral checklists, should be obtained from parents, teachers, and other significant caregivers, primarily to ascertain if the behavior is consistent over time and situations.
  - Behavior checklists should be normed, valid, and reliable for the behavior of concern. If the FP is unsure in regard to the validity and reliability of a given instrument, contact the school psychologist assigned to the child's school. Statistics, assessment, and test development are core subjects in school psychology graduate programs.
- **Observe.** Observations provide valuable data when making a behavioral diagnosis. In order to generate valid and reliable observations across settings, FPs will have to collaborate with parents, school psychologists, school nurses, teachers, and/or social workers. Observations of events, such as tantrums or defiant behaviors, should follow the ABC model:
  - What was the **antecedent** of the event?
  - Describe the **behavior.** Do not include value judgments, do not speculate on internal motivation(s), but list measurable, observable behavior.
  - What was the **consequence (good and bad)** of the behavior?
- **Test.** Psychological testing of children with behavioral problems is time-consuming and fraught with issues that reduce the validity and reliability of the testing instrument. FPs should work collaboratively with specially trained psychologists when testing is indicated.

Principles of Behavioral Intervention

- Children respond to respect from caregivers. Behavioral interventions will not be successful if the child is treated disrespectfully.
- Consistency of response is critical. Behavioral change occurs only in the context of consistent and predictable responses.
- Effective interventions include direct instruction for the child about expected behavior and its beneficial consequences, including positive reinforcement(s).
- When negative reinforcement is necessary, it should be age and behavior appropriate.
- Reassure parents that children need and want them to provide direction, and exert consistent, reasonable controls on their behavior.
- Tailor the plan to the child and the family. "One size fits all" does not apply to behavioral intervention, even in the same family. Plans must be specific—and communicated clearly to the child.
- Review progress on a regular basis and adjust the plan as needed.

Overview of Techniques for Intervention

- Most parents learned their parenting techniques from their own upbringing and lack the skills to change what can often be a cycle of dysfunctional parenting. Although poverty can be an exacerbating factor, FPs should be aware that poor parenting and the outcomes affect all socioeconomic groups. Parental training is a time-consuming process and outside the time allotment of an average office visit. FPs should be aware of community resources offered through schools, public mental health facilities, or churches, which offer free and/or reduced-cost parenting instruction.
  - **Classical and operant conditioning principles** can be effective in changing behavior permanently when used consistently. Positive and negative reinforcement and punishment, such as time-out, are effective when used properly. Children are attention-seeking beings, whether it is positive or negative attention. **Never ignore behavior!** Recognizing good behavior, even if it is expected, is one way to reinforce it. Guidelines for implementing time-out suggest that 1 minute per year of the child's life is developmentally appropriate. Although rewards can also be effective, used in isolation, the expectations of the child can escalate. As children age, and are better able to communicate, **cognitive-behavioral therapies** have also been shown to be effective in changing behavior.
  - **Addressing the cognitive component of behavior through natural and logical consequences.** When safe, parents should let children learn about their environment through exploration and experimentation. In this model, parents prepare a child-friendly environment and utilize teaching moments, including opportunities to model correct behavior and direct instruction about correct behavior. Children experience the consequences, both good and bad, of their behavior. As a child grows in intellect, parents can discuss consequences, and when necessary, alternative behavior.
  - **Therapeutic model.** In cases where behavior problems are persistent or severe and are not responding to increased parental efficacy, the FP may consider referral to a mental health professional for testing and/or counseling. This approach is most successful when the FP collaborates with mental health professionals, parents, and child (if appropriate). Children do not live in isolation, but in family and societal systems. Intervention is most successful when the system is treated as opposed to the child alone.
- **Mental health concerns in children.** Behavioral problems in children can be classified into three categories. First, there are problem behaviors that are normal for a child's age and development level, which will resolve with maturity and adequate parenting. Second, there are problem behaviors that were part of normal development, but that have persisted beyond what is age-appropriate and that will need intervention to resolve. Third, there are problem behaviors that indicate a serious underlying mental health problem. FPs should understand not only behavioral aberrations, but also normal behavioral development in order to differentiate. The American Psychological Association has compiled a classification system, which includes classifications for children with emotional/behavioral disorders in its *Diagnostic and Statistical Manual of Mental Disorders, 5th ed.* (DSM-5). Although a complete listing accompanied by diagnostic criteria can be found in the DSM-5, some common disorders that may cause behavior problems are listed here:
  - **Autism spectrum disorders (ASP):** autism, Asperger syndrome, childhood disintegration disorder, and pervasive developmental disorders. ASPs are characterized by social impairment and restricted behaviors. In addition, they may also be accompanied by language impairment, regression(s) in functioning, and mental retardation. Research studies are constantly identifying new clues to diagnosis. For example, a recent study indicated that eye-contact decline between 2 and 4 months was highly correlated with children later diagnosed with autism. Early diagnosis is important especially for children with ASPs because 50% of children that receive early intervention attend integrated kindergarten.

- **Attention-deficient and disruptive emotional/behavioral disorders:** attention-deficit/hyperactivity disorder (ADHD), oppositional defiant disorder (ODD), conduct disorder (CD), disruptive mood dysregulation disorder (DMDD).
  - ADAHD is characterized by inattention, hyperactivity, and impulsivity. These symptoms generally occur across settings, but are generally most noticeable during school and other times when seat work is required.
  - ODD is characterized by a continued pattern of defiant, disobedient, and hostile behavior.
  - CD is characterized bullying, threatening, and intimidating. In addition, rules of home, school, and society are often disregarded.
  - DMDD is new to the DSM-5. It is characterized by severe outbursts of anger and a persistent angry mood.
- **Feeding and eating disorders:** pica, rumination, anorexia nervosa, and bulimia nervosa.
- **Tic disorders:** transient tic, chronic motor or vocal tic, Tourette disorder.
- **Elimination disorders:** enuresis, encopresis.
- **Internalizing disorders:** depression, anxiety, bipolar.
  - Depression is characterized by depressed mood, irritability, and loss of interest in activities, and may also include physical symptoms. Pediatric bipolar is also a classification of depressive disorder in the DSM-5. Research is currently being conducted on this disorder, which is difficult to differentiate from ADHD and depression. Depression can also lead to suicidal ideation, which is a national crisis. A 1998 study indicated that 20.5% of high school students had seriously considered suicide during a 12-month period, whereas 7.7% of students report making at least one suicide attempt.
  - Anxiety is characterized by constant and excessive worry. Anxiety disorders may also include separation anxiety (when not developmentally appropriate), social phobias, other specific phobias, panic attacks, obsessive–compulsive disorder, and posttraumatic stress disorder.
- Bipolar disorder is characterized by manic and depressive "mood episodes."
- **Learning disabilities** are listed in the DSM-5, although they do have behavioral components as diagnostic criteria, undiagnosed or unaided learning disabilities will often lead to anxiety, depression, and frustration.
- **Oral habits** that persist beyond what is developmentally appropriate, such as nail-biting, digit-sucking, or refusal to relinquish a pacifier. These behaviors often act as self-soothing activities for children in times of stress and anxiety. By treating the underlying cause as well as the presenting problem, these behaviors may be extinguished.
- **Sleep disturbances** such as night terrors are a normal developmental stage for toddlers. However, when these disturbances persist or intensify, it may be an indication of anxiety or trauma. Other sleep disturbances may include sleepwalking and bedtime battles. Bedtime battles respond well to consistent bedtime routines and consistent expectations.
- **Gay and lesbian issues** in adolescence have been linked to increased depression and anxiety. Because of continued social stigmatism, gay and lesbian teenagers may feel isolated and without social support. Gay and lesbian teenagers are 20 times more likely to attempt a suicide. Many communities and mental health providers have developed gay and lesbian support groups to help combat this sense of isolation.
- **Early cigarette smoking and/or alcohol use** are considered problem behavior not only due to health/legal concerns, but because they are gateway drugs to more dangerous and harmful illegal drugs.
- **Working with other professionals.** Over the past decades, the time FPs have to spend with individual patients has been reduced, therefore, they must become experts in collaboration. Family/child service plans, including parenting advice/instruction, in-depth assessment, intervention planning, and counseling for mental health disorders, require interdisciplinary partnerships. Under the federal law, the IDEA, 2004 (school-aged children) and 2011 (infants and toddler), schools are required to employ school psychologists. School psychologists are experts on testing, planning interventions, and leading collaborative teams. A collaborative-minded FP, who is knowledgeable in accessing community resources, may be the most important person a child with behavioral problems encounters.

REFERENCES

1. American Psychological Association. *Diagnostic and statistical manual of mental disorders.* 5th ed. Arlington, VA: American Psychiatric Publishing; 2013.
2. Callahan SA, Panichelli-Mindel SM, Kendall PC. DSM-IV and internalizing disorders: modifications, limitations and utility. *Sch Psychol Rev* 1996;25(3):297–307.
3. Coleman MC. *Emotional and behavioral disorders: theory and practice.* 3rd ed. Needham Height, MA: Allyn & Bacon; 1996.

4. Eckert TL, Miller DN, DuPaul GJ, et al. Adolescent suicide prevention. *Sch Psychol Rev* 2003:32(1):57–76.
5. Jones W, Klin A. Attention to eyes is present but declines in 2–6 month-old infants later diagnosed with autism. *Nature* 2013;504(7480):427–431.
6. Kampaus RW, Frick PJ. *Clinical assessment of child and adolescent personality and behavior.* 2nd ed. Needham Heights, MA: Allyn & Bacon; 2005.
7. National Association of School Psychologists. *Best practices in school psychology.* 5th ed. Stratford, CT: NASP; 2008.
8. Power TJ. Promoting children's mental health. *Sch Psychol Rev* 2003;32(1):3–16.
9. Sattler JM. *Assessment of children.* 5th ed. La Mesa, CA: Jerome M. Sattler; 2006.

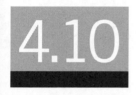

4.10 Attention-Deficit/ Hyperactivity Disorder

Deborah S. Clements

GENERAL PRINCIPLES

Attention-deficit/hyperactivity disorder (ADHD) is a condition that begins in early childhood and is characterized by symptoms of inattention, hyperactivity, and impulsivity. The symptoms broadly affect functioning in most areas of daily activity.[1] The prevalence of ADHD is estimated at between 8% and 10% of school-aged children. The condition occurs two to four times more commonly in boys than in girls and persists into adulthood in as many as 70% of cases.[2]

DIAGNOSIS
Clinical Presentation

Patients typically present as a result of concerns expressed by parents, teachers, or other caregivers during the primary grades of school. Although symptoms may not be apparent during the clinical visit, questions about school performance, behavior with friends and siblings, and completion of assignments and tasks both at home and at school are helpful in establishing a diagnosis.

• **Hyperactivity** presents as excessive talking or fidgeting, inability to remain seated during class, and difficulty playing quietly. Hyperactive features tend to predominate in the early years of childhood, peak at about 7 or 8 years of age and improve during adolescence.
• **Impulsivity** is also observed in early childhood, although tends to persist into adulthood. Commonly, these children have difficulty waiting their turn, are disruptive in the classroom, often interrupting or intruding into others' activities. Occasionally, impulsivity results in peer rejection and can later manifest in substance abuse and difficulty managing finances.
• **Inattention** is manifested by forgetfulness, losing or misplacing homework or materials from school, disorganization, failure to complete assignments or tasks, poor attention to detail, and lack of concentration. These symptoms may appear later in childhood and also persist throughout life.

Because the differential diagnosis of ADHD includes hearing or visual impairment, diabetes, thyroid disorders, fetal alcohol syndrome, and seizure disorders, a complete physical and appropriate testing should be performed.

Diagnostic Criteria

• Children ages 6 to 12 years who present with symptoms of inattention, hyperactivity, impulsivity, poor academic performance, or behavioral problems should be evaluated for ADHD. For a diagnosis to be made, the child must meet the DSM-5 criteria either in the context of the clinical visit or as observed by parents, teachers, or caregivers.[2] ADHD can be categorized into three presentations: (a) predominantly inattentive, (b) predominantly hyperactive–impulsive, and (c) combined. The presentation may change in any patient over time.

The diagnostic criteria for ADHD were established by the American Psychiatric Association in the *Diagnostic and Statistical Manual of Mental Disorders*, 5th ed. (DSM-5) and are summarized in Table 4.10-1.

Table 4.10-1	Diagnostic Criteria for ADHD/Hyperkinetic Disorder

1. Inattention: Six or more symptoms of inattention for children up to age 16, or five or more for adolescents 17 and older and adults; symptoms of inattention have been present for at least 6 months, and they are inappropriate for developmental level:
   a. Often fails to give close attention to details or makes careless mistakes in schoolwork, at work, or with other activities.
   b. Often has trouble-holding attention on tasks or play activities.
   c. Often does not seem to listen when spoken to directly.
   d. Often does not follow through on instructions and fails to finish schoolwork, chores, or duties in the workplace (e.g., loses focus, side-tracked).
   e. Often has trouble-organizing tasks and activities.
   f. Often avoids, dislikes, or is reluctant to do tasks that require mental effort over a long period of time (such as schoolwork or homework).
   g. Often loses things necessary for tasks and activities (e.g., school materials, pencils, books, tools, wallets, keys, paperwork, eyeglasses, mobile telephones).
   h. Is often easily distracted.
   i. Is often forgetful in daily activities.
2. Hyperactivity and Impulsivity: Six or more symptoms of hyperactivity–impulsivity for children up to age 16, or five or more for adolescents 17 and older and adults; symptoms of hyperactivity–impulsivity have been present for at least 6 months to an extent that is disruptive and inappropriate for the person's developmental level:
   a. Often fidgets with or taps hands or feet, or squirms in seat.
   b. Often leaves seat in situations when remaining seated is expected.
   c. Often runs about or climbs in situations where it is not appropriate (adolescents or adults may be limited to feeling restless).
   d. Often unable to play or take part in leisure activities quietly.
   e. Is often "on the go" acting as if "driven by a motor."
   f. Often talks excessively.
   g. Often blurts out an answer before a question has been completed.
   h. Often has trouble waiting his/her turn.
   i. Often interrupts or intrudes on others (e.g., butts into conversations or games).

In addition, the following conditions must be met:

- Several inattentive or hyperactive–impulsive symptoms were present before age 12 years.
- Several symptoms are present in two or more settings (e.g., at home, school or work; with friends or relatives; in other activities).
- There is clear evidence that the symptoms interfere with, or reduce the quality of, social, school, or work functioning.

The symptoms do not happen only during the course of schizophrenia or another psychotic disorder. The symptoms are not better explained by another mental disorder (e.g., mood disorder, anxiety disorder, dissociative disorder, or a personality disorder).

Based on the types of symptoms, three kinds (presentations) of ADHD can occur:

Combined Presentation: if enough symptoms of both criteria for inattention and hyperactivity–impulsivity were present for the past 6 months. (314.01 (F90.2))

Predominantly Inattentive Presentation: if enough symptoms of inattention, but not hyperactivity–impulsivity, were present for the past 6 months. (314.00 (F90.0))

Predominantly Hyperactive-Impulsive Presentation: if enough symptoms of hyperactivity–impulsivity but not inattention were present for the past 6 months. (314.01 (F90.1))

Reprinted with permission from the *Diagnostic and Statistical Manual of Mental Disorders*. 5th ed. (Copyright 2013). American Psychiatric Association.

Assessment

- Office screening tests are available and relatively straightforward. These tools may be repeated following treatment to assess effectiveness.
- Standardized questionnaires completed by teachers, parents, and other caregivers are useful in both initial diagnosis and follow-up. These include the Conners 3 Rating Scale, the AD/HD Rating Scale, BASC Monitor Rating Scale, and the Vanderbilt Assessment Scales (www.nichq.org/resources/toolkit), among others.
- Assessment may be done through progress reports submitted by teachers and caregivers.
- Safety and injury prevention should be discussed at each visit because children with ADHD are at increased risk for both intentional and unintentional injury.
- Because comorbidity is common, patients should be re-evaluated whenever new symptoms emerge or existing symptoms worsen.
- Pitfalls in accurate diagnosis:
  - Behaviors may not be observed during the office visit.
  - Assessment questionnaires may convey a false sense of validity.
  - Discrepancies may exist in reports from teachers and parents or caregivers or history may be unavailable.
  - Other diagnostic tests such as laboratory studies, computed tomography, and electroencephalogram are of little value in diagnosis of ADHD.
  - The response to stimulant medication cannot be used to confirm or refute the diagnosis of ADHD.
  - 20% to 35% of children have a comorbid psychiatric diagnosis or a learning disability.
  - Because of the potential for multiple comorbidities and overlapping conditions, accurate diagnosis may require several office visits and reassessment is needed if symptoms worsen or new concerns develop.

TREATMENT

Medications

- ADHD is a chronic condition that requires long-term treatment. Stimulants are first-line therapy for treatment of ADHD in children age 6 and older. With careful dose titration, up to 80% of children will respond to at least one stimulant without significant adverse effects.[3]
- Current medication choices include short-, intermediate-, and long-acting methylphenidate (Ritalin, Methylin, Metadate, Concerta) and dextroamphetamine (Adderall). Atomoxetine (Strattera), a non-stimulant medication, has also been approved for use in ADHD. A transdermal methylphenidate patch is also available (Daytrana) (Table 4.10-2).
- Adverse events associated with stimulant use include decreased appetite, headache, sleep disturbances, motor tics, and slowed growth velocity. Growth typically catches up during adolescence with discontinuation of medication.

Behavioral Therapy

Although behavioral therapy alone is not proven to significantly reduce the core symptoms of ADHD, behavior problems can be improved. The goal of behavioral therapy is to focus on increasing the structure of the child's daily routine and to minimize distractions. A system of positive and negative reinforcements including praise and time-outs or loss of privileges can be useful.

Alternative Therapy

Dietary modification, nutritional supplements, homeopathy, and vision therapy have been suggested as treatments for ADHD in the lay press. Studies have indicated, however, that none of these alternatives has a response better than placebo.[4]

Referral

Evaluation by a pediatric subspecialist should be considered for children less than 6 years of age. Additionally, referral is appropriate for children with comorbid psychiatric diagnoses such as oppositional defiant disorder, those with learning disabilities, speech or motor delay, and a history of abuse, of severe aggression or emotional distress, or if response to treatment remains inadequate.

Table 4.10-2 Medications Used in the Treatment of ADHD

Agent	Dose schedule	Duration of action (h)	Schedule
Stimulants			
Methylphenidate			
Ritalin, Metadate, Methylin	Two to three times daily	3–5	5–20 mg BID to TID
Ritalin SR, Metadate ER, Methylin ER	Once or twice daily	3–8	20–40 mg QD or 40 mg in morning and 20 mg in early afternoon
Concerta, Metadata CD, Ritalin LA	QD	8–12	18–54 mg QD, max 72 mg
Daytrana (patch)	Worn 9 hr/day	12–18	10–30 mg
Amphetamine			
Dexedrine, Dextrostat	BID to TID	4–6	5–15 mg BID or 5–10 mg TID
Adderall, Dexedrine spansule	QD to BID	6–8	5–30 mg QD or 5–15 mg BID
Adderall-XR	QD	8	10–30 mg QD
Focalin	BID	6–8	5–10 mg BID
Nonstimulants			
Atomoxetine			
Strattera	QD to BID	8	1.2–1.4 mg/kg/d

Adapted from Dopheide JA. ASHP therapeutic position statement on the appropriate use of medications in the treatment of attention-deficit/hyperactivity disorder in pediatric patients. *Am J Health Syst Pharm* 2005;62(14):1504, 1506.

REFERENCES

1. American Psychiatric Association. Attention-deficit/hyperactivity disorder. In: *Diagnostic and statistical manual of mental disorders.* 5th ed. Arlington, VA: American Psychiatric Association; 2013.
2. ADHD: Clinical practice guideline for the diagnosis, evaluation, and treatment of attention-deficit/hyperactivity disorder in children and adolescents. American Academy of Pediatrics. *Pediatrics* 2011;128:1007.
3. Wender EH. Managing stimulant medication for attention-deficit/hyperactivity disorder. *Pediatr Rev* 2001;22:183.
4. Baumgaertel A. Alternative and controversial treatments for attention-deficit/hyperactivity disorder. *Pediatr Clin North Am* 1999;46:977–992.

CHAPTER 5

Human Behavior and Problems of Living

Section Editor: Jessica B. Koran-Scholl

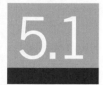

Anxiety Disorders
Michael L. Brown, Rachel Bramson

GENERAL PRINCIPLES

These groups of disorders are the most common psychiatric illnesses.[1] Patients with generalized anxiety disorder (GAD) and panic disorder (PD) present frequently in primary care. Eighty-three percent of patients with anxiety disorders present with somatic symptoms; the higher the number of symptoms, the higher the chances of an anxiety disorder. Anxiety disorders have a high public health cost with markedly decreased role functioning, reduced health-related quality of life and missed work days.[2] Failure to recognize and treat anxiety disorders in primary care results in decreased quality of life for patients and inappropriate over-utilization of health care services.[2,3] In a large study of primary care patients, 41% of those diagnosed with an anxiety disorder by study screening were not undergoing any kind of treatment.[4]

Pathophysiology

- Diminished sensitivity to γ-aminobutyric acid (GABA)/benzodiazepine complex (GABA is the main inhibitory brain neurotransmitter).
- Decreased α_2-adrenergic receptor sensitivity. This could be due to high levels of circulating catecholamines. This may be caused by an inappropriate/chronic activation of the fight or flight response.
- Studies are not uniform with regard to serotonin system, but some show abnormalities in GAD patients.
- Reduced autonomic responsiveness in GAD, possibly related to decreased vagal tone.[5]

Etiology and Mechanisms of Injury

Etiology is not known, but studies suggest familial patterns with a probable underlying genetic basis.[5] Additionally, early childhood stressors or emotional trauma may cause brain remodeling and neurochemical changes, which increase the likelihood of anxiety disorders. Neuroimaging studies suggest anatomical and functional brain differences in patients with these disorders. This area warrants further investigation.[5,6]

Diagnosis in the Primary Care Setting

Use of instruments can aid in primary care detection of anxiety disorders. The GAD-7 is readily available online and is a rapid and effective tool for screening and tracking response over time. The Zung Anxiety Scale is a brief screening instrument, whereas the Hamilton Anxiety Rating Scale and Beck's Anxiety Inventory can be used for confirmation of diagnosis and to document severity and improvement. Short 2- and 5-item (MHI-5, Mental Health Index 5) screening questionnaires for PD have high sensitivity and adequate sensitivity to merit use.[7,8] The Yale-Brown Obsessive–Compulsive Scale (YBOCS) is a standard tool for assessing the severity of symptoms and response to treatment with serial ratings. The PC-PTSD instrument is a 4-question screen suitable for use in primary care.

Definitional Changes

- A major change in DSM-5[9] involves the re-categorization of anxiety disorders into three separate categories: primary anxiety disorders, obsessive–compulsive disorders, and trauma- and stressor-related disorders. This update reflects the new understanding of the neurobiology and etiology of the disorders.
- Anxiety symptoms must be out of proportion to the actual threat or danger in the situation, and symptoms must be present for at least 6 months for all ages.

The Anxiety Disorders

- Primary anxiety disorders: GAD, PD, social anxiety disorder (social phobia), specific phobia, agoraphobia, and unspecified anxiety disorder.
- Anxiety disorders unique to childhood: separation anxiety disorder and selective mutism (other primary anxiety disorders can develop and present in childhood).
- Secondary anxiety disorders: substance/medication-induced anxiety disorder and anxiety disorder due to another medical condition.

The conditions retained in the anxiety disorders category share the common characteristic of a heightened level of anxiety and physiological arousal, whether tonically as in GAD, or episodically as in PD; they may be triggered or arise spontaneously. The obsessive–compulsive and related disorders include:

- Obsessive–compulsive disorder, body dysmorphic disorder, hoarding disorder, trichotillomania (hair-pulling disorder), excoriation (skin-picking) disorder, substance/medication-induced obsessive–compulsive and related disorder, obsessive–compulsive and related disorder due to another medical condition, other specified obsessive–compulsive and related disorder, and unspecified obsessive–compulsive and related disorder.

Obsessive–compulsive spectrum disorders share the primary feature of an unbidden, intrusive, repetitive thought, urge, or behavior, which triggers anxiety; compensatory or compulsive behaviors such as picking, pulling, touching, tapping, cleaning, and washing develop as a response to the anxiety and are an attempt to relieve it.

The Trauma- and Stressor-Related Disorders Include

- Primary trauma- and stressor-related disorders that can develop and present at any age include post-traumatic stress disorder (PTSD), acute stress disorder, adjustment disorders, other specified trauma- and stressor-related disorder, and unspecified trauma- and stressor-related disorder.
- Anxiety disorders unique to childhood: reactive attachment disorder and disinhibited social engagement disorder.

Trauma- and stressor-related disorders share the common feature of being provoked by an external event, whether traumatic as in PTSD or acute stress disorder (ASD), or a disruptive response to a nontraumatic trigger as in the case of adjustment disorders. In these disorders, the symptom of anxiety is either one of many possible responses, or part of a constellation of symptoms characteristic of the disorder. The Web site for the Anxiety and Depression Association of America has an online PTSD screen available for patients to take on their own (www.adaa.org).

Epidemiology

Forty percent of adults will have at least one anxiety disorder in their lifetime.[1] Most anxiety disorders present in the early 20s, with prevalence about two times higher in women than in men.[6] Specific phobia is the most prevalent lifetime anxiety disorder (15.5%), followed by social phobia (10.7%). Next are seasonal affective disorder (6.7%) and PTSD (5.7%), followed by GAD (4.3%) and PD (3.8%). Agoraphobia (2.5%) and obsessive–compulsive disorder have the lowest lifetime prevalence of the anxiety disorders.[1] Many adults with anxiety disorders have experienced an anxious childhood or adolescence.[10] Comorbidity with other mental health and physical disorders is common.

GENERALIZED ANXIETY DISORDER
Clinical Presentation

GAD is characterized by excessive anxiety and worry ("apprehensive expectation" is the phrase describing this in DSM-5), occurring more days than not, for at least 6 months about a number of events or activities. Associated physical symptoms include muscle tension, a feeling of being restless or "on edge," difficulty concentrating, irritability, insomnia, and fatigue.

Diagnosis (Based on DSM-5 Criteria)

GAD is based on criteria enumerated in the *Diagnostic and Statistical Manual of Mental Disorders*, 5th ed. (DSM-5).[9] The patient must experience excessive anxiety and an inability to control his or her sense of worry for at least a 6-month period and have at least three physical symptoms related to motor tension, autonomic hyperactivity, vigilance, and scanning. Motor tension and hypervigilance better differentiate GAD from other anxiety states.

Differential Diagnosis

GAD is diagnosed when the anxiety is free floating and unrelated to the specific foci of other anxiety disorders, such as worry about panic attacks (PD) or worry that focuses exclusively on health concerns (such as somatization disorder or hypochondriasis). Generalized anxiety is a frequent finding in depressive disorders; in order to make a separate GAD diagnosis, the anxiety must be present in the absence of depression. Physiological factors such as hyperthyroidism, medications, stimulant use, or abuse (including over the counter or dietary stimulants) must not be responsible for provoking and maintaining the anxiety. Exacerbations of GAD may be provoked by clearly definable psychosocial stressors, but symptoms must exceed 6 months in duration in order to be distinguished from an adjustment disorder with anxiety.

Treatment

Medical Therapy

Selective serotonin reuptake inhibitor (SSRI) medications are generally considered to be first-line interventions for GAD. **Venlafaxine extended release** (Effexor XR), **paroxetine** (Paxil), **escitalopram** (Lexapro), and **sertraline** (Zoloft) are FDA-approved for treatment of GAD. **Fluoxetine** (Prozac) is also effective.[11,12] The requirements for cardiac monitoring when using **citalopram** at doses beyond 40 mg per day make this a second-line choice within the class. This class of medicines is generally well-tolerated. Their tolerability, side-effect profile, and ease of dosing make them easy to use for the physician and easy to take for the patient. Nausea, flushing, headache, and tremor are common during the first week, and are dose-related. Insomnia is a more common side effect than somnolence, so AM dosing is recommended to start with. GAD patients are frequently more sensitive to adverse effects of medications, so lower starting doses and smaller dose increments (compared to the treatment of depression, obsessive–compulsive disorder or PD) are recommended. While **increasing the dose at 2- to 4-week intervals**, patients may begin to experience improvement as early as 2 weeks, but typically 3 to 4 weeks at a therapeutic dose is required to determine the efficacy. As with any other centrally-acting medication, tapering the dose to change or discontinue it is always necessary.

Buspirone (Buspar) is a novel medication unrelated to the SSRIs, tricyclic antidepressants (TCAs), or benzodiazepines. It is better tolerated than TCAs and can be used as a first- or second-line agent in GAD. Buspirone has been shown to be effective at total daily doses of 20 to 60 mg per day, usually divided bid or tid. Starting at 50% of the therapeutic dose (usually 7.5 mg bid), the dose is increased after a week. Dividing the dose into three, with the larger dose at night, may improve tolerability in patients who experience nausea or flushing. Like the SSRIs and TCAs, 3 to 4 weeks of treatment at a therapeutic dose are required for full response. Buspirone also has a role in augmenting SSRIs or TCAs in patients who have a partial response to monotherapy with one of these agents. As with any other centrally-acting medication, tapering the dose to change or discontinue it is always necessary.

Chronically anxious patients respond well to **benzodiazepines**, and all benzodiazepines are equally effective for the treatment of anxiety (see Table 5.1-1). The choice of one or another of these medicines is based on duration of action and pharmacokinetic factors, such as the accumulation of active metabolites, which can cause sedation or ataxia. Responders notice improvement within the first days of therapy. Benzodiazepines are appropriate in the treatment of chronic anxiety, although SSRIs are preferred since benzodiazepines may decrease alertness and psychomotor performance. Tolerance to these effects develops with consistent dosing. Absent a history of substance abuse, abuse of benzodiazepines by patients with GAD is very uncommon. However, physical dependence is to be expected. Initiating treatment with an SSRI or TCA for 1 to 2 months before attempting to taper benzodiazepines can reduce the chance of relapse. Benzodiazepines should be slowly tapered not faster than 10% to 20% of total dose per week. Many patients who are otherwise well controlled on other medications will benefit from using benzodiazepines on a prn basis for exacerbations of anxiety. Patients on benzodiazepines should not use any alcohol.

TABLE 5.1-1	Commonly Used Benzodiazepines			
Drug	Rate of onset	Usual daily dosage (mg)	Usual dose schedule	Active metabolites
Alprazolam (Xanax)	Rapid	1–6	0.5 mg TID–QID	No
Lorazepam (Ativan)	Intermediate	2–8	1 mg BID–TID	No
Clonazepam (Klonopin)	Intermediate	1–4	0.5 mg BID–TID	No
Diazepam (Valium)	Rapid	5–60	5–10 mg BID–TID	Yes
Chlordiazepoxide (Librium)	Intermediate	25–100	25 mg BID–TID	Yes
Clorazepate (Tranxene)	Rapid	7.5–60	7.5 mg BID–TID	Yes
Oxazepam (Serax)	Intermediate	30–120	10–20 mg BID–TID	No

TCAs are effective in GAD. **Imipramine** (Tofranil) has shown efficacy comparable to alprazolam. These have a greater side-effect burden, especially sedation and anticholinergic effects, compared to SSRIs or buspirone, and slower onset of action compared with benzodiazepines.

Monoamine oxidase inhibitors (MAOIs), such as **phenelzine** (Nardil) and **tranylcypromine** (Parnate), are also effective, but their complexity of drug and food interactions makes them unsuitable for general medical practice.

Other medications. Hydroxyzine (Atarax or Vistaril), an antihistamine, is superior to placebo in GAD and has a rapid onset of effect. However, its utility is limited by its sedative properties and relatively low-antianxiety properties compared to benzodiazepines. χ**-Blockers** may be helpful for symptomatic relief of tremor, but do not have antianxiety properties.

Psychotherapy
Studies clearly demonstrate that various forms of psychotherapy are helpful in treating GAD. **Cognitive behavioral therapy** (**CBT**) is superior to nondirective or supportive types of psychotherapy. **Biofeedback** and **progressive relaxation** can be helpful, especially in patients with significant complaints of muscle tension, pain, or insomnia. Referral to a psychologist or licensed counselor with specific training in these forms of psychotherapy is appropriate when considering these treatments.

Referral to a psychiatrist should be considered in cases with comorbid psychiatric disorders or when the patient has not responded to several attempts at treatment by the primary care physician. Patients with substance abuse problems should be referred to a substance abuse counselor for treatment directed at the substance abuse disorder.

PANIC DISORDER AND AGORAPHOBIA
Clinical Presentation
Panic attacks typically begin without warning. Pounding heart and dyspnea are common first symptoms, rapidly joined by dizziness or light-headedness, diaphoresis, light-headedness or faintness, chest pressure, and a sense of "impending doom," or imminent death. The symptoms typically build to a peak over 10 to 30 minutes, and resolve over the next 30 to 60 minutes, on average. When their panic attacks begin, patients most commonly present to their family physician's office or to the emergency department. Patients will most commonly describe the physical sensations first, rather than fearfulness or anxiety. With the attacks comes an intense need to escape the immediate situation, whatever it is. Phobic avoidance develops from this, as the patient gradually restricts his or her range of activities to exclude those settings in which attacks have occurred, where help might not be immediately available, or from which they might not be immediately able to escape in the event of an attack. Phobic avoidance that causes significant levels of distress or interference in the patient's life is diagnosed as agoraphobia. Up to two thirds of PD patients have some degree of phobic avoidance.[7]

Diagnosis (Based on DSM-5 Criteria)
Panic Disorder
Panic attacks are characterized by the abrupt onset of intense fear that peaks within 10 to 30 minutes of onset, and is associated with at least four autonomic symptoms, including palpitations, sweating, trembling, dyspnea, choking, chest pain, nausea, dizziness, depersonalization, paresthesias, hot or cold flashes, and fear of dying. Diagnosis requires recurrent panic attacks and either 1 month of behavior change in response to the attacks or persistent worry about additional attacks or their consequences. Panic attacks

should not be due to a general medical problem or the direct effect of a substance (e.g., amphetamines). Routine laboratory screening for general medical problems at the time of initial presentation should include basic electrolytes, calcium (hypocalcemia due to hypoparathyroidism causes tetany and tremor; can be a complication of thyroid surgery), random glucose (hypoglycemia), thyroid-stimulating hormone (hyper- and hypothyroidism), and urine drug screen. Twelve-lead EKG is usually obtained in the ED setting. This along with physical examination is generally sufficient to reassure the patient.

Sometimes however, more extensive evaluation to rule out a cardiac event may occur. Patients not reassured by extensive evaluation should be assessed for somatic symptom and related disorders. Isolated panic attacks can also occur in the context of other psychiatric conditions, most commonly other anxiety disorders and depressive disorders.

Agoraphobia

Agoraphobia is most commonly seen in patients with PD. Diagnosis requires the presence of anxiety in situations where escape is difficult or help is unavailable. Such situations are avoided, are endured with marked distress, or require a companion to be tolerated. Avoidance must not be explainable by the existence of another mental disorder. Although panic attacks are the most subjectively distressing aspect of PD to patients, severe agoraphobia can be the most disabling and the most treatment-resistant part of their illness. Patients whose agoraphobia does not improve with successful medical treatment of their panic attacks should be referred for CBT.

Treatment

In the emergency department or the office, offering patients a medical explanation and a diagnostic label for their experience can be very reassuring and therapeutic ("The workup is OK. What seems to have happened is you had a panic attack, sort of an 'adrenaline flood' in the brain"). It is not helpful to minimize or demean their experience ("it was just a panic attack")—after all, to the patient, it felt like they really were about to die! If a medical cause for the panic attack is found, management begins with treatment directed at this condition. Dietary recommendations, such as the avoidance of nicotine, caffeine, and other stimulants, are helpful.[6]

Medical Therapy

The primary goal of treating PD is preventing recurrence of spontaneous panic attacks. **Alprazolam**, because of its rapid onset, can be effective in aborting a panic attack once it has begun, especially if taken sublingually. Patients with infrequent isolated panic attacks may require only prn doses of benzodiazepines, but patients with PD typically require daily medications to prevent recurrence. Effective treatment should be continued until patients are panic free for at least 6 to 12 months. Medication should be tapered slowly to avoid withdrawal symptoms or rebound panic attacks. Recurrence rates are greater than 50% after medication discontinuation, so ongoing maintenance therapy is commonly required. Buspirone and β-blockers are not effective in PD. Many patients with PD are sensitive to the side effects of antidepressant medications such as SSRIs and TCAs, so treatment should be initiated with small doses and gradually titrated upward to therapeutic doses.

SSRIs are first-line medications in PD, alone or in combination with benzodiazepines. **Fluoxetine** (Prozac), **sertraline** (Zoloft), and **paroxetine** (Paxil) are effective. Other SSRIs, including **venlafaxine extended release** (Effexor XR) and **citalopram** (Celexa), can also be effective.[12] Full antidepressant doses are required, beginning with half of the initial dose for the first week then increasing to the first target dose. Effective doses differ for each drug (see Table 5.1-2).

The efficacy of the **TCAs** is well-established, and they are considered second-line if SSRIs fail or are not tolerated. **Imipramine** (Tofranil), **desipramine** (Norpramin), and **clomipramine** (Anafranil) are

TABLE 5.1-2	Common SSRIs in Anxiety Disorders	
Drug	**Starting dose**	**Target dose**
Fluoxetine (Prozac)	10–20 mg QAM	20–60 mg
Sertraline (Zoloft)	25–50 mg QAM	50–200 mg
Paroxetine (Paxil)	10–20 mg QAM	20–60 mg
Citalopram (Celexa)	10–20 mg QAM	20–60 mg
Escitalopram (Lexapro)	5–10 mg QAM	10–20 mg
Venlafaxine XR (Effexor XR)	37.5 mg QAM	75–225 mg

effective in PD. The initial starting dose should be 25 mg at bedtime and increased by 25 mg every 4 to 7 days as tolerated. Doses of 150 mg per day are usually required. The dosage may be slowly increased up to 300 mg per day if needed.

Nortriptyline (Pamelor) is also very effective, and may be better tolerated; doses of 75 to 150 mg per day are used. An advantage of the TCAs is the ability to monitor blood levels within defined therapeutic ranges. Three weeks of treatment at an adequate dose is usually necessary before panic suppression is achieved.

High-potency **benzodiazepines** are highly effective in the treatment of PD, with efficacy similar to that of the SSRIs and TCAs. Compared with GAD, higher doses of benzodiazepines are required in PD (see Table 5.1-1). Clonazepam is preferred for its longer duration of action, allowing less frequent doses and less risk for rebound panic between doses. As a rule, low doses should always be started, then gradually titrated upward to the lowest dose that provides the best clinical effect. For patients with severe symptoms, it may be indicated to initiate treatment with a benzodiazepine for rapid symptom relief at the same time that an SSRI or TCA is started, then gradually to reduce the benzodiazepine to prn use after a few weeks.

Most patients who take benzodiazepines maintain their therapeutic benefit on a stable dose over time. Problems of misuse or abuse of benzodiazepines are probably limited to patients with histories of alcohol or drug abuse, or who increase their too-low medication doses on their own in an attempt to self-medicate ("pseudo-addiction"). Mood symptoms should be followed, as clonazepam can sometimes cause depressed mood, and alprazolam can occasionally cause excitation or rarely mania.

MAOIs, such as **phenelzine** (Nardil) or **tranylcypromine** (Parnate), may be even more effective than the tricyclics in resistant cases. Because of the dietary restrictions and the potential for drug interactions, these drugs are not the first line of therapy and are not generally recommended in the primary care setting.

Psychotherapy
CBT is effective in the treatment of PD and has been shown to increase the likelihood that patients can eventually reduce and even discontinue benzodiazepine treatment. The primary behavioral techniques include breathing retraining, relaxation training, and exposure to somatic cues, in which the patient is taught to recognize and restructure their interpretations of their physical symptoms. This form of therapy is effective in both group and individual settings.

Treatment involving gradual exposure of the agoraphobic patient to feared situations is essential if agoraphobia is to be overcome. Focused CBT is more effective than nonspecific or purely supportive interventions in this regard. Supportive interventions and patient education are, however, helpful in encouraging the patient to undergo and work in therapy and confront these situations.

Referral to a psychiatrist should be considered in cases with comorbid psychiatric disorders or when the patient has not responded to several attempts at treatment by the primary care physician. Patients with substance abuse problems should be referred to a substance abuse counselor for treatment directed at the substance abuse disorder.

Online Provider Tools and Patient Education Resources
For clinicians, the American Psychiatric association has an extensive list of online rating scales useful for diagnosis and severity rating at their Web site http://www.psychiatry.org/practice/dsm/dsm5/online-assessment-measures

Bibliotherapy for Patients
- The Anxiety and Phobia Workbook by Edmund J. Bourne
- The Feeling Good Handbook by David R. Burns
- The Anxiety Disease by David V. Sheehan

Web Sites for Patients
- *www.healthyminds.org*—Patient Education site of the American Psychiatric Association (APA)
- *www.adaa.org*—Anxiety and Depression Association of America
- *www.nami.org*—National Alliance on Mental Illness (general information)
- *www.ocfoundation.org*—The Obsessive Compulsive Foundation (for OCD)

REFERENCES
1. Kessler RC, Petukhova M, Sampson NA, et al. Twelve-month and lifetime prevalence and lifetime morbid risk of anxiety and mood disorders in the United States. *Int J Methods Psychiatr Res* 2012;21(3):169–184.
2. Stein MB, Roy-Byrne PP, Craske MG, et al. Functional impact and health utility of anxiety disorders in primary care outpatients. *Med Care* 2005;43(12):1164–1170.

3. Katon W. Panic disorder: relationship to high medical utilization, unexplained physical symptoms, and medical costs. *J Clin Psychiatry* 1996;57(Suppl 10):11–22.
4. Kroenke K, Spitzer RL, Williams JBW, et al. Anxiety disorders in primary care: prevalence, impairment, comorbidity, and detection. *Ann Intern Med* 2007;146(5):317–325.
5. Martin EI, Ressler KJ, Binder E, et al. The neurobiology of anxiety disorders: brain imaging, genetics, and psychoneuroendocrinology. *Clin Lab Med* 2010;30(4):865–891.
6. Seedat S, Scott KM, Angermeyer MC, et al. Cross-national associations between gender and mental disorders in the world health organization world mental health surveys. *Arch Gen Psychiatry* 2009;66(7):785–795.
7. Stein MB, Roy-Byrne PP, Mcquaid JR, et al. Development of a brief diagnostic screen for panic disorder in primary care. *Psychosom Med* 1999;61(3):359–364.
8. Means-Christensen AJ, Arnau RC, Tonidandel AM, et al. An efficient method of identifying major depression and panic disorder in primary care. *J Behav Med* 2005;28(6):565–572.
9. American Psychiatric Association, DSM-5 Task Force. *Diagnostic and statistical manual of mental disorders: DSM-5*. Washington, DC: American Psychiatric Association; 2013.
10. Culpepper L. Use of algorithms to treat anxiety in primary care. *J Clin Psychiatry* 2003;64(Suppl 2):30–33.
11. Craske MG, Roy-Byrne PP, Stein MB, et al. Treatment for anxiety disorders: efficacy to effectiveness to implementation. *Behav Res Ther* 2009;47(11):931–937.
12. Baldwin D, Woods R, Lawson R, et al. Efficacy of drug treatments for generalized anxiety disorder: systematic review and meta-analysis. *BMJ* 2011;342:d1199.

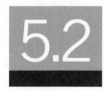

5.2 Depression

Prasad R. Padala, Kalpana P. Padala

GENERAL PRINCIPLES
Definition

Major depressive disorder (MDD) is characterized by persistent depressed mood and lack of interest and pleasure nearly every day over at least 2 consecutive weeks.[1] Depressed mood can be ascertained by either self-report or observation by a family member (Table 5.2-1). Mood may be irritable or sad in children and adolescents. The health care burden of MDD is comparable to that of cardiovascular diseases. MDD is the second leading cause of Years Lived with Disability worldwide.[2] Family physicians treat more depression than any other professional.[3]

Epidemiology

Twelve-month prevalence of MDD in the United States is approximately 7% with females experiencing 1.5 to 3 times higher rate than males.[1] Although the peak age of onset for depressive disorders is in the third decade, no age group is immune to the onset of depression. Late-life depression with vascular etiology is being increasingly recognized.

Pathophysiology

The most replicated biologic finding in depression is elevated stress levels.[4] Bioamine hypothesis postulates decreased levels or activity of norepinephrine and/or serotonin responsible for development of depressive symptoms.[4] This has resulted in developing treatment strategies targeting these two neurochemical systems. Other, less specific findings include decreased latency to first rapid eye movement sleep phase and hypoperfusion of the frontal lobes in patients with MDD.

Cerebrovascular disease is increasingly recognized to have a significant relationship to mood disorders in elderly individuals. Deep white matter hyperintensities (DWMHs) have been associated with chronicity of geriatric depression and its poor response to antidepressants.[5]

Etiology

Higher prevalence of depression in first-degree relatives of patients with major depression and higher concordance rates in monozygotic twins point to a genetic role in the etiology of depression. Exposure

TABLE 5.2-1	Patient Health Questionnaire 9

1. Over the last 2 wks, how often have you been bothered by any of the following problems?

	Not at all days 0	Several days 1	More than half the day 2	Nearly every day 3
a. Little interest or pleasure in doing things.				
b. Feeling down, depressed, or hopeless.				
c. Trouble falling/staying asleep, sleeping too much.				
d. Feeling tired or having little energy.				
e. Poor appetite or overeating.				
f. Feeling bad about yourself—or that you are a failure or have let yourself or your family down.				
g. Trouble concentrating on things, such as reading the newspaper or watching television.				
h. Moving or speaking so slowly that other people could have noticed. Or the opposite—being so fidgety or restless that you have been moving around a lot more than usual.				
i. Thoughts that you would be better off dead or of hurting yourself in some way.				

2. If you checked off any problem on this questionnaire so far, how difficult have these problems made it for you to do your work, take care of things at home, or get along with other people?

Not difficult at all	Somewhat difficult	Very difficult	Extremely difficult

to stressful life events such as the death of a child or abuse can predispose patients to develop depression. Patients with short allele of serotonin transporter gene have been found to be more susceptible to the adverse impacts of stressful life events.[6] Thus, the etiology of depression has both genetic and environmental factors.

DIAGNOSIS
Clinical Presentation
Diagnosis of depression is mainly clinical. DSM-5 criteria for MDD are easily remembered using a mnemonic "SIGMECAPS" (Table 5.2-2). For the diagnosis of MDD, one has to suffer from five (or more) of the nine symptoms nearly every day for at least 2 consecutive weeks and represent a change from previous functioning.. One of the symptoms has to be either depressed mood or markedly decreased interest in pleasurable activities. Several instruments can be used for detection of depression, including the Beck Depression Inventory,[7] Patient Health Questionnaire (PHQ-9),[8] and the Quick Inventory of Depressive Symptomatology[9] (QIDS), which not only assesses the severity of depression but also serves as a diagnostic tool.

Elderly patients often present with somatic complaints to primary care providers and often deny mood symptoms. Corroborative history from family members and friends can be invaluable in making a diagnosis in poor historians. Denial of symptoms may occur for multiple reasons, including stigma, negligence, and the fear of consequences of a diagnosis on their occupation and insurance status. Many older patients present with what otherwise looks like a depressive syndrome but steadfastly deny they have depression. This has been referred to as "masked depression" or "depression without sadness."[10]

Comorbidity is a rule rather than an exception. Anxiety disorders, substance use disorders, and other medical conditions complicate the course and treatment of depression and increase the risk for suicide.

TABLE 5.2-2	Diagnostic Criteria for MDD Based on DSM-5 Criteria[5]

Sustained low or depressed **M**ood[a]
Sleep disturbance, decreased or increased
Decreased **I**nterest or pleasure[a]
Feeling worthless or **G**uilt
Fatigue or loss of **E**nergy
Diminished **C**oncentration
Appetite disturbance, weight loss or gain (5% change in a month)
Psychomotor agitation or retardation
Recurrent thoughts of death, **S**uicidal ideation

[a]Presence of five or more of the above during the same 2-week period with at least one symptom of either depressed mood or loss of interest or pleasure.

Physical Examination

Physical examination is geared toward ruling out medical conditions such as hypothyroidism, dementia, and parkinsonism that can manifest with depression.

Classification

Depression is a heterogeneous condition and is classified into MDD, persistent depressive disorder (dysthymia), disruptive mood regulation disorder, premenstrual dysphoric disorder, depression secondary to general medical condition, substance-induced mood disorder, other specified depressive disorder, and unspecified depressive disorder. Persistent depressive disorder is a low-grade depression that is present most of the day, for more days than not, for more than 2 years. Symptoms associated with premenstrual dysphoric disorder must be present in the final week before onset of menses and start to improve within a few days after the onset of menses. Substance-induced mood disorder usually has onset within a month of intoxication or withdrawal from substance use. MDD can often be complicated with psychotic symptoms. It is also further classified into primary and secondary depression and depression with or without melancholic symptoms. Yet another classification is based on the presence or absence of atypical features such as hyperphagia, leaden paralysis, hypersomnolence, and hypersensitivity to rejection. This distinction is important as patients presenting with atypical features might respond better to monoamine oxidase inhibitors (MAOIs) such as phenelzine.

Differential Diagnosis

Bipolar disorder can manifest with depressive episodes. A history of mania in the past, family history of bipolar disorder, or past treatment with mood stabilizers alerts clinicians about the possibility of bipolar disorder. This distinction is essential to avoid the risk of switching to mania by initiating monotherapy with antidepressants in patients with bipolar disorder. Although the risk of manic switch is most robust with tricyclic antidepressants (TCAs), it is also seen with selective serotonin-reuptake inhibitors (SSRIs) and other agents such as venlafaxine and bupropion.

TREATMENT

Behavioral

The treatment of MDD includes both pharmacologic and psychologic interventions. Cognitive–behavioral therapy and interpersonal therapy are the most studied therapies for depression.[11] Patients who respond to psychologic intervention are usually in the range of mild to moderate symptom severity. The combination of psychotherapy and pharmacotherapy has resulted in better results than either treatment alone.

Medications

Several classes of antidepressants are available, including MAOIs, TCAs, SSRIs, and mixed antidepressants. SSRIs are often considered the first-line treatment for depression due to their relatively better safety profile and ease of administration. The common doses of antidepressants are outlined in Table 5.2-3.

Most of the antidepressants have comparable efficacy at 50% to 60% response rate.[11] The selection of an antidepressant is therefore dependent not on efficacy per se but on specific factors such as the side-effect profile, potential drug interactions, cost, ease of use, and formulation combined with patient-specific information such as comorbid medical conditions, and possibly the type of depressive symptomatology. TCAs should be used with caution in patients with cardiac disease. Similarly, TCAs should be avoided in people with dementia, narrow-angle glaucoma, urinary retention, and bowel obstruction because of their anticholinergic activity. The presence of a seizure disorder may preclude the use of bupropion.

Baseline symptoms often can help with selection of antidepressants. For example, "activating" antidepressants such as fluoxetine and bupropion may be prescribed for patients with hypersomnia. Likewise, mirtazapine may be of value for patients with insomnia and anorexia. Drug interactions with concomitant medications may also inform which antidepressants to avoid (Table 5.2-4).

TABLE 5.2-3	Doses of Common Antidepressants	
Medication	**Starting dose (mg/day)**	**Therapeutic dose (mg/day)**
TCAs		
Amitryptyline	25–50	100–300
Nortriptyline	25	50–200
Imipramine	25–50	100–300
SSRIs		
Citalopram	10–20	20–60
Fluoxetine	10–20	20–80
Sertraline	25–50	100–200
Paroxetine	10–20	20–50
Escitalopram	10	20
MAOIs		
Phenelzine	45	180
Tranylcypromine	20	30–60
Mixed antidepressants		
Mirtazapine	7.5–15	15–45
Venlafaxine XR	37.5	75–225
Bupropion SR	100–150	300
Duloxetine	20–30	60

TABLE 5.2-4	CYP-450 Enzyme Profiles of Commonly Used Antidepressants		
CYP-450 enzyme	**Antidepressants**	**Major inhibitors**	**Major inducers**
1A2	Fluvoxamine, mirtazapine	Ciprofloxacin, fluvoxamine, propafenone	Caffeine, carbamazepine, omeprazole
2C19	Citalopram, clomipramine	Fluvoxamine, omeprazole, ritonavir, ticlopidine	Phenytoin, valproic acid
2D6	Fluoxetine, mirtazapine, paroxetine, sertraline, venlafaxine	Fluoxetine, paroxetine, cimitidine, quinidine, ritonavir	
3A4	Citalopram, fluoxetine, mirtazapine, paroxetine, venlafaxine	Nefazodone, ciprofloxacin, ketoconazole, erythromycin, indinavir	Carbamazepine, phenobarbital, phenytoin, rifampin, ritonavir, St John wort

Special Therapy

- Electroconvulsive therapy (ECT) has been employed successfully in the management of MDD. It is known to have 80% acute response but suffers from lack of persistent effects and often necessitates maintenance treatment.[12] ECT is safe in elderly patients and often employed in patients with extreme anorexia, failure to thrive, and those with intractable suicidal thoughts.[12]
- Repetitive transcranial magnetic stimulation has recently received FDA approval for those with treatment-resistant depression.
- **Augmentation of antidepressants**: augmentation with have been used successfully in treating depression unresponsive to single antidepressants. Increasing use of atypical antipsychotics as augmentation agents is seen.

Risk Management

A major risk associated with depression is the high rate of suicide. Approximately 15% patients suffering from depression lose life due to suicide.[13] The rates of suicide are highest among white men older than 60 years of age. Direct questioning and detailed past history can inform clinicians about potential suicide risk in a patient. SADPERSONS is a useful mnemonic for assessment of suicide risk in practices (Table 5.2-5).

Patient Education

Patients need to be educated about the common symptoms of depression and the need for treatment. It must be emphasized that depression is treatable and patients should be counseled not to stop antidepressants until they consult with their physicians. Many resources are available on the internet about depression.[14,15]

Follow-Up

An increase in suicide rate is seen while recovering from an episode of depression, as the somatic symptoms of depression (sleep, appetite, and energy) are the first to improve and the cognitive symptoms (low self-esteem, guilt, and suicidal thoughts) are slower to improve. This increased risk of suicide during recovery necessitates continued monitoring while treating patients for depression.

SPECIAL CONSIDERATIONS

Late-life depression. There are several reasons depression in elderly individuals is difficult to diagnose. Older adults are less likely to endorse symptoms of depression than younger patients and often reject the diagnosis of depression. They are more likely to endorse low energy, anhedonia, and other somatic complaints, which are difficult to differentiate from general medical conditions. Likewise, there is a tendency to explain away depressive symptoms that are expressed as components of normal aging, grief, physical illness, or even dementia. Subsyndromal depression is much more common than in the elderly. To complicate matters further, suicide rates in elderly are the highest of any age group.[16] A high degree of suspicion and specific inquiry is necessary for its detection and treatment. Specific rating scales such as the geriatric depression scale are useful in screening for late-life depression (Table 5.2-6).[17] Even a four-item version of the geriatric depression scale has high sensitivity for detection of depression and could be very helpful in busy practices.

TABLE 5.2-5	Assessment Tool for Suicide Risk
S	Male sex
A	Age (young/elderly)
D	Depression
P	Previous attempts
E	ETOH
R	Reality testing (impaired)
S	Social support (lack of)
O	Organized plan
N	No spouse
S	Sickness

TABLE 5.2-6   Geriatric Depression Scale

Choose the best answer for how you have felt over the past week:

1. **Are you basically satisfied with your life?** YES/**NO**
2. Have you dropped many of your activities and interests? **YES**/NO
3. **Do you feel that your life is empty?** **YES**/NO
4. Do you often get bored? **YES**/NO
5. Are you in good spirits most of the time? YES/**NO**
6. **Are you afraid that something bad is going to happen to you?** **YES**/NO
7. **Do you feel happy most of the time?** YES/**NO**
8. Do you often feel helpless? **YES**/NO
9. Do you prefer to stay home, rather than going out, doing new things? **YES**/NO
10. Do you feel you have more problems with memory than most? **YES**/NO
11. Do you think it is wonderful to be alive now? YES/**NO**
12. Do you feel pretty worthless the way you are now? **YES**/NO
13. Do you feel full of energy? YES/**NO**
14. Do you feel that your situation is hopeless? **YES**/NO
15. Do you think that most people are better off than you are? **YES**/NO

Items in bold constitute the four-item scale.

REFERENCES

1. American Psychiatric Association. *DSM-5: diagnostic and statistical manual of mental disorders.* 5th ed. Washington, DC: American Psychiatric Association; 2013.
2. Whiteford HA, Degenhardt L, Rehm J, et al. Global burden of disease attributable to mental and substance use disorders: findings from the Global Burden of Disease Study 2010. *Lancet* 2013;382(9904): 1575–1586. doi: 10.1016/S0140-6736(13)61611-6.
3. Schumann I, Schneider A, Kantert C, et al. Physicians' attitudes, diagnostic process and barriers regarding depression diagnosis in primary care: a systematic review of qualitative studies. *Fam Pract* 2012;29(3):255–263.
4. Roy A, Campbell MK. A unifying framework for depression: bridging the major biological and psychosocial theories through stress. *Clin Invest Med* 2013;36(4):E170–E190.
5. Taylor WD, Aizenstein HJ, Alexopoulos GS. The vascular depression hypothesis: mechanisms linking vascular disease with depression. *Mol Psychiatry* 2013;18(9):963–974. doi: 10.1038/mp.2013.20.
6. Caspi A, Sugden K, Moffitt TE, et al. Influence of life stress on depression: moderation by a polymorphism in the 5-HTT gene. *Science* 2003;301(5631):386–389.
7. Rogers WH, Adler DA, Bungay KM, et al. Depression screening instruments made good severity measures in a cross-sectional analysis. *J Clin Epidemiol* 2005;58(4):370–377.
8. Kroenke K, Spitzer RL, Williams JB, et al. The patient health questionnaire somatic, anxiety, and depressive symptom scales: a systematic review. *Gen Hosp Psychiatry* 2010;32(4):345–359.
9. Rush AJ, Trivedi MH, Ibrahim HM, et al. The 16-item quick inventory of depressive symptomatology (QIDS), clinician rating (QIDS-C), and self-report (QIDS-SR): a psychometric evaluation in patients with chronic major depression. *Biol Psychiatry* 2003;54(5):573–583.
10. Undurraga J, Baldessarini RJ. Randomized, placebo-controlled trials of antidepressants for acute major depression: thirty-year meta-analytic review. *Neuropsychopharmacology* 2012;37(4):851–864. doi: 10.1038/npp.2011.306.
11. Lampe L, Coulston CM, Berk L. Psychological management of unipolar depression. *Acta Psychiatr Scand Suppl* 2013;(443):24–37. doi: 10.1111/acps.12123.
12. Lisanby SH. Electroconvulsive therapy for depression. *N Engl J Med* 2007;357(19):1939–1945.
13. Gonda X, Fountoulakis KN, Kaprinis G, et al. Prediction and prevention of suicide in patients with unipolar depression and anxiety. *Ann Gen Psychiatry* 2007;6:23.
14. http://www.nami.org.
15. American Foundation for Suicide Prevention: http://www.afsp.org/
16. Conwell Y, Duberstein PR, Caine ED. Risk factors for suicide in later life. *Biol Psychiatry* 2002;52(3):193–204.
17. Sheikh JI, Yesavage JA. Geriatric depression scale (GDS): recent evidence and development of a shorter version. In: Brink TL, ed.*Clinical gerontology: a guide to assessment and intervention.* New York, NY: Haworth Press; 1986:165–173.

5.3 Alcoholism

Robert Mallin, Brandon D. Brown

The prevalence of alcohol use disorders in primary care outpatient populations may be as high as 20%. The cost to society of these problems is staggering. Each year in the United States, alcoholism is responsible for 88,000 deaths and costs of $223.5 billion dollars.[1,2] Family physicians are in a unique position to identify and treat these problems.

GENERAL PRINCIPLES

Definition

- **Alcoholism is a primary, chronic neurobiologic disease** with genetic, psychosocial, and environmental factors influencing its development and manifestations. It is characterized by behaviors that include one or more of the following: impaired use of the drug alcohol, **compulsive use, continued use despite harm**, and **craving.**[3]
- Alcoholism or alcohol dependence is best defined by a **loss of control** over drinking.
- Because of the defense mechanism of **denial**, patients are often not consciously aware of their loss of control, and tend to minimize the amount, frequency, and consequences of their alcohol consumption.
- **Alcohol abuse** refers to the harmful use of alcohol, usually meant for patients who are having consequences for their drinking but have not yet lost the ability to control their alcohol use.
- **Physical dependence** is a state of physiologic adaptation that is manifested by a drug class-specific withdrawal syndrome that can be produced by abrupt cessation or rapid dose reduction of a drug or by administration of an antagonist.[3] In the case of alcoholism, physical dependence is sometimes but not always seen in the presence of alcoholism or alcohol dependence.
- **Low-risk drinking** is a term defined by not more than two drinks (a drink equals 1.5 oz liquor, or 12 oz beer, or 6 oz of wine) daily and no more than five in any given day for a male and no more than one drink daily for women with no more than three in any given day.
- **Exceeding these limits is considered heavy drinking.**
- **Heavy drinking is drinking in excess of maximum limits on a regular basis.**
- **At-risk drinking is heavy drinking that does not meet criteria for alcohol use disorder and places an individual at higher risk for developing alcohol-related problems.**[3]

Epidemiology

- Approximately two thirds of all American adults drink alcohol.
- Each year, 13.8 million Americans develop problems from drinking.
- Lifetime prevalence for alcoholism is 17.8% for men and 12.5% for women.[3]
- The prevalence of all alcohol use disorders is highest in young adults between the ages of 18 and 29.
- Incidence of drinking problems is greater for men than for women and declines with age.
- For those who begin drinking before the age of 15, the rate of progression to alcoholism is 15 times that of those who begin drinking at age 21. In older adults, the rates drop off precipitously.
- One-third of adolescent drinkers will transition to alcohol use disorders.
- Alcohol use disorders can occur in up to 50% of patients admitted to a community hospital and between 25% and 27% of patients seen in primary care practice visits.
- Characteristics known to influence the epidemiology of alcoholism include gender, age, family history, marital status, employment status, and occupational/educational status.
- The risk of alcoholism for the child of an alcoholic is approximately 50%. Single persons have a higher risk than those who are married. The unemployed and less educated also have a higher risk.[4]

Pathophysiology

- Alcoholism is a brain disease. A disorder in the reward system of the mesolimbic system of the brain results in dysregulated dopaminergic neurons.
- This abnormality results in craving for alcohol and impairs individuals' ability to control their use of this drug. In addition to dopamine, multiple neurotransmitter systems are involved in this process, including

the γ-aminobutyric acid system, serotonin system, N-methyl-D-asparate system, and glutamate. These systems modulate the effect of the drug, and the reward system determines the craving for it.

Etiology

- Family and twin studies show that there is a genetic component to a predisposition to alcoholism.
- Patients who develop alcoholism without a family history of the disease or those who do not develop alcoholism despite a strong family history of the disease speak to the environmental influences that must also play a part.

DIAGNOSIS

Screening

A primary screen for alcohol-related problems may be done as part of the review of systems or as part of a routine visit. Patients who drink at all, no matter how infrequently, should be asked questions from the "CAGE," a brief and practical primary screening tool for alcohol abuse. The term CAGE is an acronym for the key word in each of the four questions below. Any positive response justifies a more in-depth screen.

- Have you ever felt you should cut down on your drinking?
- Have people annoyed you by criticizing your drinking?
- Have you ever felt guilty about your drinking?
- Have you ever had a drink first thing in the morning to steady your nerves or to get rid of a hangover ("eye opener")?

A slightly longer but more accurate alternative screening test is the Alcohol Use Disorders Identification Test (AUDIT) (Table 5.3-1)[5]. AUDIT questions are provided below along with the scoring values. Typically, a total of eight points or more on the AUDIT is suggestive of alcohol dependence.

DSM-5 Diagnosis Criteria for Alcohol Use Disorder[6]

A. A problematic pattern of alcohol use leading to clinically significant impairment or distress, as manifested by at least two of the following, occurring within a 12-month period.

1. Alcohol is often taken in larger amounts or over a longer period than was intended.
2. There is a persistent desire or unsuccessful efforts to cut down or control alcohol use.
3. A great deal of time is spent in activities necessary to obtain alcohol, use alcohol, or recover from its effects.
4. Craving, or a strong desire or urge to use alcohol.
5. Recurrent alcohol use resulting in a failure to fulfill major role obligations at work, home, or school.

TABLE 5.3-1   The AUDIT Questionnaire

1. How often do you have a drink containing alcohol?
   1. Never
   2. Monthly or less
   3. Two to four times a month
   4. Two to three times a week
   5. Four or more times a week
2. How many drinks containing alcohol do you have on a typical day when you are drinking?
   1. 1 or 2
   2. 3 or 4
   3. 5 or 6
   4. 7 or 9
   5. 10 or more
3. How often do you have six or more drinks on one occasion?
   1. Never
   2. Less than monthly
   3. Monthly
   4. Weekly
   5. Daily or almost daily

TABLE 5.3-1	**The AUDIT Questionnaire** *(continued)*

4. How often during the last year have you found that you were not able to stop drinking once you had started?
   1. Never
   2. Less than monthly
   3. Monthly
   4. Weekly
   5. Daily or almost daily
5. How often during the last year have you failed to do what was normally expected from you because of drinking?
   1. Never
   2. Less than monthly
   3. Monthly
   4. Weekly
   5. Daily or almost daily
6. How often during the last year have you needed a first drink in the morning to get yourself going after a heavy drinking session?
   1. Never
   2. Less than monthly
   3. Monthly
   4. Weekly
   5. Daily or almost daily
7. How often during the last year have you had a feeling of guilt or remorse after drinking?
   1. Never
   2. Less than monthly
   3. Monthly
   4. Weekly
   5. Daily or almost daily
8. How often during the last year have you been unable to remember what happened the night before because you had been drinking?
   1. Never
   2. Less than monthly
   3. Monthly
   4. Weekly
   5. Daily or almost daily
9. Have you or someone else been injured as a result of your drinking?
   1. No
   2. Yes, but not in the last year
   3. Yes, during the last year
10. Has a relative, friend, doctor, or other health worker been concerned about your drinking or suggested that you should cut down?
    1. No
    2. Yes, but not in the last year
    3. Yes, during the last year

6. Continued alcohol use despite having persistent or recurrent social or interpersonal problems caused or exacerbated by the effects of alcohol.
7. Important social, occupational, or recreational activities are given up or reduced because of alcohol use.
8. Recurrent alcohol use in situations in which it is physically hazardous.
9. Alcohol use is continued despite knowledge of having a persistent or recurrent physical or psychological problem that is likely to have been caused or exacerbated by alcohol.
10. Tolerance, as defined by either of the following:
    a. A need for markedly increased amounts of alcohol to achieve intoxication or desired effect.

b. A markedly diminished effect with continued use of the same amount of alcohol.
  1. Withdrawal, as manifested by either of the following:
    a. The characteristic withdrawal for alcohol.
    b. Alcohol (or a closely related substance, such as a benzodiazepine) is taken to relieve or avoid withdrawal symptoms.

Clinical Presentation

- **History**
  - Typically, because of denial, alcoholism does not present straightforwardly.
  - Look for consequences from drinking in health, social, family, financial, and legal areas (Table 5.3-2).
- **Physical Examination**
  Although most patients with alcoholism will show no or only subtle physical findings, those with long-standing or severe disease will present with a variety of physical findings that are the result of alcohol-related health problems (Table 5.3-2).

Laboratory Studies

- Because the hallmark of alcoholism is a loss of control over drinking, laboratory studies are useful in determining physiologic consequences from drinking, and can be markers of excessive drinking, but are not diagnostic.
- **γ-Glutamyl transpeptidase** is a liver enzyme that may be elevated by excessive alcohol consumption. It has poor sensitivity and specificity when used alone, but may be useful when used in conjunction with other markers such as:
  - **Mean corpuscular volume** may be elevated from chronic excessive alcohol consumption.
  - **Carbohydrate deficient transferrin (%CDT)** when elevated suggests recent (7 to 14 days) heavy alcohol intake. CDT is useful for monitoring relapse to drinking.
  - **Ethyl glucuronide (EtG)** found in urine can detect even small amounts of alcohol up to 80 hours after ingestion.

TREATMENT

- Alcoholism can be treated successfully.
- **Brief interventions** have been shown to be successful. Often simply making the diagnosis of an alcohol problem and recommending a change in behavior may work.
- Once a diagnosis of alcohol dependence has been made, the appropriate recommendation is **abstinence** from alcohol and other addictive substances.
- More **formal interventions** can be designed for patients who do not respond to brief interventions, and are best handled by an addictions professional.

TABLE 5.3-2	Physical Signs of Alcohol Use Disorder
Mild	**Moderate or severe**
Hypertension	Hypertension and/or cardiomyopathy
Sudden muscle necrosis	Chronic alcoholic myopathy
Nausea, vomiting, gastritis, reflux	Chronic atrophic gastritis
Delayed gastric emptying	Pancreatitis, pseudocyst formation
Alcoholic hepatitis	Cirrhosis, alcohol ketoacidosis
Increased sputum production	Decreased platelet function
Hypothermia	Megaloblastic anemia
Hypoglycemia, lactic acidosis	Decrease in polymorphonuclear leukocytes
Nystagmus, diplopia	Decreased cell-mediated immunity and T cells
Ataxia, stupor, coma	Peripheral neuropathy, dementia
Loss of magnesium, zinc, phosphorus,	Males: breast enlargement, gonadal atrophy
calcium, potassium, thiamine, and/or folate	Females: amenorrhea, anovulation
Holiday heart syndrome: atrial or ventricular	Wernicke–Korsakoff syndrome (triad of
dysrhythmia associated with heavy drinking	confusion, ocular disturbance, and ataxia)

TABLE 5.3-3	Sample Detoxification Protocols

Basic orders
Multivitamin 1–2 qd
Quiet room with even lighting
Folate, 1 mg PO qd 3 3 d
Thiamine, 100 mg ASAP and qd for 3 d
PO fluids as tolerated; IV usually not required
Magnesium supplement 1–2 tablets PO stat and qd; may give deep magnesium sulfate IM for severe withdrawal risk (2 g q8h)

Oxazepam
Over age 55 or hepatic dysfunction. 15–30 mg PO qh until symptoms remit or sedation occurs, then repeat total dose q6–8h for first day, reducing this dosage by 25% each day. Most patients will be off medication by day 5.

Diazepam loading
Under age 55 and healthy liver. 10–20 mg PO qh until sedated. Usually no further medication is required.

Phenobarbital taper
30 mg PO qid 3 3 d, 15 mg qid 3 2 d, and 15 mg bid 3 1 d. Augment with sodium phenobarbital, 130–260 mg IM, early in treatment for severe withdrawal. Early use of IM phenobarbital for moderate to severe withdrawal is the key to success with this regimen. Use phenergan or hydroxyzine for nausea.

Severe agitation
Haloperidol, 5–10 mg, may be given PO, IM, or IV for severe agitation, in combination with any above withdrawal regimen; repeat as needed.

IM, intramuscular; IV, intravenous; PO, by mouth.
The above and other detoxification protocols may be modified for use in conjunction with instruments such as the Clinical Institute Withdrawal Assessment (CIWA-Ar) to better relate medication administration to actual withdrawal signs and symptoms.

TABLE 5.3-4	Medications to Reduce Relapse in Alcohol Use Disorders

Disulfiram	Causes flushing and vomiting when drinking alcohol	250–500 mg daily (must be taken in observed setting to be effective)
Naltrexone	Reduces craving for alcohol	50 mg daily
Acamprosate	Reduces craving for alcohol	333 mg three times daily

- **Detoxification**, treatment in an outpatient, inpatient, or residential setting, is the appropriate recommendation for those who have a diagnosis of alcohol dependence (Table 5.3-3).
- For patients who have had symptoms of withdrawal in the past, medical detoxification is recommended (Table 5.3-3).
- Medications that are approved to treat alcoholism include disulfiram, naltrexone, and acamprosate (Table 5.3-4). These medications when used in the context of a comprehensive recovery program can help reduce relapse to drinking.
- Aftercare followed by involvement in Alcoholics Anonymous improves outcome in treatment for alcoholism.

REFERENCES

1. Centers for Disease Control and Prevention (CDC). *Alcohol—related disease impact (ARDI)*. Atlanta, GA: CDC; 2014.
2. Bouchery EE, Harwood HJ, Sacks JJ, et al. Economic costs of excessive alcohol consumption in the United States, 2006. *Am J Prev Med* 2011;41:516–524.

3. Graham W, Schultz TK, eds. *Principles of addiction medicine.* 4th ed. Chevy Chase, MD: American Society of Addiction Medicine; 2009.
4. Harwood H. Updating estimates of the economic costs of alcohol abuse in the United States: estimates, update methods, and data. Report prepared by The Lewin Group for the National Institute on Alcohol Abuse and Alcoholism; 2000.
5. Babor TF, Higgins-Biddle JC, Saunders JB, et al. *The alcohol use disorders identification test, guidelines for use in primary care.* 2nd ed. Geneva, Switzerland: Department of Mental Health and Substance Dependence, World Health Organization; 2001.
6. American Psychiatric Association. *Diagnostic and statistical manual of mental disorders.* 5th ed. Arlington, VA: American Psychiatric Publishing; 2013.

Sexual Dysfunction

Jared D. Beck

Sexual problems are common. They occur in almost half of all marriages, in at least 75% of couples who seek marital therapy, and in more than half of all adults who visit primary physicians' offices.[1]

GENERAL PRINCIPLES

By definition, sexual dysfunctions are disorders in sexual desire and in the psychophysiologic changes that occur during the sexual response cycle. The *Diagnostic and Statistical Manual of Mental Disorders* (5th ed) (DSM-5) classifies them accordingly[2]:

- **Male hypoactive sexual desire disorder**—deficient (or absent) sexual fantasies and desire for sexual activity.
- **Female sexual interest/arousal disorder**—the inability to attain or maintain an adequate lubrication-swelling response of sexual excitement until sexual activity is completed.
- **Erectile disorder (ED)**—the inability to attain or maintain an adequate erection until sexual activity is completed.
- **Female orgasmic disorder**—delayed or absent orgasm following normal sexual excitement.
- **Premature ejaculation (PE)**—persistent or recurrent pattern of ejaculation during partnered sexual activity within 1 minute following penetration or before the individual wishes it.
- **Delayed ejaculation**—marked delay in ejaculation, or marked infrequency or absence of ejaculation.
- **Genitopelvic pain/penetration disorder**—persistent or recurrent difficulties with vaginal penetration during intercourse, marked vulvovaginal/pelvic pain during vaginal intercourse or penetration attempts, marked fear/anxiety about pain related to vaginal penetration, or marked tensing/tightening of pelvic floor muscles during attempted penetration.
- **Substance/medication-induced sexual dysfunction**—sexual dysfunction that develops during or within a month of substance intoxication or when related to medication use.
- **Other and unspecified sexual dysfunction**—these categories apply to presentations in which symptoms characteristic of a sexual dysfunction predominate, but do not meet full criteria for any of the previous disorders. This disorder shares its diagnosis code with the diagnosis of sexual aversion disorder from the DSM-5-TR.

DIAGNOSIS

Symptoms

Physicians should routinely ask about sexual relationships with open-ended questions, pursuing positive responses with queries directed to specific phases of the sexual response cycle.[3] A more complete history incorporates the following categories.

- **Present history**. Pursue the presenting sexual concern with specific questioning, as one would further define any other problem.
- **Sexual history**. Explore all current and past sexual experiences (including sexual abuse), relationships, attitudes, emotional reactions, knowledge, sexual identity, and body image.

- **Developmental and family history**. Discuss family attitudes toward sexuality, parental modeling, religious influences, relationships with parents and siblings, family violence, and level of family function in the couple's families of origin.
- **Nature of current relationship**. Focus on the current relationship's development and stability, changes in feelings, unresolved conflict, loss of trust, and communication problems.[3]
- **Current stressors**. Inquire about intrafamilial stresses (e.g., death, illness, problems with children, normative individual and family life cycle development transitions) and extrafamilial stresses (e.g., financial, occupational, legal).
- **Past medical history**. Identify any acute or chronic organic disease (diabetes mellitus is the most common organic cause),[1] injury, or surgery that could affect sexual functioning. Inquire about psychologic problems (depression and anxiety are most associated with sexual dysfunction).[1] Many commonly used drugs also affect sexual function, including anticholinergics, antidepressants, antihistamines, antipsychotics, anxiolytics, hormonal contraceptives, narcotics, sedative–hypnotics, and drugs of abuse (including alcohol and tobacco).
- **Self-report inventories**. The International Index of Erectile Function (IIEF) is a 15-item inventory that can help a clinician evaluate sexual functioning in men.[3] The Female Sexual Function Index (FSFI) is a 19-question inventory that helps to evaluate sexual functioning in women.[4]

Signs

A comprehensive physical examination further defines concurrent acute or chronic illness and associated physical conditions.

- **General**. Look for obesity, cachexia, and evidence of endocrine disease; determine vital signs.
- **Cardiovascular**. Search for bruits (especially femoral), peripheral pulses, evidence of venous stasis, arterial insufficiency (especially in the lower extremities), or a pulsatile epigastric mass.
- **Abdominal**. Look for pain, tenderness, mass, guarding, tympany, bowel activity, hernia, and evidence of prior surgery.
- **Neurologic**. Examine gait; coordination; deep tendon reflexes; pathologic reflexes; sensation; motor strength; integrity of the sacral reflex arc (S_2 to S_4) with perineal sensation; anal sphincter tone; and bulbocavernosus (S_2, S_3), bulbo-anal (S_3, S_4), and anal (S_4, S_5) reflexes.[3]
- Observe the **male genitalia** for testicular size and consistency, penile size, malformations, and lesions. Examine the **prostate** for size, consistency, and tenderness. Obtain **penile blood pressure measurements** on any man with ED by inflating a 3-cm pediatric blood pressure cuff around the base of the penis and auscultating the central artery of the corpora cavernosa with a 9.5-MHz Doppler stethoscope as the cuff is deflated. The ratio between the penile systolic pressure and the brachial systolic pressure should exceed 0.75. Ratios less than 0.60 indicate penile vascular insufficiency.[1]
- **Female pelvic examination**.[4] Search for the following findings:
  - **External genitalia**. Search for dermatitis, atrophy, vulvar inflammation, warts, episiotomy or other scars, and clitoral inflammation, or adhesions.
  - **Introitus**. Look for hymeneal rigidity, tags, or fibrosis, urethral caruncle, and Bartholin gland inflammation.
  - **Vagina**. Evaluate for spasm of the vaginal sphincter and adduction of the thighs with attempted vaginal examination, atrophy, discharge, inflammation, stenosis, relaxation of supporting ligaments, and tenderness along the vaginal urethra or posterior bladder wall.
  - **Bimanual examination**. Search for cul-de-sac masses or tenderness and adnexal mass or tenderness. Determine the presence, position, size, mobility, and tenderness of the uterus.
  - **Rectal examination**. Examine for hemorrhoids, fissures, constipation, and tenderness.

Laboratory Tests

- **Laboratory evaluation for systemic disease**[3] includes a complete blood count; fasting blood sugar level; urinalysis; tests for sexually transmitted diseases; lipid profiles; and tests of thyroid, liver, and renal function.
- **Evaluation for male hypoactive sexual desire disorder**.[3] Obtain an early morning serum bioavailable testosterone level in men. If levels are low or borderline, or if the low desire is associated with little or no sexual fantasy or masturbation history, then obtain a serum prolactin level.
- **Evaluation for female sexual interest/arousal disorder**.[4] Research techniques can now measure nocturnal clitoral and vaginal blood flow, and demonstrate vaginal engorgement cycles during rapid eye movement (REM) sleep, similar to erection cycles in men. Research techniques can also measure clitoral blood flow. These tools may become clinically useful to help differentiate organic from

psychogenic sexual disorders in women and to determine the role of arterial factors in affecting sexual arousal and orgasm.

- **Evaluation for male erectile disorder**[3]
  - Early morning **bioavailable serum testosterone levels** screen for hypogonadism. If the level is low, obtaining follicle-stimulating hormone (FSH), luteinizing hormone (LH), and prolactin levels can help to differentiate between primary testicular failure (high FSH and LH, normal prolactin) and secondary (pituitary–hypothalamic) failure (low FSH and LH, normal prolactin). If the FSH and LH are normal, but the prolactin is elevated, then a computed tomography (CT) scan or magnetic resonance imaging (MRI) can investigate the sella turcica for a pituitary adenoma.
  - **Nocturnal penile tumescence (NPT) evaluation** helps differentiate psychogenic interference (erections occur during sleep) from organic interference (erections do not occur). Several techniques evaluate and quantify NPT.
    - The **snap gauge** is a ring of opposing Velcro straps connected by three plastic strips. It is wrapped around the penis before sleep, and by noting whether 0, 1, 2, or 3 bands break during sleep, one can estimate the maximum erectile response.
    - The **Rigiscan** is a small computer with two cables leading to rings that encircle the base and tip of the penis. The rings detect tumescence by passively expanding and detect rigidity by actively contracting. The Rigiscan records all erectile events and measures erection duration, tumescence, and rigidity.
    - The **NEVA system** uses electrode sets attached to the corona of the glans, to the base of the penis, and to the abdominal wall. These are attached to a monitor that records impedance data, which directly correlate to changes in penile volume.
    - **NPT monitoring** is performed in a sleep laboratory where electroencephalograph (EEG) tracings detect sleep cycles. Mercury strain gauges placed around the base and tip of the penis detect tumescence. Monitoring documents all erectile events; measures duration, tumescence, and rigidity (but not as well as the Rigiscan); and correlates erections with REM sleep.
  - When a **psychogenic etiology** is suspected, the patient is evaluated for psychologic or psychiatric disorders.
  - When a **vascular etiology** is suspected, the following procedures can help to identify the cause.
    - **Intracavernous injection of vasodilators (papaverine or PGE1)** helps to screen for a vascular etiology.[3] Injections should cause an erection within 10 minutes that lasts at least 30 minutes. Delays longer than 15 to 20 minutes suggest arterial insufficiency, and a normal erection that is lost quickly suggests a cavernous leak.
    - The **Knoll/MIDUS system** is an office-based, bidirectional, continuous wave Doppler ultrasound system with spectral analysis that measures deep cavernous artery velocities. It can help to identify both arterial and venous insufficiency.
    - **Duplex ultrasound scanning** records blood flow in the cavernous arteries before and after a vasodilator (papaverine or prostaglandin E1, or PGE1) injection. Normal vessels should double in size, with an initial peak systolic flow velocity exceeding 30 cm per second.[3]
    - When no arterial flow is demonstrated, then selective **internal pudendal angiograms** can determine whether an arterial block exists that could be corrected by penile revascularization.
    - If persistent flow is present, then **cavernosometry and cavernosography** can be used to evaluate the veno-occlusive mechanisms of the corpus cavernosum. A vasoactive agent (20 mg PGE1) is injected into a corpus cavernosum to cause an erection; this is followed by a heparinized saline infusion to maintain it. Radiographic contrast is then infused, and radiographs are taken to identify leaks in specific veins and the glans-spongiosal system.
  - When a **neurogenic etiology** is suspected, the first step is a trial of an oral phosphodiesterase-5 (PDE5) inhibiting agent such as sildenafil (Viagra).[3] If the patient demonstrates no response, then the following tests may help to differentiate the problem.
    - **Bulbocavernosus reflex latency tests** measure the integrity of the sacral reflex arc (S_2 to S_4) by recording the time delay from stimulation of the glans by a pinch or squeeze to contraction of the bulbocavernosus muscle. Longer times suggest a neurologic cause for ED.
    - **Somatosensory evoked potentials** record waveforms over the sacrum and the cerebral cortex in response to dorsal penile nerve stimulation, and can help to localize neurologic lesions to peripheral, sacral, or suprasacral locations.
    - A handheld electromagnetic vibration device can be placed on the shaft of the penis to determine a threshold for **vibration perception**. Loss in perception suggests the presence of a peripheral neuropathy.

- **Perineal electromyography** can help to detect disorders in the pudendal motor tracts that could be secondary to metabolic or toxic etiologies.
- Evaluation for sexual pain disorders
  - **Office laboratory procedures** include saline and potassium hydroxide wet mounts of vaginal secretions to diagnose vaginitis or vaginosis; urinalysis, urine culture, and evaluation of prostatic secretions to diagnose associated genitourinary infections; and tests to diagnose chlamydial, herpes simplex, and gonococcal infections.
  - **Colposcopy** may diagnose specific vaginal or cervical pathology, such as human papillomavirus infections.
  - **Pelvic ultrasound** may diagnose adnexal, uterine, or cul-de-sac problems.
  - **Laparoscopy** may diagnose, and in some cases treat, adnexal or intraperitoneal pathology.
  - **Anoscopy or sigmoidoscopy** may identify associated colorectal problems.

TREATMENT

- **Medical management**
  - **Testosterone** in the form of intramuscular (IM) testosterone enanthate (200 mg every 2 to 3 weeks) is effective treatment for hypogonadal men with testosterone values less than 100 ng per dL.[5] Transdermal preparations (AndroGel, Androderm, Testoderm) applied daily will also raise testosterone levels to normal in 90% of men. Testosterone can also increase desire in women, but may produce androgenizing side effects.
  - **Bromocriptine mesylate (Parlodel)** treats hyperprolactinemia. Treatment begins with 1.25 mg daily, increasing by 2.5 mg every 3 to 7 days until the serum prolactin level is normal.[5]
  - **Yohimbine (Aphrodyne)** theoretically enhances penile erections by restricting penile venous outflow and increasing libido through a central nervous system effect. Dosage is 5.4 mg PO tid.[5]
  - The **PDE5 inhibitors** have become the drugs of choice for most men with ED. The recommended doses are as follows: sildenafil, 50 to 100 mg taken 1 hour prior to sexual activity; vardenafil (Levitra), 10 to 20 mg also taken 1 hour prior to intercourse; and tadalafil (Cialis), 10 to 20 mg taken 1 to 24 hours prior to intercourse. These drugs are contraindicated in patients taking organic nitrites because they potentiate their hypotensive effects.[6]
  - **Oral phentolamine mesylate (Vasomax)** 20 to 80 mg taken 15 minutes prior to intercourse improves erectile function in men with mild-to-moderate ED. It is available in Mexico and Brazil, but not in the United States.
  - **Intraurethrally inserted PGE1 tablets (MUSE)** in strengths of 125, 250, 500, and 1,000 mg demonstrate effectiveness in 40% of men with ED from various causes.[5]
  - **Topical nitroglycerin (Nitrol)** relaxes penile arterial smooth muscle, causing subsequent engorgement. Men with mild vascular, neurologic, or mixed arousal dysfunction may respond to 0.5 to 1.0 inches of 2% ointment applied to the penile shaft just prior to intercourse. The man must also wear a condom to avoid vaginal absorption by his partner. **Topical 2% minoxidil solution (Rogaine)** applied to the glans is reportedly as effective as nitroglycerin. Prophylactic analgesics help manage associated headache. **Topical PGE₁ (Topiglan, Alprox-TD)** is under study in men with ED. **Topical alpsrostadil (ALISTA)** may enhance clitoral arousal and vaginal lubrication in women. **Oral** and **vaginal phentolamine** are now being studied in women to determine whether they can enhance vaginal blood flow.[4]
  - **Intracavernous injection of vasoactive drugs.**[5] Patients may inject either papaverine or PGE1(alprostadil) into a corpus cavernosum with a 27-gauge needle to induce an erection. Men with neurogenic disorders, mild vascular problems, combined neurogenic and vascular disorders, and psychogenic problems for which psychosexual treatment has failed may respond well. Injections also benefit men with PE because sexual activity can continue despite the premature orgasm. Therapy begins with a low dose of either drug (10 mg papaverine; 2.5 to 5.0 mg PGE1) that is gradually increased to provide an adequate erection that lasts 1 to 2 hours. This usually requires 10 to 80 mg papaverine or 10 to 40 mg PGE1. Injections are limited to 3 per week and 10 per month. In difficult cases, these drugs may be mixed and used in combination. Bimix contains papaverine and phentolamine, and Trimix adds PGE1. Injecting vasoactive intestinal polypeptide (VIP) 0.025 mg mixed with phentolamine 2.0 mg (Invicorp) reportedly demonstrates efficacy in men who have failed other injection therapies. It is not yet available in the United States.
  - **Tricyclic antidepressants** in antidepressant doses may help treat PE because they inhibit the cholinergic component of ejaculation.

- **Thioridazine** at standard antidepressant doses may also benefit men with PE.
- **Phenoxybenzamine (Dibenzaline)** is used by men with PE in daily doses of 20 to 30 mg.[5] It should not be used by men who wish to procreate because phenoxybenzamine inhibits seminal emission.
- **Clomipramine (Anafranil)** may benefit PE by increasing the sensory threshold for genital stimuli.[5] Doses start with 25 to 50 mg 12 to 24 hours prior to sexual activity and increase until the man achieves ejaculatory control, experiences side effects, or reaches maximal recommended doses (250 mg per day).
- **Sertraline (Zoloft)** 50 to 100 mg, paroxetine (Paxil) 20 to 40 mg, and fluoxetine (Prozac) 20 to 60 mg taken 3 to 5 hours prior to sexual activity also delay ejaculation. Adding sildenafil 50 mg 1 hour prior to sexual activity increases the effectiveness of these drugs.[5]
- **Dapoxetine** may become the first Food and Drug Administration (FDA)-approved drug specifically indicated for PE. Studies indicate that 30 to 60 mg taken 1 to 3 hours before intercourse results in a three- to fourfold increase in ejaculatory latency time.[5]
- A 2.5% lidocaine–2.5% prilocaine cream (**EMLA cream**) applied to the glans and covered with a condom 30 minutes prior to intercourse also reportedly helps PE. It may also help women with introital dyspareunia and vaginismus.
- **Water-based lubricating products (K-Y Jelly, Astroglide)** applied directly to the genital area prior to intercourse may reduce discomfort associated with intercourse without increasing infection or damaging condoms.
- **Surgical management**[3]
  - **Arterial revascularization**. Successful surgery for proximal artery occlusion can improve blood flow through the hypogastric vessels. Success depends on whether the distal vessels are patent and whether surgery damages the autonomic nerves that travel over the vessels.
  - **Venous surgery**. Surgical procedures for venous incompetence have not demonstrated long-term success.
  - **Penile prosthesis**. The penile prosthesis is the most reliable surgical option in the United States, with the inflatable prosthesis implanted most frequently. Prosthesis implantation is relatively uncomplicated, but most devices require replacement after 48 to 60 months.
- **Mechanical management. Penile vacuum pumps (ErecAid)** can also aid erections. Air is withdrawn from a lubricated cylinder that the man places over his penis to create a vacuum that draws blood into the corpora cavernosum. An elastic band around the penile base maintains the erection when the cylinder is removed. A device that creates suction over the clitoris (**EROS-CTD**) is now approved by the FDA. It increases vaginal blood flow, as well as clitoral blood flow, erection, and sensitivity, and reportedly enhances sexual arousal and orgasm in women. Various **penile constriction rings (Soft Touch, Pressure Point, ACTIS Constriction Loop)** help to maintain erections in men with venous incompetence.
- **Psychosexual therapy**[3,6]
  - **Standard principles** that undergird psychosexual therapy include the beliefs that people are responsible for their own sexuality; that growth in sexual attitudes, performance, and feelings results from behavioral change; that every person deserves sexual health; that physiologic relaxation is the foundation for sexual excitement; and that boundaries must be established with the nonsexual aspects of sexual dysfunction.
  - **Cognitive–behavioral therapy** that incorporates behavioral therapy into other treatments is the treatment choice for managing most sexual dysfunctions. Behavior therapists assume that sexual dysfunction is learned maladaptive behavior that causes patients to fear sexual interaction. Therapy inhibits the learned anxious response.
  - **Sensate focus exercises** heighten sensory awareness to touch, sight, sound, and smell. As patients focus on their own sensations, they relax and overcome the barriers to their natural physiologic responses.
  - **Hypnotherapy** helps remove symptoms and alter attitudes by teaching patients to use relaxation techniques before a sexual encounter and to learn alternative ways of dealing with anxiety-provoking sexual situations.
  - **Group therapy** provides a strong support system to counteract sexual myths, correct misconceptions, and provide accurate information about sexual anatomy, physiology, and varieties of behavior.
  - **Traditional marital therapy** is also important to manage any marital or relationship problems that generate stress, fatigue, and dysphoria.

- **Specific sexual therapy techniques**
  - **Directed self-stimulation** is the most effective treatment program to date for primary orgasmic dysfunction in women.[4]
  - **The stop–start technique of Semans** and the **squeeze technique** modification of Masters and Johnson help to manage PE.
  - **Sexologic examination.** The vaginal sexologic examination helps treat women with arousal and orgasmic disorders by assisting them and their partners to identify specific erotically sensitive vaginal and genital foci. The examination is performed with the sexual partner, after the woman's signed consent.
  - **Systematic desensitization** techniques can successfully treat genitopelvic pain/penetration disorder.

REFERENCES

1. Laumann EO, Paik A, Rosen RC. Sexual dysfunction in the United States: prevalence and predictors. *JAMA* 1999;281(6):537–544.
2. American Psychiatric Association. *Diagnostic and statistical manual of mental disorders.* 5th ed. Arlington, VA: American Psychiatric Association; 2013.
3. Halvorsen JG. The clinical evaluation of common sexual concerns. *CNS Spectr* 2003;8(3):217–224.
4. Phillips NA. Female sexual dysfunction: evaluation and treatment. *Am Fam Physician* 2000;62(1): 127–136, 141–142.
5. Lue TF. Drug therapy: erectile dysfunction. *N Engl J Med* 2000;342(24):1802–1813.
6. Hellstrom WJG, ed. Treating erectile dysfunction: appropriate use of the PDE5 inhibitors. *J Fam Pract* 2005;Dec(S):2–46.

Eating Disorders
Cynthia G. Olsen, Matthew O'Neill

GENERAL PRINCIPLES

Definition

The chapter on Feeding and Eating Disorders in the 5th edition of the *Diagnostic and Statistical Manual of Mental Disorders* (DSM-5) has been updated in 2013 to better reflect the nature and continuum of anorexia nervosa and bulimia nervosa.[1] In the anorexia diagnostic criteria, the term "refusal," in regard to weight maintenance, has been removed, and amenorrhea or menstrual absence has been deleted. The DSM-5 criteria for bulimia nervosa include binge eating and compensatory behaviors (i.e., purging); the frequency has been downgraded from twice a week to once a week.

Diagnostic Criteria for Anorexia Nervosa (307.1)[1]*

- Restriction of energy intake, leading to a significantly low body weight for gender, age, developmental trajectory, and physical health or a body mass index (BMI) <17 kg per m^2.
- Intense fear of gaining weight or becoming fat or persistent behaviors that impede healthy weight gain despite being significantly underweight.
- Disturbed perception of own body weight or shape, and denial of the severity.

Diagnostic Criteria for Bulimia Nervosa (307.51)[1]*

- Recurrent binge eating, out of control, typically large amounts of food over a discrete time period (<2 hours).
- Recurrent compensatory acts to prevent weight gain (vomiting, laxatives, diuretics, enemas, fasting, diet pills, excessive exercise).

---

*Adapted from DSM-5.

- Binge–purge cycle occurs once per week for 3 months.
- Preoccupation and criticism of body weight and shape.

Epidemiology

Eating disorders affect about 4% of the U.S. population, and involve a disturbed eating behavior and distorted body image. Bulimia nervosa is three times more common than anorexia nervosa. The male-to-female prevalence of eating disorders is approximately 1 to 10. The age of onset for anorexia begins in early adolescence, and that for bulimia is in later adolescence and the twenties. Both are found predominantly in developed societies, where ideals about dieting, body size, and shape are acceptable. *Eating disorders are a fatal disease.* The mortality rate for each is significant with that for anorexia nervosa 2% to 6%, mostly from starvation, substance abuse and suicide. Low weight, poor social adjustment, and alcohol abuse are predictors of premature death.[2]

Classification

Both anorexia and bulimia may be episodic, relapsing, or chronic. The two subtypes of anorexia nervosa, *restricting type* and *binge eating/purging type*, require at least a 3-month period. Further classification includes severity based on BMI: >17 kg per m^2 *mild*; 16 to 16.9 kg per m^2 *moderate*; 15 to 15.9 kg per m^2 *severe*; 15 or less kg per m^2 *extreme*. Bulimia can be subtyped into *purging* (more common) and *nonpurging types*. Bulimia can be further categorized by severity on the basis of the average number of inappropriate episodes of compensatory behavior a week: 1 to 3 *mild*; 4 to 7 *moderate*; 8 to 13 *severe*; 14 or more *extreme*. For both types of eating disorders, remission can be classified as partial or full.[1]

DIAGNOSIS
History

Verify body perception and weight loss behaviors. When able, corroborate history with family or friends. Anorexia often presents after a stressful life event, such as a school change. Psychological features include issues of loss and separation, indifference or vigorous denial, perfectionism, dichotomous thinking, alexithymia, conflicting self-denial and hedonism, and delayed psychosocial development. The stress of starvation causes the person to appear irritable, dysphoric, anxious, and angry. Some behaviors of anorexics include impulse control problems, obsession with food and aversion to meat, cold insensitivity, other compulsive behaviors, and exhaustion due to over activity.

In the bulimic patient, careful history for binge eating and compensatory behaviors is necessary. Patients may report abdominal distention and discomfort, constipation, frequent pharyngitis, "heartburn," hematemesis, postbinge depression, and fluctuation of weight of 10 lb in a month. Patients with bulimia, unlike those with anorexia, have normal or slightly above normal body weight and admit more readily to their behaviors. Bulimia is commonly found in families with a history of rigidity, substance abuse, sexual abuse, affective disorder, and obesity. Binge eating in bulimia is often seen after a period of dieting. Psychologic features may include depressive disorders, emotional lability, low self-esteem, dissociation during the binge–purge, substance abuse (one-third), and personality disorders (one-half). Behaviors include the consumption of sweets and high caloric foods, eating before and after parties, secrecy and attempts to hide behavior, manipulation of medications, and self-induced vomiting, the most common purge method (80% to 90%). Other purge methods include regular use of laxatives, diuretics, diet pills, enemas, and syrup of ipecac (less readily available). Although anorexics might experience amenorrhea, bulimics frequently have heavy or irregular menses.

Physical Examination

Assessment includes regular monitoring of height, weight, and BMI. In the anorexia patient, findings may include emaciation and decreased muscle mass, myopathy, lanugo of the trunk, peripheral edema, dry skin, petechiae, yellowed skin from hypercarotenemia, parotid gland hypertrophy, ketotic breath, bradycardia, hypothermia, and hypotension. Patients with anorexia who engage in binge–purge behavior may also have the physical characteristics of bulimia.

In bulimia nervosa, self-induced vomiting frequently results in dental damage with posterior erosion from acidity, caries, and chips. The Russell sign is abrasions and scarring on the dorsum of the hand (typically unilateral and the dominant side) caused by scraping on the teeth. Other findings include bilateral, painless parotid and submandibular gland hypertrophy, abdominal striae, anal tears and fissures, dehydration, electrolyte disturbance, myopathy (especially proximal muscles), cardiomegaly, and arrhythmia. Complications of purging can include gastric and esophageal rupture and tears, cathartic colon, aspiration and resulting pneumonitis, cardiac arrest, tonic–clonic seizures, carpopedal spasm, and hypokalemic nephropathy.

Careful psychological evaluation should access for affective disorders, suicide risk, personality disorders, and substance abuse in both eating disorders. In starving patients, depression may be the result of metabolic disturbance and can resolve with weight gain and correction.

Laboratory and Imaging

Laboratory studies in anorexic patients may reveal normochromic normocytic anemia with leukopenia, electrolyte disturbance, hypothyroidism, low estrogen state with osteoporosis, diminished testosterone in males, increased liver enzymes due to fatty liver, hypercholesterolemia, increased growth hormone, renal insufficiency due to dehydration and hypokalemia, arrhythmias, and urine pH >7. Hypoprotienemia and vitamin deficiencies may exist. Electrocardiogram is important in severely underweight patients (<25% of baseline weight) and those using chemical purgatives, especially syrup of ipecac (emetine) to rule out potentially life-threatening arrhythmia or disturbance. Magnetic resonance imaging usually reveals a decrease in brain size with ventricular dilatation in the severely anorexic patient. In the bulimic patient, abnormal laboratory findings may include occult blood in the stool, steatorrhea, hypocalcemia or hypomagnesemia, metabolic alkalosis, hypokalemia, impaired renal function, elevated serum amylase due to vomiting (30% of patients), and elevated liver enzymes, particularly aspartate aminotransferase, lactate dehydrogenase, and alkaline phosphatase. Electrocardiographic abnormalities reflect electrolyte disturbance.

Differential Diagnosis

Psychiatric disorders that may mimic anorexia nervosa include major depressive disorder, schizophrenia, body dysmorphic disorder, substance dependency, obsessive–compulsive disorder, and social phobia. Medical conditions include colitis, carcinomas such as brain tumor, pancreatic and bronchogenic carcinoma, human immunodeficiency syndrome, superior mesenteric artery syndrome, gastric outlet obstruction, and metabolic disorders such as Addison disorder, hyperthyroidism, or thiamine deficiency.

Psychiatric disorders that may mimic bulimia nervosa include anorexia nervosa (binge eating/purging type), major depression with atypical features, borderline personality disorder, and substance abuse. Neurologic conditions that have abnormal eating features include Kleine–Levin syndrome, Kluver–Bucy-like syndromes, Parkinson disease, migraine, seizure disorders, brain tumors, and traumatic brain injury.[3] Other medical entities include gastrointestinal carcinoma, pyloric obstruction, mesenteric artery syndrome, malignant hypertension, digitalis therapy, metabolic alkalosis, opiate withdrawal, and pilocarpine therapy.

TREATMENT

The patient with an eating disorder is challenging and requires an interdisciplinary team of providers that may include the family physician, nurse, psychologist, psychiatrist, social worker, medical specialists, and nutritionist. Poorer outcome is associated with histories of sexual abuse, personality disorder, high pretreatment severity, substance abuse, poor social support, and chronicity. The first priority is to save the patient's life from complications. Medical hospitalization is required for hemodynamic or metabolic disturbance, medication overdose, and for the initiation of nutritional restoration. Psychiatric hospitalization may be required for suicidal intent depending on level of risk.[4]

Behavioral Treatment

For anorexia patients, mental health referral can help delineate the level of care needed, initiate cognitive behavioral therapy and develop an ongoing care plan. Family therapy should be included. This care is specialized, and self-help strategies should not be suggested. A nutritionist assists with learning appropriate eating behaviors, including avoiding "dietary foods" aimed at weight loss, eating in company, and developing appropriate responses to both hunger and satiety.

Patients with bulimia at normal weight need education on normal, relaxed eating behaviors, avoidance of restrictive practices, and tolerance of their body habitus. In the absence of electrolyte disorders, patients with bulimia are usually managed in an outpatient setting. Borderline personality disorder, a common comorbid condition, is characterized by self-destructive behavior, poor interpersonal relationships, and impulsive behavior, making treatment challenging. For the eating disorder patient, full-day outpatient or a residential treatment facility may be useful if the patient is seriously depressed and/or suicidal, exhibits behavior unresponsive to outpatient therapy, is partially motivated, requires help with self-control, and is in need of family therapy.[4] After care and relapse prevention, plans should be prepared upon discharge and include the family unit and the whole care team.

Medical Treatment

Medical treatment of the eating disorder patient includes stabilization of complications, reconstitution of metabolism, and refeeding. Refeeding of the anorexic person begins by increasing the daily caloric intake by 300 calories and reducing activity by 50%. "Refeeding syndrome," from overaggressive refeeding of the starving body, results in fluid and electrolyte shifts, hypophosphatemia, congestive heart failure, hyper- and hypoglycemia, diarrhea myocardial dysfunction, and neurologic dysfunction including seizures.[5] An energy intake of 1,200 kcal per day is appropriate for the first few days in severely starved, emaciated patients. Weekly weight gain expectations should be between 0.5 and 1.5 kg. Most adult females require 3,000 kcal of energy per day to achieve full-weight restoration.[6] Total parental nutrition and tube feeding are invasive, remove responsibility from the patient, are often unsuccessful, and should be used only in dire situations.

Pharmacotherapy has included prokinetic drugs for delayed gastric emptying, estrogens for osteoporosis, trace minerals and vitamins for nutritional depletion, topical fluoride and bicarbonate rinses for dental erosions, H_2 blockers for gastric reflux, and bulk fiber supplements in constipation. Psychopharmacotherapy for anorexia remains disappointing.[7] Distorted cognition does not respond to antipsychotic medications and should be used only for psychotic symptoms. Antidepressants, particularly selective serotonin–reuptake inhibitors (SSRIs), are the primary drug treatment; SSRIs with anxiolytic and antiobsessional properties are most useful. Tricyclic antidepressants should be avoided in lower-weight patients at risk for cardiovascular complications. Patients with bulimia have a better response to drug treatment than do patients with anorexia. Antidepressants can be helpful in reducing binges, even in the absence of depression. Studies with different antidepressant agents for bulimia reveal no superior agent in terms of efficacy.[8] The SSRIs (fluoxetine, paroxetine, and sertraline) have a lower risk side-effect profile and are well suited for these patients. Bupropion is listed as contraindicated in eating disorders, due to seizure risk.

REFERENCES

1. American Psychiatric Association. *Diagnostic and statistical manual of mental disorders*: DSM-5. 5th ed. Washington, DC: American Psychiatric Association; 2013.
2. Franko DL, Keshaviah A, Eddy KT, et al. A longitudinal investigation of mortality in anorexia nervosa and bulimia nervosa. *Am J Psychiatry* 2013;170:917–925.
3. Castano B, Capdevila E. Eating disorders in patients with traumatic brain injury: a report of four cases. *NeuroRehabilitation* 2010;27:113–116.
4. Williams PM, Goodie J, Motsinger CD. Treating eating disorders in primary care. *Am Fam Physician* 2008;77:187–195.
5. Hehanna HM, Moledina J, Travis J. Refeeding syndrome: what it is, and how to prevent and treat it. *BMJ* 2008;336:1495–1498.
6. Garner DM, Garfinkle PE. *Handbook of treatment for eating disorders*. 2nd ed. New York, NY: Guilford Press; 1997.
7. Bulik CM, Berkman ND, Brownlwy KA, et al. Anorexia nervosa treatment: a systemic review of randomized controlled trials. *Int J Eat Disord* 2007;40:310–320.
8. Bacaltchuk J, Hay PPJ. Antidepressants versus placebo for people with bulimia nervosa. *Cochrane Database Syst Rev* 2003;4:CD003391. doi:10.1002/14651858.CD003391.

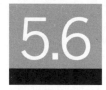

5.6 Sleep–Wake Disorders

Joshua J. Sypal, Jessica B. Koran-Scholl

INSOMNIA
General Principles

Definition

Insomnia (primary or comorbid with medical, psychiatric, or neurologic disorders) is the inability to get adequate sleep even under ideal sleep conditions. This sleep disorder results in daytime fatigue, difficulty concentrating, irritability, and depression. Adequate sleep for adults ranges from 6 to 9 hours, averaging just over 8 hours.

Epidemiology

About 10% to 20% of adult patients in primary care practices report significant insomnia symptoms, 10% to 15% experience daytime impairments, and up to 19% have chronic insomnia.[1] Women and the elderly suffer from insomnia more often than men. Insomnia is also associated with psychiatric and medical illness; poor quality of life; and poor memory, mood, and cognitive function. Because of these effects on life, 6% of the population take over-the-counter sleep aids and 6% take prescription hypnotics.[1]

Etiology

Insomnia can be caused or exacerbated by other sleep disorders; psychiatric, medical, and neurologic disorders; disruption of the sleep–wake cycle; and medications. Caffeine, alcohol, nicotine, drugs of abuse, and poor sleep hygiene also cause insomnia.

Pathophysiology

The relationship between brain function and insomnia has not been well defined.

Diagnosis

Clinical Presentation

Fatigue, impairment in daytime functioning, irritability, and depression may be a patient's presenting complaints. Patients who complain of insomnia report waking up feeling tired, waking up many times during the night, difficulty falling asleep, or waking up too early. Because the majority of patients with insomnia are not diagnosed, it is recommended that health care providers screen all patients with a brief sleep history.

History

A sleep history includes duration and frequency of symptoms of insomnia; number of hours of sleep per night; sleep conditions; medical illnesses; psychiatric illnesses; prescription and over-the-counter medications; and use of alcohol, tobacco, caffeine, and drugs of abuse. The patient's bed partner can help diagnose comorbid sleep disorders. Severe daytime drowsiness with frequent episodes of falling asleep during the day can help differentiate from narcolepsy.

DSM-5 Criteria[2]

- Predominant complaint of dissatisfaction with sleep quantity or quality with one or more of the following: difficulty initiating sleep, maintenance of sleep, or early morning awakening.
- Disturbance causes clinically significant distress of impairment in functional areas of life.
- Sleep difficulty occurs at least three nights per week and is present for at least 3 months.
- Sleep difficulty occurs despite adequate opportunity for sleep.
- Is not better explained by and does not occur exclusively during the course of another sleep–wake disorder (i.e., obstructive sleep apnea [OSA], restless legs syndrome [RLS], periodic limb movement disorder [PLMD]).
- Is not attributable to the physiological effects of a substance (i.e., steroids, antidepressants, alcohol, caffeine, etc.) and cannot be adequately explained by other coexisting mental disorders or medical conditions (i.e., bipolar disorder, depression, hyperthyroidism, pain, frequent urination, etc.).
- Classification is based upon time with <1 month considered episodic, >3 months is persistent, and >2 times per year being recurrent.

Physical Examination

A physical examination is indicated depending on the medical history.

Laboratory Studies

Ordered to rule out medical conditions on the basis of the patient's medical history and physical examination.

Diagnostic Studies

Depression and anxiety questionnaires (PHQ, Beck, Jung, or Hamilton) may be helpful in diagnosing psychiatric disorders. Sleep studies can be ordered if another sleep disorder is suspected.

Complications

Daytime drowsiness can result in poor job performance, automobile accidents, decreased quality of life, and increased depression.

Treatment

If insomnia persists after successful treatment of other disorders (another sleep disorder, psychiatric disorder, or medical condition), exacerbating pharmaceuticals have been discontinued, and proper sleep hygiene (see patient education) is maintained, then treatment with behavior therapy and/or medication is appropriate. Acute insomnia may be successfully treated with supportive counseling and a short course of hypnotic medication (which may help prevent chronic insomnia), whereas chronic insomnia is treated with behavioral therapy and a short course of hypnotic medications. Some patients may need a longer course of hypnotic or other sedating medications.

Behavioral

- **Stimulus control therapy** teaches patients to associate the bedroom only with sleep or sex. They are instructed to leave the bedroom if they are still awake after 15 to 30 minutes and return only when sleepy. This is repeated until they fall asleep.
- **Sleep restriction therapy** teaches patients to limit the time they spend in bed to their reported sleep time or a minimum of 4 hours. Daytime naps are not allowed. This state of sleep deprivation leads to more rapid sleep onset and efficient sleep.
- **Relaxation and cognitive therapies** may also be effective.
- **Bright light therapy** can help reset a disrupted sleep–wake cycle.
- **Daily exercise** may also improve sleep.

Medications

There is a risk of harm with the use of benzodiazepine and non-benzodiazepine hypnotics as well as antidepressants and other medications for insomnia. These risks must be weighed against the benefits of adequate sleep.

    Benzodiazepine and non-benzodiazepine hypnotics. Approved indications for hypnotic medications are for brief and occasional treatment. Hypnotics have been shown to be of continued benefit for up to 6 months. Over-sedation, poor coordination, and memory problems may occur early in treatment but usually resolve over time. The non-benzodiazepine hypnotics act only on the type-1 benzodiazepine receptors in the brain and do not have muscle relaxant or antiseizure properties. Short-acting agents cause less daytime drowsiness. Intermediate- and long-acting agents cause less withdrawal and rebound insomnia. Triazolam (Halcion) has been associated with pronounced anterograde amnesia, but it should be noted that all hypnotics have this potential side effect. These agents should not be used in patients with sleep apnea or active substance abuse. Half doses should be used in elderly individuals.

- **Short-acting non-benzodiazepines**—eszopiclone (Lunesta) 1 to 3 mg hs, zaleplon (Sonata) 5 to 20 mg hs, zolpidem (Ambien) 5 to 10 mg hs[3]
- **Short-acting benzodiazepines**—triazolam (Halcion) 0.125 to 0.25 mg hs, oxazepam (Serax) 10 to 15 mg hs (off-label)[3]
- **Intermediate-acting benzodiazepines**—temazepam (Restoril) 7.5 to 30 mg hs estazolam (Prosom) 0.5 to 2 mg hs[3]
- **Long-acting benzodiazepines**—flurazepam (Dalmane) 15 to 30 mg hs, clonazepam (Klonopin) 0.25 to 1 mg hs (off-label)[3]

    When patients stop taking hypnotics, they may suffer from **rebound insomnia,** which can be treated with a few days of diphenhydramine 50 mg hs, trazodone 50 to 100 mg hs, and gabapentin 100 to 300 mg hs, or by restarting the hypnotic and tapering slowly.

    Antidepressants. Antidepressants are not well studied, nor Food and Drug Administration (FDA) approved, for the treatment of insomnia. They are recommended for patients with comorbid depression, anxiety, and antidepressant-induced insomnia; however, they may help patients with primary insomnia. Insomnia often responds to treatment of the underlying disorder, even with the more activating antidepressants. Trazodone can cause daytime drowsiness, as well as orthostatic hypotension in elderly patients, and, rarely, priapism. Tricyclic antidepressants are relatively contraindicated in elderly patients and in patients who abuse drugs and alcohol or are suicidal. Tricyclic antidepressants are the least safe in overdose. Selective serotonin–reuptake inhibitors and tricyclics may exacerbate RLS and PLMD.

- Trazodone (Desyrel) 25 to 200 mg hs.
- Amitriptyline (Elavil) 10 to 25 mg hs, imipramine (Tofranil) 25 to 50, trimipramine (Surmontil) 25 to 50, nortriptyline (Pamelor) 10 to 25, doxepin (Sinequan) 25 to 50 mg hs.
- Selective serotonin–reuptake inhibitors, mirtazapine, and venlafaxine for comorbid depression.

Other Sleep Aids[3]

- Gabapentin (Neurontin) 100 to 900 mg hs.
- Diphenhydramine (Benadryl) or doxylamine (Unisom) in over-the-counter sleep preparations; however, these are not recommended. Promethazine (Phenergan) 12.5 to 25 mg hs and hydroxyzine (Atarax) 10 to 100 mg hs have sedating effects.

- Melatonin 1 to 2 mg hs may help with jet lag, shift work, and delayed sleep phase syndrome, as well as chronic insomnia.
- Ramelteon (Rozerem) 8 mg hs.
- Valerian and other herbals and L-tryptophan have little evidence to support their use.

Patient Education

Proper sleep hygiene education should include:

- Maintain a regular sleep–wake schedule, avoiding daytime naps, including weekends.
- Use the bedroom for sleeping and sex only.
- Avoid reading, watching TV, or using other electronic devices in bed.
- Make the bedroom environment quiet, dark, and comfortable.
- Establish a regular bedtime routine.
- Avoid caffeine, alcohol, and nicotine.
- Avoid heavy meals.
- Exercise regularly before 2 pm every day.

Referrals

Unless there is a history suggestive of OSA, RLS, PLMD, or narcolepsy, referral to a sleep disorder clinic for sleep studies/polysomnography is rarely necessary. Referral to a sleep disorder clinic may be appropriate for patients whose symptoms of primary or comorbid insomnia do not respond to proper sleep hygiene, hypnotic medication, and adequate treatment of their comorbid disorder.

Counseling

Hypnotic medications should be taken only when a patient can get a full night's sleep. Possible side effects of medications should be discussed with all patients. Patients should not drive or operate machinery when they initiate treatment with sedative medications.

Follow-Up

Patients who require long-term use of medications for insomnia should be reassessed frequently and referred to a sleep clinic if they do not respond to treatment.

OBSTRUCTIVE SLEEP APNEA

General Principles

Definition

OSA is the occurrence of periodic abnormal and prolonged (greater than 10 seconds) pauses in breathing due to collapse or partial collapse and occlusion of the upper airway.[4] Five or more episodes of apnea with hypopnea (decreased oxygen saturation) in 1 hour is diagnostic of sleep apnea.[4]

Epidemiology

OSA is a fairly common disorder, affecting 2% to 15% of middle age adults and more than 20% of older adults.[4] OSA occurs two to four times more in men than in women. Obesity is a risk factor, but OSA can also occur in normal-weight patients. There is also evidence of a strong genetic influence.

Etiology

OSA is influenced by many factors such as a patient's airway anatomy, stability of the respiratory control system, and their arousal threshold.

Pathophysiology

The recurrent collapse of the pharyngeal airway during sleep results in reduced, or complete, cessation of airflow despite ongoing breathing efforts. This leads to intermittent disturbances in gas exchange and fragmented sleep. The resulting hypoxia and hypercapnia is thought to lead to adverse cardiovascular outcomes, insulin resistance, and metabolic syndrome.

Diagnosis

Clinical Presentation

Patients may present with a complaint of awakening suddenly, gasping for air, morning headaches, nonrestful sleep, and daytime drowsiness.

History

The patient's bed partner may notice loud snoring and episodes of choking or gasping.

DSM-5 Criteria[2]

- Evidence by polysomnography of at least five obstructive apneas or hypopneas per hour of sleep and either of the following sleep symptoms: snoring, gasping, breathing pauses, daytime sleepiness, fatigue, or unrefreshing sleep.
  or
- Evidence by polysomnography of 15 or more obstructive apneas and/or hypopneas per hour of sleep regardless of accompanying symptoms.

Physical Examination

A physical examination is indicated depending on the medical history. Physical abnormalities in the upper airways may not be obvious on physical examination, but could include enlarged tonsils, uvula, tongue, redundant tissue in the soft palate, or nasal obstruction. The patient may also have an obese body habitus and an enlarged neck circumference.

Laboratory Studies

Laboratory studies include complete blood count for polycythemia and thyroid-stimulating hormone (TSH) for hypothyroidism.

Diagnostic Studies

Diagnostic studies include polysomnography or portable home–monitoring devices; electrocardiogram to rule out cardiac abnormalities; and a computed tomography, magnetic resonance imaging study, or endoscopy if surgery is indicated.

Classification

OSA can be separated into severity of disease by the apnea–hypopnea index (AHI). An AHI of 5 to 15 respiratory events per hour indicates mild disease, 15 to 30 per hour for moderate disease, and greater than 30 per hour as severe disease.[4] OSA can also be differentiated from central sleep apnea, which is rare, with sleep studies.

Complications

Untreated OSA can lead to hypertension, heart attack, congestive heart failure, stroke, and even death. Furthermore, daytime complications of OSA are reported as contributing to car accidents and job-related accidents.

Treatment

Comorbid conditions, including obesity, hypertension, and diabetes, should be treated. Referral to a sleep disorder clinic for nasal continuous positive-airway pressure (CPAP) therapy is usually effective and reduces morbidity and mortality.

Behavioral

Obese patients are encouraged to lose weight. All patients should avoid the supine position during sleep, stop smoking, and avoid alcohol and sedating medications including hypnotics. Patient barriers preventing compliance with nightly CPAP use should be addressed.

Medications

No medications have been shown to be effective, unless comorbid conditions exist.

Surgical

Some patients may respond to surgery to remove tissue that is obstructing the upper airways or to advance the mandible. Some patients may require tracheostomy.

Referrals

Referral to a sleep clinic for diagnosis and treatment is always indicated.

RESTLESS LEGS SYNDROME
General Principles

Definition

RLS is a neurologic disorder diagnosed by a history of an uncomfortable sensation of needing to move one's legs or arms when sitting or lying still.

Epidemiology

Approximately 2.5% to 15% of the population may have RLS, but rates vary based on different criteria.[2] Women are 1.5 to 2 times more likely to be diagnosed with RLS. There may be a genetic influence. Of patients with RLS, 80% to 90% also have PLMD.

Etiology

RLS is usually idiopathic but may be secondary to anemia, uremia, neuropathy, varicose veins, or pregnancy. RLS can also be secondary to the effects of tricyclic antidepressants, selective serotonin–reuptake inhibitors, lithium, and dopamine antagonists.

Pathophysiology

RLS may involve alterations in central dopamine mechanisms.

Diagnosis

Clinical Presentation

Patients complain of frequent uncomfortable sensations in their legs, and occasionally their arms, as well as the need to move to attempt to relieve this sensation. These symptoms are worse in the evening and while at rest. If PLMD is present, patients may complain of symptoms of insomnia.

DSM-5 Criteria[2]

- An urge to move the legs, usually accompanied by or in response to uncomfortable and unpleasant sensations in the legs, characterized by all of the following: the urge begins or worsens during periods or rest, the urge is partially or totally relieved by movement, the urge is worse in the evening or at night, or only occurs in the evening or late at night.
- Symptoms occur at least three times per week and have persisted for at least 3 months.
- Symptoms are accompanied by significant distress or impairment in one or more areas of functioning (social, occupational, educational, academic, or behavior) and are not attributable to drugs of abuse, medications, another mental disorder, or medical condition.

Physical Examination

A physical examination is indicated depending on the medical history. Check for varicose veins, neuropathy, and poor circulation.

Laboratory Studies

Laboratory studies include complete blood count and ferritin for iron deficiency anemia, chemistry panel for uremia and diabetes, and pregnancy test.

Treatment

Medications

- **Dopaminergic agents—first line[3]**
  - Pramipexole (Mirapex) 0.125 to 1.5 mg tid, Ropinirole (Requip) 0.25 to 3.0 mg tid
  - Carbidopa–levodopa (Sinemet) 12.5/50 to 25/100 bid–tid
- **Other medications[3]**
  - Gabapentin (Neurontin) 300 to 900 mg hs, Pregabalin (Lyrica) 25 mg hs, iron supplements for patients whose serum ferritin is below 50.
  - Opioids (e.g., Codeine) and benzodiazepines (e.g., Clonazepam) should not be used to treat RLS; however, they may be helpful if severe pain and insomnia are prominent symptoms.

Referrals

Sleep studies if PLMD is suspected.

PERIODIC LIMB MOVEMENT DISORDER
General Principles

Definition

PLMD is the periodic and repetitive flexion of the legs and less frequently the arms that occurs every 20 to 90 seconds for minutes to hours during sleep.

Epidemiology

PLMD occurs in 5% of people age 30 to 50 and in 44% of people over the age of 65. Most patients with RLS have PLMD (12%), but most patients with PLMD do not have RLS.

Etiology

Similar to RLS.

Diagnosis

Clinical Presentation

The patient may complain only of daytime drowsiness. The diagnosis is usually made by the history given by the patient's bed partner.

History
Similar to insomnia and RLS.

Physical Examination
Physical examination as indicated depending on medical history.

Diagnostic Workup
The diagnosis of PLMD is made using polysomnography when the periodic limb movement index is more than 15 per hour in adults and more than five per hour in children.

Complications
Same as complications listed for insomnia.

Treatment

Medications
If medical causes and RLS have been treated, and offending medications have been stopped, clonazepam (Klonopin) 0.5 to 2 mg hs or temazepam (Restoril) 15 to 30 mg hs may be helpful for continued symptoms.

Referrals
The diagnostic workup may require referral to a sleep disorder clinic.

NARCOLEPSY

General Principles

Definition
Narcolepsy is a disturbance in rapid eye movement (REM) sleep causing periods of excessive daytime drowsiness and a tendency to fall asleep at inappropriate times. Narcolepsy can be associated with sleep paralysis, cataplexy (loss of muscle tone), hypnagogic hallucinations, and disturbed sleep.

Epidemiology
Narcolepsy–cataplexy affects 1 in 2,000 people. Risk in first-degree relatives may be as high as 2%. It may affect males slightly more than females.

Etiology
Unknown

Diagnosis

Clinical Presentation
The patient complains of sleep attacks lasting minutes to hours, sometimes associated with cataplexy, paralysis, or hypnagogic hallucinations.

History
Similar to insomnia.

DSM-5 Criteria[2]
- Recurrent periods of an irrepressible need to sleep, lapsing into sleep, or napping occurring within the same day. These must have been occurring at least three times per week over the past 3 months. With at least one of the following:
  - Episodes of cataplexy occurring at least a few times per month.
  - Hypocretin deficiency measure using cerebrospinal fluid, hypocretin-1 immunoreactivity values ≤110 pg per mL.
  - Nocturnal sleep polysomnography showing REM sleep latency ≤15 minutes, or a multiple sleep latency test showing a mean sleep latency ≤8 minutes and two or more sleep–onset REM periods.
- Can be mild (<1 day a week), moderate (daily), or severe (multiple times a day).

Physical Examination
Physical examination as indicated depending on medical history.

Laboratory Studies
Laboratory and imaging studies may rule out comorbid insomnia on the basis of the patient's medical history and physical examination. Depression and anxiety questionnaires (PHQ, Beck, Jung, or Hamilton) can be used to rule out psychiatric disorders.

Complications
Dangers associated with daytime drowsiness.

Treatment

Behavioral
Taking three or four short planned naps during the day may help reduce daytime drowsiness. Patients should not drive or handle machinery.

Medications[3]
- **Daytime drowsiness**—modafinil (Provigil) 200 to 400 mg each morning, methylphenidate (Ritalin) 10 to 30 mg bid–tid 30 minutes before meals, dextroamphetamine (Dexedrine) 5 to 30 mg bid–tid.
- **Cataplexy, sleep paralysis, and hallucinations**—fluoxetine (Prozac) 20 to 60 mg qd, paroxetine (Paxil) 20 to 60 mg qd, sertraline (Zoloft) 50 to 150 mg qd, clomipramine (Anafranil) 25 to 150 mg qd, imipramine (Tofranil) 25 to 100 mg qd, nortriptyline (Pamelor) 25 to 75 mg qd, or protriptyline (Vivactil) 10 to 60 mg qd, desipramine (Norpramin) 25 to 100 mg qd, venlafaxine (EffexorSR) 75 to 225 mg qd, and atomoxetine (Straterra) 10 to 80 mg qd.
- **Insomnia**—hypnotic medications.

Referrals
Referral to a sleep clinic for diagnosis is indicated.

DELAYED SLEEP PHASE AND ADVANCED SLEEP PHASE DISORDERS

Definitions
- Delayed sleep phase disorder (DSPD) is common in teenagers and young adults who often feel more awake and productive late at night and compensate for late hours by sleeping in. DSPD generally resolves with age.
- Advanced sleep phase disorder is common in elderly individuals who fall asleep early and awaken very early. This early awakening can be particularly troublesome and potentially dangerous if the patient wanders or falls in the dark.

Treatment

Behavioral
- Bright light therapy
- Chronotherapy—delaying or advancing bedtime over time until a normal schedule is achieved
- Proper sleep hygiene

REFERENCES

1. Bonnett MH, Arand D. Overview of insomnia. http://www.uptodate.com/contents/overview-of-insomnia. Accessed March 7, 2014.
2. American Psychiatric Association. *Diagnostic and statistical manual of mental disorders.* 5th ed. Arlington, VA: American Psychiatric Publishing; 2013.
3. Ramar K, Olson E. Management of sleep disorders. *Am Fam Physician* 2013;88(4):231–238.
4. Strohl KP. Overview of obstructive sleep apnea in adults. http://www.uptodate.com/contents/overview-of-obstructive-sleep-apnea-in-adults. Accessed March 7, 2014.

5.7 Drug Misuse Disorders

Lisa Grill Dodson

Drug misuse has long been recognized as a medical and societal problem. These disorders are common, accounting for billions of dollars in medical costs, lost productivity, and years of life lost.[1] Physicians are often in the position to first recognize the signs of drug misuse in patients presenting with other common problems. Patients suffering from drug use disorders may present with acute or chronic somatic complaint: psychiatric complaints; legal, occupational, or family problems; or drug-seeking behaviors. Physicians must maintain a high level of awareness, as well as a reasonable armamentarium of screening tools to recognize and treat these disorders. This chapter addresses misuse of both illicit and prescription drugs.

DEFINITIONS

Substance abuse is a maladaptive pattern of substance use manifested by recurrent and significant adverse consequences related to the repeated use of substances. Although any use of illicit substances and misuse of prescription or over-the-counter medications can be considered at-risk use, the *Diagnostic and Statistical Manual of Mental Disorders*, 5th edition (DSM-5) combines the DSM-IV-TR categories of substance abuse and substance dependence into a single disorder measured on a continuum from mild to severe, based on the number of items endorsed from a list of 11 criteria.[2]

RECOGNITION AND SCREENING

The most important screening tool for the practicing physician is maintaining a high level of awareness of the prevalence of drug use and abuse. Local and national data and other helpful resources can be found through the SAMHSA Web site *http://www.samhsa.gov/index.aspx*. Substance abuse affects all social and economic groups and ages. Although there are a number of signs and symptoms characteristic of substance abuse, there is also wide variability in the manifestations of the disorder. In the earlier stages, the symptoms are primarily behavioral and psychological, rather than physical. Complaints of depression, irritability, anxiety, paranoia, social withdrawal, poor memory, and poor concentration can be associated with drug use. Insomnia; loss of interest in activities; and marital, legal, or occupational difficulties can also signal substance use. Physical health problems may not manifest until late in the disease course. Early recognition and intervention is associated with improved health and social outcomes.[3]

Screening Tools

There are a variety of screening tools available for use in the office setting. The gold standard for recognizing substance abuse is a careful diagnostic interview, often with appropriate use of validated screening tools. A list of validated screening tools, such as the Drug Abuse Screening Test (DAST), can be found at the Substance Abuse and Mental Health Services Administration Web site http://www.integration.samhsa.gov/clinical-practice/screening-tools#drugs

Positive screening tests should prompt additional workup or referral. Informing the patient of your level of concern about his or her drug use and offering advice regarding the consequences of drug use remains a powerful tool.

Laboratory Testing

Urinalysis remains the most commonly used and best validated method of laboratory testing for drugs of abuse. Advantages of urine testing include noninvasive collection of large sample volumes, well-established and cost-effective methodologies, and fairly standard excretion rates across populations. In addition, urine testing has been accepted for legal purposes. However, urine does not provide quantitative measures and may be adulterated by addition of external substances or forced diuresis and dilution. Blood testing offers the advantage of quantitative and qualitative measurements but is limited by invasive collection procedures and the limited sample quantities available. Other body substances, including saliva, sweat, meconium, hair, breath, and breast milk, are potentially useful for identification of drug use, but each has advantages and disadvantages.[4] Meconium may be of use in determining intrauterine drug exposure in high-risk infants but is not recommended for routine use.

Prescription Drugs

Prescription drug abuse, misuse, and diversion are a significant and increasing medical and social problem. Diversion of commonly prescribed opioids and other controlled substances is increasing. Opioid analgesics accounted for 75% of the 22,134 deaths from prescription drug overdose in 2010.[5] Many states now have Prescription Drug Monitoring Programs (PDMP), a tool which helps clinicians identify persons who may be misusing prescription drugs, deter abuse and diversion, and support access to legitimate medical use of controlled substances. Information on these programs can be found at http://www.deadiversion.usdoj.gov/faq/rx_monitor.htm. Prescribing practices that can help reduce the potential for misuse include:

- Maintaining high standards for charting, including flow sheets with prescription refills, next refill date, and diagnosis being treated
- Placing strict limits on after-hours prescribing
- Implementing prescription drug contracts with patients
- Exercising caution with brand name—only narcotic prescriptions (brand name drugs frequently have a higher street value and may offer little or no advantage in efficacy)
- Insisting on obtaining medical records from previous and concurrent providers
- Restricting controlled-substances prescription to one pharmacy per patient
- Being knowledgeable about pharmacology, abuse potential, and drug interactions
- Knowing federal and state statutes regarding controlled-substances prescription
- Carrying out appropriate diagnostic tests
- Consulting with pain or other specialists when appropriate
- Enrolling in PDMP

TREATMENT

Treatment of substance disorders is difficult and costly. Although full treatment of severe substance abuse may be outside the scope of many primary care physicians, recent regulatory changes have created new options for physicians wishing to take on the primary treatment of patients with addiction and other drug misuse disorders.[6] Previously restricted to licensed centers, federal law now allows for the office-based treatment of opioid addiction with buprenorphine.[5] The waiver program authorizes qualified physicians who have attended a minimum of 8 hours of approved training to dispense and prescribe narcotics for the purpose of treating opioid addiction. Information on this program and training is available at *http://buprenorphine.samhsa.gov.*

Primary care physicians play a crucial role in assisting the patient in recognizing problems associated with their use and the need for treatment. Brief intervention, a method of short counseling sessions focused on changing a specific behavior, has been shown to be effective in decreasing drug use.[7] The components of effective brief intervention include the following:

- Feedback to patient about effects of substance use
- Recommendations for behavioral change
- List of options to achieve behavioral change
- Discussion of patient reaction to feedback and recommendations
- Follow-up to monitor and reinforce behavioral change

The level of intervention and treatment required may exceed the limits of what is possible in the office setting. Referral to inpatient, outpatient, or residential care may be required in advanced cases. Familiarity with the principles of treatment, as well as local resources available, allows the physician to remain involved in patient care and aids in transition, following treatment. Characteristics of effective treatment programs include the following:

- An individualized treatment approach
- Treatment of multiple problems, not just drug use
- Adequate duration of treatment
- Use of behavioral methods combined with medication when appropriate
- Identification and treatment of coexisting mental disorders
- Monitoring for potential drug use while in treatment
- Multiple episodes and types of treatment as needed

Therapies include cognitive behavioral methods, such as relapse prevention therapy, individualized counseling, and motivational enhancement therapy. Twelve-step abstinence-based programs have been effectively adapted for a variety of substances and behaviors. The type of treatment that will be successful depends on a number of variables, including the motivation for entering treatment, social supports available, substance or substances of abuse, and age and gender. No one approach is universally successful. For example, adolescents, older adults, and pregnant women require substantially different approaches. Medications such as naltrexone, bupropion, and selective serotonin–reuptake inhibitors show promise in reducing additive behaviors when combined with psychosocial and behavior therapies.

CONFIDENTIALITY

Federal statutes and regulations and many state laws require strict confidentiality surrounding medical records for drug abuse, screening, assessment, and treatment. Specific authorization for release of information is required; general medical consent is not sufficient.

REFERENCES

1. Gordon AJ, Bertholet N, McNeely J, et al. 2013 Update in addiction medicine for the generalist. *Addict Sci Clin Pract* 2013;8:18.
2. American Psychiatric Association. *Diagnostic and statistical manual of mental disorders.* 5th ed. Washington, DC: American Psychiatric Association; 2013
3. Madras BK, Compton WM, Avula D, et al. Screening, brief interventions, referral to treatment (SBIRT) for illicit drug and alcohol use at multiple healthcare sites: comparison at intake and six months. *Drug Alcohol Depend* 2009;99(1–3):280–295.
4. Dolan K, Rouen, D, Kimber J. An overview of the use of urine, hair, sweat and saliva to detect drug use. *Drug Alcohol Rev.* 2004;23(2):213–217.
5. MintzerIL, Eisenberg M, Terra M, et al. Treating opioid addiction with buprenorphine-naloxone in community-based primary care settings. *Ann Fam Med* 2007;5(2):146–150.
6. Kuehn BM. Office-based treatment for opioid addiction achieving goals. *JAMA* 2005;294(7):784.
7. Krupski A, Joesch JM, Dunn C, et al. Testing the effects of brief intervention in primary care for problem drug use in a randomized controlled trial: rationale, design, and methods. *Addict Sci Clin Pract* 2012;7:27.

CHAPTER 6

Disorders of the Nervous System

Section Editor: Toby D. Free

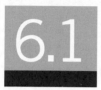

Migraine Headaches

Anne D. Walling

GENERAL PRINCIPLES
Definition

Migraine headaches are characterized by episodes of pain that last for 4 to 72 hours and are typically:
- Unilateral (predominantly temple or orbital but can extend to the occiput or neck)
- Moderate to severe in intensity
- "Pulsating," "throbbing," "piercing," or "splitting" in quality
- Exacerbated by exercise or activity and ameliorated by lying still or sleeping
- Accompanied by symptoms of photophobia (90%), phonophobia (74%), nausea (85%), vomiting (42%), or fatigue or somnolence

The diagnostic criteria require at least five attacks and exclusion of alternative diagnoses.[1]

Epidemiology

Approximately 40% of US women and 20% of men experience migraine at least once during their lifetimes.[2] The overall US migraine prevalence is about 18% of women and 9% of men.[3] The median age of onset is 24.5 years, and 75% of patients begin attacks prior to age 35.[2] The highest incidence in women (18/1,000 person-years) occurs in the 20- to 24-year age group; in men, the highest incidence (6.2/1,000 person-years) is at age 15 to 19 years.[2] In women, attacks may synchronize with menstruation and disappear during pregnancy. The number and severity of attacks tend to diminish with age.

Classification

The International Classification of Headache Disorders[1] recognizes several subtypes of migraine, based on the presence of aura before attacks or on predominant symptoms (e.g., retinal, basilar), but the same general management strategy is applicable to all migraine types. Migraine without aura is the most common subtype.

Pathophysiology

The pathophysiology of migraine is complex and incompletely understood. An inherited neurobiochemical predisposition to triggering the trigeminovascular system is certainly involved, but the roles of various factors such as neuroreceptors (especially the serotonin $5HT_1$ group) and mediators (such as calcitonin gene-related peptide) remain to be clarified.

DIAGNOSIS

The US Headache Consortium has developed evidence-based guidelines covering diagnosis, treatment, and prevention of migraine that are endorsed by American Academy of Family Physicians (AAFP) and other leading medical specialty organizations.[4]

History

The diagnosis is based on the history of typical episodes of unilateral headache plus the associated features (above). Age of onset and a family history are helpful in diagnosis. Aura (visual or neurologic symptoms prior to attacks) is pathognomonic but is present only in about 20% of cases. Many patients also describe sensitivity to certain foods (such as red wine, nitrates in smoked foods, or monosodium glutamate) or other factors (e.g., cigarette smoke, relief of stress, or menstruation) that can precipitate ("trigger") migraine attacks. The history may be complicated by the occurrence of more than one type of headache (e.g., tension or analgesic-rebound) in a migraine patient. The features of the attack (such as the severity of pain, presence of vomiting or photophobia) as well as the frequency, duration, severity, and impact on daily activities vary enormously among individual patients. Several studies have attempted to develop prediction rules to assist in migraine diagnosis. The best evidence is for a five-question screening tool with the mnemonic POUND.

- Does the headache Pulsate? (P)
- Without treatment, does it last between 4 and 72 hOurs? (O)
- Is it Unilateral? (U)
- Is the headache accompanied by Nausea? (N)
- Does the headache disrupt normal daily activities (Disabling)? (D)

If 4 or 5 questions are positive, the likelihood ratio (LR) for migraine is 24; for 3 the LR is 3.5; and for 1 or 2, it is 0.41.[5]

Differential Diagnosis

The differential diagnosis includes:

- Other recurrent headache syndromes (cluster, tension, rebound)
- Other causes of unilateral headache (temporal arteritis, carotodynia, brain or scalp conditions, including trauma)

Less than 1% of primary care patients with all types of chronic headache have serious underlying pathology. Significant adverse conditions may be indicated by "red flags," including sudden onset or accelerating symptoms, first episode after age 50, symptoms of systemic illness (e.g., fever, rash, neck stiffness), coexisting cancer, or HIV infection. Neurological symptoms and/or signs should always be fully investigated.[5]

Physical Examination

Between attacks, physical examination is normal, but a full neurologic examination is necessary to rule out alternative explanations for symptoms and to provide a baseline. During attacks, the patient looks fatigued and ill, and may be pale and vomiting. Characteristic behavior is to apply pressure and/or cold to the affected side of the head and to lie very still curled in a fetal position, in a dark, quiet room. No abnormalities are typically found on physical and neurologic examination during attacks.

Diagnostic Studies

Neuroimaging is not warranted in patients with migraine who have normal neurologic examination (Grade B recommendation).[6] The estimated prevalence of a significant intracranial abnormality in such patients is approximately 0.18%; thus, neuroimaging is unlikely to reveal a clinically significant condition.[6] Other diagnostic tests are useful only to rule out alternative diagnoses suggested by the clinical presentation.

TREATMENT

Principles

As migraine is a recurring long-term condition, patients must be encouraged to manage attacks with appropriate support from the physician. Treatment goals are to:

- Minimize the frequency, severity, and duration of attacks
- Reduce migraine-related disability and improve quality of life
- Prevent iatrogenesis or reliance on inappropriate medications
- Avoid maladaptive behaviors by the patient and others

The patient, physician, and others involved must have realistic expectations of treatment. Even with optimal, individualized treatment, migraine cannot be eliminated, but patients can minimize its impact on quality of life. Management involves optimizing general health, minimizing exposure to triggers or factors that increase the frequency or severity of attacks, considering use of prophylactic medications, and developing the optimal specific therapy for each patient's migraine attacks. Tables 6.1-1 and 6.1-2 present current evidence-based recommendations for pharmacological treatment of acute attacks and for prophylactic management, respectively. Pharmacological treatment has to be individualized as patients respond differently to the available therapies and no mechanism currently exists to predict which therapy will benefit an individual patient. Management also has to be adjusted over time as the migraine pattern evolves and the patient undergoes changes associated with age, other health conditions, and lifestyle factors. Some experts recommend using a standard assessment such as the Migraine Disability Scale (MIDAS) to help select a pharmacological treatment and monitor its effectiveness.[7]

Behavioral Therapies

During attacks, guided imagery and breathing techniques may help patients cope with pain, but the contribution of these strategies has not been assessed. Behavioral therapies have been studied in migraine prophylaxis, either alone or as adjuncts to medication. Patients vary enormously in the response to behavioral therapies. Based on a comprehensive review of behavioral and physical treatment modalities, the US Headache Consortium recommended:

TABLE 6.1-1   Pharmacological Treatments for Acute Migraine Attacks[4,12,13]

Medication class	Effective dose	Adverse effects	Quality of evidence	Comments
Analgesics				
Aspirin	500–1,000 mg	GI upset	A	May be combined with antiemetics
Ibuprofen	400–2,400	GI upset	A	First-line therapy
Naproxen Na	750–1,750	GI upset	A	First-line therapy
Acetaminophen + aspirin + caffeine	500/500/130	GI upset, insomnia	A	First-line therapy First-line therapy
Butorphanol spray	1 mg IN	Drowsiness, nausea, dizziness	A	Rescue medication only; potential rebound/abuse
Acetaminophen + codeine	400–600 + 16–25 mg	Drowsiness, nausea, dizziness	A	Severe cases; potential rebound/abuse
Ergotamines				
DHE spray	0.5–4 mg IN	Nausea, nasal discomfort, vasoconstriction	A	Avoid in heart disease, claudication
DHE SC, IM, IV	1 mg	Nausea, flushing, dysphoria, vasoconstriction	B	Use with antiemetics, moderate–severe cases, good in emergency room
Triptans				
Sumatriptan	25–100 mg (oral), 5–20 mg (nasal spray), 6 mg (SC)	Nausea, palpitations, hypertension	A	Moderate–severe cases; avoid in basilar, hemiplegic migraine, severe hypertension
Naratriptan	1–2.5 mg	As above	A	As above
Rizatriptan	5–10 mg	As above	A	As above
Zolmitriptan	2.5–5 mg	As above	A	As above
Almotriptan	12.5 mg	As above but may have lower incidence adverse effects	A	As above
Eletriptan	20–80 mg	As above	A	As above

GI, gastrointestinal.

TABLE 6.1-2	Pharmacological Treatments for Prevention of Episodic Migraine[4,10]		
Medication class	**Effective daily dose**	**Adverse effects**	**Quality of evidence**
β-Blockers			
Propranolol	80–240 mg	Fatigue, weight gain, sleep disturbance; may exacerbate depression, asthma, Raynaud, bradycardia, hypotension	A
Metoprolol	200 mg	As propranolol	A
Timolol	10 mg bid	As propranolol	A
Nadolol	20–160 mg	As propranolol	B
Atenolol	100 mg	As propranolol	B
Antiepileptics (neuromodulators)			
Divalproex sodium	500–1,500	Nausea, asthenia, somnolence, weight gain, tremor, teratogenic	A
Sodium valproate	800–1,500	As above	A
Topiramate	50–200 mg	Paresthesias, nausea, cognitive problems, weight loss	A
Antidepressants			
Amitriptyline	30–150 mg	Drowsiness, weight gain, anticholinergic effects	B
Venlafaxine	75–150 mg	nausea, vomiting, tachycardia	B
Fluoxetine	20qod–40 mg	Insomnia, fatigue, tremor	U
ACE inhibitors/ARBs			
Lisinopril	10–20 mg	Cough, dizziness	B
Candesartan	16 mg	Fatigue, muscle weakness	B
Calcium-channel blockers			
Verapamil	240 mg	Constipation, contraindicated in conduction block	C
Nimodipine	120 mg	Abdominal pain, expensive	C
Complementary therapies			
Petasites (butterbur)	50–75 mg bid	Mild gastrointestinal upset, flatulence	A
Feverfew	2.08–18.75 tid 100 mg	Gastrointestinal upset	B
Magnesium	300–600 mg	Loose stools, diarrhea	B
Riboflavin	400 mg	Mild nausea	B
NSAIDs (ibuprofen, ketoprofen, naproxen)	Not established	Gastrointestinal upset, bleeding, renal damage	B

- Relaxation training with or without thermal biofeedback, electromyographic (EMG) biofeedback, and cognitive-behavioral therapy may be considered in preventing migraine (Grade A). No recommendations could be made about which modality is best suited to specific patients.
- Relaxation therapy and biofeedback may be combined with prophylactic medications to achieve additional clinical improvement (Grade B).
- No recommendations could be made concerning hypnosis, acupuncture, transcutaneous electrical nerve stimulation, cervical manipulation, occlusal adjustment, or hyperbaric oxygen (Grade C).[8]

Medications

Migraine Prophylaxis

Preventive therapy aims to reduce migraine-associated disability by reducing the number, severity, and duration of migraine attacks. Prophylactic therapy requires adherence but should be considered when the patient perceives that the benefits of prophylaxis outweigh the disadvantages (e.g., adherence to daily medication, potential adverse effects, cost). By some estimates, nearly 40% of migraine patients could benefit from prophylactic therapy, but less than 13% currently use it.[9] Indications for prophylactic therapy include:

- Frequent, severe, prolonged, and disabling migraine attacks
- Poor response and/or adverse effects limiting use of acute migraine therapy
- Desire to reduce costs of acute therapy
- Rare migraine subtypes associated with potential neurologic damage (e.g., hemiplegic, basilar, prolonged aura)

In addition to cost and ease of use, choice of a prophylactic medication depends on efficacy plus the potential for "added benefit" for an individual patient (e.g., antihypertensive or antidepressive effect) or adverse effect such as vasoconstriction or sedation. The selected medication should be started at a low dose and increased slowly until an effective dose is established. This requires several months of monitoring for effectiveness, adherence, and potential adverse effects.

The most recent guidelines (2012)[10] made the following recommendations for migraine prevention on the basis of the evidence of efficacy:

- Effective and should be offered to suitable patients (level A)
  - β-Blockers: propranolol, metoprolol, timolol
  - Antiepileptic drugs: divalproex sodium, sodium valproate, topiramate
  - Triptans: frovatriptan (short term for menstrually-associated migraine)
- Probably effective and should be considered in suitable patients (level B)
  - β-Blockers: atenolol, nadolol
  - Antidepressants: amitriptyline, venlafaxine
  - Triptans: naratriptan, zolmitriptan (short term for menstrually-associated migraine)
- Possibly effective and may be considered in suitable patient (level C)
  - β-Blockers: nebivolol, pindolol
  - Angiotensin-converting enzyme (ACE) inhibitors: lisinopril
  - Angiotensin receptor blockers (ARBs): candesartan
  - α-Agonists: clonidine, guanfacine
  - Antiepileptic drugs: carbamazepine
- Evidence is inadequate or conflicting: cannot support or refute use for migraine prevention (level U)
  - β-Blockers: bisoprolol
  - Antiepileptic drugs: gabapentin
  - Antidepressants: fluoxetine, fluvoxamine, protriptyline
  - Calcium-channel blockers: nicardipine, nifedipine, nimodipine, verapamil
  - Acetazolamide
  - Cyclandelate

More recently, guidelines have been published concerning the use of nonsteroidal anti-inflammatory drugs (NSAIDs) and complementary treatments in migraine prevention.[11]

From the many herbs and other substances studied, evidence of reduction in frequency and severity of attacks (level A recommendation) was found only for petasites (extract of butterbur) in doses 50 to 75 mg bid. Limited evidence (level B recommendation) was found for riboflavin (400 mg), feverfew (100 mg), and magnesium (300 mg). Level B recommendations were made for naproxen sodium, fenoprofen, ibuprofen, and ketoprofen, but the benefits were perceived to be modest and based on limited data. Level C recommendations were made for flurbipofen and mefenamic acid. Aspirin and indomethacin received level U recommendations.[11]

Treatment of the Acute Attack

Goals for the management of migraine attacks include:

- Rapid and consistent relief of symptoms
- Prompt return to normal functioning

- Minimal risk of recurrence of symptoms
- Limited or acceptable adverse effects
- Minimal use of backup medications
- Cost effectiveness for patient and health systems

Individualizing therapy is essential to optimize relief of symptoms and enhance adherence with therapy. Patients and their significant others should be educated about migraine and encouraged to take responsibility for self-management. Factors in selecting therapy include:

- Targeting the most troublesome symptoms (e.g., pain, vomiting, exhaustion)
- Synchronizing medication efficacy with migraine pattern (e.g., speed of onset, time to peak symptoms, duration of symptoms, tendency to recur, time between attacks)
- Considering comorbidities and factors that limit medication choices (e.g., gastric bleeding, some forms of heart disease, potential for pregnancy, use of other medications)
- Optimizing patient confidence in medication and preference for route of administration
- Considering cost and availability of medication (including limits on number of doses per month)

The current US Headache Consortium guidelines[4,12] are due to be revised soon, but the key recommendations concur with 2009 European guidelines that incorporated more recent evidence.[13] From the many treatments studied, the US Headache Consortium found pronounced statistical and clinical benefit for some analgesics, ergotamines, and triptans.[4,12]

Analgesics and Symptomatic Medications

Analgesics such as aspirin, ibuprofen, and naproxen can effectively control migraine symptoms (especially early in the attack) if absorbed in adequate doses. Several antiemetics have some direct antimigraine effect in addition to addressing nausea and vomiting and are recommended to be given before NSAIDs or triptans in the European guidelines. In appropriate doses, the combination of aspirin and metoclopramide is as effective as sumatriptan.[14] Caffeine also has a weak antimigraine effect and appears to enhance other medications. The optimal analgesic agent (or combination of analgesics and other symptomatic agents) and dose has to be developed for each patient, but all should be counseled to treat early in the attack, control the dose and frequency of dosing to avoid rebound headache, and to report any adverse effects. Simple analgesics should not be taken for more than 15 days per month (10 days for combinations) to minimize the risk of transforming migraine into chronic daily headache from drug overuse. Both the US and European guidelines found no role but significant potential dangers in the use of butalbital for migraine. The relatively minor efficacy of opiates is more than that countered by adverse effects, principally nausea and somnolence, and the significant risk of abuse.

Ergotamines

These traditional migraine therapies are available for oral, injectable, nasal, or rectal use. The best evidence of efficacy is for dihydroergotamine (DHE) given nasally, intramuscularly, intravenously, or subcutaneously. The action is enhanced by combination with an antiemetic. The main adverse effects relate to vasoconstriction, nausea, and rebound headache. These medications must not be used during pregnancy or when vasoconstriction is contraindicated (e.g., peripheral vascular disease, coronary artery disease). Ergotamine use must be limited to under 10 days per month owing to the risk of inducing drug overdose headache.

Triptans (Serotonin 5-HT$_{1B/1D}$ Agonists)

The currently available triptans differ mainly in bioavailability, speed of effect, and duration of action. Clinical efficacy appears similar within the group, but a patient may respond well to one agent but not another. The choice of initial agent should be based on matching the pharmacologic properties of the drug (such as speed or duration of action) to the migraine pattern of an individual patient. The form of administration can also be adapted to patient needs as some triptans are available in nasal- or oral-dissolving forms and sumatriptan can be given subcutaneously. Triptans are contraindicated in basilar and hemiplegic migraine and in patients with heart disease or uncontrolled hypertension. Nausea, flushing, and palpitations may occur. About 15% to 40% of patients experience recurrence within 24 hours of taking an oral triptan. This can be reduced by giving triptans early in the attack (but not during the aura) and/or adding an NSAID (such as naproxen). A second dose of triptan is often effective for migraine recurrence. Triptan use should be restricted to up to 9 days per month to avoid development of chronic headache. Triptans are significantly more expensive than most alternative treatments.

Surgery and Procedural Interventions

Small studies report improvement in the frequency and intensity of migraine following injection of trigger areas with botulinum toxin. This treatment is advocated for patients with migraine triggered by muscle tension, those with concurrent tension headaches, and patients with migraine on 15 or more days per month in whom other treatments have been unsuccessful. One case series reported significant improvement at 5 years in 88% of 69 patients. Studies of patients treated for paradoxical cerebral embolism identified a high prevalence of migraine (especially with aura) that resolved or improved significantly after closure of patent foramen ovale.

SPECIAL CONSIDERATIONS

Migraine is a long-term condition that patients should be encouraged to manage with advice and support from their physicians. Depression and other stress-related conditions have traditionally had a high prevalence in patients with migraine. With positive coaching by physicians and individualized management utilizing the range of effective therapies, the impact of migraine on quality of life should be minimized.

REFERENCES

1. Headache Classification Subcommittee of the International Headache Society. The international classification of headache disorders: 2nd edition. *Cephalalgia* 2004;24:9–160.
2. Stewart WF, Wood C, Reed ML, et al; AMPP Advisory Group. Cumulative lifetime migraine incidence in women and men. *Cephalalgia* 2008;28:1170–1178.
3. Victor TW, Hu X, Campbell JC, et al. Migraine prevalence by age and sex in the United States: a lifespan study. *Cephalalgia* 2010;30:1065–1072.
4. Silberstein SD. Practice parameter: evidence-based guidelines for migraine headache (an evidence-based review). *Neurology* 2000;55:745–762.
5. Detsky ME, McDonald DR, Baerlocher MO, et al. Does this patient with headache have a migraine or need neuroimaging? *JAMA* 2006;296:1274–1283.
6. Frishberg BM, Rosenberg JH, Matchar DB et al. Evidence-based guidelines in the primary care setting: neuroimaging in patients with nonacute headache. US Headache Consortium 2000. http://tools.aan.com/professionals/practice/pdfs/gl0088.pdf.
7. Diamond M, Cady R. Initiating and optimizing acute therapy for migraine: the role of patient-centered stratified care. *Am J Med* 2005;118:18S–27S.
8. Campbell JK, Penzien DB, Wall EM. Evidence-based guidelines for migraine headache: behavioral and physical treatments. US Headache Consortium. http://tools.aan.com/professionals/practice/pdfs/gl0089.pdf.
9. Lipton RB, Bigal ME, Diamond M, et al.; The American Prevalence and Prevention Advisory Group. Migraine prevalence, disease burden, and the need for preventive therapy. *Neurology* 2007; 68:343–349.
10. Silberstein SD, Holland S, Freitag F, et al. Evidence-based guideline update: pharmacologic treatment for episodic migraine prevention in adults. *Neurology* 2012;78:1337–1345. http://www.neurology.org/content/78/17/1337.full.pdf+html.
11. Holland S, Silberstein SD, Freitag F, et al. Evidence-based guideline update: NSAIDs and other complementary treatments for episodic migraine prevention in adults. *Neurology* 2012;78:1346–1353.
12. Matchar DB, Young WB, Rosenberg JH, et al. Evidence-based guidelines for migraine headache in the primary care setting: pharmacological management of acute attacks. US Headache Consortium. http://tools.aan.com/professionals/practice/pdfs/gl0087.pdf. Accessed November 2013.
13. Evers S, Afra J, Frese A, et al. EFNS guideline on the drug treatment of migraine—revised report of an EFNS task force. *Euro J Neurol* 2009;16:968–981.
14. Tfelt-Hansen P. The effectiveness of combined oral lysine acetylsalicylate and metoclopramide in the treatment of migraine attacks. Comparison with placebo and oral sumatriptan. *Funct Neurol* 2000;15:196–201.
15. Guyuron B, Kriegler JS, Davis J, et al. Five-year outcome of surgical treatment of migraine headaches. *Plast Reconstr Surg* 2011;127:603–608.
16. Wahl A, Praz F, Tai T, et al. Improvement of migraine headaches after percutaneous closure of patent foramen ovale for secondary prevention of paradoxical embolism. *Heart* 2010;96:967–973.

6.2 Nonmigraine Headaches

Diego R. Torres-Russotto

GENERAL APPROACH TO THE PATIENT WITH HEADACHE

Headaches were ranked in the top three most prevalent disorders and as top ten causes of disability in the Global Burden of Disease Survey 2010. The third edition of the International Classification of Headache Disorders (ICHD-3) divides headaches into three main forms: primary headaches, secondary headaches, and other headaches. This chapter intends to review the non-migrainous primary headaches. However, differentiating primary headache syndromes such as migraine, cluster, and tension headaches from the potentially serious forms of secondary headaches caused by tumor, vascular disease, or infection is a critical task. The current recommendation is to attempt headache classification based on the patient's headache phenotype within the last year.

History

It is important to inquire about the patients' historical change of headache symptoms. This would include how many types of headaches the patient has, current age, and age of onset of different headaches. The frequency, duration, rapidity of onset, intensity, location, and character of pain are all important. One should ascertain the presence of provoking and palliating factors, including medicines (and frequency of use) that have or have not been effective. Review of associated symptoms includes nausea, vomiting, typical aura, focal neurologic and localized autonomic symptoms (such as lacrimation and rhinorrhea), and neck pain or stiffness. Red flags for secondary etiologies include presence of fever, history of any type of trauma, history of systemic infections (HIV, sepsis), changes in mental status, history of cancer, and newly diagnosed diseases as well as new drugs. New focal symptoms, pattern change, or progression in a previously stable pattern of headaches is a concern, as is onset before age 5 or after age 50. In acute settings, it is important to ask the patient if the current episode is their worst headache ever. It is rare for the patients to volunteer this critical piece of information, and its presence must prompt imaging and spinal tap considerations.

Examination

Headache with fever or neck stiffness requires exclusion of central nervous system (CNS) infection. Complete neurological exam is necessary, including strength, gait, reflexes, and Babinski sign check. Fundoscopic examination should be done on every patient to rule out papilledema and the presence or absence of spontaneous venous pulsations (reassuring if present, not pathologic if absent).

Laboratory and Imaging Studies

Most patients with typical migraine, tension headache, or other well-defined primary headache syndromes do not need further testing. Sedimentation rate, anti-nuclear antibody (ANA), and C-reactive protein should be checked in adults with new headaches. Temporal artery biopsy should be considered if concerned for temporal arteritis. Sleep study can be considered to exclude obstructive sleep apnea if headaches are worse in the morning. Since headaches are prominent in carbon monoxide poisoning, carbomethoxyhemoglobin testing could be ordered if suspected.

Neuroimaging

- **Brain magnetic resonance imaging (MRI**, preferable to head computerized tomography [CT] when possible) should be done in patients with atypical history, red flags, abnormal cognitive or neurological exam, acute hypertensive crisis, progressive symptoms, and history of cancer or trauma. New headaches associated with cough, sex, or exertion should be evaluated by imaging to exclude structural abnormalities. If brain MRI is negative, and symptoms are suggestive for cerebral venous thrombosis (CVT), MRI- or CT-venogram should be considered. Acute unilateral headaches with any focal symptom should also prompt use of magnetic resonance angiography (MRA) imaging of the neck to rule out arterial dissection. Patients with high risk of aneurysmal disease need MRA of the head also.
- **Imaging the sinuses** (usually with CT) can find occult sinusitis, especially of the sphenoid sinuses.

- **"Worst-ever" headaches** should be emergently evaluated with neuroimaging (usually CT). If CT scanning herniation does not appear to be a risk, then lumbar puncture should be performed to rule out subarachnoid hemorrhage (SAH, looking for xanthochromia).

Lumbar Puncture

Always check opening pressure to look for elevated intracranial pressures (can be seen in hydrocephalus, infections, pseudotumor cerebri, etc.).

- **Lympho- or carcinomatous meningitis** requires serial spinal taps with cytology and flow cytometry before they can be ruled out.
- **HIV and other immunocompromised patients** should be aggressively evaluated for possible CNS opportunistic infections.
- **Cerebrospinal fluid (CSF) Lyme disease tests** can occasionally be positive in the absence of positive peripheral titers. Urgent examination by an ophthalmologist is indicated if angle closure glaucoma or iritis/uveitis is suspected on the basis of a red painful eye.

CLUSTER AND OTHER TRIGEMINAL AUTONOMIC CEPHALALGIAS

Definition/Diagnosis

- Trigeminal autonomic cephalalgias (TACs) are severe unilateral headaches with ipsilateral parasympathetic features. They are differentiated by their frequency, duration, and responsiveness to certain medications.
- **Cluster headaches** consist of attacks of severe, unilateral head or face pain, lasting 15 to 180 minutes, with a frequency of 1 to 8 times per day. Attacks are associated with ipsilateral autonomic symptoms, including conjunctival injection, lacrimation, nasal congestion, rhinorrhea, eyelid edema, facial and/or forehead swelling, miosis, ptosis, with or without restlessness and agitation. Pain is excruciating, and patients are usually pacing and restless as opposed to patients with migraine. Being more common in young males, attacks occur in spells, often nocturnal, often at the same time each day on the same side of the head. Episodic cluster headaches occur in periods lasting 7 days to 1 year, separated by pain-free periods of at least 1 month. Recurrent attacks may switch sides, but side remains the same within a cluster. About 10% to 15% of patients have chronic cluster headaches, where symptoms occur for more than 1 year without remission or with remissions lasting less than 1 month.
- **Paroxysmal hemicrania** is characterized by similar attacks but lasting 2 to 30 minutes with a frequency of many times per day, and an exquisite response to indomethacin (150 to 225 mg daily).
- **Hemicrania continua** is a persistent (>3 months) unilateral headache with ipsilateral autonomic symptoms, absolutely sensitive to indomethacin.
- **Short-lasting unilateral neuralgiform headache attacks** include SUNCT (with prominent ipsilateral conjunctival redness and tearing) and SUNA (without one or neither eye symptoms).

Pathophysiology/Epidemiology

Activation of the posterior hypothalamic gray matter, vasodilation, and activation of the trigeminal parasympathetic reflexes are believed to be the underlying phenomena in TACs. Approximately 5% of cluster headaches are inherited in an autosomal dominant pattern. Cluster and the other TAC headaches are all relatively rare affecting 1% of the population or less.

Workup

Detailed headache and neurologic history, family history, and complete neurologic exam are indicated. CT/MRI/MRA imaging or carotid ultrasound may be indicated if there are findings other than the usual associated trigeminal autonomic symptoms described above or if carotid artery dissection is suspected. Eye pressure measurement is needed to rule out intermittent glaucoma.

Differential Diagnosis

Once neurological emergencies have been ruled out (SAH, CVT, carotid dissection, angle closure glaucoma, uveitis, etc.), the primary differential process is to determine the type of TAC. The importance of the differentiation between cluster and noncluster TACs is highlighted by the exquisite sensitivity to indomethacin. Trigeminal neuralgia may mimic SUNCT but lacks the associated autonomic findings.

Treatment

- **Acute treatments** for cluster headache that have shown efficacy include triptans (most often given by injection), inhaled oxygen, and the somatostatin analog octreotide. Most patients with cluster headache require prophylactic therapy.

TABLE 6.2-1   Cluster and Trigeminal Autonomic Cephalalgias Pharmacotherapy

Agent	Headache type/Rx class
Abortive treatments	
Sumatriptan injection (Imitrex)[a]	Cluster: Triptan
Sumatriptan (Imitrex), Zolmitriptan (Zomig) nasal	5HT (1B/1D) agonist
Sumatriptan (Imitrex), Zolmitriptan (Zomig), others oral	SUNCT headaches[b]
Oxygen by inhalation, high flow ~7–15 L/min	Cluster: molecular agent—mechanism of action unknown
Ergotamine and dihydroergotamine by various parenteral routes of administration (oral not generally effective for abortive treatment, but may be used as transitional agents to chronic prophylactic treatments)	Cluster: vasoconstrictor, 5HT (1B/1D) agonist and suppresses neurogenic inflammation
Octreotide injectable (expensive, considered investigational)	Cluster: somatostatin analog
Indomethacin (Indocin)	Paroxysmal hemicrania: Response to this agent is uniform and diagnostic
Preventive treatments	
Verapamil	Cluster: calcium-channel blocker
Prednisone/other steroids	Cluster: corticosteroid
Lithium	Cluster: ionic agent, class indeterminate
Methysergide (ergot derivative)—off U.S. market due to toxicity concerns	Cluster: ergot derivative
Valproic acid (Depakote)	Cluster: anticonvulsant
Topiramate (Topamax)	Cluster: anticonvulsant
Indomethacin (Indocin)	Paroxysmal hemicrania: highly effective
Cluster: possibly some degree of responsiveness

[a]Injectable triptan more effective than nasal or oral for cluster.
[b]SUNCT headaches are notably resistant to almost all treatments, some degree of response to triptans in a minority of patients has been seen.

- **Preventive therapies** that have been used with success include verapamil, prednisone, lithium, ergots, methysergide (use limited by side effects), cyproheptadine, and indomethacin; the last is also of special use in paroxysmal hemicranias and hemicranias continua (see Table 6.2-1).
- **Surgery** on the trigeminal nerve and deep brain stimulators have also been used in patients with refractory cluster headache.
- **Complications** of cluster include the risk of suicide, violent behavior, secondary depression, loss of function due to the intensity of pain, and side effects from treatments.

Patient Education

Patients with cluster headache are a highly motivated group. They need to be educated about acute treatments that can be self-administered, adherence to preventive regimens, and avoidance of triggers such as alcohol and nitrates.

TENSION-TYPE HEADACHES
Definition/Diagnosis

Tension headaches usually occur in the frontal and/or occipital areas in a bandlike pattern. They last 30 minutes to 7 days, are bilateral, and are of a non-pulsatile, tightening quality. Tension-type headaches (TTHs) are of mild to moderate intensity and do not get worse with routine exertion. Unlike migraine, they have mild (if any) nausea, and can have either photophobia or phonophobia (but not both). Cranial and muscular tenderness to palpation is the most significant finding, can be seen interictally, and helps differentiate from a migraine without aura. **Infrequent episodic TTHs** are considered benign, lasting 30 minutes to 7 days, and occurring at a frequency of less than 12 days per year. **Frequent episodic TTHs** occur more than 12 days per year, and they can evolve into **chronic TTH**, which occur more than 180 days per year.

Pathophysiology/Epidemiology

Previously TTHs were thought to be psychogenic in origin, but current data suggest peripheral nervous system mechanisms in episodic TTH, and a central mechanism in the chronic TTH subtype. TTH prevalence ranges from 30% to 78%, with a female-to-male ratio of about 1.3 to 1. However, chronic TTH prevalence is less than 5%. The more severe and chronic forms may be more common in patients with a family history of headaches.

Evaluation

Palpation of the scalp, temporalis, masseter, and paraspinal and trapezius muscles for tenderness.

Laboratory Studies and Imaging

ESR, CRP, and ANA are usually ordered to evaluate for vasculitis. Consider dissection.

Differential Diagnosis

TTHs that include either photo- or phonophobia can be mistaken for migraine. Medication-overuse headaches often complicate chronic tension headaches. Withdrawal of frequently used abortive medication can lead to reversion of chronic headaches to episodic pattern tension headaches. Chronic subdural hematoma should be suspected in elderly persons with new headaches or in those who have suffered head trauma.

Treatment

Aspirin, acetaminophen, and combinations containing one or both of these plus caffeine are often helpful for tension headaches. All nonsteroidal anti-inflammatory drugs (NSAIDs) seem to be effective. Butalbital-containing combinations can be effective but have higher risk of rebound and abuse and may decrease the effectiveness of preventive medications. Muscle relaxant can sometimes be useful. Occasional use of tramadol or mild narcotics such as acetaminophen with codeine can be considered for more intense pain. Preventive therapy for chronic headaches is often indicated. Tricyclic class medicines have been used frequently. Selective serotonin–reuptake inhibitors (SSRIs) may also be of use (Table 6.2-2). The application of heat, thermal biofeedback training, acupuncture, onabotulinum A injections, and physical modalities such as massage may all be considered.

TABLE 6.2-2	Pharmacotherapy for Tension Headaches: Frequently Used Agents
Agent	**Therapeutic class**
Abortive treatments	
Aspirin	Salicylate
Acetaminophen	NSAID-related
Ibuprofen, Naproxyn, others	NSAIDs
Toradol injectable	NSAID
Aspirin/acetaminophen/caffeine	Salicylate/NSAID-related/combination
Acetaminophen/caffeine	NSAID-related combination
Isometheptene; dichloraiphenazone, and acetaminophen (Midrin)	Vasoconstrictor, muscle relaxant, NSAID-related/combination
Butalbital/aspirin/caffeine	Barbiturate/salicylate combination
Butalbital/acetaminophen/caffeine	Barbiturate/NSAID-related combination
Tramadol (Ultram)	Atypical opioid
Acetaminophen with codeine (Tylenol #3, others)	Opioid derivative, NSAID-related combination
Preventive treatments	
Amitriptyline (Elavil), nortriptyline (Pamelor), others	Tricyclic antidepressant
Prozac, others	SSRI
Tizanidine (Zanaflex)	Antispasmodic, central α_2-adrenergic agonist

Complications

Anxiety and depression are both comorbid with chronic headaches. Whether the headaches have any causative role is unclear.

Patient Education

For mild episodic headaches, patients should be taught to use the safest effective medication on a prn basis. Education about the avoidance of medication overuse to minimize the risk of rebound headaches is warranted. Patients with chronic headaches should be taught the value of prophylactic medications. If chronic headaches persist, then patients should be given the opportunity to seek care at a specialized headache center.

OTHER IMPORTANT HEADACHE SYNDROMES

- **Chronic daily headaches.** Daily headaches occur in up to 5% of the population, and the differential includes chronic migraine (CM), chronic TTH, medication-overuse headache, new daily persistent headache and secondary headache syndromes. Both CM and chronic TTH require a headache frequency of at least 15 days per month. New daily persistent headache is daily and unremitting from the first onset (which is clearly remembered by the patient) lasting for more than 3 months. The most common cause of daily headaches is CM. CM is diagnosed as headache (tension-like or migraine-like) on more than 15 days per month for 3 months, with migrainous features at least 8 days per month. The best studied treatment paradigm for CM was through two randomized studies (PREEMPT I and II) of onabotulinum toxin A (Botox) injections in 31 prespecified sites, showing a significant reduction of headache days by about half.
- **Hypnic headaches.** These headaches are moderate to severe, occur nightly, and awaken patient from sleep, 2:1 female-to-male ratio. They last ~1 hour and are not associated with autonomic symptoms. Intracranial disorders should be excluded by neuroimaging such as MRI. Caffeine and lithium have been reported as effective treatments.
- **Neuropathic or cervicogenic headaches.** The head pain originates in cervical spine (usually C1–3) and is usually unilateral without side-shifting, ablated by treating underlying pathology or temporarily by occipital and/or upper cervical nerve blocks.
- **Posttraumatic headaches.** They resemble tension headaches but within 7 days after head trauma and are often the most prominent symptom of a whole postconcussive syndrome that may include dizziness, memory, and personality disturbances.
- **Exertional, cough-, and sex-associated headaches.** All associated with conditions that raise intra-abdominal pressure. More than 40% have some intracranial abnormality usually vascular (such as SAH), or tumor, so complete workup and imaging such as MRI/MRA is indicated. Indomethacin is often helpful. There are some reports of β-blockers being effective. Consider angina in differential of sex-associated headaches as anginal symptoms may be noted only in the head and neck in some patients.
- **Stabbing (ice-pick) headaches.** Stabbing pains last up to a few seconds to many times a day, and are felt in orbit, temple, and parietal areas in the distribution of the first division of the trigeminal nerve. There are no associated autonomic symptoms. These headaches occur more commonly in patients with other headache types such as migraine or cluster. If strictly in one area, structural lesion should be excluded by imaging.
- **Idiopathic intracranial hypertension** (formerly called pseudotumor cerebri or benign intracranial hypertension). This includes progressive diffuse headache, usually daily, non-pulsating, and aggravated by straining or cough. Papilledema, visual defects, and field defects are common. Elevated CSF pressure is detected by lumbar puncture. Typical patient is a young obese woman. Oral contraceptives, tetracycline, and many other drugs are risk factors.

REFERENCES

1. Castillo J, Munoz P, Guitera V, et al. Epidemiology of chronic daily headache in the general population. *Headache* 1999;39:190–196.
2. Diamond S. Tension-type headache. *Clin Cornerstone* 1999;1(6):33–44.
3. Dodick DW. Chronic daily headache. *N Engl J Med* 2006;354:158–165.
4. Sandrini G, Tassorelli C, Ghiotto N, et al. Uncommon primary headaches. *Curr Opin Neurol* 2006;19(3):299–304.
5. Sjaastad O, Fredriksen TA. Cervicogenic headache: criteria, classification and epidemiology. *Clin Exp Rheumatol* 2000;18(Suppl 19):S3–S6.
6. Smetana GW. The diagnostic value of historical features in primary headache syndromes. *Arch Intern Med* 2000;160:2729–2737.

7. International classification of headache disorders, 3rd edition. *Cephalalgia* 2013;33(9):1–180.
8. Bigal ME, Serrano D, Reed M, et al. Chronic migraine in the population: burden, diagnosis, and satisfaction with treatment. *Neurology* 2008;71:559–566.
9. Diener HC, Dodick DW, Goadsby PJ, et al. Chronic migraine—classification, characteristics and treatment. *Nat Rev Neurol* 2012;8:162–171.
10. Bendtsen L, Bigal ME, Cerbo R, et al. Guidelines for controlled trials of drugs in tension-type headache: second edition. *Cephalalgia* 2010;30:1–16.
11. Fernandez-de-Las-Penas C, Schoenen J. Chronic tension-type headache: what is new? *Curr Opin Neurol* 2009;22:254–261.
12. Bahra A, May A, Goadsby PJ. Cluster headache: a prospective clinical study in 230 patients with diagnostic implications. *Neurology* 2002;58:354–361.

6.3 Meningitis

Najib I. Murr

GENERAL PRINCIPLES

Definition[1,2]

Meningitis, clinically characterized by fever, headache, and meningismus, consists of inflammation of meninges and the subarachnoid space with evidence of cerebrospinal fluid (CSF) pleocytosis. Acute meningitis presents within hours to days, whereas chronic meningitis is longer than 4 weeks. Meningitis can be divided into three categories: pyogenic (bacterial), aseptic, and granulomatous.

Epidemiology and Etiology of Acute Meningitis[1–3]

Mortality from bacterial meningitis is still high (20% in adults and lower in children). The most likely pathogens causing acute bacterial meningitis depend on several factors, including age and immunocompromised status among others. Most common pathogens are:

- *Streptococcus pneumoniae*
  - Can affect all age groups
  - **Risk factors:** immunoglobulin alternative complement deficiency, asplenia, and alcoholism
  - Constitutes about 57% of meningitis cases
- *Neisseria meningitides*
  - Affects adolescents and younger adults
  - **Risk factor:** multiperson dwelling
  - 17% of meningitis
- *Listeria monocytogenes*
  - Affects neonates and adults
  - **Risk factor:** cell-mediated immunodeficiency
  - 4% of cases
- *Haemophilus influenza*
  - Affects children and adults
  - **Risk factor:** new born
  - 6% of cases
- Group B streptococcus
  - Neonates
  - **Risk factor:** age <2 months
  - 17% of cases
- Gram-negative rods
  - Affects adults
  - Mostly a nosocomial infection
  - 33% of all nosocomial meningitis
- Others such as *Staphylococcus aureus*, *Pseudomonas*, *Serratia*, and *fungi* can affect immunocompromised or neutropenic patients.

Etiology of Subacute and Chronic Meningitis[2]

- **Mycobacterial causes** include *Mycobacterium tuberculosis* and *Mycobacterium avium–intracellulare* complex (in HIV patients).
- **Spirochetal organisms** causing subacute meningitis are *Treponema pallidum* and *Borrelia burgdorferi*.
- **Fungal causes** include *Cryptococcus neoformans, Coccidioides immitis, Blastomyces dermatitidis, Histoplasma capsulatum,* and *Aspergillus.*
- **Viral organisms** (aseptic, usually acute) causing meningitis include West Nile virus, herpesvirus types 1 and 2, echovirus, Coxsackie virus types A and B, *Enterovirus,* mumps, lymphocytic choriomeningitis, Epstein–Barr virus, cytomegalovirus, and arthropod-borne viruses.
- **Parasitic organisms** include *Naegleria* and *Angiostrongylus.*

DIAGNOSIS[1–3]

Clinical Features

- The diagnosis of meningitis should be considered in patients with fever, altered mental status, and meningeal signs and symptoms. In bacterial meningitis, patients (mostly children) may have a precedent upper respiratory tract infection, otitis media, or pneumonia. The presence of rash may help defining the etiology. Meningeal signs and symptoms include the following:
  - Generalized headache (new onset), nuchal rigidity, vomiting, photophobia, and seizures (20% of acute bacterial meningitis) changes in mental status (coma being the extreme) can be signs of meningeal infection.
  - In the neonates, fever, decreased appetite, irritability, vomiting, or lassitude should alert the physician to consider meningitis. In elderly patients, signs of meningismus can be absent.
- Clinical examination in acute bacterial meningitis may reveal an ill-looking, toxic, febrile individual with neck rigidity and a positive Kernig or Brudzinski sign. Other possible signs include altered mental status and cranial nerve palsies (particularly involving nerves III, IV, VI, and VII). Focal neurologic signs include hemiparesis, monoparesis, and hemianopia among others. In subacute meningitis, these classic signs may be absent, and the patient may have fever and altered mental status only. In infections due to *N. meningitidis*, a rapidly developing, purplish skin rash may be seen.

Laboratory Diagnosis

- **CSF examination**
  - Elevated opening pressure is found in acute meningitis (greater than 18 cm H_2O), mostly of bacterial origin.
  - Purulent fluid with high polymorphonuclear cell count, increased protein, and low glucose indicates acute bacterial meningitis. Perform Gram stain and consider latex agglutination antigen testing to identify the organism. Culture of CSF will specifically identify the offending pathogen.
  - High lymphocyte count in the CSF with a normal glucose level is commonly seen in viral meningitis or partially treated pyogenic bacterial meningitis.
  - High lymphocyte count in the CSF with a low glucose level is commonly seen in tuberculosis and fungal meningitis.
- **Other laboratory tests.** Two blood cultures, complete blood count, serum electrolytes, and radiologic studies of the chest or computed tomography (CT) scanning of the sinuses may be considered in certain clinical situations. CT scanning or MRI of the brain is essential, particularly in the absence of papilledema and before performing a lumbar puncture to look for signs of increased intracranial pressure.

TREATMENT[1,2,4–6]

Empirical antimicrobial therapy should be started immediately, preferably within 30 minutes of diagnosis. In addition, corticosteroid use has been shown to reduce morbidity and mortality (bacterial meningitis in children) and improve functional outcome (adults).

Empirical Antibiotic Treatment

- Neonates (0 to 4 weeks) can be treated with ampicillin 150 to 200 mg per kg IV daily divided every 8 hours, and gentamicin 2.5 mg per kg q8–12h or cefotaxime (Claforan) 50 mg per kg IV q8h.
- Children, adolescents, and adults (5 weeks to 55 years) may be treated with one of the following regimens:
  - For children, cefotaxime 300 mg per kg of body weight IV divided every 6 hours or ceftriaxone 100 mg per kg body weight IV in two divided doses with vancomycin 60 mg per kg body weight/day IV in three divided doses.

- For adults, cefotaxime 2 g q4–6h IV or ceftriaxone 2 g q12h IV with vancomycin 30 to 45 mg per kg q12h IV.
- Patients older than 55 years can be treated with ampicillin 2 g IV q4h, vancomycin 1 g q12h IV, and cefotaxime or ceftriaxone. Patients allergic to penicillin can be treated with chloramphenicol 4 to 6 g divided every 6 hours, or trimethoprim–sulfamethoxazole (Bactrim) 10 to 20 mg/kg/day in four divided doses with gentamicin 5 mg per kg IV per day divided every 8 hours.
- **Adjunctive therapy.** Corticosteroids, such as dexamethasone 0.15 mg per kg of body weight q6h for 4 days, are recommended for patients with acute onset community acquired meningitis. Respiratory isolation for 24 hours is recommended in patients with suspected *N. meningitides* infection.
- **Specific therapy.** Once the specific pathogen is identified, specific cost-effective antibiotics should be substituted for empirical therapy.
  - *S. pneumoniae.* For infection in adults, give penicillin 4 million U IV q4h. Children should receive 0.3 million units divided every 4 to 6 hours not to exceed 24 million U. Alternatives are chloramphenicol or a third-generation cephalosporin. For penicillin-resistant pneumococci, give cefotaxime or vancomycin 1 g q12h IV.
  - *S. aureus.* For adults, give nafcillin 2 g q4h IV. For children, give 100 to 300 mg per kg of body weight IV in four divided doses. In case of methicillin-resistant *S. aureus* (MRSA) infection, give vancomycin.
  - *L. monocytogenes.* Give penicillin or ampicillin plus gentamicin. Alternative therapy is chloramphenicol or trimethoprim–sulfamethoxazole plus gentamicin.
  - *H. influenzae.* For β-lactamase-negative infections, give ampicillin; for β-lactamase-positive infections, give cefotaxime or ceftriaxone.
  - *N. meningitidis.* Give penicillin or ceftriaxone, cefotaxime, or chloramphenicol.
  - *E. coli* or **Enterobacteriaceae.** Give cefotaxime or ceftriaxone plus gentamicin.
  - **Tuberculosis.** Give a combination of isoniazid (INH), rifampin, pyrazinamide, and ethambutol, or streptomycin for 2 months, then INH and rifampin for an additional 10 months.
  - **Fungal etiology.** Give amphotericin B 1 mg per kg of body weight IV or liposomal amphotericin 5 mg per kg of body weight IV and 0.05 to 0.10 mg intrathecally of amphotericin B with or without flucytosine (5-FC, Ancobon), 150 mg per kg of body weight daily in divided doses. An alternative is fluconazole (Diflucan) 400 to 1,000 mg PO or IV, or voriconazole 200 mg PO or IV q12h, in *Cryptococcus* or *Coccidioides* meningitis.
- **Duration of therapy.** Treatment of common bacterial meningitis continues for 7 days for *H. influenzae* and *N. meningitis*, 10 to 14 days for *S. pneumoniae*, 14 to 21 days for group *B* streptococci, and 21 days for Gram-negative bacilli (other than *H. influenzae*) and 21 days or longer for *L. monocytogenes*.

Prevention

- **Meningococcal meningitis.** Contacts should be given rifampin 600 mg PO q12h for 2 days. Pregnant patients can be given 250 mg of ceftriaxone IM. Meningococcal conjugate vaccine is now recommended by the Advisory Committee on Immunization Practices (ACIP) at ages 11 to 12 years with a booster at age of 16 years. It is also recommended for travelers to countries with high incidence of meningococcal disease, patients with anatomic or functional asplenia, and patients with terminal complement deficiency.
- **H. influenzae meningitis.** Contacts younger than 12 months should receive rifampin 20 mg per kg of body weight for 4 days.

REFERENCES

1. Bratt R. Acute bacterial and viral meningitis. *Continuum (Minneap Minn)* 2012;18(6):1255–1270.
2. Zunt J, Bladwin K. Chronic and subacute meningitis. *Continuum (Minneap Minn)* 2012;18(6):1290–1315.
3. van de Beek D, de Gans J, Spanjaard L, et al. Clinical features and prognostic factors in adults with bacterial meningitis. *N Engl J Med* 2004;351:1849–1859.
4. Feigin RD, McCracken GH Jr, Klein JO. Diagnosis and management of meningitis. *Pediatr Infect Dis J* 1992;11:785–814.
5. van de Beek D, de Gans J, Tunkel AR, et al. Community-acquired bacterial meningitis in adults. *N Engl J Med* 2006;354:44–53.
6. Tunkel AR, Hartmann BJ, Kaplan SL, et al. Practice guidelines for the management of bacterial meningitis. *Clin Infect Dis* 2004;39:1275.

6.4 Seizures

Najib I. Murr

DEFINITION

A seizure is a transient event that includes symptoms and/or signs of abnormal excessive hypersynchronous activity in the brain. These symptoms/signs could manifest in the form of motor, sensory, autonomic, cognitive, or experiential phenomena. The traditional definition of epilepsy requires the occurrence of at least two unprovoked seizures.[1]

CLASSIFICATION AND CLINICAL PRESENTATION[1]

The International League Against Epilepsy (ILAE-1981) divides seizures into three major categories: partial (or focal), generalized (convulsive or nonconvulsive), and unclassified epileptic seizures. Generalized seizures can be convulsive or nonconvulsive and are divided into six types. Partial seizures can begin with a warning (aura) that reflects a focal brain onset, associated with localized symptoms (motor, sensory, autonomic, or psychic). They can remain localized (simple) or spread (secondary generalized seizure), or be associated with altered consciousness (complex). Ictal apnea, incontinence, tongue biting, or significant injury, especially a fracture or a broken tooth, or postictal headache, lethargy, confusion, or Todd paralysis, is usually suggestive of epileptic seizures instead of a nonepileptic spell. The highest incidence of seizures is in children (usually younger than 5 years) and elderly individuals. In this chapter, we will not discuss the classification of epilepsies.

Generalized Seizures

- **Tonic–clonic (grand mal):** The onset is abrupt with loss of consciousness followed by major motor activity (tonic contraction then clonic activity), apnea, and occasional cyanosis, often heralded by a brief epileptic cry but without an aura. Postictal confusion with stertorous respiration. They can represent the manifestation of idiopathic generalized epilepsy or other epileptic syndromes. Isolated provoked (hypoglycemia, prolonged sleep deprivation, others) seizures are also to be considered.
- **Clonic:** An isolated jerk or a cluster of jerks. Frequently seen in epileptic syndromes.
- **Tonic:** Usually brief (<1 minute) contraction of trunkal and/or extremity muscles.
- **Atonic seizures** cause sudden loss of muscle tone and often result in severe trauma. They can be associated with epileptic syndromes (e.g., Lennox–Gastaut).
- **Myoclonic seizures** are repetitive brief muscle contractions associated with ictal electroencephalographic (EEG) change affecting a single or multiple muscle groups (trunk, extremities). They can be seen with idiopathic generalized epilepsies or with epileptic syndromes.
- **Absence seizures**
  - Typical simple absence seizures **(petit mal)** are characterized by abrupt psychomotor arrest usually lasting less than 15 seconds with no postictal state. They typically occur multiple times a day. Complex absence seizures can be associated with minor motor manifestations (e.g., eye blinking or lip smacking). Onset of absence epilepsy is usually after age 3 years and peak incidence is between ages 5 and 10 years. Most absence seizures resolve by early adulthood.
  - Atypical absence seizures (associated with hypotonia or atonia) are common in the Lennox–Gastaut syndrome and other epileptic syndromes and conditions.

Partial Seizures

Partial seizures are always focal in onset but often spread to become generalized. Because of the possibility of an underlying central nervous system lesion, an effort to detect an aura or a sign of focal onset is required in all generalized seizure cases.

- **Simple:** Do not cause loss of consciousness. Can originate from the temporal, frontal, parietal, or occipital lobe.
  - Motor seizures can present with a Jacksonian march, aphasia, or postural. Benign Rolendic epilepsy presents with focal motor seizures (mostly involving the face) during childhood.
  - Sensory seizures can be visual, auditory, verbal, gustatory, somatic, or vertiginous.

- **Autonomic:** Nausea, vomiting, pallor, changes in heart rate, diarrhea, and diaphoresis among other manifestations.
- **Complex:** Associated with altered consciousness and most commonly are of temporal lobe origin.

DIAGNOSIS

Diagnostic evaluation varies according to clinical presentation. In general, the following tests are recommended following a single provoked or unprovoked seizure:

- **Electroencephalography.** Although it is the most useful test, the EEG is not always diagnostic. Activation procedure (hyperventilation, sleep deprivation, and photic stimulation during EEG recording), ambulatory recordings, videotaping, or repeat EEG improves diagnostic accuracy. A generalized three per second spike-and-wave discharge is diagnostic of idiopathic generalized absence epilepsy. Partial complex seizures usually show a focal abnormality on the EEG.
- **Blood tests, looking for secondary etiologies for acute seizures.** Serum electrolytes (especially sodium), calcium, magnesium, blood urea nitrogen, glucose, liver function tests—bilirubin, alkaline phosphatase, aspartate aminotransferase (serum glutamate oxaloacetate transaminase)—complete blood count, and, when indicated, toxin screens and alcohol level are sometimes diagnostic. A prolactin level is not usually considered in the workup.
- **Imaging studies.** Magnetic resonance imaging is the preferred study, but computed tomography can be done emergently looking for the possibility of intracerebral hemorrhage or other pathologies. Brain imaging should be considered in patients with focal neurological deficit and in the elderly.
- **Lumbar puncture** is indicated if infection or subarachnoid hemorrhage is suspected.
- **Anticonvulsant levels** are considered when control of seizures is poor, when drug toxicity is suspected, and within 2 weeks after drug dosage is changed or potentially cross-reacting drugs are added.

MORTALITY AND MORBIDITY

The more frequent the seizures, the higher the likelihood of secondary illness, with increased incidence of psychiatric disorders and migraine headaches with epilepsy. There is a three-time increased mortality rate compared to the general population, including the risk of sudden unexplained death in epilepsy.

TREATMENT

Treatment applies to secondary seizures (treat the underlying cause) and to epilepsy (with antiepileptic drugs, AEDs). A single unprovoked seizure does not require treatment with AEDs. The following are the general principles:

- Correction of blood chemistry abnormalities and combating inciting agents, such as drugs or infections, is essential. Identifying and avoiding triggers (such as alcohol) is also a key.
  - **Hyponatremia.** Seizures or coma occur only if serum sodium is extremely low. Hypertonic saline is best avoided. Slow correction at the rate of 12 mEq per day avoids central pontine myelinolysis.
  - **Hypocalcemia** requires one or two ampoules of calcium gluconate (90 mg per ampoule), IV over 5 to 10 minutes.
- AEDs are presented in Table 6.4-1; dosages are given below.[2-4] Drugs of choice are listed in Table 6.4-2.[2,4,5]
- Acetazolamide (Diamox), pyridoxine, adrenocorticotropic hormone (ACTH), biotin, or a ketogenic diet is useful under special circumstances.
- During pregnancy, AED treatment should be continued. Folic acid supplements may reduce birth defects.
- Rectal diazepam is useful to achieve rapid seizure control, even in the home environment, especially for febrile convulsions.
- Vagal nerve stimulation and responsive neurostimulation can improve seizure control mostly in partial epilepsy refractory to medical treatment.
- Epilepsy surgery can provide excellent outcome in selected patients with partial epilepsy refractory to medical treatment.

STATUS EPILEPTICUS

Status epilepticus is broadly defined as continuous or repetitive convulsions lasting for 30 minutes or recurrent seizures without recovery of consciousness. It is recommended that vigorous therapy for status epilepticus be initiated after 5 minutes of generalized tonic–clonic activity.

Table 6.4-1   Drugs for Seizures

| Drug | Route | Adult (mg/d) | | Pediatric (mg/kg/d) | | | Therapeutic level (µg/mL) |
		SD	MD	SD	MD	DD	
Valproic acid (Depakene)	PO	500–1,000	1,000–2,000	20	20–60	1–3	50–120
Divalproex sodium (Depakote)	PO	Same as above		Same as above		1–3	SAME
Valproate sodium (Depacon)	IV	Same at ≤20 mg/min	—	Same at ≤20 mg/min	—		SAME
Carbamazepine (Tegretol, others)	PO	200–400	400–2,000	5–20	10–30	1–3	4–12
Phenytoin (Dilantin, others)	PO IV	300–400 15–20 mg/kg at ≤50 mg/min (up to 1,500 loading)	200–700	5 15–20 mg/kg at ≤50 mg/min (up to 1,500 loading)	4–15	1–3	10–20
Phenobarbital (luminal, others)	PO, IV	90–180	90–240	2–8 PO 10–20 IV	2–8	1–2	15–40
Primidone (Mysoline)	PO	100–125	250–1,500	10 (or 50 mg)	10–30	2–3	5–12 (primidone)
Gabapentin (Neurontin)	PO	300	900–6,400	10–15	10–30	3	NA
Lamotrigine (Lamictal)	PO	25	100–700	0.15–0.6	1–15	1–2	NA
Ethosuximide (Zarontin)	PO	500	750–2,000	10–20	10–40	2	NA
Clonazepam (Klonopin)	PO	1–1.5	1.5–20	0.01–0.03	0.05–0.2	2–3	NA
Felbamate (Felbatol)	PO	600	1,200–4,800	15	15–60	3–4	30–130
Topiramate (Topamax)	PO	25–50	200–800	1–3	5–9	2	NA
Tiagabine (Gabitril)	PO	4–8	8–56	0.1	0.4–0.7	2	NA
Levetiracetam (Keppra)	PO	500	500–3,000	10–20	20–60	1–2	NA
Oxcarbazepine (Triteptal)	PO	300	600–2,400	8–10	6–50	2	NA
Zonisamide (Zonegran)	PO	100	100–600	1–2	6–8	1–2	NA
Lacosamide (Vimpat)	PO	100	200–400	NA	NA	2	NA
Perampanel (Fycompa)	PO	2	8–12	NA	NA	1	NA
Pregabalin (Lyrica)	PO	150	150–600	NA	NA	2	NA

TABLE 6.4-2	Drugs of Choice for Seizures		

Type	Seizure	First line	Alternatives (adjuncts)
Generalized	Generalized tonic–clonic	Lamotrigine Levetiracetam Topiramate Phenytoin Valproate Carbamazepine	Zonisamide, lacosamide
	Petit mal (absence)	Ethosuximide Valproate	Lamotrigine, clonazepam, zonisamide, levetiracetam
	Myoclonic	Valproate Lamotrigine Levetiracetam	Topiramate, zonisamide, clonazepam, felbamate
Partial	Simple or complex	Lamotrigine Levetiracetam Topiramate Oxcarbazepine Carbamazepine Phenytoin Zonisamide	Lacosamide, valproate, gabapentin, tiagabine, primidone, phenobarbital, pregabalin, perampanel, felbamate

Note: SD, starting dose; MD, maintenance dose.

- Treatment includes correction of abnormal findings (on diagnostic tests), urgent neurology consult, and administration of the following drugs:
  - Thiamine, 100 mg IV.
  - Dextrose, 25 to 50 g IV, is given for adults; 2 to 4 mL per kg of 25% solution for children.
  - Lorazepam (Ativan), 0.1 mg per kg IV, maximum 8 mg, given over 2 to 5 minutes. Diazepam (Valium), 0.3 mg per kg IV, maximum 20 mg, given over 2 to 5 minutes, is an alternative.
  - Lorazepam should be followed by phenytoin (Dilantin), 15 to 20 mg per kg IV infusion, is given at less than 50 mg per minute (for adults and as second choice for children). Fosphenytoin (Cerebyx) is an alternative with fewer side effects, given no faster than 150 mg per minute IV. Therapeutic level of 10 to 20 mcg per mL can be attained. Additional dose of 5 mg per kg can be considered.
  - Phenobarbital (Luminal), 10 mg per kg IV, given over 10 minutes and repeated once if needed, can be considered in case of phenytoin failure. Consider intubation and plan for transfer to intensive care unit at this stage.
  - Other AEDs available in IV formulation such as valproic acid, levetiracetam, and lacosamide can be considered.
  - For refractory status epilepticus, treatment with pentobarbital, propofol (Diprivan), or midazolam (versed) is considered in the intensive care unit and with EEG monitoring.

DRUG SIDE EFFECTS

Drug side effects are common but often controllable with serum levels. Periodic complete blood count and liver function tests are often required. Some of the common side effects are listed below:[3–5]

- Phenytoin (Dilantin) can produce stomach upset, rash, acne, gingival hyperplasia (preventable with teeth cleaning), ataxia, nystagmus, folate deficiency, drowsiness, hirsutism, sedation, and osteomalacia.
- Carbamazepine (Tegretol) can produce rash, sedation, hepatitis, bone marrow suppression, Stevens–Johnson syndrome (SJS) and hyponatremia.
- Valproic acid (Depakene) can produce hepatitis, pancreatitis, sedation, hemorrhage, tremor, weight gain, and hair loss.
- Benzodiazepines can cause sedation and respiratory depression.
- Ethosuximide (Zarontin) can cause gastrointestinal upset, ataxia, sedation, hepatitis, and generalized seizures.
- Phenobarbital and primidone (Mysoline) can cause sedation, irritability, personality change, learning disability, rash, osteomalacia, and anemia.

- Gabapentin (Neurontin) and pregabalin (Lyrica) can cause sedation, ataxia, weight gain, and nystagmus.
- Lamotrigine (Lamictal) can cause rash, SJS, sedation, blurred vision, headache, ataxia, insomnia, and vomiting.
- Topiramate (Topamax) can cause sleepiness, ataxia, psychomotor slowing, weight loss, loss of appetite, cognitive impairment, and kidney stones.
- Tiagabine (Gabitril) can produce dizziness and somnolence.
- Levetiracetam (Keppra) can cause dizziness, somnolence, mood changes anger, and suicidal ideations.
- Zonisamide (Zonegran) can produce ataxia, sleepiness, fatigue, and kidney stones.
- Lacosamide (Vimpat) can produce prolonged PR interval, sedation, dizziness, and mood changes.
- Felbamate (felbatol) can produce pancytopenia, aplastic anemia, hepatic failure, SJS, headaches, and other neurological and skin manifestations.
- Vigabatrin (Sabril) can produce vision loss, suicidality, anemia, SJS, headache, tremor, and others.
- Perampanel (Fycompa) can produce psychiatric and behavioral reactions, dizziness, somnolence, ataxia, headache, weight gain, and paresthesia.

PREVENTION

Prevention is aimed at avoidance of head trauma (e.g., with seat belts and bicycle helmets), infection (e.g., vaccines), drug abuse (e.g., drug education), stroke (e.g., blood pressure and cholesterol control), and cancer (e.g., smoking prevention). People with epilepsy should not swim alone or climb unassisted. Some states require that notification be made to driver's license authorities. Cardiopulmonary resuscitation training can reassure some family members in their ability to deal with epilepsy.

REFERENCES

1. Abou-Khalil B, Gallagher M, MacDonald R. Epilepsies. In: Darrof R, Fenichel G, Jankovic J, et al, eds. *Bradley's neurology in clinical practice.* Philadelphia, PA: Elsevier Saunders; 2012:1583–1633.
2. Drugs for Epilepsy. *Treatment guidelines from the Medical Letter* 2005;3:75–82.
3. LaRoche SM, Helmers SL. The new antiepileptic drugs: scientific review. *JAMA* 2004;291:605–614.
4. Ochoa J. Antiepileptic drugs. Medscape. http://emedicine.medscape.com/article/1187334-overview. Accessed November 14, 2013.
5. LaRoche SM, Helmers SL. The new antiepileptic drugs: clinical applications. *JAMA* 2004;291:615–620.

6.5 Transient Ischemic Attack

Sarah Parrott

GENERAL PRINCIPLES

- The American Heart Association/American Stroke Association's 2009 definition for transient ischemic attack (TIA) is "a transient episode of neurological dysfunction caused by focal brain, spinal cord, or retinal ischemia, without acute infarction." Clinicians should note that the resolution of symptoms in 24 hours is no longer included in this definition.
- **Epidemiology** of TIA is difficult to determine because some patients do not seek care for neurologic symptoms that might be diagnosed as TIA, and there is confusion among practitioners as to what constitutes TIA. **In the United States, it is estimated that 200,000 to 500,000 people suffer from TIA each year.**
- TIA **etiologies** can be classified into four categories: **large artery atherosclerosis, cardioembolism, small vessel disease, and undetermined**.

DIAGNOSIS: HISTORY AND PHYSICAL EXAMINATION

Determining the **time of onset and duration of symptoms** is an essential piece of history. **Symptoms of TIA** include any of the following: visual disturbance in one or both eyes; unilateral or bilateral weakness of the face, arm, or leg; decreased sensation or pain in the face, arm, leg, or trunk; slurring of words; difficulty pronouncing or "finding" words; clumsiness of arms or legs; loss of balance or falling to one side; apathy or inappropriate demeanor; excessive somnolence; agitation; psychosis; confusion; memory changes; and inattention to or denial of environment or body parts. The **differential diagnosis of TIA** includes seizures, migraine aura without headache, syncope, distal nerve paresthesias, vestibulopathies, and hypoglycemia. Metabolic encephalopathies (hepatic, renal, or pulmonary) can cause alterations in behavior and movement. Further description of the **symptoms** may help the clinician determine the area of the transient ischemia. A **full neurologic examination** should follow the history taking, with specific attention to cranial nerve, motor, sensory, speech, language, coordination, and cognitive functions. The decision to proceed with **outpatient versus inpatient workup** depends on stability of the patient, symptomatology, and ability to proceed with testing in a timely manner as an outpatient. The TIA **ABCD^2 score** is designed to compute a patient's short-term risk of stroke on the basis of age, blood pressure on presentation, clinical symptoms, and diabetes. The following factors are associated with the TIA score (in parentheses): age 60 years or greater (1); blood pressure 140/90 mm Hg on first evaluation (1); clinical symptoms of focal weakness with the spell (2) or speech impairment without weakness (1); duration 60 minutes (2) or 10 to 59 minutes (1); and diabetes (1). In combined validation cohorts, the 2-day risk of stroke was 0% for scores of 0 or 1, 1.3% for 2 or 3, 4.1% for 4 or 5, and 8.1% for 6 or 7. Hospitalization is reasonable in a patient with ABCD^2 score >3 presenting within 72 hours of event, indicating high risk of early recurrence, or if the outpatient workup cannot be completed expeditiously.

A **patient with TIA should undergo neuroimaging within 24 hours of symptom onset. Magnetic resonance imaging (MRI) is preferred** (including diffusion sequences). **Computed tomography (CT)** is acceptable when MRI is not readily available. **Carotid Doppler ultrasonography** can identify and quantify carotid atherosclerosis. **Transesophageal echocardiogram** with agitated saline to rule out atrial septal defect can be helpful. **Laboratory data** include a **complete blood count and chem-12**, which will rule out hematologic and metabolic causes of neurologic symptoms. Further laboratory **workup for clotting disorders** should be considered, especially if there is a family history of thrombotic events. An electrocardiogram to rule out atrial fibrillation is standard.

TREATMENT

Risk Factor Moderation

Risk factor moderation includes smoking cessation, weight loss for the obese patient, daily exercise, healthy diet including reduction/elimination of alcohol, achieving tight glycemic control, lowering lipids to acceptable range, and control of hypertension to meet the Seventh Joint National Committee (JNC-7) criteria (120/80). Please note that at the time of this book's publication, the American Heart Association/American Stroke Association has not issued a comment on JNC-8 recommendations (140/90 in patients under 60, 150/90 in patients 60 or older) as they apply to stroke prevention.

Medications

Medications include **anticoagulation** if the cause is suspected to be atrial fibrillation or related to a poorly functioning mitral valve, or **antiplatelet therapy** if the cause is vascular or unknown. Complications of antiplatelet therapy are well documented and include bleeding. The clinician may consider a medication such as a **proton pump inhibitor or H$_2$ blocker** to protect the stomach from ulcer when prescribing daily aspirin. **Oral hypoglycemics or insulin** should be used for tight control of blood glucose in patients with diabetes. Lipid control with **statin therapy**, either moderate intensity or high intensity, is recommended when there are no contraindications, as the secondary prevention benefit clearly outweighs the risks. Hormone replacement therapy using estrogen (with or without progesterone) may increase risk of clotting and should **not** be used in postmenopausal women with history of TIA.

Surgical Treatment

Surgical treatment includes carotid endarterectomy for ipsilateral stenosis >70%, carotid angioplasty and stenting for those with high risk of poor surgical outcome due to other medical illnesses, and intracranial stenting for tight, flow-limiting lesions identified by angiogram. These surgical interventions are preferably performed within 2 weeks of the TIA. There are insufficient data to support patent foramen ovale (PFO) closure for an individual who has TIA and PFO.

Patient Education

The patient should be educated on the importance of lifestyle changes, the benefits of each medicine prescribed, and the importance of medication compliance to prevent stroke. Confirmation of smoking status might be considered on an intermittent basis if initial smoking cessation is achieved. The patient should be instructed to go to the emergency room immediately by ambulance if symptoms recur, as thrombolytic medications might be used within the first 3 hours after symptom presentation in the case of stroke.

REFERENCES

1. Easton JD, Saver JL, Albers GW, et al. AHA/ASA scientific statement: definition and evaluation of transient ischemic attack. *Stroke* 2009;40:2276–2293.
2. Furie KL, Kasner SE, Adams RJ, et al. Guidelines for the prevention of stroke in patients with stroke or transient ischemic attack: a guideline for healthcare professionals from the American Heart Association/ American Stroke Association. *Stroke* 2011;42:227–276.
3. Nacije G, Gaspard N, Legros B, et al. Transient CNS deficits and migrainous auras in individuals without a history of headache. *Headache* 2014;54:493–499.
4. Purroy F, Montaner J, Molina CA, et al. Patterns and predictors of early risk of recurrence after transient ischemic attack with respect to etiologic subtypes. *Stroke* 2007;38:3225–3229.
5. Stone NJ, Robinson JG, Lichtenstein AH, et al. 2013 ACC/AHA Blood Cholesterol Guideline [published online ahead of print November 12, 2013]. *Circulation*. http://circ.ahajournals.org/content/early/2013/11/11/01.cir.0000437738.63853.7a.full.pdf+html. Accessed January 8, 2014.

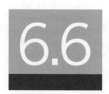

6.6 Stroke and Transient Ischemic Attack

Pierre Fayad, Najib I. Murr, Diego R. Torres-Russotto

GENERAL PRINCIPLES

Definition

Stroke is primarily a clinical syndrome of focal neurologic deficit related to a permanent brain damage from a rupture or occlusion of a blood vessel. Even silent asymptomatic infarcts are now classified as strokes reflecting the permanent brain damage. The time criteria of 24 hours for stroke has evolved, and by itself no longer sufficient to distinguish between stroke and transient ischemic attack (TIA), with supportive evidence needed from brain imaging studies.[1]

Epidemiology

Stroke is a leading worldwide cause of death and disability. In the United States, it is the fourth leading cause of death, with more than 130,000 people dying of stroke annually. Almost 800,000 Americans experience a stroke each year, resulting in substantial disability among many stroke survivors. Because of its prevalence and disability, stroke represents a high financial societal disease burden, with direct and indirect costs approaching $40 billion in 2010.[2]

Classification

Strokes are classified into two main types: hemorrhagic and ischemic.

- **Hemorrhagic strokes** (13%) occur from brain damage resulting from blood vessel rupture that can present either as ***intracerebral hemorrhage (ICH)*** (10%) when it occurs in the brain parenchyma, or as ***subarachnoid hemorrhage (SAH)*** (3%) when the bleeding occurs in the space surrounding the brain.
- **Ischemic strokes** (87%) are caused by occlusion of blood vessels supplying the brain parenchyma, resulting in ischemia and infarction. Ischemic strokes are categorized according to the underlying mechanism causing them, in ***large-vessel*** and ***small-vessel*** disease, ***cardiac embolism***, and ***undetermined*** or ***other determined etiology***.

Mechanism of Injury

- **Hypertension** is responsible for over half of all **ICH** by affecting the small vessels feeding the depth of the brain and making them prone to rupture from microaneurysm formation. Above the age of 80, and in the absence of hypertension, amyloid angiopathy becomes the most common cause of ICH, through the accumulation of amyloid in the vessel walls creating mid-size arterial fragility. In younger individuals below the age of 30, vascular malformations (arteriovenous malformations, cavernous angiomas, and aneurysms) and the use of recreational drugs become more predominant causes. Neoplasms, coagulopathies, anticoagulants, and antiplatelet medications are responsible for some of the remaining causes. The bleeding generally presents like a compact accumulation of blood that acts like a destructive mass, crushing the brain substance around it and causing mass effect.[3]

- At least 90% of spontaneous **SAHs** result from rupture of berry aneurysms that generally form in the main arteries or branches forming the circle of Willis at the base of the brain. Bleeding in such a location accumulates generally large amounts of blood filling the subarachnoid space, creating a sudden increase in intracranial pressure (ICP) with a high chance of re-bleeding and worsened outcome if the aneurysm is not isolated from the circulation. Within a few days of SAH, the blood surrounding the arteries induces vasospastic constriction (delayed SAH vasospasm) that results commonly in additional ischemic brain damage and increasing the disability.[4] SAH has one of the highest risks of early death, with up to 20% of victims dying before reaching medical care.
- Ischemic strokes are caused through various mechanisms or subtypes.
  - **Large-vessel ischemic stroke** (15%) is mostly caused by occlusive atherosclerotic plaques upon which a thrombus forms eventually causing artery-to-artery embolism. The plaques are more likely to involve the bifurcations and cervical cerebral vessels in Caucasians and cigarette smokers, whereas in African Americans, Asians, and diabetics the intracranial vessels are more likely affected. In younger adults (less than 45 years of age), large-vessel occlusions in the cervical vessels are more likely to be caused by arterial dissections.
  - **Small-vessel strokes** represent up to 26% of all strokes. They are most commonly associated with diabetes and hypertension, predominantly affecting the small blood vessels feeding the depth of the cerebral hemispheres, including the white matter and basal ganglia, and brainstem. The tiny blood vessels are affected in a way similar to the retinal and renal vessels by these conditions with the accumulation of fibrohyalinic material or microatheromas, which become eventually occlusive resulting in ischemia. Some conditions affecting the small vessels can be inherited genetically like cerebral autosomal dominant subcortical ischemic leukoencephalopathy (CADASIL).
  - **Cardioembolism** occurs in 30% of ischemic strokes. Over 50% of cardioembolic strokes are associated with atrial fibrillation. Cardiac sources of embolism can be divided into high, medium, and low risk (Table 6.6-1). High-risk cardioembolic sources include prosthetic valves, rheumatic mitral stenosis, infectious endocarditis, recent acute anterior myocardial infarction, atrial fibrillation, and cardiac neoplasms. Medium-risk cardioembolic sources include left ventricular dysfunction, congestive heart failure, bioprosthetic valves, and cardiomyopathy. Low-risk sources are represented by patent foramen ovale, atrial septal aneurysms, and spontaneous echo contrast.
  - Outside of the above categories, miscellaneous conditions that cause ischemic stroke can be identified through diagnostic investigations, and grouped under "**stroke of other determined causes**" such as sinus venous thrombosis, vasculitis, migraine-related stroke, moyamoya disease, sickle-cell disease, hypercoagulability, and radiation-induced vasculopathy.
  - In up to 30% of ischemic strokes, an etiology cannot be identified despite significant investigations. These strokes are grouped under **stroke of undetermined etiology or cryptogenic stroke**. The possibility that a proportion of these strokes may be potentially related to undocumented atrial fibrillation is emerging.

TABLE 6.6-1   Cardioembolic Sources and Risk of Embolism

High risk	Medium risk	Low/unclear risk
Atrial fibrillation	Left ventricular hypokinesia/aneurysm	Patent foramen ovale
Recent anterior myocardial infarction	Bioprosthetic valve	Atrial septal aneurysm
Mechanical valve	Congestive heart failure	Spontaneous echo contrast
Rheumatic mitral stenosis	Cardiomyopathy	
Thrombus/tumor		
Endocarditis		

DIAGNOSIS

Clinical Presentation

Patients experiencing a stroke can present with a wide variety and severity of symptoms, depending on the type, location, mechanism, and size of the stroke. Table 6.6-2 describes the major clinical symptoms of an ischemic stroke associated with a major cerebral artery. Small-vessel ischemic strokes or lacunar infarctions present in five classical syndromes described in Table 6.6-3, and more likely to present in a stuttering or progressive fashion. Embolic strokes typically have an abrupt onset of maximal clinical symptoms and deficits at onset. Large-vessel strokes are more likely to be preceded by TIAs, and may have a more stuttering course. Patients with ICH commonly experience severe headache in addition to a focal neurologic deficit, with the larger ones causing signs of increased ICP (mental status changes and vomiting). SAH classically presents with the worst abrupt headache the patient has ever experienced with or without neurologic deficits.

Stroke Code Team

An acute stroke represents an emergency where time is of the essence and should be managed accordingly. Whenever and wherever available, the Stroke Code Team should be activated as soon as possible to minimize delays in time and shorten to time to treatment with IV tPA or other interventions.[5]

History

Prompt diagnosis and treatment of stroke can improve the outcome. Note that if the patient is unable to communicate due to the neurologic deficit, other sources must be consulted. Ascertain:

- Subjective report of onset and progression and circumstances of neurologic symptoms.
- The time of onset. When stroke symptoms are discovered on awakening, the time of onset is considered the time when the patient was last known or witnessed to be normal.

TABLE 6.6-2	Major Intracranial Artery Occlusions and Clinical Syndromes		
Location	**Artery**	**Dominant**	**Nondominant**
Frontal lobe	MCA MCA: anterior division	Contralateral weakness, abulia Expressive aphasia, contralateral weakness, ipsilateral gaze deviation	Contralateral weakness, abulia Aprosodia, contralateral hemiparesis, ipsilateral gaze deviation
Parietal lobe	MCA: posterior division	Conduction aphasia, Gerstman Synd., contralateral hemianopia, sensory deficit	Anosognosia, apraxia, contralateral neglect, sensory, and hemianopia
Temporal lobe	MCA: posterior division	Receptive aphasia, contralateral hemianopia	Contralateral hemianopia
Occipital lobe	PCA	Alexia without agraphia, contralateral hemianopia	Contralateral hemianopia

TABLE 6.6-3	Major Classic Lacunar Small-Vessel Stroke Syndromes	
Lacunar syndrome	**Clinical findings**	**Location**
Pure motor stroke	Unilateral face, arm, leg No sensory, aphasia, visual defect, other cortical signs	Posterior limb internal capsule, pons
Pure sensory	Hemisensory	Thalamus, corona radiata
Sensory motor	Hemiparesis + sensory	Thalamus, adjacent internal capsule
Ataxic hemiparesis	Hemiparesis (leg worse than arm) Prominent ipsilateral dysmetria	Corona radiata, posterior limb internal capsule
Dysarthria—clumsy hand syndrome	Facial weakness, dysarthria + dysphagia Mild hand weakness and clumsiness	Corona radiata, anterior limb internal capsule

- History of prior stroke or TIA, atrial fibrillation, heart disease, diabetes, and other vascular risk factors.
- Obtain historical details that may indicate a condition other than stroke or unusual causes of stroke like alcohol or recreational drug use, trauma, seizure activity, and metabolic derangements (Table 6.6-4).

Physical Examination

The ABC (airway, breathing, and circulation) of essential emergency body functions should be assessed. Once the patient is stable, a complete medical and neurologic examination is required to assess and document the degree and localization of the deficit. Ideally, a National Institute of Neurologic Diseases and Stroke Score (NIHSS) by trained individuals, should be obtained at baseline, as it yields a quantitative score (and sub-scores) to be compared to if the patient deteriorates while reflecting the severity and potential outcome of stroke.

Laboratory Studies

Initially, complete blood count, electrolytes, creatinine and blood urea nitrogen, hepatic enzymes, prothrombin time, partial thromboplastin time, and international normalized ratio should be performed expeditiously to allow rapid eligibility evaluation for intravenous thrombolysis (Table 6.6-5). A stat finger stick blood glucose measurement is indicated to rule out hypoglycemia. An electrocardiogram (ECG) can be performed to assess for arrhythmia, concurrent cardiac ischemia, or infarct. Serial measurements of troponin are performed if there is suspicion for cardiac ischemia. Once the patient is stable, a comprehensive metabolic profile, urinalysis, fasting lipid profile and glucose, HgbA1c, and thyroid function tests, in addition to other tests as indicated according to the patient's history, should be obtained.

Imaging

Emergent noncontrast head computed tomography (CT) scan is required for patients with an acute stroke to allow the diagnosis of hemorrhage, or nonvascular causes of deficits, and assess eligibility for IV tPA. Patients presenting in the very early hours of an ischemic stroke may have a normal head CT. Magnetic resonance imaging (MRI) is far superior at imaging ischemic stroke early on, and is the preferred imaging scan if the patient is stable, not claustrophobic, and will not delay treatment with IV tPA. Adding an MRI angiogram (MRA) of the head and neck will likely help identify the vascular cause of the stroke in the specific patient, especially in young patients, and those with higher likelihood of intracranial disease. In patients where MRA cannot be obtained, CT angiography (CTA) represents an excellent alternative.

Monitoring

Patients with stroke in the acute phase can deteriorate and experience complications that worsen the outcome. Close monitoring of level of alertness, temperature, swallowing ability, and gait stability, particularly over the first few days, helps prevent complications and improve outcomes. Monitoring of multiple physiologic parameters, including vital signs, heart rhythm glucose, and electrolytes,

TABLE 6.6-4	Conditions Mimicking Stroke and Their Suggestive Features
Condition	**Suggestive features**
Psychogenic	Lack of objective cranial nerve (CN) findings, neurological findings in a nonvascular distribution, or inconsistent examination
Seizures	History of seizures, witnessed seizure activity, postictal period
Hypoglycemia	History of diabetes, low serum glucose, decreased level of consciousness (LOC)
Migraine with aura (complicated migraine)	History of similar events, preceding aura, headache
Hypertensive encephalopathy	Headache, delirium, significant hypertension, cortical blindness, cerebral edema, seizure
Wernicke encephalopathy	History of alcohol abuse, ataxia, ophthalmoplegia, confusion
CNS abscess	History of drug abuse, endocarditis, medical device implant with fever
CNS tumor	Gradual progression of symptoms, other primary malignancy, seizure at onset
Drug toxicity	Lithium, phenytoin, carbamazepine, etc.

TABLE 6.6-5	Immediate Diagnostic Studies: Evaluation of a Patient with Suspected Acute Ischemic Stroke

All patients
- Noncontrast brain CT or brain MRI
- Blood glucose
- Oxygen saturation
- Serum electrolytes/renal function tests[a]
- Complete blood count, including platelet count[a]
- Markers of cardiac ischemia[a]
- PT/INR[a]
- Activated PTT[a]
- ECG[a]

Selected patients
- TT and/or ECT if it is suspected the patient is taking direct thrombin inhibitors or direct factor Xa inhibitors
- Hepatic function tests
- Toxicology screen
- Blood alcohol level
- Pregnancy test
- Arterial blood gas tests (if hypoxia is suspected)
- Chest radiography (if lung disease is suspected)
- Lumbar puncture (if subarachnoid hemorrhage is suspected and CT scan is negative for blood
- Electroencephalogram (if seizures are suspected)

ECT, ecarin clotting time; TT, thrombin time.
[a]Although it is desirable to know the results of these tests before giving intravenous recombinant tissue–type plasminogen activator, fibrinolytic therapy should not be delayed while awaiting the results unless (1) there is clinical suspicion of a bleeding abnormality or thrombocytopenia, (2) the patient has received heparin or warfarin, or (3) the patient has received other anticoagulants (direct thrombin inhibitors or direct factor Xa inhibitors).

is essential. Level of alertness and ability to protect the airway must be followed closely. Blood pressure is commonly increased in the acute phase of stroke. In ICH and SAH, it is recommended to decrease the systolic blood pressure (SBP) below 140. In ischemic stroke, it is not recommended to decrease blood pressure initially, unless the patient is being considered for IV tPA, then SBP should be lowered below 170.

Differential Diagnosis

Numerous conditions can mimic a stroke. The most common mimickers of stroke are listed in Table 6.6-2.

MANAGEMENT OF ACUTE STROKE

The treatment of acute stroke is dependent on the underlying physiology.[5]

Acute Intensive Care and Surgical Management

Patients with ICH and SAH should be admitted to the intensive care unit and require consultation with a neurologist and neurosurgeon to assess for ventriculostomy, ICP monitoring, and possible rare surgical evacuation of hematoma. Surgical evacuation usually is reserved for cerebellar ischemic and hemorrhagic strokes with neurologic deterioration, given the smaller anatomic space and higher risk of brainstem compression and hydrocephalus. Patients with a large middle cerebral artery (MCA) infarction or "malignant MCA syndrome" are at risk for herniation, death, and severe disability, and can benefit from decompressive hemicraniectomy within the first 48 hours.

Nonoperative Acute Ischemic Stroke Management

The goals of acute stroke management are to restore and maintain blood flow to the area of ischemia, prevent further injury to this vulnerable tissue, prevent secondary complications of stroke, prevent subsequent strokes, restore function, and manage disability.

Thrombolysis and Cerebral Blood Flow Restoration
- Thrombolytic therapy requires experienced stroke teams and strict adherence to protocols and guidelines to achieve good outcomes.
- Alteplase (IV tPA) is the only FDA-approved pharmacologic agent for the treatment of acute ischemic stroke to be initiated within 3 hours of symptom onset. Additional studies documented IV tPA effectiveness in a larger time window 3 to 4.5 hours, which has not yet been approved by the FDA but applied in most institutions, and recommended in the major guidelines. IV tPA improves the odds of complete or near-complete recovery from neurologic deficits by about 11% absolute difference, compared with placebo; number needed to treat (NNT) = 19. There is no mortality benefit. There is substantial risk of symptomatic intracranial hemorrhage with absolute difference of 6% (NNH = 17), including fatal hemorrhage (NNH = 40). The therapeutic index for thrombolysis is narrow, and care must be taken to select patients in whom the benefits appear to outweigh the risks.
- Endovascular therapy for restoring blood flow through intra-arterial thrombolysis or clot retrievers, or clot fragmentation and suctioning, has demonstrated feasibility in significantly improving the chances of vessel recanalization when used within 6 to 8 hours of onset of symptoms. Some of the devices have been approved by the FDA for restoring blood flow, but have not demonstrated yet improvement of clinical outcomes after ischemic stroke, and may carry significant risk. Ongoing research studies are evaluating the newer technologies with clot stent retrievers at improving outcomes.

Acute Antithrombotic Treatment
- Early initiation of antiplatelet therapy is beneficial in patients with acute stroke at preventing death and stroke when aspirin is started within 48 hours. Aspirin 160 to 325 mg daily is recommended. Clopidogrel or Aggrenox (aspirin + extended release dipyridamole) are also good alternatives. More aggressive and early therapy with a loading dose of aspirin and clopidogrel within 24 hours in a Chinese population showed a significant decrease in the risk of deterioration and recurrent stroke.[6] Evaluation of this and other regimens in non-Chinese populations is ongoing.
- Full-dose anticoagulation with IV heparin or subcutaneously (SQ) low-molecular-weight heparins was demonstrated to be nonbeneficial in patients with acute ischemic stroke with an increased risk of bleeding. There is one exception where of full-dose anticoagulation is indicated in patients with sinus venous thrombosis, for at least a 6-month period. Subcutaneous low-dose anticoagulation is indicated for the prevention of deep venous thrombosis in patients who are immobilized or with a paralyzed leg.

Management of Acute Hypertension
- The strategy of tolerating elevated blood pressures in the setting of acute ischemic stroke (AIS), sometimes termed "permissive hypertension," maximizes collateral blood flow to the ischemic penumbra. Blood pressure reduction in the setting of acute ischemic stroke can be associated with neurologic deterioration and worse outcomes.
- Treat elevated blood pressure when:
  - Administering thrombolytics, maintain SBP <185 and diastolic blood pressure (DBP) <110.
  - SBP >220 or DBP >120 without thrombolytics.
  - Concurrent aortic dissection, congestive heart failure exacerbation, acute renal failure, and hypertensive encephalopathy.
- When *acute* blood pressure reduction is indicated, intravenous labetalol or nicardipine provide excellent options for treatment. Avoid nitrates due to potential increases in ICP.
- In contrast to ischemic strokes, hemorrhagic strokes require aggressive blood pressure lowering to minimize the volume of hemorrhage.

Supportive Care and Prevention of Secondary Complications
- Hyper- and hypoglycemia are deleterious to ischemic cells, so close attention to glycemic control is important (goal glucose 110 to 180).
- If intravenous fluid administration is required, isotonic fluids such as 0.9% saline are most appropriate to avoid precipitating intracerebral fluid shifts that can occur with hypo- and hypertonic fluids.
- Aggressively control fever with antipyretics.
- Monitor SpO_2 and provide supplemental oxygen if needed.
- Aspiration is a substantial contributor to morbidity. All patients with acute stroke should be nil per oral (NPO) with aspiration precautions until a speech and swallow evaluation is completed.
- Stroke patients have very high risk of venous thromboembolism (VTE). Pharmacologic prophylaxis with low-dose, low-molecular-weight heparin unfractionated heparin is strongly indicated in all patients unless there is specific contraindication. Mechanical VTE prophylaxis via intermittent pneumatic compression devices and graded compression stockings is recommended for patients with hemorrhagic strokes or other contraindication to low-dose heparin.

- It is prudent to order bed rest only for the first 24 hours and until neurologic status has stabilized and balance safety is assessed. Early mobilization, including passive range of motion exercises, with physical and occupational therapy helps improve function and decrease morbidity.
- Evaluation of skin integrity and use of air/circulating mattresses in bed-bound patients can help reduce the incidence of decubitus ulcers.
- Urinary retention, incontinence, constipation, and fecal impaction commonly occur after stroke and derangements of bowel and bladder function require prompt evaluation and treatment. Avoid the use of indwelling catheters due to the increased risk of urinary infections.
- Seizures occur in a small percentage of patients in the acute phase of stroke. They are more likely to occur in patients with hemorrhagic stroke, particularly those with lobar hemorrhage. In the longer term, seizures occur more commonly after 6 months to years after stroke.

Stroke Prevention

There are major updated guidelines for the primary stroke prevention,[7] before a patient develops TIA or stroke, and secondary stroke prevention,[8] after a TIA or stroke.

Prevent Subsequent Strokes

- One of the most important aspects of hospitalization for acute stroke is to identify the etiologic process to target prevention of recurrent strokes.
- Antiplatelet therapy is extremely important for secondary prevention after ischemic strokes. In patients who experience a non-cardioembolic stroke, first-line therapy is aspirin at 81 mg daily. Aspirin/ER dipyridamole (25/200 mg BID) or clopidogrel 75 mg daily are excellent alternatives to aspirin, or can be first line instead of aspirin. They can also be considered for secondary prevention in patients who have experienced a stroke while taking aspirin. The combination of aspirin and clopidogrel is contra-indicated for long-term secondary stroke prevention because of a significantly increased bleeding risk.
- Chronic anticoagulation with warfarin or other newer anticoagulants (dabigatran, apixaban, and rivaroxiban) that do not require monitoring or continuous dose adjustment is indicated exclusively when a cardioembolic source is identified as a cause of the stroke, most commonly atrial fibrillation.[9] Warfarin remains the only agent indicated in patients with prosthetic cardiac valves.
- Patients with symptomatic moderate or severe ipsilateral carotid artery stenosis (50% to 99%) should be referred for revascularization. Carotid endarterectomy (CEA) remains the procedure of choice in most patients, but stenting offers an alternative according to each individual profile. Carotid stenting is an alternative for patients with high-grade stenosis who are not candidates for CEA due to comorbid operative risk. Revascularization for asymptomatic carotid stenosis has lost some support in light of significant benefits derived from aggressive medical therapies. For patients with symptomatic or asymptomatic carotid stenosis, vertebral stenosis, or intracranial stenosis aggressive lipid management is critical to lower the risk of future stroke.[10]

Risk Factor Modification

- All patients with ischemic strokes require aggressive long-term management of modifiable risk factors.
- Controlling blood pressure clearly is effective in reducing risk of subsequent strokes. Antihypertensive therapy should be initiated during the acute hospitalization and proceed slowly with a goal blood pressure of <135/80. The optimal drug regimen remains uncertain, but available data support the use of diuretics and combination therapy with diuretics and most major antihypertensive classes.
- Lipid management is important and the majority of patients likely would benefit from statin therapy, particularly those with large-vessel atherosclerosis. Atorvastatin 80 mg daily, is the only agent studied prospectively in a randomized controlled trial (RCT) in patients with TIA or stroke and average low-density lipoprotein levels that showed a 16% relative risk reduction of stroke over and above other preventive measures. According to the new guidelines, because of the high associated cardiovascular risks, stroke would generally stratify in the high-risk group.[11]
- Optimizing glycemic control results in more favorable outcomes for cardiovascular diseases, with a target HbA1c <7%.
- Counseling about lifestyle risk factor reduction should begin prior to discharge. Provide counseling and offer tobacco cessation assistance for all smokers.
- Recommend increasing regular physical exercise to reduce cardiovascular risk by lowering blood pressure, reducing obesity, and improving glycemic control.
- It is reasonable to recommend avoidance of heavy alcohol consumption or binge drinking, and a diet rich in fruits and vegetables and low in cholesterol and cholesterol-raising fatty acids.

Referrals

- Because 40% of patients with stroke have moderate functional impairments and 15% to 30% have severe disability, early evaluation for and referral to a multidisciplinary acute rehabilitation team is extremely important. Screening for admission to a rehabilitation program should occur as soon as the neurologic and medical conditions permit safe participation.
- Depression is very common after stroke, occurring in 30% to 60% of patients. Screen all patients for depressive symptoms and counsel about the warning signs of depression that may emerge later.
- Patients who have profound disability after stroke or who had poor functional status prior to stroke may not be appropriate candidates for aggressive inpatient rehabilitation programs. These patients must continue to receive range of motion exercises, monitoring and treatment of contractures, and aggressive prevention of decubitus ulcers.

Patient Education

Counsel all patients with stroke about the warning signs of stroke and the importance of medication adherence. Family members play an important role in poststroke recovery and require education as to the nature of their loved one's neurologic deficit, prognosis for recovery, and plan for rehabilitation. All patients discharged on anticoagulation should receive intensive teaching about signs of bleeding, dietary issues, and activity modification.

Follow-Up

All patients who have experienced a stroke require follow-up care with primary care providers for long-term blood pressure management, lipid lowering, diabetes management, dietary and exercise counseling, smoking cessation, and management of anticoagulation if indicated. Clinicians also should monitor progress with rehabilitation therapy, changes in physical functional capacity, social functioning, and emergence of new cardiovascular symptoms or medication side effects. Given the high prevalence, patients should be screened for depression at follow-up appointments.

REFERENCES

1. Sacco RL, Kasner SE, Broderick JP, et al. An updated definition of stroke for the 21st century: a statement for healthcare professionals from the American Heart Association/American Stroke Association. *Stroke* 2013;44:2064–2089.
2. Go AS, Mozaffarian D, Roger VL, et al. Heart disease and stroke statistics—2014 update: a report from the American Heart Association. *Circulation* 2014;129:e28–e292.
3. Morgenstern LB, Hemphill JC 3rd, Anderson C, et al. Guidelines for the management of spontaneous intracerebral hemorrhage: a guideline for healthcare professionals from the American Heart Association/American Stroke Association. *Stroke* 2010;41:2108–2129.
4. Connolly ES Jr, Rabinstein AA, Carhuapoma JR, et al. Guidelines for the management of aneurysmal subarachnoid hemorrhage: a guideline for healthcare professionals from the American Heart Association/american Stroke Association. *Stroke* 2012;43:1711–1737.
5. Jauch EC, Saver JL, Adams HP Jr, et al. Guidelines for the early management of patients with acute ischemic stroke: a guideline for healthcare professionals from the American Heart Association/American Stroke Association. *Stroke* 2013;44:870–947.
6. Wang Y, Wang Y, Zhao X, et al. Clopidogrel with aspirin in acute minor stroke or transient ischemic attack. *N Engl J Med* 2013;369:11–19.
7. Goldstein LB, Bushnell CD, Adams RJ, et al. Guidelines for the primary prevention of stroke: a guideline for healthcare professionals from the American Heart Association/American Stroke Association. *Stroke* 2011;42:517–584.
8. Furie KL, Kasner SE, Adams RJ, et al. Guidelines for the prevention of stroke in patients with stroke or transient ischemic attack: a guideline for healthcare professionals from the american heart association/american stroke association. *Stroke* 2011;42:227–276.
9. Culebras A, Messe SR, Chaturvedi S, et al. Summary of evidence-based guideline update: prevention of stroke in nonvalvular atrial fibrillation: report of the Guideline Development Subcommittee of the American Academy of Neurology. *Neurology* 2014;82:716–724.
10. Brott TG, Halperin JL, Abbara S, et al. 2011 ASA/ACCF/AHA/AANN/AANS/ACR/ASNR/CNS/SAIP/SCAI/SIR/SNIS/SVM/SVS guideline on the management of patients with extracranial carotid and vertebral artery disease: executive summary. *Stroke* 2011;42:e420–e463.
11. Stone NJ, Robinson JG, Lichtenstein AH, et al. 2013 ACC/AHA guideline on the treatment of blood cholesterol to reduce atherosclerotic cardiovascular risk in adults: a report of the American College of Cardiology/American Heart Association Task Force on Practice Guidelines. *Circulation* 2014;129:S1–45.

Movement Disorders

Danish E. Bhatti, Diego R. Torres-Russotto

GENERAL PRINCIPLES
Definition

Parkinsonism is the presence of bradykinesia with resting tremor, rigidity, or postural instability. Most common causes are idiopathic Parkinson disease (IPD)[1] and medication-induced Parkinson's. While essential tremor (ET) is a familial action and posture tremor condition, involving hand and head. ET patients commonly have ataxia and hearing loss.[2] *Dystonia* is an involuntary, sustained contraction of muscles resulting in abnormal postures or jerky tremor. Dystonia can be focal or generalized and is caused by many conditions.[3] Finally, *restless leg syndrome (RLS)* is characterized by an irresistible urge to move the legs to alleviate the presence of crawly sensations, commonly worse in the evening.[4]

Epidemiology

Mean age of onset in Parkinsonism is 70 years. Disease prevalence increases with age, with 1% at age 65 increasing to 4% to 5% by 85 years of age, and 2% to 6% of population (prevalence 305/100,000; incidence 23/100,000 per year) are affected. Onset peaks occur during early adulthood (second decade) and late adulthood (sixth decade). Dystonia has an incidence of 4.47/10[5]. Most common locations are blepharospasm and cervical and laryngeal dystonia. Its prevalence has been likely underestimated to be 16.43/10[5.4] RLS prevalence in general population ranges from 7.2% to 11.5%; however, about 3% are severe enough to require treatment.

Pathophysiology

The pathological hallmark of IPD is accumulation of "Lewy bodies" inside the neurons, composed of α-synuclein protein which spreads caudocranically.[5] Synucleinopathies include IPD, multiple system atrophy (MSA) and dementia with Lewy Bodies (DLB). Tau-pathies (with microscopic tubular aggregations) include progressive supranuclear palsy (PSP) and cortico-basal degeneration (CBD). ET pathophysiology includes possible involvement of the cerebellum, the Guillain–Mollaret triangle, and GABA-ergic mechanisms.[2] Dystonia involves basal ganglia dysfunction, excessive neuroplasticity, abnormal sensory-motor processing, and generalized decreased inhibition[6] RLS has an unclear pathophysiology although it involves an abnormality of dopamine transmission. RLS has been linked to iron deficiency, pregnancy, and renal failure.[4]

DIAGNOSIS
Clinical Presentation

Parkinsonism may present with rigidity, decreased dexterity of the hand, resting tremor, small handwriting, decreased arm swing when walking, or a hand or foot dystonia. An acute onset is concerning for secondary etiologies, including dopamine-blockers use.[7]

ET has a gradual onset of postural and action tremor in both hands and forearms, worse with stress or fatigue. Two thirds improve with alcohol. ET worsens over years and can involve head, voice, jaw, trunk, and legs.[2]

Dystonia presents as focal (most common neck and eyes), segmental, or generalized. It is usually painless (except cervical dystonia). Severity fluctuates based on stress, fatigue, and activity.[8]

RLS utilizes the mnemonic URGE to describe symptoms: **U**rge to move the legs (usually accompanied by creepy-crawly sensations), **R**est makes the symptoms worse, **G**etting up and moving makes symptoms better, and **E**venings are worse. It has been associated with periodic limb movements of sleep (PLMS) and PD. When severe, symptoms can spread to the upper extremities.[4]

Physical Examination

In Parkinsonism, resting tremor is usually distal. PD patients might have a tremor during arm posture-holding (so-called reemergent tremor). A useful feature to diagnose resting tremor is that its amplitude decreases or disappears as soon as the muscle involved with the tremor gets voluntarily contracted.

Bradykinesia is characterized by decreased amplitude and speed of movements. Rigidity is an increase in tone irrespective of the speed of passive movement. A cog-wheel sign may be felt when tremor is associated with it.

Postural and action tremors in ET are those that appear or which amplitude increases as soon as the muscles involved get contracted. Intention tremor is also common in ET, a kinetic tremor which amplitude increases with target-directed movements. ET tremor is regular and rhythmic (jerky and irregular suggest dystonia or myoclonus), distal, and does go away with rest (tremor at rest suggests PD, dystonia, or myoclonus). Head tremor can be vertical or horizontal, and voice tremor is rhythmic and regular.[2]

With dystonia, one should document areas of involvement, posturing, effect of activity and distraction, and presence of tremors and associated disorders (PD). Blepharospasm is the most common focal dystonia, causing excessive blinking, squinting and difficulty keeping eyes open. Cervical dystonia causes torticollis (chin to one side), anterocollis (chin pulled down), retrocollis (chin pulled up), and laterocollis (head to one side); and is commonly associated with a jerky head tremor.

Clinical examination is usually normal in RLS. It is important to look for signs of secondary causes of RLS, including anemia, pregnancy, renal failure, neuropathy, and Parkinsonism.

Laboratory and Imaging

Laboratory includes blood tests to look for secondary etiologies such as Wilson disease (serum copper and ceruloplasmin), autoimmune disorders (ANA panel), iron abnormalities, heavy metals, vitamin deficiencies, renal failure, and metabolic profile.

Imaging with brain MRI is reserved to rule out structural etiologies such as stroke, tumors, depositions (like iron), and specific signs of certain disorders. Dopamine transporter scan (DaTscan) is a nuclear test recently approved by the FDA to differentiate Parkinson from ET. However, an evaluation by a Movement Disorders specialist remains the Gold Standard in difficult-to-diagnose phenomenology.

Differential Diagnosis

Drug-induced Parkinsonism is commonly seen with the use of anti-dopaminergic drugs like antipsychotics and antiemetics (metoclopramide, etc.). Strokes can cause Parkinsonism. Other rare but treatable etiologies include excess mineral deposition in the brain (copper, manganese), metabolic, autoimmune disorders, and toxic chemicals (heavy metals, MPTP+, etc.).

Neurodegenerative Parkinsonism is loosely classified as typical (IPD) and atypical (MSA, PSP, CBD). In addition, Parkinsonism may also be seen in primary dementias such as Alzheimer disease and DLB, and Huntington disease. Genetic causes include monogenic Parkinson diseases, autosomal dominant and recessive ataxias, etc.

ET needs to be differentiated from resting, dystonic, ataxic, physiologic, rubral, myoclonic, and medication-induced action tremors.

Dystonia may be confused with ET, ataxic tremor, neck pain from orthopedic causes and Parkinson disease (which may or may not be present with it).

RLS may be confused with akathisia (generalized restlessness and urge to move, commonly tardive or medication-induced), neuropathy, and myoclonus.

TREATMENT

Movement disorder treatments offer measurable improvements of quality of life.

Ancillary Management

Speech therapy can be highly effective for hypophonia and voice tremor; occupational therapy (OT) and physical therapy (PT) are extremely helpful in keeping patients independent. ET patients benefit from tools and modifications to improve functioning, for example, weighted utensils and pens, tremor neutralization devices (lift PULSE), etc. Gait and balance therapy will help PD and ET patients with postural instability to decrease falls and improve walking.

Medical Management

Dopamine replacement can be useful in PD, RLS, and some dystonias (Table 6.7-1). Other drugs target GABA-ergic, cholinergic, and other systems (Table 6.7-2).

Initial Monotherapy

Most commonly used drugs in Parkinsonism for initial monotherapy are levodopa (with carbidopa), Rasagiline, dopamine agonists, and occasionally anti-cholinergics. There is no known long-term toxicity of using levodopa as initial therapy (ELLDOPA trial);[9] however, minimum effective doses should be used to avoid long-term complications (STRIDE-PD trial).[10]

TABLE 6.7-1 | Common Medications for Parkinson Disease

	MOA	Starting dose	Common SE	Warnings
Amantadine	Likely DA and NE	100 mg/day	Dizziness, insomnia	Death, suicidality, seizures, cardiac failure
Carbidopa/levodopa	Increase DA	25/100 mg 0.5 tabs TID, slow titration	Nausea, vomiting, dyskinesia	Suddenly stopping Sinemet can cause a severe withdrawal reaction
Entacapone	Reversible COMT inhibitor	200 mg TID with levodopa doses	Dyskinesia, drowsiness and dizziness	Warning against concomitant use of COMT and MAO inhibitors
Pramipexole	Dopamine receptor agonist	0.125 mg TID (IR) or 0.375 mg/day (ER)	ICD, peripheral edema	Sleep attacks without warning. Hallucinations, orthostatic hypotension
Rasagline/Selegline	Irreversible MAO-B inhibitor	0.5–1 mg/day (Rasag) 5 mg BID (Seleg)	Headache, GI, depression, and dyskinesia	Risk of serotonin Syndrome with some drugs including some antidepressants
Ropinirole	Dopamine receptor agonist	0.25 mg TID (IR); 2 mg/day (ER)	ICD, peripheral edema	Sleep attacks without warning. Hallucinations, orthostatic hypotension
Rotigotine	Dopamine receptor agonist	2 mg/day (patch only)	ASR, drowsiness and somnolence	Tachycardia, sleep attacks, orthostatism, ICD, rash

PD drugs are pregnancy category C.
IR, immediate release; ER, extended release; ICD, impulse control disorder.

TABLE 6.7-2 | Medications for RLS, ET, and Dystonia

	Mechanism of action	Starting dose	Common side effects	Warnings (including black box)
Clonazepam	GABA agonist	0.5 mg QHS	Drowsiness, ataxia	Cognitive impairment, suicidality, fetal malformation
Gabapentin	Voltage gated Ca^+ channel	100–300 mg TID	Somnolence, cognitive SE, dizziness	Effects on driving, sedation, suicidal behavior or ideation, multiorgan hypersensitivity
Pregabalin	As above	50 mg BID	Blurred vision, weight gain	As above and angioedema, PR interval prolongation, decreased platelet count
Primidone	GABA agonist	50 mg QHS	Ataxia, Vertigo	CI: porphyria suicidal ideation or behavior
Propranolol	β-Adrenergic blocker	80 mg daily (XL)	Fatigue, SOB dizziness, depression	WPW, cardiac failure, bradicardia, bronchospasm, hypoglycemia, erectile dysfunction
Topiramate	GABA and sodium channel	Titration from 25 mg BID	Cognitive dysfunction, fatigue	Glaucoma, visual field defects, oligohydrosis and hyperthermia, met. acidosis
Trihexyphenidyl	M1 Ach R antagonist	2 mg q day	Blurred vision, dizziness	Glaucoma, bradycardia, oligohydrosis

For dopaminergic drugs for RLS, see Table 6.7-1.
RLS, restless leg syndrome; ET, essential tremor, BID, twice daily; QHS, once every night; Ach R, acetylcholine receptor; WPW, Wolf–Parkinson–White syndrome.

Drugs with most robust evidence for treatment of ET include propranolol, primidone, and topiramate. Drug choice is based on side-effect profile (Table 6.7-2).

Most effective oral drugs in dystonia include clonazepam, trihexyphenidyl, and baclofen. Treatment of choice for most focal dystonias is chemodenervation with botulinum toxin injections, which act by blocking the release of acetylcholine at the neuromuscular junction. Chemodenervation is highly effective, with sustained, safe benefit expected through many years of therapy.[6]

Gabapentin and pregabalin are effective first-line therapy for RLS.[11] Because of long-term complications and significant side effects, it is suggested to avoid dopaminergic therapy as first line of treatment, although they are extremely effective.

Add-On Therapies (Long-Term Complications)

With Parkinsonism, motor fluctuations occur when the benefit from levodopa goes away before the next scheduled dose, producing an OFF time. This OFF time can be decreased by increasing the frequency of dosing, giving dopamine agonists, using controlled-release preparations, or adding drugs that slow down the destruction of the dopamine (MAOi, COMT inhibitors). Medication-induced dyskinesias are an indication of overshooting the therapeutic threshold. Dyskinesias are handled by reducing least-effective medications or adding amantadine. Deep brain stimulation (DBS) surgery improves drug-resistant tremor, motor fluctuations, ON time and dyskinesias. Parkinson disease psychosis is associated with the use of anti-Parkinsonian medications, but many other drugs can induce it. Rivastigmine and similar cholinergics can be used for dementia. Overall, antipsychotics should be avoided.[12]

ET symptoms worsening may require multiple medications or DBS.

Dystonia symptoms worsening may require chemodenervation or DBS.

RLS augmentation is characterized by symptoms spreading to the rest of the body, starting earlier in the day, and requiring higher doses. This is seen with long-term use of dopaminergic and other medications. Treatment often requires exchanging dopaminergic drugs into other medications. Use of opioids like methadone is reserved for severe cases.

Surgical Treatment

DBS surgery is the standard of care in patients with PD, ET, and dystonia, with poorly controlled symptoms on medical management. The brain targets include thalamus (primarily for tremor any cause), subthalamic nucleus (PD), and globus pallidus (PD and systonia).[13,14] DBS is highly effective in controlling symptoms and has been shown to significantly improve quality of like. With a low mortality and morbidity rate, it is considered very safe in surgical centers with enough experience. DBS usually does not lose its efficacy over the years, and can be programmed so to adapt to new needs.

Prognosis

IPD has a good prognosis with an average life expectancy close to normal. Atypical Parkinsonisms have a shorter life expectancy of 10 to 15 years from diagnosis.

ET has a normal life expectancy with some gradual worsening of symptoms, with many patients developing significant disabilities.

Referral

Referral to a neurologist could be useful to handle difficult cases. Referral to a Movement Disorder specialist could be considered any time the diagnosis is uncertain, DBS or chemodenervation might be indicated, or the patient is responding poorly to medications.

Patient Education

American Parkinson Disease Association (APDA) has chapters in every state and support groups in every major city. The APDA and the American Academy of Neurology (AAN) Web sites have many useful patient education resources.[15]

REFERENCES

1. Fahn S. Description of Parkinson disease as a clinical syndrome. *Ann NY Acad Sci* 2003;991:1–14.
2. Sullivan KL, Hauser RA, Zesiewicz TA. Essential tremor. Epidemiology, diagnosis, and treatment. *Neurologist* 2004;10(5):250–258.
3. Steeves T, Dykeman J, Jette N, et al. The prevalence of primary dystonia: a systematic review and meta-analysis. *Mov Disord* 2012;27(14):1789–1796.
4. Bogan R, Cheray J. Restless legs syndrome: a review of diagnosis and management in primary care. *Postgrad Med* 2013;125(3):99–111.

5. Braak H, Del Tredici K, Rub U, et al. Staging of brain pathology related to sporadic Parkinson's disease. *Neurobiol Aging* 2003;24(2):197–211.
6. Torres-Russotto D, Perlmutter J. Task-specific dystonias: a review. *Ann NY Acad Sci* 2008;1142:179–199.
7. Rao G, Fisch L, Srinivasan S. Does this patient have Parkinson disease? *JAMA* 2003;289(3):347–353.
8. Jinnah HA, Berardelli A, Comella C, et al; Dystonia Coalition Investigators. The focal dystonias: current views and challenges for future research. *Mov Disord* 2013;28(7):926–943.
9. Fahn S, Oakes D, Shoulson I, et al; The Parkinson Study Group. Levodopa and the progression of Parkinson's disease. *N Engl J Med* 2004;351:2498–2508.
10. Stocchi F, Rascol O, Kieburtz K, et al. Initiating levodopa/carbidopa therapy with and without entacapone in early Parkinson disease: the STRIDE-PD study. *Ann Neurol* 2010;68(1):18–27.
11. Garcia-Borreguero D, Ralf Kohnen M, Silberd M, et al. The long-term treatment of restless legs syndrome/ Willis–Ekbom disease: evidence-based guidelines and clinical consensus best practice guidance: a report from the International Restless Legs Syndrome Study Group. *Sleep Med* 2013;14(7):675–684.
12. Bhatti D, Torres-Russotto D. Pharmacological management of psychosis in Parkinson disease: a review. *Curr Drug Ther* 2012;7(3):151–163.
13. Follett K, Torres-Russotto D. Deep brain stimulation of globus pallidus interna, subthalamic nucleus, and pedunculopontine nucleus for Parkinson's disease: which target? *Parkinsonism Relat Disord* 2012;18(Suppl 1):S165–S167.
14. Martinez-Ramirez D, Okun M. Rationale and clinical pearls for primary care doctors referring patients for deep brain stimulation. *Gerontology* 2014;60(1):38–48.
15. American Parkinson Disease Association (APDA). Information & Referral Center. http://www.apdaparkinson.org/information-referral-centers/. Accessed August 3, 2014.

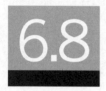

6.8 Alzheimer's Disease

Kalpana P. Padala, Prasad R. Padala

GENERAL PRINCIPLES

Definition

Alzheimer's disease (AD) is the leading cause of dementia in the elderly population. This progressive neurodegenerative disease presents with global cognitive decline, personality changes, behavioral complications, and functional impairment. This was first described in 1907 by Alois Alzheimer who found progressive loss of neurons and abnormal clumps and bundles of fibers in the brain of a woman who presented with disorientation, memory problems, paranoid delusions, and hallucinations.[1]

Epidemiology

Prevalence of AD in the United States is 11% in people over age 65 years and increases to 13.9% in those above age 71 years and 32% in those above age 85 years. Currently, there are 5.2 million Americans with AD in 2014.[2] Conservative estimates project tripling of this number to 16 million by 2050.[3] The annual cost of caring for patients with AD in the United States is estimated to be around 150 billion dollars ranking third after heart disease and cancer.[3] This cost includes direct costs such as medications, physician visits, day care, hospitalization, and nursing home costs; and indirect costs such as the time caregivers spend with patients and associated loss of productivity in the workplace.

Pathophysiology

Intracellular deposition of neurofibrillary tangles and extracellular deposition of β-amyloid plaques are diagnostic of AD at autopsy.[4] Degree of cognitive impairment in AD is more closely related to the burden of the neurofibrillary tangles than the plaques. Hippocampus, basal forebrain, entorhinal, and temporal cortices, areas important in the processing of memory, have profound neuronal loss in AD.

Etiology

There is no single known etiology. Increasing age and positive family history are the two greatest risk factors for AD. Presence of ApoE4 allele increases the risk of AD. ApoE4 allele is present in 40% to

65% of patients with AD. Inheritance of one allele of ApoE4 increases the chances of developing AD twofold, whereas inheriting both alleles increases the chances 10-fold.[5]

DIAGNOSIS
Clinical Presentation
The diagnosis of AD is clinical and based on exclusion of common causes of memory dysfunction. The following criteria are outlined in the *Diagnostic and Statistical Manual of Mental Disorders*, 5th edition (DSM-5):[6]

Probable AD is diagnosed if either of the following is present, otherwise Possible AD should be diagnosed.

1. Evidence of a causative AD genetic mutation from family history or genetic testing.
2. All three of the following is present.
   i. Clear evidence of decline in memory and learning and at least one other cognitive domain: aphasia, apraxia, agnosia, and executive dysfunction.
   ii. The cognitive decline is gradual in onset and steadily progressive without extended plateaus.
   iii. No evidence of mixed etiology (i.e., absence of other neurodegenerative or cerebrovascular disease or other neurological, mental, or systemic disease or condition likely to contribute to cognitive decline).

The earliest symptom reported is impairment in recent memory. Other common deficits include learning deficits, language deficits, word-finding difficulty, repetitiveness, disorientation, and misplacing items (Table 6.8-1). Behavioral problems include apathy, agitation, anxiety, depression, disinhibition, hallucinations, irritability, paranoid delusions, and sleep disturbances. Functional decline such as difficulty cooking, handling finances, and driving often necessitate involvement of social services such as daycare programs and later institutionalization.

Physical Examination
A complete physical and neurologic examination is important to rule out systemic (such as hypothyroidism) and neurologic (such as cerebrovascular disease, Huntington disease, Parkinson disease) conditions. Frontal lobe release signs and anosmia are common neurologic findings in AD.

Laboratory Tests
Laboratory workup is necessary to rule out reversible and other causes of dementia. This includes a complete blood count, vitamin B_{12} and folic acid levels, comprehensive metabolic panel, thyroid-stimulating hormone, and serologic tests for syphilis. In some cases, toxicology screen, cerebrospinal fluid exam, and chest x-ray may be necessary.

Imaging
A non-contrast computerized tomographic imaging of the brain is routinely done to rule out other causes of dementia such as normal pressure hydrocephalus. Other neuroimaging techniques, such as magnetic resonance imaging (MRI), are indicated with sudden deterioration of cognition, headaches, head injury, or abnormal neurologic examination.

Differential Diagnosis
• **Vascular dementia:** It is the second most common form of dementia comprising 10% to 20% of all dementias. Cognitive decline is usually noted after a cerebrovascular event, followed by a plateauing of cognition until the next cerebrovascular event. This is often referred to as stepwise deterioration

TABLE 6.8-1	Ten Warning Signs of AD
Memory loss	Challenges in planning or solving problems
Difficulty performing familiar tasks	Disorientation to time and place
Trouble understanding visual images and spatial relationships	Problems with language
Misplacing things	Poor or decreased judgment
Withdrawal from work or social activities	Changes in mood and personality

Source: http://www.alz.org/AboutAD/Warning.asp.

in cognition. Corresponding changes in MRI or computed tomography (CT) are usually seen. There is also evidence of decline in complex attention and executive function.

- **Dementia with Lewy bodies:** This neurodegenerative dementia is associated with Parkinsonism, fluctuations in cognition, autonomic dysfunction, visual hallucinations, and neuroleptic sensitivity. It is characterized by the presence of Lewy bodies in brainstem and cortex on postmortem pathologic examination.
- **Frontotemporal dementia:** This is a heterogeneous group of rapidly progressive dementias, commonly seen in younger age group. Focal atrophy of frontal and temporal lobes is a characteristic finding. Inappropriate social behavior is an early clinical feature. Language dysfunction and behavioral abnormalities are the main clinical manifestations.
- Reversible causes of dementia include medication use, alcohol use, depression, thyroid disease, vitamin B_{12} deficiency, renal and hepatic dysfunction, hyponatremia, hypercalcemia, normal pressure hydrocephalus, subdural hematomas, chronic meningitis, and cerebral neoplasms.

TREATMENT

Referrals/Counseling

A multidisciplinary team approach is necessary for the diagnosis and management of dementia. Referral to a geriatric evaluation clinic will often provide assessment from a geriatrician, geriatric psychiatrist, social worker, pharmacist, and nurse specialist. Several assessment tools can be used to monitor the progress of AD when such referrals are not available: Mini Mental State Examination[7] and AD Assessment Scale-cognitive subscale[8] can be used for assessment of cognition. Activities of Daily Living scale and Instrumental Activities of Daily Living scale reliably assess the functional status of a patient. Neuropsychiatric inventory is a caregiver report of common behavioral problems seen in AD.[9]

Behavioral Management

Nonpharmacologic interventions are crucial in the management of behavioral problems in AD and include several strategies such as structured activities, environmental interventions, sensory enhancement and relaxation techniques, social contact, and behavior therapy. Structured activities, such as outdoor walks, physical activities, and recreational activities, and environmental interventions, such as having wandering areas and reduced stimulation, avoiding confrontations, and monitoring personal comforts, go a long way in and management of many behavioral problems.

Medications

Although there is no cure for AD, two classes of medications are used to manage cognitive problems. Cholinesterase inhibitors increase the availability of acetylcholine, a neurochemical essential for memory. Three drugs are currently marketed in the United States and include donepezil, galantamine, and rivastigmine. Donepezil is administered once daily, usually started at 5 mg a day and titrated to 10 mg at 4 to 6 weeks. Donepezil is also available in 23 mg strength. Galantamine is usually started at 4 mg twice daily and titrated to 8 mg twice daily at 4 to 6 weeks. Maximum approved dose is 12 mg twice daily, although clinical studies have shown no superiority of this dose over 8 mg twice daily dose. Extended release tablets of galantamine are available at 8, 16, and 24 mg strengths. Rivastigmine is usually started at 1.5 mg twice daily and titrated up every 2 weeks in 1.5-mg increments to reach 6 mg twice daily dose. Transdermal patches of rivastigmine are useful in those with polypharmacy. Transdermal patch of rivastigmine is usually started at 4.6 mg/24 hour patch, which could be increased after 4 weeks to 9.5 mg/24 hour patch or 13.3 mg/24 hour patch. Although well tolerated, some patients experience gastrointestinal side effects. Several strategies such as starting at a lower dose, slower titration, and taking the medications with food can be helpful.

The second class of drugs targets the glutamate receptors and prevents death of neurons by excessive influx of calcium (excitotoxicity). Memantine is an uncompetitive N-methyl-D-aspartate receptor antagonist. It is started at 5 mg a day and titrated by increments of 5 mg weekly to reach the target dose of 10 mg twice daily. It can be used in combination with a cholinesterase inhibitor due to the different mechanisms of action.

Although mainly used for cognitive decline, cholinesterase inhibitors have been found to be helpful in the management of behavioral problems such as hallucinations and agitation. Specific treatments for behavioral problems, such as selective serotonin–reuptake inhibitors for depression and atypical antipsychotics for hallucinations and delusions, are sometimes used (Table 6.8-2). Given the increased

TABLE 6.8-2	Medications for Behavioral Problems in AD	
Medication	**Indication**	**Dose/day**
Citalopram, Paroxetine, Fluoxetine	Depression, anxiety, and agitation	10–20 mg
Sertraline	Irritability	25–100 mg
Methylphenidate	Apathy	5–10 mg

death associated with use of atypical antipsychotics in this population, it is important to educate the family and patient about the potential and get informed consent.

Risk Management

Detailed evaluation of safety risks is essential at the intake and at each follow-up visit. Common safety concerns include cooking, driving, firearm safety, financial mismanagement, wandering in hazardous weather, and abuse. Involvement of family and social services can often help in management of these safety concerns. Practical interventions such as involving meals on wheels, disabling the car, taking away the firearms or the ammunition, family involvement in fiscal management, wander guards can be life-saving. It is also crucial to establish advance directives and health care power of attorney.

Patient Education

Education about the disease, course of the illness, and the need for multiple interventions is essential. Family members need to be educated about various manifestations of dementia in different stages such as the cognitive problems, behavioral problems, and functional decline, all stemming from one disease process rather than multiple entities. It is also essential to educate about what to expect from medications used to treat dementia. Furthermore, educating about respite, accessing local support network such as the local chapter of Alzheimer Association, Area Office of Aging (AOA) can reduce caregiver burden. In the later stages of AD, families of patients need to be provided information on nursing homes in the local community and also about terminal care.

REFERENCES

1. Fuller SC. Alzheimer's disease (senium praecox): the report of a case and review of published cases [Translated from Alzheimer's originally published notes]. *J Nerv Ment Dis* 1912;39:452–454.
2. Hebert LE, Weuve J, Scherr PA, et al. Alzheimer disease in the United States (2010–2050) estimated using the 2010 census. *Neurology* 2013;80(19):1778–1783.
3. http://www.alz.org/alzheimers_disease_alzheimer_statistics.asp.
4. Perl DP. Neuropathology of Alzheimer's disease and related disorders. *Neurol Clin* 2000;18:847.
5. Roses AD. Apolipoprotein E alleles as risk factors in Alzheimer's disease. *Annu Rev Med* 1996;47:387–400.
6. American Psychiatric Association. *Diagnostic and statistical manual of mental disorders.* (4th ed., text rev.). Washington, DC: American Psychiatric Association; 2000.
7. Folstein MF, Folstein SE, McHugh PR. Mini-mental state: a practical method for grading the state of patients for the clinician. *J Psychiatr Res* 1975;12:189–198.
8. Mohs RC, Rosen WG, Davis KL. The Alzheimer's disease assessment scale: an instrument for assessing treatment efficacy. *Psychopharmacol Bull* 1983;19(3):448–450.
9. Cummings JL, Mega M, Gray K, et al. The neuropsychiatric inventory: comprehensive assessment of psychopathology in dementia. *Neurology* 1994;44(12):2308–2314.

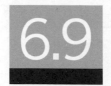

Peripheral Neuropathy

J. Americo M. Fernandes Filho

GENERAL PRINCIPLES

Peripheral nerves contain motor, sensory, and autonomic fibers alone or in combination. Peripheral nerves may be damaged by various causes, including hereditary, toxic, nutritional, ischemic, inflammatory, metabolic, infectious, and paraneoplastic disorders. Peripheral neuropathies vary widely in their presentation, depending on the specific fibers involved, as well as on whether the axon itself or the myelin sheath is primarily affected.

DIAGNOSIS

- **Signs and symptoms.** Patients with peripheral neuropathy may present with altered sensation, pain, weakness, or autonomic symptoms. In the early stages, patients may experience only pain or other subjective symptoms. Measurable sensory deficits may be less appreciable. Motor dysfunction, if present, may range from mild to severe weakness, and usually more pronounced distally. Decreased muscle stretch reflexes may be an early objective sign of nerve dysfunction and may help localizing the process in the peripheral nervous system. Stumbling, tripping, or clumsiness of either hands or feet may also be reported. Autonomic dysfunction is most often associated with diabetes (see Chapter 17.2).
- **Approach to the patient.** If particular symptoms are thought to represent a peripheral neuropathy, the identification of treatable causes or underlying medical conditions (particularly diabetes, alcoholism, and nutritional deficiencies) should be the first priority. It is important to establish if the involvement is focal, multifocal, or diffuse (asymmetric or symmetric). The onset pattern (acute or chronic) and progression in time and space, combined with if axons or myelin are primarily affected, will be very important in differentiating between hereditary and acquired disorders as well as in guiding evaluation and treatment. History of recent viral illnesses or any new medications should be obtained. Work and hobbies should be reviewed for activities that cause repetitive nerve trauma as well as any potential toxic exposures. Hereditary neuropathies are common. A detailed family history is often helpful in previously unrecognized or long-standing distal neuropathies.

MONONEUROPATHIES

Mononeuropathies are usually due to entrapment, compression, or other physical injuries of peripheral nerves deep to fibrous bands (where they pass through bony openings or arch across bony prominences). Repetitive work or cumulative trauma may also be implicated. Electrodiagnostic studies are useful to confirm the diagnosis and quantify the injury. Treatment is generally conservative, including work or activity modification. Surgical exploration should be reserved for more chronic mononeuropathies that have begun to show evidence of weakness or atrophy. **Mononeuropathy multiplex** results from multifocal involvement of individual peripheral nerves; the clinical picture is highly variable and potentially confusing. Ischemic diabetic neuropathy, as well as vasculitides and chronic inflammatory demyelinating polyradiculoneuropathy (CIDP), account for most cases.

- **Trigeminal neuralgia** (tic douloureux) is relatively common and usually idiopathic. Magnetic resonance imaging can help differentiate from secondary causes such as multiple sclerosis, a brain tumor, or vascular anomaly. Trigeminal neuralgia is characterized as brief paroxysmal attacks of severe, lancinating facial pain in the maxillary or mandibular divisions of the trigeminal nerve (the ophthalmic division is rarely involved). Many patients report trigger points sensitive to even mild stimuli, such as light touch, chewing, tooth brushing, shaving, or talking. Antiepileptic drugs like carbamazepine (200 to 300 mg three times a day) and oxcarbazepine, with slow dose escalation, are usually effective. Carbamazepine can be started on 100 mg at bedtime and increased by 100 mg every 1 to 3 days until symptoms are relieved. Some patients may require doses of up to 400 mg tid. Other agents like phenytoin (Dilantin), lamotrigine, or baclofen may be a useful alternative or an adjunct to carbamazepine. Referral to specialist or surgical evaluation is considered in patients refractory to medical treatment.
- **Bell palsy** (idiopathic facial paralysis), an acute onset of isolated facial nerve paralysis, is common. It occurs at any age, and the etiology remains unclear. Although still somewhat controversial, evidence

is accumulating that reactivated herpes viruses (simplex type 1 or zoster) in cranial nerve ganglia are the most common cause of Bell palsy. The prognosis, with or without specific treatment, is excellent, as almost all patients have spontaneous recovery in 1 to 3 weeks. However, 15% of patients (particularly those who are older or more severely affected) may show some residual weakness for several months or even permanently. Bilateral Bell palsy is rare and potentially more worrisome, with causes like Lyme disease, human immunodeficiency (HIV) infection, leukemia, syphilis, infectious mononucleosis, or sarcoidosis.

- **Clinical presentation.** Symptoms typically develop overnight and the patient notices a facial droop on awakening. Many patients recall sitting in a draft or report a recent viral illness. The degree of impairment is widely variable, ranging from mild weakness and a delay in blinking to complete paralysis and inability to close the eye. Forehead muscles are involved in Bell palsy. Frontal sparing indicates a central nervous system lesion. Corneal sensation is intact. Food may catch in the cheek on the affected side.

- **Therapy.** Patient education about careful eye care is essential. The eye should be kept moist and lubricated with artificial tears or an ophthalmic ointment (Lacrilube). It may also be necessary to protect the eye with a shield or to tape it shut during sleep. If no strong contraindications to steroids exist, prednisone, 60 to 80 mg daily for 5 to 10 days may be helpful, especially if started within the first 2 or 3 days. Although antivirals alone are not indicated, adding an antiviral agent like acyclovir or valacyclovir to prednisone therapy may improve recovery rates compared with prednisone alone (however, strong evidence for use of combined therapy is lacking).

- **Brachial plexus neuropathies** are usually due to blunt or penetrating trauma. Any injury that is directed to the axilla or that forcibly stretches the head and shoulder may result in numbness and paresthesias of the arm and diffuse weakness of the arm and shoulder. Direct extension of apical lung tumors (Pancoast tumor) or metastatic brachial plexopathy, particularly from breast cancer, is common. Radiation therapy is also known to cause plexopathies. Neuralgic amyotrophy (Parsonage–Turner syndrome), an inflammatory disorder of the peripheral nervous system, may affect brachial plexus or, less often, extraplexal nerves. It is characterized by severe pain of sudden onset, followed by muscle weakness and atrophy.

- **Carpal tunnel syndrome** (CTS) is the most common of all entrapment neuropathies. Any process that encroaches on the median nerve, either intrinsically or extrinsically, can cause CTS (Chapter 15.5).

- **Ulnar nerve entrapment** at the elbow, in either the ulnar groove or the cubital tunnel, is the most common site. It usually results in chronic mechanical compression or stretch of the ulnar nerve. Trauma and subsequent arthritic changes at the elbow joint, often long before clinical presentation can result in the "tardy ulnar palsy." Patients who lean on their elbows at work or who have had prolonged elbow pressure after coma or general anesthesia, or who have been immobilized because of surgery, are susceptible. Patients experience intermittent paresthesia in the fourth and fifth fingers, as well as medial aspect of the hand. They may also experience generalized weakness of grip and clumsiness of the hand and fingers, especially with fine manipulation. The ulnar nerve may occasionally be compressed at the wrist (Guyon canal). It may occur as result of trauma, mass lesion (often a ganglion cyst) or in individuals with certain occupations with repetitive movement or pressure against the ulnar nerve, like in long-distance bicyclists. Motor symptoms are more pronounced with fewer, if any, sensory symptoms.

- **Radial nerve injuries** are less common than in median and ulnar nerves. Most common entrapment sites are in the mid-arm as it wraps around the spiral groove and axilla. It can also be affected more distally in the posterior interosseous and superficial sensory radial nerves. It most often occurs after external compression, rarely by internal structures. While lesions at the spiral groove will clinically cause wrist-drop and of finger extensors along with mild weakness of supination and elbow flexion (with sensory disturbance in the superficial sensory nerve distribution), lesions that more proximal (axilla) will also cause arm extension (triceps) weakness and sensory disturbance, extending into the posterior forearm and arm. Entrapment of the posterior interosseus nerve (radial tunnel syndrome) at the level of the supinator muscle causes wrist and finger drop with a wrist radial deviation on attempt to extent the wrist due to sparing of radial-innervated muscles proximal to the takeoff of the posterior interosseous nerve and no sensory loss.

Lumbosacral Neuropathies

- **Meralgia paresthetica** is a compression neuropathy of the lateral femoral cutaneous nerve of the thigh. It is commonly seen in obese or diabetic individuals. Patients experience numbness, pain, paresthesia, and decreased sensation of the anterolateral thigh. There is no objective weakness.

- **Femoral neuropathy** is most commonly iatrogenic from direct nerve trauma or poor leg positioning during surgical procedures. It results in weakness of knee extension and paresthesia of the anteromedial thigh and the medial aspect of the lower leg and foot. The previously called diabetic femoral neuropathy is a misnomer. Patients with diabetes may present with a subacute process consistent with a radiculoplexopathy, also known as diabetic amyotrophy, where there is also involvement of muscles not innervated by the femoral nerve.

- **Peroneal neuropathy** may be caused by pressure at the level of the fibular head exerted by an ill-fitting cast, trauma, or improperly positioned delivery room stirrups. Diabetic and patient with an underlying peripheral polyneuropathy may have a higher incidence. Patients present with a foot-drop and sensory changes of the dorsum of the foot and ankle.
- **Tibial neuropathy** (tarsal tunnel syndrome) most often is attributable to compression of the tibial nerve in the tarsal tunnel at the medial malleolus. This results in burning and paresthesias of the sole of the foot, and may be aggravated by walking or prolonged standing. Proximal tibial nerve lesions are also rare and most are located near the popliteal fossa, usually related to compression like by a Baker's cyst.

POLYNEUROPATHIES

Polyneuropathies are characterized by diffuse, bilateral, and symmetrical damage, producing a distal, stocking or glove pattern of paresthesias and sensory loss, later followed by decreased muscle stretch reflexes and muscle weakness.

- **Diabetic neuropathy** is the most commonly encountered polyneuropathy. Some form of neuropathy develops in over one half of all people with diabetes (also see Chapter 17.2). It usually develops after many years, although it may occasionally be the presenting feature of diabetes. Strict glycemic control and good daily foot care are key to preventing complications of diabetic neuropathy. Early recognition of diabetic neuropathy may decrease the incidence of lower extremity complications.
  - **Clinical presentation.** The primary types of diabetic neuropathy are sensorimotor and autonomic. A patient may have only one type of neuropathy or might develop different combinations of neuropathies. Most commonly, patients with diabetes experience a distal, symmetrical polyneuropathy with predominantly sensory involvement and mild motor signs. Initially, the patient may not perceive pain, thus initiating a cascade of events that may ultimately lead to the development of diabetic ulcers with potential for infection or amputation. Later, the patient may also experience severe burning discomfort or dysesthesias, particularly of the plantar surfaces of the feet. Involvement of large myelinated fibers may cause decreased joint position sense, leading in more severe cases to both sensory ataxia and secondary arthropathy (Charcot joints). Some patients with diabetes may have purely autonomic signs and symptoms. Postural hypotension is probably most common, but gastrointestinal (diabetic gastroparesis, intestinal hypomotility, and constipation or diarrhea) and genitourinary (impotence and atonic bladder) symptoms may also occur. Myocardial infarction is commonly silent in patients with diabetes because of loss of small pain fibers in the cardiac sympathetic system. Patients with diabetes frequently develop single as well as multiple mononeuropathies. These patients are more prone to both ischemic and entrapment neuropathies.
  - **Therapy.** Optimal glycemic control is most important for both prevention and treatment. Patient education about daily foot care is essential for preventing complications of diabetic neuropathy. The American Diabetes Association (ADA) recommends a thorough annual foot examination by a health care professional for all patients with diabetes. For pain control, the tricyclics, especially amitriptyline, 10 to 150 mg at bedtime, may be helpful. Either desipramine or nortriptyline, 75 to 150 mg, may be a useful alternative in patients unable to tolerate amitriptyline. Duloxetine, an antidepressant, in the doses of 60 to 120 mg was approved for the treatment of diabetic neuropathic pain (60 mg daily had similar benefits compared to twice a day dose with better tolerability). Pregabalin, an antiepileptic drug, was also approved for use. Other antiepileptic medications including gabapentin, carbamazepine, phenytoin, lamotrigine, topiramate, oxcarbazepine, and lancosamide may also be attempted. Topical capsaicin 0.075% applied once daily or 5% lidocaine may also help relieve diabetic neuropathy. Referral to pain clinic should be considered in refractory cases.

Inflammatory neuropathies

- **Herpes zoster** (shingles) is a painful rash that is caused by the reactivation of latent varicella virus in the distribution of the affected nerve (see Chapter 19.8). The characteristic vesicular eruption is unilateral and most often involves a thoracic dermatome. Risk factors of developing herpes zoster include increasing age, underlying malignancy, and immunosuppression.
  - **Clinical presentation.** The prodrome of herpes zoster includes malaise, headache, photophobia, abnormal skin sensation, and occasional fever. These may precede the eruption by several days. Vesicles on the tip of the nose may indicate ophthalmic zoster. If there is eye pain, redness, or

photophobia, the patient should refer to an ophthalmologist. Involvement of the geniculate ganglion of the facial nerve may result in an acute facial nerve paralysis, accompanied by an eruption on the ear and within the ear canal (Ramsay Hunt syndrome). Weakness or paralysis, especially of the facial nerves, or disseminated zoster is more likely to occur in elderly individuals or in patients immunocompromised by HIV or malignancy.

- **Therapy.** High-dose acyclovir (Zovirax) 800 mg five times daily for 7 days, valacyclovir (Valtrex) 1,000 mg tid, or famciclovir (Famvir) 500 mg tid, also for 7 days have been shown to decrease both the duration and severity of acute symptoms if started early (within the first 72 hours of symptoms in all patients older than 50 years). There is evidence to support using antiviral therapy and possibly low-dose tricyclic antidepressants to prevent postherpetic neuralgia. Combination therapy of antivirals with corticosteroids may decrease the pain of acute herpes zoster and speed lesion healing and could be considered in older patients with no contraindications. For established postherpetic neuralgia, there is good evidence to support treatment with anticonvulsant like gabapentin, pregabalin, tricyclic antidepressants, and topical agents.
- **Lyme disease.** Bell palsy, which may be bilateral, or a polyradiculopathy may be seen in the early disseminated phase of Lyme disease (see Chapter 19.9).
- **Leprosy.** Despite its low incidence in the United States, leprosy remains the most common cause of treatable peripheral neuropathy in the world. Leprosy must be included in the differential diagnosis whenever a patient from a high-risk group presents with a peripheral neuropathy. As leprosy and its attendant skin lesions progress, increasing anesthesia, with the potential for breakdown and injury, occurs in the lesions. Some degree of sensory loss is always present in leprosy. It is not unusual for symptoms of neuropathy to occur long before other manifestations of the disease.
- **Acute inflammatory demyelinating polyradiculopathy** or **Guillain–Barré syndrome (GBS).** GBS is a syndrome of symmetrical, rapidly progressive, ascending muscle weakness with decreased or absent muscle stretch reflexes. Epidemiologic studies have linked it to infection with *Campylobacter jejuni* in addition to other viruses including cytomegalovirus and Epstein–Barr virus. *Campylobacter jejuni* gastroenteritis is the most frequent antecedent infection. All patients should be hospitalized to carefully monitor their cardiac and respiratory status, neurologic consultation and testing, and to initiate either plasmapheresis or immunoglobulin therapy. Most patients make a good recovery. Prognosis is worse in elderly patients and also in patients with more rapid progression of muscle weakness or evidence of axonal involvement.
- **CIDP.** This disorder is a relatively common neuropathy that often goes unrecognized. Clinical and electrophysiologic diagnostic criteria have been established, allowing clinicians to distinguish CIDP from other acquired neuropathies. The usual clinical picture is of motor and sensory symptoms with an elevated cerebrospinal fluid (CSF) protein value. A minority may present with predominantly motor or sensory symptoms. Specifically, effective immunotherapies are available for CIDP.
- **HIV** (see Chapter 19.4). The initial presentation of HIV infection may be as GBS or CIDP. HIV testing is indicated in these patients. In later stages, secondary opportunistic infections of the peripheral nervous system, primarily by herpes zoster or cytomegalovirus, or secondary malignancies may involve the peripheral nerves. A painful distal symmetric polyneuropathy occurs in about 30% of AIDS patients.
- **Nutritional neuropathies** are more often related to deficiency of multiple rather than a single vitamin. This seems to be true in cases of polyneuropathy related to alcoholism, bariatric surgery. Patients with anorexia or bulimia, malabsorption, and food faddists may also experience vitamin deficiencies. A symmetrical distal polyneuropathy is common to most the nutritional neuropathies.
  - **Alcoholic neuropathy** is clinically indistinguishable from nutritional neuropathies due to vitamin deficiencies. In a few alcoholic patients, a neuropathy may occur despite an adequate diet. The prognosis for ultimate, but slow, recovery is good for patients who are able to stop drinking and resume a proper diet with multivitamin supplements (see Chapter 5.3).
  - **Vitamin B$_1$ (thiamine) deficiency,** or beriberi, most commonly occurs in chronic alcoholics. Although its primary form is a Wernicke–Korsakoff encephalopathy, a typical distal polyneuropathy may also occur. Both entities are treated with parenteral injection of thiamine 100 mg daily for several days, followed by 100 mg daily PO.
  - **Vitamin B$_6$ (pyridoxine) deficiency** is caused by certain drugs that interfere with pyridoxine metabolism, notably isoniazid and dapsone. These drugs are used in the treatment of leprosy, which itself causes a sensory neuropathy—the clinical picture is potentially confusing. Hydralazine is chemically related to isoniazid and may also cause pyridoxine deficiency. Pyridoxine supplements, 50 to 100 mg per day may prevent this complication. Pyridoxine deficiency may also be seen in the setting of malnutrition and in hemodialysis patients. However, excessive amounts of pyridoxine ($>$ as little as 200 mg daily) may cause a severe sensory neuronopathy.

- **Vitamin B$_{12}$ deficiency** may present initially with only vague paresthesias without objective signs. In older patients, hematologic abnormalities may not be apparent until the neurologic complications have become irreversible. As the disease evolves, patients develop weakness, hyperreflexia, and abnormalities in the posterior column as noticed by loss of vibration and position sense and ataxia. The pattern of corticospinal tract and posterior column of spinal cord involvement prompted the use of the term "subacute combined degeneration of the cord." Diagnosis of vitamin B$_{12}$ deficiency is typically based on measurement of serum vitamin B$_{12}$ levels; however, about 50% of patients with subclinical disease have normal B$_{12}$ levels. A more sensitive method of screening for vitamin B$_{12}$ deficiency is measurement of serum methylmalonic acid and homocysteine levels, which are increased early in vitamin B$_{12}$ deficiency. Copper deficiency may cause a clinical syndrome similar to vitamin B$_{12}$ deficiency.
- **Vitamin E deficiency** may be observed in disorders with lipid malabsorption and in hereditary conditions. Clinical features are of a spinocerebellar ataxia associated with a polyneuropathy.
- **Toxic neuropathies** develop over several weeks to months as a result of continued exposure to certain drugs, industrial toxins, or heavy metals. A progressive, symmetrical, ascending polyneuropathy is most frequently seen with occupational exposures. The most commonly implicated drugs include anticancer agents, particularly cisplatin and vinca alkaloids, as well as isoniazid, dapsone, nucleoside analogues, and amiodarone. Rare incidents of arsenic poisoning, either intentional or resulting from insecticide exposure, may cause a late-onset progressive polyneuropathy. Chronic lead exposure causes a predominantly motor neuropathy, typically beginning in the upper limbs primarily involving the wrist and finger extensors. Management is supportive care and avoidance from or removal of the offending toxin. The majority of toxic neuropathies are self-limited and improves gradually after toxin elimination.
- **Hereditary neuropathies,** generally showing a slowly progressive and indolent course, are common. They are typically associated with high-arched feet (pes cavus) and hammertoe deformity, as well as slowly progressive weakness and wasting of peroneal muscle groups. Current therapy is limited to symptom relief. The ultimate prognosis is fairly good, with a manageable degree of disability.
- **Miscellaneous.** Patients with peripheral neuropathies are occasionally found to have one of the dysproteinemias, most often monoclonal gammopathy of unknown significance. Multiple myeloma rarely causes a polyneuropathy. Monoclonal proteins may be detected by serum or urine protein electrophoresis or immunofixation. Patients with distant, occult malignancy may present with a paraneoplastic sensory motor neuropathy or sensory neuronopathy. It is most commonly associated with small-cell lung carcinomas. Antineuronal nuclear antibodies may serve as serologic markers of these paraneoplastic syndromes, preceding detection of cancer by months or even years.

REFERENCES

1. Poncelet AN. An algorithm for the evaluation of peripheral neuropathy. *Am Fam Physician* 1998;57:755–764.
2. Aring AM, Jones DE, Falko JM. Evaluation and prevention of diabetic neuropathy. *Am Fam Physician* 2005;71(11):2123–2128.
3. Gronseth G, Paduga R. Evidence-based guideline update: steroids and antivirals for Bell palsy: report of the Guideline Development Subcommittee of the American Academy of Neurology. *Neurology* 2012;79:2209–2213.
4. Baugh RF, Basura GJ, Ishii LE, et al. Clinical practice guideline: Bell's palsy. *Otolaryngol Head Neck Surg* 2013;149:S1–S27.
5. Shapiro BE, Preston DC. Entrapment and compressive neuropathies. *Med Clin North Am* 2009;93:285–315.
6. Habib AA, Brannagan TH. Therapeutic strategies for diabetic neuropathy. *Curr Neurol Neurosci Rep* 2010;10:92–100.
7. Argoff CE, Backonja MM, Belgrade MJ, et al. Diabetic peripheral neuropathic pain: consensus guidelines for treatment. *J Fam Pract* 2006;55:1–20.
8. Said G. Diabetic neuropathy- a review. *Nat Clin Pract Neurol* 2007;3:331–340.
9. Fashner J, Bell AL. Herpes zoster and postherpetic neuralgia: prevention and management. *Am Fam Physician* 2011;83:1432–1437.
10. Hughes RA, Cornblath DR. Guillain-Barre syndrome. *Lancet* 2005;366(9497):1653–1666.
11. Oh R, Brown DL. Vitamin B$_{12}$ deficiency. *Am Fam Physician* 2003;67:979–986.
12. Hammond N, Wang Y, Dimachkie MM, et al. Nutritional neuropathies. *Neurol Clin* 2013;31:477–489.
13. Grogan PM, Katz JS. Toxic neuropathies. *Neurol Clin* 2005;23(2):377–396.

CHAPTER 7

Eye Problems

Section Editor: Shou Ling Leong

7.1 Conjunctivitis and Other Causes of a Red Eye

Sean M. Oser, Syed M. Atif, Tamara K. Oser

The most common causes of "red eye"—conjunctivitis, trauma, allergies, and subconjunctival hemorrhage—are usually benign. Some conditions, however, require urgent evaluation and treatment; these include keratitis, episcleritis, scleritis, iritis, orbital cellulitis, and acute angle closure glaucoma. Signs and symptoms requiring urgent referral to an ophthalmologist include severe pain despite topical anesthetics, proptosis, perilimbal injection, photophobia, tenderness, and decreased vision.[1]

INFECTIOUS CONJUNCTIVITIS (BACTERIAL, VIRAL)

General Principles

Infectious conjunctivitis is the most common cause of red eye. Outbreaks are not uncommon in schools, childcare centers, and military bases, but the condition is quite common in the general population as well.[1-3]

Diagnosis

History

Patients with bacterial conjunctivitis present with burning, irritation, eyes "pasted shut" in the morning, and copious purulent discharge that may become bilateral within 2 days. Viral conjunctivitis may be accompanied by burning discomfort, but there may also be a gritty sensation. It is associated with a more watery discharge and is often epidemic. Chlamydial conjunctivitis is more common in younger patients and tends to be subacute in nature. It tends to present with watery discharge, but this progresses to become mucopurulent, and is often associated with urethritis or vaginitis.[1-3]

Physical Examination

Visual acuity should be assessed and should remain normal unless the cornea is involved, as with keratitis. Diffuse hyperemia involving the bulbar and tarsal conjunctiva is present, with sparing of the limbal conjunctiva. Corneal staining with fluorescein should be performed, using topical anesthetic drops, cobalt blue filter, sterile irrigation fluid, and magnification. The cornea should be examined for a poor surface light reflex, infiltrate, ulcer, or ciliary or perilimbal injection. The presence of small papillae is common with viruses, and lid vesicles suggest herpesvirus infection. In herpes simplex, corneal involvement is usually dendritic.[1,2]

Laboratory Studies

Bacterial cultures should be obtained in neonates and in patients who have severe inflammation or chronic or recurrent conjunctivitis. Results most commonly reveal *Staphylococcus epidermidis, Staphylococcus aureus, Haemophilus influenzae,* or *Streptococcus pneumoniae.* Viral studies are rarely performed. Immunofluorescent tests on ocular scrapings for *Chlamydia trachomatis* and culture for *Neisseria gonorrhoeae* are required when either of these agents is suspected. Urethral or cervical cultures may be indicated.[2,3]

Treatment

Contact lens use should be discontinued and eye makeup discouraged until symptoms have resolved. Frequent hand hygiene and patient education reinforcing it are essential to limit transmission.[1,2]

Bacterial conjunctivitis is mostly a self-limiting disorder, but treatment results in earlier clinical remission and reduces transmission.[2,4] Topical antibiotics (drops or ointment) should be applied every 2 to 4 hours. Coverage should include Gram-positive organisms. Choices include bacitracin, sulfacetamide, gentamicin, tobramycin, a fluoroquinolone, and erythromycin; or combination agents, such as bacitracin–neomycin–polymyxin B, gramicidin/neomycin/polymyxin B, trimethoprim–polymyxin B, and bacitracin–polymyxin B. Neomycin preparations are more likely to invoke a hypersensitivity reaction. Gentamicin or one of the topical fluoroquinolones (ciprofloxacin, levofloxacin, gatifloxacin, moxifloxacin, besifloxacin, and ofloxacin) is the treatment of choice in contact lens wearers, where *Pseudomonas* infection is more likely.[2]

When *N. gonorrhoeae* is present in adults, systemic therapy is indicated due to the sight threatening nature of this condition.[2,3] Recommended treatment is ceftriaxone, 1 g IM or IV, administered as a single dose and augmented by topical antibiotics and frequent topical saline irrigation in areas with endemic penicillin-resistant gonorrhea. Empiric treatment for chlamydia is also recommended, as there is frequent coinfection. Chlamydial adult inclusion conjunctivitis should be treated orally with azithromycin 1 g as a single dose or with doxycycline 100 mg twice daily for 7 days.[3]

Viral conjunctivitis is usually due to adenovirus, herpes zoster, or herpes simplex infection. In adenoviral conjunctivitis, treatment is supportive and includes cold compresses, artificial tears, and antihistamines.[3] This is an extremely contagious condition for up to 14 days and may not resolve for up to 3 weeks. Topical ophthalmic antibiotics are often utilized because of difficulty distinguishing between viral and bacterial infection.[1] Ophthalmology referral is indicated for corneal involvement with herpes zoster.[1] If the trigeminal nerve is involved, treat with oral acyclovir, famciclovir, or valacyclovir for 7 to 10 days.[2,3] Ophthalmology referral is also indicated for corneal involvement with herpes simplex, which should also be treated for 7 to 10 days with acyclovir, famciclovir, or valacyclovir.[1,3]

NEONATAL CONJUNCTIVITIS

General Principles[2]

It is imperative to diagnose the specific etiologic agent in neonatal conjunctivitis. Chemical irritation presents within 24 hours of birth and is most commonly caused by prophylactic erythromycin, tetracycline, or silver nitrate. It is important to rule out maternal sexually transmitted infections such as gonorrhea and chlamydia. More commonly, staphylococci or streptococci are the etiologic agents. Gonococcal infection should be managed in an inpatient setting. Another common condition to differentiate is congenital nasolacrimal duct obstruction, which usually causes ocular discharge without redness. The presence of pseudomonal infection or herpes simplex type 2 infection requires consultation.[2]

Diagnosis

A detailed maternal history is important. Physical examination should assess for systemic illness. Culture is recommended in all cases and may be accompanied by Gram stain and immunofluorescent antigen detection.[1–3]

Treatment

Topical therapy includes gentamicin for Gram-negative and erythromycin for Gram-positive organisms. Oral erythromycin is recommended for chlamydial involvement. For gonococcal infection (gonococcal ophthalmia neonatorum), inpatient observation and a single dose of IV or IM ceftriaxone are recommended.[2] Supportive treatment alone is needed for chemical conjunctivitis. Most nasolacrimal duct obstructions resolve spontaneously by the age of 1 year; persistence past this age should prompt ophthalmology referral.

ALLERGIC CONJUNCTIVITIS

General Principles

Seasonal allergic conjunctivitis (SAC) and perennial allergic conjunctivitis (PAC) are common immediate hypersensitivity reactions. Vernal keratoconjunctivitis (VKC) and atopic keratoconjunctivitis (AKC) are chronic and more severe, and may lead to sequelae.[5]

Diagnosis

History

SAC and PAC are characterized by pathognomonic bilateral itching, tearing, and mild eyelid swelling and may be associated with other allergy symptoms, such as rhinitis. VKC occurs in children and adolescents with more severe symptoms, including photophobia. This is most frequently seasonal, recurrent, and also associated with other allergy symptoms. AKC is associated with dermatitis and cataracts. There is typically a personal or family history of atopy.[5]

Physical Examination

Bilateral irritation and watery or mucoid discharge occur in SAC and PAC, and may be accompanied by mild erythema and edema. In atopic disease, corneal involvement and blepharitis are common. Giant papillae are found on the conjunctiva in VKC and in contact lens–associated conjunctivitis.[1,2,5]

Treatment

Cold compresses, saline irrigation, and ocular lubricants may provide symptomatic relief. Elimination or reduction of the allergen exposure should be attempted when the trigger can be identified.[1,2,5] Contact lens use should be discontinued until symptoms resolve. Topical ophthalmic vasoconstrictors such as naphazoline induce symptom relief quickly, but rebound hyperemia is possible with prolonged use. The combination of naphazoline and pheniramine is more effective than either agent alone. Topical ophthalmic antihistamines (azelastine, emedastine) and mast cell stabilizers (lodoxamide, nedocromil, cromolyn) can be effective as well.[1–3] Olopatadine, azelastine, and ketotifen have multimodal effects and may offer the advantage of both immediate and long-lasting benefits.[3,5] Topical ophthalmic ketorolac (a nonsteroidal anti-inflammatory drug [NSAID]) has been shown to provide effective relief from allergic conjunctivitis symptoms as well.[1,3] Topical ophthalmic corticosteroids may be used in severe cases, but long-term use has been associated with cataracts and glaucoma, and should be administered under the direction of an ophthalmologist.[1,3]

KERATITIS

General Principles

Keratitis involves inflammation of the cornea. Bacterial keratitis is usually caused by *Staphylococcus* and *Streptococcus* species, with *Pseudomonas aeruginosa* more common among contact lens wearers;[1,2] bacterial corneal ulcer is a manifestation of bacterial keratitis.[6] Herpes simplex is the most common cause of viral keratitis. Ultraviolet radiation exposure can also lead to keratitis.

Diagnosis

History

Bacterial keratitis is associated with severe pain, photophobia, and foreign body sensation.[1,2] Pain, photophobia, blurred vision, tearing, and redness are seen with HSV-associated keratitis.[7] In keratitis resulting from UV radiation, symptoms include severe pain 6 to 12 hours after exposure, redness, decreased vision, and usually a lack of discharge.[2]

Physical Examination

Erythema, corneal infiltrate, and a fluorescein-staining opacity are seen with bacterial keratitis.[2] Dendritic lesions revealed by fluorescein staining are characteristic of viral involvement.[2,7] With UV exposure leading to keratitis, a hazy, punctate fluorescein-staining pattern can be seen.[2]

Treatment

Topical antibiotics, pain control, and same-day ophthalmology referral are indicated for bacterial keratitis.[2] Viral keratitis is usually self-limited, but antiviral therapy reduces duration of infection, and prompt ophthalmology referral within a few days is recommended.[2,8] For keratitis caused by UV exposure, treatment recommendations include ophthalmology referral, pain relief with topical cycloplegic drops, and oral pain medication.[2]

EPISCLERITIS

General Principles

Episcleritis is a superficial inflammation of the scleral lining. It affects the episcleral tissue lying between the conjunctiva and sclera. Episcleritis is usually idiopathic, but a significant proportion of patients may have underlying systemic and/or collagen vascular disease, such as rheumatoid arthritis, systemic lupus erythematosus, polyarteritis nodosa, inflammatory bowel disease, or ankylosing spondylitis.[1,2]

Diagnosis

Symptoms include photophobia, tearing, and blurred vision. Patients may note moderate discomfort, but discomfort may also be absent.[1,2] Physical examination reveals episcleral edema (which may be patchy), episcleral vascular congestion, and/or tenderness. The differential diagnosis of episcleritis includes viral conjunctivitis and scleritis.

Treatment

Since episcleritis is self-limited, medication is usually not needed, though topical NSAIDs and artificial tears may be helpful for symptomatic relief.[1]

SCLERITIS
General Principles

Scleritis is an acute, severe, vision-threatening inflammation of the sclera that may be diffuse (more common) or nodular (more severe). Scleritis is often idiopathic, but there is a high incidence (33% to 50%) of associated systemic immune-mediated collagen vascular disease, including rheumatoid arthritis, systemic lupus erythematosus, polyarteritis nodosa, ankylosing spondylitis, granulomatosis with polyangiitis (Wegener's), and sarcoidosis.[1,2,9] If untreated, the nodular form may progress to a necrotizing form, with associated loss of scleral tissue.

Diagnosis

History

Symptoms include acute onset of severe, boring ocular pain which may radiate to the periorbital area; diurnal variation of pain with increased severity at night; and prominent photophobia and watering from the eye. Additionally, patients may complain of decreased vision.[1,2]

Physical Examination

Tenderness to palpation, diffuse erythema, scleral edema, and decreased visual acuity are usually present on physical examination.[1] Comprehensive examination to evaluate for other underlying systemic illness should be undertaken, including examination of the skin, joints, heart, and lungs in particular.

Laboratory and Imaging

Laboratory testing should include antinuclear antibodies (ANAs), anti-neutrophil cytoplasmic antibodies (ANCAs), rheumatoid factor (RF), C-reactive protein (CRP), erythrocyte sedimentation rate (ESR), and urinalysis.[2] When ankylosing spondylitis is suspected, radiography of the sacroiliac joints can be useful as well.

Differential Diagnosis

Differential diagnosis of scleritis includes episcleritis (more redness, less pain), conjunctivitis (discharge present), and uveitis (by slit-lamp exam).

Treatment

Oral NSAIDs are most useful in cases of milder disease.[2] For more severe cases, prompt ophthalmology referral is necessary. Topical corticosteroids may be used,[2] as may systemic corticosteroids and/or immunosuppressive agents, often with rheumatologic consultation. There is emerging evidence supporting the use of biologic agents as well.[9]

IRITIS
General Principles

Iritis, or inflammation of the anterior uvea, can be caused by trauma, infection, malignancy, systemic autoimmune/inflammatory disease, syphilis, HIV infection, and sarcoidosis.[1,2]

Diagnosis

Symptoms may include pain, blurred vision, erythema, tearing, and photophobia.[1,2] Physical examination reveals pupillary constriction and decreased pupillary reactivity. Iritis is usually unilateral, but it can be bilateral with associated chronic disease.[1,2] Consider chest X-ray to detect sarcoidosis and serologic testing for syphilis and HIV infection.[2]

Treatment

Prompt ophthalmologic consultation should be obtained to determine treatment, which should include topical cyclopegics and oral analgesia, and may include corticosteroids.[2]

SUBCONJUNCTIVAL HEMORRHAGE

General Principles

Subconjunctival hemorrhage is benign bleeding just beneath the conjunctiva. It may result from straining (such as with constipation, severe coughing, sneezing, vomiting, or during labor), trauma, hypertension, bleeding disorders, or anticoagulant medications.[1] If seen in an infant or child, physical abuse should be considered.[10]

Diagnosis

This is a clinical diagnosis, with patients usually asymptomatic other than noticing an area of redness. Examination reveals normal vision, pupils, and corneas, with a well-demarcated red patch on white sclera.[1]

Treatment

No treatment is necessary, as like ecchymoses elsewhere, subconjunctival hemorrhages resorb spontaneously over the course of days to weeks.[1]

REFERENCES

1. Cronau H, Kankanala RR, Mauger T. Diagnosis and management of red eye in primary care. *Am Fam Physician* 2010;81:137–144.
2. Deibel JP, Cowling K. Ocular inflammation and infection. *Emerg Med Clin North Am* 2013;31:387–397.
3. Azari AA, Barney NP. Conjunctivitis: a systematic review of diagnosis and treatment. *JAMA* 2013;310:1721–1729.
4. Sheikh A, Hurwitz B, van Schayck CP, et al. Antibiotics versus placebo for acute bacterial conjunctivitis. *Cochrane Database Syst Rev* 2012;9:CD001211.
5. La Rosa M, Lionetti E, Reibaldi M, et al. Allergic conjunctivitis: a comprehensive review of the literature. *Ital J Pediatr* 2013;39:18.
6. Srinivasan M, Mascarenhas J, Rajaraman R, et al. The steroids for corneal ulcers trial (SCUT): secondary 12-month clinical outcomes of a randomized controlled trial. *Am J Ophthalmol* 2014;157:327–333.
7. Rowe AM, St Leger AJ, Jeon S, et al. Herpes keratitis. *Prog Retin Eye Res* 2013;32:88–101.
8. Newman H, Gooding C. Viral ocular manifestations: a broad overview. *Rev Med Virol* 2013;23(5):281–294.
9. Wakefield D, Di Girolamo N, Thurau S, et al. Scleritis: immunopathogenesis and molecular basis for therapy. *Prog Retin Eye Res* 2013;35:44–62.
10. DeRidder CA, Berkowitz CD, Hicks RA, et al. Subconjunctival hemorrhages in infants and children: a sign of nonaccidental trauma. *Pediatr Emerg Care* 2013;29:222–226.

7.2 Age-Associated Eye Diseases: Cataracts, Glaucoma, and Macular Degeneration

F. Samuel Faber, Anthony M. Cheng, David Richard

CATARACTS

General Principles

- **Definition:** Cataracts are opacifications that form in the lens of the eye. Larger cataracts and those close to the visual axis may result in visual complaints.
- **Epidemiology:** The self-reported incidence of cataract among those over age 50 in the United States is 31.8% in diabetics and 21.2% in non-diabetics.[1] The prevalence of any type cataract in the Blue Mountain Eye Study (Australia, 1992–1994 and 1997–2000) of residents 49 and older was 46.8%.[2]

- **Etiology:** Risk factors for cataract include age; smoking; alcohol use; sunlight exposure; diabetes mellitus; hypoparathyroidism (sic); Down's syndrome; ocular trauma; uveitis; and the use of medications like corticosteroids, oral or topical β-blockers,[3] and allopurinol.[4]

Diagnosis

- **Clinical presentation:** Asymptomatic cataracts are commonly noted by the family physician. Most cataracts are painless and develop slowly. Posterior subcapsular cataracts are the exception and may develop rapidly. Trouble with driving is the most common presenting complaint. Glare or halos around oncoming headlights, blurred vision, and decreased distance vision may make night driving especially difficult. Trouble reading fine print can also occur.
- **Physical examination:** Visual acuity should be measured. A non-dilated ophthalmoscopic examination will frequently confirm a suspected cataract. A milky discoloration of the lens may be seen by illuminating the pupil with an ophthalmoscope held at 45 degrees to the patient's eye. Changes in the red reflex or difficulty clearly seeing the retina on direct ophthalmoscopy may also indicate the presence of a cataract. A slit-lamp examination will confirm the cataract and the specific location within the lens. Glare testing can quantitatively test the functional impact of the cataract.

Monitoring

No specific monitoring is required as a delay in therapy does not alter overall prognosis. Patients should be referred to an ophthalmologist when visual changes begin to interfere with daily activities like reading and driving.

Treatment

- **Prevention:** Tobacco smoking cessation reduces the relative risk of developing cataracts.[5] Antioxidant vitamins β-carotene, C, and E do not appear to prevent cataract.[6]
- **Surgery**
  - **Preoperative considerations:** Aspirin and warfarin do not need to be stopped prior to surgery.[7] α-Blockers, especially tamsulosin, are associated with intraoperative floppy iris syndrome and may make cataract surgery more difficult.[8]
  - Removal of the lens is the definitive therapy for cataracts. It is a low-risk procedure that is usually done under local anesthesia.
  - In most cases, an artificial lens is inserted to replace the native lens. It is supported by the posterior lens capsule, which is left in place. Monofocal intraocular lenses will improve vision as a prescribed focal length, usually distant. Multifocal intraocular lenses may improve both distant and near vision, but there is an increased risk of halos and glare compared with monofocal lenses. Toric artificial intraocular lenses may improve visual acuity in patients with astigmatism.

Results

A postoperative acuity of 20/40 is seen in about 90% of patients. Preexisting ocular comorbidities reduce the effect of lens replacement in a significant minority of patients.

Complications

Posterior capsule opacification is the most common complication and may cause significant visual loss in up to 50% of patients.[9] It is treated relatively easily with laser capsulotomy. The risk of macular degeneration appears to be about fivefold higher in eyes that have had the native lens removed than in controls.[10] The association is confounded by the fact that cataracts and macular degeneration have several common risk factors. Rare complications (<2%) include endophthalmitis, bullous keratopathy, lens malposition, cystoid macular edema, and retinal detachment.

AGE-RELATED MACULAR DEGENERATION

General Principles

- **Definition:** Age-related macular degeneration (AMD) is an idiopathic process that disrupts the normal microarchitecture of the macula, resulting in central vision loss.
- **Epidemiology:** The prevalence in the United States is between 3.1% and 5.4% of persons older than 50 years.[11] AMD increases with age: in a large cohort over the age of 65, the prevalence of AMD increased from 5% to 27.1% over 8 years.[12] The rate of visual impairment due to AMD rises from 6% between ages 65 and 74 to nearly 20% over age 75.

- **Classification:** Early AMD is characterized by any combination of small or medium-sized drusen (focal deposits) and hypo- or hyperpigmentation of the retina, and intermediate AMD by at least one large or numerous medium-sized drusen. There are two types of late or advanced AMD. Non-neovascular AMD includes drusen and geographic atrophy of the retinal pigmented epithelium extending to the center of the fovea. Neovascular AMD is characterized by choroidal neovascularization that is associated with sub-retinal fluid, lipid deposition, hemorrhage, retinal pigmented epithelium detachment, and fibrotic scar.[13]
- **Etiology:** The pathophysiology is incompletely understood but is thought to be interplay between oxidative stress and gene polymorphisms. Damage to Bruch membrane and the retinal pigmented epithelium are thought to lead to development of disease. The strongest risk factor is age (see Epidemiology).[14] Other risk factors include smoking (OR 2.15, 95% CI 1.42 to 3.26),[15] heavy alcohol use (OR 1.47, 95% CI 1.1 to 1.95),[16] sunlight exposure (OR 1.38, 95% CI 1.09 to 1.47),[17] cataract surgery (RR 3.81, 95% CI 1.89 to 7.69),[18] and gene polymorphisms.[19] Family history increases risk: genetic factors are estimated to account for 47% of overall AMD risk, whereas environmental factors account for 37% of overall AMD risk.[20] Possible risk factors include aspirin use and hypertension.

Diagnosis

- **Clinical presentation:** Gradual loss of vision in one or both eyes generally accompanies AMD. It may take place over months to years. Patients may complain about perceived distortion of objects. Patients often report resorting to bright lights or magnifying lenses to read fine print or perform tasks that require fine visual acuity. Acute or rapidly progressive vision loss suggests neovascular AMD.
- **Physical examination:** Retinal dysfunction can be confirmed in the family physician's office using a Snellen chart at 20 feet or a standard pocket card. The patient should wear his usual corrective lenses. If acuity is poor, the tests should be repeated with the patient looking through a pinhole card, which will compensate for common refractive errors but not for retinal disease. A retinal examination may reveal the presence of drusen (which appear as yellow dots), hemorrhage, sub-retinal fluid, or a grayish discoloration of the macula due to neovascularization. Presence of small drusen in both eyes is associated with a very low risk of progression (0.4% to 3.0% over 5 years). Large drusen and pigmentary abnormalities confer a higher risk of progression (around 47.3%).[21]
- **Imaging:** Fluorescein angiography or optical coherence tomography are used in the evaluation of neovascular AMD to confirm neovascularization and to monitor therapeutic response.

Monitoring

Amsler grids are used to monitor for retinal deformation or detachment. An Amsler grid looks like a sheet of graph paper with a dot in the middle. Patients are asked to look at the dot daily and report immediately if the grid lines appear curved. The sensitivity of test is limited by patient compliance and its subjective nature. Other tests such as preferential hyperacuity perimetry, macular mapping test, and noise-field capimetry are more sensitive and quantitative.

Treatment

- **Referrals:** Patients with acute visual changes should be immediately referred to an ophthalmologist. Patients with symptoms or findings of early AMD may be referred on a routine basis.
- **Medications:** Antioxidants slow the progression of AMD and reduce the chance of legal blindness in patients with intermediate or advanced disease. A daily combination of the following has been shown to be effective: β-carotene 15 mg, vitamin C 500 mg, vitamin E 400 IU, zinc 80 mg, and copper 2 mg.[22] Be aware that β-carotene is associated with an increased risk of lung cancer in smokers.
- **Special therapy:** Antivascular endothelial growth factor antibodies (ranibizumab, bevacizumab, pegaptanib) are recommended for subfoveal choroidal neovascularization. They have been shown to reduce vision loss and improve visual acuity. There is a risk of ocular adverse events, including endophthalmitis, uveitis, retinal detachment, retinal tear, retinal hemorrhage, and traumatic lens damage.[23] Nonocular risks include gastrointestinal hemorrhage, traumatic subdural hematoma, and duodenal ulcer hemorrhage.[23]
- **Photodynamic therapy** can be combined with antivascular endothelial growth factor antibodies in patients with choroidal neovascularization. A photo-activated dye is injected intravenously and the abnormal vascular bed exposed to a cool laser. The light activates the dye, which then scleroses the abnormal vessels.

- **Conventional laser therapy** coagulates abnormal new blood vessels. Although it causes disappearance of drusen, it may not decrease the development of choroidal neovascularization or geographic atrophy or vision loss.
- **Macular translocation surgery, cataract surgery, retinal transplantation, and implantable miniature telescope** are still being studied, and their roles are not well defined.
- **Patient education**
  - Recommend smoking cessation.
  - Discourage high dietary fat intake as it may increase the risk of progression of AMD.
  - Counsel all patients about the need to report acute changes in vision and how to use an Amsler grid.
  - Reassure patients that a high degree of independence and self-sufficiency is possible even though AMD is not currently curable or reversible. Because the disease tends to spare peripheral vision, many people, even those with advanced central vision loss, retain the ability to move about safely in their environments.
- **Community resources:** Vision rehabilitation can improve functional ability. Low vision aides (including large print books, print projectors, and large font computer screens) all work by allowing an image to fall on a larger area of retina, but may not improve reading performance.
- **Follow-up:** Patients with neovascular AMD should be encouraged to obtain regular follow-up with their ophthalmologist. Annual follow-up for non-neovascular AMD with an ophthalmologist if available or with a family physician otherwise is considered.
- **Family physicians** should be aware of the risk of comorbid depression.

PRIMARY OPEN-ANGLE GLAUCOMA
General Principles
- **Definition:** Glaucoma is a group of eye diseases characterized by a chronic and progressive optic neuropathy, resulting in loss of retinal ganglion cells and their axons, leading to visual field loss and ultimately blindness.[24,25] Glaucoma is commonly associated with an elevation of intraocular pressure (IOP); however, this is not a defining criterion of the disease.[25] Types of primary glaucoma include primary open-angle glaucoma (POAG), angle-closure glaucoma, and congenital glaucoma (often hereditary). Secondary causes of glaucoma include trauma, medication, and other disease states. POAG is the most common type of glaucoma, accounting for two-thirds of all cases of glaucoma. POAG causes gradual, asymptomatic loss of peripheral vision in a characteristic pattern, followed by central vision loss if untreated.
- **Epidemiology:** Glaucoma is seen in 2.5% of the population (1.9% POAG) over the age of 40 and increases with age to an estimated 7.8% over the age of 80.[26] No gender predilection has been established although some studies indicate a higher prevalence in men.[27]
- **Etiology:** In addition to advancing age, other risk factors for the development of glaucoma include ethnicity (higher in African American (7.5% prevalence) and Hispanic (2% to 5%) populations,[26,27] increased intraocular pressure, a positive family history (7.7%), and severe myopia (11% if myopia greater than six diopters).[26] Several studies indicate a possible relationship between developing POAG and underlying hypertension and type 2 diabetes mellitus, but the data remain inconsistent.[27]

Diagnosis
- **Clinical presentation:** Visual complaints are a late finding of the disease process. Because the vast majority of patients with POAG are asymptomatic, it is estimated that 50% of glaucoma sufferers in the United States and 90% worldwide are undiagnosed.[25] A comprehensive history should look for a family history of glaucoma, a medical history of diabetes, hypertension or a disease requiring use of oral steroids (asthma, connective tissue diseases, and others), a medication history (especially corticosteroids), and an ocular surgery history (falsely lower IOP can occur after LASIK surgery).[24]
- **Physical examination:** A complete ocular examination is important, including visual acuity, pupillary and fundoscopic examination. The finding of an optic cup-to-disc ratio (CDR) of ≥ 0.7. CDR asymmetry and disc hemorrhage are associated with an increased risk of POAG.[26]

Intraocular pressure (IOP) measurement of 22 mm Hg or greater is considered the threshold, with increasing IOP above 22 mm Hg associated with greater likelihood of POAG. The current standard for measuring IOP is Goldmann applanation tonometry, which measures the force required to flatten the cornea.[24,26,28] Shiotz tonometers may be used by some family physicians to measure IOP. The tonometer base is placed against the anesthetized eye to take a reading, so excellent cleaning between uses is critical. Other forms of tonometry, including air puff tonometry, rebound tonometry, and palpation, are also used.

TABLE 7.2-1	American Academy of Ophthalmology Recommended Frequency for Eye Examinations

	Frequency based on risk factors (yr)	
Age (yr)	No risk factors	Risk factors[a]
<40	Every 5–10	Every 5–10
40–54	Every 2–4	Every 1–3
55–64	Every 1–3	Every 1–2
≥65	Every 1–2	Every 1–2

[a]Risk factors were not specifically defined by the American Academy of Ophthalmology. On the basis of the results of this study, historical risk factors include increasing age (especially older than 80 years), family history of POAG, black race, and increasing myopia.

Other forms of testing include visual field testing, preferably by automated static threshold perimetry. Serial measurement of visual fields is another means beside IOP to judge treatment and may be required before changing management.[24,25] Other testing including central corneal thickness measurements are being looked at as screening tools and as aiding the measurement of IOP in helping to stratify treatment for patients with POAG.[24]

Monitoring

Follow-up ophthalmologic visits vary but generally are every 6 months for those with recent disease, yearly if stable, and every 1 to 2 months if there is evidence of progression.[24] Risk factors for progression in those with known POAG include intraocular pressure, older age, disc hemorrhage, increasing CDR, thinner central cornea, and β-zone peripapillary atrophy. Further, when such changes are noted in one eye, it increases the likelihood of future damage in the other eye. Indications for adjusting therapy include inability to achieve the target IOP; progressive optic nerve damage regardless of IOP; or intolerance, contraindication, or nonadherence to medication.

Screening

Screening for POAG is controversial. According to the American Academy of Ophthalmology (AAO), screening for glaucoma should be a part of every eye professional's comprehensive adult eye evaluation, starting at age 18, with a risk-based frequency (see Table 7.2-1[26]). The U.S. Preventive Services Task Force (USPSTF) found insufficient evidence to recommend for or against screening adults for glaucoma.[29]

Treatment

- **Overview:** The treatment of POAG can take the form of topical medication or surgical intervention. Either way, the goals of treatment should be to control IOP in the target range, stabilize visual fields, stabilize optic nerve fiber layer status, and preserve vision.[24] Treatment of glaucoma suspects should be limited to those with abnormal examinations with the same goals as listed above.[24]
- **Medications:** Topical medications are used to lower IOP and may be given alone or in combination. Family physicians treat many patients with POAG and therefore need to be aware of the potential side effects of the medications being utilized as well as their benefits. The use of prostaglandin analogs (increase out flow of intraocular fluid from the eye) or β-adrenergic antagonists (β-blockers decrease fluid production) are first-line topical treatment for POAG and are the most common initial intervention. The AAO recommends starting with prostaglandin analogs as they are more effective in lowering IOP (AAO level of evidence A:I). The target decrease in IOP should be 25% below baseline[24] as a 50% reduction in visual field loss progression occurs with a decrease in IOP between 20% and 40%.[25] Other commonly used medications include carbonic anhydrase inhibitors (decrease production of intraocular fluid) and α-adrenergic agonists (decrease fluid production and increase drainage) (see Table 7.2-2[24,30,31]). Cholinergic agents (increase fluid drainage) such as Pilocarpine will not be discussed owing to their limited use due to their side-effect profile. Regardless of the medication used, it is vital that the physician and patient come up with a shared decision-making plan that addresses the dosage, cost, and patient tolerance issue as one-third of patients do not utilize the medications for POAG as prescribed at 1 year.[32] Efforts to simplify eye drop regimens, teaching drop installation techniques, and providing adequate patient information may all help to improve

| TABLE 7.2-2 | Medications to Treat Glaucoma |

Medication name (brand name)	Formulation	Dosage	Common side effects	Cost-wholesale acquisition cost
Prostaglandin analogs				
Latanopost (Xalatan)	0.005% soln	1 drop qPM	Change in eye color (increase in brown pigment), burning, itching, stinging, blurred vision in treated eye, Pregnancy Cat: C	$17.00 ($109.00)
Bimatoprost (Lumigan)	0.01% soln	1 drop qPM		$105.00
Travaprost (Travatan Z)	0.004% soln	1 drop qPM		$77.00 ($96.00)
Tafluprost (Zioptan)	0.0015% soln	1 drop qPM		$104.00
β-Blockers				
Betaxolol (Betoptic S)	0.25% susp	1 drop qAM/bid	Hypotension, bradycardia, fatigue, bronchoconstriction, CHF, exacerbation, depression. Use with caution: asthma, CHF. Contraindicated: uncompensated CHF, severe COPD, all contact lenses, pregnancy Cat: C	$51.00 ($172.00)
Carteolol	1% soln	1 drop qAM/bid		$13.00
Levobunolol	0.5% soln 0.25%/0.5% (generic)	1 drop qAM/bid		$14.00 ($40.00)
Metipranolol	0.3% soln	1 drop qAM/bid		$21.00
Timolol				
Betimol	0.25%/0.5% soln	1 drop qAM/bid		$61.00
Istalol	0.5% soln	1 drop qAM/bid		$100.00
Timoptic ocudose	0.25%/0.5% soln	1 drop bid		$285.00
Timpotic/generic	0.25%/0.5% soln	1 drop bid		$3.00 ($109.00)
Carbonic anhydrase inhibitors				
Brinzolamide (Azopt)	1% susp	1 drop tid	Stinging, burning, eye discomfort, blurred vision, dermatitis. Use with caution: severe hepatic or renal impairment. Pregnancy Cat: C	$131.00
Dorzolamide (Trusopt)	2% soln	1 drop tid		$40.00 ($77.00)

TABLE 7.2-2	Medications to Treat Glaucoma (Continued)			
Medication name (brand name)	Formulation	Dosage	Common side effects	Cost-wholesale acquisition cost
α-Agonists				
Apraclonidine (lopidine)	0.5%/1% soln	1 drop tid	Burning, stinging in treated eye, fatigue, headache, drowsiness, dry mouth/nose. Use with caution. History of CAD, vasovagal syncope. Contraindications: MAOI use. Pregnancy Cat: C	$68.00 ($115.00)
Brimonidine (Alphagan P)	0.1%/0.15% soln	1 drop bid/tid also 0.2% soln (generic)		$17.00 ($93.00)
Combinations				
Brinzolamide/ Bromonidine (Simbrinza)	1%/0.2% soln	1 drop tid	See individual components	$88.00
Bromonidine/ Timolol (Combigan)	0.2%/0.5% soln	1 drop bid	See individual components	$94.00
Timolol/Dorzolamide (Cosopt)	0.5%/2% soln	1 drop bid	See individual components	$60.00 ($141.00)

CHF, congestive heart failure; COPD, chronic obstructive pulmonary disease; CAD, coronary artery disease; MAOI, monoamine oxidase inhibitors.

adherence. Techniques to reduce systemic absorption include refrigeration of the medications to increase viscosity, and finger occlusion of the nasolacrimal duct for 5 minutes after instillation.

• **Surgery:** Surgery is generally used when medical treatment fails to appropriately lower IOP; however, surgery may be utilized as initial therapy for POAG, especially if patients are unable to use or prefer not to use eye drops. Laser trabeculoplasty is the surgery of choice (AAO A:1 evidence), lowering IOP by increasing aqueous outflow. Laser surgery is highly successful, lowering the IOP sufficiently about 75% of the time. Surgery may be repeated or medication added if the drop in IOP is insufficient.[28] Other surgical interventions are incisional in nature and include trabeculectomy or aqueous shunts, both of which should be reserved for those who fail medication or laser trabeculoplasty. Other treatments including acupuncture/acupressure and herbal medication lack direct evidence of success.

REFERENCES

1. Centers for Disease Control and Prevention (CDC). Prevalence of visual impairment and selected eye diseases among persons aged >/=50 years with and without diabetes—United States, 2002. *MMWR* 2004;53(45):1069–1071.
2. Tan AG, Wang JJ, Rochtchina E, et al. Comparison of age-specific cataract prevalence in two population-based surveys 6 years apart. *BMC Ophthalmol* 2006;6:19.
3. Kanthan GL, Wang JJ, Rochtchina E, et al. Use of antihypertensive medications and topical beta-blockers and the long-term incidence of cataract and cataract surgery. *Br J Ophthalmol* 2009;93:1210.
4. Garbe E, Suissa S, LeLorier J. Exposure to allopurinol and the risk of cataract extraction in elderly patients. *Arch Ophthalmol* 1998;116(12):1652–1656.

5. Kelly SP, Thornton J, Edwards E, et al. Smoking and cataract: review of causal association. *J Cataract Refract Surg* 2005;31(12):2395–2404.

6. Mathew MC, Ervin AM, Davis RM. Antioxidant vitamin supplementation for preventing and slowing the progression of age-related cataract. *Cochrane Database Syst Rev* 2012;6:CD004567.

7. Katz J, Feldman MA, Bass EB, et al. Risks and benefits of anticoagulant and antiplatelet medication used before cataract surgery. *Ophthalmology* 2003;110(12):2309.

8. Bell CM, Hatch WV, Fischer HD, et al. Association between tamsulosin and serious ophthalmic adverse events in older med following cataract surgery. *JAMA* 2009;301(19):1991–1996.

9. Clark DS. Posterior capsule opacification. *Curr Opin Ophthalmol* 2000;11(1):55–64.

10. Wang JJ, Med M, Klein R, et al. Cataract surgery and the 5-year incidence of late stage age-related maculopathy: pooled findings from the Beaver Dam and Blue Mountains eye studies. *Ophthalmology* 2003;110:1960–1967.

11. Bailey RN, Indian RW, Zhang X. Visual impairment and eye care among older adults—five States, 2005. *MMWR* 2006;55(49):1321.

12. Lee PP, Feldman ZW, Ostermann J, et al. Longitudinal prevalence of major eye diseases. *Arch Ophthalmol* 2003;121(9):1303–1310.

13. Chakravarthy U1, Evans J, Rosenfeld PJ. Age related macular degeneration. *BMJ* 2010;340:c981.

14. van Leeuwen R, Klaver CC, Vingerling JR, et al. The risk and natural course of age-related maculopathy: follow-up at 6 1/2 years in the Rotterdam study. *Arch Ophthalmol* 2003;121(4):519–526.

15. Seddon JM, George S, Rosner B. Cigarette smoking, fish consumption, omega-3 fatty acid intake, and associations with age-related macular degeneration: the US Twin Study of Age-Related Macular Degeneration. *Arch Ophthalmol* 2006;124(7):995–1001.

16. Chong EW, Kreis AJ, Wong TY, et al. Alcohol consumption and the risk of age-related macular degeneration: a systematic review and meta-analysis. *Am J Ophthalmol* 2008;145(4):707–715.

17. Sui GY, Liu GC, Liu GY, et al. Is sunlight exposure a risk factor for age-related macular degeneration? A systematic review and meta-analysis. *Br J Ophthalmol* 2013;97(4):389–394.

18. Klein R, Klein BE, Wong TY, et al. The association of cataract and cataract surgery with the long-term incidence of age-related maculopathy: the Beaver Dam eye study. *Arch Ophthalmol* 2002;120(11):1551–1558.

19. Seddon JM, Francis PJ, George S, et al. Association of CFH Y402H and LOC387715 A69S with progression of age-related macular degeneration. *JAMA* 2007;297(16):1793–1800.

20. Bressler SB, Muñoz B, Solomon SD, et al; Salisbury Eye Evaluation (SEE) Study Team. Racial differences in the prevalence of age-related macular degeneration: the Salisbury Eye Evaluation (SEE) Project. *Arch Ophthalmol* 2008;126(2):241–245.

21. Age-Related Eye Diseases Study Group. A simplified severity scale for age-related macular degeneration. AREDS report 18. *Arch Ophthalmol* 2005;123:1570–1574.

22. Age-Related Eye Disease Study Research Group. A randomized, placebo-controlled, clinical trial of high-dose supplementation with vitamins C and E, beta carotene, and zinc for age-related macular degeneration and vision loss. AREDS report no. 8. *Arch Ophthalmol* 2001;119(10)1417–1436.

23. Schmucker C, Loke YK, Ehlken C, et al. Intravitreal bevacizumab (Avastin) versus ranibizumab (Lucentis) for the treatment of age-related macular degeneration: a safety review. *Am J Ophthalmol* 2011;95(3):308–317.

24. American Academy of Ophthalmology Glaucoma Panel. *Primary open-angle glaucoma suspect.* San Francisco, CA: American Academy of Ophthalmology; 2010.

25. Quigley HA. Glaucoma. *Lancet* 2011;377(9774):1367–1377.

26. Holland H, Johnson D, Hollands S, et al. Do findings on routine examination identify patients at risk for primary open-angle glaucoma? *JAMA* 2013;309(19):2035–2042.

27. Leske MC. Open-angle glaucoma—an epidemiologic overview. *Ophthalmic Epidemiol* 2007;14:166–172.

28. Open-Angle Glaucoma. *DynaMed* September 11, 2013. http://web.b.ebscohost.com.medjournal.hmc .psu.edu:2048/dynamed

29. Screening for Glaucoma. United States Preventive Services Task Force Recommendation Statement, July 9, 2013. http://www.uspreventiveservicestaskforce.org/Page/Topic/recommendation-summary/glaucoma-screening

30. Brinzolamide/brimonidine (Simbrinza) for glaucoma. *Med Lett Drugs Ther* 2013;55(1421):57.

31. Medication Guide. Glaucoma Research Foundation. July 6, 2012. http://www.glaucoma.org/treatment/medication-guide.php

32. Waterman H, Evans JR, Gray TA, et al. Interventions for improving adherence to ocular hypotensive therapy. *Cochrane Database Syst Rev* 2013;4:CD006132.

Ocular Emergencies
Ahad Shiraz, Timothy D. Riley

OCULAR EMERGENCIES DUE TO INJURY
Chemical Injury

Presentation

Chemical injuries are a true ocular emergency with potentially severe sequelae. Most injuries are caused by acidic or alkalotic substances.[1] Acid burns are generally less severe than those caused by alkalotic agents. Patients commonly present with severe pain, epiphora, and blepharospasm after the agent comes into contact with the eye.[2] Injuries typically take place in industrial settings, often despite the use of protective eyewear.

Diagnosis

A detailed history and physical examination regarding the exposure event is critical for an accurate diagnosis. While an attempt should be made to know the exact substance that caused the injury, treatment should not be delayed in so doing. There are four classes of chemical burn injuries as per the Roper-Hall scale, with class I having the best prognosis and IV the worst.

Management

Copious irrigation with isotonic saline or lactated Ringer's is needed immediately until the pH of eye surface reaches a normal range of 7.2 to 7.4. Thereafter, pH should be rechecked every 15 to 30 minutes to confirm stabilization. This is followed by an examination, which should include a sweep of the fornices with eyelid eversion to check for hidden particles. Fluorescein examination should be performed to inspect for damage to cornea and conjunctiva. Evaluation of intraocular pressure is also important since chemical burns may cause significant ocular pressure abnormalities.[1] Topical antibiotics (usually fluoroquinolones) are recommended if the epithelial defect is significant. Topical steroids limit local inflammation and promote healing.[2]

Follow-Up

Close ophthalmology follow-up is needed for further assessment of healing and intraocular pressure, and to monitor for corneal melting.

Corneal Abrasion

Presentation

This common ocular injury consists of a defect in the epithelial surface of the cornea often caused by trauma, foreign bodies, and contact lenses. Key elements of the history and presentation include photophobia, pain, and foreign body sensation.[3]

Diagnosis

Pen light examination, visual acuity, and special staining are all part of the evaluation. Penlight examination should include inspection for evidence of trauma, signs of which include a dilated or nonreactive pupil. Visual acuity must be tested to determine whether there is need for referral. Careful examination should be performed, including visualization of the red reflex and eyelid eversion for foreign bodies. Epithelial defects can be visualized with fluorescein staining viewed under a cobalt blue or Wood's lamp.[3]

Management

Treatment includes topical nonsteroidal anti-inflammatory drugs (such as diclofenac solution) and topical antibiotics (with pseudomonal coverage in the setting of contact lens use). Level A evidence suggests that patching delays healing and is not recommended.[3]

Hyphema

Presentation

Hyphema results from a direct blow to the eye or orbit, and is often related to sports activities. Afflicted patients develop pain in the eye, decreased visual acuity, and injection of the globe.

Diagnosis

Blood in the anterior chamber confirms the diagnosis. This finding may be delayed for hours to days following injury if bleeding is gradual. A noncontrast CT scan of the orbit is recommended if open globe, intraocular foreign body, or intraorbital hemorrhage is suspected.[4,5]

Management

Strict bed rest with head elevated at least 20 degrees and bilateral eye patches to minimize eye movement are recommended. Atropine 1% two drops bid reduces ciliary spasm. Dilation of the eye with cyclopentolate or scopolamine also provides pain relief and aids with examination of the posterior segment.[6-8] If an ophthalmologist is not readily available, intraocular pressure should be reduced by the use of oral acetazolamide or mannitol. Oral analgesics that are free of aspirin may also be considered.

Follow-Up

Immediate ophthalmologic referral is indicated in all cases of hyphema.[9] Vitrectomy has been described for clotted hyphema.

Retinal Detachment

Presentation

Retinal detachment occurs with an incidence of 12 in 100,000.[10] Lifetime risk through age 85 is 3%.[11] Risk factors include trauma, increasing age, myopia, history of cataract surgery, diabetic retinopathy, and family history of retinal detachment.[11] Typical symptoms include unilateral flashing lights, floaters, blurry vision, distorted images, loss of vision, and peripheral field defect.[10,11]

Diagnosis

Fundoscopic examination typically shows retinal distortion.[10,11] Slit lamp examination may show pigmented granules in the anterior vitreous.[12]

Management

Patients with suspected retinal detachment should be instructed to lay on the side opposite the visual defect to minimize risk of progression to the macula.[12] Immediate referral to ophthalmology is critical to preserve vision if signs of retinal tear are noted.[10-12] Even in the absence of physical examination signs, a suggestive history is sufficient for an urgent referral. Ophthalmologic surgical techniques have a high degree of success at preserving vision. Scleral buckling, pars plana vitrectomy, and pneumatic retinopexy are techniques used to relieve vitreoretinal traction and repair tears, holes, or detachments.[10-12]

Follow-Up

Patients may need to spend a period of days to weeks face down if gas was instilled into the eye, and are typically prescribed topical antibiotics and steroids postoperatively. Vision and pain should improve, and worsening of these symptoms should be reported immediately.[12]

OCULAR EMERGENCIES DUE TO SYSTEMIC ILLNESS
Central Retinal Artery Occlusion

Presentation

The chief symptom is typically sudden onset painless loss of monocular vision. Consider predisposing conditions such as hypertension, diabetes, giant cell arteritis, and sickle cell disease. Outcomes are related to acuity of presentation and duration of visual impairment.[11]

Diagnosis

Fundoscopic examination findings of an infarcted retina with resultant whitish discoloration and a classic "cherry-red spot" on the macula are diagnostic.[13] If the diagnosis is uncertain, fluorescein angiography of the fundus is recommended.[11]

Management

Goals of therapy are to increase the perfusion pressure of the retinal circulation and to remove the obstruction, which may be a thrombus or embolus. Commonly used treatments include acetazolamide 500 mg IV, ocular massage (to encourage mechanical disintegration of clot), and when appropriate local fibrinolytic therapy.[11]

Follow-Up

Follow-up with ophthalmology is important to monitor for retinal and iris neovascularization, which may occur months later.

Acute Angle Closure Crisis

Presentation

Acute angle closure crisis occurs when drainage from the anterior chamber of the eye is suddenly reduced. Optic nerve damage and subsequent visual loss can occur within hours. Signs and symptoms on presentation can include a red and painful eye, mid-dilated pupil with relative afferent pupillary defect (Marcus Gunn pupil), blurred vision, halos around lights, headache,[14] and nausea.[11]

Diagnosis

Intraocular pressure should be measured as soon as possible. Findings of intraocular pressure >30 mm Hg, conjunctival injection, corneal edema or haziness, mid-dilated pupil, decreased visual acuity, and shallow anterior chamber suggest the diagnosis.[11]

Management

Immediate treatment to reduce intraocular pressure is indicated. Initial treatment consists of oral acetazolamide 500 mg, as well as timolol 0.5%, apraclonidine 1%, and pilocarpine 2%, one drop each in the affected eye, one minute apart, then repeated three times at 3- to 5-minute intervals. Eye pressure should be rechecked at least hourly until the patient can be seen by an ophthalmologist.[11] Definitive treatment is surgical.[15]

Follow-Up

Postoperatively, steroid eye drops are recommended. Because half of patients who suffer from unilateral acute angle closure will develop the condition in the contralateral eye within 5 years, prophylactic surgery is recommended for the unaffected eye.[14]

Temporal Arteritis (Giant Cell Arteritis)

Presentation

Temporal arteritis (TA) is a subset of giant cell arteritis involving the temporal, ophthalmic, and basilar arteries.[16] It can cause blindness due to ophthalmic artery ischemia, with visual disturbances occurring in 35% and visual loss in 16% on presentation.[17] Because visual loss can occur within hours of the onset of symptoms,[16] rapid recognition and appropriate treatment are critical. Presentation can vary significantly, from fatigue and fever to visual blurring, amaurosis fugax, or complete blindness.[16] Predictive signs and symptoms include temporal artery beading, temporal artery prominence, and jaw claudication.[18]

Diagnosis

Any suspicion for TA should be thoroughly investigated. Physical examination should include constitutional, ocular, musculoskeletal, and neurologic assessment, including palpation for temporal artery beading or tenderness superior to the tragus.[16] A normal erythrocyte sedimentation rate (ESR) makes the diagnosis unlikely,[18] and 89% of patients with TA will have an ESR above 50.[16] Temporal artery biopsy is diagnostic, and an immediate, urgent referral for biopsy is indicated. Additional testing may include blood counts, urinalysis, metabolic panel, and chest X-ray.[16]

Management

Immediate initiation of high-dose corticosteroids (typically 40 to 60 mg oral prednisolone) can prevent the catastrophic complications of TA. Complicated cases should be hospitalized for IV steroids. Treatment should not be delayed, as histologic findings of TA have been found after 14 days of oral steroid.[17] Rheumatology should be consulted for co-management throughout the course of the illness. Low-dose aspirin can prevent cerebral ischemia. Prednisolone should be tapered slowly: reduce 10 mg every 2 weeks to 20 mg; then by 2.5 mg every 4 weeks to 10 mg; then by 1 mg every 1 to 2 months.[16]

Follow-Up

Return visit should be within 1 week with frequent follow-up through the following 12 months thereafter to monitor for vascular disease and complications from steroid use.[16]

REFERENCES

1. Hemmati HD, Colby KA. Treating acute chemical injuries of the cornea. *EYE NET Magazine*. October, 2012.
2. Fish R, Davidson RS. Management of ocular thermal and chemical injuries including amniotic membrane therapy. *Curr Opin Ophthalmol* 2010;21:317–321.
3. Wipperman J, Dorsch J. Evaluation and management of corneal abrasions. *Am Fam Physician* 2013;87:114–120.

4. Harlan JB Jr, Pieramici DJ. Evaluation of patients with ocular trauma. *Ophthalmol Clin North Am* 2002;15:153.

5. Arey ML, Mootha VV, Whittemore AR, et al. Computed tomography in the diagnosis of occult open globe injuries. *Ophthalmology* 2007;114:1448.

6. Walton W, Von Hagen S, Grigorian R, et al. Management of traumatic hyphema. *Surv Ophthalmol* 2002;47:297.

7. Sankar PS, Chen TC, Grosskreutz CL, et al. Traumatic hyphema. *Int Ophthalmol Clin* 2002;42:57.

8. Brandt MT, Haug RH. Traumatic hyphema: a comprehensive review. *J Oral Maxillofac Surg* 2001;59:1462.

9. Hamill MB. Current concepts in the treatment of traumatic injury to the anterior segment. *Ophthalmol Clin North Am* 1999;12:457.

10. Gelston CD. Common eye emergencies. *Am Fam Physician* 2013;88(8):515–519.

11. Pokhrel PK, Loftus SA. Ocular emergencies. *Am Fam Physician* 2007;76(6):829–836.

12. Kang HK, Luff AJ. Management of retinal detachment: a guide for non-ophthalmologists. *BMJ* 2008;336(7655):1235–1240.

13. Beatty S, Au Eong KG. Acute occlusion of the retinal arteries: current concepts and recent advances in diagnosis and management. *J Accid Emerg Med* 2000;17:324–329.

14. American Academy of Ophthalmology Glaucoma Panel. *Primary angle closure.* San Francisco, CA: American Academy of Ophthalmology; 2010:29.

15. Emanuel ME, Parrish RK IInd, Gedde SJ. Evidence-based management of primary angle closure glaucoma. *Curr Opin Ophthalmol* 2014;25(2):89–92.

16. Caylor TL, Perkins A. Recognition and management of polymyalgia rheumatica and giant cell arteritis. *Am Fam Physician* 2013;88(10):676–684.

17. Ezeonyeji AN, Borg FA, Dasgupta B. Delays in recognition and management of giant cell arteritis: results from a retrospective audit. *Clin Rheumatol* 2011;30(2):259–262.

18. Smetana GW, Shmerling RH. Does this patient have temporal arteritis? *JAMA* 2002;287(1):92.

CHAPTER 8

Ear, Nose, and Throat Problems

Section Editor: Jason M. Patera

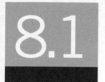

Acute Otitis Media
Carey Christiansen Ford

GENERAL PRINCIPLES
Definition

Acute otitis media (AOM) is an acute suppurative infection of the middle ear, often occurring in the setting of an upper respiratory infection. AOM may occur in adults, although more frequently develops in children. Generally short-lived, AOM in a healthy child has a self-limited course and only in some cases needs antibiotic therapy.[1]

Anatomy and Pathophysiology

The much higher propensity of children for AOM is in part due to the less steeply angled, shorter eustachian tube, which allows reflux of organisms and debris from the nasopharynx into the middle ear. With congestion of the tube from an upper respiratory infection, secretions can accumulate and bacterial pathogens can multiply, leading to inflammation and clinical symptoms.[1]

Epidemiology

AOM is the most common bacterial infection of children, with 5 million cases diagnosed per year. An estimated 30 million clinic visits for AOM are made each year.[1] It is also the most common reason for antibiotic use in children, and is the reason for 50% of antibiotics prescribed to preschool-age children.[2] However, office visits for AOM decreased in number between 1995–1996 and 2004–2005, with a resulting decrease in antibiotic prescriptions.

Risk may be reduced by breastfeeding for at least 6 months, ceasing pacifier use after 6 months of age, avoidance of "bottle-propping," and elimination of secondhand smoke exposure.[2] Other risk factors that are not modifiable include genetic predisposition, male gender, premature birth, Native American or Inuit ethnicity, family history, the presence of siblings in the home, and low socioeconomic status.[2]

Administration of influenza and pneumococcal vaccines may be of some benefit for reduction of the incidence of AOM and are recommended.[2]

Etiology

Streptococcus pneumoniae, non-typable *Haemophilus influenzae*, and *Moraxella catarrhalis* are the most commonly found pathogens found on culture of middle ear fluid obtained by tympanocentesis.[2,3]

S. pneumoniae has been found in middle ear fluid in 25% to 50% of children with AOM, *H. influenzae* has been found in 15% to 30%, and *M. catarrhalis* has been found in 3% to 20%.[2]

The microbiology of AOM may be changing due to the administration of the pneumococcal conjugate vaccine to infants, with an increase in *H. influenzae*.[2]

Viruses, including respiratory syncytial virus, rhinovirus, coronavirus, parainfluenza, adenovirus, and enterovirus, have been found in respiratory secretions and/or middle ear effusion (MEE) in 40% to 75% of AOM cases and in 5% to 22% of MEE without bacteria.[4] Viruses may be the causative pathogen when antibiotic treatment is ineffective. However, viruses are the only pathogen in AOM in only 10% of cases.[2]

In 16% to 25% of cases of AOM, no organism can be found in middle ear fluid.[2]

DIAGNOSIS

AOM must be carefully distinguished from otitis media with effusion (OME) to avoid over diagnosis and inappropriate antibiotic use. Although OME may precede AOM, or occur as a consequence of eustachian tube dysfunction, OME does not necessitate antibiotics.

Elements of the definition of AOM are all of the following: recent, usually abrupt, onset of signs and symptoms of middle ear inflammation and MEE. Changes from the 2004 guideline include the description of more specific otoscopic findings. The diagnosis of AOM should be made in children with moderate to severe bulging of the tympanic membrane (TM) or new onset of otorrhea not due to another cause, such as otitis externa. It can also be made in the presence of a mildly bulging TM plus either less than 48 hours of ear pain or intense erythema of the TM.[5] Children without MEE should not be diagnosed with AOM.

1. The presence of MEE is indicated by any of the following:
   a. Bulging of the TM
   b. Limited or absent mobility of the TM
   c. Air-fluid level behind the TM
   d. Otorrhea

Clinical Presentation

Signs and symptoms of AOM are nonspecific and may vary with age group. Cough, nasal discharge, and other upper respiratory symptoms are common and nonspecific. Fever, vomiting, otalgia, otorrhea, and hearing loss are variably present, with ear pain present only in 50% to 60% of children with AOM.[5]

Infants may present with irritability, fever, pulling on the ear, or anorexia. Clinical history alone is poorly predictive of the presence of AOM.[1]

Physical Examination

The position of the TM is key for differentiating AOM from OME; a red TM alone is inadequate for diagnosis. Importantly, AOM must be distinguished from OME.[5]

- **Pneumatic otoscopy.** Evaluation of the TM for position, color, translucency, and mobility provides predictive information. In one Finnish study, a cloudy-appearing, bulging TM with impaired mobility was the strongest predictor of AOM, with impaired mobility having the highest sensitivity and specificity. Cloudiness was the next best, with bulging of the membrane having high specificity but lower sensitivity.[6] It has also been reported that a bulging TM is highly associated with the presence of a bacterial pathogen, another indicator of the importance of this physical finding.[7]
- Care must be taken to ensure an adequate examination. Important factors include adequate illumination, a functioning bulb, and obtaining a tight seal with the external auditory canal. A crying child's TM may appear pink or red, impairing the examination. Excess cerumen in the canal can also impair the examination and should be removed.[1]
- **Tympanometry.** It is an adjunctive diagnostic technique to determine the pressure of the middle ear space. In one study, the sensitivity and specificity of a flat tympanogram for the presence of an MEE were 90% and 86%, respectively.[8] A seal must be made with the external canal for an accurate reading.
- **Acoustic reflectometry.** A seal does not need to be made, an advantage over tympanometery. Like tympanometry, acoustic reflectometry relies on measuring sound waves returning from the TM to measure the middle ear pressure.[8]
- **Tympanocentesis.** It is the gold standard for diagnosis of an MEE. Culture of fluid may be done to direct antibiotic use. This is not routinely used, but is an excellent diagnostic tool used by a specialist for refractory or recurrent AOM.[8]

Differential Diagnosis

- OME
- Eustachian tube dysfunction
- Otitis externa
- Temporomandibular junction pain
- Dental pain
- Pharyngitis
- Upper respiratory infection

TREATMENT

Medications

Pain may be significant with AOM, persisting even after treatment; as antibiotics do not provide symptomatic relief in the first 24 hours, it is important to use analgesics as necessary. Antipyretics, including acetaminophen and ibuprofen, are the mainstays of pain control in AOM, and should be given for fever and pain as necessary. Home remedies, such as oil drops in the ear canal, or the external application of heat or cold, have not been directly evaluated and may have limited effectiveness but are unlikely to cause harm. Topical agents such as benzocaine drops are beneficial in patients over 5 years of age, but short-acting.[5]

There are no data supporting the use of decongestants and antihistamines for AOM; children treated with these medications have an increased risk of medication side effects.[6]

Observation Versus Antibiotic Use

The decision to observe a patient without prescribing antibiotics is directed by the patient's age and the severity of symptoms. A major change from the 2004 guideline includes the elimination of a caveat allowing observation in the case of uncertain diagnosis; greater emphasis is now placed on accurate diagnosis and complete visualization of the TM. Initial treatment can consist of observation in children aged 24 months or older with bilateral AOM with non-severe symptoms (mild otalgia for less than 48 hours, temperature less than 102.2°F).[5] A system must be established to follow up and begin antibiotic therapy in the case of worsening symptoms or lack of improvement within 48 to 72 hours of diagnosis. Additionally, for children aged 6 months to 2 years, initial observation may be offered for children with unilateral AOM with mild symptoms. Symptomatic treatment with antipyretics/analgesics is still indicated with the decision to observe. In the first 24 hours of observation, the patient should experience a stabilization of symptoms, possibly after a period of worsening. By 72 hours if no improvement is noted, antibiotics are indicated.[2,5]

If antibiotic use is indicated, amoxicillin at high dose (80 to 90 mg/kg/day) is recommended for most children. If amoxicillin has been given in the past 30 days, there is a history of recurrent AOM unresponsive to amoxicillin, or the child has concurrent purulent conjunctivitis, an antibiotic with additional β-lactamase coverage should be used (e.g., amoxicillin–clavulanate 90 mg/kg/day of amoxicillin with 6.4 mg/kg/day of clavulanate).[5] If antibiotics are given, within 48 to 72 hours the child's symptoms, including fever, irritability, and discomfort, should improve. If the patient is not improved, either the causative bacteria is resistant to the therapy or an additional viral infection may be present.

- Amoxicillin allergy
  - **Cefdinir:** 14 mg/kg/day in one to two doses
  - **Cefpodoxime:** 10 mg/kg/day in one dose
  - **Cefuroxime:** 30 mg/kg/day in two doses
  - **Ceftriaxone:** (50 mg IM or IV per day for 1 or 3 days)
- Alternative treatment[5]
  - **In case of failure of initial antibiotic:** amoxicillin–clavulanate (90 mg/kg/day of amoxicillin with 6.4 mg/kg/day of clavulanate in two doses), or clindamycin 30 to 40 mg/kg/day in three doses (concurrent prescription for third-generation cephalosporin should be given in case of failure of second antibiotic), or parenteral treatment with ceftriaxone.
  - Substantial resistance exists to erythromycin–sulfisoxazole, azithromycin, and sulfamethoxazole–trimethaprim, a change from the 2004 guideline.
  - If patient does not tolerate oral medication, a single dose of parenteral ceftriaxone (50 mg per kg) may be used, although a 3-day course is more effective.
- Duration of therapy
  - A 10-day course of therapy is recommended for children under age 2 years, whereas children 2 to 5 years of age may be prescribed a 7-day course. For children 6 years and older with mild to moderate symptoms, 5 to 7 days of antibiotic therapy is sufficient.[5]

Referral

For refractory or recurrent AOM, a referral to an otolaryngologist may be warranted for tympanocentesis and placement of tympanostomy tubes. Tympanostomy tubes may be offered for recurrent AOM (defined as three episodes in 6 months or four episodes in 1 year, with one episode in the preceding 6 months).[5]

Complications

Complications of AOM are rare, even without antibiotics or with delaying antibiotics, but include acute mastoiditis, intracranial abscess, bacterial meningitis, epidural abscess, brain abscess, lateral sinus thrombosis, cavernous sinus thrombosis, subdural empyema, and carotid artery thrombosis.[7] A more common complication is perforation of the TM, resulting in purulent otorrhea. Infrequently, chronic suppurative otitis media may develop.[7] Complications of chronic or recurrent otitis may include school absenteeism, decreased hearing, and speech delay. MEE may persist for weeks after resolution of AOM, leading to transient hearing loss, which should be monitored if it occurs.[2]

Prognosis

Prognosis is excellent; most children with AOM recover without sequelae.

REFERENCES

1. Rothman R, Owens T, Simel D. Does this child have acute otitis media? *JAMA* 2003;290:1633–1640.
2. American Academy of Pediatrics and American Academy of Family Physicians, Sub-committee on Management of Acute Otitis Media. Diagnosis and management of acute otitis media. *Pediatrics* 2004;113:1451–1465.
3. Berman S. Otitis media in children. *N Engl J Med* 1995;332:1560–1565.
4. Heikkinen T, Thint M, Chonmaitree T. Prevalence of various respiratory viruses in the middle ear during acute otitis media. *N Engl J Med* 1999;340:260–264.
5. Lieberthal AS, Carroll AE, Chonmaitree T, et al. The diagnosis and management of acute otitis media. *Pediatrics* 2013;131(3):e964–e999.
6. Karma PH, Penttila MA, Sipila MM, et al. Otoscopic diagnosis of middle ear effusion in acute and non-acute otitis media. The value of otoscopic findings. *Int J Pediatr Otorhinolaryngol* 1989;12(1):37–49.
7. McCormick DP, Lim-Melia E, Saeed K, et al. Otitis media: can clinical findings predict bacterial or viral etiology? *Pediatr Infect Dis J* 2000;19(3):256–258.
8. Pichichero M. Acute otitis media: part I. Improving diagnostic accuracy. *Am Fam Physician* 2000;61(7):2051–2056.
9. Flynn CA, Griffin GH, Schultz JK. Decongestants and antihistamines for acute otitis media in children. *Cochrane Database Syst Rev* 2004;3:CD001727.
10. Klein JO, Pelton S. Epidemiology, pathogenesis, clinical manifestations, and complications of acute otitis media (online). http://www.uptodate.com.

8.2 Chronic Otitis Media

Russell G. Maier

GENERAL PRINCIPLES

Chronic otitis media (COM) encompasses a broad area of ear disease that is discussed as three main clinical entities: otitis media with effusion (OME), chronic suppurative otitis media (CSOM), and COM. OME is defined as the presence of fluid in the middle ear without signs or symptoms of infection. Controversy exists regarding the diagnosis and treatment of OME. OME has been studied by several evidence-based panels since the 1990s that have developed objective treatment recommendations.[1,2] Much of the discussion on OME is based on these panels' recommendations for ages 2 to 12. CSOM is defined as chronic (6-week) otorrhea through a tympanic membrane (TM) that is not intact. COM is defined as a perforation lasting longer than 1 month without drainage.

OTITIS MEDIA WITH EFFUSION
Clinical Presentation

In children and adults, the presentation is similar; commonly there are no complaints. The diagnosis is made on a screening examination or follow-up for acute otitis media (AOM). If symptoms are present, they include behavioral changes, parental or patient complaints of diminished hearing, or a fullness or discomfort in one or both ears. Historically, the most common cause of OME is a prior ear infection.

Risk Factors

Risk factors of OME include recurrent AOM, group childcare, passive smoke exposure, absence of breastfeeding as an infant, craniofacial abnormalities, and possibly allergies.

Clinical Examination

The diagnosis of OME is primarily clinical. There are few useful tests and no laboratory studies that aid in the diagnosis. It is important to document whether the effusion is unilateral or bilateral.

Physical Examination

By definition, a middle ear effusion is present, and there is no evidence for acute infection. The external auditory canal should appear normal. The TM may appear normal or thickened. A middle ear effusion may be noted as an air–fluid level, bubbles, or serous or serosanguinous fluid in the middle ear. If fever, a bulging erythematous eardrum, or drainage is present, the diagnosis of OME cannot be made.

Additional Tests

- *Pneumatic otoscopy.* Pneumatic otoscopy should be used as the primary diagnostic method, as a TM that appears normal may have fluid behind it.[1] For pneumatic otoscopy to be accurate, a complete seal must be obtained in the ear canal. When slight positive and negative pressure is applied to the TM, it should move briskly back and forth. An effusion inhibits this movement.
- *Tympanometry.* If following clinical examination and pneumatic otoscopy the clinician is unsure about the diagnosis, tympanometry provides a useful adjunct and is accurate for infants 4 months and older. An effusion produces a flat, type B tympanogram.

Treatment

Treatment for adults and children is primarily medical but varies depending on the examination and underlying illnesses.

- *Children at risk.* Children at risk, those with sensory, physical, cognitive, or behavioral issues, should be considered for earlier evaluation. These children may be less tolerant of hearing loss. A hearing and, if necessary, speech and language assessment should be performed.
- Normal child with OME for less than 3 months:
  - *Watchful waiting.* In a variety of studies, the spontaneous resolution of OME ranges from 75% to 90% over 3 months. Given that approximately two thirds of all children improve without any treatment and with no risk to the child, watchful waiting is the recommended treatment course. Interval visits are optional after the initial diagnosis. At 3 months, the child should be reassessed for resolution by pneumatic otoscopy and/or tympanometry.
  - *Antibiotics.* In the past, antibiotics have been an option for treatment during the first 3 months. Given the increasing difficulties and risks with resistant organisms, watchful waiting is now the preferred course.
  - *Antihistamines and decongestants.* These are ineffective and have no role.[1]
  - *Steroids.* Steroids are not recommended because they show no benefit, especially in this early period.[3]
- *Risk factor reduction.* In all patients, there are several modifiable risk factors that contribute to OME. The child should not be exposed to any secondary smoke. Any smoking by family members or relatives should be done outside of the home or car, not in a different room. Group childcare is a risk factor that rarely can be modified.
- OME for 3 months or more in normal children
  - *Hearing evaluation.* At 3 months, all children with bilateral effusions should receive a hearing evaluation. If the hearing loss is 20 decibels (dB) or greater, the patient should have language testing.
  - *Watchful waiting.* Children at low risk who pass their hearing test may be reassessed at 3- to 6-month intervals. Asymptomatic OME tends to resolve spontaneously. If on reassessment the OME is present and the hearing evaluation is >39 dB, then surgery is recommended. From 21 to 39 dB of hearing loss, a comprehensive audiologic evaluation is indicated. Treatment options depend upon the child's situation and parental preference. If the hearing loss is <21 dB, a repeat test should be done in 3 to 6 months.
  - *Antibiotics.* Antibiotics have no benefit beyond 1 month. For parents averse to surgery, a single course may be tried. A 10- to 14-day course of amoxicillin or trimethoprim–sulfamethoxazole would be first-line treatment, with amoxicillin doses at 40 to 80 mg/kg/day in three divided does. Repeat courses are not recommended.[1]

- *Surgery.* Candidates for surgery have OME for 4 months or longer with persistent hearing loss, recurrent or persistent OME in children at risk (regardless of hearing status), or OME with structural damage to the TM or middle ear. Tympanostomy tubes are the recommended surgical option. If repeat tube placement is needed, adenoidectomy is recommended. Myringotomy or tonsillectomy provides no benefit over watchful waiting. Of note, although studies show a quicker resolution of the effusion, an intermediate endpoint, no study has demonstrated an improvement in language or school performance.[4]
- *Patient education.* Resources include patient handouts at http://familydoctor.org/330.xml, http://www.cdc.gov/drugresistance/community/files/GetSmart_OME.pdf, and for ear tubes http://www.entnet.org/healthinfo/ears/Ear-Tubes.cfm.

CHRONIC SUPPURATIVE OTITIS MEDIA AND CHRONIC OTITIS MEDIA
Clinical Presentation
CSOM often presents with drainage from an ear. Usually the individual feels fine or otherwise appears healthy. The patient may complain of otalgia, state that he or she is "out of sorts," or complain of hearing loss or difficulty hearing from the affected ear. COM is usually painless.

Risk Factors
Risk factors include recurrent AOM, immune impairment (e.g., from diabetes or chronic illness), allergies, craniofacial abnormalities, and certain subpopulations, including Eskimos and Native Americans. The use of tympanostomy tubes results in an approximately 1.6% to 3.0% incidence of chronic otorrhea.

Physical Examination
Clear otorrhea is unusual, and a cerebrospinal fluid leak should be considered. Especially in children, one needs to rule out a foreign body with secondary otitis externa as the cause of otorrhea. In adults as well, a careful examination and possibly a therapeutic trial must be done to rule out otitis externa as the cause of otorrhea. Once the external auditory canal has been cleaned, the TM should be examined. Often a large central perforation is seen, with an abnormal middle ear noted. Marginal perforations are more often associated with cholesteatomas and other severe complications. If a cholesteatoma is noted, the patient should be referred to an otolaryngologist. CSOM with cholesteatoma is primarily a surgical disease.

Laboratory Studies
If possible, cultures should be obtained. Material from the middle ear is most helpful. Drainage from the external auditory canal is acceptable, but the canal should be sterilized and the culture obtained from newly accumulated fluid. Culture should include both aerobes and anaerobes.

- *Tympanometry.* If a perforation is suspected but not seen, a tympanogram will show a large canal volume but flat tracing or will fail to make a seal.
- *Audiologic evaluation.* Because many patients complain of hearing abnormalities, it is helpful to document this finding so as to follow it during treatment. A conductive hearing loss of more than 30 dB is suggestive of disruption of the ossicular chain.
- *Imaging studies.* The diagnosis of CSOM and COM is primarily clinical. If a cholesteatoma is suspected, if the diagnosis is uncertain, or if intracranial extension is suspected, computed tomography or magnetic resonance imaging should be performed.[5]
- *Immediate referral.* Patients with a facial palsy, labyrinthitis, or suspected intracranial suppuration should be referred immediately.

Treatment
Chronic Suppurative Otitis Media
Initial management is medical and involves removing the debris. If the practitioner does not have an operating microscope or suction, treatment may be better referred to an otolaryngologist. Following removal of debris, the preferred treatment in children and adults with topical fluoroquinolones is recommended.[6] The long-term goal is a dry ear and involves aural toilet.[7] In a patient with systemic signs and symptoms with concern for invasive disease, systemic antibiotics are indicated.

- *Aggressive medical management.* For CSOM refractory to topical treatment and aural toilet consideration of a fungal infection, referral to an otolaryngologist should be considered.
- *Surgery.* If aggressive medical management fails, tympanomastoid surgery should be considered as the next step.

Chronic Otitis Media

A dry, uninfected middle ear does not require acute treatment other than being kept dry. Definitive repair is done electively in adults or at age 9 to 12 years in children.

Patient Education

Resources include http://www.nlm.nih.gov/medlineplus/ency/article/007010.htm for OME and http://www.nlm.nih.gov/medlineplus/ency/article/003042.htm (accessed on 15 March, 2014) for the acute draining ear.

REFERENCES

1. American Academy of Family Physicians; American Academy of Otolaryngology-Head and Neck Surgery; American Academy of Pediatrics Subcommittee on Otitis Media with Effusion. Otitis media with effusion. *Pediatrics* 2004;113:1412–1429. http://pediatrics.aappublications.org/content/113/5/1412.full.html. Accessed March 15, 2014.
2. National Institute for Health and Clinical Excellence. Surgical management of otitis media with effusion in children. 2008. http://publications.nice.org.uk/surgical-management-of-otitis-media-with-effusion-in-children-cg60. Accessed March 15, 2014.
3. Mandel EM, Casselbrant ML, Rockette HE, et al. Systemic steroid for chronic otitis media with effusion in children. *Pediatrics* 2002;110:1071–1080.
4. Roberts JE, Rosenfeld RM, Zeisel SA. Otitis media and speech and language: a meta-analysis of prospective studies. *Pediatrics* 2004;113:e238–e248.
5. Kimmelman CP. Office management of the draining ear. *Otolaryngol Clin North Am* 1992;25:739.
6. Hannley MT, Denneny JC IIIrd, Holzer SS. Use of ototopical antibiotics in treating 3 common ear diseases. *Otolaryngol Head Neck Surg* 2000;122:934.
7. Acuin, J. Chronic suppurative otitis media. Burden of illness and management options. World Health Organization. http://www.who.int/pbd/publications/Chronicsuppurativeotitis_media.pdf. Accessed March 15, 2014.

8.3 Otitis Externa

Paul Evans

Otitis externa is an inflammatory condition, usually self-limiting, of the external auditory canal (EAC). It is commonly seen in primary care because it affects all age groups. The incidence increase in summertime owing to water exposure in swimming, especially in fresh water, increased humidity, and related activities that reduce cerumen protection.[1,2] Otitis externa can be diffuse or circumscribed, can be acute or chronic, or can have eczematous features. Rarely, it can progress to necrotizing or "malignant" otitis externa in diabetics or other immunocompromised patients, leading to serious illness, cranial nerve palsies, or death.[3] Risk factors include anatomic abnormalities such as EAC stenosis; cerumen obstruction; foreign bodies; trauma; instrumentation; swimming or moisture exposure; use of a hearing aid or ear plugs; soap; stress; and predisposing skin disorders, such as eczema, seborrhea, or psoriasis.[1]

I. Clinical Presentation

  A. **Symptoms.** The most frequently described symptoms are itching, purulent discharge, otalgia, plugging of the ear, mild hearing loss, ear fullness, and tinnitus. Pain is often increased by chewing or pinnal pressure.[4]

  B. **Signs.** On examination, there is tragal or pinnal tenderness, an erythematous and edematous EAC, and discharge. Pinnal eczema is often present. Otorrhea, crusting, and lymphadenopathy (late) may also occur.[3]

II. Diagnosis

  A. **Acute otitis externa.** It is usually infectious in origin, with *Pseudomonas aeruginosa* or *Staphylococcus aureus* being the most common isolates. Fungi such as *Aspergillus, Candida,* and others have also been infrequently implicated. Anaerobes may also play a role.[3,5,6] Cultures in acute otitis should be reserved for therapeutic failures because most patients respond to first-line therapy. Noninfectious causes, such as contact dermatitis, eczema, psoriasis, or trauma, should be sought.

B. Chronic otitis externa. Chronic otitis is defined by symptoms lasting longer than 2 months. Causes similar to acute otitis externas are seen, but chronic otitis may be the result of failure to correctly diagnose and treat the pathogen initially. Predisposing factors remain contributory.

C. Necrotizing or "malignant" external otitis. This is a rare but important infection seen most commonly in elderly diabetics and the immunocompromised. Severe ear pain and systemic signs and symptoms may be present along with cranial nerve palsies. If not detected early and treated aggressively, this condition may progress to skull base osteomyelitis with possible erosion to the central nervous system. *Pseudomonas* is the most common pathogen.[5]

III. Management

A. Acute otitis externa

1. Clean out exudates and debris by gently suctioning or swabbing. Use of irrigation is controversial.

2. Initial culture is not necessary.

3. Topicals using four to five drops per dose three or four times per day may be used for 7 to 14 days or 3 days after symptom relief. Mild acids (Domeboro Otic, VolSol HC) lower pH to inhibit *Pseudomonas* growth.[7]

4. Antibiotics with and without hydrocortisone have been effective. Neomycin solutions or suspensions, such as polymyxin B HC (Cortisporin or Coly-Mycin S), and quinolone otic solutions, such as ofloxacin 0.3% (Floxin Otic or Cipro HC), are beneficial. Ophthalmic solutions of quinolones such as ofloxacin 0.3% (Ocuflox) and ciprofloxacin 0.3% (Ciloxan) as well as aminoglycoside ophthalmic solutions such as gentamycin sulfate 0.3% (Garamycin) or tobramycin sulfate 0.3% (Tobrex) or some with antibiotic and topical steroids such as tobramycin 0.3% plus dexamethasone (Tobrex) or ciprofloxacin 0.3% with dexamethasone 0.1% (Ciprodex) have gained in popularity. These must be avoided in perforated tympanic membranes.[1–3,5]

5. Antifungals such as amphotericin B 3% (Fungizone), tolnaftate 1% (Tinactin), or clotrimazole 1% (Lotrimin) are used for otomycosis.[2,3,5,7]

6. If infection spreads to the concha or to the preauricular or infra-auricular area, systemic antibiotics should be considered. If a fungal etiology is suspected, topical nystatin and clotrimazole have been successful first-line agents.[7]

7. Cotton wicks for a severely swollen EAC assist in reducing swelling and more effectively getting topical therapy to targeted tissue.[1,5] After 48 to 72 hours, the wick can usually be removed, with continuation of drops for the full 7 to 14 days.

8. Pain control with a topical anesthetic (e.g., benzocaine, antipyrine, and dehydrated glycerin [Auralgan], 2 to 4 drops q1–2h as required), acetaminophen, or ibuprofen is usually successful. Occasionally, short-term narcotic analgesics may be necessary.

B. Chronic otitis externa

1. Maintain cleanliness of the EAC.

2. Because initial treatment has failed for 2 months or longer, bacterial and fungal cultures should now be done. A screening potassium hydroxide (KOH) preparation can rapidly detect fungal elements, which indicates otomycosis.

3. Reexamine for other conditions, such as chronic purulent otitis media with perforation, furunculosis, eczema, seborrhea, or psoriasis.

4. Carefully evaluate for contact dermatitis due to prior therapies. Common sensitivities to neomycin and other agents in topical preparations must be kept in mind.

5. If compliance has been ensured with an appropriate regimen for the cultured pathogen, a change to another antibiotic is indicated. Mixed bacterial and fungal infections may require multiple drug therapy. Addition of topical steroids reduces inflammation and the accompanying symptoms.

6. If all medical therapy fails, surgical consultation is appropriate for consideration for conchomeatoplasty or another procedure as a last resort.

C. Necrotizing or malignant otitis externa. All elderly diabetics and immunocompromised patients with external otitis should be monitored for this serious complication. This rare condition requires early and aggressive therapy, including consultation with an otolaryngologist. Initial outpatient antimicrobials such as ciprofloxacin 500 to 1,000 mg q12h, or long-term antipseudomonal β-lactam antibiotics (piperacillin, ticarcillin, or cegtazidime) as well as aminoglycosides (e.g., tobramycin) can be used.[3] Treatment periods may be up to 8 weeks or more. If this is clinically ineffective, hospitalization with antipseudomonal parenteral antibiotics (e.g., ceftazidime and gentamicin), careful debridement, and computed tomography or magnetic resonance imaging to delineate the extent of bony or soft-tissue erosions are recommended.[3,5]

IV. Prevention

A. Infection causes. Because most of the bacterial and fungal organisms thrive on moist tissues, attention to drying the EAC and lowering the growth of pathogens with a mildly acidic environment is important. Over-the-counter preparations for preventing swimmer's ear that contain a drying agent and a mild acid such as Vosol, SwimEar, or StarOtic are effective; similar home remedies can be made with a mixture of 50% isopropyl alcohol and 50% vinegar (5% acetic acid). When applied after moisture exposure, such a mixture is both efficacious and cost effective. Drying the ear with a hair dryer on low setting may also be helpful.[1]

B. Noninfectious causes. Maintaining good aural hygiene and getting early treatment of dermatologic problems lowers the incidence of otitis externa. Use of topical steroids for eczematous conditions as well as for allergic or contact dermatitis is helpful. Patients who use occlusive EAC devices, such as hearing aids, earpieces, or stethoscopes, must maintain a high level of attention to cleanliness to avoid bacterial or fungal contamination.

REFERENCES

1. Schaefer P, Baugh RF. Acute otitis externa: an update. *Am Fam Physician* 2012;86(11):1055–1061.
2. Silverberg M, Lucchesi M. Common disorders of the external, middle, and inner ear. In: Tintinalli JE, Stapczynski J, Ma O, et al, eds. *Tintinalli's emergency medicine: a comprehensive study guide.* 7th ed. New York, NY: McGraw-Hill; 2011.
3. Brown KD, Banuchi V, Selesnick SH. Diseases of the external ear. In: Lalwani AK, ed. *Current diagnosis and treatment in otolaryngology-Head and neck surgery.* 13th ed. New York, NY: McGraw Hill; 2010: chap 47.
4. Yoon PJ, Kelley PE, Friedman NR. Ear, nose, & throat. In: William Hay WW, Levin MJ, Deterding RR, et al, eds. *Current diagnosis and treatment: pediatrics.* 21st ed. New York, NY: McGraw Hill; 2012:chap 18.
5. Lustig LR, Schindler JS. Lustig LR, et al. Ear, nose, & throat disorders. In: Papadakis MA, McPhee SJ, Rabow MW, et al, eds. *Current medical diagnosis & treatment 2014.* New York, NY: McGraw-Hill; 2014:chap 8.
6. Lee H, Kim L, Nguyen V. Ear infections: otitis externa and otitis media. *Prim Care* 2013; 40(3):671–686.
7. Fort GG. Otitis externa. In: Ferri FF, ed. *Ferri's clinical advisor 2014: 5 books in 1.* Philadelphia, PA: Elsevier Mosby; 2014: 812–813.

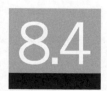

8.4 Pharyngitis
John L. Smith

GENERAL PRINCIPLES

Epidemiology

Acute pharyngitis is one of the more common illnesses seen by primary care physicians. Only about 10% of adults and 15% to 30% of children presenting with pharyngitis will have group A β-hemolytic streptococcal (GABHS) infection.[1] Most pharyngitis, both viral and streptococcal, is transmitted by hand contact with nasal discharge and not oral contact.[2]

Etiology

Pharyngitis has both viral and bacterial causes, but GABHS is the only commonly occurring bacterial etiology.[1] Group C and G β-hemolytic *Streptococcus*, *Neisseria*, *Chlamydia*, and *Mycoplasma* are much less likely bacterial causes.

DIAGNOSIS

Up to 70% of adults in the United States who present with a main complaint of sore throat are treated with antibiotics;[3] only about 10% have streptococcal pharyngitis. For this reason, various guidelines have been recommended using clinical and laboratory criteria to improve the accuracy of diagnosis and limit the inappropriate usage of antibiotics. The major problem in the diagnosis and treatment of adults with pharyngitis is not which of the multiple guidelines to follow, but that clinicians usually fail to follow any guideline at all.[4]

History

Although the symptoms of GABHS may be mild, frequent complaints are sudden onset of sore throat, headache, pain with swallowing, and fever. Abdominal pain, nausea, and vomiting may also be present.

Physical Examination

Frequent signs of GABHS are pharyngeal erythema, exudate, palatal petechiae, and anterior cervical lymphadenopathy. Sometimes a beefy red uvula is also present.[1] An associated sandpaper-like exanthem consisting of erythematous papules and located in the groin, neck, and axilla may be present, and the rash is referred to as scarletiniform (scarlet fever).

Laboratory Studies

The two tests most commonly used in the diagnosis of GABHS pharyngitis are a throat culture and one of a number of rapid antigen detection tests (RADTs). The various RADTs have very good specificity at about 95%, but the sensitivities vary at about 80% to 90% depending on the specific tool.[5] With that in mind, guidelines support a backup throat culture (gold standard) in children and adolescents with a negative RADT because of the small risk of acute rheumatic fever, but it is not necessary in adults as the risk is substantially less.[6,7] Culture is also unnecessary with a positive RADT because of its high specificity.

Classification

Clinical scoring systems are no longer recommended for use in differentiating the etiology of pharyngitis because of the broad overlap between the signs and symptoms of group A strep (GAS) and non-streptococcal causes—mostly viral.[6] Even when all the GAS criteria in a scoring system are present (e.g., fever, lack of cough, tender anterior cervical adenopathy, and tonsillar exudates), GABHS infection is found only 35% to 50% of the time. With identification of a streptococcal infection based on clinical grounds generally so poor, a laboratory test should be utilized in determining the presence of the infection, except when very obvious viral features such as conjunctivitis, hoarseness, cough, coryza, or oral ulcers are present. Additionally, diagnostic studies are not recommended for children less than 3 years old because of a low incidence of streptococcal pharyngitis and the rarity of acute rheumatic fever. An exception might be a symptomatic child with a school-aged sibling with a documented GABHS infection.[6]

Differential Diagnosis

A sore throat can have other noninfectious etiologies such as gastroesophageal reflux disease, postnasal drainage, thyroiditis, seasonal allergies, a foreign body, and smoking.[2]

TREATMENT

The goals of therapy of GABHS are to prevent suppurative complications and rheumatic fever (which is now very rare in most developed countries), decrease the length and severity of symptoms (may decrease symptoms by 1 to 2 days), and to limit the length of infectivity, allowing earlier return to work or school.[1] Treatment with antibiotics does not decrease the rate of poststreptococcal glomerulonephritis. Untreated GABHS may be infectious for up to 1 week after the acute illness,[2] and antibiotic treatment shortens that to 24 hours after the initiation of antibiotic treatment.[8]

Medications

The treatment of choice for GABHS continues to be penicillin because of its efficacy, narrow spectrum, and cost. Recommended regimens in adults are 250 TID–QID or 500 mg BID for 10 days, or 1.2 million units of benzathine penicillin G intramuscularly × 1. Children can be given 250 mg BID or TID for 10 days, or 600,000 units intramuscularly × 1 if less than 27 kg. Erythromycin and first-generation cephalosporins can be used in penicillin-allergic patients, although cephalosporins should not be used if the allergic response was an immediate-type hypersensitivity reaction.[6] Cephalosporins of varying generations have been shown to be twice as likely to give a bacteriologic cure for a GABHS infection in adults compared with penicillin, but 19 patients would need to be treated for one additional cure.[9]

Azithromycin and a number of broader spectrum cephalosporins have been effective in treating GABHS infections with a once-daily dosage; however, the expense and broad spectrum make this option less desirable. Shortened courses of therapy of some of these same antibiotics may be effective, but also have the same disadvantages noted.[6] Once-daily amoxicillin has been shown effective at 50 mg per kg up to 1,000 mg daily for 10 days.[10]

If a patient has a recurrent episode shortly after treatment, noncompliance or reexposure is more likely than treatment failure. Frequent, recurrent episodes of GABHS confirmed by culture or RADT in a symptomatic patient may be viral infections in a strep carrier (the *Streptococcus* is present in the pharynx with no immunologic response to it), or real GABHS infections. Amoxicillin/clavulanate or clindamycin has shown high rates of clearance of bacteria in this circumstance.

Other

Although not recommended in the clinical practice guidelines of the Infectious Diseases Society of America,[6] oral and intramuscular steroids have been shown to decrease duration and severity of pain in both children and adults with moderate to severe pharyngitis including GABHS infections.[11]

Operative

Clinicians should recommend watchful waiting for recurrent throat infections if there have been fewer than seven episodes in the past year or fewer than five episodes per year in the past 2 years or fewer than three episodes per year in the past 3 years.[12]

Risk Management

It is not necessary to test asymptomatic family contacts.[5] GABHS carriers are unlikely to infect close contacts, or develop secondary complications themselves. Up to 20% of school children in the winter/spring in temperate climates may be carriers.[6]

Follow-Up

It is not necessary to do a test of cure on asymptomatic patients.[5]

Complications

The suppurative complications are peritonsillar abscess, retropharyngeal abscess, mastoiditis, sinusitis, and otitis media. Nonsuppurative complications are rheumatic fever, which is rare in the United States and Europe, and poststreptococcal glomerulonephritis. There is no firm evidence that treating streptococcal pharyngitis will prevent glomerulonephritis.[1] Scarlet fever is a GABHS infection that produces an exotoxin, which induces the associated scarletiniform rash.[10]

REFERENCES

1. Bisno AL. Acute pharyngitis. *N Engl J Med* 2001;344(3):205–211.
2. Vincent MT, Celestin N, Hussain A. Pharyngitis. *Am Fam Physician* 2004;69(6):1465–1470.
3. Linder JA, Stafford RS. Antibiotic treatment of adults with sore throat by community primary care physicians: a national survey 1989–1999. *JAMA* 2001;286:1181–1186.
4. Linder JA, Chan JC, Bates DW. Evaluation and treatment of pharyngitis in primary care practice. The difference between guidelines is largely academic. *Arch Intern Med* 2006;166:1374–1379.
5. Humair JP, Revaz SA, Bovier P, et al. Management of acute pharyngitis in adults. Reliability of rapid streptococcal tests and clinical findings. *Arch Intern Med* 2006;166:640–644.
6. Shulman ST, Bisno AL, Clegg HW, et al. Clinical practice guideline for the diagnosis and management of group A streptococcal pharyngitis: 2012 update by the Infectious Diseases Society of America. *Clin Infect Dis* 2012;55(10):e86–e102.
7. Bisno AL, Gerber MA, Gwaltney JM Jr, et al. Practice guidelines for the diagnosis and management of group A streptococcal pharyngitis. *Clin Infect Dis* 2002;35:113–125.
8. Snellman LW, Stang HJ, Stang JM, et al. Duration of positive throat cultures for group A streptococci after initiation of antibiotic therapy. *Pediatrics* 1993;91(6):1166–1170.
9. Casey JR, Pinichero ME. Meta-analysis of cephalosporins versus penicillin for treatment of group A streptococcal tonsillopharyngitis in adults. *Clin Infect Dis* 2004;38(11):1526–1534.
10. 9. Andrews M, Condren M. Once-daily amoxicillin for pharyngitis. *J Pediatr Pharmacol Ther* 2010;15(4):244–248.

11. Hayward GI, Thompson MJ, Perera R, et al. Corticosteroids as stand alone or add-on treatment for sore throat. *Cochrane Database Syst Rev* 2012;10:CD008268.
12. Baugh RF, Archer SM, Mitchell RB, et al. Clinical practice guideline: tonsillectomy in children. *Otolaryngol Head Neck Surg* 2011;144(1 Suppl):S1–S30.

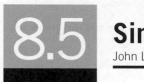

Sinusitis
John L. Smith

GENERAL PRINCIPLES
Definition

Rhinosinusitis is the term proposed by many authorities to replace the more commonly used term sinusitis.[1,2]

Anatomy

The frontal, ethmoid, and maxillary sinuses drain through the osteomeatal complex.

Classification

Acute bacterial rhinosinusitis (ABRS) by definition has less than a 4-week duration.[3] Chronic sinusitis is diagnosed with signs and symptoms lasting greater than 4 weeks.

Pathophysiology

The term rhinosinusitis more accurately reflects the pathophysiology of infection of the nasal and sinus cavities, because these cavities are contiguous. Impaired mucociliary clearance and osteomeatal obstruction contribute to the development of ABRS as well as chronic sinusitis.

Etiology

The majority of viral upper respiratory infections (URIs) ("common cold") also affect the sinus cavities[4] and therefore could be termed rhinosinusitis. Adults experience two to three colds per year and children from three to eight episodes.[5,6] Between 0.5% and 2% of URIs in adults and 5% and 10% in children develop into ABRS. The majority of community-acquired rhinosinusitis in adults and children is caused by *Streptococcus pneumoniae*, *Haemophilus influenzae*, and *Moraxella catarrhalis*.[1] One half to two thirds of patients with sinus symptoms who visit a family medicine clinic are unlikely to have bacterial infection.

Chronic sinusitis, when cultures are performed, often reveal a mixture of anaerobic and aerobic bacteria to include *Prevotella*, *Fusobacterium*, anaerobic streptococci, staphylococci, as well as those bacteria usually responsible for ABRS.[3] Chronic sinusitis is often secondary to noninfectious causes such as allergy, non-eosinophilic rhinosinusitis, gastroesophageal reflux disease, cystic fibrosis, immunodeficiencies, and anatomic considerations such as nasal septal deformities, polyps, and malignancies.[3]

DIAGNOSIS
History

In the office, clinicians rely on patient history and physical examination to make the diagnosis. A typical URI has an initially clear nasal discharge, which is often followed by a few days of an increased mucoid or purulent characteristic and then returns to clear or disappears.[7] A change in the color of the nasal discharge (so often reported by patients or caregivers) is, therefore, not a specific sign of bacterial infection, and may be due to the influx of neutrophils that may occur after a few days of viral infection.[1] Most often the constitutional symptoms and fever abate in the first couple of days.[7] The diagnosis of sinusitis (ABRS), consequently, is most often based on a departure from the typical viral course. URI symptoms not improving after 10 days or worsening after 5 to 7 days have an increased likelihood of a bacterial infection.[1,3,7,8] The diagnosis of ABRS is also made when symptoms of severe illness with a temperature >39°C or 102.2°F accompanied by purulent rhinorrhea or facial pain with signs and symptoms not improving after 3 days.[7,8] The likelihood of bacterial disease also increases with a history of facial pain, purulent rhinorrhea, and postnasal drainage. Other frequent symptoms are congestion, facial and maxillary pain, headache, and cough. The symptoms of ABRS are less specific in children than in adults. Symptoms include persistent nasal congestion, discharge of any color, and cough lasting more than 10 days.[7] Children are less likely to present with facial pain or headache. Many have vomiting from the mucous drainage.

Physical Examination

Erythema of the nasal mucosa, sinus tenderness, and orbital swelling are indicative of bacterial disease, with purulent drainage at the middle meatus even more predictive.[2] Pain is often a less prominent symptom in chronic sinusitis.

Laboratory

Results of blood studies, such as elevated sedimentation rate and C-reactive protein, are nonspecific indications of sinusitis. Nasal cultures are of limited value because the mixed flora does not correlate with bacteria aspirated directly from the sinuses.

Imaging

When necessary, contrast enhanced CT scan of the paranasal sinuses is the recommended imaging study.[7–9] CT scan is usually reserved for confirmatory evidence when the patient's signs and symptoms are vague or uncertain, for signs of orbital or CNS complications, or when the response to treatment is poor.[3,7–9] Classically, standard radiography has been used to detect acute sinusitis with the Caldwell (anterior–posterior) view used for assessing the frontal sinuses and the Water (occipitonasal) view for the maxillary sinuses, but they are not particularly sensitive.[10] A limitation of CT scanning is that it cannot differentiate bacterial from viral disease.[10]

Differential Diagnosis

The differential diagnosis of ABRS includes protracted viral URI, dental disease, nasal foreign body, migraine or cluster headaches, temporal arteritis, tension headaches, and temporomandibular disorders.

TREATMENT
Medications

Antibiotic therapy for ABRS is associated with improved outcomes, and is therefore recommended and based on the most likely etiologic agents and their susceptibilities. Indiscriminate use of antibiotics for URIs has resulted in an increase in resistance to the point that almost 40% of *S. pneumoniae* have at least intermediate resistance.[1,9] Resistance of pneumococci to penicillin is usually based on alterations in the penicillin-binding proteins, which leads to decreased affinity[1] and therefore can often be overcome with an increased dose. *H. influenzae* and *M. catarrhalis* resistance to penicillins is primarily secondary to β-lactamase production.[1,5,11] Given the high rate of viral disease and also the spontaneous remission rate of ABRS that is 50% to 70%,[5] standard antibiotic regimens with amoxicillin are 83% to 88% efficacious, while high-dose amoxicillin/clavulanate may reach 90% to 92%.[4,5]

Recent clinical practice guidelines have diverged on the initial empiric treatment of choice for mild sinusitis. The Infectious Diseases Society of America (IDSA) recommends amoxicillin with clavulanic acid, but admits this is a weak recommendation.[8] Pediatrics guidelines, as well as those from the University of Michigan Health System (UMHS), continue to recommend amoxicillin.[8,9] In keeping with the latter recommendations:

- In patients with mild severity illness, no antibiotic treatment in last 4 to 6 weeks, older than 2 years, and not in daycare, low-dose amoxicillin may be used. Amoxicillin 500 to 1,000 BID (in children 45 mg/kg/day) is used.
- In areas with a high prevalence of non-susceptible pneumococcus, high-dose amoxicillin (90 mg per kg) may be used up to 2,000 mg BID.
- In patients not meeting these criteria, high-dose amoxicillin with clavulanic acid is recommended with the amoxicillin component dosed at 90 mg/kg/day (maximum 4 g) and the clavulanate at 6.4 mg/kg/day divided BID.[7,9]

UMHS guidelines consider trimethoprim/sulfamethoxazole an alternative first line option, and in PCN allergic patients would allow macrolides, respiratory fluoroquinolones (not ciprofloxacin), and doxycycline. UMHS and Pediatrics also recommend cefuroxime, cefpodoxime, and cefdinir for patients who are allergic to penicillin without a type 1 hypersensitivity reaction. In children with a history of type 1 hypersensitivity reactions, a combination of cefixime and clindamycin or, if necessary, a respiratory fluoroquinolone may be used.[7,8] In adults, second-line therapies are respiratory fluoroquinolones and amoxicillin/clavulanate.[8,9]

The usual duration of treatment is 10 to 14 days; however, shorter courses of 5 to 7 days have been recommended by some,[8] and longer courses may be necessary in chronic sinusitis. If there is a lack of response after 3 to 5 days, reevaluate the antibiotic regimen and consider other options. Treatment with a macrolide after inadequate response to a cephalosporin may result in antibiotic failure 60% of the time.[4]

Topical and oral decongestants and antihistamines are not recommended.[7–9] Guaifenesin has not been shown to be useful in treating sinusitis. Nasal corticosteroids, such as mometasone, have been shown to be efficacious in improving the symptoms of rhinosinusitis.[6] Oral corticosteroids do not have proven efficacy, but may be helpful in patients who fail to respond to initial antibiotic therapy or have marked mucosal edema.

Special Therapy

Saline lavage or spray may help to liquefy secretions and improve drainage (1/4 tsp of salt in 8 oz of water).[3]

Surgery

Removing the adenoids has shown an improvement in rhinosinusitis in 70% to 80% of children.[2]

REFERENCES

1. Anon JB, Jacobs MR, Poole MD, et al. Antimicrobial treatment guidelines for acute bacterial rhinosinusitis [Review]. *Otolaryngol Head Neck Surg* 2004;130(1 Suppl):1–45.
2. Goldsmith A, Rosenfeld RM. Treatment of pediatric sinusitis. *Pediatr Clin North Am* 2003;50:413–426.
3. Slavin RG, Spector SL, Bernstein IL. The diagnosis and management of sinusitis: a practice parameter update. Joint Council of Allergy, Asthma, and Immunology. *J Allergy Clin Immunol* 2005;116:S13–S47.
4. Poole MD, Portugal LG. Treatment of rhinosinusitis in the outpatient setting. *Am J Med* 2005;118(7A):45S–50S.
5. Poole MD. Acute bacterial rhinosinusitis: clinical impact of resistance and susceptibility. *Am J Med* 2004;117(3A):29S–38S.
6. Meltzer EO, Bachert C, Staudinger H. Treating acute rhinosinusitis: comparing efficacy and safety of mometasone furoate nasal spray, amoxicillin, and placebo. *J Allergy Clin Immunol* 2005;116(6):1289–1295.
7. Wald ER, Appelgate KE, Bordley C, et al. Clinical practice guideline for the diagnosis and management of acute bacterial sinusitis in children aged 1–18 years. *Pediatrics* 2013;132:e262–e280.
8. Chow AW, Benninger MS, Brook I, et al. IDSA clinical practice guideline for acute bacterial rhinosinusitis in children and adults. *Clin Infect Dis* 2012;54(8):e72–e112.
9. University of Michigan Health System. Acute rhinosinusitis in adults. Ann Arbor (MI): University of Michigan Health System; 2011 August:9.
10. Mafee MF, Tran BH, Chapa AR. Imaging of rhinosinusitis and its complications: plain film, CT, and MRI. *Clin Rev Allergy Immunol* 2006;30(3):165–186.
11. Piccirillo JF. Acute bacterial sinusitis. *N Engl J Med* 2004;351:902–910.

8.6 Allergic Rhinitis

Denise K.C. Sur

GENERAL PRINCIPLES

- Allergic rhinitis is a common condition affecting approximately 20% of the US population and ranking as the sixth most prevalent chronic illness in the United States. Patients with this condition can be severely restricted in their daily activities and spend excessive time away from work and school.

DIAGNOSIS

History

- The history is the major diagnostic tool in recognizing allergy as a cause of rhinitis. The most common symptoms of allergic rhinitis are paroxysms of sneezing, rhinorrhea, nasal and palatal pruritus, ocular symptoms, and nasal obstruction. Allergic rhinitis can be either seasonal or perennial, with the seasonal type primarily related to pollen and the perennial type related to indoor allergens such as molds, dust mites, cockroaches, and animal dander.
- Other types of rhinitis include eosinophilic nonallergic rhinitis, vasomotor rhinitis, and rhinitis medicamentosa. Patients with eosinophilic nonallergic rhinitis or vasomotor rhinitis usually do not experience pruritus or paroxysms of sneezing. Patients with rhinitis medicamentosa usually have a history of repetitive topical decongestant use.
- Nasal congestion associated with headache, purulent rhinorrhea, postnasal discharge, and halitosis suggests sinusitis (see also Chapter 8.5). Persistent unilateral obstruction suggests the presence of polyps or other structural obstructions.
- Risk factors for allergic rhinitis include a family history of atopy, exposure to indoor allergens such as dust mites, birth during the pollen season, early antibiotic use, and maternal smoking exposures in the first year of life.[1]

Physical Examination

- Patients with allergic rhinitis, whether seasonal or perennial, often have pale, bluish, boggy mucosa and clear secretions. Children may have darkening under the eyes and a nasal crease resulting from rubbing the nose. Conjunctivitis may or may not be present. The nonallergic patient, especially the patient with vasomotor rhinitis, is more apt to have erythematous mucosa with secretions of any color or consistency.

Laboratory Testing

- Skin testing (epicutaneous [prick] testing) with appropriate antigens and positive- and negative-control substances is the most useful procedure for detection of allergic triggers in allergic rhinitis, but is not necessary for the diagnosis or treatment of allergic rhinitis. Skin testing is specific and sensitive, and can assist in management by either avoidance or immunotherapy. It is important to note that food allergies need not be routinely tested because they rarely play a role in allergic rhinitis.
- A specific serum immunoglobulin E (IgE) radioallergosorbent test (RAST) should be used in lieu of skin testing only when the patient has severe eczema or dermatographism. RAST testing is less sensitive and more expensive than skin testing.

TREATMENT

Three approaches may be used: avoidance, medication, and immunotherapy.

Avoidance

- Avoidance of allergen exposure is always indicated but may be difficult to achieve.
- Patients with allergic rhinitis should avoid exposure to cigarette smoke, pets, and allergens to which they have known sensitivity. Although measures that help control indoor allergen exposure include placement of dust-proof covers over pillows and mattresses, frequent dusting of surfaces and floors with a damp mop, and maintenance of an indoor humidity below 50% have been

TABLE 8.6-1	Commonly Used Antihistamines
Antihistamine	**Usual dosage**
First-generation antihistamines	
Bropheniramine	12–24 mg PO q12h
Chlorpheniramine maleate (Chlor-Trimeton)	4 mg PO q4–6h
Diphenhydramine (Benadryl)	25–50 mg PO q4–6h
Promethazine (Phenergan)	12.5 mg PO q12h
Second-generation antihistamines	
Cetirizine (Zyrtec)	5–10 mg PO daily
Desloratadine (Clarinex)	5 mg PO daily
Fexofenadine	180 mg PO daily
Loratadine	10 mg PO daily

proposed, studies have not found any benefit.[2–4] Measures that help control outdoor allergens include closing of windows, running of air conditioners, and avoidance of lawn mowing and leaf raking may be helpful.

Medications

- **Antihistamines.** These medications relieve sneezing, itching, and rhinorrhea but not congestion. They are less efficacious than nasal steroids but equally or more effective than cromolyn.[5,6] Their most common adverse effects are sedation, performance/learning impairment, and anticholinergic effects (dry mouth, constipation, urinary retention, and abdominal pain). Because they cross the blood–brain barrier easily and therefore increase the likelihood of sedative side effects, first-generation antihistamines have limited usefulness in the treatment of allergic rhinitis. Compared with first-generation antihistamines, second-generation medications are equally or more effective, have fewer adverse effects, and are, therefore, preferred. Of the second-generation antihistamines, both loratadine and fexofenadine have FDA approval on labeling as non-sedating. Cetirizine does not have this labeling because it produces a higher incidence of somnolence and fatigue than placebo. Cetirizine and fexofenadine are appropriate for use in children >6 months of age. Azelastine, an intranasal antihistamine preparation, offers acute symptomatic relief with minimal sedation. Its main drawback is that it leaves a bad taste in the mouth. Commonly used antihistamines are listed in Table 8.6-1.
- **Decongestants.** Oral decongestants are α-adrenergic agonists. They have been shown to be effective but can cause side effects, including hypertension, nervousness, insomnia, irritability, headache, palpitations, and urinary obstruction and are contraindicated in patients with glaucoma or using monoamine oxidase inhibitors. Increasing abuse of pseudoephedrine has led to the substitution of phenylephrine in many over-the-counter preparations. Unfortunately, phenylephrine is less effective for the treatment of rhinitis. Finally, nasal decongestants should be used for only 2 to 3 days because prolonged use can lead to rebound congestion and rhinitis medicamentosa.
- The most commonly used decongestant is pseudoephedrine (Sudafed), 60 mg PO q4–6h.
- **Inhaled steroids.** Topical nasal corticosteroids are the **most potent medical treatment** currently available for allergic rhinitis and should be first-line therapy. They have been proven safe for long-term use but can occasionally cause nasal irritation, burning, and bloody nasal discharge. Rare reports of septal perforation have been made. Some nasal corticosteroids are approved for use in children older than 2 years and one formulation, Nasacort, just became available for over-the-counter use. Commonly used inhaled steroids are listed in Table 8.6-2.
- **Anti-leukotriene agents.** Montelukast is the only allergic rhinitis agent in this class approved for the management of allergic rhinitis. It is less effective than intranasal glucocorticoids and antihistamines but may have a role in patients not tolerating nasal sprays. Its adverse effects include insomnia, anxiety, and depression, which limit its use in patients with mood disorders.
- **Inhaled mast cell stabilizers.** Nasal cromolyn sodium (Nasalcrom) is available over-the-counter and has been shown to be beneficial in treating allergic rhinitis in both adults and children. Its full effect may take up to 3 to 4 weeks, and adherence may be decreased secondary to need for use four times a day, but its use may eliminate the need for antihistamines and decongestants in the long term.

TABLE 8.6-2 Commonly Used Inhaled Agents

	Dosage
Steroid	
Beclomethasone	1–2 sprays each nostril bid
Budesonide (Rhinocort)	2 sprays each nostril bid or 4 sprays each nostril qd
Flunisolide (Nasalide)	2 sprays each nostril bid
Fluticasone propionate (Flonase)	2 sprays each nostril qd or 1 spray each nostril bid
Triamcinolone acetonide (Nasacort)	2 sprays each nostril qd
Mometasone furoate	2 sprays each nostril qd
Dexamethasone sodium phosphate	2 sprays each nostril bid–tid
Antihistamine	
Azelastine	1–2 sprays each nostril bid
Olopatadine	2 sprays in each nostril bid
Mast cell stabilizers	
Cromolyn (Nasalcrom)	1 spray each nostril tid–qid

On the basis of its human and animal safety profiles, cromolyn should be the first drug considered for the management of allergic rhinitis in pregnant women and may be preferred in patients with allergic rhinitis and asthma.

- **Inhaled antihistamines.** Two topical antihistamines, azelastine and olopatadine are now available. They are shown effective in placebo-controlled studies and, like oral antihistamines, can cause sedation.
- **Inhaled anticholinergics.** Ipratropium bromide relieves rhinorrhea only and is appropriate for patients 6 years of age or older with rhinorrhea not controlled with other medications.

Immunotherapy

- Subcutaneous immunotherapy is the administration of increasing doses of allergens to which the patient is sensitive and is the only available treatment that has a disease-modifying effect. It is indicated when severe symptoms are present that do not respond to avoidance or medication. Allergy injections given over a 3- to 5-year period may reduce symptoms in approximately 85% of cases but requires multiple injections that must be administered in a medical office.
- Sublingual immunotherapy is used extensively throughout Europe but is not yet approved for use in the United States. A systematic review of 63 randomized, placebo-controlled trials, including 5,131 children and adults with allergic rhinitis and asthma yielded good support of sublingual immunotherapy for asthma and moderate support for rhinitis and conjunctivitis.[7]

REFERENCES

1. Gendo K, Larson EB. Evidence-based diagnostic strategies for evaluating suspected allergic rhinitis. *Ann Intern Med* 2004;140:278.
2. Koopman LP, van Strien RT, Kerkhof M, et al; Prevention and Incidence of Asthma and Mite Allergy (PIAMA) Study. Placebo-controlled trial of house dust mite-impermeable mattress covers effect on symptom in early childhood. *Am J Respir Crit Care Med* 2002;166(3):307–313.
3. Terreehorst I, Hak E, Oosting AJ, et al. Evaluation of impermeable covers for bedding in patients with allergic rhinitis. *N Engl J Med* 2003;349(3):237–246.
4. Sheikh A, Hurwitz B, Shehata Y. House dust mite avoidance measures for perennial allergic rhinitis. *Cochrane Database Syst Rev* 2007;(1):CD001563.
5. van Bavel J, Findlay SR, Hampel FC Jr, et al. Intranasal fluticasone propionate is more effective than terfenadine tablets for seasonal allergic rhinitis. *Arch Intern Med* 1994;154:2699.
6. Welsch PW, Stickerk WE, Chu CP, et al. Efficacy of beclomethasone nasal solution, flunisolide, cromolyn in relieving symptoms of ragweed allergy. *Mayo Clin Proc* 1987;62:125.
7. Agosti JM, Sanes-Miller CM. Novel therapeutic approaches for allergic rhinitis. *Immunol Clin North Am* 2000;20:401.

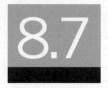

Head and Neck Malignancies

Jason M. Patera

INTRODUCTION

Head and neck cancer encompasses cancer of the paranasal sinuses, nasal cavity, oral cavity, salivary glands, pharynx, larynx, and thyroid. This chapter focuses on squamous cell carcinomas of the head and neck (HNSCC) as they account for more than 90% of head and neck cancers.[1] Thyroid disorders are discussed elsewhere in the text.

DEFINITION

The head and neck consist of the above-mentioned areas that are defined as follows:

- Paranasal sinuses—maxillary, frontal, sphenoid, ethmoid sinuses
- Nasal cavity—passageway ending posteriorly at nasopharynx, bordered by paranasal sinuses
- Oral cavity—floor of the mouth, anterior tongue, lips, buccal mucosa, hard palate, retromolar trigone, and gingiva
- Nasopharynx—posterior to the nasal cavity, from the base of the skull to the soft palate
- Oropharynx—posterior tongue, epiglottis, tonsils, soft palate, and associated pharyngeal wall
- Hypopharynx—pyriform sinuses, posterior larynx, posterior pharyngeal wall (from the level of the epiglottis superiorly to the level of the cricoid inferiorly)
- Larynx—vocal cords and epiglottis

EPIDEMIOLOGY

Head and neck cancer is estimated to account for 55,070 new cases and 12,000 deaths in the United States in 2014.[2] These cancers occur at a much increased incidence in men, which is especially true with the increasing incidence of HPV-associated squamous cell carcinoma (SCC).[3] While decreased tobacco use has resulted in a decrease in related HNSCC, the increasing prevalence of HPV has created an offsetting increase in HNSCC.[3] Increasing age is also a risk factor of development of HNSCC, but human papilloma virus (HPV)-related cancers are associated with a relatively earlier age of onset.[4] A recent cross-sectional study of adults 14 to 69 years of age revealed an HPV prevalence of 6.9%. HPV was most common between the ages of 30–34 and 60–64, and three times more common in men versus women.[5]

HPV-related HNSCC most commonly involves the oropharynx, with HPV subtypes 16 and 18 being the most common. These HNSCCs are occurring at a younger age and at a disproportionately higher rate in males. Fortunately, these also carry a more favorable prognosis.[3]

Tobacco (smoked and smokeless) is a well-known risk factor for HNSCC with a powerful impact; smokers are 10 times more likely to develop HNSCC than non-smokers.[6] Alcohol consumption is associated with HNSCC development and has been found to play a synergistic role with tobacco, creating a 30-fold increased risk in individuals that smoke and drink.[2]

DIAGNOSIS

History

Most head and neck cancers occur in men, usually older than 50 years of age. However, with increasing incidence of HPV-related HNSCC, the diagnosis is commonly made earlier. The symptoms are largely dependent on the location of the primary tumor. Because of the complexity of the anatomy and lack of cancer-specific symptoms, early recognition of head and neck cancers requires a thorough history and evaluation. Persistent symptoms in the head and neck area warrant further investigation.

Cancers of the nasopharynx commonly present with nasal obstruction, epistaxis, headaches, and neck masses from metastases. Obstruction of the nasopharynx and eustachian tube can lead to unilateral serous otitis media. Persistent or recurrent otitis media can be due to obstruction from a nasopharyngeal carcinoma.

Cancers of the oral cavity often present as non-healing ulcers, lesions, or masses. They can lead to poorly fitting dentures and dental changes. Tongue and lip lesions present as exophytic or ulcerative lesions often with associated pain and bleeding. Premalignant findings, such as erythroplakia or leukoplakia, can be present. Bleeding, referred otalgia, and dysarthria can also occur with oral cavity cancer.

Cancer of the oropharynx can lead to decreased tongue mobility and altered speech. Often times, lesions in the posterior oropharynx and hypopharynx do not present with early symptoms. Symptoms can include sore throat and ear pain. The cancers can also contribute to obstructive sleep apnea and present with snoring.

Laryngeal cancer can present in several ways depending on the location. Persistent hoarseness is a common presentation, and is why a full ENT evaluation is indicated if hoarseness persists beyond 2 weeks without another clear cause. Other common symptoms include dysphagia, chronic cough, hemoptysis, and stridor. When the cancer presents late, palpable lymph nodes may be the presenting complaint.

Head and neck cancers can cause a variety of nonspecific and chronic symptoms. Symptoms of hoarseness, otalgia, odynophagia, and chronic cough warrant significant concern. Any mass that is noted deserves a complete evaluation.

Physical Examination and Workup

The physical examination for initial evaluation consists of thorough inspection and palpation. The family physician should inspect the external auditory canals and tympanic membranes. The skin and mucosal surfaces of the head and neck should be carefully inspected. Palpation of the tongue, palate, and floor of the mouth should be performed. Lymph nodes in the head and neck should be thoroughly and systematically palpated. A complete examination includes indirect mirror examination of the oropharynx, hypopharynx and larynx, and direct endoscopy.

An examination under anesthesia is performed to enable biopsies, further endoscopic evaluation, and better characterize the location and extent of the tumor. Fine needle aspiration is commonly used to establish the diagnosis of cancer when a patient presents with a suspicious mass or lymph node. Head and neck imaging (CT, MRI) is commonly done to assess for lymph node involvement and the extent of invasion. Panendoscopy (laryngoscopy, bronchoscopy, and esophagoscopy) and positron emission tomography scanning can help find distant metastases, most commonly occurring in lungs, liver, and bone, as well as second primary malignancies, which occur most commonly in the head and neck, lungs, and esophagus. Distant metastases are found in less than 10% of patients at diagnosis and are most commonly found in patients with advanced nodal involvement at presentation. Tumor staging with the TNM staging system is site dependent.

TREATMENT

With HNSCC, about one-third of patients present with stage I or II disease, providing them with a 70% to 90% 5-year survival. Treatment at this early stage is typically surgical excision or definitive radiation therapy.[7] The decision between modalities is often based on accessibility, lending the oral cavity to better outcomes with surgical excision than the rest of the head and neck. It should be noted that patients with tobacco- and alcohol-related cancers are at an increased risk of recurrence and careful monitoring is required.

When cancers of the head and neck present at an advanced stage, treatment options become more numerous and varied. A multidisciplinary approach utilizing chemotherapy, radiation and surgery, in various combinations and sequences, is key to providing favorable outcomes. For example, SCC of the tongue base is an aggressive cancer that commonly presents with stage III or IV disease. These tumors are routinely treated with radiation therapy, which maximizes preservation of anatomy and function. With the increasing incidence of HPV-related cancers of the tonsils and tongue base, these tumors are having a more favorable prognosis and improved response to treatment.

REFERENCES

1. Tribius S, Hoffman M. Human papilloma virus infection in head and neck cancer. *Dtsch Arzteb Int* 2013;110:184–190.
2. American Cancer Society. *Cancer Facts & Figures 2014*. Atlanta: American Cancer Society; 2014.
3. Bose P, Brockton NT, Dort JC. Head and neck cancer: from anatomy to biology. *Int J Cancer* 2013;133(9):2013–2023.
4. Chaturvedi AK, Engels EA, Pfeiffer RM, et al. Human papillomavirus and rising oropharyngeal cancer incidence in the United States. *J Clin Oncol* 2011;29(32):4294–4301.

5. Gillison ML, Broutian T, Pickard RK. Prevalence of oral HPV infection in the United States, 2009–2010. *JAMA* 2012;307(7):693–703.

6. Sturgis E M, Cinciripini PM. Trends in head and neck cancer incidence in relation to smoking prevalence: an emerging epidemic of human papillomavirus-associated cancers? *Cancer* 2007;110(7):1429–1435.

7. Vokes EE. Head and neck cancer. In: Longo D, Fauci A, Kasper D, et al, eds. *Harrison's manual of medicine*. 18th ed. New York, NY: McGraw-Hill Medical; 2013.

CHAPTER 9

Cardiovascular Problems

Section editor: Douglas J. Inciarte

9.1 Hypertension

Oscar O. Perez Jr, Michael R. King

GENERAL PRINCIPLES

Systemic hypertension (HTN) in adults is defined as systolic blood pressure (SBP) of 140 mmHg or higher or diastolic blood pressure (DBP) of 90 mmHg or higher, based on the average of at least two readings taken with the patient comfortable and at rest. Prehypertension is defined as SBP 120 to 139 mmHg or DBP 80 to 89 mmHg.

The accuracy of the blood pressure (BP) determination rises with the number of BP readings averaged. Borderline readings should be averaged over at least three visits. Abnormal readings should be initially confirmed in the contralateral arm.

HTN is the most common diagnosis recorded during adult visits to primary care physicians. The prevalence of HTN rises with age, affecting more than 35% of American residents ages 40 to 59 years and 65% of those 60 or older, with an increasing prevalence that at age >75 years, approaching 80% of the population.

Risk factors for developing HTN include prehypertension, obesity, a family history of HTN, African American heritage, type 2 diabetes mellitus, and increasing age. Although common, it is not normal for BP to increase with age in adults, but the absolute health risks from HTN increase with age.

HTN is a powerful risk factor for myocardial infarction (MI), congestive heart failure (CHF), stroke, kidney failure, and premature death. The risk of developing cardiovascular disease doubles with each 20 mmHg increment of SBP or each 10 mmHg increment of DBP above 115/75 mmHg. In controlled clinical trials, treatment of HTN reduces the risk of CHF by 50%, stroke by 35% to 40%, and MI by 20% to 25%.

DIAGNOSIS

Clinical Presentation

HTN is usually asymptomatic until it produces morbid sequelae such as angina, MI, stroke, or CHF. Some patients get HTN-related headaches at malignant levels of high BP, but it is often hard to determine whether the headache was a cause or an effect of elevated BP. However, emerging research from Norway hints that patients with HTN suffer from less headache frequency than do patients with normal BP. These findings paralleled earlier research that found that people with elevated, untreated high BP were as much as 50% less likely to suffer a headache than were patients with similar health profiles but normal BP.

Target organ damage (TOD) refers to symptomatic or asymptomatic hypertensive injury to the heart, brain, kidneys, eyes, or large arteries. TOD is common, but may be missed unless evidence for it is sought.

HTN is classified according to severity as Stage 1 (SBP 140 to 159 mmHg or DBP 90 to 99 mmHg) or Stage 2 (SBP 160 to 179 mmHg or DBP 100 to 109 mmHg). Classification is defined by either SBP or DBP, whichever falls into the higher stage.

History

The history should be obtained with three general aims in mind:

- Detection of exacerbating conditions or reversible causes of HTN
- Diagnosis of morbid sequelae from HTN
- Assessment of other risk factors for cardiovascular and renal disease

For each of these aims, history should be followed by careful physical examination and a few well-chosen tests.

The history should include assessment of lifestyle factors, comorbidities, and medications, which may cause or exacerbate HTN. The clinician should probe for alcohol or drug abuse, sleep apnea, pregnancy, renal artery stenosis (atherosclerotic if HTN began after age 50, congenital if onset was before age 30), hyperthyroidism or hypothyroidism, primary renal disease, panic disorder, primary hyperaldosteronism, and medication side effects (e.g., oral contraceptives, corticosteroids, stimulants). Although many patients may have one or more of these factors contributing to their HTN, only about 5% of patients have a solely reversible cause for their HTN.

The most common symptomatic morbid sequelae of HTN are angina, MI, stroke, transient ischemic attack (TIA), and CHF. Hypertensive renal failure is relatively rare, as is visual loss. Hypertensive TOD underlies each of these sequelae. Asymptomatic TOD is even more common and must also be considered, including chronic kidney disease (CKD) or acute kidney injury, left ventricular hypertrophy, silent coronary artery disease, hypertensive retinopathy, and peripheral arterial disease (such as carotid stenosis or abdominal aortic aneurysm).

Risk stratification includes assessment of TOD and other major cardiovascular risk factors, including family history; tobacco use; and history of diabetes, dyslipidemia, or renal insufficiency. Their presence and severity increase the clinical risk for HTN, and the importance of its control.

Physical Examination

The diagnosis of HTN depends on accurate BP readings that reflect the patient's usual BP. Readings taken when a patient is acutely ill or in pain should not be used to diagnose HTN. Routine BP measurements should be taken with the patient seated, after at least 5 minutes of rest, with the arm and back supported and the arm at the level of the heart with uncrossed feet, both flat on the floor. Note the index marks on the BP cuff to ensure proper placement and fit. SBP should be recorded at the onset of sounds, and DBP at their disappearance. At least two readings are recommended at each visit. Falsely elevated readings may occur if the BP cuff is too small or if severe atherosclerosis is present. If the radial artery is still palpable as a "cord" after inflating the cuff until the pulse is obliterated, then systolic readings are probably not reliable.

Home BP measurements are typically about 5 to 10 mmHg lower than those taken in the medical office, and average home BP levels above 135/85 mmHg should be considered hypertensive. Understanding this caveat, home BP readings can improve the accuracy of diagnosis and classification, and enhance patients' commitment to controlling their HTN. A consistent and significant discrepancy between BP levels at home and in the medical office beyond 10 mmHg may warrant further investigation, including ambulatory BP monitoring.

Automatic ambulatory BP monitoring improves diagnostic and prognostic accuracy. But for reasons of practicality, it should be reserved for patients in whom a significant "white-coat" response is highly suspected, or for patients with symptoms of paroxysmal hypotension or paroxysmal HTN.

The remainder of the physical examination should include height, weight, and assessments of cardiovascular and neurologic status. The latter include:

- Fundoscopic examination to look for signs of atherosclerosis and hypertensive retinopathy
- Auscultation of the heart and the lungs to detect rales, heart murmurs, gallops, and arrhythmias
- Palpation and auscultation of the carotid arteries and major peripheral arteries to detect diminished pulses and bruits as signs of atherosclerosis
- Assessments for peripheral edema and jugular venous distension that may indicate CHF
- A neurologic survey examination to screen for signs of a past stroke

Laboratory Studies

Laboratory studies should be used to aid in assessments for TOD, to identify other cardiovascular risk factors, and to diagnose conditions that may exacerbate BP elevation or be reversible causes for HTN.

Unless the history and physical examination suggest otherwise, initial laboratory testing can be limited to:

- Serum electrolytes, blood urea nitrogen (BUN), and creatinine
- Complete blood count
- Fasting blood glucose level or HbA1c
- Fasting serum lipid profile
- Urinalysis and a spot urine albumin/creatinine ratio

A standard 12-lead resting electrocardiogram (ECG) should be performed as a baseline study and to assess for conduction abnormalities that may have implications for antihypertensive medication choices. ECG signs of left ventricular hypertrophy or ischemic heart disease should be given attention, but the resting ECG is not a good screening test for these problems.

TREATMENT
Behavioral

Beneficial lifestyle changes (diet, exercise, and alcohol restriction) should be included in the management of all hypertensive patients. These can suffice as the sole therapy for asymptomatic patients with Stage 1 HTN who have no evidence of TOD or diabetes, if BP can be kept lower than 140/90 mmHg. In patients with CKD or diabetes, there no longer remains a recommendation to treat to a more aggressive target (previously 130/80). It is recommended that these patients have their BP targets mirror those of the uncomplicated hypertensive patient (140/90). If the lifestyle changes suggested below do not control BP after 6 months, drug therapy should be added for most patients. For patients with *no TOD and no other cardiovascular risk factor*, giving lifestyle changes up to 12 months is reasonable. Most patients with TOD or diabetes will require antihypertensive medication to achieve target BP. Nonpharmacologic treatment can be expected to lower BP on the order of 4 to 15/2 to 8 mmHg. The same lifestyle alterations are also recommended for the primary prevention of HTN.

The nonpharmacologic treatments for HTN supported by evidence from controlled trials are as follows:

- **Weight loss:** Patients who are at least 10% above ideal body weight, or whose body mass index exceeds 27, should be instructed on a regimen of diet and exercise that can be sustained indefinitely. Gradual and maintained weight loss is the goal.
- **Low-sodium diet:** The average American consumes 4 to 5 g of sodium (9.5 to 12 g of salt) daily, mostly in processed foods. Limiting dietary sodium to less than 2 g per day is recommended. Patients should be taught to use food labels and to make healthy choices in restaurants.
- **DASH diet:** A low-fat diet rich in fruits, vegetables, low-fat dairy, fish, poultry, whole grains and nuts, with little red meat, sweets, or sugary drinks, is recommended. This diet also emphasizes potassium-rich foods such as bananas, citrus, tomatoes, broccoli, squash, and green leafy vegetables.
- **Moderation of alcohol** to less than two standard drinks per day: One drink equals 12 oz of beer, 5 oz of wine, or 2 oz of liquor. Some patients (especially women) may be sensitive enough to alcohol that further restriction is necessary.
- **Regular aerobic activity:** Regular activities such as brisk walking, jogging, cycling, and tennis pursued on most days lower BP and overall cardiovascular risk independently of weight loss. Aerobic exercise also reduces overall cardiovascular risk by other mechanisms. A regular walking routine is a reasonable exercise regimen for most patients.

Adherence to treatment for a generally asymptomatic condition, whether behavior change or medication use, is often difficult for patients. The physician should set a schedule of regular follow-up and encourage open dialog with sensitivity to patient views, values, and culture.

Medications

There are more than 70 different drugs approved for use in the United States for treating HTN. Grouping these drugs into pharmacologic classes aids in therapeutic decision making. The major classes and subclasses of antihypertensive drugs available in the United States, with one example of each, are shown in Table 9.1-1. Preparations containing two antihypertensive drugs are also available. Table 9.1-1 shows only starting doses; full prescribing information should be read and reviewed before prescribing.

| TABLE 9.1-1 | Antihypertensive Drug Classes with Example Drugs |

Class/subclass/drug name (trade name)	Starting dose[a]
Diuretics	
Thiazides	
Hydrochlorothiazide (HydroDIURIL, others)	25 mg qd
Potassium sparing	
Amiloride (Midamor)	5 mg qd
Loop	
Furosemide (Lasix)	20 mg bid
β-Blockers	
Without ISA	
Atenolol (Tenormin)	50 mg qd
With ISA	
Acebutolol (Sectral)	200 mg bid
α–β-Blocker	
Labetalol (Normodyne, Trandate)	100 mg bid
Angiotensin-converting enzyme inhibitors	
Lisinopril (Prinivil, Zestril)	10 mg qd
Calcium-channel blockers	
Dihydropyridines	
Amlodipine (Norvasc)	5 mg qd
Diltiazem (Cardizem, others)	120 mg qd (b)
Verapamil (Calan, others)	180 mg qd[b]
Angiotensin receptor blockers	
Losartan (Cozaar)	50 mg qd
Aldosterone antagonists	
Spironolactone (Aldactone)	25 mg qd
α₁-Blockers	
Doxazosin (Cardura)	1 mg qd
Central α₂-agonists	
Clonidine (Catapres)	0.1 mg bid
Peripheral antiadrenergics	
Reserpine (Serpasil)	0.1 mg qd
Direct vasodilators	
Hydralazine (Apresoline)	10–25 mg qid
Direct renin inhibitors	
Aliserken (Tekturna)	150 mg qd

ISA, intrinsic sympathomimetic activity.
[a]Review of full prescribing information is strongly advised.
[b]Sustained-release formulations recommended.

Medication regimens should be individualized for each patient based on the following:

- Evidence that the drug(s) will improve the patient's long-term health (not just lower BP)
- The patient's comorbidities and other cardiovascular risk factors
- The patient's past responses or reactions to medications
- Potential drug interactions
- Factors (such as cost and dosing convenience) that will affect the patient's ability to adhere to the prescribed treatment

African Americans and elderly patients tend to respond better to thiazide diuretics and calcium-channel blockers (CCBs) than they do to other classes of medications, but the other considerations above should take precedence over age and race.

High-quality evidence from controlled clinical trials has led to compelling indications for certain classes of antihypertensive drugs in the presence of certain types of TOD or comorbidity, as shown

TABLE 9.1-2	Guidelines for Choosing Initial Drugs for Hypertension Based on Comorbidities

	Coexisting medical condition								
Drug	Pregnancy	CAD	CHF	LVH	↓HR	DM	COPD	Gout	CKD
Diuretics									
Thiazide	—	—	Yes	—	—	Yes	—	No	No
Loop	—	—	Yes	—	—	—	—	No	Yes
Potassium sparing	—	—	Yes	—	—	—	—	—	No
β-Blockers									
Without ISA	—[b]	Best	Yes[c]	—	No	Yes[a]	No	—	—
With ISA	—	—	—	—	—	—[a]	No	—	—
Labetalol	Yes	—	No	—	No	—	No	—	—
ACE inhibitors	No	Yes	Yes	—	—	Best	—	—	Best[d]
Calcium blockers									
Diltiazem	—	—	No	—	No	—	—	—	Yes
Verapamil	—	—	No	—	No	—	—	—	Yes
Dihydropyridines	—	—	—	—	—	Yes	—	—	Yes
α$_2$-Agonist	—	—	—	—	—	—	—	—	—
Aldosterone antagonists	No	—	Yes	—	—	—	—	—	—
Angiotensin blocker	No	—	Yes	Yes	—	Yes	—	—	Best[d]
Methyldopa	Yes	—	—	—	—	—	No	—	No
Direct renin inhibitors									
Tekturna	—	—	—	—	—	—	—	—	—

Combined therapy with two drugs from different classes should be considered in most cases.
Best, first choice; Yes, drug is preferred; No, drug is relatively contraindicated; —, drug is acceptable but evidence is insufficient to rank treatment options.
ACE, angiotensin-converting enzyme; CAD, coronary artery disease; CHF, congestive heart failure; COPD, chronic obstructive pulmonary disease; CKD, chronic kidney disease; DM, diabetes mellitus; HR, bradycardia; ISA, intrinsic sympathomimetic activity; LVH, left ventricular hypertrophy.
[a]Caution in diabetes: β-Blockers may blunt awareness of hypoglycemia.
[b]Avoid atenolol in pregnancy.
[c]Combine with diuretic and ACE inhibitor for systolic CHF.
[d]ACE inhibitors and angiotensin blockers are contraindicated in bilateral renal artery stenosis, or if serum creatinine is >3.0 mg/dL. The combination is no longer recommended in patients with or without heart failure.

in Table 9.1-2. For all other patients, first-line medications are based on the strength of evidence that they reduce cardiovascular risk.

The first-line antihypertensive drug classes are thiazide diuretics (TZD), angiotensin-converting enzyme inhibitors (ACEIs), CCBs, and angiotensin receptor blockers (ARBs). β-Receptor blockers no longer enjoy a first-line status in the treatment of HTN, indicated by national guidelines released by the AHA in 2013. Among the remaining choices, a TZD should be included in most patients' regimens because of low cost of TZDs and consistent evidence for their high efficacy across multiple controlled trials. Caution: TZD can precipitate gout attacks, and should be avoided in patients with known gout.

For most patients, each medication should be started at the lowest recommended dosage and titrated upward, if necessary, at 2- to 8-week intervals, depending on the severity of the HTN. Elderly patients may require even lower doses. Begin with a single-drug or a low-dose combination. More than one half of patients will require at least two medications to control their HTN. Dose titration and switching of medications are often both necessary. Patient education about this is important to engender trust and realistic expectations.

Follow-Up

Well patients with Stage 1 HTN should have follow-up visits every 1 to 2 months until the BP goal is reached without significant medication side effects (i.e., side effects that are unacceptable to the patient or the physician). Patients with Stage 2 HTN and/or complicating comorbidities should be seen every 2 to 4 weeks until the BP is clearly coming under control without unacceptable side effects. Once the BP goals are reached and stable on a given therapeutic regimen, follow-up can be stretched out to 6 months, unless other conditions dictate more frequent visits.

Goal BP levels should be SBP <140 mmHg and DBP <90 mmHg for most patients. However, in patient >59 years of age, the JNC-8 now has given the strongest of recommendations (Grade A evidence from randomized controlled trials), to treat to a goal of SBP of <151 and a DBP of <91. As mentioned previously, neither diabetics nor patients with CKD require any more aggressive BP goals than those of the uncomplicated hypertensive patient (140/90). Many clinicians choose to set target BP levels below these threshold because in population-based studies cardiovascular risk rises steadily with BP level, starting at SBP >115 mmHg or DBP >75 mmHg. However, care should be taken to avoid overly aggressive BP reduction in elderly patients, because they are at higher risk for orthostasis, tend to have stiffer arteries, and are at higher risk for stroke from episodic hypotension.

If treatment goals have not been met at the prescribed follow-up intervals, the medication dose should be changed, a different class of drug should be tried, or a second drug from another class should be added (see Table 9.1-1). Combining two first-line drugs from different classes at low to moderate doses is often effective, and including a diuretic is desirable. However, the exception to this is the use of a dual blockade method of the renin–angiotensin–aldosterone system. Several new randomized trials and a meta-analysis all showed that there was no benefit to the use of dual blockade (an ACE + an ARB), and indeed, may harm patients with or without heart failure. Avoid unwanted drug interactions, especially those that have cardiac and electrolyte effects. β-Blockers, central sympatholytics, α_1-blockers, and peripheral antiadrenergics are best reserved as second-line drugs (except in pregnancy, as discussed below). Direct vasodilators are useful for patients failing treatment with first- and second-line drugs, but they should be combined with a diuretic.

Laboratory tests at follow-up are determined by the type of therapy, comorbid conditions, and the baseline values.

Special Therapy

Hypertensive crises are rare clinical emergencies in which high BP must be lowered immediately to prevent or limit a morbid complication. The situation, not the BP level alone, constitutes the emergency. Examples include:

- Acute pulmonary edema
- Acute MI
- Hypertensive encephalopathy
- Eclampsia
- Dissecting aortic aneurysm

In these situations, a controlled reduction of BP by 20% to 25% over a few minutes to a few hours is indicated.

Hypertensive urgencies are situations in which BP should be lowered to 160 to 170/100 to 110 mmHg within 24 hours to prevent complications. These include:

- Severe perioperative HTN
- Accelerated malignant HTN (BP >220/120 mmHg and rising)

Precipitous decreases in BP should be avoided. The goal is clinical stabilization, not normalization of BP. Relatively short-acting parenteral (IV) antihypertensives, followed by oral therapy, usually work best. Suggested IV drugs and doses are listed in Table 9.1-3. If IV therapy is not an option, oral captopril (Capoten), 25 mg, clonidine (Catapres), 0.1 to 0.2 mg, or labetolol (Normodyne), 200 to 400 mg, can be used; each has a hypotensive effect within 1 hour. Sublingual administration is not more effective than oral.

In the setting of acute cerebrovascular attack, HTN should generally not be treated unless SBP is greater than 220 mmHg or unless there are signs of progressive intracranial bleeding. Quiet bed rest often results in a significant decrease in BP.

Complications

Antihypertensive medications have variable effects on cardiac conduction, cardiac contractility, arterial and venous tone, renal function, and electrolyte metabolism (especially potassium). The prescriber must be aware of these potential side effects when deciding on therapy and during follow-up

TABLE 9.1-3	Parenteral Drugs for Hypertensive Crisis

Drug name (trade name)	Dose for hypertensive crisis[a]
Labetolol (Normodyne)	20–40 mg IV q10 min
Methyldopa (Aldomet)	250–500 mg IV q6 h
Hydralazine (Apresoline)	20–40 mg IV q1–2 h nonpregnant
	5–10 mg IV q20 min in pregnancy
Diazoxide (Hyperstat)	50–150 IV q15 min
Enalaprilat (Vasotec IV)	1.25 mg IV q6 h
Nitroprusside (Nipride)	0.2–10 µg/kg/min IV
	(use low dose in pregnancy)

[a]Review of full prescribing information is strongly advised.

examinations. Drug interactions may potentiate or ameliorate symptomatic or metabolic side effects. New signs or symptoms of cardiac arrhythmia, dyspnea with exertion, edema, or fatigue should be thoroughly investigated. The serum electrolyte panel, BUN, and creatinine should be checked at least once per year; abnormalities should be addressed and followed up. Patients with existing cardiac disease, renal disease, or diabetes, and those on multiple medications, are at the highest risk for complications. Such patients also are likely to gain more absolute benefit from control of HTN than are patients without diabetes or TOD.

SPECIAL CONSIDERATIONS
Hypertension in Pregnancy

HTN occurs in 6% to 8% of pregnancies in the United States. It is associated with significant maternal morbidity, including seizure, stroke, encephalopathy, and hemorrhage. Additionally, HTN in pregnancy is a major contributor to uteroplacental insufficiency, placental abruption, prematurity, and fetal demise. Recently, the increasing prevalence of worldwide obesity and metabolic syndrome has led to concern for increasing numbers or women that could develop HTN in their childbearing years and pregnancy.

HTN in pregnancy is classified as either chronic or gestational. Criteria for diagnosis of either form are similar to the nonpregnant state:

- **Mild chronic or gestational HTN** is defined as SBP of 140 mmHg greater or DBP of 90 mmHg or greater
- **Severe chronic HTN is** defined as SBP of 180 mmHg or greater or DBP of 110 mmHg or greater
- **Severe gestational HTN** is defined as SBP of 160 mmHg or greater or DBP of 110 mmHg or greater

HTN in pregnancy should be diagnosed only after an elevated BP is documented on at least two readings taken 6 hours apart with the patient in the sitting position after a 10-minute rest. The HTN is considered chronic if the patient was diagnosed prior to conception or prior to the 20th week of gestation. Women with no recent BP readings who present for prenatal care after the 20th week, and who meet the criteria for HTN, should be considered to have gestational HTN. If HTN persists beyond the usual postpartum period, a diagnosis of chronic HTN can be made in retrospect.

Pre-eclampsia is a pregnancy-induced, multisystem disease defined by gestational HTN with proteinuria (2+ on dipstick on two occasions 6 hours apart or >3 g/24-hour urine collection). Given the increased risk of morbidity and mortality associated with pre-eclampsia, all women diagnosed with HTN during pregnancy should have a 24-hour quantitative urine protein measured. For those women with chronic HTN, a baseline measurement will document possible pre-existing renal disease that may influence subsequent diagnosis of pre-eclampsia. Chronic HTN is a known risk factor for the development of pre-eclampsia, with 20% to 30% of women with chronic HTN developing pre-eclampsia. The classification of pre-eclampsia as well as its treatment is covered in Chapter 14.8.

Treatment for chronic HTN in pregnancy and gestational HTN (without proteinuria) is dictated by the known effects of antihypertensive medications on uteroplacental blood flow and fetal outcome studies. Because numerous controlled trials have failed to demonstrate fetal or maternal benefit from treating *mild* HTN in pregnancy, the American College of Obstetrics and Gynecology (ACOG) recommends *not starting* antihypertensive medication for mild chronic or gestational HTN in pregnancy, unless there are comorbid conditions such as HTN-associated headaches, TOD, or rising BP levels.

For women already taking antihypertensive medication at the time of pregnancy diagnosis, current data support stopping therapy if HTN is mild, or switching treatment to the smallest effective dose of a first-line antihypertensive drug for use in pregnancy.

- **First-line antihypertensive drugs for HTN during pregnancy**
  - Methyldopa 250 to 500 mg PO tid–qid
  - Labetolol 100 to 400 mg bid–tid
- **Acceptable second-line choices**
  - Other β-blockers (*excluding* atenolol that has been associated with growth restriction)
    - Metoprolol 50 to 200 mg bid
    - Pindolol 5 to 15 mg bid
  - CCBs
    - Nifedipine 10 to 30 mg tid
    - Nicardipine 20 to 40 mg tid
  - Hydrochlorothiazide 25 to 50 mg qd
  - Hydralazine 10 to 50 mg qid
- **Contraindicated in pregnancy**
  - ACE inhibitors
  - ARBs
  - Aldosterone antagonists

The use of ACE inhibitors during pregnancy is associated with a variety of renal and pulmonary toxicities in the fetus.

Treatment of acute, severe HTN in pregnancy should occur expeditiously to reduce the risk of maternal stroke and placental abruption.

Hydralazine has been the preferred agent in the United States due to its long history of safety and rapid onset of action; however, thrombocytopenia has been rarely reported in neonates born to women treated in the third trimester.

- **Recommended antihypertensive drugs for acute severe HTN in pregnancy**
  - Hydralazine 5 to 10 mg IV every 15 to 20 minutes
  - Labetalol 20 mg IV bolus with 20 to 40 mg every 15 minutes as needed
  - Nifedipine* 10 mg PO q15 minutes, max 30 mg
  - Nicardipine* 5 mg per hour IV, increase at 2.5 mg per hour q5 to 15 minutes up to 15 mg per hour
  - Sodium nitroprusside 0.25 µg/kg/minute IV, increase 0.25 µg/kg/min q5 minutes up to 5 µg/kg/minute

REFERENCES

1. James PA, Oparil S, Carter BL, et al. Evidence based guidelines for the management of high blood pressure in adults. Report from the panel members appointed to the Eighth Joint National Committee. *JAMA* 2014;311:503–520.
2. National High Blood Pressure Education Program. *The seventh report of the Joint National Committee on prevention, detection, evaluation and treatment of high blood pressure (JNC 7).* Bethesda, MD: NIH National Heart, Lung, and Blood Institute; 2003. Publication 03–5233.
3. ALLHAT Collaborative Research Group. Major outcomes in high-risk hypertensive patients randomized to angiotensin-converting enzyme inhibitor or calcium channel blocker vs diuretic: the Antihypertensive and Lipid-Lowering Treatment to Prevent Heart Attack Trial (ALLHAT). *JAMA* 2002;288(23):2981–2997.
4. Tronvik E, Stovner LJ, Hagen K, et al. High pulse pressure protects against headache: prospective and cross-sectional data (HUNT study). *Neurology* 2008;70(16):1329–1336.
5. Appel LJ, Champagne CM, Harsha DW, et al. Effects of comprehensive lifestyle modification on blood pressure control: main results of the PREMIER clinical trial. *JAMA* 2003;289(16):2083–2093.
6. New England Journal of Medicine. JW Gen. Med. December 31, 2013.
7. Dahlof B, Devereux RB, Kjeldsen SE, et al. Cardiovascular morbidity and mortality in the Losartan Intervention for Endpoint reduction in hypertension study (LIFE): a randomised trial against atenolol. *Lancet* 2002;359(9311):995–1003.

Caution must be exercised with the concomitant use of calcium-channel blockers and magnesium as the combination has been reported to cause neuromuscular blockade and severe hypotension.

8. Demers C, McMurray JJ, Swedberg K, et al. Impact of candesartan on nonfatal myocardial infarction and cardiovascular death in patients with heart failure. *JAMA* 2005;294(14):1794–1798.
9. Casaa P, Weiliang C, Stavros L, et al. Effect of inhibitors of the renin-angiotensin system and other antihypersensitive drugs on renal outcomes: systematic review and meta-analysis. *Lancet* 2005;366;2026–2033.
10. Report on National High Blood Pressure Education Program Working Group on High Blood Pressure in Pregnancy. *Am J Obstet Gynecol* 2000;183:S1–S22.
11. Sibai BM. Diagnosis and management of gestational hypertension and preeclampsia. *Obstet Gynecol* 2003;102:181–192.
12. Lowe SA, Brown, MA, Dekken GA, et al. Guideline for the management of hypertension disorders in pregnancy 2008. *J Obstet Gynecol* 2009;49(3):242–246.
13. Yoder SR, Thornberry MD, Bisognano JD. Hypertension in pregnancy and women of childbearing age. *Am Med J* 2009;122:890–895.
14. Chronic hypertension in pregnancy. ACOG Practice Bulletin No. 29. July 2001.
15. American College of Obstetricians and Gynecologists. Task Force on Hypertension in Pregnancy. Hypertension in pregnancy. Report of the American College of Obstetricians and Gynecologists' task force on hypertension in pregnancy. *Obstet Gynecol* 2003:122(5):1122–1131.

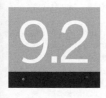

9.2 Ischemic Heart Disease

Douglas J. Inciarte

GENERAL PRINCIPLES

- Ischemic heart disease (IHD) is a chronic medical condition prone to acute exacerbations and affecting a sizable percentage of the adult population. The manifestations may be broad and have impact on inpatient and outpatient care. This chapter focuses on outpatient diagnosis and management.
- IHD is a term interchangeable with coronary artery disease (CAD), coronary heart disease (CHD), and atherosclerotic heart disease (ASHD). Although in the most precise sense the terms are not identical, generally they all refer to a condition of obstructed blood flow in the coronary arteries that may result in ischemia or infarction of the myocardium. Clinically, patients with IHD may be asymptomatic, may have chronic stable angina, may present with an acute coronary syndrome (ACS; see below), or may present with sudden death as their initial symptoms.

Classification

- The estimated prevalence of CHD is 13,200,000, and one in three American adults is estimated to have some type of cardiovascular disease (CVD).[1] Since 1900, CVD has been the number 1 cause of death every year except 1918.[1] It is also the most costly medical condition in the United States.[1]
- ACSs are classified as unstable angina (UA), non-ST segment elevation myocardial infarction (NSTEMI) or ST segment elevation MI (STEMI) depending on serologic evidence of myocardial damage and on electrocardiographic (ECG) findings.
- Several classification schemes exist for grading stable angina, although the most commonly utilized may be the Canadian Cardiovascular Society system commonly referred to as CCSS.

Canadian Cardiovascular Society[2] Class Description	
I	Ordinary physical activity does not cause angina
II	Slight limitation of ordinary physical activity
III	Marked limitation of ordinary physical activity
IV	Inability to perform any physical activity without discomfort

- Most commonly in IHD, an obstruction develops due to atherosclerosis. Atherosclerotic plaques may be stable and result in a pattern of chronic angina precipitated when myocardial oxygen demand exceeds the supply that is available across a coronary artery obstruction. ACS typically occurs when an unstable coronary artery plaque ruptures, promoting thrombus formation on the surface and acutely obstructing the vessel lumen.
- The degree of coronary obstruction does not necessarily correlate with the likelihood of an acute coronary event; high-grade stenosis may never progress to infarction while less obstructive plaques may rupture and cause infarction. Some patients with angina have normal appearing coronary arteries. This situation can occur when the etiology of the symptoms is not cardiac, but it can also occur among patients who develop cardiac ischemia from coronary artery vasospasm (Prinzmetal angina). Those with Prinzmetal angina are typically younger and have fewer traditional IHD risk factors. The etiology is unclear and the prognosis (absent concomitant CAD) is favorable. Other patients may have microvascular disease or diffuse disease that is hard to detect on routine catheterization. These patients are more commonly women and may still have a substantial risk for progression to MI.
- Atherosclerosis is a chronic inflammatory disease resulting from a complex interplay between cellular and chemical factors affecting the vascular endothelium. The atherosclerotic process occurs over years; is triggered by traditional IHD risk factors such as smoking, obesity, diabetes, hypertension, hyperlipidemia, and genetics; and results in the formation of obstructing plaques. Investigation into other contributor factors continues, but the most recent evidence shows that 80% to 90% of patients with IHD have traditional risk factors[3] and 87% to 100% of patients who suffer fatal IHD events have at least one traditional risk factor.[4]
- A number of novel serum markers have been found to be associated with heart disease. Some are risk factors and others are only markers of disease. High-sensitivity C-reactive protein (hs-CRP) has derived the most attention and appears to be an independent risk factor for heart disease. Lipoprotein-a is a nonmodifiable risk factor that is genetically programmed and signifies risk for early-onset heart disease. In contrast, elevated homocysteine elevates risk for heart disease, but lowering homocysteine levels does not reduce the risk of heart disease and is thus considered only a risk marker.
- IHD is associated with obstructive sleep apnea and snoring, but the nature and direction of this association are not yet clear.

DIAGNOSIS
Clinical Presentation

- An ACS may present with "typical" chest pain, atypical angina, sudden fatigue, congestive heart failure symptoms, or even nausea and vomiting. Diagnostic and management decisions must be made quickly and implemented immediately because the efficacy of many of the available treatments declines rapidly with time from onset of ischemia. Patients presenting with symptoms consistent with ACS should be classified very rapidly as having probable noncardiac pain, stable angina, UA/NSTEMI, or STEMI meeting reperfusion criteria.
- Stable angina commonly presents as exertional chest pain, tightness, shortness of breath, or fatigue. It has often been occurring for weeks or months before the patient consults a physician.
- IHD presents in enough ways and across a broad enough spectrum of patients that it would be misleading to describe a "typical" patient or presentation. Rather, a high index of suspicion should be maintained for IHD among men over 40 and women over 50, with a rapidly increasing prior probability with advancing age.
- Primary prevention of IHD is an important part of a primary care physician. Baseline risk among asymptomatic adults should be estimated using the National Cholesterol Education Program (NCEP) framework,[5] either by counting risk factors or by calculating risk using the Framingham equation (accessible at http://cvdrisk.nhlbi.nih.gov/calculator.asp). The NCEP framework does overestimate risk among low-prevalence populations and can underestimate risk in some high-prevalence groups (e.g., Indian and other south Asian populations) by as much as 50%, so clinical judgment is required.

History

History is the most important information in the decision process for suspected IHD. It should address the following parameters:

- *The location, character, and time course of the symptoms.* Chest or left arm pressure or pain of a steady, dull nature is classic for cardiac ischemia. The feeling may be profound but vague and not even termed pain or pressure by the patient. Alternatively, some patients will insist that the sensation is one only of pressure, not pain. Occasionally pain may be present only in the jaw or scapular area. Sharp or pleuritic pain weighs against the diagnosis, as does pain that can be localized with one finger. Paresthesias (especially perioral tingling) suggest panic attack. Water brash has high specificity for gastroesophageal reflux. Reduced pain upon sitting up and leaning forward suggests pericarditis. Women may frequently present with vague symptoms that may be considered "atypical."

• Prior history of IHD.
• Classic epidemiologic risk factors are smoking, hyperlipidemia, hypertension, obesity, and family history. These have little or no diagnostic value for ACS,[6] but should be assessed in evaluating chronic angina. Those that are modifiable are key points in primary and secondary prevention.
• *Diabetes*. Patients with long-standing diabetes often lack the characteristic pain of acute ischemia.
• A complete listing of current medications including over-the-counter and alternative or herbal preparations and a list of any illicit drugs being used, especially cocaine.

A full cardiac and vascular review of systems should be included in the history for suspected chronic angina, but gathering this information should not be allowed to delay the rapid evaluation of ACS.

Physical Examination

• Physical examination in cases of suspected ACS should be expeditiously conducted and directed to key findings, which include pulmonary edema, particularly sudden or "flash" edema; mitral valve murmur, particularly if of new onset; marked hypertension; hypotension or shock; confusion or other mental status changes; other neurologic deficits consistent with stroke; and hypoxia. These findings can be detected by a careful assessment of the ABCs (airway, breathing, and circulation), review of vital signs, as well as a heart, lung, and focused neurologic examination.
• For patients with suspected chronic angina, a more complete directed physical examination emphasizing cardiovascular findings should be carried out. Carotid, abdominal, and renal bruits; pedal pulses (and ankle-brachial indices if pulses are diminished); and jugular venous waveform should be included. Chest tenderness to palpation that completely reproduces the presenting pain may make ACS less likely but does not exclude the possibility, and this finding must be interpreted within the context of other clinical data.

Laboratory Studies

• ECG is, with history, the foundation of diagnosis and risk stratification for suspected ACS. Certain crucial features are important:
  • ST segment elevation of at least 1 mm in two contiguous leads
  • New-onset left bundle branch block
• Either of the above findings on an ECG in a patient with chest pain is diagnostic of STEMI, and the patient should be triaged appropriately and emergently for reperfusion therapy via either thrombolytic therapy or emergent percutaneous coronary intervention (PCI). Patients with ST segment depression in the anterior leads in a pattern consistent with a posterior MI may also benefit from emergent reperfusion. Patients meeting these criteria must be identified immediately and emergently triaged from the outpatient setting to appropriate facilities to receive thrombolysis within 30 minutes or PCI within 90 minutes. Patients not meeting these criteria should not receive reperfusion therapy as it worsens outcomes.[7]
• Other ECG findings such as Q waves of 1 mm or greater not known to be present previously, T-wave inversion, hyperacute T waves ($\geq$50% of the maximal QRS amplitude), ST segment depression, and new conduction abnormalities or arrhythmias may also be important markers of ischemia.
• Cardiac troponins T and I are more than 90% sensitive and similarly specific at 8 or more hours from the onset of pain.[8] Either or both may be assayed, generally for levels >0.1 ng per mL. Positive troponins with normal ECG can distinguish NSTEMI from UA and help identify patients who are at increased risk for infarction or sudden death.
• All patients suspected of IHD should have a fasting lipid profile, glucose, complete blood count (CBC), estimated glomerular filtration rate (GFR), and electrolytes measured. Evaluation of ACS should not be delayed to obtain them; lipids may be measured fasting up to 24 hours after symptom onset.[7]

Imaging

• Patients suspected of IHD should have a chest radiograph performed for pulmonary edema and cardiac enlargement. Evaluation of patients with ACS and initiation of reperfusion therapy, however, should not be delayed for radiography.

TABLE 9.2-1 Comparison of Stress Test Options[9]

	Sensitivity	Specificity	Advantages	Disadvantages/Cautions
Stress ECG	67	72	Cost effective Readily available Good measure of function	Not reliable with baseline ECG changes or for patients on digoxin High false-positive rate among women
Stress myocardial perfusion (thallium or sestamibi)	89	76	Very sensitive Good measure of function	Costly No assessment of structure
Stress echocardiogram	85	86	Good measure of function Very specific Good measure of cardiac structure More affordable than myocardial perfusion	Images may be compromised by obesity
Adenosine myocardial perfusion (thallium or sestamibi)	90	70	Very sensitive	Costly Caffeine ingestion may lead to false negatives Adenosine may cause bronchospasm No assessment of structure
Dobutamine echocardiogram	82	85	Very specific Good measure of cardiac structure More affordable than myocardial perfusion	Dobutamine may induce tachyarrhythmias Images may be compromised by obesity

- Stress testing is employed to assess cardiac structure and function. It is commonly used to assess the probability of significant coronary artery disease among those who have anginal symptoms or who are preparing for noncardiac surgery. A number of different stress and imaging modalities are available. The advantages and disadvantages of the most commonly utilized forms are displayed in Table 9.2-1. If stress testing is to be used for this purpose, pretest probability needs to be considered before ordering an examination. If the pretest probability is very low, the result of a stress test may not influence decision making. If the risk is very high, then a negative test may not influence the decision whether a catheterization is necessary but may be helpful in targeting vessels for future revascularization.
- Stress testing may also be useful for assessing a patient's functional capacity, assessing myocardial viability post-MI, and occasionally for guiding medical management of IHD.
- Left heart catheterization is the gold standard for evaluating coronary artery anatomy. It is generally safe and is appropriate for identifying the location and extent of obstructive disease. If suspicion for Prinzmetal or vasospastic angina is high, a heart catheterization may also be used with ergonovine to assess for the presence of coronary artery spasm.
- Computed tomography (CT) scan has evolved as an emerging technology that may have significant potential for heart disease. Multidetector CT and CT angiography are both being utilized and investigated, but the role that these emerging technologies will ultimately play in the diagnosis and management of heart disease is not yet clear.

Differential Diagnosis

- Patients presenting with chest pain and related complaints have ACS in a minority of cases, approximately 30% in the emergency department setting[8] and less than 5% in the primary care physician's office setting.[10] Other high-probability diagnoses that should be considered are panic attack, gastroesophageal reflux disease, musculoskeletal pain, and pleurisy. Panic attack and gastroesophageal reflux disease are often close mimics of angina, and both are more common than angina in primary care settings. Both can result in morbidity, if misdiagnosed as angina, from inappropriate cardiac workups and from failure to treat the patient's real condition. Also consider other life-threatening diagnoses such as aortic dissection, pulmonary embolus, pneumothorax, or perforating ulcer, among others.

TREATMENT

- Outpatient management of ACS focuses on rapid identification and risk stratification, immediate transport of reperfusion candidates to properly equipped facilities, and appropriate referral and transport of moderate- and high-risk patients. Patients without known true hypersensitivity or active bleeding should receive 325 mg of aspirin stat and be placed on 2 L per minute of oxygen by nasal cannula or mask while awaiting transport. If ECG monitoring is available, it should be in place. Nitroglycerine can be administered sublingual every 5 minutes as tolerated by blood pressure for pain relief. A defibrillator should be ready, and personnel trained in its use should be with the patient continuously. Time is of the essence in ACS. American College of Cardiology/American Heart Association (ACC/AHA) standards are to keep total ischemic time to less than 120 minutes.[7] Patients with evidence of STEMI should be transported rapidly to a facility capable of providing appropriate reperfusion—thrombolysis or PCI.
- Outpatient management of IHD consists of primary and secondary prevention. Inpatient management of ACS is outside the scope of this chapter. Common to both primary and secondary intervention is risk factor reduction—weight loss; smoking cessation; and good control of hypertension, hyperlipidemia, and diabetes (in order of absolute benefit) if present. Risk factor reduction occurs through both behavioral and medical interventions. Treatment of hypertension should be to a BP goal of <140/90 for all patients including those with renal disease or diabetes. Lipid lowering should be achieved with a statin, if tolerated, and in conjunction with the NCEP goals as described below.[5] National treatment goals for diabetes are for a HbA1c <7.0, though available evidence does not clearly demonstrate reduced ACS risk for such tight diabetes control.

Population	Goal
<2 risk factors	Low-density lipoprotein (LDL) <160 mg/dL
2 or more risk factors	LDL <130 mg/dL
Known IHD or diabetes	LDL <100 mg/dL
Very high-risk patients	Optional LDL target of 70 mg/dL (recent ACS, IHD plus diabetes; metabolic syndrome)

- Operative interventions, for example, coronary artery bypass grafting (CABG) or percutaneous intervention (PCI) with stent placement, are available for treatment of disease in appropriate patients.

Behavioral

- Smoking is the most powerful modifiable risk factor for IHD, and smoking cessation is essential for both primary and secondary prevention. Physicians should ask about smoking habits at each visit, counsel the patient to quit, assess the willingness to quit, and assist the patient in quitting smoking.
- Depression is thought to be an independent risk factor for IHD and ACS and is associated with a worse prognosis. Treatment with selective serotonin-reuptake inhibitors (SSRIs) improves depression morbidity though not cardiac outcomes.[11] Current expert opinion is to use SSRIs among patients with IHD as needed in a manner consistent with how they would be used in the absence of heart disease.
- Weight loss is an important component of reducing risk for MI. Body mass index (BMI) has traditionally been used as a measure of risk with the goal being <25, but waist-to-hip ratio has emerged as a more reliable measure of risk. Weight loss should target a waist circumference of <40 inches in men and <35 inches in women.[12]
- Exercise both reduces risk directly and is an important component of weight loss. A written exercise prescription should be given for 30 to 60 minutes of activity, defined as brisk walking, 5 to 7 days

per week,[12] and progress toward that goal should be monitored and reinforced at every visit. Patients may opt for more vigorous activity based on stress test results.

Medications

- Medical management of IHD can involve a diverse array of medications. The most common are described in Table 9.2-2. The three medications in bold type are recommended to all patients unless contraindicated, with regular assessment of compliance. Intensive medical therapy is capable of achieving regression of coronary plaques and reducing ACS events.

Surgery

- Emergent reperfusion therapy reduces mortality and morbidity, and is the standard of care for STEMI meeting the criteria above. PCI is preferred in high-volume centers if door-to-balloon times of 90 minutes or less can be achieved. Thrombolysis should be initiated (with a target door-to-needle time of 30 minutes) if suitably skilled PCI is not available in that time frame.[13] The primary care physicians must honestly assess the procedure volume and skills of their referral facility and the realistically likely time to initiation of therapy in making referral decisions.
- Among stable angina patients, CABG improves survival for patients with left main disease, severe proximal left anterior descending (LAD) disease, or three-vessel disease with diminished left ventricular (LV) function. (A vessel is considered diseased if it has ≥50% obstruction on coronary angiography.) Recent improvements in angioplasty technology, particularly stenting, may make percutaneous revascularization an appropriate alternative for some such patients. Patients with diabetes do not fare as well with percutaneous revascularization as with CABG.
- Anginal pain, ability to exercise, and daily role function are important patient-oriented outcomes. Consultation and evaluation for revascularization (either percutaneous or by CABG) to reduce pain and improve function is appropriate for many patients with stable IHD, even if mortality is unlikely to be reduced.

Special Therapy

- Yearly influenza vaccine is indicated among patients with IHD. Also, patients with IHD should have a pneumovax once, which is to be repeated when the patient is older than 65 if the first pneumovax was administered before the patient was 65 years old.

SPECIAL CONSIDERATIONS

- The prevalence and the magnitude of impact of IHD have made appropriate management of this condition a high priority among groups following the quality of care for chronic diseases. Physicians should follow quality standards such as aspirin, statins, and β-blockers for secondary prevention and should develop systems for identifying and tracking patients with IHD.

REFERENCES

1. Thom T, Haase N, Rosamond W, et al. Heart disease and stroke statistics 2006 update. A Report from the American Heart Association Statistics Committee and Stroke Statistics Subcommittee. *Circulation* 2006;113:e85–e151.
2. Goldman L, Hashimoto B, Cook EF, et al. Comparative reproducibility and validity of systems for assessing cardiovascular functional class: advantages of a new specific activity scale. *Circulation* 1981;64:1227–1234.
3. Khot UN, Khot MB, Bajzer CT, et al. Prevalence of conventional risk factors in patients with coronary heart disease. *JAMA* 2003;290(7):898–904.
4. Greenland P, Knoll MD, Stamler J, et al. Major risk factors as antecedents of fatal and nonfatal coronary heart disease events. *JAMA* 2003;290(7):891–897.
5. National Cholesterol Education Program. National Heart, Lung, and Blood Institute. http://www.nhlbi.nih.gov/guidelines/cholesterol/atp_iii.htm. Accessed June 30, 2006.
6. Jayes RL, Beshansky JR, D'Agostino RB, et al. Do patients' coronary risk factor reports predict acute cardiac ischemia in the emergency department? A multicenter study. *J Clin Epidemiol* 1992;45:621.
7. Antman EM, Anbe DT, Armstrong PW, et al. ACC/AHA guidelines for the management of patients with ST-elevation myocardial infarction; a report of the American College of Cardiology/American Heart Association Task Force on Practice Guidelines (Committee to Revise the 1999 Guidelines for the Management of Patients with Acute Myocardial Infarction). *J Am Coll Cardiol* 2004;44(3):E1–E211.
8. Ebell MH, Flewelling D, Flynn CA. A systematic review of troponin T and I for diagnosing acute myocardial infarction. *J Fam Pract* 2000;49:550.

TABLE 9.2-2	Drugs Used Commonly in the Treatment of IHD			
Intervention	Dose	Primary prevention	Secondary prevention	Comments[a]
ACE inhibitors	Drug dependent	N/A	Only for high risk or for LVSD	Class effect May substitute ARB if intolerant of ACE Contraindicated if allergic, renal failure, hyperkalemia, hypotension, renal artery stenosis, pregnancy
Aspirin	75–162 mg daily	Moderate or high risk (e.g., Framingham 10-yr risk estimate >6%)	Standard of care; withhold only for documented hypersensitivity or active bleeding	Higher doses associated with increased risk, but no benefit Contraindicated if allergic or if significant bleeding risk
α-Blockers	Drug dependent	Hypertension	Standard of care; withhold only for proven intolerance (asthma and patients with COPD should receive cautious trial)	Class effect except for LVSD Use only bisoprolol, carvedilol, or metoprolol succinate with LVSD Contraindicated in heart block, hypotension, severe reactive airway disease
Calcium-channel blockers	Drug dependent	N/A	Angina relief	Avoid short-acting non-DHPs, e.g., verapamil, diltiazem Non-DHPs may cause heart block if combined with β-blockers Non-DHPs are not to be used with LVSD Contraindicated in hypotension, heart block
Eplerenone	25–50 mg daily	N/A	<14 days post-MI if also with LVSD or diabetes	Aldactone in the same class but never tested for this indication Contraindicated with renal failure, hyperkalemia
Nitroglycerine	Drug dependent	N/A	Angina relief	Contraindicated in hypotension or within 24 h after PDE inhibitor use (e.g., Viagra)
Clopidogrel	300 mg load 75 mg daily	Possible harm	If ASA intolerant + ASA post-PCI or UA/NSTEMI[b]	Contraindicated if allergic or if significant bleeding risk
Statins	Drug dependent	Based on NCEP recommendations per risk profile	Standard of care; withhold only for documented intolerance	Class effect for secondary prevention, titrate to LDL <100 or optional, to LDL <70 in high-risk patients

DHPs, dihydropyridines; LVSD, left ventricular systolic dysfunction (ejection fraction <40%).
[a]Assume contraindications considered before any medication given; the list of contraindications described here is not exhaustive; please consult a drug reference for a more comprehensive list.
[b]Clopidogrel should be administered for 1 to 12 months post-PCI with bare metal stent or post-UA/NSTEMI without stenting. It should be administered for at least 12 months post–drug-eluting stent.

9. Murthy TH, Bach DS. Comparative review of stress tests. *Clin Fam Pract* 2001;3(4):814.
10. Klinkman MS. Episodes of care for chest pain. *J Fam Pract* 1994;38:345.
11. Agency for Healthcare Research and Quality. Post-myocardial infarction depression (Evidence report/technology assessment report 123). Rockville, MD: U.S. Government Printing Office; 2005. AHRQ publication 05-E018-02.
12. Smith SC, Allen J, Blair SN, et al. AHA/ACC guidelines for secondary prevention for patients with coronary and other atherosclerotic vascular disease: 2006 update. *Circulation* 2006;113:2363–2372.
13. Van de Werf F, Gore JM, Avezum A, et al; GRACE Investigators. Access to catheterisation facilities in patients admitted with acute coronary syndrome: multinational registry study. *BMJ* 2005;330:441–444.

9.3 Murmurs and Valvular Heart Disease

Douglas J. Inciarte

GENERAL PRINCIPLES

A heart murmur may have no pathologic significance—simply a representation of physiologic increases in blood flow. However, a murmur may be an important indicator of the presence of valvular abnormalities. The history and physical examination is the critical screening tool for all patients. In certain instances, further evaluation with electrocardiogram, chest x-ray, echocardiogram, and heart catheterization is required. Diagnosis is important in valvular heart disease in order to achieve timely management prior to the onset of irreversible damage. Timing of surgical intervention correlates with good outcome. Generally, patients with stenotic valvular lesions can be monitored clinically until symptoms appear. On the other hand, patients with regurgitant valvular lesions require careful echocardiographic monitoring for left ventricular function and may require surgery even in the absence of symptoms. A brief discussion of some basic diagnostic tools is listed below. In addition, the most common valvular heart diseases as well as murmurs in pregnancy, murmurs in athletes, and murmurs in infants and children are reviewed in the following text.

DIAGNOSIS

History

History suggesting valvular heart disease is directed at symptoms potentially related to dysfunction of a valve. These symptoms can be thought of as relating to diminished forward flow (fatigue and decreased exercise tolerance) and symptoms relating to pulmonary congestion (paroxysmal nocturnal dyspnea and orthopnea).

Physical Examination

The physical examination focuses on the location, timing, duration, and quality of the murmur. In addition to these cardinal elements, various provocative maneuvers can cause changes in the murmur, changes that aid diagnosis. The Valsalva maneuver and standing decrease preload. Squatting or raising the legs increases preload. Handgrip increases afterload. There is no maneuver that decreases afterload. The beat after the long pause associated with a premature beat may also give clues to the etiology of a murmur by causing increased filling of the left ventricle.

On cardiac physical examinations, murmurs need to be described and characterized to predict prompt management; for this reason, murmurs needs to be described as below.

Murmur description: A murmur is described by different number of features, including intensity (grade), frequency, timing, shape, location, and radiation.

Intensity: The intensity of a murmur is primarily determined by the quantity and velocity of blood flow at the site of its origin, the transmission characteristic of the tissues between the blood flow and stethoscope, the site of auscultation or recording, and the distance of transmission. In general, the intensity declines in the presence of obesity, emphysema, and pericardial effusion.

Murmurs are usually louder in children and in thin individuals.
Six grades are used to classify the intensity of a murmur:

- Grade I is the faintest murmur that can be heard (with difficulty)
- Grade II murmur is also a faint murmur but can be identified immediately
- Grade III murmur is moderately loud
- Grade IV murmur is loud and is associated with a palpable thrill
- Grade V murmur is very loud, could be heard placing the edge of the diaphragm of stethoscope over the patient's chest, and is associated with a palpable thrill
- Grade VI murmur is the loudest and can be heard without a stethoscope

Pitch: The frequency of the murmur determines the pitch, which may be high or low. It can be described as harsh, rumbling, scratchy, grunting, blowing, squeaky, and musical. Quality and pitch are closely related.

Configuration: The time course of murmur intensity corresponds to the "shape" of a diagram of murmur intensity over time, as in a phonocardiogram. A number of configurations or shapes of murmurs are recognized:

- Crescendo
- Decrescendo
- Crescendo–decrescendo (diamond shaped)
- Plateau (unchanged in intensity)

Location: The location on the patient's chest where the murmur is loudest is typically described as apical or parasternal. Parasternal murmurs are further described by the intercostal space and right or left side of the sternum.

Timing: The duration of a murmur is assessed by determining the length of systole or diastole that the murmur occupies. The murmur can be long (e.g., it occupies most of systole or diastole) or brief. The following classification is useful[2]:

- For systolic murmurs:
  - Midsystolic (or systolic ejection)
  - Holosystolic (or pansystolic)
  - Early systolic
  - Late systolic
- For diastolic murmurs:
  - Early diastolic
  - Mid-diastolic
  - Late diastolic (or presystolic)

Laboratory Studies

- **Electrocardiogram (ECG)**. The ECG is not a specific tool for the diagnosis of valvular heart disease. Findings such as atrial enlargement or left ventricular hypertrophy (LVH) often occur late in the course of valvular heart disease.
- **Chest x-ray (CXR)**. Like the ECG, the CXR does not offer early or specific diagnostic clues to valvular heart disease. Radiographic evidence of cardiomegaly or pulmonary congestion is a late finding.
- **Echocardiogram**. The echocardiogram is the definitive indicator that rules in or rules out the presence of valvular heart disease. It should be used when there is moderate clinical suspicion of valvular heart disease.

SPECIFIC DIAGNOSIS AND TREATMENT BASED ON VALVULAR DISEASE OR CONDITION

Aortic Stenosis (AS)

General Principles
Pathophysiology. Left ventricular outflow obstruction leads to increased left ventricular pressure. In order to maintain normal wall stress, the left ventricle undergoes concentric hypertrophy. Subsequently, a decrease in contractile performance and in ejection fraction is noted.

Etiology of Valvular AS. Senile AS (age-related degenerative calcific changes), congenitally bicuspid vale with superimposed calcification, rheumatic heart disease.

Diagnosis

Clinical presentation. Exertional dyspnea, angina pectoris, syncope, congestive heart failure, and sudden death.

Physical Examination

- **Murmur**: Harsh, diamond-shaped **systolic** murmur. AS murmur is heard best in second right intercostal space and radiates into neck vessels. It gets softer with maneuvers that increase afterload (handgrip).
- Diminished intensity (or absence) of aortic valve closure
- Weakened (**parvus**) and delayed (**tardus**) upstroke of carotid artery pulsation
- **Narrow** pulse pressure

Treatment

Management. Asymptomatic AS management includes close clinical follow-up to monitor aortic valve area (normal is 3 to 4 cm^2). In addition, patients require endocarditis antibiotic prophylaxis and avoidance of medication that could result in hypotension. Symptoms occur late in the course of disease and are an ominous sign. Onset of symptoms triggers the need for surgical evaluation.

    Surgery. Aortic valve replacement is indicated if the patient becomes symptomatic, if there is evidence of left ventricular dysfunction, or if the patient has an expanding poststenotic aortic root. Percutaneous balloon aortic valvuloplasty is preferable in children and young adults with congenital, noncalcific AS.

Special Considerations: Subvalvular Aortic Stenosis

Hypertrophic cardiomyopathy (with outflow obstruction). This is a familial disease characterized by marked hypertrophy of the left ventricle, most commonly the interventricular septum. The murmur is similar to valvular AS, but differs in that any maneuver that will make the left ventricle larger in diastole with make the subvalvular AS murmur softer. Conversely, any maneuver that will decrease the left ventricular size in diastole will make the murmur louder. This is the most common cardiac abnormality found in young athletes who die suddenly during vigorous physical activity.

- **Special therapy:** β-Blockers are the standard of therapy, whereas calcium-channel blockers are sometimes useful.
- The guidelines for surgical intervention (myomectomy) are not well defined.
- The incidence of sudden death is 2% to 4% per year in adults and 4% to 6% per year in children and adolescence.

Mitral Stenosis

General Principles

Pathophysiology. Thickening and immobility of the mitral valve leaflets cause obstruction of blood flow from the left atrium to left ventricle and increased pressure within the left atrium, pulmonary vasculature, and right heart. A decreased mitral valve orifice (normal 4 to 6 cm^2) requires an abnormally elevated left atrioventricular pressure gradient to move blood from the left atrium to the left ventricle. The elevated pulmonary venous and pulmonary arterial wedge pressures reduce pulmonary compliance, contributing to clinical symptoms.

    Etiology. Mitral stenosis (MS) and mixed MS and mitral regurgitation (MR) are generally rheumatic in origin. Other etiologies include infective endocarditis and mitral annular calcifications. Rarely, congenital defects, endomyocardial fibroelastosis, malignant carcinoid syndrome, and systemic lupus erythematosis cause MS.

Diagnosis

Clinical presentation. Many patients deny symptoms because patients gradually reduce activity with the slow progression of disease. Clinical presentation includes:

- Exertional dyspnea (most common and often only symptom)
- Hemoptysis
- Thromboembolism
- Chest pain
- Infective endocarditis
- Right-sided heart failure

Physical Examination
- *Murmur*: Low-pitched, rumbling, diastolic murmur, heard best at the apex with the patient in the left lateral decubitus position. (Duration of the murmur corresponds with the severity.)
- Accentuated S1
- Opening snap
- Prominent "a" wave in jugular venous pulsations with normal sinus rhythm

Treatment

Management. An annual history and physical examination, as well as a CXR and ECG, are recommended in asymptomatic patients. Endocarditis prophylaxis is indicated in patients with MS; however, no further medical therapy is indicated. When mild symptoms develop, diuretics may be helpful in reducing left atrial pressure and decreasing symptoms. If symptoms are more than mild or if there is evidence of pulmonary hypertension, mechanical intervention is warranted and delaying intervention worsens prognosis.

Surgery. Mitral balloon valvotomy is indicated in symptomatic patients with isolated MS whose valve orifice is <1.7 cm². Balloon valvotomy is the procedure of choice in individuals with mobile, thin leaflets with no or little calcium. If balloon valvotomy is not possible, a surgical ("open") valvotomy can be performed. Mitral valve replacement is indicated in individuals with MS and significant associated MR.

Aortic Regurgitation

General Principles

Etiology
- *Abnormalities of valve leaflets*: Rheumatic heart disease, endocarditis, congenital
- *Aortic root disease*: Aortic dilation/dissection, syphilitic aortitis, Marfan syndrome, rheumatoid spondylitis

Pathophysiology. In AS, an abnormal regurgitation of blood from the aorta to the left ventricle occurs during diastole. As a result, the left ventricle must pump the regurgitant volume in addition to the normal volume returning from the left atria. An increase in left ventricular end-diastolic volume is the main hemodynamic compensation. The left ventricle undergoes adaptive change, namely dilation and eccentric hypertrophy.

Diagnosis

Clinical presentation. Symptoms of dyspnea on exertion, fatigue, and decreased exercise tolerance appear due to left ventricular failure. Also, patients with AR may experience an uncomfortable sensation associated with large pulse pressure.

Physical Examination
- *Murmur*: Blowing diastolic murmur which is best heard with the patient leaning forward, after exhaling. The murmur may get louder with increased afterload (handgrip).
- Bounding pulse
- Widened pulse pressure
- Displaced cardiac impulse (down and to patient's left)

Treatment
- **Management.** Asymptomatic patients require regular clinical evaluation, assessment of left ventricular function, and endocarditis antibiotic prophylaxis. The mainstays of medical management in symptomatic patients are afterload reduction (vasodilators), which reduces the amount of aortic regurgitations. Long-acting nifedipine has been shown to delay the need for valve surgery.
- **Surgery.** Compelling evidence supports surgical correction before the onset of permanent left ventricular damage, even in asymptomatic patients. AR should be corrected in patients who remain symptomatic despite optimal medical therapy. Aortic valve replacement should also be performed with progressive left ventricular dysfunction and a left ventricular ejection fraction <55% or left ventricular end-systolic volume >55%—"55/55 Rule" (even if asymptomatic).

Mitral Regurgitation

General Principles
- **Pathophysiology** A portion of the left ventricular output is forced backward into the left atrium (LA) leaving the forward cardiac output into the aorta reduced. In acute MR, the LA is normal size

and relatively noncompliant. LA pressure rises dramatically with subsequent pulmonary edema and right heart failure. In chronic MR, dilation and eccentric hypertrophy of the LA occur, making the LA more compliant; therefore, pulmonary edema is less likely to develop.

Etiology
- *Acute MR*: Endocarditis, ruptured chordae, papillary muscle dysfunction
- *Chronic MR*: Rheumatic heart disease, myxomatous degeneration, congenial anomaly, infective endocarditis, hypertrophic cardiomyopathy

Diagnosis
Clinical presentation. The most common symptoms with chronic, severe MR include fatigue, exertional dyspnea, and orthopnea. Patients with pulmonary vascular disease can develop right-sided heart failure. In acute, severe MR, left ventricular failure with acute pulmonary edema is common.

Physical Examination
- *Murmur*: Apical, holosystolic murmur at apex with radiation to left axilla. The murmur of MR will become louder with increased afterload (handgrip).
- Presence of S_3, which indicates severe disease
- Laterally displaced cardiac impulse

Treatment
- **Management.** Asymptomatic patients require regular clinical evaluation, assessment of left ventricular function, and endocarditis antibiotic prophylaxis. In a normotensive patient with acute severe MR, nitroprusside can be utilized to diminish the amount of MR, in turn increasing forward output and reducing pulmonary congestion. For the asymptomatic patient with chronic MR, there is no generally accepted medical therapy. There are no large long-term studies to indicate that the use of vasodilators are beneficial in chronic MR. Heart rate should be controlled with digitalis, rate-lowering calcium-channel blockers, or β-blockers if atrial fibrillation develops.
- **Surgery.** The optimal timing of surgery in patient with chronic MR can be a difficult decision. Routine echocardiographic evaluation should be performed in individuals with severe MR. Surgery is recommended when a patient is symptomatic despite optimum medical management. Surgery should also be considered when left ventricular dysfunction is progressive, with left ventricular ejection fraction declining below 60% (even if asymptomatic).

Special Considerations
- **Mitral valve prolapse (MVP).** MVP is an exceedingly common condition and often asymptomatic. Patients may present with symptomatic arrhythmia, atypical chest pain, or exaggerated autonomic symptoms. Physical examination reveals a click (with or without a murmur), which move toward S_2 with increased preload and increased afterload. Some patients require endocarditis antibiotic prophylaxis. The degree of pathology is related to the degree of MR. β-Blockers can be used for symptomatic treatment of chest pain.

Valvular Heart Disease in the Athlete
Preparticipation Physical
The preparticipation physical should focus on a family history of heart disease; sudden death; personal history suggesting syncope, near syncope, or arrhythmia; and evaluation of heart murmurs in supine, sitting, standing, squatting, and postsquatting positions.

High-Risk Murmurs
Most common causes of serious valvular heart disease in athletes causing sudden death are mitral prolapse and subaortic stenosis (caused by hypertrophic cardiomyopathy).

Risk Assessment
The main issue with MVP is the degree of ectopy present, especially with exercise. In hypertrophic cardiomyopathy, the most significant problem is the degree of outflow obstruction, which is usually related to the thickness of the septum.

Valvular Heart Disease in Pregnancy
Etiology
Most murmurs in pregnancy are physiologic as there is a 50% increase in circulating blood volume during pregnancy.

Preexisting Disease

Preexisting valvular heart disease often is exacerbated by pregnancy. The increased blood volume and enhanced cardiac output associated with normal pregnancy can accentuate the murmurs associated with **stenotic** heart valve lesions (e.g., MS, AS), whereas murmurs of AR or MR may actually ease in the face of lowered systemic vascular resistance.

Valvular Lesions With Increased Maternal and Fetal Risk

- Severe AS with or without symptoms
- MR or AR with NYHA functional Class III to IV symptoms
- MS with NYHA functional Class II to IV symptoms
- Valve disease resulting in severe pulmonary hypertension (pulmonary pressure >75% of systemic pressures)
- Valve disease with severe left ventricular dysfunction (EF <0.40)
- Mechanical prosthetic valves requiring anticoagulation
- AR in Marfan syndrome

Valvular Heart Disease in Infants and Children

Etiology

The physician must consider valvular heart disease as a subset of congenital heart disease. In diagnosis of murmurs in infants and children, think of congenital problems and then rule in or out a valvular etiology.

- **Left to right** shunts, for example, ventricular septal defect (VSD) or atrial septal defect (ASD)
- **Obstructive lesions**, such as AS, pulmonic stenosis, coarctation of the aorta
- **Valvular insufficiency**

Relative frequency of pathologic murmurs in infants: Of murmurs in congenital heart disease, 63% are caused by the six most common congenital defects:

- Pulmonic stenosis > PDA > ASD > Coarctation of the aorta > Aortic stenosis

Diagnosis

Findings more common in infants and children than in adults include grunting, poor feeding, sweating, poor weight gain, wheezing, decreased exercise tolerance, cough, and squatting after exercise (to increase preload). Cyanosis and edema are very late findings.

Treatment

- **Referrals.** Pediatric cardiologists do not order echocardiograms in a large percentage of patients seen in referral for murmur. This makes the strategy of referring all questionable murmurs to a pediatric cardiologist more cost-effective than ordering echocardiograms and referring only the pediatric patients with positive findings on echo.
- **Surgery.** Children who have congenital heart disease that might require surgery should be treated with input from a pediatric cardiologist. Reasons not to operate include the fact that some structural problems, such as VSD and PDA, sometimes resolve on their own. Other reasons not to operate include the fact that younger children are poorer operative candidates and that artificial valves will need to be replaced as the child grows. Reasons not to wait too long include irreversible processes (such as pulmonary hypertension) and irreversible structural damage (such as dilatation or hypertrophy of the ventricles).

REFERENCES

1. Bonow RO, Carabello B, de Leon AC, et al. Guidelines for the management of patients with valvular heart disease: executive summary. A report of the American College of Cardiology/American Heart Association Task Force on Practice Guidelines (Committee on Management of Patients with Valvular Heart Disease). *Circulation* 1998;98:1949–1984.
2. Boon NA, Bloomfield P. The medical management of valvular heart disease. *Heart* 2002;87:395–400.
3. Carabello BA, Crawford FA. Valvular heart disease. *N Engl J Med* 1997;337:32–41.
4. Davies MK, Gibbs CR, Lipp GYH. ABC of heart failure—investigation. *BMJ* 2000;2730:297–300.
5. Liberthson RR. Sudden death from cardiac causes in children and young adults. *N Engl J Med* 1996;334:1039–1044.
6. Rosenhek R, Binder T, Porenta G, et al. Predictors of outcome in severe asymptomatic aortic stenosis. *N Engl J Med* 2000;343:611–617.

7. Scognamiglio R, Rahimtoola SH, Fasoli G, et al. Nifedipine in asymptomatic patients with severe aortic regurgitation and normal left ventricular function. *N Engl J Med* 1994;331:689–694.
8. Shipton B, Wahba H. Valvular heart disease: review and update. *Am Fam Physician* 2001;63:2201–2208.
9. Spirito P, Bellone P, Harris K, et al. Magnitude of left ventricular hypertrophy and risk of sudden death in hypertrophic cardiomyopathy. *N Engl J Med* 2000;342:1778–1785.
10. Stapleton JF. Natural history of chronic valvular heart disease. *Cardiovasc Clin North Am* 1986;16:105–149.
11. Chatterjee K. Auscultation of Heart Murmurs. Up to date. http://www.uptodate.com/contents/auscultation-of-cardiac-murmurs. Accessed April 23, 2014.

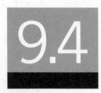

9.4 Heart Failure

Jenny Papazian, Denise Barnard

GENERAL PRINCIPLES

Definition

Heart failure (HF) is a complex clinical syndrome deriving from cardiac dysfunction that may be either acute or chronic in its presentation. The "classic" presentation of acute, severe HF evokes an image of a dyspneic patient sitting upright due to pulmonary edema with poor peripheral perfusion. However, identical or more severe hemodynamic abnormalities are commonly found in the patient with chronic HF without extreme symptoms or dramatic physical examination signs, reflecting a slower, insidious onset. Therefore, while acute HF is readily diagnosed, signs and symptoms of chronic HF are frequently overlooked in clinical practice.

The syndrome of HF can result from congenital or acquired abnormalities of cardiac muscle (endocardium, myocardium) or from valvular, great vessel, or pericardial disorders. HF results when the heart is unable to generate cardiac output sufficient to meet and maintain the metabolic requirements of the body without a marked elevation in filling pressure (at rest, upon exertion, or under other physiologic demands). This chapter focuses on the diagnosis, evaluation, and treatment of the patient with chronic HF due to left ventricular (LV) dysfunction. This working definition of chronic HF still does not identify disease physiology in terms of the degree of systolic (ejection-related) or diastolic (relaxation-related) LV dysfunction, nor infer disease etiology. Chronic HF may be associated with a wide spectrum of LV functional abnormalities, which may range from patients with normal LV size and preserved ejection fraction (EF) to those with severe LV dilatation and/or markedly reduced EF. In most patients, abnormalities of systolic and diastolic dysfunction coexist, regardless of LV EF.

Patients with an LV EF ≤40% are classified as having heart failure with reduced EF (HF-rEF), whereas those with EF ≥50% are classified as heart failure with preserved EF (HF-pEF). Patients with HF-pEF are further classified as *borderline* HF-pEF if EF is 41% to 49% or *improved* HF-pEF if EF has improved to greater than 40%, respectively.[1] The latter two categories represent a heterogeneous and intermediate group of patients in whom the optimal treatment and clinical outcomes are undefined and understudied.

Epidemiology

HF is an invariably progressive syndrome affecting over 5 million persons in the United States. It is the only cardiovascular disorder with increasing prevalence, especially among elderly individuals and in women. More than 550,000 new cases of HF are diagnosed annually, and both HF-pEF and HF-rEF appear equal in frequency. The incidence of HF approaches 10 per 1,000 population after age 65 and approximately 80% of patients hospitalized with HF are more than 65 years old.[1–4] By the year 2050, one in five Americans will be over 65 years of age.[4] HF is the primary diagnosis in more than 1 million hospitalizations annually.[3] Patients hospitalized for HF are at high risk for recurrent hospitalizations, with a 1-month readmission rate of 25%.[2]

At the age of 40 years, the lifetime risk of developing HF in Americans is 20%.[3] This common, yet generally preventable, syndrome is characterized by high mortality, frequent hospitalization, and reduced quality of life. It is the most common Medicare diagnosis-related group, and more Medicare dollars are spent for the diagnosis and treatment of HF than for any other diagnosis. The total cost of HF care in the United States exceeds $30 billion annually, with over half of these costs spent on hospitalizations.[2-4] Despite marked advances in medical and surgical therapy over the past two decades, the morbidity and mortality from HF remain unacceptably high, averaging 10% mortality at 1 year and 50% mortality at 5 years.[3]

Pathophysiology

HF commonly results from a single acute event, or due to chronic or repetitive cardiac injury. Inciting factors include conditions as disparate as myocardial infarction (MI) and myocardial damage due to viral myocarditis, alcohol, or a chemotherapeutic agent. This can be explained by the observation that regardless of the nature of the cardiac injury, the adaptive systemic response to altered cardiac function and hemodynamics as well as the resultant cardiac structural changes and cellular processes that develop within the heart itself are remarkably consistent. The characteristic pathophysiology of HF derives from systemic and local cardiac neurohormonal activation designed to be compensatory in nature, but results in deleterious changes in myocardial structure and cellular function in areas that were previously normal.[5] This process is termed "*cardiac remodeling*," whose key features include the following:

- Remodeling is initiated by a threshold-reaching injury to the heart, resulting in systemic and local neurohormonal activation—renin–angiotensin–aldosterone (RAAS) and sympathetic nervous systems.
- Neurohormonal activation results in additional myocardial damage that continues after resolution of the initiating event and tends to progress over time.
- Cardiac remodeling therefore results in increased cardiac chamber volumes and muscle mass (eccentric LV hypertrophy), increased extracellular matrix deposition, and myocardial fibrosis.

Etiology

The most common etiology of HF in the United States is ischemic heart disease.[1] Hypertensive or valvular heart disease and primary cardiomyopathy (familial or idiopathic) are also common. Myocardial dysfunction can be secondary to infectious, metabolic, endocrine, nutritional, or toxic causes (notably alcohol and anthracyclines); acute stress (Takotsubo cardiomyopathy); connective tissue or pericardial diseases; neuromuscular or autoimmune disorders; as well as infiltrative diseases (amyloidosis, iron overload, sarcoidosis) or undiagnosed congenital heart disease. This chapter will not address the category of high-output HF (due to thyrotoxicosis, sepsis, severe anemia, beriberi, Paget disease, myeloma, pregnancy, or significant arteriovenous shunting).

Classification

The American College of Cardiology and the American Heart Association adopted an innovative approach to the classification of HF beginning in 2001. This classification scheme emphasizes risk factors for both the development and progression of the disease.[1] Four well-defined stages comprise the HF syndrome. The first two stages (A and B) were devised to assist health care providers to more easily identify patients *at risk* for developing HF with the goal of disease prevention in mind. Stage C denotes the majority of patients who have been diagnosed with clinical HF, and Stage D denotes patients who have developed refractory HF despite optimal therapy (Table 9.4-1).

Within Stage C, the New York Heart Association (NYHA) classification system is traditionally employed to categorize HF symptoms and estimate prognosis in clinical trials. To be useful in practice, one must consider the patients' baseline subjective symptoms in reference to a normal or expected activity level for someone their age. The NYHA Symptom classification is as follows:

- Class I patients have no perceived symptoms or limitations in performing ordinary physical activities.
- Class II patients have symptoms of HF with slight or moderate levels of physical activity.
- Class III patients have a marked limitation of exercise tolerance, symptoms with simple activities of daily living but remain comfortable at rest.
- Class IV patients have symptoms of HF at rest.

DIAGNOSIS
Clinical Presentation

The clinical presentation of a patient with HF can be subtle, and patients with significant degrees of LV dysfunction may remain asymptomatic for some time. Because early diagnosis and treatment reduce morbidity and mortality, successful therapy depends on a high level of clinical suspicion and

TABLE 9.4-1   **AHA/ACC Classification System for Chronic HF in the Adult**

	Stage A	Stage B	Stage C	Stage D
Stage descriptor	High risk for developing HF but does NOT have structural heart disease or symptoms of HF.	Has structural heart disease but does NOT have signs or symptoms of HF.	Has structural heart disease AND either current or previous symptoms of HF.	Has structural heart disease with refractory HF symptoms that requires special interventions.
Patient profile	Hypertension, diabetes, atherosclerotic disease, obesity or metabolic syndrome. Exposure to cardiotoxins, or with a family history of cardiomyopathy.	Left ventricular hypertrophy, prior myocardial infarction, valvular, or other structural heart diseases are present, yet patient remains asymptomatic.	Any structural heart disease with symptoms or signs of HF. Even if symptoms resolve on medical therapy, patient remains Stage C.	Symptoms at rest despite maximal medical therapy, recurrent HF hospitalizations, or requiring special interventions such as heart transplantation, mechanical circulatory assistance, or hospice care.
Key point	Heart failure is generally preventable at this stage.	Overt heart failure is still preventable at this stage.	Guideline derived HF treatment slows disease progression and reduces morbidity and mortality at this stage.	End-stage HF has limited therapeutic options.

screening for signs and/or symptoms of HF in all patients at risk for its development (Stages A and B).[1] The clinical presentation of a patient with Stage C (overt) HF may be acute but often is more insidious and progressive. Acute or sudden-onset HF symptoms (minutes to hours) should prompt evaluation for myocardial ischemia/infarction, arrhythmia, acute valvular or LV structural deterioration, or hypertensive urgency producing a rapid, abrupt change in LV pressure or volume-loading conditions. Slow or gradual onset HF symptoms (days to weeks) is more common, as mild symptoms of HF are often unrecognized or ignored by the patient until they become severe or persistent at rest.

History and Symptoms

- Pertinent **historical elements** should include information regarding the risk factors for HF, the type and/or the extent of cardiac structural abnormalities present and the temporal nature or duration of the cardiac injury.[6] Risk factors include hypertension, diabetes, dyslipidemia, coronary or peripheral vascular disease, skeletal or cardiac myopathy, valvular heart disease, rheumatic fever, mediastinal irradiation, sleep-disordered breathing, exposure to cardiotoxic agents, current/past alcohol, cocaine or amphetamine abuse, smoking, collagen vascular diseases, HIV infection, thyroid or other metabolic disorders, pheochromocytoma, other systemic diseases (e.g., sarcoidosis, amyloidosis, hemosiderosis) and morbid obesity. In addition, a family history of sudden cardiac death, cardiomyopathy, or tachyarrhythmia should be sought. If familial cardiomyopathy is suspected, a more detailed family history should be obtained, preferably including three generations.[1]
- Symptoms *strongly suggesting* a diagnosis of HF include dyspnea at rest or with exertion, orthopnea, paroxysmal nocturnal dyspnea (PND), nocturnal or recumbent cough or other sleep disturbance, pedal or scrotal swelling, impaired exercise capacity or endurance. Less specific presentations of HF include early satiety, nausea and vomiting, abdominal discomfort or bloating, exertional wheezing, unexplained fatigue, weakness, or malaise, mental confusion or impaired concentrating ability, and daytime oliguria with recumbent nocturia. The spectrum of symptoms in a given patient reflects

the relative extent of systemic and/or pulmonary venous congestion related to fluid overload versus reduced cardiac output (hypoperfusion).

- In a patient with known LV dysfunction and previously diagnosed HF, provocative and exacerbating factors should be reviewed.[1] Serial monitoring of weight gain or loss, medication and diet adherence, appetite, activity tolerance and sleep quality may reveal pitfalls to the most optimal therapeutic plan. Common precipitants of decompensation are excess dietary sodium, medication noncompliance or errors, drug interactions or side effects, use of over-the-counter medications such as nonsteroidal anti-inflammatory drugs (NSAIDs), substance abuse, uncontrolled diabetes or hypertension, infection, thyroid dysfunction, arrhythmias, myocardial ischemia, renal or hepatic insufficiency, pregnancy, and other physical or emotional stressors. At each visit, an assessment of the severity and triggers of dyspnea, fatigue, chest discomfort, palpitations, or presyncope should be performed.

Physical Examination

- **Acute decompensated HF.** The classic findings of acute decompensated "congestive" HF include a resting tachycardia, tachypnea, diffuse pulmonary rales, and an abnormal apical impulse (enlarged, diffuse, displaced, dyskinetic, or sustained).[7] In acute, decompensated "low output" HF, particularly HF-rEF, systemic hypoperfusion may be manifest as by hypotension, a reduced pulse pressure or pulsus alternans, diminished carotid upstroke volume, Cheyne–Stokes respirations, cool extremities, and altered mentation. Whether this is a new onset diagnosis, or an acute decompensation of chronic HF, these patients will generally require acute hospitalization.
- **Chronic HF.** In chronic HF, it is very common to find fairly clear lung fields with coarse breath sounds or reduced respiratory diaphragmatic excursion.[7] Bibasilar or diffuse rales are observed typically when filling pressures are rapidly or markedly elevated. Pleural effusions, when present, are more right-sided than left, or bilateral. The greater the number of symptoms and signs observed in a given patient, the more reliable is the diagnosis of HF. The most specific physical findings are an elevated jugular venous pressure, an S_3, a laterally displaced apical impulse, pulmonary rales that do not clear with cough, and peripheral edema not due to primary venous insufficiency. Nonspecific physical findings include cardiomegaly or an abnormal apical impulse, an S_4, and tachypnea.
- Signs of biventricular or predominant "right-heart" failure include an elevated jugular venous pressure, right ventricular (RV) parasternal lift or subxiphoid tap, RV gallop, loud P_2 (pulmonary hypertension), abdominojugular reflux, pulsatile or tender hepatomegaly, ascites, and peripheral (dependent) edema. Signs of right-sided HF without signs of LV dysfunction may redirect your attention to primary or secondary pulmonary vascular diseases. Murmurs may reveal the cause of HF (valvular stenosis or regurgitation, hypertrophic cardiomyopathy with outflow tract obstruction) or in the case of mitral regurgitation, a possible consequence of LV remodeling and enlargement.[7]

Diagnostic Testing—Laboratory and Imaging

- **Electrocardiography.** The baseline electrocardiogram should be assessed for signs of prior infarction, ischemia, arrhythmia, conduction delays, and chamber enlargement or hypertrophy as these may provide clues to the underlying etiology of LV dysfunction. Low QRS voltage may indicate an occult primary or secondary infiltrative myocardial disease such as amyloidosis or a pericardial effusion. Nonspecific ST-T wave abnormalities are common. The QT/QTc interval may be prolonged, can reflect electrolyte abnormalities, myocardial disease, and drug effects, and confers an increased risk of ventricular arrhythmia.
- **Chest radiography.** It is important to note that a normal chest radiograph does not rule out the diagnosis of HF, but may afford a differential diagnosis. The chest x-ray can yield information on HF etiology and the degree of fluid overload or hemodynamic compensation. The cardiothoracic ratio and silhouette show that cardiac chambers are grossly enlarged. The amount of pulmonary vascular crowding, upper lobe redistribution, edema, Kerley B lines, or pleural effusions points more to volume status in the chronic setting and to the time course of hemodynamic alterations in the acute setting.
- **Laboratory tests.** The HF treatment guideline of the ACC/AHA recommends that all patients with HF initially undergo complete laboratory evaluation, including a complete blood count (CBC), serum electrolytes (including calcium, magnesium), blood urea nitrogen and serum creatinine, glucose, liver function tests, a fasting lipid profile, thyroid-stimulating hormone, and a urinalysis.[1] Other laboratory tests such as HIV or other viral serologies, serum transferrin and iron saturation, and rheumatologic markers are obtained only if indicated by the history and physical examination. Serial measurements of electrolytes and renal function are typically advisable during medication titration.

- **Serum biomarkers.** For outpatients with complaints of dyspnea, measurement of brain natriuretic peptide (BNP) or N-terminal pro-BNP (NT-pro-BNP or BNPP) are well validated and useful tests to support the diagnosis of HF, as these peptides are synthesized and released by the heart primarily in response to hemodynamic perturbations.[1] The level of BNP or BNPP correlates with disease severity and prognosis in both ambulatory outpatients and acute decompensated hospitalized patients, such that its measurement is a class 1 recommendation in HF treatment guidelines.[1] However, natriuretic peptides have not been shown to be effective in screening and identifying asymptomatic patients with ventricular dysfunction. Elevations in plasma BNP levels are seen in acute, decompensated and chronic HF, acute MI, myocardial ischemia, and LV hypertrophy. The normal ranges for BNP and NT-proBNP are higher in women than in men, and in both sexes increase with age and/or declining renal function.[8] In contrast, in the setting of morbid obesity, BNP levels may be disproportionately low. Marked elevations in BNP levels correlate with symptoms and the degree of LV systolic dysfunction (EF). However, a modestly elevated BNP level can occur in other settings, such as post-cardioversion, cardiac surgery, anemia, pulmonary embolism, pulmonary hypertension, renal failure, bacterial sepsis, severe burns, and other critical illnesses. Cardiac troponin levels can be elevated in decompensated HF patients without evidence of active myocardial ischemia or acute coronary syndromes, including patients without coronary artery disease (CAD). Measurement of this indicator of myocardial injury is recommended as part of the evaluation of patients with acute decompensated HF.[1] Troponin elevations are usually mild but when present are associated with impaired hemodynamics, more severe LV dysfunction, worse clinical outcomes, and higher mortality rates.[1,8–10] Newer, emerging biomarkers of myocardial fibrosis such as soluble ST-2 and galectin-3 are predictive of both hospitalization and death in HF and may be additive to natriuretic peptide levels. Multimarker assessment strategies as a means to guide treatment are being evaluated for relative efficacy in predicting change in prognosis over time in HF patients.[8–10]
- **Echocardiography.** The most valuable and cost-effective test in the diagnosis of HF is two-dimensional echocardiography with Doppler imaging, which facilitates the detection of abnormalities in myocardial, valvular, and pericardial structure and function.[11] One major determinant of the appropriate course of therapy for HF is whether the LV EF is preserved or reduced. This information is quantified by echocardiography, along with cardiac chamber dimensions and/or volumes, LV wall thickness, and ventricular diastolic filling dynamics. Further, echocardiography provides an estimation of intracardiac hemodynamics, an evaluation of chamber geometry and assesses regional wall motion. The preference for echocardiography as an imaging modality is based upon its nearly ubiquitous availability and imaging quality without the use of ionizing radiation. Alternatively, the LV or RV EF and ventricular filling dynamics can also be determined by radionuclide imaging techniques. Cardiac magnetic resonance (CMR) imaging and cardiac computed tomography (CT) are also increasingly useful modalities in evaluating ventricular size, function and mass, detecting intracardiac shunts, RV dysplasia and other anatomical abnormalities. Given their cost, inherent radiation exposure, and imaging limitation at elevated heart rates, the routine use of these modalities has been limited. CMR and CT can be protocoled in order to distinguish viable myocardium from ischemic, infarcted, or fibrotic scar tissue. Ischemia and viability assessments by these techniques may be an important tool in determining whether to refer HF-rEF patients with known CAD for surgical revascularization.[12]
- **Other diagnostic testing.** Once the clinical diagnosis of HF is confirmed with supportive data from echocardiography, the remainder of diagnostic testing is directed at determining the underlying etiology. Irrespective of LV EF, in all patients with HF, the etiology that is most important to consider and exclude is CAD. Strategies involving noninvasive stress ischemia evaluation or coronary angiography are best chosen based on symptoms, signs, and CAD risk factors. With respect to acute decompensated HF, the use of invasive hemodynamic monitoring is recommended for those patients with poor perfusion and/or severe dyspnea in whom clinical assessment is unable to assess fluid status, hemodynamics, and cardiac output.[1]

Prognostic Assessment

An assessment of prognosis should be considered an integral part of the evaluation of a patient with HF. Risk assessment is recommended at the time of diagnosis and periodically thereafter. There are a number of well-validated multivariable risk scores available to help estimate an individual patient's risk of mortality, both in the ambulatory and acute care settings, for both HF-rEF and HF-pEF populations, although their utilization is considered a class IIA guideline recommendation.[1] In the absence of access to these score models or nomograms, each of the following is an easy-to-measure variable that lends independent, additive prognostic information.[13]

- **Extent of LV dysfunction**. LV EF less than 0.35 with lower values worse, significant LV enlargement, dilation, or concomitant restrictive filling dynamics (significant diastolic dysfunction) denote an extremely high-risk patient. Concomitant RV enlargement or dysfunction worsens prognosis further.
- **Symptom class**. Risk worsens with higher NYHA class, with NYHA IV having a 30% to 50% annual mortality risk. Persistent moderate to severe HF symptoms despite standard medical therapy warrants consideration of patient referral to an HF specialist.
- **Hemodynamics**. Clinical, echocardiographically estimated or measured pulmonary hypertension in the setting of LV systolic dysfunction carries a worse prognosis and is an indication for more aggressive therapy.
- **Exercise capacity**. Although age dependent, the inability to walk more than 300 m in a 6-minute walk test (for any reason) infers substantially greater annual risk of death or morbidity compared with a patient who can walk 450 m or more. Markedly impaired oxygen consumption with exercise, measured as a VO_2 max <15 mL/kg/minute, or achieving less than 4 to 5 metabolic equivalents (METS) of work on bicycle or treadmill cardiopulmonary exercise test has a markedly adverse prognosis. Significant exercise impairment corresponds to a 1-year mortality rate of 20% or higher.
- **Arrhythmia**. Atrial fibrillation, atrial or ventricular tachyarrhythmias, or evidence of other conduction system disease such as arteriovenous (AV) nodal block or left bundle branch block worsen prognosis. Any family history of sudden death is associated with worse prognosis. Approximately 50% to 70% of patients with low EF and symptomatic HF have episodes of nonsustained ventricular tachycardia on routine ambulatory electrocardiographic monitoring; this is generally not indicated for screening purposes in the absence of symptoms.
- **Hyponatremia**. Serum sodium concentration of 135 mg per dL or less is generally related to intense renin–angiotensin system activation and denotes a higher-risk patient.
- **Chronic kidney disease.** Significant renal insufficiency not due to expected (reversible) medication effects is associated with worse outcomes in HF. Worsening renal function typically defined as an increase in serum creatinine ≥0.2 mg per dL or a corresponding decrease in estimated glomerular filtration rate ≥5 mL × min × 1.73 m² is an adverse sign predicting substantially higher rates of mortality and hospitalization in patients with HF.
- **Anemia.** Anemia is present in up to 35% of HF patient populations. In studies that analyzed hemoglobin as a continuous variable, a 1-g per dL decrease in hemoglobin was independently associated with significantly increased mortality risk. Anemia can worsen cardiac ischemia, impair cardiac function and is associated with poor outcomes, including a higher risk of hospitalization, decreased exercise capacity, and poor quality of life.

Assessment of Comorbidities

Patients and practitioners often underestimate the substantial influence of comorbid diagnoses or conditions on the clinical course and stability of patients with HF. These common conditions include atherosclerosis, diabetes, hypertension, hyperlipidemia, thyroid dysfunction, anemia, obstructive sleep apnea, depression, and obesity. Concurrent infections can trigger HF decompensation due to fever and physiologic stressors and should be treated early and aggressively. Treating these conditions optimally may reduce ongoing or limit additional myocardial injury as well as reduce hospitalizations and improve outcomes. In particular, sleep-disordered breathing and depression are very common in HF populations and worsen clinical outcomes and quality of life. Immunizations and general health care maintenance should be kept up to date.

Differential Diagnosis

The differential diagnosis of a patient with prominent *dyspnea* ± *edema* includes pulmonary parenchymal disease (obstructive vs. interstitial), pulmonary thromboembolic disease, cor pulmonale, pulmonary veno-occlusive disease, primary or other secondary pulmonary arterial hypertension, exertional asthma, severe anemia, mitral stenosis, neuromuscular disease, constrictive pericarditis, or metabolic causes (i.e., acidosis). The differential diagnosis of a patient with predominant *edema* ± *dyspnea* includes severe venous insufficiency, nephrotic syndrome, cirrhosis, lymphedema, combined vascular insufficiency, and adverse medication effects (i.e., dihydropyridine calcium-channel blockers).

TREATMENT
Pharmacologic Management of Chronic HF-rEF

The majority of clinical research trials that have established the foundation of traditional medical therapy have focused on HF with systolic LV dysfunction (LVD). The implicit goals of treating chronic HF are to (a) improve patient symptoms and quality of life, (b) slow or reverse the progression of cardiac dysfunction, and (c) reduce HF mortality, morbidity, and therefore the cost burden of acute care. Since the pathophysiology of HF is complex, so follows the pharmacologic regimen. Angiotensin-converting enzyme inhibitors (ACE-I) and β-blockers have become the cornerstone of therapy to delay, halt, or reverse cardiac remodeling and improve mortality. In addition, the roles of diuretic therapy, aldosterone inhibition, digoxin, and other vasodilator therapy are reviewed.

Angiotensin-Converting Enzyme Inhibitors

Contemporary treatment guidelines for systolic LVD mandate that an ACE-I be utilized as primary therapy unless contraindicated.[1,14] ACE-I improve hemodynamics by reducing afterload and attenuate the vasoconstrictor activity of angiotensin II (Ang II). Ang II also has thrombogenic, atherogenic, profibrotic, and other effects that contribute to progressive LV remodeling. ACE-I improve HF symptoms and quality of life. The progression of HF is slowed by ACE-I therapy, as evidenced in clinical trials by a survival benefit and fewer hospitalizations. ACE-I are indicated for use in the primary prevention of HF in patients at risk, post-MI patients regardless of EF, and in patients with documented LVD regardless of symptoms (AHA Stages A to D).[1]

ACE-I are typically initiated at low dose and uptitrated over days to weeks until side effects are noted or the dose reaches the equivalent of those used in the HF trials (Table 9.4-2). In general, higher achieved doses result in greater reductions in morbidity and hospitalization for HF, but mortality reduction is seen at virtually all doses. Electrolytes and renal function should be checked before initiation, after every dose increase, and after addition of other medications. Hypotension is seen most frequently during the first few days of initiation or dose increase, particularly in patients with hypovolemia, a recent large diuresis, or severe hyponatremia (serum sodium under 130 mmol per L). ACE-I lower blood pressure and alter intra-renal hemodynamics, inducing a predictable increase in serum creatinine. A modest elevation and plateau in blood urea nitrogen and serum creatinine concentration are expected with the use of diuretics and/or vasodilator therapy in HF. Progressively worsening renal function, however (i.e., serum creatinine increase of more than 0.3 mg per dL over a normal baseline, or a serum creatinine >2.5 to 3.0 mg per dL, may represent renal hypoperfusion due to a reduction in cardiac output or renal perfusion pressure.

In the absence of hyperkalemia, most HF experts will still initiate ACE-I therapy in a patient with a serum creatinine ≤3 mg per dL, employing an agent that is hepatically cleared to prevent drug or

TABLE 9.4-2	Angiotensin-Converting Enzyme Inhibitors and Angiotensin Receptor Blockers Commonly Used for the Treatment of Chronic HF (Generic Names Listed)	
	Starting dose	**Maximum dose**
ACE-I		
Captopril	6.25 mg 3 times daily	50 mg 3 times daily
Enalapril	2.5 mg twice daily	10–20 mg twice daily
Fosinopril	5–10 mg daily	40 mg daily
Lisinopril	2.5–5 mg daily	20–40 mg daily
Perindopril	2 mg daily	8–16 mg daily
Quinapril	5 mg twice daily	20 mg twice daily
Ramipril	1.25–2.5 mg daily	10 mg daily
Trandolapril	1 mg daily	4 mg daily
ARBs		
Candesartan	4–8 mg daily	32 mg daily
Irbesartan	75 mg daily	150–300 mg
Eprosartan	300 mg daily	800 mg daily
Losartan	25–50 mg daily	50–100 mg daily
Olmesartan	10 mg daily	20–40 mg daily
Telmesartan	20 mg daily	40–80 mg daily
Valsartan	20–40 mg twice daily	160 mg twice daily

metabolite accumulation and profound hypotension. Other possible side effects of ACE-I include orthostatic hypotension, dizziness, hyponatremia, cough, and angioedema. Cough develops in 5% to 10% of patients on an ACE-I but is much more common, up to 50%, in Asian/Chinese populations. Cough represents the most common reason for drug withdrawal. It should be noted that cough might also represent worsening HF or other conditions, so if not resolved after a temporary discontinuation of the drug, the ACE-I should be restarted. Angioedema can be mild, or life-threatening in severe cases. Its prevalence is estimated at <1%, but is more common in black populations.

Angiotensin Receptor Blockers

This class of drugs has become an acceptable alternative to ACE-I for both the prevention and treatment of HF.[1] The most convincing data regarding the efficacy of angiotensin receptor blockers (ARBs) in HF therapy derives from the recent Candesartan in Heart Failure Assessment of Reduction in Mortality and Morbidity Trial (CHARM). The CHARM study had three placebo-controlled arms, one evaluating candesartan as an alternative to an ACE-I, the second as added therapy, and the third as therapy in patients with HF-pEF. In each arm, a therapeutic benefit from the ARB was observed.[15,16]

Like ACE-I, ARBs are also initiated at low dose and uptitrated over days to weeks (Table 9.4-1). An ARB is the best substitute for an ACE-I when the latter induces cough. The risk of angioedema is much lower with ARBs, but has been observed in approximately 8% of patients given an ARB *after* developing angioedema to the former drug. Other ARB side effects are quite similar to those of the ACE-I class of agents. Aside from the pathway of drug metabolism, little difference exists between the available ACE-I and ARBs, the choice of agent becomes clinician or formulary preference.

β-Blockers

The pivotal trials that provided incontrovertible evidence of the efficacy of β-blocker therapy in patients with chronic HF were the U.S. Carvedilol Trials Program, Cardiac Insufficiency Bisoprolol Study-2 (CIBIS-II), and the Metoprolol CR/XL Randomized Intervention Trial in Congestive Heart Failure (MERIT-HF) study.[17–19] HF guidelines state that only carvedilol, sustained release metoprolol succinate, or bisoprolol should be added to background ACE-I or ARB therapy (Table 9.4-3). The reason for this is that β-blockers are a very heterogeneous group of agents, exhibiting variable selectivity for β-receptors, marked differences in pharmacokinetics, and many have ancillary vasodilating or additional antioxidant properties. First, the patient should be carefully evaluated for clinical stability and should be considered euvolemic.

β-Blockers should be started at low dose and in general, uptitrated approximately every 2 weeks, with target doses reached in about 8 to 12 weeks. Patients should be followed carefully for signs of impending decompensation or side effects (fluid retention, hypotension, dyspnea, fatigue, bradycardia, or heart block). Patients who manifest worsening HF symptoms or fluid retention should have diuretic medications adjusted. A temporary dose reduction in ACE-I, ARB, or other vasoactive medications may be necessary when symptomatic hypotension is present. With careful observation the vast majority of patients can tolerate β-Blockers therapy and achieve target doses. In general, patients on chronic β-Blockers therapy experiencing an acute decompensation should remain on their β-blocker, or be given a reduced dose and uptitrated again following symptomatic resolution. Avoid abrupt discontinuation, especially in patients with underlying ischemic heart disease. If the initiation or uptitration of β-blockers to target doses proves difficult, consider referral to an HF specialist.

TABLE 9.4-3	β-Adrenergic Blocking Drugs Approved for the Treatment of Chronic HF-rEF	
β-Blocker	Initial dose and typical increment during uptitration	Treatment dose goal in clinical trials
Bisoprolol	1.25 mg daily	10 mg daily
Carvedilol	3.125 mg twice daily	25 mg twice daily
		50 mg twice daily if >85 kg
Metoprolol CR/XL	12.5–25 mg daily	200 mg daily

Other Vasodilators

For patients with HF and LV systolic dysfunction intolerant of ACE-I or ARB therapy (due to renal dysfunction or hyperkalemia), the combination of hydralazine (H) and isosorbide dinitrate (ISDN) is recommended.[1,20] The mortality benefit with H-ISDN is not as great as that seen with ACE-I or ARB but is significantly better than those of placebo or vasodilatory α-blockers (prazosin). The H-ISDN combination is appealing in chronic kidney disease, as it tends to increase renal cortical blood flow. Side effects including headache, dizziness, diarrhea, tachycardia, and somnonence are significant with this regimen; up to 25% of patients will discontinue one or both. The benefit of nitrates is presumed to be related to enhanced nitric oxide bioavailability. Hydralazine is a direct-acting vasodilator, but also reduces nitrate tolerance. Nitrate therapy is useful in decreasing orthopnea and PND and tends to improve exercise tolerance in patients who have persistent limitations despite optimization of other therapies.

The African-American Heart Failure Trial (A-HeFT) enrolled 1,050 self-identified African American patients who had NYHA class III or IV HF with LV dilation and systolic dysfunction.[21] A new fixed-dose combination of H-ISDN (or placebo) was utilized in addition to background therapy of an ACE-I or ARB, a β-blocker, and a loop diuretic. Many patients were also taking digoxin and an aldosterone antagonist. Patients receiving the H-ISDN combination demonstrated a 43% reduction in all-cause death and a 33% reduction in first HF hospitalizations and a significant improvement in quality of life. The fixed-dose combination (BiDil) includes 37.5 mg H and 20 mg ISDN, and was titrated to 225/120 mg per day in three divided doses in this study.

The Prospective Randomized Amlodipine Survival Evaluation Trial-2 (PRAISE-2) added amlodipine or placebo to background HF therapy of an ACE-I, digoxin, and diuretics in nonischemic cardiomyopathy and symptomatic HF.[22] There was no survival advantage (or disadvantage) attributable to amlodipine administration in this population, and very little data regarding patients also taking β-blockers. Calcium-channel blockers are not indicated as routine treatment for HF in patients with current or prior symptoms of HF and reduced LV EF, but amlodipine could be considered for the management of hypertension.[1]

Aldosterone Inhibitors

The Randomized Aldosterone Evaluation Study (RALES) demonstrated a beneficial effect on mortality due to progressive HF from low-dose spironolactone in patients with a recent hospitalization, and continued moderate to severe HF symptoms (NYHA class III or IV) on ACE-I or ARB therapy.[23] The Eplerenone in Mild Patients Hospitalization and Survival Study in Heart Failure (EMPHASIS-HF) found a reduction in the rate of death from any cause or hospitalization for HF in patients with NYHA class II symptoms.[24]

Clinical guidelines recommend aldosterone receptor antagonists in normokalemic patients with serum creatinine less than 2.5 mg per dL with NYHA class II to IV HF and LV EF less than 0.35. Aldosterone receptor antagonists are also recommended to reduce morbidity and mortality following an acute MI in patients with LV EF of less than 0.40 who develop symptoms of HF based on findings in the EPHESUS trial.[1,23] Serum sodium and potassium should be checked at 1 week, frequently thereafter, including any time there is a change in dosage of any medication that may influence potassium balance or renal function. Strong consideration should be given to lowering or eliminating supplemental potassium when spironolactone is added to the regimen, to lessen the risk of potentially fatal hyperkalemia.

Digitalis

Digoxin remains a controversial drug in HF with systolic LVD two centuries after its initial use. Digoxin withdrawal from patients with stable chronic HF on an ACE-I contributes to decompensation requiring treatment or hospital admission, reduced exercise capacity, and lower quality-of-life scores.[25] In the Digitalis Investigation Group (DIG) trial, the addition of digoxin to baseline therapy had a neutral effect on mortality but decreased hospitalizations for HF. Digoxin increases EF by 3% to 5% due to its positive inotropic effects mediated by sodium–potassium pump inhibition.[26] More importantly, digoxin improves rest and exercise LV hemodynamics, and is sympathoinhibitory, attenuating the neurohormonal and baroreceptor abnormalities seen in chronic HF. This latter role as neurohormonal antagonist may be the more important mechanism of action, as all other agents with positive inotropic activity have increased HF mortality in clinical trials.

Digoxin therapy may be limited by renal insufficiency and conduction abnormalities (heart block, slow atrial fibrillation) but is generally well tolerated, with few side effects at recommended doses. Current guidelines state its use should be considered if HF symptoms remain after ACE-I and β-blockers

TABLE 9.4-4	Commonly Used Diuretic Drugs for the Treatment of Sodium and Fluid Retention in Chronic HF	
	Initial oral dose	**Recommended maximal oral dose**
Thiazide class		
Chlorothiazide	250 mg daily	500 mg daily
Hydrochlorothiazide	25 mg daily	50–100 mg daily
Metolazone	2.5 mg daily	10 mg daily
Loop diuretics		
Furosemide	10–40 mg daily or twice daily	200 mg daily or twice daily
Bumetanide	0.5–1.0 daily or twice daily	4–5 mg daily or twice daily
Torsemide	10 mg daily	200 mg daily

titration when the EF remains less than 0.40 or for patients with severe symptoms who have not yet responded symptomatically to optimal medical therapy.[1] Loading doses are unnecessary, and most patients should be prescribed a dose of 0.125 mg daily. Current guidelines suggest doses of digoxin that achieve a plasma concentration of drug in the range of 0.5 to 0.9 ng per mL. There have been no prospective, randomized studies of the relative efficacy or safety of different plasma concentrations of digoxin. Overt digoxin toxicity is commonly associated with serum digoxin levels greater than 2 ng per mL but can occur at lower levels, especially in the setting of hypokalemia, hypomagnesemia, or hypothyroidism.[26,27] Digoxin trough levels should be obtained if there is clinical suspicion of toxicity due to signs or symptoms and to determine whether dose (or dose frequency) reduction is indicated in the setting of worsening renal function or loss of lean body mass. The initiation of medications with known or possible interactions that may increase digoxin concentrations (verapamil, quinidine, amiodarone, spironolactone, and certain antibiotics) should be coupled with measurement of digoxin level within 1 week of initiation of the drug to ensure the digoxin level does not exceed 1 ng per mL.[1]

Diuretics

Diuretic therapy is indicated for symptoms or signs of systemic or pulmonary congestion due to volume overload.[28–30] Diuretics relieve congestive symptoms by promoting excretion of excess sodium and therefore water (Table 9.4-4). There are no controlled clinical trial data prospectively evaluating the overall impact of diuretic therapy on mortality in patients with HF. Diuretics promote activation of the RAAS, potentiate the hypotensive effects of ACE-Is/ARBs, and may decrease cardiac output, especially in patients with diastolic LVD. Chronic diuretic therapy can be limited by the development of diuretic resistance or refractoriness. Diuretics also induce hypokalemia, hypomagnesemia, and hyperuricemia, and promote calciuria. Electrolytes require close monitoring when diuretics are used.[30]

Thiazide diuretics should be used if fluid retention is mild, but are effective only when the glomerular filtration rate is greater than 30 mL per minute. Loop diuretics are the mainstay of diuretic therapy in HF when congestion is moderate. When fluid retention is extreme or the patient has become refractory to loop diuretics, intravenous administration of a loop diuretic or the addition of the thiazide-like agent metolazone (1 to 5 mg 30 minutes to 1 hour prior to loop agent) can dramatically increase natriuresis and induce severe electrolyte loss. Potassium-sparing diuretics should be used with caution in patients on ACE-Is or ARBs and in patients with diabetes prone to type IV renal tubular acidosis.

Pharmacologic Management of Chronic HF-pEF

Trials using comparable and efficacious agents for HF-rEF have generally been disappointing when used in patients with HF-pEF.[1,31–33] Therefore, most of the recommended therapies for HF with diastolic LVD are directed at symptoms, especially comorbidities, and risk factors that may worsen cardiovascular disease. CAD and hypertension should be aggressively treated, if present. Blood pressure control remains the most important recommendation in patients with HF-pEF as it has been shown to reduce hospitalizations for HF.[34] β-Blocking agents, ACE and ARBs are all reasonable to employ for this purpose.[1]

Diuretics are typically necessary for congestive symptoms, but excessive preload reduction (nitrates, diuretics) can impair cardiac output and exacerbate hypotension and should be used with caution. There is no recommended role for digoxin therapy in a patient with HF-pEF. Patients with atrial fibrillation and rapid ventricular response intolerant of or refractory to β-blocker or amiodarone therapy should be referred to an electrophysiologist for possible catheter ablation.

Nonpharmacologic HF Therapies

Patient Education/Behavioral Interventions

Discuss with the patient *and family* the diagnosis and reason(s) for the development of HF, including estimated prognosis and intended treatment plan. Symptoms referable to HF should be reviewed and patients instructed to call if symptoms are noted or increased, particularly rapid weight gain or loss. Emphasize sodium restriction to 1,500 mg per day, along with daily weight monitoring. Stress the importance of medication adherence, good nutrition, and physical activity. Fluid restriction is generally necessary only when excessive or when volume status is difficult to manage with diuretics and sodium restriction. Fluid restriction is advisable in the setting of severe hyponatremia, however. Smoking cessation should be advocated.[1]

Guidelines recommend that patients' literacy, cognitive status, psychological state, culture, and access to social and financial resources be taken into account for optimal education and counseling.[1] It is also recommended that providers frequently assess for medication nonadherence or dietary noncompliance (sodium, alcohol, excess fluids), drug abuse, and medication additions by other providers (calcium-channel blockers in HF-rEF, NSAIDs, glitazones, remicade, and certain over-the-counter medications or supplement use[35]). It is important to confirm and treat uncontrolled hypertension, diabetes, paroxysmal arrhythmias, depression, or sleep apnea. Surveillance laboratory testing is helpful in detecting decreasing renal or hepatic function, new or worsening anemia, and occult infection.

Written educational materials are quite useful and downloadable from the Heart Failure Society of America Web site (www.hfsa.org or www.abouthf.org) and the American Heart Association Get with the Guidelines program. Consider referral to a dietician or disease management program when patient understanding is an impairment to the success of your plan of care. Such disease management programs have been shown to significantly reduce HF hospitalizations, produce shorter lengths of stay, lower health care costs, and improve both quality of life and survival.[36]

Exercise and Cardiac Rehabilitation

Several controlled trials have shown that exercise training can reduce symptoms, increase exercise capacity, and improve the quality of life of patients with chronic HF. Exercise prescriptions (aerobic and light resistance training) are generally safe in compensated HF. In the Heart Failure: A Controlled Trial Investigating Outcomes of Exercise Training (HF-ACTION) trial, 2,331 medically stable outpatients with HF with reduced EF were randomized to exercise training for 3 months or to standard medical therapy. When adjusted for CAD risk factors, patients assigned to the exercise group had a significant reduction in all-cause mortality, cardiovascular mortality, and hospitalizations.[37] On the basis of clinical guidelines, cardiac rehabilitation is recommended in clinically stable patients with HF in order to improve functional capacity, exercise duration, health-related quality of life, and mortality.[1]

Treatment of Sleep Disorders

Sleep disorders are common in patients with HF. A study of adults with chronic HF treated with evidence-based therapies found that 61% had either central or obstructive sleep apnea.[38]

The primary treatment of obstructive sleep apnea (OSA) is nocturnal continuous positive airway pressure (CPAP). In a major trial, CPAP for OSA was effective in decreasing the apnea–hypopnea index, improving nocturnal oxygenation, increasing LV EF, lowering norepinephrine levels, and increasing the distance walked in 6 minutes. These benefits were sustained for up to 2 years.[39] Clinical guidelines therefore recommend maintaining a high index of suspicion for sleep disorders in HF patients and referring patients for a sleep study when indicated.[1]

Biventricular Pacemakers

Dyssynchronous contractions between the LV and RV can be improved by electrically activating the right and left ventricles in a sequential manner with a biventricular pacemaker device. Cardiac resynchronization therapy (CRT) appears to improve EF, reduce secondary mitral regurgitation, and improve HF symptoms (when moderate to severe), as well as enhance exercise capacity and quality of life.[40–42] There is strong evidence to support the use of CRT to improve survival and to decrease hospitalizations in patients with persistently symptomatic HF receiving optimal medical therapy who have cardiac dyssynchrony (evidenced by a prolonged QRS duration greater than 120 ms) and an EF of 0.35 or less. Based on the Multicenter Automatic Defibrillator Implantation Trial-Cardiac Resynchronization Therapy (MADIT-CRT) trial, CRT may also be considered for patients with class I symptoms greater than 40 days after MI with EF less than 0.30, sinus rhythm, left bundle branch block, and QRS duration greater than 150 ms.[43] CRT should not be considered as "rescue" therapy for Stage D HF.[1]

Automated Implanted Cardiac Defibrillators

Patients with HF-rEF are at increased risk for ventricular tachyarrhythmias leading to sudden cardiac death. Current guidelines recommend prophylactic implantation of automated implanted cardiac defibrillators (AICD) in patients with nonischemic cardiomyopathy or ischemic heart disease with an EF less than 35% and mild to moderate HF symptoms (NYHA II or III) when at least 1-year survival with good functional capacity is expected.[1] AICD implantation is also recommended in patients at least 40 days post-MI with EF less than 0.30 and NYHA class I symptoms.[40,43] Again, optimal medical therapy should be previously employed and demonstrate a persistent reduction in EF. AICDs are generally not warranted in patients with refractory HF (Stage D) or in patients with concomitant diseases that shorten life expectancy independent of HF. AICDs have bradycardia and anti-tachycardia pacing capabilities as well. Although highly effective in preventing sudden death, frequent shocks (appropriate or inappropriate) reduce quality of life and increase patient anxiety. Of note, antimicrobial prophylaxis is not recommended before dental, gastrointestinal, or genitourinary procedures to prevent device infection.[44]

Mechanical Circulatory Support Devices and Cardiac Transplantation

Cardiac transplantation is considered the gold standard for the treatment of refractory (Stage D) HF. Since the first cardiac transplantation in 1967, advances in immunosuppressive therapy have greatly improved the long-term survival of transplant recipients as well as their functional status and health-related quality of life.[45] Selected patients with Stage D HF and poor prognosis should be referred to an advanced HF treatment program or cardiac transplantation center for evaluation.[46]

Mechanical circulatory support (MCS) devices have emerged as a viable therapeutic option for patients with advanced Stage D HF with reduced EF refractory to optimal medical therapy. MCS can be used as (a) bridge to transplantation and a decision regarding transplantation candidacy and for (b) "destination" or permanent therapy. Bridge to transplantation and destination therapy have the strongest database with regard to survival, functional capacity, and health-related quality of life benefits. Use of nondurable or temporary MCS (i.e., percutaneous or extracorporeal ventricular assist devices) is reasonable as a "bridge to recovery" or "bridge to decision" for carefully selected unstable patients with low EF with acute, profound hemodynamic compromise.[47,48]

Advanced Directives and End-of-Life Care

It is mandatory that discussions about advance directives occur in context with prognosis. These conversations are best performed in the office setting following the initial HF diagnosis, and after hospitalizations or change in clinical status. Including the spouse or a close family member is preferable. Use of prognosis modeling algorithms previously discussed is often helpful.[49] Referral to an Advanced Heart Failure Treatment Program or Palliative Care Program for a confirmatory opinion is considered. Palliative care focuses on relief of pain and discomfort, provides emotional support for patient and family, and assists with transitions of care when quality of life can no longer be maintained. Patients with advanced (Stage D) HF can be enrolled in palliative care yet receive life-prolonging therapies such as inotropic drug infusions or destination therapy MCS.[50] Hospice care focuses on symptom management while discontinuing life-prolonging medicine or treatment that does not improve patients' quality of life. Some patients may choose deactivation of their AICD to avoid the discomfort of frequent shocks. Utilization of end-of-life care services such as hospice should occur after full and appropriate application of evidence-based pharmacologic and nonpharmacological treatments.[51]

REFERENCES

1. Yancy CW, Jessup M, Bozkurt B, et al. 2013 ACCF/AHA guideline for the management of heart failure: a report of the American College of Cardiology Foundation/American Heart Association Task Force on Practice Guidelines. *J Am Coll Cardiol* 2013;62(16):e147–e239.
2. Krumholz HM, Merrill AR, Schone EM, et al. Patterns of hospital performance in acute myocardial infarction and heart failure 30-day mortality and readmission. *Circ Cardiovasc Qual Outcomes* 2009;2:407–413.
3. Go AS, Mozaffarian D, Roger VL, et al. Heart disease and stroke statistics–2013 update: a report from the American Heart Association. *Circulation* 2013;127:e6–e245.

4. Curtis LH, Whellan DJ, Hammill BG, et al. Incidence and prevalence of heart failure in elderly persons, 1994–2003. *Arch Intern Med* 2008;168:418–424.

5. Cohn JN, Ferrari R, Sharpe N. Cardiac remodeling-concepts and clinical implications: a consensus paper from an international forum on cardiac remodeling. *J Am Coll Cardiol* 2000;35:569–582.

6. Greenberg B, Hermann D. *Contemporary diagnosis and management of heart failure.* 3rd ed. Newtown, PA: Handbooks in Healthcare; 2005.

7. Chatterjee K. Physical examination in heart failure. In: Hosenpud JD, Greenberg BH, eds. *Congestive heart failure, pathophysiology, diagnosis and comprehensive approach to management.* 3rd ed. Philadelphia, PA: Lippincott Williams & Wilkins; 2007:615–627.

8. Maisel AS, Bhalla V, Braunwald E. Cardiac biomarkers: a contemporary status report. *Nat Clin Pract Cardiovasc Med* 2006;3(1):24–34.

9. Horwich TB, Patel J, MacLellan WR, et al. Cardiac troponin I is associated with impaired hemodynamics, progressive left ventricular dysfunction, and increased mortality rates in advanced heart failure. *Circulation* 2003;108:833–838.

10. Januzzi JL Jr. Use of biomarkers to "guide" care in chronic heart failure: what have we learned (so far)? *J Card Fail* 2011;17:622–625.

11. Vitarelli A, Tiukinhoy S, Di LS, et al. The role of echocardiography in the diagnosis and management of heart failure. *Heart Fail Rev* 2003;8:181–189.

12. Fihn SD, Gardin JM, Abrams J, et al. 2012 ACCF/AHA/ACP/AATS/PCNA/SCAI/STS guideline for the diagnosis and management of patients with stable ischemic heart disease: a report of the American College of Cardiology Foundation/American Heart Association Task Force on Practice Guidelines, and the American College of Physicians, American Association for Thoracic Surgery, Preventive Cardiovascular Nurses Association, Society for Cardiovascular Angiography and Interventions, and Society of Thoracic Surgeons. *Circulation.* 2012;126:e354–e471.

13. Hermann DD, Greenberg BH. Prognostic factors In: Poole-Wilson P, Colucci W, Massie B, et al, eds. *Heart failure: scientific principles & clinical practice.* New York, NY: Churchill Livingstone; 1997:439–454.

14. Garg R, Yusuf S. Overview of randomized trials of angiotensin-converting enzyme inhibitors on mortality and morbidity in patients with heart failure. Collaborative Group on ACE Inhibitor Trials. *JAMA* 1995;273(18):1450–1466.

15. Granger CB, McMurray JJ, Yusuf S, et al. Effects of candesartan in patients with chronic heart failure and reduced left-ventricular systolic function intolerant to angiotensin-converting-enzyme inhibitors: the CHARM-Alternative Trial. *Lancet* 2003;362:772–776.

16. McMurray JJ, Ostergren J, Swedberg K, et al. Effects of Candesartan in patients with chronic heart failure and reduced left-ventricular systolic function taking angiotensin-converting-enzyme inhibitors: the CHARM-Added Trial. *Lancet* 2003;362:767–771.

17. MERIT-HF Study Group. Effect of metoprolol CR/XL in chronic heart failure: metoprolol CR/XL randomized intervention trial in congestive heart failure. *Lancet* 1999;353:2001–2007.

18. Packer M, Bristow MR, Cohn JN, et al. The effect of carvedilol on morbidity and mortality in patients with chronic heart failure. *N Engl J Med* 1996;334:1349–1355.

19. CIBIS Investigators and Committees. The Cardiac Insufficiency Bisoprolol Study II (CIBIS II): a randomized trial of beta-blockade in heart failure. *Lancet* 1999;353:9.

20. Cohn JN, Johnson G, Ziesche S, et al. A comparison of enalapril with hydralazine-isosorbide dinitrate in the treatment of chronic congestive heart failure. *N Engl J Med* 1991;325:303–310.

21. Taylor AL, Ziesche S, Yancy C, et al. Combination of isosorbide dinitrate and hydralazine in blacks with heart failure. *N Engl J Med* 2004;351:2049–2057.

22. Packer M, O'Connor CM, Ghali JK, et al. Effect of amlodipine on morbidity and mortality in severe chronic heart failure. *New Engl J Med* 1996;335:1107–1114.

23. Packer M, Gheorghiade M, Young JB, et al. Withdrawal of digoxin from patients with chronic heart failure treated with angiotensin-converting enzyme inhibitors. RADIANCE Study. *N Engl J Med* 1993;329:1.

24. The Digitalis Investigation Group. The effect of digoxin on mortality and morbidity in patients with heart failure. *N Engl J Med* 1997;336:525.

25. Pitt B, Zannad F, Remme WJ, et al; Randomized Aldactone Evaluation Study Investigators. The effect of spironolactone on morbidity and mortality in patients with severe heart failure. *N Engl J Med* 1999;341:709–717.

26. Zannad F, McMurray JJ, Krum H, et al; for the EMPHASIS-HF Study Group. Eplerenone in patients with systolic heart failure and mild symptoms. *N Engl J Med* 2011;364:11–21.

27. Rathore SS, Curtis JP, Wang Y, et al. Association of serum digoxin concentration and outcomes in patients with heart failure. *JAMA* 2003;289:871–8.

28. Adams KF Jr, Patterson JH, Gattis WA, et al. Relationship of serum digoxin concentration to mortality and morbidity in women in the Digitalis Investigation Group trial: a retrospective analysis. *J Am Coll Cardiol* 2005;46:497–504.

29. Brater DC. Diuretic therapy. *N Engl J Med* 1998;339:387–395.
30. Dormans TJ, Gerlad PG, Russell FM, et al. Combination diuretic therapy in severe congestive heart failure. *Drugs* 1998;55(2):165–172.
31. Leier CV, Cas LD, Metra M. Clinical relevance and management of the major electrolyte abnormalities in congestive heart failure: hyponatremia, hypokalemia and hypomagnesemia. *Am Heart J* 1994;128:564–574.
32. Philbin EF, Rocco TA Jr. Use of angiotensin-converting enzyme inhibitors in heart failure with preserved left ventricular systolic function. *Am Heart J* 1997;134(2 pt 1):188–195.
33. Yusuf S, Pfeffer MA, Swedberg K, et al. Effects of candesartan in patients with chronic heart failure and preserved left-ventricular ejection fraction: the CHARM-Preserved Trial. *Lancet* 2003;362:777–781.
34. Edelmann F, Wachter R, Schmidt AG, et al. Effect of spironolactone on diastolic function and exercise capacity in patients with heart failure with preserved ejection fraction: the Aldo-DHF randomized controlled trial. *JAMA* 2013;309:781–791.
35. Piller LB, Baraniuk S, Simpson LM, et al. Long-term follow-up of participants with heart failure in the antihypertensive and lipid-lowering treatment to prevent heart attack trial (ALLHAT). *Circulation* 2011;124:1811–1818.
36. Hermann DD. Naturoceutical agents and cardiovascular medicine—the hope, hype and the harm. *ACC Curr J Rev* 1999;8(5):53–57.
37. Fonarow GC, Stevenson LW, Walden JA, et al. Impact of a comprehensive heart failure management program on hospital readmissions and functional status of patients with advanced heart failure. *J Am Coll Cardiol* 1997;30:725–732.
38. O'Connor CM, Whellan DJ, Lee KL, et al. Efficacy and safety of exercise training in patients with chronic heart failure: HF-ACTION randomized controlled trial. *JAMA* 2009;301:1439.
39. MacDonald M, Fang J, Pittman SD, et al. The current prevalence of sleep disordered breathing in congestive heart failure patients treated with beta-blockers. *J Clin Sleep Med* 2008;4:38–42.
40. Bradley TD, Logan AG, Kimoff RJ, et al. Continuous positive airway pressure for central sleep apnea and heart failure. *N Engl J Med* 2005;353:2025–2033.
41. Bristow MR, Saxon LA, Boehmer J, et al. Cardiac-resynchronization therapy with or without an implantable defibrillator in advanced chronic heart failure. *N Engl J Med* 2004;350:2140–2150.
42. Cleland JG, Daubert JC, Erdmann E, et al. The effect of cardiac resynchronization on morbidity and mortality in heart failure. *N Engl J Med* 2005;352:1539–1549.
43. Moss AJ, Hall WJ, Cannom DS, et al. Cardiac-resynchronization therapy for the prevention of heart-failure events. *N Engl J Med* 2009;361:1329–1338.
44. Zareba W, Klein H, Cygankiewicz I, et al; MADIT-CRT Investigators. Effectiveness of Cardiac resynchronization Therapy by QRS Morphology in the Multicenter Automatic Defibrillator Implantation Trial–Cardiac Resynchronization Therapy (MADIT-CRT). *Circulation* 2011;123:1159–1166.
45. Baddour LM, Epstein AE, Erickson CC, et al. Update on cardiovascular implantable electronic device infections and their management: a scientific statement from the American Heart Association. *Circulation* 2010;121:458–477.
46. Butler J, Khadim G, Paul KM, et al. Selection of patients for heart transplantation in the current era of heart failure therapy. *J Am Coll Cardiol* 2004;43:787–793.
47. Mehra MR, Kobashigawa J, Starling R, et al. Listing criteria for heart transplantation: International Society for Heart and Lung Transplantation guidelines for the care of cardiac transplant candidates2006. *J Heart Lung Transplant* 2006;25:1024–42.
48. Feldman D, Pamboukian SV, Teuteberg JJ, et al. The 2013 International Society for Heart and Lung Transplantation Guidelines for mechanical circulatory support: executive summary. *J Heart Lung Transplant* 2013;32:157–187.
49. Slaughter MS, Rogers JG, Milano CA, et al. Advanced heart failure treated with continuous-flow left ventricular assist device. *N Engl J Med* 2009;361:2241–2251.
50. Adler ED, Goldfinger JZ, Kalman J, et al. Palliative care in the treatment of advanced heart failure. *Circulation* 2009;120:2597–2606.
51. Goda A, Williams P, Mancini D, et al. Selecting patients for heart transplantation: comparison of the Heart Failure Survival Score (HFSS) and the Seattle heart failure model (SHFM). *J Heart Lung Transplant* 2011;30:1236–1243.

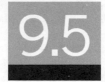

Atrial Fibrillation and Other Supraventricular Tachycardias

Yaowen Eliot Hu, Thomas M. Howard

ATRIAL FIBRILLATION
General Principles

Epidemiology

Atrial fibrillation (AF) is one of the most common cardiac dysrhythmias. There are about 2.5 million patients with this condition in the United States. The prevalence of AF is strikingly related to age, affecting as many as 10% of those older than 75 years. As the median age of the U.S. population continues to increase, so does the prevalence of AF. AF is a considerable health burden in that it increases total mortality twofold, heart failure threefold, and stroke rates fivefold. It is responsible for 10% to 15% of all strokes in the United States.[1-3]

Classification

The following classification has been proposed by the 2001 American College of Cardiology/American Heart Association/European Society of Cardiology Board Task Force. Management of AF is dependent on recognition of the appropriate classification:

- **Paroxysmal AF** is self-terminating and lasts less than 7 days and usually less than 48 hours. It can further be subdivided into first-episode paroxysmal AF and recurrent paroxysmal AF. Therapy here should focus on prevention of recurrence.
- **Persistent AF** is not self terminating and lasts longer than 7 days. This can again be first episode or recurrent. Therapy should focus on modulation of heart rhythm or rate and preventing recurrence.
- **Permanent or chronic AF** has been present for more than 1 year, and cardioversion either has not been attempted or has failed. Control of ventricular rate is the usually preferred therapeutic option.

Over a 5-year period, about 25% of patients with paroxysmal AF will progress to persistent AF; the likelihood is increased in patients with other risk factors that are discussed below.[1-3]

Etiology

Besides age, other independent risk factors for AF include valvular heart disease, heart failure, coronary heart disease, obesity, obstructive sleep apnea, hypertension, and diabetes. Some other potentially **reversible causes** of AF include any cause of arterial hypoxemia; hypokalemia; hypomagnesemia; acute alcohol consumption; pericarditis; myocardial infarction (MI); and hyperadrenergic states such as postoperative period, including postcardiac surgery, theophylline, or other stimulant toxicity and endocrinopathies (hypo/hyperthyroidism, pheochromocytoma). About 10% of patients with AF have none of the above identifiable risk factors; they are considered to have **"lone" AF**, which necessitates further classification according to the system listed above.[1-4]

Pathophysiology

The pathogenic property common to all risk factors for AF is diastolic dysfunction of the left ventricle, which in turn leads to left atrial dilatation, stretch, and fibrosis and subsequent vulnerability to AF.[1]

Diagnosis

Clinical Presentation

Symptoms can often be vague and include fatigue, lightheadedness, palpitations, breathlessness, and exercise intolerance. Younger and more active patients and those with paroxysmal AF are more likely to report symptoms. Acute presentations may include decompensated congestive heart failure and angina.

History and Physical Examination

Initial evaluation of the patient with AF includes a careful history and physical examination to assess for presence of symptoms, other comorbidities, and potentially reversible causes as noted above. An irregularly irregular pulse that is usually greater than 100 beats per minute (bpm) is characteristic of AF. **"Slow" AF** may indicate associated disease of the conduction pathway. It is important to assess if the patient is **hemodynamically stable** or **unstable** as this would dictate further course of management.

Laboratory Studies

- Basic laboratory workup, including screening thyroid tests, complete blood count, and comprehensive metabolic panel, are warranted, especially for a first episode of AF. Urine drug screening and medication levels in the blood may also be considered.
- All patients with AF should have an **electrocardiogram (ECG)** and a **transthoracic echocardiogram (TTE)** to help identify AF and quantify any underlying cardiovascular disease and guide subsequent management.
- The **ECG** demonstrates chaotic electrical activity with an irregularly irregular rate and rhythm. This is evidenced by constantly changing R–R intervals and no discernible P waves before the QRS complexes. The fibrillation waves are best seen in leads II, III, aVF, and V_1. The fibrillation pattern may be fine or coarse. A few patients have fine AF with little evidence on the ECG. The irregular ventricular pattern should allow determination of AF. Some patients have coarse fibrillation waves, making it difficult to distinguish from atrial flutter. This can again be distinguished by the erratic ventricular response. The QRS complexes are narrow unless there is aberrant ventricular conduction. The ECG may also reveal evidence of acute myocardial ischemia, pre-excitation, sinus node or conduction system disease, or QT prolongation (Figure 9.5-1).[1]
- The **TTE** determines left atrial size (a predictor for AF recurrence), presence of any valvular and/or pericardial heart disease, and can also detect left ventricular hypertrophy and ventricular dysfunction that will influence management decisions. **Transesophageal echocardiogram (TEE)** is more sensitive for identifying atrial thrombi.
- Intracardiac **electrophysiologic studies** may be useful in young patients with idiopathic lone AF to detect underlying pre-excitation or conduction pathway disease.
- **Stress testing** is indicated only if the initial evaluation suggests the presence of ischemic heart disease.

Treatment

Immediate management of AF depends on the hemodynamic status of the patient. If unstable, immediate synchronized cardioversion is indicated. If stable, management decisions that need to be made when managing AF include:

- Whether to attempt to restore and then **maintain sinus rhythm,** that is, **adopt a rhythm-control strategy,** or

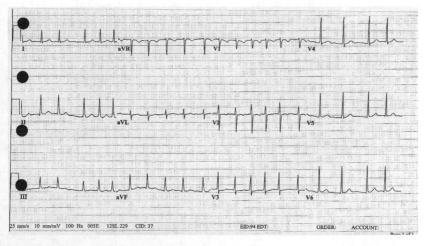

Figure 9.5-1. Atrial fibrillation: Note the characteristic irregularity in the R–R intervals and the absence of well-defined P waves preceding the QRS complexes.

- How to optimally **control ventricular rate** both acutely and long-term, that is, **adopt a rate-control strategy,** and
- How to **minimize the risk of thromboembolism** both in the peri-cardioversion and long-term settings

Depending on a patient's age, presenting symptoms, medical history, comorbidities, and previous response to AF therapy, the following questions can help guide individual treatment decisions:

- Does the patient have symptoms that would benefit from maintenance of sinus rhythm?
- Is he or she a candidate for anticoagulation therapy?
- What are the potential long-term risks of antiarrhythmic drug therapy versus the risks of focusing on rate control and allowing the arrhythmia to persist?

For many years, the accepted strategy to manage AF was to routinely restore sinus rhythm with cardioversion and then maintain it with antiarrhythmic drugs. Recent studies (AFFIRM, RACE, PIAF, STAF, CAFE) have, however, shown that rhythm- and rate-control strategies were equivalent with respect to mortality and stroke rates.[5] There were fewer hospitalizations, fewer adverse drug effects, and lower costs with rate-control strategy. The patients included in these studies were primarily elderly patients with recurrent or persistent AF or at high risk for recurrent AF who were minimally symptomatic and without significant heart failure. These trials also demonstrated that rhythm control does not prevent AF-related stroke. Based on these studies, the following extrapolations as to the **goals of treatment** can be made:

- Rate control is to be considered the first-line strategy in elderly patients with persistent or recurrent AF who are at high risk for thromboembolic events.
- Rhythm-control strategy may be appropriate in younger patients with a first episode of AF or paroxysmal AF, in patients at low risk for thromboembolism, patients with persistent AF that remain symptomatic despite rate control, and in patients with heart failure.
- Patients at **high risk for thromboembolism need to be anticoagulated with warfarin or other anticoagulants,** unless contraindicated, regardless of whether a rhythm- or rate-control strategy is pursued.[1,4–8]

Rate Control

Rate control may be achieved by either pharmacologic or nonpharmacologic means. The recommended ventricular rate in patients with AF is 60 to 80 bpm at rest and less than 110 bpm with daily activities. Despite optimal control of the resting ventricular rate, some patients with AF will have excessive tachycardia and symptoms of palpitations and dyspnea with their usual daytime activities.

- **Pharmacologic rate control.** For patients with AF in acute settings who do not have decompensated heart failure or the Wolff–Parkinson–White (WPW) syndrome, atrioventricular (AV) nodal blocking agents such as β-blockers, diltiazem, and verapamil are the most effective drugs.
  - **β-Blockers** are preferred in patients with ischemic heart disease and those with high sympathetic tone such as in the postoperative period, hyperthyroidism, alcohol withdrawal, pulmonary embolism, pericarditis, or systemic infection.
  - **Diltiazem or verapamil** may be useful particularly in patients with contraindication to β-blocker use such as reactive airways disease.
  - **Digoxin** is less useful in acute settings because of its slow onset of action. However, in patients with decompensated heart failure, it is the initial drug of choice due to the negative inotropic effect of β-blockers and calcium-channel blockers.

Patients with minimal symptoms may initially be treated with **oral short-acting preparations** with dose titration and then converted to the appropriate dose of an extended-release preparation once their ventricular rate is controlled. Acutely symptomatic patients may require **intravenous administration** of one of these medications that can later be converted to an extended-release preparation. Intravenous dosages for β-blockers and calcium-channel blockers are described in the latter section on supraventricular tachycardias. Loading regimens for digoxin vary between 0.25 and 0.50 mg intravenously in repeated doses up to 1.0 to 1.5 mg over 8 to 24 hours. Usual maintenance doses range between 0.125 and 0.5 mg PO daily. Caution needs to be exercised in patients with renal dysfunction to avoid digoxin toxicity.[1,2,5]

- **Nonpharmacologic rate control.** Surgical measures are indicated in patients with permanent AF who do not respond or continue to be symptomatic with pharmacologic rate/rhythm control. These include AV node ablation with placement of a pacemaker, burst or dual-site atrial pacing and implantable atrial defibrillator, maze procedure to interrupt re-entrant circuits in the left atrium and percutaneous radiofrequency ablation of arrhythmogenic foci around the junction of the pulmonary veins and left atrium.[1-3]

Rhythm Control

The main advantages to restoring sinus rhythm are that it returns the heart to normal functioning and prevents the progressive atrial remodeling associated with persistent AF, in addition to alleviating symptoms of AF.

- **Restoration of sinus rhythm.** About 50% to 60% of patients whose duration of AF is less than 48 hours will cardiovert spontaneously. An attempt to restore sinus rhythm in patients who do not do so may be made by either electrical cardioversion or the use of antiarrhythmic drugs. Cardioversion is to be preceded and followed by adequate anticoagulation as discussed in the following section.[1,2]
- **Electrical cardioversion.** This is performed using synchronized direct current (DC) cardioversion starting with low energy levels. Before cardioversion, all antiarrhythmic drug levels should be titrated to their therapeutic ranges, digoxin levels should be checked to exclude digoxin toxicity, and patients with hyperthyroidism should be functionally euthyroid to limit the likelihood of recurrence. This is usually the treatment of choice in patients with AF who are hemodynamically unstable.[1,3,5]
- **Pharmacologic cardioversion.** This can be achieved using class IA (procainamide, quinidine), IC (flecainide, propafenone), and III (amiodarone, sotalol) drugs. This is usually reserved for patients with highly symptomatic, persistent AF. Because of the propensity for proarrhythmic effects, initiation of antiarrhythmic agents is preferably done in the inpatient setting with continuous ECG monitoring, especially in the presence of structural heart disease of left ventricular (LV) dysfunction. Some of the commonly used antiarrhythmic drugs are as follows:[1-3,5]
  - Quinidine usage has markedly decreased due to the associated risk of torsades de pointes. When used, the dose is 300 to 600 mg SR every 8 to 12 hours.[1,3,5]
  - Propafenone is usually started at a dose of 150 mg every 8 hours and may be gradually increased to a maximum daily dose of 900 mg. It is contraindicated in patients with LV dysfunction and conduction defects.[1,3,5]
  - Flecainide has a 1-year efficacy rate of about 50% in preventing AF. The initial dose is 50 mg twice daily to a maximal daily dose of 400 mg. It is also contraindicated in the presence of LV dysfunction and heart failure.[1-3,5]
  - Amiodarone is relatively slow acting and is useful in the setting of acute ischemia, acute MI, or LV dysfunction. It has a 1-year efficacy rate of about 70% in preventing AF. It has a long half-life of 2 months that makes it hard to reverse its toxicity. Long-term use may be associated with bradycardia, pulmonary, liver, optic nerve, and thyroid toxicity. Lower maintenance doses of 200 to 400 mg per day are preferred.[1-3,5]
  - Dofetilide is a new antiarrhythmic drug and is complicated to administer but offers an alternative if amiodarone is contraindicated.[1,3,5]
  - Sotalol is commonly used for AF prophylaxis rather than cardioversion. Efficacy varies widely depending on the severity of heart disease. It is started at a dose of 80 mg twice daily to a maximal daily dose of 500 to 600 mg.[1-3,5]
  - Dronedarone was approved by the FDA in 2009 for treatment of paroxysmal AF and persistent AF after the ATHENA trials showed decreased death in patients with non-permanent AF.[9] It is started at 400 mg twice daily without a loading dose or the need for titration. However, in 2010 to 2011, the FDA issued multiple warnings for dronedarone use in AF as there were risks of heart failure, liver failure, arrhythmias such as torsades de pointes, and interactions with warfarin. Extreme caution must be taken when prescribing dronedarone as preliminary results of the PALLA trials in 2011 also showed increased risk of death, stroke, and heart failure.[10]
- **Maintenance of sinus rhythm.** This may be achieved by continuing antiarrhythmics as noted above or by surgical means. The main risks linked to pharmacologic rhythm-control strategies are a lack of efficacy with ongoing AF that goes undetected and potentially lethal proarrhythmic effects, including torsades de pointes. The former is linked to the increase in stroke risk associated with the discontinuation of anticoagulation when sinus rhythm was believed to have been restored.[1-3,5]
  - **Nonpharmacologic** measures to rhythm control that are being currently used include:
    - Burst or dual-site **atrial pacing and implantable atrial defibrillation**
    - **Maze procedure** to surgically interrupt re-entrant circuits in the left atrium that requires open heart surgery

○ **Percutaneous radiofrequency ablation** is a catheter-based procedure that uses radiofrequency energy for **pulmonary vein isolation (PVI)** from the left atrium and ablation of arrhythmogenic foci in and around the junction of the pulmonary veins and left atrium. Despite its high efficacy rate and low recurrence of AF, its use is still limited by the associated complications.[1,3,5]

Minimizing Thromboembolic Risk

Prevention of thromboembolism in patients with AF undergoing cardioversion:

- **Step 1.** For patients with AF of ≥48 hours or of unknown duration and are hemodynamically stable, anticoagulation (INR 2.0 to 3.0) is recommended for at least 3 weeks prior to and 4 weeks after cardioversion, regardless of the method (electrical or pharmacologic) used to restore sinus rhythm.[6–8]
- **Step 2.** As an alternative to Step 1 above, it is reasonable to perform transesophageal echocardiography (TEE) to rule out left atrial thrombus. For patients with no identifiable thrombus, cardioversion is reasonable immediately after anticoagulation with unfractionated heparin administered by an initial intravenous bolus injection followed by a continuous infusion in a dose adjusted to prolong the activated partial thromboplastin time to 1.5 to 2 times the reference control value. This is continued until successful transition to oral anticoagulation with warfarin to a target INR of 2.0 to 3.0 oral anticoagulation is then continued for at least 4 weeks post-cardioversion. For patients in whom atrial thrombus is identified by TEE, oral anticoagulation (INR 2.0 to 3.0) is recommended for at least 3 weeks after restoration of sinus rhythm, and a longer period of anticoagulation may be appropriate even after apparently successful cardioversion, because the risk of thromboembolism often remains elevated in such cases.[6–8]
- **Step 3.** For patients with AF of more than 44-hour duration requiring immediate cardioversion because of hemodynamic instability, heparin should be administered concurrently (unless contraindicated) as mentioned in Step 2. Thereafter, oral anticoagulation (INR 2.0 to 3.0) should be provided for at least 4 weeks, as for patients undergoing elective cardioversion.[6–8]
- **Step 4.** For patients with AF of less than 48-hour duration associated with hemodynamic instability (angina pectoris, MI, shock, or pulmonary edema), cardioversion should be performed immediately without delay for prior initiation of anticoagulation.[6–8]

Chronic Anticoagulation Therapy

- **Step 1.** Anticoagulation recommendations for atrial flutter are the same as those for AF.[6–8]
- **Step 2.** Antithrombotic therapy, using antiplatelet agents or vitamin K antagonists, to prevent thromboembolism is recommended for all patients with AF, except those with lone AF or contraindications.[6–8]
- **Step 3.** The selection of the antithrombotic agent should be based upon the absolute risks of stroke and bleeding and the relative risk and benefit for a given patient. Warfarin has historically been the first-line oral anticoagulant used in AF.[6–8] Recent studies have introduced the use of direct thrombin inhibitors and factor inhibitors such as apixaban, rivaroxaban, and dabigatran as first-line oral anticoagulants in AF due to elimination of INR monitoring with use of these medications.[11,12] However, extreme caution must be used when prescribing these medications as severe irreversible bleeding have been reported as a potential side effect.[13] Estimation of stroke risk in the patient can be summarized with a scoring system known as CHADS2 (congestive heart failure, hypertension, age >75, diabetes mellitus, and previous history of stroke), which identifies and categorizes different risk factors for stroke in AF. The CHA2DS2-VASc score is another formula to estimate the risk of stroke in patient with AF as an attempt at the lower end of the risk stratum of CHADS2, with the inclusion of patients age 65 to 74 years, in addition to age ≥75, recognizing that stroke risk increases across the age spectrum, and also includes gender such as female sex has a risk factor in some but not all studies. The presence of vascular disease is least well established as an independent risk factor for stroke in patients with AF. The two scoring systems have been compared in multiple cohorts in a largest study of nearly 80,000 individuals with modest ability to predict stroke, again when compared (c-statistic 0.69 vs. 0.67, respectively). The CHADS2 score is considered a simple and most studied scoring system to guide the clinician to select the thromboembolic agent for the prevention of strokes on patients with AF.[17–19]

The current guideline recommendations for risk stratification and antithrombotic drug prescription incorporates the CHADS2 scoring system and are as follows:[14,15]

Low risk	No risk factors
Aspirin, 81–325 mg daily	
Intermediate risk	One moderate-risk factor
Aspirin, 81–325 mg daily	
or Warfarin (INR 2.0–3.0)	
or new oral anticoagulant	
High risk	Any high-risk factor or >1 moderate-risk factor
Warfarin (INR 2.0–3.0)	
or new oral anticoagulant	

High-risk factors: prior stroke, TIA, or systemic embolism.
Moderate-risk factors: age >75 years, hypertension, diabetes mellitus, and heart failure or impaired left ventricular systolic function.
Excluded populations include patients with reversible causes of AF, pregnant patients, and patients with prosthetic valves or mitral stenosis and contraindications to antithrombotic therapy.

SUPRAVENTRICULAR TACHYCARDIAS

General Principles

Supraventricular tachycardia (SVT) refers to arrhythmias with three or more complexes at a rate exceeding 100 bpm, where the focus originates in the AV junctional area above the Bundle of His. Re-entry phenomena account for the majority of these dysrhythmias.[1]

Diagnosis

Clinical Presentation

Patients often describe sensations such as heart pounding or racing. They have regular or skipping beats and may become anxious. There is generally no association with activity. Episodes are usually well tolerated in young people in the absence of any coexistent heart disease. In elderly individuals and in those with pre-existing cardiac disease, the clinical presentation can be acute with hypotension, angina, and pulmonary edema.

Physical Examination

A complete physical examination should be undertaken with emphasis on the cardiovascular system. Evaluation is identical to that described for AF.

Laboratory Studies

• **Electrocardiographic findings.** Patients in whom SVT is suspected should have a 12-lead ECG with a rhythm strip lasting at least 2 to 3 minutes. If P waves are difficult to distinguish due to the rate of the tachycardia, leads aVF and V^1 may be helpful.
• **Ambulatory 24-hour electrocardiographic monitoring (Holter monitoring).** A Holter monitor or event monitor may be considered if the resting ECG is normal and the history is suggestive of a dysrhythmia.
• **Additional studies.** Laboratory studies may also include the following depending on the clinical situation—electrolytes, calcium, magnesium, hemoglobin, arterial blood gases, thyroid function, urine drug screen, and medication level.
• **A TTE** to determine structural heart disease as discussed before.

Classification of SVT

SVT may be classified according to the regularity of the rhythm, the width of the QRS complex, and the relationship of the P waves to the QRS complex. SVT can be narrow (QRS complexes less than 120 ms) or wide (QRS complexes greater than 120 ms). Wide-complex SVT arises when ventricular activation occurs with bundle branch block aberrancy or in the presence of pre-excitation. SVT can further be classified into regular or irregular SVT based on the R–R interval.[1]

- **Regular rhythm SVT.** The R–R interval is consistent and equal. A differential diagnosis of tachycardia mechanisms can further be generated on the basis of the **R–P interval**, the time interval between the peak of an R wave and the subsequent P wave, during the tachycardia. Identification of the specific type of SVT assists in therapy.[1]
- **Short RP tachycardias** have an R–P interval that is less than 50% of the R–R interval. These include:
  - **"Typical" AV nodal re-entrant tachycardia (AVNRT).** This occurs in patients who have functional dissociation of their AV node into "slow" and "fast" pathways. Conduction proceeds anterograde down the slow pathway, with retrograde conduction up the fast pathway. Atrial and ventricular excitation occurs concurrently with every tachycardia circuit. On a 12-lead ECG, P waves are often hidden within the QRS complexes and are not visible, or they are buried at the end of the QRS complexes. This is usually an abrupt-onset tachycardia lasting seconds to hours; it accounts for 50% to 60% of all regular narrow QRS tachycardia.[1]
  - **Orthodromic AV re-entrant tachycardia (O-AVRT)** is an accessory pathway–mediated re-entrant rhythm that occurs when anterograde conduction to the ventricle takes place through the AV node and retrograde conduction to the atrium occurs through an accessory pathway. P waves are seen shortly after the QRS complexes.[1]
  - **Sinus tachycardia or ectopic atrial tachycardia** associated with first-degree AV block. The two rhythms differ with respect to the P-wave axis and morphology. Here, the P wave after each QRS complex is actually conducting to the subsequent QRS complex with a prolonged PR interval.[1]
  - **Junctional tachycardia** arises from the AV junction. The electrical impulses conduct to the atrium and ventricle simultaneously and therefore, as in typical AVNRT, P waves may not be easily discernible. This is commonly seen in children after surgical correction of congenital heart defects. In adults, it is commonly seen after mitral or aortic valve surgery, with acute MIs or in digitalis toxicity.[1]
- **Long R–P tachycardias** have an R–P interval that is greater than 50% of the R–R interval. These include:
  - **Sinus tachycardia.** The P waves conduct to the subsequent QRS complexes with normal PR intervals. Typically it does not exceed 170 bpm. Onset and termination are gradual. It is often a reflection of extra-cardiac abnormalities, such as infection, hypovolemia, anxiety, pain, hyperthyroidism, acute severe anemia, and fecal impaction.[1]
  - **"Atypical" AVNRT** occurs when anterograde conduction proceeds over the fast AV nodal pathway with retrograde conduction over the slow AV nodal pathway in patients with dual AV nodal physiology. As the retrograde conduction to the atrium is slow, the P wave is inscribed well after the QRS complex.[1]
- **WPW syndrome** includes the presence of pre-excitation on a 12-lead ECG with symptoms or documentation of SVT. This results from anterograde activation of the ventricle via an accessory pathway as well as the AV node, resulting in a short PR interval together with a delta wave slurring the upstroke of the QRS complex. The most common form seen is an **orthodromic AVRT**. This can at times degenerate into AF.[1]
- **Atrial flutter.** Atrial flutter is often a regular, narrow QRS tachycardia. It is a rhythm characterized by an atrial rate of 240 to 350 bpm, commonly with variable AV block (2:1, 3:1, or 4:1) causing a ventricular response of 70 to 150 bpm. The characteristic flutter waves (sawtooth) are best seen in leads II, II I, aVF, and V_1.[1]

Irregular Rhythm SVT
- AF (refer to previous section)
- Multifocal atrial tachycardia is an irregular SVT characterized by three or more different P-wave morphologies on a 12-lead ECG. Frequently, PR intervals are variable. It is often associated with chronic obstructive pulmonary disease and heart failure, and may be potentiated by concomitant therapy with theophylline. Therapy is targeted at the underlying pathology.[1]

Treatment

- **Regular, narrow-complex SVT**
  - **Vagal maneuvers.** Carotid sinus massage, Valsalva maneuver, gagging, and a baroreceptor reflex may be tried. If carotid sinus massage is used, auscultation should be performed first to rule out the presence of a carotid bruit. Massage should not exceed 10 seconds and should be done unilaterally.[1,3]

- **Pharmacotherapy** with drugs that slow or block the AV node can be used to acutely terminate SVTs that require the AV node as an integral part of the re-entrant tachycardia and to slow the ventricular rate in AF, atrial flutter, and atrial tachycardias.
  - Adenosine is very effective in the treatment of SVTs (excluding AF and atrial flutter). It is given by rapid (1 to 3 seconds) IV push (6 mg) via an antecubital vein followed by a 10- to 30-mL saline flush. A lower initial dose (3 mg) should be used if a central vein is used. If this is not successful, a 12-mg dose may be given in 1 to 2 minutes and repeated if the patient still does not respond. Toxicities include prolonged asystole in patients with sick sinus syndrome and second- or third-degree AV block. Side effects such as facial flushing, dyspnea, and chest pressure are usually of brief duration.
  - Verapamil is dosed at IV boluses of 5 to 10 mg over 2 to 3 minutes and can be repeated in 15 to 30 minutes if necessary.
  - Diltiazem can be given as an IV bolus of 0.25 mg per kg over 2 minutes, with a repeat bolus of 0.35 mg per kg if needed. This can be followed with a continuous infusion initiated at 10 mg per hour that can then be titrated to the desired effect.
  - Metoprolol is dosed at 5 mg intravenously and may be repeated in 5 minutes.[1,3]
- **Electroconversion.** For patients who do not respond to pharmacotherapy or vagal maneuvers and who are unstable (i.e., hypotensive), synchronized cardioversion is recommended. Electrical conversion recommendations are identical to AF.[1,3]
- **Radiofrequency ablation** offers definitive cure for many SVTs and, given their high success rate and low complication rates, antiarrhythmic drugs are now rarely indicated for the treatment of SVTs.[1,3,16]
- **WPW:** AV nodal blocking agents must be avoided, as they may facilitate conduction over the accessory pathway and increase the ventricular rate paradoxically, initiating VF. Hemodynamic compromise should be treated with prompt DC cardioversion. The therapy of choice is ablation of the accessory pathway. Pharmacologic therapy is reserved for patients who are unable to undergo an ablation procedure and is targeted at slowing conduction and prolonging refractoriness of the accessory bypass tract with class Ia, Ic, and III antiarrhythmic agents.[1,3]

ACKNOWLEDGMENT

The authors wish to acknowledge Kavitha K. Arabindoo for previous contributions to this chapter.

REFERENCES

1. Green, GB, Harris, IS, Lin, GA, and Moylan, KC, *The Washington Manual of Medical Therapeutics 31st Edition*, 2004: 158–169.
2. Glatter K, Herweg B, Jaffe C. Atrial fibrillation. *Patient Care*. 2006:58–66.
3. Zipes DP, Camm AJ, Broggrefe M, et al. Atrial fibrillation. *J Am Coll Cardiol* 2006;48(5):e247–e346.
4. Salem DN, Daudelin HJ, Levine HJ, et al. Antithrombotic therapy in valvular heart disease. *Chest* 2001;119(1 Suppl):207S–219S.
5. Stulz B. Atrial fibrillation: a therapeutic update. *Emergency Medicine*. 2006:35–43.
6. European Atrial Fibrillation Trial Study Group. Optimal oral anticoagulant therapy in patients with nonrheumatic atrial fibrillation and recurrent cerebral ischemia. *N Engl J Med* 1995;333:5.
7. Fihn SD, McDonell MB, Vermes D, et al. A computerized intervention to improve timing of outpatient follow-up: a multicenter randomized trial in patients treated with warfarin. *J Gen Intern Med* 1994;9:131.
8. Go AS, Hylek EM, Borowsky LH, et al. Warfarin use among ambulatory patients with nonvalvular atrial fibrillation: the anticoagulation and risk factors in atrial fibrillation (ATRIA) study. *Ann Intern Med* 1999;131:927–934.
9. Hohnloser SH, Crijns HJ, van Eickels M, et al. Effect of dronedarone on cardiovascular events in atrial fibrillation. *N Engl J Med* 2009;360:668–678.
10. Connelly SJ, Camm AJ, Halperin JL, et al. Dronedarone in high-risk permanent atrial fibrillation. *N Engl J Med* 2011;365:2268–2276.
11. Dabigatran and atrial fibrillation: the alternative to warfarin for selected patients. *Prescrire Int* 2012;21(124):33–36.
12. Adam SS, McDuffie JR, Ortel TL, et al. Comparative effectiveness of warfarin and new oral anticoagulants for the management of atrial fibrillation and venous thromboembolism: a systematic review. *Ann Intern Med* 2012;157(11):796–807.
13. Eerenberg ES, Kamphuisen PW, Sijpkens MK, et al. Reversal of rivaroxaban and dabigatran by prothrombin complex concentrate: a randomized, placebo-controlled, crossover study in healthy subjects. *Circulation* 2011;124(14):1573–1579.

14. Eckman MH, Singer DE, Rosand J, et al. Moving the tipping point: the decision to anticoagulate patients with atrial fibrillation. *Circ Cardiovasc Qual Outcomes* 2011;4(1):14–21.
15. Gage BF, Waterman AD, Shannon W, et al. Validation of clinical classification schemes for predicting stroke: results from the National Registry of Atrial Fibrillation. *JAMA* 2001;285(22):2864–2870.
16. Lesh MD, Van Hare GF, Epstein LM, et al. Radiofrequency catheter ablation of atrial arrhythmias: results and mechanisms. *Circulation* 1994;89(3):1074–1089.
17. Lip GY, Nieuwlaat R, Pisters R, et al. Refining clinical risk stratification for predicting stroke and thromboembolism in atrial fibrillation using a novel risk factor-based approach: the euro heart survey on atrial fibrillation. *Chest* 2010;137(2):263.
18. Van Staa TP, Setakis E, Di Tanna GL, et al. A comparison of risk stratification schemes for stroke in 79,884 atrial fibrillation patients in general practice. *J Thromb Haemost* 2011;9(1):39.
19. Manning WJ, Singer DE. Risk of embolization in atrial fibrillation. UpToDate. Last topic review November 11, 2014. Accessed February 06, 2014. http://www.uptodate.com/contents/risk-of-embolization-in-nonvalvular-atrial-fibrillation.

9.6 Ventricular Dysrhythmias

Julie Jeter, Daniel E. Brewer

GENERAL PRINCIPLES

Patients with frequent premature ventricular contractions (PVCs) or nonsustained ventricular tachycardias (VTs) but no other evidence of heart disease should be reassured that they have an excellent prognosis. If treatment is needed for symptomatic palpitations, β-blockers should be used.

Patients with complex ventricular dysrhythmias after myocardial infarction and those with diminished ventricular systolic function and either sustained VT or inducible VT (on electrophysiologic study, or EPS) are at high risk for cardiac death. They should be investigated for reversible ischemia and other factors that may exacerbate their rhythm disturbances. These patients should all receive β-blockade if tolerated. Those at highest risk should receive EPS and consideration of an implantable cardiac defibrillator (ICD). Empirical therapy with antiarrhythmic medications is almost never appropriate because of the increased mortality associated with these agents.

Definition

Ventricular dysrhythmias are abnormal electrical conductions that arise in the ventricle. They range from simple premature ventricular beats to VT to ventricular fibrillation (VF).

Epidemiology

Almost all people have some premature ventricular beats. Complex dysrhythmias are most common in patients with cardiomyopathies, with those having the lowest ejection fractions at greatest risk.[1] Ventricular dysrhythmias are estimated to cause around 300,000 deaths per year in the United States, equaling one-half of the cardiac mortality.

Classification

VTs are characterized by their morphology and duration.

- Morphology
  - **Monomorphic VT:** Each ventricular beat is identical.
  - **Pleomorphic VT:** More than one pattern of monomorphic VT is present.
  - **Polymorphic VT:** The shape of the ventricular beat changes from beat to beat.
- Duration
  - **Salvos:** three to five beats.
  - **Nonsustained VT:** more than six consecutive beats, less than 30 seconds.
  - **Sustained VT:** more than 30 seconds or any time period with hemodynamic compromise.

Pathophysiology

VTs may be the result of a re-entrant conduction mechanism or due to abnormal automaticity of ventricular myocytes. This may occur due to hypoxia, electrolyte abnormality, or scarring from myocardial infarction.

Etiology

The most common etiology of VT/VF in developed nations is ischemic cardiomyopathy. Other cardiomyopathies, as well as congenital diseases such as Brugada syndrome or the long QT syndrome can also cause VT/VF.[2] Surgical repair scars from congenital structural cardiac disorders can also lead to ventricular dysrhythmias. Electrolyte disturbances, infection, illicit drugs, and cardiac agents are causes as well.

DIAGNOSIS

Clinical Presentation

Patients with VT/VF may be resuscitated survivors of a sudden death episode. Many asymptomatic or minimally symptomatic patients are identified while being monitored in the hospital for ischemia, infarction, or for congestive heart failure. Palpitations and syncope/presyncope are the most common symptoms.

History

Palpitations

Patients frequently present to family physicians complaining of palpitations. A very small minority of these will have a serious ventricular dysrhythmia as the underlying cause. Historical features that make an underlying cardiovascular cause more likely include corresponding chest pain or dyspnea, a known history of coronary or structural heart disease, or multiple risk factors for atherosclerosis.

In a patient with palpitations, a careful history of the character, timing, and associated symptoms should be taken. A history of prescription (Table 9.6-1) and over-the-counter drugs, caffeine intake, alcohol and tobacco use, and anxiety is often very helpful. Illicit drugs such as amphetamines and cocaine may cause palpitations.

Syncope

A careful history of any syncopal episode may give a clue to the underlying cause. In general, syncope of cardiac origin is more likely to be sudden and associated with an injury at the time of the fall, whereas vasovagal syncope is usually preceded by warning symptoms of nausea, warmth, or lightheadedness. In vasovagal syncope, protective reflexes usually remain intact during the fall. Vasovagal syncope is much more common than syncope on the basis of VT/VF.

Exercise-associated syncope in a young person should prompt an investigation for hypertrophic cardiomyopathy. This is the most common cause of sudden death in young athletes. Studies have

TABLE 9.6-1	Some Common Drugs that Lengthen the QT Interval
Phenothiazines, especially chlorpromazine	
Tricyclic antidepressants	
Selective serotonin reuptake inhibitors	
Serotonin and norepinephrine reuptake inhibitors	
Fluoroquinolone and macrolide antibiotics	
Long-acting β_2-agonists	
Triptans	
Class IA cardiac drugs	
Quinidine, procainamide, disopyramide	
Class IC cardiac drugs	
Flecainide, encainide, sotalol	

confirmed that a positive family history of sudden cardiac death is an independent predictor of risk for sudden cardiac death and ventricular dysrhythmia.

Physical Examination

Physical examination in the patient who is suspected of having VT/VF should focus on **evidence of heart failure, ventricular outflow obstruction, and atherosclerotic vascular disease.** This examination should include careful palpation and auscultation of the heart searching for an **S_3 gallop or murmur.** The regularity of the cardiac rhythm should be assessed. The pulmonary examination may show evidence of pulmonary edema (rales in the dependent fields). The general examination should include evaluation for jugular venous distention and dependent peripheral edema. The character of peripheral arterial pulses should be assessed.

Laboratory Studies

- **Electrolytes.** Electrolyte disturbances can cause VT/VF. Hypokalemia is the most common abnormality, but hypocalcemia and hypomagnesemia have also been implicated in causing this problem.
- **Drug levels.** Any patient who takes digoxin should have the drug level and electrolytes checked. Digoxin toxicity most commonly causes pleomorphic VT, and this is much more common in the presence of hypokalemia. Theophylline toxicity can also cause VT. In suspected cases of accidental ingestion or intentional overdose, toxicology screens may be helpful to check for tricyclic antidepressants, methamphetamines, and cocaine.
- **Metabolic parameters.** Hypoxemia and metabolic acidosis can cause or aggravate ventricular dysrhythmias, particularly in acutely ill patients.
- **Cardiac assays.** Evaluate for myocardial ischemia, infarction, or inflammation with serial troponin levels.

Imaging

- **Electrocardiography.** It is unusual to capture VT on a 12-lead electrocardiograph (ECG), but an office ECG during an asymptomatic period may give important clues to the underlying diagnosis of palpitations and syncope and is indicated in all patients who are evaluated for VT. [Level A evidence] **A resting ECG cannot rule out serious disease.** The tracing should be examined for signs of ventricular irritability (PVCs), pre-excitation (a delta wave of early ventricular depolarization), ventricular hypertrophy, and ischemic disease. PVCs are characterized by premature wide complexes (more than 120 ms) followed by a compensatory pause before the next ventricular beat. Patients with a preexisting bundle branch block pattern or Wolf–Parkinson–White syndrome may have a wide-complex supraventricular tachycardia (SVT), so prior tracings should be examined if they are available. The QT interval should be carefully measured and the QTc calculated as well.
- **Distinguishing ventricular tachycardia from SVT.** If the ECG shows a wide-complex (>QRS 120 ms) tachycardia, a systematic approach may be taken to determine whether the tachycardia is of supraventricular or ventricular origin (an example of VT is shown in Figure 9.6-1):
  - Is there an absence of RS complex in all precordial leads (V1–V6)?
  - If there is an RS complex, is the RS interval greater than 100 ms in any precordial lead?
    - This is measured from the start of the R wave to the nadir of the S wave.
  - Is there AV dissociation?
    - Evidenced by independent P waves or fusion beats.
  - Are any of the three morphologic criteria for VT present in leads V1, V2?
    - R wave longer than 30 ms in V_1 or V_2. Notched S wave.
    - More than 60 ms to nadir of S wave.
  - An affirmative answer to any of these questions suggests VT rather than SVT with aberration.
- **Evaluation for ischemia.** A majority of patients with VT/VF have ischemic cardiac disease as the underlying etiologic factor (see Chapter 9.2). For this reason, most patients should undergo an evaluation for reversible ischemic disease. The specific test (exercise stress test, exercise or pharmacologic stress with nuclear imaging or echocardiography, cardiac catheterization, cardiac CT or MRI or positron emission tomography) should be chosen on the basis of the patient's level of risk, ability to exercise, and baseline ECG as well as the expertise and preference of the performing physician.
- **Echocardiography.** Some measure of left ventricular function is required in assessing the patient with VT/VF who is potentially at high risk for complications. The most commonly used and readily accessible test in most settings is the calculated ejection fraction obtained from an echocardiogram.

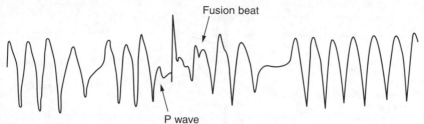

Figure 9.6-1. Ventricular tachycardia. (Courtesy of Freeman Rawson, MD, University of Tennessee, Knoxville.)

The echocardiogram can also evaluate possible valvular heart disease and show focal wall motion abnormalities suggestive of ischemic cardiac disease or inherited cardiac disorders associated with sudden death or VT.

Monitoring

Holter Monitor/Event Monitor
Holter monitoring is often the first step in evaluation of palpitations. This test creates a continuous ECG recording for 24 hours and allows the physician to see the cardiac rhythm that is present at the time of the patient's symptoms. It is important that the patient fills out the diary of symptoms that occur while wearing the monitor. A normal Holter tracing at the time of symptomatic palpitations has an excellent negative predictive value (it nearly rules out serious VT/VF as the cause). On the other hand, PVCs are a very common finding on a Holter monitor, and minor abnormalities, especially if the patient is asymptomatic, should not be overinterpreted.

If the patient's symptoms are infrequent and there is concern that they will not occur during the time a Holter monitor is worn, an event monitor can be used. This device is triggered at the time the patient's symptoms occur and provides a continuous ECG. This increases the likelihood of capturing a symptomatic episode, but event monitoring is significantly more expensive than Holter monitor testing.

Critical Care Telemetry Monitoring
Many serious ventricular dysrhythmias are diagnosed in the hospital while monitoring a patient in the first few days after a myocardial infarction. Routine monitoring of continuous ECGs for such patients is now standard and the immediate treatment of VT/VF in the postinfarct period has been a major part of the reduced mortality of myocardial infarction since the introduction of coronary care units. Patients with acute myocardial infarction should have routine continuous electrocardiographic monitoring in the initial stage of their hospital care.

Patients in the hospital for exacerbation of congestive heart failure should also receive continuous monitoring. They are at increased risk for VT/VF, and they often have asymptomatic dysrhythmias.

Surgical Diagnostic Procedures
- **Cardiac catheterization.** Cardiac catheterization is often required to delineate the extent of coronary disease. The cardiac output and pressure measurements obtained at the time of catheterization are generally considered to be the most accurate measurements of left ventricular function available. Cardiac catheterization and EPS can be performed at the same time.
- **EPS.** The gold standard for evaluating a patient with known or suspected VT/VF is an EPS. Current guidelines recommend patients with a history of myocardial infarction and symptoms of syncope, presyncope, or palpitations undergo EPS testing. This is an invasive test similar to a cardiac catheterization in which multiple electrical leads are threaded to the endocardium to map electrical impulses and to induce dysrhythmias with applied electrical impulses. VTs are characterized as inducible or noninducible and suppressible or nonsuppressible (with medication) at the time of EPS. Inducible sustained VT is an indication of increased risk for sudden death in patients with reduced ejection fraction. Some VTs can be cured by ablation at the time of EPS.

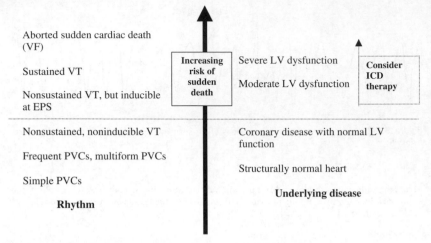

Figure 9.6-2. Risk stratification of patients with ventricular dysrhythmias.

Staging

- **Risk stratification.** Strategies to define which patients are at highest risk for death from VT/VF are still being refined. The most effective treatment is prevention by placement of an ICD, but this is expensive and has significant morbidity associated with it. Reduced ejection fraction and known prior episodes of symptomatic VT/VF are clearly high-risk factors. For other patients, it is still unclear if inducibility at EPS, abnormal signal averaged ECG (SAECG), or other factors will be best at identifying those at highest risk (Figure 9.6-2). Imaging-based (cardiac CT and MRI) risk stratification parameters are promising but not developed enough to use in clinical practice.

TREATMENT

- **Emergency treatment.** Patients who present with VT/VF in an emergency setting (cardiac arrest, sustained VT with hemodynamic compromise) should be treated according to current Advanced Cardiac Life Support (ACLS) protocols. The 2010 revisions of the ACLS protocol emphasize chest compressions and proceeding rapidly to the initial defibrillation. The protocol recommends one shock followed by cardiopulmonary resuscitation (CPR) for 2 minutes regardless of rhythm after shock.[3]
- **Hemodynamically unstable patients.** Patients with witnessed cardiac arrest or VT/VF and hemodynamic instability should be electrically defibrillated without delay with power according to the manufacturer's recommended settings. After the first attempt at cardioversion/defibrillation, effective CPR should be instituted regardless of rhythm. Those who have been unconscious for an unidentified period of time may receive five cycles of CPR (about 2 minutes) prior to attempted defibrillation.[3]
- **Patients with polymorphic ventricular tachycardia (Torsades de pointes)** should be given an intravenous infusion of 1 to 2 g of magnesium and prepare for pacing.[3]
- **Patients with wide-complex tachycardia but adequate blood pressure.** Patients with a wide-complex tachycardia who maintain an adequate blood pressure should be treated as though they have VT unless it is known with certainty that the rhythm is supraventricular. There are many guidelines that attempt to distinguish between VT and supraventricular tachycardia (SVT) with aberrant conduction on the basis of ECG criteria, but physicians caring for patients in emergency situations should ignore this distinction and manage all wide-complex tachycardias as if they are VT.[3]
  - The 2010 guideline recommends **amiodarone 150 mg** as the first agent for a stable patient with a wide-complex tachycardia that is believed to be VT. This is given as an IV infusion over 10 minutes. Alternative agents include procainamide and sotalol. Lidocaine is no longer considered to be a first-line agent in VT/VF. It is particularly important to remember to **go immediately to electrical cardioversion if the patient's hemodynamic status begins to deteriorate or** if the rhythm deteriorates to VF.[3]

Behavioral

Patients with palpitations should be instructed to reduce caffeine and eliminate smoking. They should discontinue any medications that may be contributing to the symptoms if possible. Such medications include theophylline and sympathomimetic agents such as pseudoephedrine.

Medications

β-Blockers

β-Blockers have significant antiarrhythmic properties and have been shown to reduce mortality for patients with ischemic heart disease and congestive heart failure. The benefit of β-blockade increases with the patient's risk for adverse events. β-Blockers also may have the effect of decreasing symptomatic palpitations in low-risk patients. They should be the first pharmacologic treatment considered for both symptomatic palpitations in patients with structurally normal hearts and for patients with life-threatening ventricular dysrhythmias. All patients with known coronary disease and/or congestive heart failure should receive β-blockers unless there is intolerance or a specific contraindication.

Antiarrhythmics

Patients whose dysrhythmias are not controlled with β-blockers may be candidates for amiodarone. **Amiodarone** is a type III antiarrhythmic and is the only antiarrhythmic other than β-blockers that has been shown to be no worse than placebo in causing excess mortality in clinical trials. Recent studies have shown no survival benefit from amiodarone versus placebo. Amiodarone is associated with significant complex drug–drug interactions and many adverse side effects for the lung, liver, thyroid, and skin. Its effects on overall survival in high-risk patients are uncertain, however. Amiodarone and/or β-blockers are sometimes used to help reduce the number of inappropriate activations of ICDs.[4,5]

There are many other antiarrhythmic medications that are available, but they all have potential for proarrhythmic effect and may cause increased mortality in treated patients. For these reasons, their use has fallen out of favor.[4,6] These should be used only with caution in carefully selected patients. The classification of antiarrhythmics is shown in Table 9.6-2.

Surgery

Patients with ischemic heart disease and VT/VF may benefit from revascularization (either angioplasty or bypass surgery) to correct the ischemia.

Special Therapy

Implanted Cardiac Defibrillators

ICDs are used in the treatment of patients with life-threatening ventricular dysrhythmias who are at high risk for sudden death. These devices are physically similar to pacemakers. They have an implanted power source beneath the skin of the chest and electrical leads connected to the heart, which can sense VT/VF and deliver either overdrive pacing or electrical defibrillator shocks in response to sustained dysrhythmias. **In clinical trials that have randomized patients to ICDs or antiarrhythmic drugs, the ICDs have consistently been better at improving survival in high-risk patients.** ICDs have been shown to be better even in patients who appear to have adequate suppression of their dysrhythmias with medication.[7,8]

The disadvantages of ICDs are that they are invasive, expensive, and occasionally may give shocks to patients who are still conscious. They may also increase the incidence of severe heart failure.

Referrals. Patients who are potential candidates for ICD therapy should be referred to an electrophysiologist for further evaluation.

TABLE 9.6-2	**Classification of Antiarrhythmic Drugs**
Type 1A	Quinidine, disopyramide, procainamide
Type 1B	Lidocaine, tocainide, mexiletine, phenytoin
Type 1C	Flecainide, encainide
Type II	β-Blockers
Type III	Amiodarone
Type IV	Calcium-channel antagonists

The American College of Cardiology and the American Heart Association list the following as **Class 1 recommendations for ICD therapy:**

- Secondary prevention in patients with heart failure and reduced left ventricular ejection fraction (LVEF) who have a history of cardiac arrest, VF, or hemodynamically destabilizing ventricular tachycardia.[9]
- Primary prevention in patients with an LVEF ≤35% and New York Heart Association (NYHA) functional Class 2 or 3 symptoms while undergoing optimal medical therapy, and a reasonable expectation of survival with good functional status for at least 1 year. Those patients with ischemic etiology should be at least 40 days post-MI.[10]

Counseling. Patients with risk for VT/VF should receive aggressive cardiac risk factor management according to their underlying disease(s) and risk profile. This may include counseling about exercise, smoking cessation, and low-fat diet. Aggressive management of lipids, blood pressure, congestive heart failure, and diabetes are also warranted.

Patient education. Patients with a device should be educated about topics such as air travel, use of various types of power equipment, and keeping emergency information on their person at all times. Extensive educational material is typically available from the manufacturer.

Follow-up. Patients who have had an ICD placed need a routine schedule of follow-up to investigate the correct functioning of the device. Some of this follow-up can typically be accomplished by telephonic monitoring. Patients who do not receive a device need close monitoring of their underlying illness(es). Those who take amiodarone need specific monitoring for adverse drug effects.

Results. Patients at high risk for VT/VF who are treated with an ICD have a relative risk reduction for death of about 30% compared to placebo or antiarrythmic medications alone.

Complications. Potential complications of amiodarone include bradycardias, pulmonary fibrosis, and thyroid dysfunction. Complications of ICDs include inappropriate shocks, operative morbidity, and a possible increase in severity of heart failure.

REFERENCES

1. Yancy CW, Jessup M, Bozkurt B, et al. 2013 ACCF/AHA guideline for the management of heart failure: a report of the American College of Cardiology Foundation/American Heart Association Task Force on Practice Guidelines. *Circulation* 2013;128:e240–e327.
2. Yancy CW, Jessup M, Bozkurt B, et al. 2013 ACCF/AHA guideline for the management of heart failure: a report of the American College of Cardiology Foundation/American Heart Association Task Force on Practice Guidelines. *Circulation* 2013;128:e240–e327.
3. Neumar RW, Otto CW, Link MS, et al. Part 8: adult advanced cardiovascular life support: 2010 American Heart Association guidelines for cardiopulmonary resuscitation and emergency cardiovascular care. *Circulation* 2010;122:S729–S767.
4. Kutyifa V, Kloppe A, Zareba W, et al. Impact of carvedilol and metoprolol on inappropriate implantable cardioverter-defibrillator therapy: the MADIT-CRT trial (Multicenter Automatic Defibrillator Implantation Trial With Cardiac Resynchronization Therapy). *J Am Coll Cardiol* 2013;62(15):1343–1350.
5. Packer DL, Prutkin JM, Hellkamp AS, et al. Impact of implantable cardio-defibrillator, amiodarone, and placebo on the mode of death in stable patients with heart failure. *Circulation* 2009;120:2170–2176.
6. Echt DS, Liebson PR, Mitchell LB, et al. Mortality and morbidity in patients receiving encainide, flecainide or placebo. The Cardiac Arrhythmia Suppression Trial. *N Engl J Med* 1991;324:781–788.
7. Bardy GH, Lee KL, Mark DB, et al; Sudden Cardiac Death in Heart Failure Trial (SCD-HeFT) Investigators. Amiodarone or an implantable cardioverter-defibrillator for congestive heart failure. *N Engl J Med* 2005;352:225–237.
8. Tracy CM, Epstein AE, Darbar D, et al. 2012 ACCF/AHA/HRS focused update incorporated into the ACCF/AHA/HRS 2008 guidelines for device-based therapy of cardiac rhythm abnormalities: a report of the American College of Cardiology Foundation/American Heart Association Task Force on Practice Guidelines and the Heart Rhythm Society. *Circulation* 2013;127:e283–e352.
9. Smith SC, Benjamin E, Bonow R, et al. AHA/ACC guidelines for secondary prevention for patients with coronary and other atherosclerotic vascular disease: 2011 update. *Circulation* 2011;124:2458–2473.
10. Moss AJ, Zareba W, Hall WJ, et al; Multicenter Automatic Defibrillator Implantation Trial II Investigators. Prophylactic implantation of a defibrillator in patients with myocardial infarction and reduced ejection fraction. *N Engl J Med* 2002;346:877–883.

9.7 Venous Thrombosis and Thrombophlebitis

Mitchell S. King, Linda F. Chang

GENERAL PRINCIPLES

Deep venous thrombosis (DVT) and subsequent embolism of clot to the pulmonary circulation, termed pulmonary embolism (PE), are potentially life-threatening conditions that require prompt diagnosis and treatment to limit the associated morbidity and mortality. Venous thromboembolism (VTE) constitutes both DVT and PE and the annual incidence is estimated to be between 300,000 and 600,000 cases per year in the United States.[1] Recent data reported an average of 547,596 hospitalizations with VTE between the years 2007 and 2009 among those aged ≥18 years in the United States.[2] The mortality risk is 10% to 30% of all VTE patients within 30 days if untreated.[1] The recurrence risk could be up to 53% within 10 years for patient with idiopathic VTE.[3]

Venous thrombosis most commonly affects the veins of the lower extremities under conditions associated with Virchow triad—namely venous stasis, endothelial injury, or a hypercoagulable state. Locally, the acute formation of clot can be associated with pain and edema and long term with chronic venous stasis, edema, and leg ulcerations. Embolism of the clot can lead to obstruction of the pulmonary arteries, acute right heart failure, cardiovascular collapse, and death. Superficial thrombophlebitis, although generally not life-threatening, can arise under similar conditions and pose a risk for development of DVT as well as cause considerable patient discomfort. Risk factors for VTE include hospitalization, surgery, trauma, immobility, pregnancy, malignancy, hormonal therapy and contraceptives, thrombophilia, previous VTE, age, and obesity (Table 9.7-1).[4,5]

DEEP VENOUS THROMBOSIS
Clinical Presentation

A high index of clinical suspicion is necessary for the diagnosis of DVT.

- **The history** may include lower extremity aching, swelling, or feeling of warmth. A search for risk factors, such as obesity, trauma, surgery, recent hospitalizations or travel, family history or personal history of DVT, congestive heart failure, pregnancy, and oral contraceptive pill (OCP) use, should be included.
- **The physical examination** may be normal or may include findings of lower extremity swelling, tenderness, warmth, or palpable venous "cords."

TABLE 9.7-1	Risk Factors for Deep Venous Thrombosis[4,5]
Risk factor	**Odds ratio**
Major surgery (general, spinal cord, orthopedic)	Greater than 10
Trauma or joint replacement	Greater than 10
Previous VTE	2–9
Arthroscopic knee surgery	2–9
Congestive heart or respiratory failure	2–9
Malignancy	2–9
Pregnancy	2–9
Medications (e.g., oral contraceptives, tamoxifen, and related medications)	2–9
Immobility	Less than 2
Advanced age and obesity	Less than 2

Diagnostic Testing

Laboratory Findings

- d-Dimer laboratory testing may be used to exclude DVT in patients without risk factors (95% sensitive and negative predictive value 94%) or in higher-risk patients along with a negative venous duplex scan (99% sensitive, specificity 50%).[5,6] A complete blood count (CBC), prothrombin time (PT), and partial thromboplastin time (PTT) should be obtained in anticipation of starting anticoagulant therapy.
- In patients younger than 40 years, without apparent risk factors, or with recurrent or family history of DVT, consider assessment for protein C deficiency, protein S deficiency, antithrombin III deficiency, lupus anticoagulant, hyperhomocysteinemia, and the genetic mutations for factor V Leiden and prothrombin 20210. Interpretation of these laboratory results must take into account current usage of heparin, warfarin (Coumadin), or OCPs as well as the presence of renal or liver disease, disseminated intravascular coagulation, pregnancy, and acute arterial or venous thrombosis.

Venous Imaging

- Duplex venous scanning has become the test of choice to assess the patient for DVT. This test is noninvasive and less sensitive for calf vein thrombi, which are not thought to be clinically significant unless they propagate proximally, which occurs approximately 20% of the time. Serial testing over several days can be done to evaluate the patient for the possibility of proximal propagation of calf vein thrombosis.[5-8] Computed tomography (CT) venography provides comparable results but requires administration of contrast materials and exposure to radiation.[8]
- Venography is the standard by which the other tests are measured, but it is invasive and carries with it a risk of contrast sensitivity and of developing DVT as a result of the procedure. Consider using venography in the setting of a high clinical suspicion when the noninvasive test results are negative or when the clinical suspicion is very low and the noninvasive test results are positive.

PULMONARY EMBOLISM

Clinical Presentation

- **History.** A patient with PE may present with nonspecific symptoms, such as dyspnea, palpitations, and a sense of impending doom, or with more classic symptoms of chest pain, cough, hemoptysis, symptoms consistent with DVT, or cardiovascular collapse.
- **Physical findings** are also nonspecific. The most common physical findings are tachypnea, tachycardia, and signs consistent with DVT.

Diagnostic Testing

Laboratory Findings

- Arterial blood gases should be obtained and may reveal a low or normal pO_2 and pCO_2.
- A CBC, PT, and PTT should be ordered in anticipation of use of anticoagulants.
- d-Dimer laboratory testing may be used to exclude PE in patients without risk factors or in higher-risk patients along with a negative chest CT scan or ventilation–perfusion (V/Q) scan.
- See above for workup of the hypercoagulable state.

Imaging

- **Chest radiography** findings with PE are nonspecific and may show effusions, atelectasis, localized infiltrates, or decreased vascular markings, or they may be normal.
- **Spiral CT** scan of the chest (sensitivity 87%, specificity 91%) has become the preferred test in most centers because of its availability and ability to examine other structures within the chest. It is the test of choice in patients with abnormal chest x-rays who would be expected to have abnormal V/Q scans. With high-risk patients and normal CT scans, additional testing should be considered to exclude DVT/PE.[7,8]
- **Ventilation–perfusion scanning** is valuable in diagnosing or "ruling out" PE in patients with normal chest x-rays and absence of underlying pulmonary disease. Findings are reported as normal, low, intermediate, or high probability of PE based on the presence or absence of mismatched wedge-shaped perfusion defects. If the findings are nonconfirmatory or discordant with the level of clinical suspicion, d-dimer testing and duplex scanning may be helpful, or invasive testing with pulmonary arteriography may be indicated.
- **Pulmonary arteriography** is the gold standard test for diagnosing PE, and, if positive, shows clot obstruction of one or more pulmonary arteries. This invasive test exposes the patient to contrast material and may be less readily available, depending on the availability of personnel.

TREATMENT OF DVT AND PE

Goal of therapy is to prevent complications and reduce VTE reoccurrences. Oxygen, intravenous fluids, ventilator support, and other supportive measures should be provided as indicated by the clinical status of the patient.

Anticoagulants

Initial Treatment

- **Parenteral** anticoagulation therapy with low-molecular-weight heparin (LMWH), fondaparinux, unfractionated heparin (UFH), or SC heparin is the immediate drug of choice for treating acute VTE and should be initiated when the diagnosis is suspected, unless there are contraindications to its use, such as increased risk of bleeding or heparin sensitivity.[9,10]
- **Oral** anticoagulation with rivaroxaban is another immediate option for treatment of acute VTE.[9]
- **Vitamin k** antagonist such as warfarin can be initiated along with rapid-acting anticoagulants (heparin, fondaparinux, or rivaroxaban). Combination therapy should be used for a minimum of 5 days and until the patient's international normalized ratio (INR) is greater than 2 (commonly between 2 and 3) for at least 24 hours before discontinuing rapid-acting anticoagulants.
- Table 9.7-2 provides an overview of anticoagulants dosing for acute DVT.
  - With use of UFH, it is critical to achieve a therapeutic aPTT within 24 hours of diagnosis to minimize the chances of thrombus extension or recurrent DVT or PE.
- **Therapeutic** range should be adjusted to recommended aPTT based on the responsiveness of the test reagent and coagulometer used.[9,11] For example:
  - aPTT goal is based on corresponding level of heparin concentration of 0.2 to 0.4 units per mL by protamine titration, or
  - an antifactor Xa level of 0.3 to 0.7 unit per mL
- Unfractionated heparin can be given IV or SC administration and a weight-based nomogram has been developed to assist with attaining recommended therapeutic goal (Table 9.7-2).
  - LMWH can be dosed once or twice a day without laboratory monitoring for most patients. For obese, pregnant, renal compromised individuals, dose adjustment based on the antifactor Xa level.[12,13] LMWH-anti-Xa activity peaks at 4 hours after the SC administration of a weight-adjusted dose regimen; therefore, the assay should be performed at this time.
- **Laboratory monitoring UFH.** aPTT monitoring every 6 hours until therapeutic and a stable PTT has been attained for continuous administration. For SC administration, aPTT should be drawn at 6 hours after the morning administration and adjust the dose to achieve institution therapeutic goals. While the patient is on heparin, a CBC should be obtained every 2 to 3 days to monitor for thrombocytopenia. Mild degrees of thrombocytopenia (more than 100,000 platelets per high-power field) occur commonly with heparin therapy. More severe degrees of thrombocytopenia may be associated with arterial thrombosis and may require cessation of heparin therapy.[10,13]
- Duration of therapy with UFH or LMWH should be at least 5 days and can be discontinued after the INR is in the therapeutic range for 2 days.
- Adverse reactions and management.[13,14]
  - **Bleeding**. Major bleeding occurred in 1.1% of patients treated with LMWH and 1.9% of patients treated with UFH.
    - Intravenous protamine sulfate at 1 mg per 100 units of UFH up to a maximum of 50 mg or 1 mg per 100 antifactor Xa units of LMWH should be given for major bleeds.
  - **Thrombocytopenia**. Platelet counts drop to less than 150,000 in up to 30% of patients on UFH therapy and it usually occurs within the first 5 days of therapy. This will level back to normal with continued therapy. However, heparin-induced thrombocytopenia (HIT) is a serious adverse drug reaction and requires immediate intervention. It is mediated by immunoglobulin antibodies directed against the heparin–platelet factor 4 complex. Patients should be evaluated for HIT when platelet counts drop by more than 50% or below 100,000. HIT occurs in 3% of patients receiving UFH and less than 1% of patients on LMWH.[7] Platelet counts should be monitored every 2 to 3 days.
  - Other adverse effects associated with heparin therapy are osteoporosis, skin reactions, alopecia, and hypersensitivity.
- **Pregnancy**. Drug of choice is adjusted-dose LMWH throughout pregnancy or IV UFH (usual bolus and maintenance protocol) for at least 5 days, followed by adjusted-dose UFH or LMWH for the remainder of the pregnancy.[12] Neither UFH nor LMWH is secreted into breast milk and can be safely administered to nursing mothers if prolonged anticoagulation is needed.

TABLE 9.7-2 . Heparin Dosing and Nomogram for Adjustment of IV Heparin[9]

Intravenous UFH

Initial dose	80 units/kg bolus, then 18 units/kg/h
aPTT, <35 s	80 units/kg bolus, then increase 4 units/kg/h
aPTT, 35–45 s	40 units/kg bolus, then increase 2 units/kg/h
aPTT, 46–70 s	No change
aPTT, 71–90 s	Decrease infusion rate by 2 units/kg/h
aPTT, >90 s	Hold infusion 1 h, then decrease infusion rate 3 units/kg/h
Subcutaneous UFH	Initial dose 333 units/kg, then 250 units/kg bid

LMWHs

Enoxaparin (Lovenox)	1 mg/kg every 12 h or 1.5 mg/kg once daily
Dalteparin (Fragmin)	200 IU/kg as single daily dose or divided into bid dosing
Tinzaparin (Innohep)	175 units/kg daily

Others

Fondaparinux (Arixtra)	<50 kg is 5 mg SC daily, 50–100 kg is 7.5 mg SC daily, >100 kg is 10 mg SC daily
Rivaroxaban (Xarelto)	15 mg q12 h for 21 days, then 20 mg daily with food

Outpatient DVT Management

With the availability of LMWH, outpatient DVT management has been found to be safe and cost-effective.[9,15,16] The protocol is similar to inpatient therapy, using LMWH for short-term anticoagulation until warfarin is within the therapeutic range. Candidates must be hemodynamically stable, without renal failure, not at high risk for bleeding, adequate home circumstances (well-maintained living conditions, strong family/friend support, phone access), and access to daily clinical laboratory monitoring until the INR is therapeutic.

Other agents such as dabigatran or rivaroxaban may be used and has been found to be safe and efficacious.

Other Treatments

- **Other anticoagulants**. Direct thrombin inhibitors such as lepirudin, argatroban, and bivalirudin are approved as an alternative for patients with or at high risk for HIT. Danaparoid is a factor Xa inhibitor and another alternative to the management of patients with HIT.[9]
- Thrombolytic therapy is not recommended for the treatment of DVT or PE in most patients. The exception is for patients with massive ileofemoral thrombosis or hemodynamically unstable PE patients and low risk for bleeding. The recommended means to administer the thrombolytic is intravenously.[9]
- Inferior vena caval filter is recommended in patients with a contraindication to anticoagulant therapy.
- Pulmonary embolectomy should be considered in unstable patients with massive PE who may not be candidates for thrombolytics.

Long-Term Treatment

Warfarin is preferred over LMWH for long-term therapy in patients with VTE who do not have comorbid cancer. LMWH is preferred over warfarin for patients with cancer who develop VTE. Both warfarin and LMWH are recommended as first-line agents over dabigatran or rivaroxaban for long-term therapy.[9,18]

Warfarin initial dose is 10 mg daily for 2 days, then dosing based on INR results for most patients. A lower dose is recommended for elderly patients because of their increased pharmacodynamic response.[17]

- **Laboratory monitoring**. PT should be obtained daily initially. After a therapeutic value has been achieved, PT INR may be obtained twice weekly until stabilized and thereafter weekly to monthly.
- **Duration of therapy**. The range can be from 3 to 12 months with a target INR of 2.5 (INR range 2.0 to 3.0) for the majority of patients. If the INR is outside of the desired therapeutic range, the

TABLE 9.7-3 **Recommended Duration of Anticoagulation for DVT/PE[9,18]**

Patient conditions	Duration
First episode due to reversible risk factor	3 mo
First episode of unprovoked VTE	3 mo, then evaluate risk-benefit ratio for extended therapy
Second episodes of unprovoked VTE	Low to moderate bleeding risk, extended anticoagulant therapy
	High bleeding risk, 3 mo of anticoagulant therapy
Active cancer	Low to moderate bleeding risk, extended anticoagulant therapy
	High bleeding risk, extended anticoagulant therapy is still suggested

Yearly assessment of the risk-benefit of continuing anticoagulation is recommended for patients on extended therapy.

TABLE 9.7-4 **Management of Elevated INR Values[18]**

Elevated INR but <4.5; no significant bleeding	Lower or omit dose; if only minimally elevated, no dose reduction may be needed
INR ≥4.5 and <10.0; no significant bleeding	Omit 1–2 doses; monitor frequently; when therapeutic, resume at lowered dose; if urgent surgery planned, vitamin K1 may be given (<5 mg orally) with expected reduction in INR in 24 h. Additional 1–2 mg in 24 h if needed.
INR ≥10.0; no significant bleeding	Hold warfarin; administer vitamin K1 (2.5–5 mg orally even if not bleeding) with expected drop in INR in 24–48 h; monitor INR frequently; when INR therapeutic, resume warfarin at lowered dose.
Serious or life-threatening bleeding with any INR value	Hold warfarin; administer fresh frozen plasma (FFP) or prothrombin complex concentrate (PCC) along with vitamin K1 (5–10 mg by slow IV infusion); PCC suggested over FFP. Repeat FFP or PCC as needed based on INR; may repeat vitamin K1 if needed.

recommendation is to adjust the dose up or down in increments of 5% to 20% of the total weekly dose of warfarin. Tables 9.7-3 and 9.7-4 present specific duration of therapy and management of suboptimal therapeutic values.
- **Complications**. Bleeding and warfarin-induced skin necrosis are the two major complications. Warfarin has many clinically significant drug–drug or drug–food interactions and these can affect PT values.
- **Pregnancy**. Warfarin is absolutely contraindicated in pregnancy.

DVT Prophylaxis
- **Risk factors** for development of DVT include obesity, trauma, surgery (particularly lower extremity orthopedic surgery), prior history of or family history of DVT, OCP use, congestive heart failure, malignancy, and pregnancy. Identifying risk factors and assessing the degree of risk for the patient are the first steps in providing appropriate prophylactic therapy (Tables 9.7-1 and 9.7-5).
- **Recommendations** are shown in Table 9.7-6.[19–21] Consideration for prophylactic therapy needs to balance the risk of VTE and risk of bleeding for each patient.

Superficial Thrombophlebitis

Superficial thrombophlebitis generally occurs in the lower extremity in association with trauma, infection, or varicose veins. It manifests as a tender cord or knot with some surrounding erythema. In the upper extremity, it is most commonly seen with intravenous cannulation. In the absence of inciting

TABLE 9.7-5	Risk for DVT Without Prophylaxis[1,19–21]

Patient group	DVT prevalence, %
Medical patients	10–20
General surgery	15–40
Major gynecologic surgery	15–40
Major urologic surgery	15–40
Neurosurgery	15–40
Stroke	20–50
Hip/knee arthroplasty, hip fracture surgery	40–60
Major trauma	40–80
Spinal cord injury	60–80
Critical care patients	10–80

TABLE 9.7-6	Recommendations for Deep Venous Thrombosis Prophylaxis[19–21]

Low-risk medical and surgical patients	No need to use any specific prophylaxis other than early and persistent ambulation
Moderate-risk medical and surgical patients	Not at risk for major bleeding complications: LMWH, low-dose unfractionated heparin, or mechanical prophylaxis
	At risk for major bleeding complications: Mechanical prophylaxis
High-risk patients (includes knee and hip surgery)	Not at risk for major bleeding complications: LMWH or low-dose unfractionated heparin along with mechanical prophylaxis
	At risk for major bleeding complications: Mechanical prophylaxis with intermittent pneumatic compression
Patient NOT candidate for LMWH or unfractionated heparin and NOT at risk for major bleeding	Low-dose aspirin, fondaparinux, or mechanical prophylaxis

causes, consideration should be given to evaluation for malignancy or an underlying hypercoagulable state. Treatment involves use of heat, elevation, and nonsteroidal anti-inflammatory medications. If the process appears to be extending to the thigh and the saphenofemoral junction, anticoagulation and ligation or excision of the vein may be necessary. If extension into the deep system is a concern, duplex scanning should be performed to assess the need for additional anticoagulant therapy.

REFERENCES

1. Beckman MG, Hooper WC, Critchley SE, et al. Venous thromboembolism-A public health concern. *Am J Prev Med* 2010;38(4S):S495–S501.
2. *Morb Mortal Wkly Rep* 2012;61(22). http://www.cdc.gov/mmwr. Accessed December 2013.
3. Galioto NJ, Danley DL, Van Mannen RJ. Recurrent venous thromboembolism. *Am Fam Physician* 2011;83(3):293–300.
4. Gurza EJ, Lingam P. Deep vein thrombosis. Essential Evidence Plus 2012. www.essentialevidenceplus.com. Accessed December 2013.
5. Bates SM, Jaeschke R, Stevens SM, et al. Diagnosis of DVT: antithrombotic therapy and prevention of thrombosis, 9th ed: ACCP evidence-based practice guidelines. *Chest* 2012;141(2 Suppl):e351S–e418S.
6. Wilbur J, Shian B. Diagnosis of deep venous thrombosis and pulmonary embolism. *Am Fam Physician* 2012;86(10):913–919.

7. Quiroz R, Kucher N, Zou KH, et al. Clinical validity of a negative computed tomography scan in patients with suspected pulmonary embolism. *JAMA* 2005;293:2012.
8. van Strijen MJ, de Monyé W, Kieft GJ, et al. Diagnosis of pulmonary embolism with spiral CT as a second procedure following scintigraphy. *Eur Radiol* 2003;13:1501.
9. Kearon C, Akl EA, Comerota AJ, et al. Antithrombotic therapy for venous thromboembolic disease: antithrombotic therapy and prevention of thrombosis, 9th ed: ACCP evidence-based clinical practice guidelines. *Chest* 2012;141(2 Suppl):e419S–494S.
10. Spinler SA. New concepts in heparin-induced thrombocytopenia: diagnosis and management. *J Thromb Thrombolysis* 2006;21(1):17.
11. Vandiver JW, Vondracek TG. Antifactor Xa levels versus activated partial thromboplastin time for monitoring unfractionated heparin. *Pharmacotherapy* 2012;32(6):546–558.
12. Bates SM, Greer IA, Middeldorp S, et al. VTE, thrombophilia, antithrombotic therapy, and pregnancy: Antithrombotic Therapy and Prevention of Thrombosis, 9th ed: American College of Chest Physicians Evidence-Based Clinical Practice Guidelines. *Chest* 2012;141(2 Suppl):e691S–e736S.
13. Garcia DA, Baglin TP, Weitz JI, et al. Parenteral anticoagulants: antithrombotic therapy and prevention of thrombosis, 9th ed: American College of Chest Physicians Evidence-Based Clinical Practice. *Chest* 2012;141(2 Suppl):e24S–e43S.
14. Erkens PMG, Prins MH. Fixed dose subcutaneous low molecular weight heparin versus adjusted dose unfractionated heparin for venous thromboembolism. *Cochrane Database Syst Rev* 2010;(9):CD001100.
15. Segal JB, Bolger DT, Jenckes MW, et al. Outpatient therapy with low molecular weight heparin for the treatment of venous thromboembolism: a review of efficacy, safety, and costs. *Am J Med* 2003;115:298.
16. Merli G. Anticoagulants in the treatment of deep vein thrombosis. *Am J Med* 2005;118(8A):13S.
17. American Geriatrics Society Guideline. The use of oral anticoagulants (warfarin) in older people. *J Am Geriatr Soc* 2002;50:1439.
18. Ageno W, Gallus AS, Wittkowsky A, et al. Oral anticoagulants: antithrombotic therapy and prevention of thrombosis, 9th ed: ACCP Evidence-based Clinical Practice Guidelines. *Chest* 2012;141(2 Suppl):e44S–e88S.
19. Kahn SR, Lim W, Dunn AS, et al. Prevention of VTE in nonsurgical patients: antithrombotic therapy and prevention of thrombosis, 9th ed: ACCP Evidence-based Clinical Practice Guidelines. *Chest* 2012;141(2 Suppl):e195S–e226S.
20. Gould MK, Garcia DA, Wren SM, et al. Prevention of VTE in nonorthopedic surgical patients: antithrombotic therapy and prevention of thrombosis, 9th ed: ACCP Evidence-based Clinical Practice Guidelines. *Chest* 2012;141(2 Suppl):e227S–e277S.
21. Falck-Ytter Y, Francis CW, Johanson NA, et al. Prevention of VTE in orthopedic surgical patients: antithrombotic therapy and prevention of thrombosis, 9th ed: ACCP Evidence-based Clinical Practice Guidelines. *Chest* 2012;141(2 Suppl):e278S–e325S.

9.8 Peripheral Arterial Disease

Ferdinando Andrade

GENERAL PRINCIPLES

Definition

The American Heart Association defines peripheral arterial disease (PAD) as atherosclerosis affecting the lower extremities. PAD is a manifestation of systemic atherosclerosis and carries significant morbidity and mortality. Patients with PAD have the same relative risk of death as patients with known coronary artery disease (CAD) or cerebrovascular disease. Thus, they need to be treated aggressively to reduce the risk of cardiovascular events.

Anatomy

Disease that affects lower extremities involves the following arteries: aortoiliac, aortic bifurcation, common iliac, external iliac, femoral, popliteal, tibial, and dorsalis pedis.

- Following the anatomical distribution of blood flow, PAD affecting the aortoiliac arteries causes pain in buttocks and hips; disease of the common femoral or aortoiliac arteries causes pain in the thighs; disease of the superficial femoral arteries causes pain in the upper two thirds of the calves; and disease of the popliteal vessels affects the lower third of the calves. PAD in the tibial and peroneal arteries causes foot pain.
- Vessel location, anatomy, as well as severity of disease affect the options for revascularization.

Epidemiology

It is estimated that PAD affects 8 to 12 million people in the United States. PAD is underdiagnosed and undertreated due to disease unawareness and because symptoms may mimic other common conditions.

Classification

Arterial vascular disease (AVD) refers to noncoronary atherosclerosis, which includes cerebrovascular disease, aortic disease, renal disease, and PAD.

Etiology

The risk factors for PAD are the same as for atherosclerosis.

- *Traditional risk factors*: The presence of CAD or cerebrovascular disease makes patients more prone to PAD. Cigarette smoking and diabetes carry the highest risk for PAD. Hypertension, dyslipidemia, particularly low high-density lipoprotein (HDL) and high triglycerides, and hypercoagulability are important risk factors.
- *Novel risk factors for atherosclerosis*: Lipoprotein (a), apolipoprotein (apo) A-1, apo B-100, high-sensitivity C-reactive protein (CRP), fibrinogen, and homocystine are new identifiable risks for atherosclerosis. Their roles in PAD are being investigated.
- Genetic predisposition for collagen synthesis (Marfan syndrome, Ehler–Danlos IV syndrome) and inflammatory diseases (Takayasu arteritis) are rare, but carry significant risks for PAD.

Mechanism of Injury

The development of atherosclerosis is a complex process. Many factors are at play and interact in the process of plaque formation. Lipid abnormality leads to fatty deposition in the vessel's intima. Local vessel conditions such as oxidative stress, vascular smooth muscle activation, activation of the inflammation cascade, release of mediators of inflammation, endothelial dysfunction, vessel damage by shearing forces, all contribute to plaque rupture, platelet activation, and thrombosis. Eventually, blood vessel injury ensues, leading to vessel remodeling, thrombosis, compromised blood flow, and ischemia to tissues.

DIAGNOSIS

Clinical Presentation

About 30% of patients present with classic symptoms of claudication, which is the development of pain triggered by exercise and resolved by rest. Some patients have no symptoms while the majority present with vague and nonspecific symptoms: leg heaviness, achiness, fatigue when walking, numbness, etc. Occasionally, patients present with acute occlusion (a cold, cyanotic, and pulseless extremity); when they do, it is a medical emergency.

History

Medical history is focused on assessing symptoms, functional capacity, and determining the existence of PAD risk factors: presence of cardiovascular disease (myocardial infarction, stroke, transient ischemic attack), cigarette smoking, hypertension, diabetes mellitus, dyslipidemia, and family history of arterial disease. The American College of Cardiology/American Heart Association (2005 guidelines) has identified the following groups, which are at risk for lower extremity PAD:

- Age ≥70 years
- Age 50 to 69 years with a history of smoking or diabetes
- Age 40 to 49 with diabetes and at least one other risk factor for atherosclerosis
- Leg symptoms suggestive of claudication with exertion or ischemic pain at rest
- Abnormal lower extremity pulse examination
- Known atherosclerosis at other sites (e.g., coronary, carotid, renal artery disease)

Physical Examination

A complete physical examination is warranted, with special attention to cardiovascular system: blood pressure in both arms. *Cardiac examination*: heart rate, rhythm, presence of murmurs, jugular venous distention (JVD), and carotid bruits. *Lungs*: auscultation. *Abdomen*: palpation and auscultation for bruits. *Evaluation of peripheral circulation*: palpation of all peripheral pulses, assessment of capillary refill and presence of signs of circulatory compromise (skin atrophy, loss of hair, nail changes), and presence of skin ulceration or coolness.

Diagnostic Studies

- *Routine studies*: Complete blood count (CBC), comprehensive metabolic panel, fasting blood sugar, and lipid profile. If the suspicion of PAD exists, an ankle brachial index (ABI) is the first and most useful test to order.
- The ABI is the ratio of the systolic ankle blood pressure to the systolic brachial artery pressure, both measured in the supine position using Doppler.
  - A normal ABI is 0.9 to 1.3. ABI correlates well with disease severity and patient functional state. An ABI <0.9 has a 90% sensitive and 95% specificity for PAD. An ABI <0.4 correlates with pain at rest and ulceration and an ABI <0.2 is associated with ischemic gangrenous extremities.
  - ABI can also be measured during a treadmill test (5 minutes at 2 mph and 12 degree incline). Ankle pressure <50 mmHg indicates PAD.
  - A normal ABI does not completely rule out PAD (patients may have an abdominal aneurysm or may have toe disease).
  - The presence of significant media arterial calcinosis makes ABI not reliable due to decreased compressibility of the vessel. Medial calcinosis is common in patients with diabetes. ABI >1.3 is suspicious for medial calcinosis. In these patients, toe pressures and Doppler waveforms are more useful.
- *Toe systolic pressure index* (TSPI). Measured by strain-gauge or plethysmographic technique. Normally, TSPI should be >0.60 ± 0.17. Absolute values <30 mmHg in patients with ulcers predict poor healing prognosis.
- *Segmental pressures*. It is the serial measurement of pressures along the leg. A drop of 20 mmHg compared to opposite leg is significant.

Imaging Studies

- Duplex ultrasound and Doppler
  - It measures the velocity of flowing blood in arteries and veins and provides quantification of the degree of stenosis. As a vessel narrows, the velocity increases. It identifies stenosis and occlusion with 92% to 95% sensitivity and 97% to 99% specificity. Vessels are classified as normal; 1% to 19% stenosis, 20% to 49% stenosis, 50% to 99% stenosis, and occluded.
  - It allows measurement of intima-media wall thickness, which correlates with atherosclerosis.
  - *Doppler waveform*. Blood flow in normal vessels has a triphasic waveform: forward systolic peak, reverse flow (early diastole), and forward flow (late diastole). As vessels narrow, the reverse flow is lost.
  - It is also useful in monitoring aneurysm progression as well as surveillance of graft patency.
- Angiography and magnetic resonance angiography (MRA) are considered the gold standard as diagnostic tools and in the planning for revascularization.
  - *Angiography*. It is invasive, uses contrast material, carries higher morbidity, and is more expensive than MRA. However, it allows immediate angioplasty if indicated.
  - *MRA*. It is noninvasive, uses contrast agents that are not nephrotoxic, it does not use ionizing radiation, and it provides detailed anatomy of disease. It is superior to computed tomography (CT) angiography but cannot be used in patients with pacemaker or other metallic objects.
  - Recent advances in MRA, such as "time of flight" techniques, which allows removal of background tissue signals, and new three-dimensional (3D) MRA provide images close to the angiograms.
  - 3D MRA is currently used only in patients with collagen vascular disease and vascular inflammatory conditions.
- CT angiography provides good images and is used to diagnose aortic dissecting aneurysm as well as postoperative surveillance for leaks. It uses ionizing radiation and nephrotoxic contrast agents.

TREATMENT

The goals of treatment are (a) to decrease risks factors for PAD and (b) to improve functional status by decreasing claudication, improving exercise tolerance, decreasing limb pain, preventing skin ulceration, and amputation.

Behavioral Therapy

- *Smoking cessation.* All efforts must be made to help patients stop smoking. Smoking cessation decreases pain and slows disease progression. Patients must be counseled at each visit about cessation and be offered nicotine replacement therapies, alone or in combination with Wellbutrin (bupropion).
- *Exercise.* Prescribed walking regimen of 30 minutes three times a week significantly improves symptoms of claudication and improves functional status. The benefit of exercise is not fully understood; it is not just due to development of collateral circulation, but due to improved muscle biochemistry (energy utilization, endothelial function) and gait.

Medications

- *Antiplatelet drugs.* Aspirin 81 to 325 mg daily or Clopidogrel 75 mg per day reduces the risk of fatal and nonfatal cardiovascular events in patients with PAD.
- *Cilostazol.* A phosphodiesterase III inhibitor that inhibits platelet aggregation and improves quality of life of patients with PAD. Usual dose is 100 mg bid, and 50 mg bid if patient takes calcium-channel blockers. It cannot be used in patients with heart failure.
- Pentoxifylline, 1.2 g per day has been used in patients with PAD. It is thought to improve rheology of red blood cells (RBCs), but its benefits are questionable.

Treatment of Risk Factors

- *Hyperlipidemia.* Lipid reduction using statins decreases disease progression. The benefit is likely due to plaque stabilization and improvement of endothelial function. The National Cholesterol Education Program Adult Treatment Panel III (NCEP/ATPIII) recommends treatment with target goal of low-density lipoprotein (LDL) <100 mg per dL and triglycerides <150 mg per dL.
- Blood pressure reduction
  - Angiotensin-converting enzyme inhibitors (ACEIs) have positive effect on PAD beyond blood pressure lowering effect and are recommended in patients with PAD.
  - β-Blockers reduce cardiovascular events, so their use is encouraged in patients with PAD, except in patients with severe disease.

Endovascular Intervention

- Percutaneous transluminal angioplasty (PTA). It is the reopening of blood vessel via balloon angioplasty that causes "a controlled" medial artery dissection. Advances in techniques, wires, and stents have expanded the role of PTA in treating PAD.
  - *Indication*: loss of tissue, rest pain, persistent symptoms in spite of conservative therapy, or progressive disease.
  - It is generally done in patients who have localized disease, short segment, noncalcified lesions in large vessels, and most commonly used in vessels above the inguinal canal such as aortoiliac vessels. It can be done with or without stent placement.
  - Indicated in patients not able to tolerate surgery and for those who need saphenous vein for cardiac revascularization.
  - Not recommended for popliteal or femoral disease due to risk of dissection and restenosis.
  - *Risks*: Dissection, restenosis, groin hematoma, and pseudoaneurysm.
- PTA can be repeated, and it does not preclude subsequent surgical revascularization if needed.

Surgery

- Arterial bypass surgery is considered the gold standard in revascularization due to long-term patency.
  - It carries significant morbidity and mortality due to its invasiveness and need for general anesthesia.
  - Outcomes are affected by patient's age, gender, smoking, and comorbid conditions, particularly diabetes and hypertension.
  - Indicated in patients with disabling claudication and to prevent limb loss due to ischemia.
  - Indicated for patients with diffuse disease and long lesions, and those who have severe and progressive disease.
  - It is the best choice for infrainguinal vessel disease.

Patient Education and Counseling

Patients need to be educated on the deleterious effects of smoking and sedentary lifestyle. All efforts must be made to improve patient's compliance with treatment of blood pressure, lipids, and diabetes.

Monitoring

The progression of PAD is variable and unpredictable. However, the higher the risk factors, the higher the likelihood of progression. Patients with disease need to be monitored for disease progression in order to identify and treat complications promptly.

Referral

Patients with severe and progressive disease should be referred to a vascular surgeon.

SPECIAL CONSIDERATIONS

• Patients with known history of Marfans syndrome and Ehler–Danlos syndrome, and those affected by Takayasu arteritis need to be screened regularly for the development of aneurysms and other symptoms of PAD. Patients with these conditions need to be under the care of a cardiologist and followed closely.

REFERENCES

1. ACC/AHA Guidelines for the management of patients with peripheral arterial disease (lower extremity, renal, mesenteric, and abdominal aortic). *J Am Coll Cardiol* 2004;109:2595. http://www.acc.org/clinical/guidelines/pad/summary.pdf.
2. Graeme J, Norman PE, Eikelboom JW. Medical treatment of peripheral arterial disease. *JAMA* 2006;295:547–553.
3. Belch J, Topol EJ, Agnelli G, et al. Critical issues in peripheral arterial disease detection and management: a call to action. *Arch Intern Med* 2003;163:884.
4. Hiatt W. Medical treatment of peripheral arterial disease and claudication. *N Engl J Med* 2001;344:1608.
5. van den Bosch M, Mali WP, Bloemenkamp DG, et al. Peripheral arterial disease. *Lancet* 2002;359(9311):1070.
6. Lesho E. Management of peripheral arterial disease. *Am Fam Physician* 2004;69:525–533.
7. Lawson G. The importance of obtaining ankle-brachial indexes in older adults: the other vital sign. *J Vasc Nurs* 2005;23(2):46–51.
8. Third Report of the National Cholesterol Education Program (NCEP) Expert Panel on Detection, Evaluation, and Treatment of High Blood Cholesterol in Adults (Adult Treatment Panel III). Third Report of the National Cholesterol Education Program (NCEP) Expert Panel on detection, evaluation, and treatment of high blood cholesterol in adults (Adult Treatment Panel III) final report. *Circulation* 2002;106:3143.
9. Schillinger M, Exner M, Mlekusch W, et al. Statin therapy improves cardiovascular outcome of patients with peripheral artery disease. *Eur Heart J* 2004;25(9):742–748.
10. Yusuf S, Sleight P, Pogue J, et al. Effects of an angiotensin-converting-enzyme inhibitor, ramipril, on cardiovascular events in high-risk patients. The Heart Outcomes Prevention Evaluation Study Investigators. *N Engl J Med* 2000;342:145.
11. Stewart K, Hiatt W, Regensteiner J, et al. Exercise training for claudication. *N Engl J Med* 2002;347:1941.
12. Tucker De Sanctis J. Percutaneous interventions for lower extremity peripheral vascular disease. *Am Fam Physician* 2001;64:1965.
13. Hirsch AT, Haskal ZJ, Hertzer NR, et al. ACC/AHA 2005 guidelines for the management of patients with peripheral arterial disease (lower extremity, renal, mesenteric, and abdominal aortic): executive summary a collaborative report from the American Association for Vascular Surgery/Society for Vascular Surgery, Society for Cardiovascular Angiography and Interventions, Society for Vascular Medicine and Biology, Society of Interventional Radiology, and the ACC/AHA Task Force on Practice Guidelines (Writing Committee to Develop Guidelines for the Management of Patients With Peripheral Arterial Disease) endorsed by the American Association of Cardiovascular and Pulmonary Rehabilitation; National Heart, Lung, and Blood Institute; Society for Vascular Nursing; TransAtlantic Inter-Society Consensus; and Vascular Disease Foundation. *J Am Coll Cardiol* 2006;47:1239.

CHAPTER 10

Respiratory Problems

Section Editor: David Harnisch Sr.

10.1 Asthma

Elisabeth L. Backer

GENERAL PRINCIPLES
Definition

Asthma is a chronic inflammatory disorder of the airways involving various cells (especially mast cells, eosinophils, and T lymphocytes), which is marked by recurrent episodes of wheezing, chest tightness, breathlessness, and cough, occurring particularly at night or in the early morning. Asthma is associated with an increase in airway responsiveness to a variety of stimuli, leading to widespread, but variable airflow limitation, which may revert spontaneously or with treatment.[1–3]

Pathophysiology

- A genetic predisposition has been recognized although atopy is the strongest identifiable predisposing factor. Obesity is increasingly recognized as a risk factor. Episode triggers include airway inflammation and hyperresponsiveness of sensitive patients to inhaled allergens (house dust mites, cockroaches, cats, seasonal pollens).
- Nonspecific precipitators include exercise, upper respiratory tract infections, rhinitis/sinusitis, postnasal drainage, aspirations, gastroesophageal reflux disease (GERD), weather changes, and stress, while selected individuals react to aspirin and nonsteroidal anti-inflammatory drugs.[3]
- Exposure to environmental tobacco smoke (or to various agents in the workplace) is a common trigger.

DIAGNOSIS
Clinical Presentation

Patients may present with intermittent or chronic symptoms of airway obstruction (breathlessness, cough, wheezing, chest tightness). Symptoms and signs may vary widely in terms of intensity and frequency. The classic triad consists of cough, shortness of breath, and wheezing.[2] Symptoms may occur infrequently or continuously, spontaneously, or secondary to triggers. There may be a circadian rhythm with symptoms worse at night, nadir between 3 and 4 A.M.

Physical Findings

Patients may present with diffuse wheezing (varying pitches, tones, and timing) heard bilaterally and prolonged expiration. There may be contributing findings, which would include allergic rhinitis, nasal polyps, hives, eczema, and atopic dermatitis. Patients may use accessory muscles, be found to have pulsus paradoxus, and present with globally reduced breath sounds in severe airway obstruction.[2,3]

Classification of Severity

- **Mild intermittent asthma:** Symptoms equal or less than twice a week; otherwise asymptomatic and normal peak expiratory flow (PEF) between exacerbations; nocturnal symptoms equal or less than twice a month; use of short-acting β-agonists for symptom relief less than twice a week; forced expiratory volume in 1 second (FEV_1) or PEF equal or greater than 80% of predicted; and one or no exacerbations requiring oral glucocorticoids per year.

- **Mild persistent asthma:** Symptoms more than twice a week, but less than once a day; nocturnal symptoms more than twice a month; minor interference with normal activity; FEV_1 or PEF greater than 80% of predicted; and two or more exacerbations requiring oral glucocorticoids per year.
- **Moderate persistent asthma:** Daily symptoms; daily use of inhaled short-acting β_2-agonist; nocturnal symptoms more than once a week; some limitation in normal activity; FEV_1 or PEF greater than 60% but less than 80% of predicted.
- **Severe persistent asthma:** Continual symptoms; limited physical activity; frequent exacerbations; frequent nocturnal symptoms; need for short-acting β-agonists for symptom relief several times per day; extreme limitations in normal activity; FEV_1 or PEF equal or less than 60% of predicted.

Laboratory Tests and Imaging

Peak Flow

Peak flow is a simple test measuring airflow during maximal exhalation. It is important to have establishment of baseline and zone scheme (red <50%, yellow 50% to 80%, green >80% of predicted/personal value). PEF is usually lowest upon awakening, highest before midpoint of waking day (diurnal variation). PEF <200 mL per minute indicates severe airflow obstruction.[3] PEF is used to monitor trends in lung function.[2]

Spirometry Measures FEV_1 and Forced Vital Capacity

The degree of airway obstruction defined by percent of predicted FEV_1 achieved:
- >80%: borderline obstruction
- 60% to 80%: mild obstruction
- 40% to 60%: moderate obstruction
- <40%: severe obstruction

An increase in FEV_1 $\geq12\%$ (or increase in forced vital capacity $\geq15\%$) postbronchodilator therapy suggests reversible airway obstruction/asthma.[2]

Bronchoprovocative Testing

This test is useful if asthma is suspected and spirometry is nondiagnostic, or if patient presents with atypical asthma symptoms. It is done in pulmonary function test laboratories, using metacholine or histamine. A negative metacholine challenge argues against asthma diagnosis.

Other Tests

- Chest x-ray (CXR) is almost always normal, but may show hyperinflation/bronchial wall thickening. It is indicated in patients with atypical symptoms, or to exclude complications.[3]
- Blood tests are used to investigate allergic basis of disease (elevated eosinophil count/immunoglobulin E).
- Allergy testing consists of skin testing (most accurate for aeroallergens, not for foods) or radioallergosorbent test (more expensive, lesser sensitivity).[2]
- **Other:** Further evaluations for GERD or sinusitis may be helpful.

Differential Diagnosis

In children, consideration should be given to foreign body aspiration, cystic fibrosis, viral bronchiolitis, and tracheomalacia. In young adults, the differential includes bronchiectasis, pulmonary embolism, GERD, sarcoidosis, and vasculitides. In older adults, the common diagnoses of chronic obstructive pulmonary disease and congestive heart failure should be considered. Psychiatric causes that mimic asthma include conversion disorder. Vocal cord dysfunction should be considered in all age groups.

The differential diagnosis of persistent cough in case of normal CXR and lung functions includes postnasal drip, GERD, postviral tussive syndrome, medication-induced cough (angiotensin-converting enzyme inhibitors, ACE-I). These conditions are normally not associated with diffuse wheezing.

Comorbid conditions commonly include seasonal allergic rhinitis/conjunctivitis, perennial rhinitis, recurrent/chronic sinusitis, postnasal drip, and nasal polyps.

TREATMENT

Treatment includes initial spirometry and follow-up testing every 6 to 12 months; routine monitoring of symptoms and lung functions (PEF) is done at home. It is important to control trigger factors (allergens, respiratory infections, irritants, chemicals, physical activity, emotional stress). Consideration should be given to pneumococcal vaccination and annual influenza vaccinations. Goals of asthma treatment include reduction in impairment, as well as reduction in risk.

Pharmacologic Treatment[2]

A stepwise approach to therapy is recommended by the 2007 update of the National Asthma Education and Prevention Program Expert Panel Report III.[4] The aim of treatment is to maintain control of asthma with minimum amount of medication, thereby decreasing the risk of adverse effects.

Mild Intermittent Asthma
- Short-acting bronchodilator (inhaled β_2-agonist) as needed for symptom relief[5]
- Mast cell–stabilizing agents (cromolyn/nedocromil) can be used prior to exercise to prevent bronchoconstriction[6,7]

Mild Persistent Asthma
- Low-dose inhaled steroids, metered-dose inhalers versus multidose dry powder inhalers[8]
- Use of spacer device to optimize delivery and minimize oropharyngeal deposition
- Reduction of dose by 25% to 50% over several months if patient remains asymptomatic
- Short-acting inhaled bronchodilator as needed for symptom relief[9]
- Trial of leukotriene-modifying agents (montelukast)—response may vary
- Long-acting inhaled β_2-agonists (salmeterol)—less efficacious than inhaled steroids;[10] use if incomplete response to low-dose inhaled steroids
- **Alternative choice to inhaled steroids:** Mast cell–stabilizing agents (less effective)

Moderate Persistent Asthma
- Medium-dose inhaled steroids (fluticasone, budesonide)
  - Side effects possible; limit oropharyngeal/gastrointestinal absorption via mouth rinses
  - Use lowest dose needed to maintain asthma control[2]
- Low-dose inhaled steroid in combination with long-acting inhaled bronchodilator (salmeterol) if needed[2]
- Trial of leukotriene-modifying agents as additional "controller" agent; patients may be able to reduce inhaled steroid dose
- Alternative strategies include use of theophylline, but frequent side effects and narrow therapeutic window limit usefulness

Severe Asthma
- Medium- or high-dose inhaled steroids and long-acting inhaled bronchodilators
- Possible addition of theophylline and leukotriene modifiers—dosage limitations due to toxicity risk
- Oral corticosteroids if needed, at minimum dosage
- Optimal use of multiple concomitant "controllers"—no data available[2]

Management of Acute Asthma Exacerbation[11]
- Inhaled β_2-agonist (and inhaled anticholinergic)
- Systemic corticosteroid (oral or intravenous)
- Oxygen
- Monitor FEV_1 or PEF, O_2 saturation, pulse
- Hospitalization if severe exacerbation, high-risk patient, or incomplete/poor response to initial treatment

SPECIAL CONSIDERATIONS
- Complications include exhaustion, dehydration, airway infection, cor pulmonale, tussive syncope, pneumothorax, and acute respiratory failure (hypercapnea/hypoxia). The death rate is increasing worldwide (especially in urban minorities).
- Patient education leads to decreased hospitalizations, improved daily functioning, and increased patient satisfaction linked to:
  - Active comanagement and use of asthma action plan (monitoring of symptoms and lung functions)
  - Understanding of and adherence to medication
  - Knowledge of treatment plan for deteriorating condition or emergency situation[2,12]

REFERENCES
1. Global Initiative for Asthma Management and Prevention. NHLBI/WHO Workshop Report, U.S. Department of Health and Human Services. Bethesda, MD: NIH; 1995. Publication 95–3659.
2. http://www.uptodate.com/contents/an-overview-of-asthma-management?source=search_result&search=asthma&selectedTitle=1%7E150. Accessed December 12, 2014.

3. Tierney LM, McPhee SJ, Papadakis MA. *Current medical diagnosis and treatment*. New York, NY: Lange Medical Books, McGraw-Hill; 2002:278–290.
4. National Asthma Education and Prevention Program: Expert Panel Report III: guidelines for the diagnosis and management of asthma. Bethesda, MD: NHLI; 2007. NIH publication no. 08–4051. www.nhlbi.nih.gov/guidelines/asthma/asthgdln.htm.asthma/asthgdln.pdf. Accessed December 12, 2014.
5. Nelson HS. Adrenergic bronchodilators. *N Engl J Med* 1995;333:499.
6. Woolley M, Anderson SD, Quigley BM. Duration of protective effect of terbutaline sulfate and cromolym sodium. *Chest* 1990;97:39.
7. Bundgaard A, Enehjelm SD, Schmidt A, et al. A comparative study of the effects of two different doses of nedocromil and placebo. *Allergy* 1988;43:493.
8. Barnes PJ. Inhaled glucocorticoids for asthma. *N Engl J Med* 1995;332:868.
9. Drazen JM, Israel E, Boushey HA, et al. Comparison of regularly scheduled with as-needed use of alb-uterol in mild asthma. Asthma Clinical Research Network. *N Engl J Med* 1996; 335:841.
10. Verberne AA, Frost C, Roorda RJ, et al. One year treatment with salmeterol compared with beclometha-sone in children with asthma. *Am J Respir Crit Care Med* 1997;156:688.
11. Cline DC. Practical approaches to treating acute bronchospasm. *Postgrad Med* 2005;118:9–17.
12. Gibson PG, Powell H, Coughlan J, et al. Self-management education and regular practitioner review for adults with asthma. *Cochrane Database Syst Rev* 2000;CD001117.

10.2 Acute Bronchitis and Pneumonia

William J. Hueston

ACUTE BRONCHITIS

General Principles

Acute bronchitis is one of the most common diagnoses made in primary care practices. Symptoms of acute bronchitis can mimic asthma in acute stages. For patients in the early stages of acute bronchitis, pulmonary function tests may be indistinguishable from those of patients with asthma. As the bronchitis improves, patients are sometimes left with a lingering postbronchitic syndrome that may resemble asthma or, more specifically, cough-variant asthma (see Chapter 10.1).

Diagnosis

Clinical Presentation

Patients with either acute bronchitis or pneumonia usually present with a productive cough but may also complain of pleuritic chest pain, shortness of breath, occasional hemoptysis, and fever (usually less than 101°F). In most cases, acute bronchitis symptoms are preceded or accompanied by symptoms of an upper respiratory tract infection. On physical examination, wheezes or diffuse rhonchi may be present. The presence of localized rales should raise the possibility of pneumonia.

Laboratory or Radiologic Evaluation

Unless the patient has an underlying chronic pulmonary disease or appears seriously ill, there is little benefit from evaluating arterial blood gases, white blood cell counts, sputum Gram stains or culture, or routine chest radiograph.

Differential Diagnosis

In addition to suspecting pneumonia in patients with a cough, one should consider sinusitis and asthma in patients presenting with a productive cough and wheezing. Particularly in younger patients, symptoms of recurrent or chronic cough may be indicators of underlying asthma and warrant further evaluation. Prolonged cough may occur with pertussis. Testing with either culture or polymerase chain reaction testing for *Bordetella pertussis* may be indicated for patients whose cough persists beyond 30 days and who can potentially expose infants to this bacterium.

Treatment of Acute Bronchitis

Antibiotic Use

There is little evidence to support the use of routine antibiotics in previously healthy patients with acute bronchitis. Patients with underlying asthma, cystic fibrosis, chronic obstructive pulmonary disease (COPD), or another illness that would predispose to immunoincompetence may benefit from antibiotic administration using such medications as azithromycin 500 mg once followed by 250 mg a day for four additional days, trimethoprim–sulfamethoxazole (Bactrim, Septra) one double-strength tablet bid, or cephalexin (Keflex), 250 mg qid.

Bronchodilators

Because patients with acute bronchitis often present with wheezing and have reversible changes on pulmonary function tests, the use of aerosolized bronchodilating agents, such as albuterol (Proventil), one to two puffs qid for 7 to 10 days, may be useful for reducing the duration of symptoms and returning patients to their usual activity earlier.

Complimentary Alternative Medication Therapy

Pelargonium sidoides, an extract from flowering plants in the Geranium family, has been evaluated in some studies for symptomatic treatment of acute bronchitis and has been shown to reduce symptom durations by 1 to 2 days.[1] Originally developed in eastern Europe, Pelargonium is now available without a prescription in the United States in several over-the-counter preparations.

Treatment of Postbronchitic Syndrome

Patients who have experienced acute bronchitis may continue to cough for several months following their acute illness. This cough is usually unproductive and may be exacerbated by exercise, changes in temperature or humidity, or other factors that instigate airway reactivity. In these patients, continued treatment with albuterol or a similar β_2-agonist agent may help the airway reactivity and reduce the cough. Eventually, these symptoms subside totally and the bronchodilator can be discontinued.

PNEUMONIA

General Principles

Many bacterial organisms are responsible for pneumonia in ambulatory patients, although in most cases a specific bacterium is not found. The morbidity of pneumonia in patients with bacterial etiologies and the increased mortality among older patients and those with underlying pulmonary diseases make the timely diagnosis and proper management of pneumonia in ambulatory patients important.

Diagnosis

Clinical Presentation

Patients with pneumonia present with a productive cough, sometimes with hemoptysis. Pleuritic chest pain, shortness of breath, tachypnea, and fever may also accompany the cough. Some patients, especially children and the elderly, may not have a cough and may exhibit vague, poorly defined symptoms, such as fever, nausea, or abdominal pain. Patients often have rales in the affected area, although with consolidation rales may not be present. With consolidation, the only physical findings may be decreased breath sounds and egophony. Decreased breath sounds may also be noted in patients with associated pneumonic pleural effusions.

Laboratory and Radiologic Evaluation

The diagnosis of pneumonia is confirmed by chest radiography. Both posteroanterior and lateral views should be taken when possible to help localize the area of infiltrate. A sputum specimen for Gram stain and culture can often be helpful in directing the selection of antibiotic. In patients with underlying pulmonary diseases, arterial blood oxygen concentration should be evaluated by blood gas analysis or pulse oximetry. For patients who appear ill, a white blood cell count and differential may be useful for following the progress of recovery, and a blood culture should be strongly considered.

Presentation in Elderly Patients

Older patients may not exhibit any of the usual signs and symptoms of pneumonia. Many older individuals have nonspecific symptoms, such as anorexia, confusion, or falls, as early signs of pneumonia. Because of the high mortality in the geriatric population, pneumonia should be considered in all older patients who are exhibiting acute changes in their mental status or general health.

Treatment

Individualizing Management

Many previously healthy individuals with acute pneumonia can be managed on an outpatient basis. However, based on the increased mortality from pneumonia among patients with certain risk factors, hospital admission should be strongly considered for patients with chronic pulmonary diseases, patients with cirrhosis, those showing significant hypoxia or hypotension, elderly patients, and those with impaired immunocompetence. In addition, patients with signs of compromise, such as tachypnea (respiratory rate over 30) or hypotension, should be hospitalized.

Antibiotic Selection

The difficulty in obtaining sputum specimens from some patients makes empirical treatment with antibiotics the recommended management of all pneumonias encountered in the primary care setting. In addition, recent growth in the number of *Streptococcus pneumoniae* strains that are resistant to penicillin and other commonly used antibiotics makes antibiotic selection very important.

- **Treatment with low risk for drug-resistant *Streptococcus pneumoniae* (DRSP).** Initial antibiotic selection should be based on Gram stain results. In the absence of an adequate specimen, for previously healthy patients, antibiotics should be chosen to cover the most common community-acquired agents. For ambulatory patients, empirical therapy with an extended spectrum macrolide such as azithromycin (Zithromax), 500-mg single dose followed by 250 mg daily, or a fluoroquinolone with enhanced pneumococcal activity (such as gatifloxicin, levofloxacin, or moxifloxacin) will be effective against the most common bacterial organisms as well as atypical agents. In heavy smokers and patients with underlying COPD, consideration should be given to using a drug that is also effective against *Haemophilus influenzae*, such as second-generation cephalosporins or clarithromycin (Biaxin, 500 mg bid), or a fluoroquinolone with enhanced pneumococcal activity all of which are effective against *Mycoplasma*, *S. pneumoniae*, and *Legionella*. In cases where fever and symptoms persist, a follow-up chest film may be useful to evaluate for a potential empyema. In addition, patients who are not improving with empirical therapy should be suspected of having DRSP and should be treated accordingly (see below).

- **Inpatient treatment in patients with healthcare-associated pneumonia (HCAP) or other high risks for methicillin-resistant *Staphylococcus aureus* (MRSA) infection.** Patients who have pneumonia and were hospitalized in the past are 10 times more likely to become infected with MRSA than those with community-acquired pneumonia.[2] In addition, patients who live in a nursing home or have been getting routine care in a dialysis center are at higher risk for MRSA. In these patients, initial antibiotic coverage should include a β-lactam (such as piperacillin–tazobactam) along with vancomycin or linezolid for potential MRSA infection. In severely ill patients or those who have an increased likelihood of possible Pseudomonas infection, the addition of a second anti-pseudomonal drug such as a fluoroquinolone or aminoglycoside is recommended.

- **Inpatient treatment for patient at high risks for DRSP.** Risk factors for infection with DRSP include recent hospitalization; use of β2-lactam antibiotics in the previous 3 months; severe underlying illness such as malignancy, chronic renal failure, or advanced liver disease. In patients with higher risk for DRSP, initial therapy should be started with either a fluoroquinolone with enhanced pneumococcal activity (such as levofloxacin or ofloxacin) or, in critically ill patients, vancomycin. Fluoroquinolones with enhanced *S. pneumococcus* activity demonstrate good activity against intermediate-resistant *Streptococcus* but not against highly resistant strains. Vancomycin should be used for highly resistant strains or in critically ill patients where resistance status is unknown.

Follow-Up

In patients with lobar or segmental pneumonias that do not clear with antibiotic therapy, further evaluation with computed tomography may be advisable to evaluate for an obstructing tumor. In addition, because of the increased possibility of an underlying tumor associated with pneumonia in patients older than 40 years, a follow-up chest film is indicated in 4 to 6 weeks in such individuals.

Special Consideration

Because of the increased morbidity associated with pneumonia in certain risk classes, patients with underlying asthma, COPD, and threatened immunocompetence (including prior splenectomy, cardiac or renal disease, or age greater than 65) should receive a pneumococcal vaccine and yearly influenza vaccinations (see Chapter 1.4). *Smoking cessation should be discussed with patients with asthma, COPD, or other conditions placing them at risk for bronchitis and pneumonia.*

REFERENCES

1. Albert RH. Diagnosis and treatment of acute bronchitis. *Am Fam Physician* 2010;82:1345–1350.
2. Hospital-Acquired Pneumonia Guideline Committee of the American Thoracic Society and Infectious Diseases Society of America. Guidelines for the management of adults with hospital-acquired, ventilator-associated, and healthcare-associated pneumonia. *Am J Respir Crit Care Med* 2005;171:388–416.

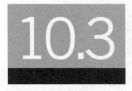

10.3 Chronic Obstructive Pulmonary Disease

Kevin J. Berg, Joshua J. Raymond

GENERAL PRINCIPLES

Chronic obstruction of airflow is the culmination of obstructive bronchiolitis and parenchymal destruction (emphysema) and results in the disease process chronic obstructive pulmonary disease (COPD). Airway dilatation, reduction of bronchial inflammation and secretions, and relief of hypoxia are key aspects of management, as well as avoiding noxious environmental exposures such as cooking/heating fuels, occupational chemicals, and tobacco inhalation. For most, tobacco smoking cessation is the key to avoid disease progression. Tobacco smoking causes 99% of COPD, though only 20% of smokers will develop COPD. The differing susceptibility of smokers to COPD is thought to relate, in part, to variability in their adaptive response to cumulative oxidative stress.[1,2] COPD is currently the 4th leading cause of U.S. mortality and the 12th leading cause of chronic disability. By 2020, COPD is estimated to be the third leading cause of disability worldwide.[3]

DIAGNOSIS

Clinical Findings

The clinical features of COPD are cough, wheezing, chest tightness, sputum production, weight loss, and progressive dyspnea. Unlike the dyspnea caused by the short-term airway obstruction occurring in asthma, COPD obstructive changes are less reversible. Important psychologic symptoms and functional limitations include withdrawal, isolation, and depression.

Airflow obstruction results in progressive hyperresonance on lung field percussion. Prominent accessory muscle use is accompanied by diminished breath sounds on auscultation.[4]

Right-sided heart failure caused by hypoxemia and pulmonary hypertension leads to peripheral edema and dyspnea in chronic bronchitis. Failing respiratory muscles and parenchymal destruction cause patients to make prolonged puffing efforts and pursed lip breathing to attempt to maintain lung expansion (to increase their extrinsic positive-end expiratory pressure).[5,6]

Laboratory Test

COPD is diagnosed in a patient over the age of 40 and may present or be suspected in patients with the proceeding clinical indicators: chronic cough (may be intermittent and unproductive), chronic sputum production (any pattern), history of environmental exposure to risk factors, family history COPD, and daily dyspnea that worsens over time or with exercise. Spirometry is needed to ultimately confirm the clinical diagnosis.[3] Testing that might be used in the diagnosis or management of COPD is outlined below:

- Spirometric testing demonstrates a characteristic pattern of reduced airflow, with a post-bronchodilator forced expiratory volume at 1 second (FEV_1)/forced vital capacity (FVC) ratio of less than 70% of the predicted value. This is the disease standard for confirmation and monitoring progression of the disease. One caveat to remember is that spirometric cutoff points are not clinically validated and depend on the patient population. For instance, a fixed ratio of <0.7 for FEV_1/FVC may overdiagnose elderly patients due to age-related changes in lung volumes and may underdiagnose adults <45 years old.[3] One method to standardize the diagnosis of COPD is to use the National Institute for Health and Care Excellence COPD guidelines or Global Initiative for Chronic Obstructive Lung Disease (GOLD) assessment tool. Another tool, The Combined Assessment of

COPD (CAT) combines objective data from spirometric results, and validated subjective patient symptom scores in a matrix; identifying COPD severity as GOLD stage 1 (mild) to stage 4 (severe). This in turn assists the practitioner in stepwise management of COPD symptoms.[7,8]

GOLD Classification for Severity of Airflow Limitation

Severity	Post-bronchodilator FEV1
GOLD 1 (mild)	≥80% predicted
GOLD 2 (moderate)	≥50% and <80% predicted
GOLD 3 (severe)	≥30% and <50% predicted
GOLD 4 (very severe)	<30% predicted

- Complete blood count to detect anemia or polycythemia.
- An arterial blood gas (ABG) to evaluate a patient that is decompensating. That is to say, for patients with any of the following: forced expiratory volume in 1 second <35% predicted, clinical signs of respiratory failure, clinical signs of right heart failure, and oxygen saturation <92% (as measured by pulse oximetry). ABG may reflect acute-on-chronic respiratory failure with partial pressure of oxygen (PaO_2) <60 mmHg (8 kilopascal [kPa]), or partial pressure of carbon dioxide ($PaCO_2$) >50 mmHg (6.7 kPa).
- Radiographic findings on chest x-ray maybe normal or can include[9] bronchial wall thickening (indicated by ring shadows and parallel line shadows), increased lung markings (small ill-defined opacities in parenchyma), prominent vessels (large central pulmonary arteries if pulmonary hypertension), increase in the anteroposterior (AP) diameter of the chest cavity, hyperlucency of peripheral lung fields, signs of hyperinflation (obtuse costophrenic angle, low diaphragm, diaphragmatic flattening), Saber-sheath trachea (trachea normal to level of thoracic inlet, then narrows in coronal plane), increased retrosternal airspace (>2.5 cm between sternum and ascending aorta), increased length of lung (>30 cm), bullae, and signs of arterial deficiency in outer lung fields (reduced number and size of pulmonary vessels and branches, vessels distorted and may have increased branching angles).

Patients with chronic bronchitis may also have infiltrates during periods of active infection; atelectasis related to mucus trapping; and pneumothorax or pneumo-mediastinum can also be seen in critical hypoxic presentations. Testing for α_1-antitrypsin deficiency should be considered in younger patients with COPD without a smoking history or if a family history of this is elicited.

Differential Diagnosis Considerations

During acute exacerbations, decompensated congestive heart failure, pneumonia, and pulmonary embolism are considered. During insidious presentations options may include α_1-antitrypsin deficiency and cystic fibrosis. Other presentations include obliterative bronchiolitis, bronchiectasis, and tuberculosis.

TREATMENT

Smoking cessation is the most critical intervention proven to slow the accelerated decline in lung function causing COPD. Overall treatment goals relieve symptoms, decrease pulmonary inflammation, and improve oxygenation.[10] Generally, treatment follows in a stepwise fashion adding longer acting agents as disease severity and symptomatology dictate, with addition or subtraction of agents as exacerbations or improvements occur.

Medication, Oxygen, and Surgery

- Bronchodilator therapy with sympathomimetic agents such as β_2-receptor agonists relax airway smooth muscle and relieve air hunger.[10]
  - Short-acting β_2-agonists such as albuterol (Proventil, others) provide immediate relief from acute bronchospasm and are recommended for use as initial and rescue agents delivered by either metered-dose inhalers or nebulizers.
  - Long-acting β_2-agonist preparations such as salmeterol (Serevent) are given twice daily and decrease the frequency of acute exacerbations.
- Anticholinergic bronchodilators inhibit the parasympathetic drive to the bronchial smooth muscle, resulting in bronchodilation. Examples include:
  - Ipratropium (Atrovent) is a short-acting anticholinergic agent available in both inhaler and nebulizer forms that can be combined with β-agonists for enhanced bronchodilation.
  - Tiotropium bromide (Spiriva) is a once-daily inhaled agent that achieves 24-hour muscarinic blocker blockade for prolonged improvement in lung volume preservation.

- Phosphodiesterase-4 inhibitors (Roflumilast) are oral daily medications used in conjunction with a long-acting bronchodilator or a long-acting anticholinergic. Used alone they have no bronchodilator activity but in combination they have been shown to improve FEV_1. The exact mechanism is unknown, but they are thought to reduce inflammation by inhibiting the breakdown of intracellular cyclic AMP.[3] Phosphodiesterase-4 inhibitors have inconsistent results regarding reduction of COPD exacerbation rates. Used in patients with severe COPD, studies have demonstrated improvement in FEV_1 but inconsistent results regarding reduction of exacerbation rates.[11,12]
- Corticosteroid administration, by inhalation (Pulmicort, others), oral (Prednisone, others), or parental routes (Decadron, others) is controversial in COPD treatment; guidelines recommend inhaled corticosteroid be considered for patients with moderate to severe airflow limitation whose symptoms persist despite optimal bronchodilatory therapy.[13]
- Theophylline may be added if symptoms continue despite triple therapy or for those who cannot afford inhaler therapy. Theophylline improves lung function but requires frequent monitoring of drug levels and concerns for adverse reactions and drug–drug interactions often limit theophylline use. Its effects on exacerbations are uncertain.[14]
- Vaccination against pneumococcal and influenza should be offered to all patients.
- Correction of hypoxia is critical for morbidity reduction in COPD management.[10] Long-term oxygen therapy is recommended for patients with COPD and severe hypoxemia (oxygen saturation less than 88% or partial arterial oxygen pressure less than 55 mmHg). Supplemental oxygen improves endurance and exercise capacity in patients with moderate to severe COPD.[15] A multicenter randomized trial with 203 patients who had hypoxemia and COPD demonstrated that continuous oxygen therapy had benefits on survival rates compared with nocturnal oxygen therapy.[16] The goal oxygen saturation should be approximately 90% to avoid respiratory acidosis.[17] Current Medicare continuous oxygen supplementation reimbursement guidelines require an arterial pO_2 of 55 mmHg or less on room air, clinically diagnosed cor pulmonale plus a room air pO_2 of 55 to 59 mmHg, or a hematocrit of 55% or greater. Nighttime use is critical to prevent cardiac arrhythmias and pulmonary hypertension. Oxygen can be supplied through compressed gas, liquid reservoirs, or room air concentration devices and delivered via mask or nasal cannuli that incorporate demand-flow devices.
- Surgical interventions, such as lung volume reduction surgery (surgical removal of hyperinflated but poorly perfused areas of lung) or single lung transplantation, have resulted in improved measures of quality of life and function in highly selected patients, and improved 5-year survival rates in patients with severe COPD and heterogeneous distribution of emphysema with upper lobe predominance.[18] Conversely, patients with severe COPD and FEV_1 less than 20%, homogenous emphysema, or low carbon monoxide diffusion capacity have an increased 30-day mortality after lung volume reduction surgery.[19]

Supplemental Therapies

- Pulmonary rehabilitation, an important nonpharmacologic therapeutic intervention can improve exercise capacity, reduce dyspnea, and decrease the number and length of hospitalizations for acute exacerbations.[20] It is underutilized by providers. Typical components include patient assessment, exercise training, education, nutritional intervention, and psychosocial support. Several studies have demonstrated that pulmonary rehabilitation therapy has positive impacts on health-related quality of life, reduced symptoms, improved peripheral muscle strength, exercise endurance, reduced number of hospital days, and improved psychosocial status. Recent results from a large, randomized 1-year trial of a comprehensive disease management program at five Veterans Affairs medical centers demonstrated a reduction in hospitalizations and emergency room visits.[21,22]
- Nutritional support for the increased respiratory effort of labored breathing, especially in the undernourished, may increase weight and exercise capacity in stable COPD.[15,23,24]
- Complications include respiratory failure leading to progressive hypercapnea and decreased mental alertness. Hypoxemia leads to increasing pulmonary vascular pressures, secondary polycythemia, and ischemia complications of extremities and internal organs.
- Patient education including smoking cessation is by far the single most important educational element in COPD management. It is important that the patient know the proper inhaler technique for each of the differing medication devices. Facilitating expectoration to reduce fatigue and breathing exercises can improve airflow between exacerbations.[25]

SPECIAL CONSIDERATIONS

Screening and treatment for comorbidities should include cardiovascular disease, metabolic syndrome, osteoporosis, depression, and lung cancer. Close communication between patient, family, and health care provider reduces unnecessary hospitalizations.[26] Facilitating the frank discussions between the patient and the family about the use of mechanical ventilation, cardiopulmonary resuscitation, and other advance treatment wishes by the health care provider team during periods of relative disease stability can help guide the treatment intensity decisions during periods of clinical decompensations when communication with the patient directly may be compromised.

REFERENCES

1. Fabbri LM, Hurd SS. Global strategy of the diagnosis, management and prevention of COPD. *Eur Respir J* 2003;22:1–12.
2. Wright JL, Levy RD, Churg A. Pulmonary hypertension in COPD: current theories of pathogenesis and their implications for treatment. *Thorax* 2005;60:605–609.
3. Global Initiative for Chronic Obstructive Lung Disease. http://www.goldcopd.com/guidelines-global-strategy-for-diagnosis-management.html. Accessed February 2, 2014.
4. Stephens MB, Yew KS. Diagnosis of chronic obstructive pulmonary disease. *Am Fam Physician* 2008;78(1):87–92.
5. Spahija J, de Marchie M, Grassino A. Effects of imposed pursed-lips breathing on respiratory mechanics and dyspnea at rest and during exercise in COPD. *Chest* 2005;128:640–650.
6. Martin A, Davenport P, Extrinsic threshold PEEP reduces post-exercise dyspnea in COPD patients: A Placebo-controlled, Double-blind Cross-over Study. *Cardiopulm Phys Ther J* 2011;22(3):5–10.
7. Lee H, Kim, J, Tagmazyan K. Treatment of stable chronic obstructive pulmonary disease: the GOLD guidelines. *Am Fam Physician* 2014;88:655–663.
8. Gruffydd-Jones K, Loverridge C. The 2010 NICE COPD guidelines: how do they compare with the GOLD guidelines? *Prim Care Respir J* 2011;20(2):199–204.
9. Shaker SB, Dirksen A, Bach KS, et al. Imaging in chronic obstructive pulmonary disease. *COPD* 2007;4(2):143.
10. National Collaborating Centre for Chronic Conditions. Chronic obstructive pulmonary disease. National clinical guideline on management of chronic obstructive pulmonary disease in adults in primary and secondary care. *Thorax* 2004;59(Suppl 1):1–232.
11. Calverley PM, Rabe KF, Goehring UM, et al; M2-124 and M2-125 study groups. Roflumilast in symptomatic chronic obstructive pulmonary disease: two randomised clinical trials [published correction appears in *Lancet* 2010;376(9747):1146]. *Lancet* 2009;374(9691):685–694.
12. Fabbri LM, Calverley PM, Izquierdo-Alonso JL, et al; M2-127 and M2-128 study groups. Roflumilast in moderate-to-severe chronic obstructive pulmonary disease treated with longacting bronchodilators: two randomised clinical trials. *Lancet* 2009;374(9691):695–703.
13. Bonay M, Bancal C, Crestani B. The risk/benefit of inhaled corticosteroids in chronic obstructive pulmonary disease. *Expert Opin Drug Saf* 2005;4:251–271.
14. Ram FS, Jardin JR, Atallah A, et al. Efficacy of theophylline in people with stable chronic obstructive pulmonary disease: a systematic review and meta-analysis. *Respir Med* 2005;99(2):135–144.
15. Bradley JM, O'Neill B. Short-term ambulatory oxygen for chronic obstructive pulmonary disease *Cochrane Database Syst Rev* 2005(4):CD004356.
16. Nocturnal Oxygen Therapy Trial Group. Continuous or nocturnal oxygen therapy in hypoxemic chronic obstructive lung disease: a clinical trial. *Ann Intern Med* 1980;93(3):391–398.
17. Celli BR, MacNee W; ATS/ERS Task Force. Standards for the diagnosis and treatment of patients with COPD: a summary of the ATS/ERS position paper. *Eur Respir J* 2004;23(6):932–946.
18. Sanchez PG, Kucharczuk JC, Su S, et al. National emphysema treatment trial redux: accentuating the positive. *J Thorac Cardiovasc Surg* 2010;140(3):564–572.
19. National Emphysema Treatment Trial Research Group. Patients at high risk of death after lung-volume-reduction surgery. *N Engl J Med* 2001;345(15):1075–1083.
20. Griffiths TL, Burr ML, Campbell IA, et al. Results at 1 year of outpatient multidisciplinary pulmonary rehabilitation: a randomized controlled trial. *Lancet* 2000;355:362–368.
21. Ries AL, Bauldoff GS, Carlin BW, et al. Pulmonary rehabilitation: joint ACCP/AACVPR evidence-based clinical practice guidelines. *Chest* 2007;131(5 Suppl):4S–42S.
22. Rice KL, Dewan N, Bloomfield HE, et al. Disease management program for chronic obstructive pulmonary disease: a randomized controlled trial. *Am J Respir Crit Care Med* 2010;182 (7):890–896.
23. Nutritional guidelines for people with COPD: Cleveland Clinic Foundation Health Information Center. http://my.clevelandclinic.org/health/diseases_conditions/hic_Understanding_COPD/hic_Coping_with_COPD/hic_Nutritional_Guidelines_for_People_with_COPD. Accessed February 10, 2006.
24. Collins PF, Stratton RJ, Elia M. Nutritional support in chronic obstructive pulmonary disease: a systematic review and meta-analysis. *Am J Clin Nutr* 2012;95(6):1385–1395.
25. Pulmonary health/exercise and care: National Emphysema Foundation. http://www.nef-usa. org/pulhthex.jsp.
26. Pulmonary rehabilitation: a team approach to improving the quality of life: American College of Chest Physicians. http://www.chestnet.org/patients/guides/pulmonary/.

10.4 Tuberculosis

Michelle Anne Bholat, Patrick T. Dowling

GENERAL PRINCIPLES

Tuberculosis (TB) is an infectious disease caused by *Mycobacterium tuberculosis, a slow-growing, aerobic, rod-shaped bacterium* that can live only in humans. Second to HIV/AIDS as the foremost cause of death due to a single infectious agent, it is spread primarily through an airborne route when an individual with pulmonary **disease** coughs or sneezes. Its hallmark is the ability to persist as a long-term asymptomatic infection, known as latent **TB infection (LTBI).** In the competent host, cellular immunity is able to maintain the latent status in most patients infected, allowing them to remain symptomatic and noninfectious throughout their lifetime. However, there is a 10% lifetime risk of progressing to the disease state, often decades later, primarily in persons with compromised immune systems, such as those living with HIV, or in elderly patients with malnutrition or diabetes, and tobacco users.

A classic disease of poverty, over 90% of all cases occur in the developing world. Currently one-third of the world's population has **LTBI.** And although the TB death rate worldwide has dropped 45% since 1990, almost 9 million people developed active **disease** worldwide in 2013, resulting in 1.3 million deaths.[1,2] Approximately 60% of all new cases globally occur in Asian countries.

In 2013, a total of 9,588 new TB cases were reported in the United States, a decrease of 4.2% from 2012. Of these patients, 6.8% were HIV positive and 5.7% homeless. The highest rates in the United States are found among recent immigrants, the elderly and ethnic and racial minorities. Asians have the highest incidence—25.9 times higher than whites, among all racial/ethnic groups. Among U.S.-born persons, the incidence among blacks was 6.2 times higher than that among whites. Although **foreign-born (FB)** persons account for only 13% of the U.S. population, they represent almost 65% of all patients with active disease. Four states, all with large immigrant populations, California, Texas, New York and Florida, accounted for 51% of all TB cases in 2013. The TB incidence per 100,000 by race or ethnicity were Asian 18.7, blacks 5.3, Hispanics 5.0, and whites 0.7 in 2013. Among persons with TB, 95% of Asians, 75% of Hispanics, 40% of blacks, and 23% of whites were FB. Five countries of origin account for the greatest number of cases among FB: Mexico (26%), Philippines (12%), Vietnam (8%), India (8%), and China (5%). **These epidemiologic data are important for screening and diagnostic purposes.**[1-4]

Although pulmonary disease is the most common clinical presentation, 15% of the patients have an extrapulmonary form of disease. Patients with HIV infection have an extremely high rate of both pulmonary and extrapulmonary disease. Moreover, extrapulmonary involvement tends to increase in frequency **in the setting of a compromised immune system.**

Endogenous reactivation of **LTBI** as opposed to new primary infection **(exogenous re-infection)** accounts for the majority of active disease cases in the United States. Individuals with advanced HIV infection are the exception to this because they have unusually high rates of primary infection. Chronic medical conditions, outlined in Table 10.4-1, as well as corticosteroid use and immunocompromised states (HIV) are important predisposing factors for reactivation.[3]

An 85-year-old live attenuated vaccine, the bacillus Calmette-Guerin **(BCG),** derived from *Mycobacterium bovine,* is still administered to over half the infants in the world, including Mexico. Although it does not prevent TB disease, it can reduce **TB meningitis** and **military TB** in young children.

Targeted Testing and Treatment of LTBI

Although one-third of the world's population has **LTBI**, 90% will live a lifetime without developing active disease. Since the epidemiological risk factors for the 10% that progress to disease are known, targeted testing to identify those at high risk is indicated as treatment can reduce the risk of progressing from the latent infectious state to active disease. This remains the cornerstone of the U.S. strategy for TB elimination.

Individuals at high risk of developing TB who would benefit by treatment of LTBI include those at risk for recent infection (lower socioeconomic status or recent immigrant from high-incidence country) and those who are at risk for progression to active TB (based on the presence of medical conditions). The CDC recommends that tuberculin skin testing (TST) **be performed only in persons**

TABLE 10.4-1	Relative Risk for Developing Active Tuberculosis by Selected Clinical Conditions

Clinical conditions	Relative risk (%)
Silicosis	30
Diabetes mellitus	2.0–4.1
Chronic renal failure/hemodialysis	10.1–25.3
Gastrectomy	2–5
Jejunoileal bypass	27–63
Solid-organ transplantation	20–74
Carcinoma of head or neck	16

who belong to at least one of the high-risk groups noted (Table 10.4-2) as "a decision to test is a decision to treat." Routine screening of other persons, including children not belonging to high-risk groups, is discouraged. A notable exception is individuals receiving antitumor necrosis factor-α products (anti-TNFs) such as infliximab (Remicade) for rheumatoid arthritis or Crohn disease. They should be screened for LTBI before anti-TNFs is initiated. Anergic patients with HIV infection should be treated if they are close contacts, previously had a positive skin test, or are members of a group in which the prevalence of TB is at least 10% (Table 10.4-2).[3,4]

Tuberculin skin testing. For more than a century, the Mantoux test, which involves the injection of 0.1 mL of intermediate-strength purified protein derivative (PPD) intradermally, has been used in the diagnosis of TB. It cannot distinguish between past infections and current disease, or reactions due to previous BCG vaccination. The test is interpreted at 48 to 72 hours by measuring the degree of maximum induration, not erythema; it is acceptable to read the skin test up to 96 hours. A negative test result does not exclude the disease. Active disease must be ruled out before treating for LTBI. Although anergy testing may provide prognostic information for immunocompromised individuals, it is no longer recommended. Unless additional diagnostic testing is employed, a positive reaction in those who previously received BCG should be assumed to be secondary to exposure as opposed to the BCG as reactivity to that vaccine wanes with time. There are three cutoff levels for determining a positive TST reaction based on sensitivity, specificity, and prevalence of TB in different groups:

- A ≥5-mm induration is a positive result for HIV-positive individuals, recent contacts with persons with active TB, individuals whose chest x-ray (CXR) findings are consistent with old healed TB (fibrotic changes), and patients with organ transplants and other immunosuppressed patients receiving more than 15 mg per day of prednisone for more than 1 month.
- A ≥10-mm induration is positive for recent immigrants (within the last 5 years) from high-prevalence countries; low-income minority populations; residents and employees of correctional facilities, nursing homes, and shelters; health care workers; injection drug users, individuals with chronic medical conditions (see Table 10.4-1); and children <4 years or infants, children, and adolescents exposed to adults in high-risk categories.
- A ≥15-mm induration is positive for persons with no risk factors for TB.

TABLE 10.4-2	LTBI Treatment Regimens

Drugs	Duration	Interval	Minimum doses
Isoniazid	9 mo[b]	Daily	270
		Twice weekly[a]	76
Isoniazid	6 mo	Daily	180
		Twice weekly[a]	52
Isoniazid and rifapentine	3 mo	Once weekly[a]	12
Rifampin	4 mo	Daily	120

[a]Use DOT.
[b]Use 9 months for HIV-positive patients on treatment and children 2 to 11 years old.

Diagnostic Blood Tests for TB

Within the last decade, two interferon gamma release assays (IGRAs) have been developed as new diagnostic tests for TB. They are the QuantiFERON–TB Gold In-Tube test (QFT–GIT) and the T–SPOT.TB test (T–Spot).

Although a positive IGRA means that the person has been infected with TB bacteria, it cannot distinguish if the person has LTBI or TB disease. However, it is not subject to reader bias as the case may be with the **TST** and is not affected by prior **BCG** vaccination. They are the preferred method testing for LTBI for anyone who has received the BCG shot or will have a difficult time returning for a second appointment to read the TST.[3,5–7]

Treatment Regimens for LTBI

Although 90% of active cases of TB in non-HIV-infected individuals are secondary to endogenous reactivation, treatment that diminishes or eradicates the bacterial population in "healed" or radiographically invisible lesions is an important means of reducing progression to active disease. There are several treatment regimens available for the treatment of LTBI and providers should choose the appropriate regimen based on the following: drug susceptibility results of the presumed source case (if known), coexisting medical illness and potential for drug–drug interactions, who are at especially high risk for TB disease and are either suspected of nonadherence or given an intermittent dosing regimen, and directly observed therapy (DOT) for LTBI should be considered.

Isoniazid Regimen

Since 1965, isoniazid (INH) for 6 to 12 months has been the mainstay of therapy of individuals with LTBI infection, as it can reduce the rate of reactivation by at least 70%. However, adherence to therapy has been problematic because of the long duration of therapy and concerns about toxicity. The current CDC recommendations for treatment with INH **include a 6- and 9-month regimen**.

The 9-month regimen is preferred because it is more efficacious. However, treatment for 6 months may be more cost-effective and result in greater adherence by patients. Accordingly, health care providers may prefer to implement the 6-month regimen rather than the 9-month regimen. Every effort should be made to ensure that patients adhere to LTBI treatment for at least 6 months. The preferred regimen for children aged 2 to 11 years is 9 months of daily INH.[3]

New: 12-Dose Weekly Isoniazid and Rifapentine

Rifapentine (RPT) is a rifamycin derivative with a long half-life and greater potency against *M. tuberculosis* than *rifampin*. A new directly observed 12-dose, once-weekly regimen of INH and RPT for 3 months is recommended as an option equal to the standard INH 9-month daily regimen for treating LTBI in otherwise healthy people, age 12 or above, who had recent contact with infectious TB, or had tuberculin skin test or blood test for TB infection recent conversions of a TST or IGRA, or those with radiologic findings consistent with healed pulmonary TB.[5,8]

The regimen may be used in otherwise healthy HIV-infected persons, 12 years of age and older, who are **not on antiretroviral medications.** Further, it may also be considered for children aged 2 to 11 years if completion of 9 months of INH is unlikely and hazard of TB disease is great.

The 12-dose regimen is NOT recommended for the following individuals:

• Children younger than 2 years of age
• People with HIV/AIDS who are taking antiretroviral therapy (ART)
• People presumed to be infected with INH or rifampin-resistant *M. tuberculosis*
• Pregnant women or women expecting to become pregnant while taking this regimen

Rifampin (RIF) Regimen

A 4-month regimen of up to 600 mg daily can be considered for persons who cannot tolerate INH or who have been exposed to INH-resistant TB. It should not be used to treat HIV-infected persons taking some combinations of ART. The choice between the 12-dose regimen and other recommended LTBI treatment regimens depends on several factors, including:

• Feasibility of DOT
• Resources for drug procurement and patient monitoring
• Considerations of medical and social circumstances that could affect patient adherence
• Preferences of the patient and prescribing health care provider

Anergic patients or those with a previous history of a positive PPD and HIV infection should be treated if they are close contacts. Before initiating treatment, physicians must ensure that active disease is ruled out with a normal CXR. After that the decision to treat hinges on an analysis of risks and benefits.[3,5]

- **For pregnant, HIV-negative women,** INH given daily or twice weekly for 9 months is recommended. For women at risk for progression of LTBI to disease, especially those who are infected with HIV or who have likely been infected recently, initiation of therapy should not be delayed on the basis of pregnancy alone, even during the first trimester. For women whose risk for active TB is lower, some experts recommend waiting 3 months postpartum because of the risk of INH hepatotoxicity.
- **Risk of therapy.** Treatment of LTBI is usually indicated, regardless of age, in patients who belong to high-risk groups. INH is associated with age-related hepatitis, beginning after age 19 and increasing significantly after age 35. Extensive use of alcohol enhances this association. Fatal INH-associated hepatitis has been reported. The risk is highest among women, particularly black and Hispanic women; it may also be increased during the postpartum period. **Baseline studies** are indicated in individuals at high risk for hepatotoxicity, such as those with HIV infection, alcoholism, chronic liver disease, pregnancy, or postpartum status. These patients should be monitored **monthly** and liver function tests (LFTs) obtained if clinically indicated. INH should be discontinued if liver enzymes reach **THREE times** the upper limit of normal levels in symptomatic patients or **five times the** upper limit of normal levels in asymptomatic patients. Because INH may increase the serum level of phenytoin (Dilantin), a decreased dosage of the latter may be necessary. Women receiving RIF and oral contraceptives should be advised to use a backup method of contraception to avoid pregnancy. Pyridoxine, **25 to 100 mg per day**, is recommended in high-risk **adults to reduce the risk of INH-induced peripheral neuropathy.**[3]

DIAGNOSIS AND TREATMENT OF TB DISEASE

Initiation of a diagnostic evaluation for TB is usually based on suspicion for TB on epidemiologic, clinical, and radiographic grounds.

History and Physical Examination

- Although some patients may be asymptomatic, most present with chronic nonspecific symptoms, such as cough, fever, night sweats, weight loss, lassitude, and hemoptysis.
- Extrapulmonary disease may present as a fever of unknown origin. On examination, patients often appear chronically ill with weight loss.

Laboratory Studies

- Diagnosis depends on CXR findings and identification of the acid-fast bacillus (**AFB**) in the sputum.
- **Radiographic findings.** Classically, the CXR reveals fibrocavitary lesions of the upper lobes; however, a varied picture may be present, with infiltration, miliary nodules, or an effusion. Conversely it may be normal, especially with disseminated disease. HIV-infected patients tend to have atypical CXRs or normal CXRs **as immunosuppressed individuals may lack the cellular immune response that causes cavitations.**

Bacteriologic evaluation. The detection of AFB on microscopic examination of stained smears is the most rapid and inexpensive TB diagnostic tool. In many countries, smears are the only diagnostic test used. Stained sputum smears are not as sensitive as sputum cultures as at least 5,000 to 10,000 bacilli per mL are needed for detection of bacteria in stained smears; in contrast, 10 to 100 organisms are needed for a positive culture.

The sensitivity and positive predictive value of AFB smear microscopy is approximately 45% to 80% and 50% to 80%, respectively. AFB visualized on a slide may represent *M. tuberculosis* or nontuberculous mycobacteria, so species identification requires culture and/or nucleic acid amplification. A nucleic acid amplification system test (**NAAT**) provides rapid confirmation that the infecting mycobacteria are *M. tuberculosis*. In the setting of high clinical suspicion for TB, initiation of empiric therapy based on preliminary acid-fast staining results is appropriate.

Culture. All clinical specimens suspected of containing mycobacteria should be cultured. A culture is required for drug susceptibility testing; it can also be used for species identification. The sensitivity and specificity of sputum culture are about 80% and 98%, respectively. Cultures, which typically take 6 to 8 weeks, have a sensitivity of 81% and a specificity of 98%; **these percentages are lower** with noncavitary disease. The use of a liquid medium system can provide information in 7 to 14 days. A 2-hour test has been developed that detects *M. tuberculosis*, and resistance to rifampin. The test, known as the **Xpert MTB/RIF** assay, is an automated test that works directly from a patient's sputum without requiring a lengthy bacterial culture. This rapid diagnostic assay is as sensitive as currently available culture methods.[9] It enables patients to receive their diagnosis **during a single clinic visit.**

- **Reporting and public health.** TB is a reportable disease in the United States. As such, persons with confirmed or suspected TB must be reported to a state or local public health authority promptly; in many states, this period is 24 hours.
- **Surgical and invasive diagnostic tools.** Transbronchial biopsy can provide immediate diagnosis in smear-negative cases, but because of its risks and expense it should be reserved for selected cases (e.g., HIV-infected patients), primarily to exclude other diagnoses.

Treatment of Active Tuberculosis

Empiric Therapy

A presumptive clinical diagnosis is sufficient for initiation of treatment pending diagnostic laboratory results when the clinical suspicion for TB is considered likely. Outpatient management of individuals suspected of **active** TB should be considered. Hospitalization is recommended if the patient is incapable of self-care or poses an infectious risk to others. Hospitalized patients suspected of having TB should be placed in respiratory isolation until **sputum** results become available or they have completed 2 weeks of treatment with clinical response. Public health officials **MUST** be notified **to locate any contacts and to ensure their compliance and follow-up.**

Chemotherapy

Successful treatment requires multidrug therapy aimed at the *Mycobacterium* species susceptible to the chosen drugs; they must be taken on a regular basis for a sufficient period of time. It is now recommended that all patients be treated initially with **four drugs for 2 months daily**. The drugs include isoniazid (INH), rifampin (RIF), pyrazinamide (PZA), and ethambutol (ETH) or streptomycin. **Children, pregnant women, and adults at risk for INH-induced neuropathy should receive pyridoxine (vitamin B$_6$) daily.** Because compliance over long periods of time with several drugs is difficult, **DOT** should be considered. Consultation with public health is strongly recommended; reporting of active disease cases is mandatory. The following are current national recommendations:

- **Confirmed or suspected active TB cases.** These should be treated with a four-drug regimen until the results of mycobacterial cultures and sensitivities have been obtained. Administer daily INH:[10] children, 10 mg per kg; adults, 300 mg; RIF: children, 10 to 20 mg/kg/day; adults, 10 mg/kg/day to a maximum dose of 600 mg per day; PZA: children 20 to 30 mg/kg/day; adults, 25 mg/kg/day to a maximum of 2 g per day; ETH: children and adults, 15 to 25 mg/kg/day. Streptomycin should be substituted for ETH in very young children. If there is no resistance to INH and RIF, both PZA and ETH are discontinued after 2 months if repeat sputum cultures are negative and there is improvement in the patient's clinical condition. INH and RIF are continued for an additional 4 months for a total treatment course of 6 months. If the patient remains symptomatic, or if a follow-up smear or culture result remains positive after 2 months of therapy, therapy with INH/RIF should be continued for total of 9 months and consultation is recommended. (See joint document ATS/CDC in references for detailed discussion of options.)
- **HIV-infected patients.** Three possible regimens that include RIF-based treatments have been recommended by the CDC. However, RIF is contraindicated when the patient is receiving protease inhibitors (PIs) or nonnucleoside reverse transcriptase inhibitors (NNRTIs). In its place are 6-month rifabutin-based treatments and 9-month streptomycin-based regimens, which may be used on such patients. The use of streptomycin is contraindicated in pregnant women. **(Consult the public health department for recommendations.)**
- **Multidrug-resistant (MDR) TB.** This is disease that is resistant to both INH and RIF. Patients should be treated with a regimen that includes three or four drugs to which the TB isolate is susceptible. Combinations with levofloxacin and moxifloxacin appear promising. Consultation with public health department and CDC is recommended.
- **Extrapulmonary disease.** Treatment is the same as above for active TB but is continued for 9 months. Because of a paucity of data, the recommendation is that miliary TB, bone or joint TB, and TB meningitis in children and infants require 12 months of therapy with public health consultation.
- **Pregnancy and lactation.** Use INH, RIF, and ETH for 9 months with pyridoxine, 25 mg per day. Streptomycin should be avoided because of ototoxicity to the fetus; PZA is not recommended because its teratogenicity is unknown. Lactating women who are taking antituberculous medication should breastfeed before ingesting their medication. Bottle supplementation should be used for the first feeding after dosing. (For infants whose mothers were treated for active TB during pregnancy and who are themselves on INH for treatment of LTBI, bottle-feeding is recommended.)

Monitoring for Adverse Reactions

Liver enzymes, bilirubin, creatinine, and a complete blood count/platelet count should be obtained as baseline information before implementing the standard regimens. If PZA is to be used, uric acid should be obtained. If ETH is included in the regimen, obtain baseline and monthly visual acuity as well as red–green perception testing to detect drug-induced optic neuritis. Patients should be **seen monthly** and monitored clinically for adverse effects. For individuals with abnormal baseline studies, follow-up studies are indicated. In those with normal baseline studies, follow-up laboratory testing should be done only if drug toxicity is suspected.

Evaluation of Response to Treatment

Repeated sputum examinations, beginning with weekly smear quantitation, are desirable until sputum conversion is documented. More than 85% of patients on INH and RIF with positive cultures convert to negative after 2 months. If sputum remains positive after 2 months, drug susceptibility studies should be repeated, and DOT should be implemented. CXRs are less valuable than sputum examinations for evaluation and should not be routinely performed.

NONTUBERCULOUS MYCOBACTERIUM

Nontuberculous mycobacteria **(NTM)** are ubiquitous and are responsible for producing cutaneous, pulmonary, lymphatic, and disseminated disease.

- **Disseminated *Mycobacterium avium* complex (MAC) disease** is the most common bacterial infection in patients with AIDS, occurring in 20% to 40% and is the most common cause of NTM pulmonary disease worldwide. In those with HIV, it is rare with CD4 counts greater than 100; it should be suspected in HIV-infected persons with CD4 counts below 50. The prognosis of patients with MAC, like other opportunistic infections, has improved significantly due to several factors, including the use of highly active antiretroviral therapy (HAART) regimens. Prophylaxis with a macrolide agent such as clarithromycin or azithromycin is indicated in patients with CD4 counts below 50.
- ***Mycobacterium kansasii*,** the second most common nontuberculous mycobacteria pulmonary disease, presents with variable and nonspecific signs and symptoms. Diagnosis is based on clinical, radiographic, and bacteriologic criteria as well as measures to exclude other pulmonary disease, including TB. Pulmonary disease caused by *M. kansasii* responds to most TB regimens. Consultation with local health department experts is recommended.

REFERENCES

1. Reves R, Schluger NW. Update in tuberculosis and nontuberculous mycobacterial infections 2013. *Am J Respir Crit Care Med* 2014;189(8):894–898.
2. Herbert N, George A, Baroness Masham of Ilton, et al. World TB Day 2014: finding the missing 3 million. *Lancet* 2014;383(9922):1016–1018.
3. Hartman-Adams H, Clark K, Juckett G. Update on Latent Tuberculosis Infection. *Am Fam Physician* 2014;89(11):889–896..
4. Walter ND, Painter J, Parker M, et al. Persistent LTBI reactivation risk in United States immigrants. *Am J Respir Crit Care Med* 2014;189(1):88–95.
5. Sterling TR, Villarino ME, Borisov AS, et al. Three months of rifapentine and isoniazid for latent tuberculosis infection. *N Engl J Med* 2011;365(23):2155–2166.
6. Painter JA, Graviss EA, Hai HH, et al. Tuberculosis screening by TST or QuantiFERON-TB Gold In-Tube Assay among an immigrant population with a high prevalence of TB and BCG vaccination. *PLoS One* 2013;8(12):e82727.
7. LoBue PA, Castro KG. Is it time to replace the tuberculin skin test with a blood test? *JAMA* 2012;308(3):241–242.
8. Shepardson D, Marks SM, Chesson H, et al. Cost-effectiveness of a 12-dose regimen for treating latent tuberculous infection in the United States. *Int J Tuberc Lung Dis* 2013;17(12):1531–1537. doi: 10.5588/ijtld.13.0423.
9. Centers for Disease Control and Prevention (CDC). Availability of an assay for detecting Mycobacterium tuberculosis, including rifampin-resistant strains, and considerations for its use—United States, 2013 [Erratum in: *MMWR* 2013;62(45):906]. *MMWR* 2013;62(41):821–827.
10. Francis J. Curry National TB Center. Excellent comprehensive site with teaching modules. www.nationaltbcenter.edu/.

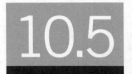

10.5 Lung Cancer
Daniel G. Hunter-Smith, James E. Hannigan

GENERAL PRINCIPLES
Epidemiology and Pathology

Primary cancer of the lung is the leading cause of cancer mortality in the United States in both men and women, with estimated cancer deaths in 2013 of 118,080 men and 110,110 women. The median age for lung cancer diagnosis is rising and is now about 71. The incidence of lung cancer has been falling among men for two decades and recently began falling among women.[1] Cigarette smoking is estimated to be the cause in 85% of all lungs cancers; women are more likely than men to develop lung cancer not associated with tobacco use.[2]

Histologically, primary lung cancer is divided into two categories, small-cell lung cancer (SCLC) and non–small-cell lung cancer (NSCLC). Adenocarcinoma and squamous cell carcinoma are the two major types of NSCLC. This categorization is useful for clinical staging, treatment, and prognosis. Histological types vary between men and women as follows: SCLC: 15% versus 18%; NSCLC: adeno-carcinoma 31% versus 38%, squamous cell 27% versus 18% (data from United States, 1998–2002).[3]

- **Screening.** The U.S. Preventive Services Task Force (USPSTF) recommends annual screening with low-dose computed tomography (LDCT) in adults aged 55 to 80 years who have at least a 30 pack-year smoking history and currently smoke or have quit within the past 15 years. (B recommendation) LDCT was judged to provide moderate net benefit to asymptomatic persons who are at high risk for lung cancer when the accuracy of image interpretation is similar to that found in the National Lung Screening Trial (NLST), and the resolution of most false-positive results occurs without invasive procedures. The NLST demonstrated a 20% reduction in lung cancer mortality and a 7% overall mortality reduction, as many smokers die of related causes other than lung cancer. It is estimated that 320 people would have to be screened annually with LDCT for 3 years to prevent one lung cancer death.[4]
- **History and clinical presentation.** Risk factors, especially active or passive smoking exposure must be obtained. Industrial or home exposure to radon, asbestos, and other airborne particulate matter may also be relevant. Family members who are first-degree relatives of a patient with lung cancer have been shown to have a 2.4-fold increase in risk for developing lung cancer. The most common presenting signs and symptoms of lung cancer are cough, hemoptysis, dyspnea, chest pain, bone pain, and weight loss. Many lung cancers have few or subtle symptoms.

DIAGNOSIS
Physical Examination

Frequently, the examination is unremarkable. However, patients may present with bronchial obstruction causing fever, coarse rales, egophony, decreased breath sounds, and dullness to percussion over the obstructed area. Patients presenting with an unexplained pleural effusion have a 45% chance of malignancy.

Special Studies and Staging

Spread to regional or distant sites is present in three quarters of patients at the time of diagnosis. The histologic diagnosis is obtained by trans-thoracic fine needle or bronchoscopic biopsy. Abdominal CT and bone scans are performed to identify or rule out distant metastases. One of four stages for NSCLC is determined (I, II, IIIA, IIIB, and IV) based on the tumor, nodal, and metastatic status. Because of its propensity for brain metastases, a brain magnetic resonance imaging (MRI) is obtained as part of the staging workup of SCLC, and often in NSCLC that is widespread.

COMPLICATIONS OF LUNG CANCER
- **Complications due to tumor extension or metastasis.** Paralysis of the cervical sympathetic nerve due to tumor invasion resulting in upper eyelid ptosis, pupillary constriction, anhydrosis, and flushing of the affected side of the face is known as **Horner syndrome.** A tumor near the apex of the lung

can involve the brachial plexus resulting in Horner syndrome plus muscle atrophy and neurotic arm pain on the affected side. This is known as **Pancoast syndrome.** Compression of bronchial tubes by tumor extension commonly causes obstructive pneumonia. Compression of the superior vena cava causes facial swelling, rubor, and neck vein distention, and is called superior vena cava syndrome.

- **Paraneoplastic syndromes associated with NSCLC**
  - **Hypercalcemia.** This is most commonly seen with squamous cell carcinoma. It can be caused by ectopic secretion of parathormone-like substances as well as bone metastases and results in polyuria, dehydration, constipation, and mental confusion. Treatment consists of vigorous saline hydration to restore a urinary output of 2 L per day. Furosemide is added if fluid overload results. Thiazide diuretics should be avoided. Zolderdronic acid (Zometa) or pamidronate (Aredia) should also be given to lower serum calcium.
  - **Hypertrophic pulmonary osteoarthropathy.** This is associated with adenocarcinomas. Manifestations include clubbing of the fingers, joint and bone pain, and elevated alkaline phosphatase. The condition improves with nonsteroidal anti-inflammatory drugs (NSAIDs) and treatment of the tumor.
  - **Spinal cord compression.** Severe back pain associated with motor and sensory loss related to the spinal cord level of compression. Treatment with IV dexamethasone (4 to 6 mg q6 hours) should be given urgently, followed by radiation therapy or surgical decompression.
- **Paraneoplastic syndromes associated with SCLC**
  - **The syndrome of inappropriate excretion of antidiuretic hormone (SIADH).** The initial therapy includes fluid restriction with the possible addition of demeclocycline (Declomycin) 150 to 300 mg qid. SIADH improves with treatment of the tumor.
  - **Eaton Lambert syndrome.** This presents with myasthenia-like neurologic changes. Sensory neuropathies or limbic encephalopathies may also occur.

TREATMENT
Surgical
Curative surgery is possible only for the earlier stages of NSCLC (Stages 0, I, II, and possibly IIIA). Patients with the following complications are not surgical candidates: superior vena cava syndrome; tumors closer than 2 cm to the carina; low pulmonary reserve; comorbid disease with unacceptable surgical risk; involvement of the pericardium, heart, esophagus, or great vessels; and SCLC unless discovered as an isolated pulmonary nodule. Patients who are candidates for surgery should be evaluated with preoperative pulmonary function tests.

Radiation
This therapy is reserved for patients with Stage IIIA or IIIB NSCLC and for palliation of bone or spinal metastases. Radiation is also part of the definitive treatment of limited SCLC (see below).

Chemotherapy
A combination of two chemotherapy drugs is more active than a single agent, but no additional benefit is seen when a third agent is added. Several doublets of chemotherapy appear to be equally active.[5] A new class of drugs, the epidermal growth factor receptor (EGFR) inhibitors, can cause a dramatic regression of NSCLC in 10% to 20% of patients. Patients who are most likely to respond to EGFR inhibitors such as erlotinib (Tarceva) are women, nonsmokers, patients of Asian ethnicity, and those with bronchiolar alveolar cancer. Response rates have been correlated with specific mutations in the EGFR gene. The most common side effect is an acneiform rash, and patients who develop a severe rash are more likely to respond to the treatment. A monoclonal antibody to the vascular endothelial growth factor (VEGF), called bevacizumab (Avastin), is commercially available. In patients with advanced NSCLC, the addition of bevacizumab to chemotherapy results in an improvement in survival. Patients with squamous cell histology were excluded because of an increased incidence of fatal hemoptysis with bevacizumab. They are mostly treated with carboplatin and paclitaxel at the outset. The chemotherapy for adenocarcinoma often begins with carboplatin (a derivative of the metal, platinum) and pemetrexed, a multitargeted antifolate that interferes with the tumor cells ability to synthesize DNA.[6]

When planning treatment of SCLC, oncologists generally recognize two stages: limited stage, which can be encompassed in a single radiation treatment field, and extensive stage, which cannot. The former may be treated with concomitant chemoradiation if patients have good performance status, while extensive stage is treated solely with chemotherapy, reserving radiation for local problems.

The family physician should be kept constantly apprised of the patient's status and the next steps taken in their care.

Follow-Up

On the basis of data from the National Cancer Institute's Surveillance, Epidemiology, and End Results of patients diagnosed between 1998 and 2000, the estimated overall 5-year survival rates for patients with NSCLC by stage are IA, 49%; IB, 45%; IIA, 30%; IIB, 31%; IIIA, 14%; IIIB, 5%; and IV, 1%. The 5-year survival rates of SCLC by stage are I, 31%; II, 19%; III, 8%; and IV, 2%.[1]

REFERENCES

1. What are the key statistics about lung cancer? American Cancer Society Web site. http://www.cancer. org/cancer/index. Revised July 12, 2013. Accessed March 21, 2014.
2. Wakelee HA, Chang ET, Gomez SL, et al. Lung cancer incidence in never smokers. *J Clin Oncol* 2007;25:472–278.
3. Youlden DR, Cramb SM, Baade, PD. The international epidemiology of lung cancer: geographical distribution and secular trends. *J Thorac Oncol* 2008;3:819–831.
4. Campos-Outcalt D. Lung cancer screening: USPSTF revises its recommendation. *J Fam Prac* 2013;62:733–740.
5. Pisters KMW. Adjuvant chemotherapy for non-small-cell lung cancer—the smoke clears. *N Engl J Med* 2005;352:2640–2642.
6. Cataldo VD, Gibbons DL, Perez-Soler R, et al. Treatment of non-small-cell lung cancer with erlotinib or gefitinib. *N Engl J Med* 2011;364:947–955.

CHAPTER 11

Gastrointestinal Problems

Section Editor: Michael A. Malone

Peptic Ulcer Disease and Gastritis

Stephanie A. Gill, Jay Zimmermann, Alan M. Adelman

PEPTIC ULCER DISEASE

General Principles

Peptic ulcers may involve any portion of the upper gastrointestinal (GI) tract, but most ulcers are found in the stomach and the duodenum. Duodenal ulcers are approximately three times as common as gastric ulcers. *Helicobacter pylori* (HP) is the major cause of peptic ulcer disease (PUD). Non-HP PUD is frequently caused by nonsteroidal anti-inflammatory drugs (NSAIDs). A rare cause of PUD is Zollinger–Ellison syndrome.

Diagnosis

Clinical Presentation

Although PUD may occur or recur in the absence of pain, epigastric discomfort, also called dyspepsia, is the most common presenting symptom. Associated symptoms may include fullness, belching, bloating, heartburn, food intolerance, nausea, or vomiting. Severity and description of the pain is variable and correlates poorly with size or number of ulcers. The clinical presentation of PUD overlaps with that of other causes of epigastric discomfort (gastroesophageal reflux disease, nonulcer or functional dyspepsia, gastric cancer, cholelithiasis, and coronary artery disease).

   Physical examination usually reveals only epigastric tenderness. Findings such as a succussion splash (gastric outlet obstruction), abdominal rigidity (perforation), or heme-positive stools (bleeding) are suggestive of complications of PUD.

Laboratory Studies[1]

- **Initial testing for *H. pylori.*** There are several noninvasive ways to test for HP that avoid the need for an endoscopy. Initial testing to determine the presence of HP, if available, should be with either the stool antigen or urea breath test. Stool antigen for HP is easy to perform. Its average sensitivity is 91% to 98% and specificity is 94% to 99%. Urea breath testing requires a breath sample, but the availability of the testing can be limited. The average sensitivity is 90% to 96% and specificity is 88% to 98%.
  - Serologic testing should be performed if the stool antigen or urea breath tests are unavailable. Finger-stick testing, quantitative serologic testing, and enzyme-linked immunosorbent assay (ELISA) testing are the available serologic tests. Quick serologic or finger-stick testing is a qualitative procedure for office use but is not recommended as first-line testing. The average sensitivity is 67% to 88% and specificity is 75% to 91%. ELISA testing is a quantitative assay. Its average sensitivity is 86% to 94% and specificity is 78% to 95%.
  - Upper endoscopy is recommended as the initial study in patients with complications of PUD, patients with signs of systemic disease, patients ≥55 years of age, and patients who have failed empiric therapy. The main advantage of endoscopy is its capacity to obtain biopsy specimens for pathology and testing for HP. If an ulcer is diagnosed endoscopically, a rapid urease test (*Campylobacter*-like organism, or CLO) is the quickest means to determine the presence of HP. The average sensitivity is 88% to 95% and specificity is 95% to 100%. Histologic testing requires special stains.

Its average sensitivity is 93% to 96% and specificity is 98% to 99%. Culture can also determine the presence of HP. The average sensitivity is 80% to 98% and specificity is 100%. Culture and drug sensitivities are important when drug resistance is suspected.

- Double-contrast upper GI studies can reliably diagnose both duodenal and gastric ulcers, but the false-negative rate can exceed 18%, whereas the false-positive rate is 13% to 35%.
- **Follow-up testing.** Follow-up testing is not generally recommended, but it can be performed for patients with persistent symptoms. Stool antigen for HP (as early as 7 days after completion of treatment) or a falling ELISA titer (1, 3, and 6 months after therapy) are the easiest methods for a test of cure. However, the ELISA may remain elevated in successfully treated individuals for up to 18 months. A serologic test cannot document eradication of HP. A CLO at repeat endoscopy or a urea breath test (4 weeks after therapy) can also be used.

Therapy

General Approach to the Assessment of PUD[2,3]

First, patients with complications of PUD (bleeding, gastric outlet obstruction, perforation), signs of systemic disease (anemia, unexplained weight loss, lymphadenopathy, abdominal mass), persistent or recurrent symptoms, or a family history of GI cancer should be evaluated by upper endoscopy and managed immediately (see Chapter 11.3). Patients ≥55 years of age should also be considered for prompt endoscopy and management. Second, medications that can cause epigastric discomfort should be discontinued. In particular, patients should be questioned about the use of NSAIDs, both prescription and over the counter. In all other patients with dyspepsia symptoms, clinicians may consider two approximately equivalent management options: (a) test for HP and if positive treat with HP-eradicating agents; or (b) use an empiric trial of acid suppression with proton pump inhibitor (PPI) for 4 to 8 weeks. The test-and-treat option is preferred in populations with HP infection ≥10%. The empiric PPI strategy is preferred in low-prevalence populations.

In the test-and-treat strategy, therapy is determined by the presence or absence of HP. Antibiotic treatment is given to patients who are positive for HP. The addition of a PPI or histamine receptor antagonist (H_2RA) hastens relief of pain. PPIs also have anti-HP action and are included in some anti-HP regimens. Patients with HP-negative ulcers are treated with traditional acid suppression agents alone. The value of treating nonulcer dyspepsia patients with HP infection remains to be determined.

- **Regimens for *H. pylori*.**[1] Multiple regimens have been shown to be equally effective with eradication rates 70% to 85%. The following regimens are given for 10 to 14 days. The PPI or H_2RA is to be given for a total of 4 weeks.
  - PPI (standard dose), amoxicillin 1,000 mg bid, and clarithromycin (Biaxin) 500 mg bid (the combination of lansoprazole, clarithromycin, and amoxicillin is available as Prevpac)
  - Bismuth 2 tabs qid, metronidazole 500 mg tid, tetracycline 500 mg qid, PPI daily or H_2RA as directed
- **Traditional acid suppression agents**
  - **PPIs.** Omeprazole (Prilosec) 20 mg daily, pantoprazole (Protonix) 40 mg daily, lansoprazole (Prevacid) 15 mg daily, and rabeprazole (Aciphex) 20 mg daily are first-line treatment for acid suppression.
  - **H_2RA.** Ranitidine (Zantac) 150 mg bid, famotidine (Pepcid) 20 mg bid, nizatidine (Axid) 150 mg bid, and cimetidine (Tagamet) 400 mg bid are equally effective. Cimetidine appears to be associated with the highest incidence of side effects and drug interactions.
  - Sucralfate (Carafate), 1 g qid, is effective in healing peptic ulcers. There are no significant side effects, but the size of the tablet and frequency of administration are potential drawbacks.
- **Antacids.** Antacids are effective in healing ulcers, but their use is limited by the number of doses required. Aluminum hydroxide/magnesium hydroxide/simethicone antacids (Maalox extra strength, Mylanta double strength), 2 tablets qid, are unlikely to produce constipation or diarrhea. Phosphate depletion can occur with antacid use in malnourished patients, and hypermagnesemia can result in patients with chronic renal failure.
- Dietary therapy is limited to the elimination of foods that exacerbate symptoms, and the avoidance of alcohol and coffee (with or without caffeine). Both alcohol and coffee increase gastric acid secretion.
- Cessation of cigarette smoking speeds ulcer healing. In HP-negative ulcers, smoking cessation decreases the risk of recurrence.
- **Combination therapy.** There is no evidence that combination therapy of traditional agents (e.g., sucralfate and an H_2RA) hastens healing.

Special Consideration

Refractory or Recurrent Ulcers

Eradication of HP reduces the rate of recurrence of peptic ulcers in individuals with HP-positive ulcers. In patients with a refractory or recurrent ulcer and documented HP, several issues should be considered. Any NSAID should be discontinued. Compliance with medication should be reviewed. Resistant HP has been reported, necessitating retreatment with a different antibiotic regimen. In patients with a gastric ulcer, cancer should be considered. Zollinger–Ellison syndrome should be considered in patients with severe or multiple ulcers, large gastric mucosal folds, or unexplained diarrhea and steatorrhea.

Maintenance Therapy

Smokers, patients with recurrent non-HP ulcers, elderly patients, and patients with a history of a bleeding ulcer should receive maintenance therapy with a daily PPI.

GASTRITIS/GASTROPATHY

General Principles

Gastritis/gastropathy is a collection of disorders characterized by damage to the gastric mucosa. Gastritis represents the presence of inflammation, whereas in gastropathy inflammation is absent. These disorders can be either acute (associated with acute injury secondary to NSAID use, stress, alcohol, bile acids) or chronic (autoimmune, HP). Since gastropathy associated with NSAID use is the most common form encountered by physicians, this section deals specifically with NSAID-related gastropathy.

Diagnosis

Presentation

Pain is much less common than in PUD. Usually patients are asymptomatic unless blood loss is appreciable. Life-threatening GI bleeding may be the initial presentation. Anorexia, nausea, or vomiting may be present, although dyspeptic symptoms do not correlate well with endoscopic findings.

Risk factors for development of NSAID gastropathy include age older than 60 years, previous history of ulcers with or without complications, concomitant use of corticosteroids, high doses of NSAIDs, and extended use of NSAIDs. Other potential factors may include alcohol consumption and smoking. Concurrent use of anticoagulants increases the risk of GI complications.

Physical examination. Physical findings are usually absent unless the patient presents with bleeding.

Laboratory studies. Although not common, anemia can be the initial finding, prompting further radiologic or endoscopic evaluation.

Treatment[4]

- **Discontinue use of NSAID.** Reduce or discontinue other risk factors.
- **Medication.** H_2RA and PPI have been shown to be effective in healing gastric ulcers secondary to NSAID use. PPI is the drug of choice as co-therapy if the NSAID cannot be discontinued.
- If the patient has PUD and is found to be positive for HP, then treatment for HP is recommended.

Special Consideration

Prevention

Avoid NSAIDs when feasible or minimize the dose of NSAID. Two prophylactic agents are available. Misoprostol is used in patients who have a history of ulcers, especially with bleeding as a complication. A PPI may be used as an alternative for individuals who cannot tolerate misoprostol.

REFERENCES

1. Chey WD, Wong BC; Practice Parameters Committee of the American College of Gastroenterology. American College of Gastroenterology guideline on the management of Helicobacter pylori infection. *Am J Gastroenterol* 2007;102:1808–1825.
2. Loyd RA, McClellan DA. Management of functional dyspepsia. *Am Fam Physician* 2011;83(5):547–552.
3. Ford AC, Moayyedi P. Clinical review: dyspepsia. *BMJ* 2013;347:f5059.
4. Lanza FL, Chan FK, Quigley EM; Practice Parameters Committee of the American College of Gastroenterology. Guidelines for the prevention of NSAID-related ulcer complications. *Am J Gastroenterol* 2009;104:728–738.

11.2 Gastroesophageal Reflux Disease

Sumaira Iqbal, George G.A. Pujalte

Gastroesophageal reflux disease (GERD) has troublesome symptoms, or complications, resulting from the reflux of gastric contents. It is the most common diagnosis among all gastrointestinal (GI) complaints, with 10% to 30% of the U.S. population affected with symptoms weekly.[1] GERD accounts for about 4% of all visits in family practice.[2] It can be further classified based on symptoms, and on the presence or the absence of erosions in the intestinal cavity. The two categories are (a) nonerosive reflux disease (NERD) or symptoms without erosions and (b) erosive reflux disease (ERD).

ETIOLOGY

The physiological causes for reflux are the following: (a) increased number of transient lower esophageal sphincter (LES) relaxations; (b) ineffective esophageal motility; and (c) reduced LES tone. All these factors contribute to increased exposure to gastric content. Symptoms become apparent with exposure to a lower pH, a longer clearance time, and a higher total acid exposure. Bile acid and pancreatic secretions are also components of the refluxate in individuals suffering from GERD.[2]

The risk factors and conditions associated with GERD are obesity, hiatal hernia, use of estrogen and nitrates, anticholinergics, and tobacco use. Hiatal hernia may separate the LES from the crural diaphragm, resulting in a weakened gastroesophageal barrier. Obesity poses risks by the same mechanism, because it increases the predisposition to hiatal hernia via an increase in intragastric pressure.

CLINICAL PRESENTATION

"Heartburn" and regurgitation are the two cardinal symptoms of GERD. Heartburn is the common term for the discomfort or the burning sensation felt by GERD sufferers that starts behind the sternum and rises to the neck. This condition usually becomes worse after meals or with reclining. Regurgitation is the process of refluxing gastric content into the mouth.

A strong association exists between GERD and a history of a nocturnal cough and chest pain.[3] The cardiac causes of chest pain, however, must be ruled out first and foremost. Other common symptoms include dysphagia, dyspepsia, and hoarseness.

DIAGNOSIS

There are no standard criteria for the diagnosis of GERD. Once a clinical syndrome is apparent, empiric suppression using a short course of proton pump inhibitors (PPIs) may be used as a diagnostic test. The test is positive if the symptoms of GERD improve more than 50% to 70% after the trial of PPIs.[3] There is variability in the dose and duration of PPIs used. Current U.S. treatment guidelines are congruent with this practice, recommending treatment without invasive diagnostic testing, unless weight loss, GI bleeding, or anemia is present.[2] Questionnaires, such as the GERD questionnaire, have been formulated that are based on symptoms, assessing their frequency and duration to help predict the likelihood of the presence of GERD.

An upper endoscopy is not first in the diagnosis of GERD; however, it is indicated when alarming symptoms indicate a complication of GERD. These symptoms include dysphagia, odynophagia, involuntary weight loss, GI bleed, and nonresponse to PPIs.[4] Endoscopy is specific to finding abnormalities of the mucosa, such as esophagitis, strictures, masses, ulcers, and Barrett's esophagus. A normal endoscopic examination does not rule out NERD.

A double-contrast barium esophagram is not used for the diagnosis of GERD.[4] This test is indicated when dysphagia is present and evaluating the anatomy of the esophagus is necessary. The esophagram can aid in the detection of strictures, rings, and other complications of GERD.

Esophageal manometry has limited value in the diagnosis of GERD and can be used to assist in the placement of a pH-measuring device.[3] Manometry assesses peristalsis and the contractile pressure in the body of the esophagus. In addition, it can measure the resting tone and the relaxation of the lower and upper esophageal sphincters. Based on these abilities, manometry is clinically indicated to rule out achalasia or severe hypomobility in a scleroderma-like esophagus.

Ambulatory reflux monitoring is used to test for the presence of abnormal esophageal acid exposure, reflux frequency, and associated symptoms. It is done either through transnasal catheters or by a pH-measuring capsule. It is indicated for patients with refractory GERD or preoperatively for NERD prior to fundoplication.[3] The transnasal catheter is passed through the nose to be positioned above the LES. It is possible to monitor the pH for 24 hours safely and inexpensively.[3] The capsule is placed in the same region where endoscopy is used. Since it is wireless, it is tolerated better and provides a longer duration of pH monitoring, from 48 to 96 hours.[3] However, the use of the capsule is limited because of the associated cost.

TREATMENT OPTIONS

Symptomatic relief, disease prevention, and management of complications are the goals of treatment for GERD. Lifestyle modifications should include weight loss for those patients who are overweight or have had a recent weight gain. Head-of-bed elevation with meals, and avoidance of meals 2 to 3 hours prior to bedtime should be recommended.[4] Other modifications should include smoking cessation and avoidance of fatty or spicy meals.

PPIs are the mainstay of the treatment for GERD. An 8-week course of PPIs is the choice for symptomatic relief and for healing erosive esophagitis.[4] As the disease has a tendency to return, it is not surprising that patients do relapse after discontinuing medication; long-term PPI use may be indicated. PPIs should be started and maintained at the lowest daily dosage that provides relief. The patient should be directed to take PPIs before the first meal of the day. Those individuals with a partial response to PPIs can switch to twice-daily therapy. No major difference in efficacy exists in different PPIs.[4] Overall, PPIs are well tolerated and safe in pregnancy when indicated.[3] However, PPIs can be a risk factor for the *Clostridium difficile* infection and should be used with care in patients at risk. Those individuals with GERD refractory to optimal PPIs should undergo endoscopy to rule out other etiologies. A negative endoscopic evaluation implies the possible need for ambulatory pH monitoring to confirm GERD. If reflux is present and refractory to PPIs, additional anti-reflux therapies, including surgery, should be considered.

Antacids and mucosal protective agents provide rapid symptomatic relief; however, their effect is short-lived. They have not been shown to adequately heal erosive esophagitis.[2]

Histamine H_2–receptor antagonists are effective in healing mucosa in milder forms of the disease. They have been associated with tachyphylaxis after several weeks of use; hence, long-term use has not been recommended.[1]

Prokinetic medications, such as cisapride and metoclopramide, are options in patients with delayed gastric emptying. Symptom relief is short term, lasting only 4 to 8 hours. The side effects of these medications include fatigue, tremor, tardive dyskinesia, and cardiac events.[2]

Surgical intervention is an option for long-term therapy. The procedure used often is laparoscopic fundoplication, where the fundus of the stomach is wrapped around the esophagus, reinforcing the gastroesophageal junction. It is indicated in patients who want to discontinue medications, who are noncompliant, who have side effects from medical therapy, and who have refractory GERD. Preoperative ambulatory pH monitoring is mandatory prior to the procedure. Surgical therapy has symptomatic relief efficacy similar to that of medical therapy.[1] Efficacy is also dependent on the surgeon's experience[1] and should be offered on the basis of a patient's preference.

Alternative and nontraditional therapies are also being studied for individuals with GERD. Although large-scale studies are lacking, some evidence indicates that a low-carbohydrate diet may alleviate the symptoms of GERD.[2] Acupuncture improves esophageal motility, limits LES relaxation, and reduces esophageal pain perception; these effects may be beneficial in relieving GERD symptoms.[2] Melatonin has been recognized to signal gut motility, inhibit gastric acid secretion, and increase gastrin.[2] Gastrin contracts the LES; combined with the other actions of melatonin, it decreases the overall contact of the refluxate with the esophageal mucosa.

Certain botanicals may benefit individuals suffering from GERD. The Chinese honeysuckle flower has antioxidant properties; peppermint oil has been reported to accelerate gastric emptying; *Iberogast*, consisting of nine botanicals, may provide symptomatic relief, although the mechanism of action is unknown.[2]

COMPLICATIONS

Untreated, persistent GERD can have a deleterious health impact. The potential complications include esophagitis, esophageal ulcerations, bleeding, strictures, Barrett's esophagus, and esophageal adenocarcinoma. The incidence of esophageal adenocarcinoma has increased significantly over the past

20 years from 200% to 600%, despite the use of PPIs.[2] Individuals with nocturnal symptoms were noted to have a higher likelihood of complications.[1] Complications of GERD should be detected early and require prompt referral to a gastroenterologist or surgeon.

REFERENCES

1. Fock KM, Poh CH. Gastroesophageal reflux disease. *J Gastroenterol* 2010;45:808–815.
2. Patrick L. Gastroesophageal reflux disease (GERD): a review of conventional and alternative treatments. *Altern Med Rev* 2011;16(2):116–133.
3. Lacy BE, Weiser K, Chertoff J, et al. The diagnosis of gastroesophageal reflux disease. *Am J Med* 2010;123:583–592.
4. Katz P, Gerson L, Vela M. Guidelines for the diagnosis and management of gastroesophageal reflux disease. *Am J Gastroenterol* 2013;108:308–328.

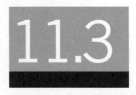

11.3 Upper Gastrointestinal Bleeding

Mel P. Daly

GENERAL PRINCIPLES

Definition

Upper gastrointestinal (UGI) bleeding occurs from the UGI tract.

Epidemiology

UGI bleeding is a common clinical problem, with an annual incidence of 50 to 150 per 100,000 of the population. The incidence is twice as common in males and increases with age. Mortality from UGI bleeding is about 10% and may reach 35% in patients hospitalized for another medical condition. Patients over age 80 account for 25% of all UGI bleeds and 33% of UGI bleeds occurring in hospitalized patients. The prognosis for patients with upper gastrointestinal bleeding appears to be improving. Most episodes of nonvariceal bleeding (80%) are self-limited and require only supportive therapy, but if bleeding is continuous or recurrent, the mortality is 30% to 40%. Surgery may be required in 15% to 30% of patients.[1]

Etiology of UGI Bleeding (Table 11.3-1)

Peptic ulcers, gastritis/duodenitis, esophageal varices, gastroesophageal mucosal tears, and esophagitis account for 90% of cases. Other causes include gastric tumors, hematobilia, hiatal hernia, aortointestinal fistula, vascular malformations, vasculitis, and Dieulafoy lesion (submucosal arterial malformation).[2]

- **Peptic ulcer disease (PUD)** is the most common cause of UGI bleeding. Duodenal or gastric ulcers caused by *Helicobacter pylori* are common causes of UGI bleeding. There is a synergistic risk of ulcer bleeding in patients using nonsteroidal anti-inflammatory drugs (NSAIDs). Other risks factors for PUD include physiologic stress and excess gastric acid production. Although pain is the usual presenting symptom, 10% of patients present with UGI bleeding.
- **Gastritis** is associated with using NSAIDs (and selective cyclo-oxygenase inhibitors) and alcohol, severe systemic disease, major trauma, burns, and ventilator use. These conditions also increase the risk of bleeding from underlying PUD. Patients with these secondary episodes of bleeding have a higher mortality than those admitted with primary upper gastrointestinal bleeding.
- **Esophageal varices** occur in patients with cirrhosis (alcoholic and non–alcohol-related) who have portal hypertension. Bleeding is more likely in patients with advanced cirrhosis and large varices. Concomitant PUD, gastritis, or Mallory–Weiss tears in alcoholic patients may also cause hemorrhage.
- **Gastroesophageal (GE) mucosal tears (Mallory–Weiss).** Hemorrhage results from mucosal laceration of the GE junction induced by retching or vomiting. Patients are often heavy alcohol users,

TABLE 11.3-1	Causes of Upper Gastrointestinal Bleeding

Common
Gastritis (erosive due to NSAIDs)
Esophagitis
Peptic ulcer disease
Esophagogastric varices with or without portal hypertensive gastropathy
Gastroesophageal mucosal tears
Cancer (carcinoma, lymphoma, polyps)
Dieulafoy lesions (active arterial bleeding or an adherent clot on an underlying vessel in the absence of an ulcer)

Rare
Infections (CMV, herpes, *Candida*)
GERD
Aortoenteric fistula
Blood dyscrasia
Vasculitis
Hemorrhagic telangiectasia
Pancreatic cancer
Uremia

and 30% use aspirin or NSAIDs. Tears may also occur from violent coughing, severe asthma attacks, seizures, cardiopulmonary resuscitation, and straining at stool.
- **Other causes.** Blood dyscrasias, vasculitis, connective tissue diseases (CTDs), and hereditary hemorrhagic telangiectasia (Osler–Rendu–Weber disease) may rarely be the cause of UGI bleeding. Hematobilia occurs secondary to trauma, injury, or vascular malformations of the liver or biliary tree. Aortoduodenal fistulas and large ectatic submucosal arteries (Dieulafoy lesion) or arteriovenous malformation (AVMs) may cause massive hemorrhage. Gastroesophageal reflux disease (GERD), cancer, and infections such as cytomegalovirus (CMV), herpes, or *Candida* may cause UGI bleeding but more usually cause chronic blood loss. Rarely, large hiatal hernias may cause blood loss as a result of linear mucosal tears. Even more rarely, gastric cancer, lymphoma, polyps, and other tumors of the stomach or small intestine may cause UGI bleeding.

DIAGNOSIS
Clinical Presentation
Clinical presentation depends on the location, source, and acuity of the bleed.[2]

- Acute UGI bleeding often presents with bloody vomiting. Blood from a recent bleed is usually bright red. Bleeding from varices is usually abrupt and massive. Melena (black, tarry, malodorous stools) usually is the result of UGI bleeding or lesions of the small intestine if GI transit time is prolonged. Melena can be seen with variable degrees of blood loss, being seen with as little as 50 mL of blood. Hematochezia (maroon or bright red blood per rectum can be the presenting symptom in a small proportion of cases of UGI bleeding. A history of alcohol abuse, cigarette smoking, or NSAID use may often exist. In these cases, bleeding is typically brisk and may be accompanied by hemodynamic instability.
- Chronic or unrecognized UGI bleeding may present with pallor, dizziness, dyspnea, iron deficiency anemia, or occult blood in stool.
- Physiologic responses to UGI bleeding
  - In acute UGI bleeding, the physiologic response depends on the rate and extent of hemorrhage. Blood loss less than 500 mL is usually asymptomatic, except in elderly patients with coronary artery or chronic lung disease.
  - Rapid blood loss results in decreased cardiac output reflex, and orthostatic hypotension indicating a reduction in blood volume of more than 20%. Lightheadedness, confusion, nausea, sweating, fainting, and thirst are commonly associated with symptoms.

- When blood loss approaches 40% of blood volume, shock occurs, with tachycardia, hypotension, pallor, and cold clammy extremities.
- Initial hemoglobin levels do not give a useful estimate of the volume of hemorrhage in the acute setting, and levels may be normal despite significant blood loss.
- Chronic blood loss may be asymptomatic or present with signs and symptoms of anemia, hyponatremia, and hypoalbuminemia as a result of retention of hypotonic fluid to replenish intravascular volume.

History and Physical Examination

These identify the cause in only 50% of cases.

- **Prior history** of PUD or dyspepsia may suggest ulcer bleeding. A history of medication (NSAIDS, clopidogrel, and anticoagulants) and alcohol use should be elicited. Symptoms of cirrhosis may suggest variceal bleeding. Bleeding from other sources (e.g., frequent nosebleeds, bruising) may suggest a coagulopathy. Patients with renal disease, aortic stenosis, and hereditary hemorrhagic telangiectasia are more likely to have angiodysplasia. Odynophagia, dysphagia, or gastric reflux may occur in patients with esophageal ulcer. Retching or violent coughing may occur prior to bleeding in patients with Mallory–Weiss tears.[3]
- **Examination.** Epigastric tenderness is suggestive of PUD. Hepatosplenomegaly may occur in liver disease or malignancy. A rectal examination may reveal melena, but stool may be normal in patients with minimal or recent bleeding.
- **Laboratory studies.** If blood loss is rapid, the hematocrit may not reflect the magnitude of loss because equilibration with hemodilution requires 8 hours. Initial laboratory tests should include a complete blood count, serum chemistries, liver tests, and coagulation studies. The blood urea nitrogen may be elevated due to blood protein breakdown to urea by intestinal bacteria and reduced glomerular filtration rate. A ratio of blood urea nitrogen to serum creatinine of greater than 20 is predictive of a bleed coming from an upper GI source.

TREATMENT

Always begins with resuscitation, restoration of intravascular volume, correction of hemoglobin loss, and treatment of pathophysiologic changes.

- **Resuscitation.** Vital signs should be monitored frequently and fluid replaced rapidly. Intravenous access using two wide-bore cannulae should be gained. Crystalloids (normal saline or Ringer solution) or fresh frozen plasma (especially in patients with coagulopathy) should be used until blood is available. Military antishock trousers may be required to correct shock. For unstable cardiac patients, central venous or pulmonary wedge pressures should be measured, with a goal of keeping blood pressure and pulse stable and maintaining urinary output at more than 40 mL per hour. Blood transfusions should be initiated if hemoglobin is <7 g per dL with a goal of maintaining a level of ≥9 g per dL. Blood replacement is especially important in elderly patients and those intolerant of hypoxia (coronary artery disease, pulmonary disease). Intravenous proton pump inhibitor therapy may reduce the risk for rebleeding when endoscopy is also performed. Transfusing patients with suspected variceal bleeding to hemoglobin >10 g per dL should be avoided as it can precipitate worsening of the bleeding.
- **Gastric lavage through a nasogastric (NG) tube** can localize bleeding proximal to the ligament of Treitz. NG suction removes gastric fluid, blood, and swallowed air and can control nausea and vomiting. It is helpful when patients are suspected to have ongoing bleeding and who may benefit from early endoscopy. It has, however, been shown to be ineffective in achieving hemostasis and is **no longer** recommended as a first-line intervention. The presence of blood or "coffee-grounds" on NG aspiration confirms an UGI source, whereas a clear aspirate reduces the likelihood of an UGI source. If endoscopy is to be scheduled in the next several hours, then NG placement is not necessary.

Specific Therapeutic Interventions

Peptic Ulcer Bleeding

- *Medications*: Antacids should be with pantoprazole or omeprazole. Prokinetics such as erythromycin or metoclopramide are effective in facilitating gastric emptying, allowing better visualization at endoscopy. If *H. pylori* infection is diagnosed, treatment with regimens that include a protein pump inhibitor/bismuth, amoxicillin/clarithromycin/tetracycline, and metronidazole are usually effective (see Chapter 11.1).[4]

- Endoscopy is the diagnostic modality of choice for acute upper GI bleeding and once a bleeding lesion has been identified, therapeutic interventions under direct visualization can achieve hemostasis and prevent recurrent bleeding in most patients. Risks of endoscopy include aspiration, adverse reaction to conscious sedation, perforation, and causing bleeding.
- Laser photocoagulation and electrocautery under direct endoscopic visualization may rapidly control active ulcer bleeding.
- Infusion of epinephrine in quadrants around the bleeding point and then into the bleeding vessel achieves hemostasis in 95% of cases (if endoscopic hemostasis fails). Fibrin glue and human thrombin may be the most effective injection materials.
- Mechanical devices "endoclips" may be an option for major bleeding ulcers, especially for arterial tears.
- Surgery is indicated if hemorrhage is brisk or sustained for longer than 6 to 12 hours, or if shock is not controlled by resuscitation. Patients with rapidly bleeding or recurring gastric ulcers may be surgical candidates. Surgery usually involves underrunning the ulcer and pyloroplasty.

Gastritis and Gastric Erosions

Antacids and H_2 receptor blockers reduce the incidence of hemorrhage from stress ulcers. Misoprostol is effective in preventing gastritis due to NSAIDs. Sucralfate and proton pump inhibitors are also effective for patients with prior UGI bleeding who require continued NSAIDs. Laser and electrocautery under direct visualization may control persistent bleeding.

Variceal Bleeding

Only 50% of patients with variceal hemorrhage stop bleeding spontaneously; however, following cessation of acute bleeding, there is a high risk of recurrent hemorrhage.[5] Variceal bleeding may be completely controlled by endoscopic injection of a sclerosing agent, thrombin, epinephrine, or other agents. Noninvasive pharmacologic treatment aimed at causing splanchnic vasoconstriction and thus reducing portal pressure (vasopressin, somatostatin, propranolol). In patients with suspected variceal bleeding, octreotide is given by intravenous bolus of 20 to 50 mcg, followed by continuous infusion at rate of 25 to 50 mcg per hour. Thermal modalities or mechanical (banding, sewing, hemoclips, and endoloop) techniques often effectively control bleeding. Acute bleeding may be abated by balloon occlusion with a Sengstaken–Blakemore tube followed by definitive therapy within 48 hours. Antibiotic prophylaxis with intravenous ciprofloxacin or cephalexin should be instituted in any patient with cirrhosis and GI hemorrhage. Recurrent bleeding may be prevented by periodic endoscopic sclerotherapy. Propranolol given twice daily (at a dose that reduces the heart rate by 25%) decreases portal pressure, although the response is nonuniform.

Arteriovenous Malformations

When actively bleeding, AVMs are best treated with electrocautery. Mallory–Weiss tears usually stop bleeding spontaneously but may require cautery or injection therapy.

Interventions. Esophagogastroduodenoscopy (EGD) has replaced barium studies for diagnosing UGI bleeding because of its greater accuracy and the potential for therapeutic interventions.[6]

- In stable patients, EGD is usually indicated to locate the bleeding source, arrest hemorrhage, and make a definitive diagnosis. Early endoscopy (within 24 hours) is usually recommended for most patients with acute UGI bleeding.
- Persistent UGI hemorrhage is an indication for immediate EGD. If bleeding is heavy, the source may not be identified. Patients with cirrhosis should have EGD because there may be more than one source of hemorrhage. Patients with visible bleeding vessels or varices are candidates for endoscopic treatment.
- *Angiography.* If bleeding continues and EGD fails to reveal the source, angiography may be useful in diagnosing bleeding from varices, vascular ectasias, and aneurysms. Angiography may also be useful in the management of esophageal varices and Mallory–Weiss tears and in the embolization of bleeding ulcers or tumors in patients who are not surgical candidates.
- Colonoscopy is generally required for patients with melena and a negative upper endoscopy.

SPECIAL CONSIDERATIONS

Bleeding from varices has a high recurrence rate and mortality (50% to 70%). Peptic ulcers with visible vessels have a rate of rebleeding of up to 50%. Other prognostic indicators include severity of the initial bleed, hemodynamic instability, hemoglobin <10 g per dL, active bleeding at the time of endoscopy, age (older patients have a higher mortality), concomitant disease, ulcer diameter greater than 2 cm, and the requirement for emergency surgery.[7] The risk of rebleeding is reduced by treating

H. pylori, prescribing proton pump inhibitors, co-treating patients who are prescribed NSAIDs with a proton pump inhibitor, prescribing β-blockers for patients with varices, and consideration of using somatostatin or octreotide.

REFERENCES

1. Esrailain E, Gralnek IM. Nonvariceal gastrointestinal bleeding: epidemiology and diagnosis. *Gastroenterol Clin North Am* 2005;34:589.
2. Rockney DL. Major causes of upper gastrointestinal bleeding in adults. http://www.uptodate.com/contents/major-causes-of-upper-gastrointestinal-bleeding-in-adults? Updated August 14, 2013.
3. Saltzman JR. Approach to acute upper gastrointestinal bleeding in adults. http://www.uptodate.com/contents/approach-to-acute-upper-gastrointestinal-bleeding-in-adults? Updated October 03, 2014.
4. Saltzman JR. Overview of the treatment of bleeding peptic ulcers. http://www.uptodate.com/contents/overview-of-the-treatment-of-bleeding-peptic-ulcers? Updated October 03, 2014.
5. Bajaj JS, Sangual AJ. Management of acute variceal hemorrhage. www.uptodate.com. 2014.
6. Barkun AN, Bardou M, Kuipers RJ, et al. International consensus recommendations on the management of patients with nonvariceal upper gastrointestinal bleeding. *Ann Intern Med* 2010;152:101–113.
7. Srygley FD, Geradao CJ, Tran T, et al. Does this patient have a severe upper gastrointestinal bleed. *JAMA* 2012;307:1072–1079.

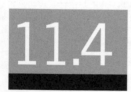

11.4 Cholelithiasis and Cholecystitis

Cayce Onks, Eric M. Pauli

ASYMPTOMATIC CHOLELITHIASIS
Background

Definition
- Asymptomatic gallstones are those discovered incidentally by abdominal imaging (ultrasonography [US] or computed tomography [CT]) being performed for unrelated symptoms or diseases. Patients will have no symptoms attributable to the presence of cholelithiasis.

Anatomy
- The gallbladder is an elongated pear-shaped sac (7 to 10 cm long, 2.5 to 3.5 cm wide) that stores and concentrates bile and releases it in response to a meal.
- A moderately distended gallbladder can contain 50 to 60 mL of bile, but may become much larger (300 mL) with pathological processes.
- The gallbladder is lined by simple columnar epithelium that is responsible for the active absorption of water used to concentrate bile.

Epidemiology
- The prevalence of asymptomatic gall stones varies with age, sex, race, and ethnicity. Screening ultrasound studies of select populations suggests an overall incidence of 5% to 21%.[1,2] Overall rates are higher in females, individuals in the seventh decade of life and in individuals of Hispanic descent (as compared to white, black, or Asian).[3]

Pathophysiology
- Conjugated bile salts, lecithin, and cholesterol comprise 80% to 95% of solids dissolved in bile.
- Cholesterol solubility depends on the relative concentration of cholesterol, bile salts, and phospholipids.
- Imbalances in these concentrations result in precipitation of cholesterol crystals, which, over time, results in gallstone formation.
- Gallstones may occur due to high biliary cholesterol concentration, defective formation of micelles, cholesterol crystal nucleation factor excess (e.g., calcium), deficiency of anti-nucleating factors (e.g., lecithin), delayed gallbladder emptying, or excessive biliary excretion of bile (hemolytic anemia).[4]

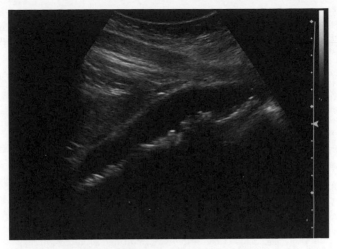

Figure 11.4-1. Longitudinal ultrasound view of the gallbladder demonstrating multiple dependent hyperechoic structures with posterior shadowing artifact consistent with multiple small gallstones.

Diagnosis

Clinical Presentation
- Asymptomatic gallstones are usually discovered incidentally on abdominal imaging (x-ray, US, or CT) or at the time of surgery for nonbiliary tract disease.

History
- Unremarkable, except for the risk factors noted above.

Physical Examination
- Generally unremarkable; however, stigmata of associated diseases may be found (cirrhosis, obesity, anemia, diabetes, etc.).

Laboratory Studies
- Generally unremarkable; however, abnormalities of associated diseases may be found (e.g., anemia from hemolysis).

Imaging
- Abdominal US, CT scan, or x-ray demonstrates gallstones (Figure 11.4-1).

Monitoring
- The majority of patients with asymptomatic cholelithiasis can be managed expectantly, no additional testing or follow-up is warranted.[5]
  - Only 1% to 4% becomes symptomatic each year.[6]
  - 60% to 70% of patients will never develop symptoms.[5]

Treatment

Medications
- Medical therapy for gallstones with oral bile acid therapy is generally not recommended for asymptomatic patients.

Protocol
- Recommendations for the treatment of gallstones have been developed by the Society for Surgery of the Alimentary Tract (http://www.ssat.com/cgi-bin/chole7.cgi) and by the Society of American Gastrointestinal and Endoscopic Surgeons (http://www.sages.org/publications/guidelines/guidelines-for-the-clinical-application-of-laparoscopic-biliary-tract-surgery/).

Surgery
- Prophylactic cholecystectomy is not indicated for asymptomatic patients, including patients with hemolytic anemia, patients undergoing bariatric surgery, and those with comorbid conditions (diabetes, cirrhosis, hemolytic anemia).
- Surgical referral is appropriate once symptoms begin, as recurrent symptoms develop in 70% to 80%.[5] Biliary colic is the presenting symptom in the majority of patients (see Symptomatic Cholelithiasis below).
- Complications (acute cholecystitis, cholangitis, and pancreatitis) generally occur after symptom onset; these are uncommonly the initial presenting symptom.
- Cholecystectomy for asymptomatic patients with a calcified ("porcelain") gallbladder or with gallstones larger than 3 cm should be considered due to a higher risk of gall bladder cancer in these patients.

Counseling
- Patients should be reassured that no surgery is indicated for asymptomatic cholelithiasis.
- Patients should be advised to seek medical care if they develop symptoms of acute cholecystitis, cholangitis, or pancreatitis (see below).

Patient Education
- American Academy of Family Physicians: http://familydoctor.org/familydoctor/en/diseases-conditions/gallstones.html
- American Gastroenterological Association: http://www.gastro.org/patient-center/digestive-conditions/gallstones
- National Institutes of Health, National Digestive Diseases Information Clearinghouse: http://digestive.niddk.nih.gov/ddiseases/pubs/gallstones/index.aspx

SYMPTOMATIC CHOLELITHIASIS
General Principles
Definition
- The term symptomatic cholelithiasis is applied to gallstones to which patient symptoms can be attributed. Although this definition is somewhat simplistic, determining whether a patient's foregut symptoms are the result of gallstones or alternate pathophysiology (e.g., peptic ulcer disease, reflux esophagitis, gastroparesis, etc.) can be challenging.

Epidemiology
- As noted above, the majority of patients with cholelithiasis have no symptoms; however, the 15-year cumulative probability of developing symptoms (biliary colic or other complications) is 18% of initially asymptomatic patients.[5] Patients with symptomatic cholelithiasis are at a higher risk for developing gallstone-related complications (acute cholecystitis, biliary pancreatitis) than those without symptoms.[7]
- Patients with symptomatic cholelithiasis follow one of the following three clinical courses:
  1. Resolution of symptoms is seen in >50% of patients in one study, and is facilitated by avoiding exacerbating factors (i.e., fatty foods).[8]
  2. Symptoms may persist or worsen.
  3. Patients may develop gallstone-related complications, including choledocholithiasis, acute cholelithiasis, cholangitis, and acute biliary pancreatitis. Acute cholecystitis is the most common severe complication of gallstones, developing in 1% to 3% of patients with symptomatic cholelithiasis per year.[9]

Pathophysiology
- Pain related to gallstones typically occurs when a stone transiently obstructs the infundibulum–cystic duct junction, resulting in a partial obstruction of the gallbladder.
- Cholecystokinin-induced gallbladder emptying is inhibited, and contraction in the setting of an obstruction results in pain from significant increases in pressure within the gallbladder.

Diagnosis
Clinical Presentation
- The classic description of biliary colic is sudden onset right upper quadrant (RUQ) or epigastric pain that radiates to the back or right shoulder.

- Pain typically lasts less than 1 hour, and is commonly associated with nausea, vomiting, and diaphoresis.
- Pain is usually described as an intense dull pressure and is less commonly identified as true colic (sharp, intermittent, or spasmodic pain).
- Pain usually occurs postprandial (especially meals with high fat content) or at night.

History
- Patients may have a known history of asymptomatic cholelithiasis or may present with biliary colic as their initial presenting symptom of cholelithiasis.

Physical Examination
- Generally unremarkable; however, stigmata of associated diseases may be found. Patients may have residual RUQ pain on palpation.
- Fever or tachycardia suggests the development of complicated gallstone disease.

Laboratory Studies
- Generally unremarkable; however, abnormalities of associated diseases may be found (e.g., anemia from hemolysis).
- Leukocytosis, transaminitis, or elevations in amylase and lipase suggest the development of complicated gallstone disease.

Imaging
- Ultrasound has an 84% sensitivity and a 99% specificity for detecting gallstones and is the diagnostic test of choice for diagnosing gallstones and their complications (Figure 11.4-1).[10]

Monitoring
- Patients with symptomatic cholelithiasis should be referred to a surgeon for consideration of elective cholecystectomy.
- Patients who elect to undergo observation of their symptomatic cholelithiasis (rather than surgery) require no additional monitoring or testing in the absence of new or changing symptoms.

Pathologic Findings
- Gallstones will be seen on pathologic examination of the gallbladder (Figure 11.4-2). Pathological alterations of the gallbladder itself, including chronic inflammation and wall thickening, may also be noted.

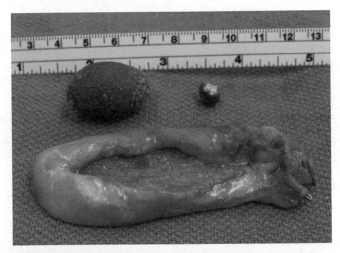

Figure 11.4-2. Operative photo of a large and a small gallstone from a patient with postprandial biliary colic undergoing cholecystectomy. The opened gallbladder with a thickened wall is in the foreground.

Differential Diagnosis
- The differential diagnosis of symptomatic cholelithiasis should include any upper abdominal and foregut disease, including gastroesophageal reflux, peptic ulcer disease, pancreatitis, complicated gallstone disease, and hepatitis. Small bowel and colon pathology (such as irritable bowel or inflammatory bowel disorders) should also be considered.

Treatment

Medications
- Pain management
  - Nonsteroidal anti-inflammatory drugs (NSAIDs) have a proven benefit in alleviating pain associated with gallstones.[11]
    - Oral ibuprofen or intravenous (IV) ketorolac can be utilized in the chronic and acute setting settings, respectively.
  - Narcotics are also utilized in the management of symptomatic cholelithiasis.
    - Oral oxycodone or IV morphine can be utilized in the chronic and acute settings, respectively.
- Dissolution therapy
  - Oral bile salt therapy with ursodeoxycholic acid works best on pure cholesterol stones. The presence of calcium (and calcium salts) within the stones limits the effectiveness of dissolution therapy.
  - Oral dissolution therapy works best with:
    - Patients with minimal symptoms, small, non-calcified stones (<1 cm) and an otherwise normal functioning gallbladder.[12]

Surgery
- Laparoscopic cholecystectomy is recommended for patients with symptomatic cholelithiasis.
- Newer methods of laparoscopic surgery, including robotic assisted laparoscopy, single-incision laparoscopy or natural orifice (transvaginal) surgery, may be offered to select patients.
- Open cholecystectomy may be necessary in some patients due to previous surgical history or due to problems encountered during an attempted laparoscopic cholecystectomy.

Results
- 92% of patients with symptomatic cholelithiasis will have resolution of their symptoms following cholecystectomy.[13]
  - Patients with atypical gallstone symptoms (gas bloat, belching, lower abdominal pain) are less likely to have complete symptom resolution.

Counseling
- The decision to perform surgery for symptomatic cholelithiasis depends on the degree of symptoms, the patient's surgical risk (age, body mass index, comorbid conditions, and past surgical history), and their willingness to tolerate risk.
  - Risk of surgical complications from cholecystectomy (~2%, one time).
  - Risk of developing an acute gallstone-related problem (~3% per year) that may require a more complex series of procedures.

Special Considerations
- Expectant observation, dietary modification, or medical dissolution therapy may be recommended for patients who are poor surgical candidates.
- Pregnant patients with symptomatic cholelithiasis are generally managed expectantly unless their symptoms are severe or result in failure to gain weight as the pregnancy progresses. In these cases, elective cholecystectomy should be performed during the second trimester.

Patient Education
- Society of American Gastrointestinal and Endoscopic Surgeons: http://www.sages.org/publications/patient-information/patient-information-for-laparoscopic-gallbladder-removal-cholecystectomy-from-sages/

ACUTE CHOLECYSTITIS
General Principles

Definition
- Sudden onset inflammation and infection resulting from complete obstruction of gallbladder emptying.

Epidemiology
- Develops in 1% to 3% of patients with symptomatic cholelithiasis per year.[9]

Pathophysiology
- Obstruction of the cystic duct with a gallstone results in acute inflammation and infection of the gallbladder.

Etiology
- Obstruction of the cystic duct results in gallbladder distention and bile stasis. Propagation of a cytokine cascade furthers the inflammatory process. Some (but not all) patients develop an infection within the gallbladder itself, typically with enteric organisms.

Diagnosis

Clinical Presentation
- Patients complain of fever and RUQ or epigastric pain radiating to the back or shoulder. They may have associated nausea, vomiting, and diaphoresis. Pain may be more intense and longer (hours) in duration than prior bouts of biliary colic.

History
- The majority of patients will have a history of symptomatic cholelithiasis (although a formal diagnosis may or may not have been made).

Physical Examination
- A wide variety of findings may be present depending on the degree of the systemic inflammatory response.
  - Fever, tachycardia, and focal RUQ peritoneal signs are common findings.
  - Hypotension and diffuse peritoneal signs suggest sepsis from a severe infection (gangrene or perforation of the gallbladder).
- Cessation of inspiration during palpation over the gallbladder (Murphy's sign) is sensitive (97%) but not specific (48%) for acute cholecystitis.[14]

Laboratory Studies
- Leukocytosis with a left shifted differential is common.
- Mild transaminitis, hyperbilirubinemia, and alkaline phosphatase elevations are common and non-specific.

Imaging
- US will demonstrate gallstones, gallbladder wall edema and thickening (>4 mm), and pericholicystic fluid. The sonographer may also elicit a "sonographic Murphy's sign" during the examination.
- Scintigraphy using 99mTc-hepatic iminodiacetic acid (HIDA) scan is utilized when the diagnosis is not clear following US. In acute cholecystitis, the gallbladder will not be visualized because radiotracer will not enter it due to cystic duct obstruction.
- Many patients have a CT scan performed, although this is generally unnecessary unless it is being used to evaluate for alternative pathologic diagnoses. The scan may demonstrate pericholicystic fluid, inflammatory stranding, gallbladder wall thickening, and possibly gallstones (Figure 11.4-3).

Monitoring
- Acute cholecystitis warrants urgent medical treatment. Patients should be referred to an acute care facility for diagnostic studies, medical management, and surgical consultation.

Pathologic Findings
- Gallstones, gallbladder wall thickening, edema, inflammation, and ischemia are all common pathologic findings on gallbladder specimens.

Differential Diagnosis
- Perforated viscus, acute appendicitis, cholangitis, hepatitis, acute pancreatitis, pelvic inflammatory disease (with peri-hepatitis), and diverticulitis should all be in the differential diagnosis of acute cholecystitis.

Treatment

Medications
- Narcotic pain medications are the preferred mode of analgesia.
- While there are data to suggest that NSAIDs may reduce the inflammatory reaction, many of these agents (e.g., ketorolac) increase the bleeding risk during operative intervention, and therefore should be avoided.

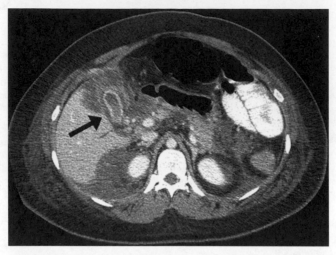

Figure 11.4-3. CT scan of a patient with acute cholecystitis. There is fluid and stranding surrounding the gallbladder (*arrow*) with gallbladder wall thickening.

- Broad-spectrum penicillins or cephalosporins are the empiric antibiotics of choice and have been shown to reduce septic complications.[15]

Surgery
- Laparoscopic cholecystectomy remains the procedure of choice for acute cholecystitis, although the risk for conversion to an open procedure is somewhat higher in the setting of an acute inflammatory response.

Results
- Mortality following cholecystectomy for acute infection is 0.5%, whereas morbidity ranges from 5% to 20%.[16]

Special Considerations
- Patients who are unfit surgical candidates should undergo percutaneous decompression of the gallbladder with a cholecystostomy tube, which may be placed under local anesthesia only.
- Pregnant patients with acute cholecystitis should undergo cholecystectomy.

CHRONIC CHOLECYSTITIS
General Principles
Defined
- Recurrent inflammatory process involving the gallbladder.[16]

Epidemiology
- Approximately 25% of persons with gallstones eventually develop chronic cholecystitis, although most remain asymptomatic.[2]

Pathophysiology
- Subepithelial fibrosis and mononuclear cell infiltrate with resultant scarring and dysfunction of the gallbladder.[16]

Etiology
- Thought to be intermittent obstruction of the cystic duct by gallstone.[16]

Diagnosis
Clinical Presentation
- Many times asymptomatic or with radiographic evidence of gallstones.

History
- Episodic RUQ pain with radiation to the back or right scapula. Nausea and vomiting associated 60% to 70% of the time.[16]
- Episodes lasting 1 to 5 hours distinguishing it from acute cholecystitis.
- May be associated with pain after meals, dyspepsia, flatulence, and fatty food intolerance although this is less specific for gallbladder disease.[17]
- Patient feels well between attacks.

Physical Examination
- Usually a normal physical examination when not having attacks.
- May have mild RUQ tenderness.

Laboratory Studies
- Liver function test is typically normal in asymptomatic disease.

Imaging
- US—study of choice due to its high sensitive (95% to 98%) for gallstones.
- Abdominal radiographs are less helpful; only 10% to 15% of gallstones will be calcified enough to be identified.
- CT—only 50% of gallstones are identified due to the fact that most are isodense with bile.[16]

Differential Diagnosis
- Acute cholecystitis, asymptomatic cholelithiasis, peptic ulcer disease, biliary dyskinesia, pancreatitis, acute hepatitis, appendicitis, hepatic abscess, acute renal pathology, right-sided pneumonia, myocardial infarction

Treatment

Medications
- Dissolution therapy can be considered in nonsurgical candidates or patients who refuse surgery.
- Bile acid salts may provide dissolution (as described above).
  - 40% to 60% success after 12 to 24 months with carefully selected patients.
  - 25% to 50% will recur within 5 years. Therefore, should consider maintenance therapy.[17]

Surgery
- Elective laparoscopic cholecystectomy is the treatment of choice.

Results
- Mortality <0.3% in the United States.
- <10% of patients with complications.
- 90% will be symptom free following surgery.[13]

Special Considerations
- Persistent RUQ pain, chills, or fevers suggestive of choledocholithiasis, cholangitis, or other biliary diseases.
- Pregnancy with chronic cholecystitis is managed conservatively until delivery unless severe metabolic changes or symptomatology exist.
- Patients with chronic cholecystitis undergoing other surgical procedures should have consideration given to concomitant cholecystectomy if appropriate.

ACALCULOUS CHOLECYSTITIS
General Principles

Definition
- Acute or chronic signs and symptoms of biliary colic or cholecystitis in the absence of gallstones.

Epidemiology
- A slim minority (<1%) of patients with presentation of cholecystitis.

Pathophysiology
- Unclear for acute acalculous cholecystitis but appears that gallbladder stasis and progression to ischemia can play a causative role and course typically complicated with gangrene, perforation, and peritonitis.[16]

- Association with critically ill individuals who have had major surgeries, trauma, and burns, or who have required long-term parenteral nutrition.[16]
- Chronic acalculous cholecystitis may be associated with biliary dyskinesia.[16]

Diagnosis
Clinical Presentation
- Acute acalculous cholecystitis—acute RUQ pain and fever almost exclusively in a critically ill patient.
- Chronic acalculous cholecystitis—intermittent biliary colic (RUQ pain, food intolerance, and nausea).
- Presentation may be severely delayed due to the critical illness of the patient or due to atypical symptoms.

Physical Examination
- Fever.
- RUQ pain may be difficult to elicit in the critically ill patient.
- May be normal in chronic acalculous cholecystitis.

Laboratory Studies
- Leukocytosis.
- Could have complicated picture with associated critical illness.
- Abnormal metabolic studies and coagulation panel in septic shock and multiorgan failure.
- May be normal in chronic acalculous cholecystitis.

Imaging
- US and CT findings with gallbladder wall thickening and pericholecystic fluid in the absence of gallstones.[16]
- HIDA scan has a controversial roll in chronic acalculous cholecystitis, but an ejection fraction <35% at 20 minutes felt to be abnormal.[16]

Treatment
Medication
- Same as for acute calculous cholecystitis.
- Recognized high incidence of gangrene and empyema (>50%) warrants broad-spectrum antibiotic coverage.[16]

Surgery
- Cholecystectomy is warranted for a high suspicion or confirmed diagnosis.
- Timing of surgery is highly dependent on clinical scenario of a critical ill patient.
- Cholecystostomy tube should be placed in patients unfit for surgical cholecystectomy.

Results
- Mortality for acute acalculous cholecystitis is high at 40% typically because of concomitant disease as well as the delayed diagnosis of gallbladder infection.[16]

CHOLEDOCHOLITHIASIS
General Principles
Definition
- The presence of a gallstone within the biliary tree (e.g., common bile duct [CBD], common hepatic duct, etc.)

Anatomy
- The CBD is formed by the junction of the common hepatic duct and cystic duct. It is 3 to 4 cm in length passing commonly through the pancreas to its insertion into the second portion of the duodenum. Its diameter is 5 to 13 mm.[18]

Epidemiology
- Incidence of CBD stones seen before or during cholecystectomy is approximately 12%.[19] Fifteen percent of CBD stones are found in combination with gallstones.[20] It is felt that 73% will pass spontaneously.[20]

Pathophysiology
- Stones can become obstructive in the lower end of the CBD and the tapered portion within the pancreas and ampulla. A ball-valve mechanism can also occur where the stone falls back into the CBD after failing to pass.[19]

• Complete or partial obstruction can cause accumulation of bacteria, ischemia, and necrosis. Infection can lead to as ascending cholangitis. Ischemia and necrosis lead to chronic stricture formation.

Diagnosis

History and Clinical Presentation

• RUQ pain or biliary colic radiating to the back or scapula.[19]
• More commonly can be found silent or at the time of cholecystectomy.
• Patients can present with complications such as obstructive jaundice, pancreatitis, or ascending cholangitis. Presentation can be biliary pain (steady, increasing, >4 to 6 hours, right scapular radiation), jaundice, and fevers. Progression to mental status changes and hypotension may represent acute suppurative cholangitis.[19]
• Predictors of CBD stone: cholangitis, ultrasound findings (stone, CBD dilation), jaundice, hyperbilirubinemia, elevated alkaline phosphatase, pancreatitis, cholecystitis, elevated amylase, or lipase.[21]

Physical Examination

• Typically normal unless complication. Depending on the complication, patients could present with fevers, hypotension, tachycardia, jaundice, RUQ pain, epigastric pain, pruritus, tea-colored urine, and acholic stools.

Laboratory Studies

• Elevated serum bilirubin, alkaline phosphatase, transaminases, and γ-glutamyl transpeptidase. Because liver function assays can be elevated in a variety of diseases, the positive predictive value of these tests is overall low, but the negative predictive value of normal tests is high and is useful to exclude choledocholithiasis.
• Leukocytosis.
• Positive blood cultures are possible in cholangitis.
• Elevated pancreatic enzymes in suspected biliary pancreatitis.
• Urine bilirubin.

Imaging

• Ultrasound—23% to 80% detected depending on body habitus and operator experience.[22]
• CT—75% sensitivity for showing CBD stones with obstruction.[23]
• Endoscopic ultrasound—93% sensitive and 97% specific.[24]
• MRI cholangiopancreatography is 95% sensitive and 89% specific for choledocholithiasis.[25]

Surgical Diagnostic Procedures

• Intraoperative cholangiography (IOC) is useful for diagnosing CBD stones in patients undergoing cholecystectomy. It has a high sensitivity and specificity, but is highly operator dependent.
• Endoscopic retrograde cholangiopancreatography (ERCP) is uncommonly used solely as a diagnostic tool for choledocholithiasis due to the risk of post-ERCP pancreatitis.

Treatment

Medication

• No medical treatment regimens recommended specifically for the treatment of choledocholithiasis.
• Medical management of symptomatic CBD stone revolves around clinical scenario.
• Pain management—IV opioid analgesics.
• Preoperative—NPO, IV fluids, electrolyte correction, anticoagulant recognition, and management.
• Cholangitis—broad-spectrum antibiotics with coverage for Enterobacteriaceae (68%), Enterococci (14%), Bacteroides (10%), and Clostridium (7%); anti-pseudomonal penicillin β-lactamase inhibitor (e.g., piperacillin/tazobactam); or in life-threatening scenarios carbapenems.[26]

Surgery

• The mode of stone removal depends on when the stone is discovered.
  • If choledocholithiasis is identified before or after cholecystectomy, ERCP is generally considered the therapeutic procedure of choice (Figure 11.4-4).
  • If choledocholithiasis is identified on an IOC, treatment will depend on surgeon's preference, clinical scenario, and health care facility resources.
    • Options include laparoscopic or open CBD exploration (transcystic or via a choledochotomy) or an ERCP performed intraoperatively or postoperatively.

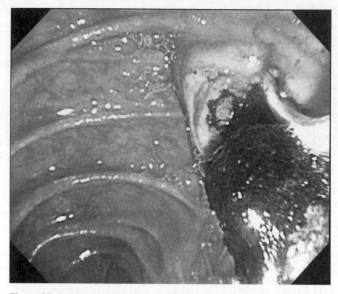

Figure 11.4-4. Endoscopic view of balloon extraction of common bile duct stone extraction from the ampulla of Vater during ERCP.

Special Considerations
- Mortality rate of cholangitis in association with CBD stones is 2% to 5%.[16]
- CBD stones account for 50% of all cases of pancreatitis.[16]

REFERENCES

1. Barbara L, Sama C, Morselli Labate AM, et al. A population study on the prevalence of gallstone disease: the Sirmione Study. *Hepatology* 1987;7:913–917.
2. Glambek I, Kvaale G, Arnesjö B, et al. Prevalence of gallstones in a Norwegian population. *Scand J Gastroenterol* 1987;22:1089–1098.
3. Everhart JE, Khare M, Hill M, et al. Prevalence and ethnic differences in gallbladder disease in the United States. *Gastroenterology* 1999;117:632–639.
4. Venneman NG, Erpecum K. Pathogenesis of gallstones. *Gastroenterol Clin N Am* 2010;39:171–183.
5. Gracie WA, Ransohoff DF. The natural history of silent gallstones: the innocent gallstone is not a myth. *N Engl J Med* 1982;307:798–800.
6. Beckingham IJ. Gallstone disease. *BMJ* 2001;322:91–94.
7. Friedman GD, Raviola CA, Fireman B. Prognosis of gallstones with mild or no symptoms: 25 years of follow-up in a health maintenance organization. *J Clin Epidemiol* 1989;42:127–136.
8. Festi D, Reggiani ML, Attili AF, et al. Natural history of gallstone disease: Expectant management or active treatment? Results from a population-based cohort study. *J Gastroenterol Hepatol* 2010;25:719–724.
9. Friedman GD. Natural history of asymptomatic and symptomatic gallstones. *Am J Surg* 1993;165:399–404.
10. Shea JA, Berlin JA, Escarce JJ, et al. Revised estimates of diagnostic test sensitivity and specificity in suspected biliary tract disease. *Arch Intern Med* 1994;154:2573–2581.
11. Colli A, Conte D, Valle SD, et al. Meta-analysis: nonsteroidal anti-inflammatory drugs in biliary colic. *Aliment Pharmacol Ther* 2012;35:1370–1378.
12. Tomida S, Abei M, Yamaguchi T, et al. Long-term ursodeoxycholic acid therapy is associated with reduced risk of biliary pain and acute cholecystitis in patients with gallbladder stones: a cohort analysis. *Hepatology* 1999;30:6–13.
13. Berger MY, Olde Hartman TC, Bohnen AM. Abdominal symptoms: do they disappear after cholecystectomy? *Surg Endosc* 2003;17:1723–1728.
14. Singer AJ, McCracken G, Henry MC, et al. Correlation among clinical, laboratory, and hepatobiliary scanning findings in patients with suspected acute cholecystitis. *Ann Emerg Med* 1996;28:267–272.

15. Indar A, Beckingham I. Acute cholecystitis. *BMJ* 2002;325:639–643.
16. Pitt H, Ahrendt S, Nakeeb A. Calculous biliary disease. In: Mulholland M, Lillemoe K, Doherty G, et al., eds. *Greenfield's surgery-principles and practice.* 5th ed. Philadelphia, PA: Lippincott Williams & Wilkins; 2011:960–980.
17. Vincent E. Cholelithiasis and cholecystitis. In: Paulman P, Paulman A, Harrison J, eds. *Taylor's manual of family medicine.* 3rd ed. Philadelphia, PA: Lippincott Williams & Wilkins; 2008:373–380.
18. Strasberg S. Hepatic, biliary, and pancreatic anatomy. In: Garden O, Parks R, eds. *Hepatobiliary and pancreatic surgery.* 5th ed. Edinburgh: Saunders Elsevier; 2014:17–38.
19. Nathanson L. Gallstones. In: Garden O, Parks R, eds. *Hepatobiliary and pancreatic surgery.* 5th ed. Edinburgh: Saunders Elsevier; 2014:174–195.
20. Bellows C, Berger D, Crass R. Management of gallstones. *Am Fam Physician* 2005;72:637–642.
21. Abboud BA, Malet PF, Berlin JA, et al. Predictors of common bile duct stones prior to cholecystectomy: a meta-analysis. *Gastrointest Endosc* 1996;44:450.
22. Lindsel DR. Ultrasound imaging of pancreas and biliary tract. *Lancet* 1990;335:390–393.
23. Baroll RL. Common bile duct stones. Reassessment of criteria for CT diagnosis. *Radiology* 1987;162:419–424.
24. Prat F, Amouyal G, Amouyal P, et al. Prospective controlled study of endoscopic ultrasonography and endoscopic retrograde cholangiography in patients with suspected common bile duct lithiasis. *Lancet* 1996;347:75–79.
25. Hochwalk SN, Dobransky M, Rofsky NM, et al. Magnetic resonance cholangiopancreatography accurately predicts the presence or absence of choledocholithiasis. *J Gastrointest Surg* 1998;2:573–579.
26. Chambers H, Gilbert D, Eliopoulos G, et al. *The sanford guide of antimicrobial therapy v.3.09.* 43rd ed. In-App Subscription. Accessed February 28, 2014.

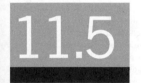

11.5 Viral Hepatitis

Jarrett K. Sell, Abraham R. Taylor

GENERAL PRINCIPLES

Definition

Hepatitis is defined as inflammation of the liver and can be caused by many etiologies. This chapter explores viral causes of hepatitis, which can cause both acute and chronic liver diseases. Differentiation of the exact viral cause is essential in the management of viral hepatitis, since each virus varies significantly in its mode of transmission, prevention, treatment, and clinical course.

Epidemiology and Classification

Hepatitis A

The hepatitis A virus (HAV) is a ribonucleic acid (RNA) enveloped picornavirus that has greatly declined in incidence to less than 10% of viral hepatitis infections since the introduction of progressive U.S. vaccine recommendations in 1996. The virus is spread via the fecal–oral route, and the average incubation period is 28 days (range, 15 to 50 days). As many as 70% of children under 6 years of age may be asymptomatic with a minority of young children presenting with jaundice. Adults and older children, on the other hand, are typically symptomatic, with approximately 70% presenting with jaundice. HAV infection is a self-limited disease with symptom resolution typically in 2 months without progression to chronic infection.

The virus is shed in the stool and primarily spread by contaminated water or food, personal contact, and drug use. Sexual contact, particularly in men who have sex with men (MSM), can also transmit the virus. The incidence rate of hepatitis A infection is 0.4 cases per 100,000 persons and accounted for an estimated 2,800 new infections in 2011.[1] Rates of infection are slightly higher in Hispanics and Asian/Pacific Islanders, but men and women have similar rates. Although travel, household contacts, daycare centers, and intravenous drug use are risk factors for infection, over half of reported infections report no risk behaviors or exposures for hepatitis A during the 2 to 6 weeks prior to infection.

Hepatitis B

Hepatitis B virus (HBV) is a DNA double-stranded hepadnavirus that is present in blood and other bodily fluids. HPV is very efficiently transmitted via contact with infected serum, with needle-stick exposures to HBV-contaminated needles, resulting in disease in 6% to 24% of cases.[2] Relatively resilient, HBV can survive for up to 7 days outside of a human host.[3] The incubation period for HBV is typically 2 to 3 months (range of 6 weeks to 6 months), which can then result in acute, symptomatic illness in 30% to 50% of all individuals. However, children younger than 5 years and immunosuppressed persons are more likely to be asymptomatic.[3] Risk of progression from acute to chronic infection is typically inversely proportional to age with the greatest risk occurring in infants at 90%; likewise, the risk of chronic infection after acute infection reduces to about 5% in individuals over 5 years of age.[3]

Since the implementation of a national vaccination program for HBV in the 1990s, the incidence of acute HBV infection in the United States has significantly declined. Specifically, reported annual incidence of acute HBV dropped from 11.5 cases per 100,000 population in 1985 to 1.6 cases per 100,000 population in 2006.[3,4] At a 98% reduction, the decline was highest for those under 15 years old, for whom universal infant vaccination or childhood catch-up vaccination was recommended.[4] Notwithstanding this success in primary prevention, the burden of chronic infection with HBV still affects an estimated 800,000 to 1.4 million members of the United States.[3] Prior to HBV vaccination, about 30% to 40% of these cases occurred through maternal–fetal transmission, particularly in women of Asian descent where disease prevalence is high. In the United States, estimated annual deaths due to chronic HBV from associated liver diseases such as failure, cirrhosis, and hepatocellular cancer range from 2,000 to 4,000 deaths per year.[3] For acute infection, case fatality rates in the United States are approximately 1% due to fulminant hepatic failure.[4]

Hepatitis C

Approximately 3.2 million persons in the United States are chronically infected with the hepatitis C virus (HCV), making it the most common blood-borne infection in the nation. Prevalence is highest at 3.25% in those of the "baby boomer generation" born between 1945 and 1965, which accounts for three-fourths of all HCV infections and 73% of HCV-associated mortality.[5] Those with additional risk factors and higher prevalence also include those with a history of intravenous drug use, 20 or more lifetime sexual partners, blood transfusion before 1992, men, non-Hispanic blacks, and prison inmates. Fifty-seven percent of patients aged 20 to 59 years who had ever used injection drugs were found to have antibodies to HCV, making it the greatest predictor of risk.[6] However, over half of patients infected with HCV are unaware of their infection and have never been tested for HCV.[7]

Sixty to 70% of persons newly infected with the HCV are typically asymptomatic or have mild symptoms that do not prompt them to seek medical attention, making reporting of acute HCV infections and risk for chronic infection, which develops in 75% to 85% of acutely infected persons, challenging. The incidence of HCV infection increased steadily in the 1980s with a peak incidence of 380,000.[8] Subsequently, the incidence has declined as HCV was identified in 1988 and sensitive blood screening was developed and implemented in 1992. According to the Centers for Disease Control and Prevention[1] in 2011, there were 1,229 reported cases of acute HCV, representing an estimated 16,500 (7,200 to 43,400) actual acute cases.[1] This is a 45% increase in 2011 compared with 2010 after 6 years of little change in incidence. The increase is attributed to increase HCV infections among adolescents and young adults with risk factors that include persons who have used injection drugs or opioids, are white, and live in nonurban areas. Unfortunately, lack of diagnosis, linkage to care, and treatment for those that are chronically infected allow for continued transmission of HCV and continued morbidity and mortality due to hepatitis C infection. By 2007, HCV infection superseded human immunodeficiency virus (HIV) as a cause of death in the United States, and HCV infection is currently the number one cause for liver transplantation.[9]

The HCV is most efficiently transmitted though percutaneous exposure to blood, with transfusion of unscreened blood or use of injection drugs presenting the greatest risk. Infection can also occur less commonly via occupational, perinatal, and sexual transmission. Healthcare workers are at particular occupational risk, with a 1.8% risk of HCV infection after a needle injury[10] and greatest risk with deep injuries and procedures, which involve placement of a hollow-bore needle in the source patient's vein or artery. The risk of maternal–fetal vertical transmission has been estimated to be 4.3% in mothers with HCV RNA present, with a higher rate of 19.4% in HIV-coinfected mothers.[11] Method of delivery and breast feeding has not been shown to affect risk.

Sexual transmission has traditionally been thought to be rare. However, persons with multiple sex partners, MSM, or those who are coinfected with HIV are at higher risk for sexual transmission.[12,13] Therefore, sexual transmission of HCV can occur but is much less efficient than by the percutaneous route.

Hepatitis D

Dependent on the viral mechanisms of HBV to replicate, the hepatitis D virus (HDV) infection must have requisite HBV coinfection. HDV interferes with HBV replication, making viral burden of HBV typically less. In the United States, HDV infection is predominantly in those receiving multiple blood products and users of intravenous drugs; however, HDV is endemic in the Mediterranean, Asia, and the Pacific islands. Approximately 5% of HBsAg-positive individuals are coinfected with HDV.[14] HDV complicates HBV disease and can lead to earlier disease progression and a more complicated clinical course.

Hepatitis E

Hepatitis E virus (HEV) is a single-stranded RNA virus transmitted via fecal–oral transmission that typically causes only acute liver inflammation; however, immunosuppressed persons may have difficulty with clearance. To date, chronic HEV infection has been shown only in developing countries in persons who are immunosuppressed from solid organ transplantation.[15] This disease is typically most prevalent in Asia, Africa, Middle East, and Central America. Incubation times vary from 15 to 60 days postexposure (mean of 40 days). Serologic evidence of exposure in the United States may be around 21%, and reasons why clinically meaningful symptomatic infection is not more frequently recognized are unclear.[16]

Other Viral Etiologies of Hepatitis

Multiple other viruses can cause liver inflammation as part of a broader viral syndrome and can be classified as non-hepatotropic, meaning they do not have particular predilection for hepatic tissue. Some alternative viral etiologies include herpes-type viruses such as Epstein–Barr virus (EBV), cytomegalovirus (CMV), varicella zoster virus (HZV), and herpes simplex. Other alternative viral etiologies include flaviviruses such as yellow fever virus and Dengue fever virus; non-polio enteroviruses such as cocksackie and echovirus; filioviruses including Ebola virus and Marburg virus; adenoviruses; Parvovirus B19; severe acute respiratory syndrome (SARS) virus; influenza virus; measles; rubella; and others. Only several of these warrant special attention.

Of the herpes viruses, EBV typically causes a syndrome referred to as mononucleosis, common in adolescents, which can cause hepatosplenomegaly with rash, fatigue, and exudative pharyngitis. Diagnosis is confirmed with predominance of atypical lymphocytes on complete blood count and the presence of heterophile antibodies. CMV can cause a similar syndrome that is heterophile-negative and plays an important role in hepatitis post-solid-organ transplant, where the immunosuppressant medications allow CMV infection to not infrequently cause acute/chronic graft injury and dysfunction. For instance, in liver transplant patients, antivirals and immunoglobulin may help prevent organ failure during CMV hepatitis of a liver graft. CMV infections in transplant recipients may be primary—CMV-seronegative patients receiving donor organ from CMV-seropositive patients—or secondary—CMV-positive recipients with reactivation after immunosuppression. Superinfection is also possible where reinfection occurs in CMV-seropositive recipients.

DIAGNOSIS

History

Initial evaluation of persons with suspected viral hepatitis infection should include a thorough discussion about ethnicity, country of birth, occupation, travel, close contacts, potential food or water exposures, and past and future high risk behaviors. Particular focus should be placed on drug use, receipt of blood products or an organ transplant before 1992, history of incarceration, previous sexually transmitted infections, HIV testing, and sexual practices. Prior or present symptoms of acute or chronic liver disease such as fever, fatigue, anorexia, abdominal pain, nausea, vomiting, dark urine, clay-colored stools, jaundice, rash, or arthralgias should be obtained. Acute infection may be asymptomatic depending on the viral etiology and age of the patient. Chronic infection is initially asymptomatic; but, as cirrhosis and subsequent liver failure develops, symptoms may include malaise, weight loss, abdominal swelling, jaundice, pruritus, bruising, bleeding, edema, or confusion. In addition, patients should be screened for alcohol use and questioned regarding hepatotoxic drugs or supplements. Those being considered for treatment should also have a thorough psychological evaluation and assessment for cardiopulmonary disease as well as other comorbidities.

Physical Examination

During a comprehensive physical examination, particular attention for signs of acute or chronic HCV infection would include a detailed skin examination looking for jaundice, nail changes, ecchymosis, petechiae, palmar erythema, or spider hemangiomata, which are typically found on the chest or shoulders. Men should be examined for gynecomastia or hypogonadism. During the abdominal examination, it is important to detect the signs of portal hypertension such as hepatic or splenic enlargement, epigastric venous hum, ascites, or caput medusa with a rectal examination to detect rectal varices. Neurological examination would focus on determination of asterixis or altered mental status.

Laboratory and Imaging

Hepatitis A

The diagnosis of acute hepatitis A viral infection is confirmed by serum immunoglobulin M (IgM) anti-HAV testing, which has high sensitivity and specificity. Anti-HAV IgM is typically positive once symptoms develop and remain positive for up to 6 months. A false-positive result, prior immunity, or asymptomatic infection may be diagnosed in the setting of a patient without typical symptoms of acute hepatitis A infection with a positive anti-HAV IgM result. Serum immunoglobulin G (IgG) anti-HAV is present several weeks after the onset of acute infection and typically remains present indefinitely. Prior immunization or infection can be measured by total anti-HAV (IgM and IgG). Stool or serum detection is not commonly used in clinical practice for the detection of HAV.

Less specific serum laboratory findings include elevated transaminase levels, total and direct bilirubin, and alkaline phosphatase. The alanine transaminase (ALT) level is typically higher than the aspartate transaminase (AST) level, with transaminase levels in the several hundred to several thousand U per L range. Transaminase levels peak in elevation before the peak in bilirubin levels, which often rises above 10 mg per dL. Imaging is not routinely required in the absence of atypical features or other medical risk factors.

Hepatitis B

According to the United States Preventative Services Task Force (USPSTF), screening for HBV is most highly supported in pregnant women, where treatment of infants with neonatal HBV vaccination and hepatitis B immune globulin significantly reduces the rates of infant chronic infection.[17] Screening is also recommended by the Centers for Disease Control and Prevention (CDC) for infants who are born to HBsAg positive; persons born in countries with HBsAg seropositivity $\geq 2\%$; unvaccinated, U.S.-born persons with a parent born in countries with HBsAg seropositivity rates $\geq 8\%$; persons infected with HIV; MSM; users of intravenous drugs; household, needle-sharing, or sexual contacts of persons who are HBsAg positive; persons initiating hemodialysis; persons undergoing evaluation for immunosuppressive therapy prior to treatment; donors of biologic material; persons whose blood or bodily fluids are the source of exposures that may have indications for postexposure prophylaxis; and persons with AST/ALT elevation of uncertain cause.[3] Screening is performed by measurement of HPV surface antigen (HBsAg), HPV surface antibody (HBsAb), and HBV core antibody (HBcAb).

For acute hepatitis B infections, HBsAg, HBV envelope antigen (HBeAg), and HBcAb IgM are initially positive and then gradually sero-convert to HBV surface antibody (HBsAb), HBV envelope antibody (HBeAb), and HBV core immunoglobulin G antibody (HBcAb IgG). In addition to these serologic markers of infection, sensitive polymerase chain reaction (PCR) analysis of serum, and in some cases hepatic tissue via biopsy, can detect levels of HBV DNA. Hepatitis B serology is summarized in Table 11.5-1. HBsAg is indicative of current, active infection and, other than detection of HBV DNA, is the first serologic test to become positive after exposure. Evidenced by HBsAb, immunity can be gained either through vaccination or through resolved prior exposure and resolution of acute infection. HBcAb IgM is present early in acute infection and remains positive during the window period of seroconversion when HBsAg and HBsAb may be not detected. Because HBcAb can only be gained from exposure to HBV, it can identify patients who have been exposed to virus in the past and can help differentiate immunity of vaccination from immunity of resolved infection. HBeAg is an important test in those infected with HBV, since HBeAg is associated with replication and degree of infectivity and positively correlates with HBV DNA levels.

HBV disease surveillance involves monitoring of patients with established infection for development of cirrhosis and liver failure as well as periodic screening for hepatocellular carcinoma (HCC) in those at increased risk. Confirmed HBsAg-positive patients should undergo surveillance testing for HBeAg, viral DNA levels, and alanine aminotransferase (ALT) levels, and occasionally biopsy to identify HBeAg-negative infections and to determine prognosis, disease surveillance schedules, and indications for treatment. Additional testing involves monitoring of complete blood counts, prothrombin and partial thromboplastin times, and other liver function tests. Those persons at increased risk for HCC include persons who have family history of HCC, who are of Asian or African descent, who are older, and who have known cirrhosis. Estimates suggest that 15% to 40% of cases of chronic HBV infection develop hepatic complications.

TABLE 11.5-1	Serologic Testing for Hepatitis B Virus

	HBsAg	HBsAb	HBeAg	HBeAb	HBcAb IgM	HBcAb IgG	HBV DNA
Acute infection Early	+	−	+	−	+	−	Typically >20,000 IU/mL
Acute infection window	−	−	+/−	+/−	+	+/−	Detectable or undetectable
Resolved infection/immune	−	+/−	−	+/−	−	+	Undetectable
Chronic carrier	+ (>6 mo)	−	+/−	+/−	−	+	<2,000 IU/mL
Chronic infection	+ (>6 mo)	−	+	−	−	+	Typically >20,000 IU/mL
Chronic infection precore mutant	+ (>6 mo)	−	−	+	−	+	Typically 2,000–20,000 IU/mL
Occult HBV	−	−	+/−	+/−	−	+	Typically >20,000 IU/mL
Vaccination	−	+/−	−	−	−	−	Undetectable

To screen for HCC, ultrasound is more sensitive and specific than serum α-fetoprotein levels and is considered the test of choice for surveillance of HCC. Clinicians may choose to add α-fetoprotein levels to ultrasound if there are concerns about the interpretation or the validity of this operator-dependent test; additionally, where ultrasound is not locally available or when cost is prohibitive, α-fetoprotein is an acceptable alternative to ultrasonography. Frequency of monitoring is recommended to be every 6 to 12 months. Although HCC surveillance is a standard of care in management of HBV hepatitis, a Cochrane review of this practice found insufficient evidence to support its use to reduce mortality.[18]

Hepatitis C

In 2012, the Centers for Disease Control and Prevention (CDC) released the recommendation that persons born between 1945 and 1965 should be offered a test at least once for HCV infection regardless of HCV risk factors. The USPSTF in 2013 agreed to the same recommendation based on reliable available testing, benefits of detection and early intervention, and the prevalence of undiagnosed HCV infection in the "baby boomer" age group. These new screening recommendations are a change from the 1998 CDC guidelines, which only recommended testing for those with HCV risk factors. Risk-based screening of persons not born between 1945 and 1965 should be considered in intranasal drug users, those on long-term dialysis, those with unregulated tattoos, recipients of transfusions or organ transplants before July 1992, recipients of clotting-factor concentrates before 1987, and those that were ever incarcerated. Screening should also be considered for patients with unexplained elevated ALT levels. Annual HCV screening should be considered among persons who inject drugs and HIV-infected MSM.

Antibodies to the HCV (anti-HCV) testing are recommended for initial screening. FDA-approved tests for anti-HCV, which detect antibodies to HCV-encoded antigen, include laboratory-based enzyme immunoassays (EIAs) and a point-of-care immunoassay that can be done at home. The average time to detection of anti-HCV after exposure is 8 to 9 weeks, with >97% of persons testing positive 6 months after exposure. A positive anti-HCV test indicates current or past HCV infection or a false-positive result and should be confirmed with quantitative PCR testing for HCV RNA. HCV RNA can be detected in blood within 1 to 3 weeks after exposure, and may be the only positive test in those who are immunocompromised (e.g., those receiving chronic hemodialysis).

Acute hepatitis C can be distinguished from chronic hepatitis C infection based on testing both anti-HCV and HCV RNA. Acute hepatitis C infection is highly likely if HCV RNA is positive with negative anti-HCV. In chronic hepatitis C, both tests will remain positive. Acute HCV infection does not progress to chronic infection in 15% to 25% of cases and would result in positive anti-HCV and negative HCV RNA testing. A false-positive anti-HCV result is most likely in persons with no risk factors, and repeat HCV RNA testing 6 months later can be used to confirm the absence of chronic infection if suspicion is high.

Once the diagnosis of current HCV infection is made, additional laboratory testing can be helpful to guide treatment. A quantitative HCV RNA test provides a baseline from which to measure response to treatment, but it is neither an accurate measurement of duration of infection nor a predictor of progression to cirrhosis. The HCV genotype test is critical for determination of the optimal treatment regimen, duration, and likelihood of response. The HCV comes in six genotypes, with additional subtypes, that vary in prevalence by region. Genotype 1, which is the hardest to treat, is the most common in the United States and comprises 60% to 70% of HCV infections in this area. Genotypes 2 and 3 are also present in the United States with genotypes 4, 5, and 6 being rare. Before treatment, testing of renal function, hepatic synthetic function (bilirubin, prothrombin time, and albumin), a complete blood count, thyroid-stimulating hormone, and serum aminotransferases are also necessary as a baseline to monitor drug toxicities and to assess readiness for treatment.

Unfortunately, the quantitative HCV RNA viral level, HCV genotype nor the degree of amino-transferase level elevation is able to fully describe or predict the degree of liver damage, the development of HCC, or the progression to cirrhosis in an individual infected with the HCV. Approximately 30% of patients with chronic hepatitis C have persistently normal serum ALT levels, which often predict less risk for development of cirrhosis, but up to 29% of patients with normal ALT levels can have late-stage cirrhosis.[19] Ultrasound can be useful for evaluation of the liver parenchyma, to screen for carcinoma, and look for extrahepatic manifestations of cirrhosis, but also cannot always determine the degree of fibrosis or presence of cirrhosis. CT is not routinely used since it is not significantly better than ultrasonography and adds radiation and contrast exposure. Liver biopsy, which is invasive and not without risk, remains the gold standard for determining the degree of liver fibrosis, which is useful in the decisions to proceed with treatment. Subsequently, noninvasive serologic (e.g., aspartate aminotransferase to platelet ration [APRI], Fibrotest/FiroSure, Hepascore) and radiologic tests (e.g., ultrasound elastography, magnetic resonance elastography) continue to be developed for use individually or in combination to better predict the degree of fibrosis.

Differential Diagnosis

The differential diagnosis of patients presenting with symptoms or signs of liver disease or mildly elevated liver enzymes, which may be the only initial laboratory finding in chronic infections, is very broad and may include other viral and nonviral infectious causes, alcoholic hepatitis, nonalcoholic steatohepatitis, autoimmune hepatitis, cholangitis, cirrhosis, drug-induced liver injury, hemochromatosis, hereditary metabolic disorders (e.g., Wilson disease, α_1-antitrypsin deficiency), and HCC.

TREATMENT
Medications/Immunizations

Hepatitis A

Since hepatitis A viral infection is a self-limited disease, the treatment is supportive with a minority of patients requiring hospitalization or progressing to fulminant hepatic failure. In 2011, 43% of patients with reported hepatitis A infection required hospitalization and 0.7% died.[1] Hepatic failure and death is more common in those with advanced age and chronic hepatitis C infection,[20] although in the United States only approximately 3% of cases of acute liver failure between 1998 and 2007 were due to HAV.[21]

Immunization against the HAV has been extremely effective along with handwashing, water treatment and proper food handling at preventing the spread of hepatitis A infection. Initial 1996 Centers for Disease Control and Prevention (CDC) recommendations for vaccination targeted those at highest risk for disease transmission: international travelers, illicit drug users, MSM, persons with chronic liver disease, those with clotting-factor disorders, persons with occupational risk for infection, and children in areas with high rates of hepatitis A infection. The CDC's Advisory Committee on Immunization Practices (ACIP) expanded these recommendations in 2006 to include all children starting at 12 months of age.

HAV vaccination, which is an inactivated vaccine, is recommended in two doses spread a minimum of 6 months apart, with a higher adult dose for those greater than 18 years of age. Vaccination is approved only for those 12 months of age or older and may be given to those who are immunocompromised. Postvaccination testing is not generally recommended since the vaccine is highly effective.

Postexposure prophylaxis for hepatitis A is also an effective treatment strategy to minimize the spread during outbreaks. Initially, intravenous immune globulin (IVIG) was the only method for the protection of exposed individuals. However, in 2007, the CDC updated their recommendations to include the use of a single dose of HAV vaccine within 2 weeks after exposure for those healthy persons aged 1 to 40 years.[22] Vaccination is typically preferred in this group due to ease of administration, long-term protection, and equivalent efficacy to IVIG.[23] Infants under 12 months of age, older persons, those who are immunocompromised, and persons with chronic liver disease should be given IVIG prior to travel to an endemic area or after exposure. Postexposure prophylaxis is needed only for close personal contacts (e.g., household and sex contacts, persons sharing illicit drugs, and child-care center staff, attendees and attendees' household members) of those with confirmed hepatitis A infection.

Hepatitis B

Primary prevention of HBV through immunization plays an important role in population management of disease. The CDC recommends standard immunization schedule for all children under 18 years old with three-dose series at 0, 1, and 6 months. For adults, immunization is recommended for those at highest risk of contracting the virus or of having complications—healthcare workers, those at risk for sexual exposure, others at risk of needle exposure to HBsAg-positive individuals, HIV-positive individuals, intravenous drug uses, close personal/household contacts of those with HBV infection, those with end-stage renal disease or otherwise considering dialysis, those other chronic liver diseases, and those traveling to countries with endemicity >2%. Immunity postvaccination may be indefinite with immunological memory persisting even after HBsAb levels are no longer detectable.[24] Postexposure prophylaxis is indicated for infants born to HBsAg-positive mothers; for persons, including healthcare workers, recently exposed to a needle of serum from an HBsAg-positive individual; or for persons with recent sexual exposure to an HBsAg-positive partner. Postexposure prophylaxis involves vaccination of all unvaccinated individuals and intramuscular administration of one dose of hepatitis B immune globulin at a dose of 0.06 mL per kg of body mass.

For chronic HBV infection, the main goals of treatment are to reduce viremia and to preserve liver function because chronic infection is not universally curable. The paragon of all treatment outcomes, delayed HBsAg seroconversion is only rarely achieved. Secondary goals of therapy are seroconversion of HBeAg and reduction of HBV DNA levels. Integral to evaluating risk of progression, testing is indicated for HIV and HCV coinfection for all patients and for HDV only in intravenous drug users in persons from countries with high HDV prevalence. All patients with HBV should also be vaccinated for HAV.

General hepatitis B treatment recommendations include treatment of persons with high levels of HBV DNA in HBeAg-negative infection, active hepatitis ascertained either by very high ALT levels or by biopsy if treatment indications are equivocal, and compensated or decompensated cirrhosis. Management options for chronic HBV include pegylated interferon α-2A (pegIFN), which maintains the best long-term response rates, as well as five other oral antiviral agents that inhibit viral reverse transcriptase. Table 11.5-2 summarizes these available treatment options. Treatment duration with pegIFN lasts 6 to 12 months with monitoring ALT and aspartate aminotransferase for response as well as monitoring complete blood counts. Lamivudine, adefovir, entecavir, tenofovir, and telbivudine comprise the available oral options. Recommended first-line treatment options are for pegIFN, entecavir, and tenofovir.[25] Drug treatment typically is no more likely to result in seroconversion than no treatment when ALT levels are less than two times the upper limit of normal (ULN).[25] Treatment is generally indicated due to much greater increased risk of liver disease and progression when HBeAg-negative patients with confirmation of sustained, active hepatitis through documentation of elevated ALT levels (>2× ULN) and with HBV DNA greater than 20,000 IU per mL.

Hepatitis C

With acute management of hepatitis C being supportive for the few symptomatic patients who seek medical care during acute infection, treatment of hepatitis C is focused on prevention of liver damage and cirrhosis. Historically, it has been challenging to accurately predict who is at greatest risk for progression to cirrhosis and who would most benefit from treatment, which has not been universally curative nor without risk. Predictors of greater likelihood of treatment response include genotypes 2 and 3, baseline viral load <800,000 IU per mL, Caucasian race, IL28B polymorphisms, and treatment adherence. Proper patient selection with an individualized patient-centered approach has been essential to care.

Historically, the backbone of hepatitis C treatment has been pegylated interferon-α (IFN-α), which is given in a weekly injection, and ribavirin, which is given orally, for 24 to 48 weeks for most

TABLE 11.5-2   Treatment Options for Hepatitis B Viral Hepatitis

Drug	Dose	Advantages	Disadvantages	Bottom line
Pegylated IFN-α	180 mcg/wk	• Weekly dosing • Finite treatment duration • Durability of viral suppression improved • No resistance	• Increased side effects • Contraindicated in decompensated cirrhosis	• First line
Lamivudine	100 mg/d	• Oral • Low cost • Clinical experience in pregnancy (category C)	• High rates of resistance	• Years of clinical experience and low cost • Good combo for HBV with HIV coinfection when lamivudine is part of HIV treatment
Adefovir	10 mg/d	• Oral • Active against lamivudine-resistant HBV • Less drug resistance than lamivudine	• Poor potency for viral suppression • Least potent drug	• Good combo for lamivudine resistance
Entecavir	0.5 mg/d	• Oral • More potent than lamivudine • Low drug resistance in nucleoside-naïve patients	• Some inducible cross resistance with lamivudine resistance	• First line • Poor option after development of nucleoside resistance
Telbivudine	600 mg/d	• Oral • Slightly more potent than lamivudine	• High rates of resistance • Cross resistance with lamivudine • More expensive than lamivudine	• Only slightly more potent than lamivudine at increased cost
Tenofovir	300 mg/d	• Oral • More potent than lamivudine • Effective against lamivudine-resistant HBV • Very low rates of drug resistance		• First line • Good combo for any nucleoside resistance

patients. These agents inhibit HCV replication. This drug regimen has provided cure rates of 20% to 80% depending on genotype and other host factors. Adverse effects from interferon and ribavirin are common, limiting completion of therapy. A majority of patients develop flu-like symptoms with other common side effects such as anemia, neutropenia, thrombocytopenia, rash, hair loss, thyroid dysfunction, and significant depression.

Fortunately, since 2011 there have been a number of new treatment options to improve the efficacy and tolerability of hepatitis C treatment. Boceprevir and telaprevir, which are protease inhibitors, were the first of newer direct acting antiviral agents that were FDA approved in 2011 for triple therapy in combination with interferon and ribavirin to improve the sustained viral response for patients with genotype 1, which had lower cure rates with traditional therapy. The rapidly evolving future treatment of HCV with direct acting antiviral agents, such as sofosbuvir, which was FDA approved in 2013, is expected to provide interferon-free treatment options, shorter courses of therapy, cure rates above 90%, and greater tolerability, but not without greater cost. The costs of current therapy must be weighed against future benefits in the reduction of cirrhosis and need for liver transplantation. Cost and access to care will likely be limiting factors that will need consideration if significant reduction in the disease burden of hepatitis C in the United States is desired.

There is currently no available vaccination for HCV, but patient infected with hepatitis C should be screened for and immunized against hepatitis A and B if they are not already infected or immune.

Hepatitis D

The only approved treatment for HDV is IFN-α with a meta-analysis of HDV treatment with IFN suggesting modest benefit.[26,27] Additional options include substitution of standard IFN-α with pegylated interferon; limited evidence suggests that this treatment may be more efficacious.[28] Additional treatment options for HDV have been discouraging. Response rates to treatment are low but are better if treatment is begun soon after acquisition of HDV.[27] Because of low response rates, the primary means of prevention of HDV-related disease would be avoidance of exposure to HDV and vaccination against HBV.

Hepatitis E

Because infections are self-limiting, supportive care is the standard of care for HEV; recently, a published article from a retrospective multicenter cohort study in chronic HEV in solid organ recipients suggested that 3 months of ribavirin is effective.[29]

Referrals

Initially, referral may be needed for patients with atypical, complex or advanced symptoms, comorbid disease, or if diagnosis is unclear. Patients with acute viral hepatitis infection who are developing hepatic failure should be ideally managed in a liver transplant center. All patients with chronic hepatitis B or C should be considered for referral to a physician competent in the evaluation, management, and treatment of chronic hepatitis.

Patient Education

Patient education should focus particular attention on the natural course of the disease, risk of transmission, treatment options, and prevention. All patients should be counseled regarding appropriate vaccinations, blood precautions and avoidance of high risk behaviors, alcohol, illicit drugs, and other hepatotoxic agents.

REFERENCES

1. CDC. Surveillance for Viral Hepatitis—United States, 2011. http://www.cdc.gov/hepatitis/Statistics/2011Surveillance. Accessed April 1, 2014.
2. Diakun KR. Review of Hepatitis B for the Clinical Laboratory Scientist. Med TechNet Online services. 1997. http://www.medtechnet.com/public_pdf/mtc18.pdf. Accessed February 2, 2014.
3. Weinbaum CM, Williams I, Mast EE, et al. National Center for HIV/AIDS, Viral Hepatitis, STD, and TB Prevention, Division of Viral Hepatitis. Center for the Centers for Disease Control and Prevention (CDC). Recommendations for identification and public health management of persons with chronic hepatitis B virus infection. *MMWR Recomm Rep* 2008;57(RR-8):1–20.
4. Wasley A, Grytdal S, Gallagher K. CDC. Surveillance for acute viral hepatitis—United States, 2006. In: CDC. Surveillance Summaries, March 21, 2008. *MMWR* 2008;57(No. SS-2). http://www.cdc.gov/mmwr/preview/mmwrhtml/ss5702a1.htm. Accessed February 2, 2014.
5. Smith BD, Morgan RL, Beckett GA, et al. Recommendations for the identification of chronic hepatitis C virus infection among persons born during 1945–1965. *MMWR Recomm Rep* 2012;61(43):886.
6. Armstrong GL, Wasley A, Simard EP, et al. The prevalence of hepatitis C virus infection in the United States, 1999 through 2002. *Ann Intern Med* 2006;144(10):705–714.
7. Denniston MM, Jiles RB, Jan Drobeniuc J, et al. Chronic hepatitis C virus infection in the United States, National Health and Nutrition Examination Survey 2003 to 2010. *Ann Intern Med* 2014;160(5):293–300.
8. Armstrong GL, Alter MJ, McQuillan GM, et al. The past incidence of hepatitis V virus infection: implications for the future burden of chronic liver disease in the United States. *Hepatology* 2000;31(3):777–782.
9. Ly KN, Xing J, Klevens RM, et al. The increasing burden of mortality from viral hepatitis in the United States between 1999 and 2007. *Ann Intern Med* 2012;156:271–278.

10. CDC. Hepatitis C Information for Health Professionals. http://www.cdc.gov/hepatitis/HCV. Accessed April 1, 2014.
11. Yeung LT, King SM, Roberts EA. Mother-to-infant transmission of hepatitis C virus. *Hepatology* 2001;34(2):223–229.
12. Terrault NA, Dodge JL, Murphy EL, et al. Sexual transmission of hepatitis C virus among monogamous heterosexual couples: the HCV partners study. *Hepatology* 2013;57(3):881–889.
13. Yaphe S, Bozinoff N, Kyle R, et al. Incidence of acute hepatitis C virus infection among men who have sex with men with and without HIV infection: a systematic review. *Sex Transm Infect* 2012;88(7):558–564.
14. Rizzetto M, Ponzetto A, Forzani I. Epidemiology of hepatitis delta virus: overview. *Prog Clin Biol Res* 1991;364:1–20.
15. Kamar N, Selves J, Mansuy JM, et al. Hepatitis E virus and chronic hepatitis in organ-transplant recipients. *N Engl J Med* 2008;358:811–817.
16. Thomas DL, Yarbough PO, Vlahov D, et al. Seroreactivity to hepatitis E virus in areas where disease is not endemic. *J Clin Microbiol* 35:1244–1247.
17. Lin K, Vickery J. Screening for hepatitis B virus infection in pregnant women: evidence for the U.S. Preventive Services Task Force reaffirmation recommendation statement. *Ann Intern Med* 2009;150:874–876.
18. Wun YT, Dickinson JA. Alpha-fetoprotein and/or liver ultrasonography for liver cancer screening in patients with chronic hepatitis B. *Cochrane Database Syst Rev* 2003;(2):CD002799.
19. Bacon BR. Treatment of patients with hepatitis C and normal serum aminotransferase levels. *Hepatology* 2002;36(5 Suppl 1):S179–S184.
20. Vento S, Garofano T, Renzini C, et al. Fulminant hepatitis associated with hepatitis A virus superinfection in patients with chronic hepatitis C. *N Engl J Med* 1998;338(5):286.
21. Lee WM, Squires RH, Nyberg SL, et al. Acute liver failure: summary of a workshop. *Hepatology* 2008;47(4):1401–1415.
22. Advisory Committee on Immunization Practices (ACIP) Centers for Disease Control and Prevention (CDC). Update: prevention of hepatitis A after exposure to hepatitis A virus and in international travelers. Updated recommendations of the Advisory Committee on Immunization Practices (ACIP). *MMWR Morb Mortal Wkly Rep* 2007;56(41):1080–1084.
23. Victor JC, Monto AS, Surdina TY, et al. Hepatitis A vaccine versus immune globulin for postexposure prophylaxis. *N Engl J Med* 2007;357(17):1685–1694.
24. Petersen KM, Bulkow LR, McMahon BJ, et al. Duration of hepatitis B immunity in low risk children receiving hepatitis B vaccinations from birth. *Pediatr Infect Dis J* 2004;23(7):650–655.
25. Lok ASF, McMahon BJ. Chronic hepatitis B: Update 2009. AASLD Practice Guideline Update. http://www.aasld.org/practiceguidelines/pages/default.aspx. Accessed March 27, 2014.
26. Abbas Z, Khan MA, Salih M, et al. Interferon alpha for chronic hepatitis D. *Cochrane Database Syst Rev* 2011;(12):CD006002.
27. Lau JY, King R, Tibbs CJ, et al. Loss of HBsAg with interferon-alpha therapy in chronic hepatitis D virus infection. *J Med Virol* 1993;39:292.
28. Niro GA, Ciancio A, Gaeta GB, et al. Pegylated interferon alpha-2b as monotherapy or in combination with ribavirin in chronic hepatitis delta. *Hepatology* 2006;44:713.
29. Kamar N, Izopet J, Tripon S, et al. Ribavirin for chronic hepatitis E virus infection in transplant recipients. *N Engl J Med* 2014;370:1111–1120.

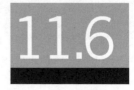

11.6 Pancreatitis and Pancreatic Cancer

Abdul Waheed, Cynthia Rizk, Lena Jafilan

PANCREATITIS
General Principles

Definition

Pancreatitis typically presents with abdominal pain due to inflammation of the pancreas. Acute abdominal pain is a common presentation in the outpatient and emergency department setting, and distinguishing pancreatitis can pose a significant diagnostic challenge. Abdominal pain is the presenting complaint in 1.5% of office-based visits and in 5% of emergency department visits.[1] Pancreatitis is always one of the top differential diagnoses when considering a painful acute abdominal process.

Pancreatitis is an inflammatory process involving the retroperitoneal organ—the pancreas. Acute pancreatitis may occur as an isolated attack, or may be recurrent.[2] Recurrent pancreatitis may, over time, lead to chronic pancreatitis. Chronic pancreatitis is a progressive fibroinflammatory process of the pancreas that results in permanent structural damage. This can lead to the impairment of exocrine and endocrine functions.[3] There are various aspects that help distinguish chronic from acute pancreatitis.

Classification

The classification of acute pancreatitis is divided as follows:[2,4]

- Mild acute pancreatitis, which is characterized by the absence of organ failure and local or systemic complications.
- Moderately severe acute pancreatitis, which is characterized by transient organ failure (resolved within 48 hours) and/or local or systemic complications without persistent organ failure (>48 hours).
- Severe acute pancreatitis, which is characterized by persistent organ failure that may involve one or multiple organs.

There are many scoring systems and clinical predictor pathways suggested in the classification of acute pancreatitis in above categories as given in diagnosis and management section below.

Epidemiology

Acute pancreatitis is a leading cause of hospitalization in the United States. The reported annual incidence of acute pancreatitis has ranged from 4.9 to 35 per 100,000 of the population. Some patients may require brief hospitalization, whereas others may be critically ill with multiple-organ dysfunction requiring intensive care monitoring.[2] Mortality in acute pancreatitis is usually due to systemic inflammatory response syndrome (SIRS) and organ failure in the first 2-week period, while after 2 weeks it is usually due to sepsis and its complications. Approximately 15% to 25% of all patients with acute pancreatitis develop severe acute pancreatitis. Fagenholz and colleagues reported that mortality from acute pancreatitis decreased from 12% to 2% between 1998 and 2003 in United States. This is largely because of early recognition and better treatment. However, morbidity and mortality still remain high in subgroups of severe disease.[5]

Pathophysiology

The exact pathophysiology of pancreatitis is not completely understood. Acute pancreatitis is characterized by severe inflammatory reaction that usually extends beyond the pancreas, leading to systemic inflammatory response. In severe cases, this results in multiple-organ failure and death. Several pathways have been suggested. This includes increased intracellular calcium level and intracellular activation of exocrine digestive enzymes, including trypsin in the acinar cells leading to parenchymal cell death. There is increasing vasospasm and subsequent tissue ischemia along with neurogenic mechanisms causing vasoconstriction and edema. This is associated with rising levels of digestive enzymes in blood prosystemic inflammatory response.[4]

Chronic pancreatitis is characterized by endocrine and exocrine secretory dysfunction and structural damage. Both animal models and humans have led to many different attempts to theorize the pathophysiology of chronic pancreatitis including the toxic-metabolic theory, the oxidative stress hypothesis, the stone and duct obstruction theory, and the necrosis–fibrosis hypothesis. The secretory dysfunction is the basis for diagnostic use of secretin.[6]

Etiology

Many different etiologic mechanisms have been implicated in acute pancreatitis as summarized below:

- Mechanical obstruction in the biliary system includes gall stones, biliary sludge, ascariasis, periampullary diverticulum, pancreatic or periampullary cancer, ampullary stenosis, strictures of the bile duct or duodenum, and duodenal obstruction.
- Toxic includes alcohol including methanol and ethanol, organophosphate poisoning, and scorpion venom.
- *Metabolic*: hypercalcemia, hyperlipidemia.
- A large number of drugs have been implicated but the common ones include didanosine, pentamidine, metronidazole, stibogluconate, tetracycline furosemide, thiazides, sulphasalazine, 5-ASA, L-asparaginase, azathioprine, valproic acid, sulindac, salicylates, calcium, and estrogen.

- Infections include viruses (like mumps, coxsackie, hepatitis B, cytomegalovirus, varicella zoster, herpes simplex, HIV), bacteria (like Mycoplasma, Legionella, Leptospira, Salmonella), fungi (like Aspergillus), and parasites (like Toxoplasma, Cryptosporidium, Ascaris).
- Trauma includes iatrogenic injury during endoscopic retrograde cholangiopancreatography (ERCP) or other hepatobiliary procedures and blunt or penetrating abdominal injuries.
- Congenital/genetic include familial and sporadic mutations syndromes like CFTR and α_1-antitrypsin deficiency, choledococele type V, pancreatic divisum.
- Vascular factors include ischemia from any reason, including atheroembolism or vasculitis (like polyarteritis nodosa and systemic lupus erythematosus).

Of the above, gall stones and alcohol abuse account for majority of the cases (60% to 70%). The remainder of acute cases associated with a variety of causes, including post-ERCP, drug induced, hypertriglyceridemia, trauma, and postsurgical.[7]

Alcohol accounts for majority, nearly 70% of cases, of the cases in chronic pancreatitis. Another 20% are considered idiopathic, whereas the rest are associated with diseases such as cystic fibrosis, pancreatic tumors, autoimmune diseases, genetic defects, and congenital anomalies.[3]

Diagnosis

Clinical Presentation and History

Typically, patients present with acute-onset severe epigastric or right upper quadrant (RUQ) abdominal pain with or without radiation to the back or flank. It generally presents rapidly with peak 30 to 60 minutes after onset, or may present more gradually depending on the cause. Nausea and vomiting are commonly present. Sitting up or leaning forward may help alleviate the symptoms.[1-4]

A complete history should explore all possible factors as listed in etiology section above, especially enquiring and searching electronic records for the presence of cholelithiasis, alcoholism, or lipid disorders (particularly familial hypertriglyceridemias); recent surgeries and procedures; and reviewing medication list.

Physical Examination

One must pay particular attention to vital signs as patient may present with sepsis or septic shock. They may be febrile, tachycardic, and/or hypotensive secondary to third spacing. Patient may present with icterus depending on the cause, pleural effusions, epigastric and abdominal tenderness and/or distension, and decreased bowel sounds in the presence of ileus. Skin should be examined for erythema nodosum (erythematous skin nodules from fat necrosis) and Grey Turner and Cullen signs. These are associated with severe hemorrhagic pancreatitis, are ecchymosis in the flank and periumbilical areas, respectively.[1-4]

Laboratory Studies

Initial evaluation of pancreatitis should include a complete blood count with differential, complete metabolic count, including calcium, bilirubin and liver enzymes, amylase, lipase, C-reactive protein, lipid profile with triglycerides, and arterial blood gases if patient is hypoxic. Patient may present with leukocytosis depending on severity, hypocalcemia, hemoconcentration secondary to third spacing, and elevated liver enzymes if the etiology involves cholestasis. Both serum amylase and lipase are still the mainstay in helping establish the diagnosis of pancreatitis, although lipase is more sensitive and specific than amylase.[1,2,8] Lipase rises faster and remains elevated longer than amylase, which only has a half-life of about 10 hours; therefore, lipase is more useful in patients presenting more than 24 hours after onset of symptoms. It is also more specific and sensitive than amylase. Amylase may be positive in conditions other than pancreatitis; however, an amylase level more than three times the level of normal can be considered more reliable for diagnosis.[2,8] One must keep in mind that patients with alcoholic pancreatitis or hypertriglyceridemia induced pancreatitis may not be able to make amylase.[8,9]

Diagnostic Criteria

A three-point diagnostic criterion was developed by Japanese Ministry of Health, Labor and Welfare.[10] It is widely practiced as adapted by practice guidelines by Banks and Freeman[11] in 2006 and modified by Kiriyama et al.[12] in 2010. In order to make diagnosis, two out of three criteria are required to diagnose pancreatitis. These criteria are (a) abdominal pain characteristic of pancreatitis, (b) serum amylase and/or lipase level greater than or equal to three times the normal limit, and (c) characteristic imaging findings on ultrasound, computed tomography (CT), or MRI.[12]

Imaging

Although ultrasound, CT, or MRI has been suggested by the practice guidelines as mentioned in the above section, the best modality of imaging remains controversial. American College of Radiology (ACR) proposes an evidence-based approach toward diagnostic image of choice with regularly reviewed ACR Appropriateness Criteria accessible from their webpage.[13] It suggests RUQ ultrasound as the choice of diagnostic imaging for first time acute presentation of pancreatitis of less than 48 to 72 hours, with typical abdominal pain and appropriately increased amylase and/or lipase. A CT performed at this time will not likely change management, and will also likely miss any necrosis. However, if amylase and lipase levels are equivocal and clinical symptoms are atypical, then a CT with contrast is recommended. In moderate to severe cases of pancreatitis, including critically ill patients with sepsis or septic shock, signs, or symptoms greater than 7 to 21 days, known necrotizing pancreatitis CT with contrast is recommended. CT without contrast may be considered as an alternative in cases where contrast is inadmissible. MRI and magnetic resonance cholangiopancreatography (MRCP) with contrast are preferred over CT without contrast in patients who are critically ill and cannot have contrast for confounding acute kidney injury (AKI).[13]

The need for follow-up imaging depends upon severity and patient's clinical progress. American Gastroenterology Association recommends the use of rapid-bolus CT scan at 72 hours of onset for patients who have severe disease with end organ damage or who get progressively sicker instead of resolution to look for extent of necrosis.[7]

Assessment of Severity

Assessment of severity of clinical condition requires review of several factors in history, physical examination, laboratory data, and imaging. Several scoring systems have been proposed to categorize severity initially as well as through the course of illness. These are useful tools for management (like determining the level of care) and prognosis. Ranson's criteria[14] (Table 11.6-1) is the easiest and widely used but has limited utility because it cannot be used until the 48-hour point where multiorgan failure may have already developed. C-reactive protein (CRP) is one of the acute phase reactants made by the liver in response to interleukin-1 and interleukin-6. At 48 hours, CRP above 150 mg per L has a sensitivity, specificity, positive predictive value, and negative predictive value of 80%, 76%, 67%, and 86%, respectively, for severe acute pancreatitis.[15] This is why several clinical, laboratory, and radiologic risk factors have been suggested to be used in a systematic approach. Many of these have been incorporated into scoring systems such as the SIRS score.[16] (Table 11.6-2), the APACHE II score (several online calculators are available), the bedside index of severity in acute pancreatitis (BISAP) score,[17] and the CT severity index (Table 11.6-3).[18] American Gastroenterology Association (AGA) recommends the use of APACHE II system to predict severity of disease with a more cutoff.[6] Those with predicted severe disease and moderate disease with severe comorbid conditions should be admitted to intensive care unit or intermediate care unit. Those with mild to moderate disease and comorbid conditions should be considered for intermediate care unit or intensive care unit.[7] APACHE III was developed after the AGA guidelines but has not been shown to be superior to APACHE II.[19]

SIRS score or APACHE II scores can both be reasonable approach for their ease of use, ready availability, and cost effectiveness.

Treatment

Treatment for interstitial edematous acute pancreatitis, or the typical presentation of pancreatitis, is mainly supportive care, including pain control, fluid resuscitation, and monitoring of nutritional

TABLE 11.6-1	Ranson's Criteria		
0 hours		**48 hours**	
Age	>55 yr	Hematocrit fall	>10%
White blood cell count	>16,00	Blood urea nitrogen	>5 increase despite fluid
Blood glucose	>200	Serum calcium	<8 mg/dL
Lactate dehydrogenase	>350	PO$_2$	<60 mmHg
AST	>200	Base deficit	>4 meq/L
		Fluid sequestration	>6 L

TABLE 11.6-2 **SIRS Score Criteria**

Two or more of the following conditions

Temperature	>38.3°C or <36°C
Heart rate of more	>90 bpm
Respiratory rate	>20
WBC count	4,000 > 12,000 or <

TABLE 11.6-3 **CT Severity Index**

Grade	Findings on CT scan	Score
A	Normal pancreas, normal size, sharply defined, smooth contour, homogenous enhancement, retroperitoneal perinephric fat without enhancement	0
B	Focal or diffuse enlargement of pancreas, irregular contour, enhancement may be homogenous but peripancreatic fat enhancement is present	1
C	Peripancreatic inflammation with intrinsic pancreatic abnormalities	2
D	Intrapancreatic or extrapancreatic fluid collection	3
E	Two or more collections of gas in the pancreas or retroperitoneum	4
	0% necrosis on contrast enhanced CT	0
	<33% necrosis on contrast enhanced CT	2
	33–50% necrosis on contrast enhanced CT	4
	>50% necrosis on contrast enhanced CT	6

CT severity index = CT scores + necrosis score on contrast (max = 10); score >6 indicates severe disease.

status. One study showed that early and aggressive resuscitation (receiving at least one-third of their cumulative 72 hours total of fluids within the first 12 to 24 hours) helped decrease morbidity and mortality.[20] Generally patients may begin tolerating oral nutrition within 24 to 48 hours if their pain and nausea are well controlled and there are no other contraindications like ileus. A soft, low-fat, low-residue diet is recommended with advancement as tolerated. Some patients may feel well enough to try solids right away, and there is no evidence to suggest this may be contraindicated, provided it is tolerated. In more severe pancreatitis especially involving patients in the critical care unit, parenteral or enteral feedings may be necessary.[21] There have been studies stating that enteral feedings are more preferred.[2,21] Close monitoring of hemodynamic and nutritional status is especially warranted in critical care patients as they may quickly develop third spacing with subsequent hypotension, and aggressive volume repletion may be needed with close monitoring for complications.[2,20,21]

Pain control is generally with opioids such as fentanyl pump, meperidine, morphine, and dihydromorphone. Some controversy exists over the use of morphine sphincter of Oddi spasm, leading to worsening of pancreatitis; however, there is no high-quality patient-oriented evidence to suggest that it is contraindicated. In fact, all narcotics have the capability to increase this pressure, and meperidine causes an increased risk in seizures.[22]

Antibiotics are not indicated for routine management of acute pancreatitis. There is some evidence that antibiotics might be helpful in the presence of necrosis; however, this is controversial. Clinical judgment should be used to determine the presence of infection and the need for treatment. Electrolyte and metabolic abnormalities including calcium, magnesium, and glucose should be addressed as well.

In every patient at each admission, aggressive search for the etiology is recommended, and based upon the etiology, actions for further prevention should be taken. The initial steps could be taken while the patient is still in the hospital. For example, in case of alcoholism, talk should be started on behavioral change and rehabilitation while the patient is still in the hospital. Patients with gall stone pancreatitis would ultimately need cholecystectomy. Insulting medications should be stopped right away. Any significant hypertriglyceridemia should be treated appropriately.

We suggest early consult with surgery for the presence of necrosis, presentation after 48 hours, and presence of gall stones or higher SIRS score or APACHE II scores.

PANCREATIC CARCINOMA

Pancreatic carcinoma is one of the aggressive cancers with poor prognosis in majority of the cases. It is one of the leading causes of cancer death in United States.[23] A 2-year survival rate is close to 10%.[24] Unfortunately, there are no good screening tests available for the general population.

General Principles

Definition

Malignancy in pancreas can arise from either of the parenchymal parts, exocrine or endocrine; however, vast majority of adenocarcinomas are from the exocrine part. Most of these arise from the pancreatic ductal system.[25]

Pathophysiology

There is no single theory that can explain the pathophysiology of pancreatic cancer. However, as with any oncologic process, pancreatic cancer is thought to have a fine interplay of oncogenes and environmental factors. The Notch and Hedgehog pathways are an active area of research both for understanding of the disease and for potential future treatment.[26]

Risk Factors

Pancreatic cancer has two distinct varieties, with one variety having familial aggregation and the other just arising with newer mutations. Clinical risk factors include cigarette smoking, familial history, chronic pancreatitis, and type II diabetes, and family history of pancreatic and other gastrointestinal (GI) malignancies. Germline gene mutations in known cancer-causing genes such as BRCA1, BRCA2, and STK11 (gene responsible for Putz–Jegher syndrome) have also been associated with pancreatic cancer.[27] Risks not firmly established due to inadequate data include obesity, gallbladder disease, dietary factors, physical inactivity, and occupational exposures.[25] Intraductal papillary mucinous neoplasm, also referred as IPMN, of the pancreas is a cystic neoplasm of the pancreas with malignant potential.

Diagnosis

History

Patients usually present with general nonspecific symptoms of weight loss, pain, anorexia, nausea, vomiting, and weakness with or without jaundice. Classically these symptoms are associated with dark-colored urine and clay-colored stools.[23]

Physical Examination

Physical examination may be completely normal. In an appropriate setting, jaundice and easy bruising may be present. Painless jaundice with weight loss is classic for hepatobiliary and pancreatic malignancies. A nontender, distended, palpable gallbladder may also be present. Sometimes nonspecific signs of liver obstruction, left supraclavicular lymphadenopathy, and recurrent superficial thrombophlebitis may also be present. Widespread or migratory thrombophlebitis also known as Trousseau syndrome may also be present.

Laboratory Evaluation

Biochemistry and serologic markers are very nonspecific. Serum bilirubin and alkaline phosphatase levels may be elevated, but have no diagnostic role. Similarly elevated CA 19-9 levels are not diagnostic but may increase the index of and highly useful in prognostication. These are also useful for postsurgical disease surveillance.[23]

Imaging

Initial imaging modality for painless jaundice is ultrasonography. The ACR Appropriateness Criteria for imaging a patient with painless jaundice is eight for ultrasonography, MRI with contrast, MRCP, and CT scan. Dual-phase helical CT is becoming more popular in diagnosis of pancreatic cancer, with sensitivity at 98% in detecting both pancreatic cancers and distant metastases. It also helps in staging. If clinical suspicion is high and CT is negative, endoscopic ultrasonography should be performed next, with a sensitivity of 92% and a specificity of 100%.[23]

Treatment

Surgical resection of the tumor involves extensive surgery and is the only potentially curative treatment for pancreatic cancer. Unfortunately, only 15% to 20% patients are candidates for surgery because of late-stage presentation of the disease.

Whipple procedure involves extensive surgery with the gastric antrum, the entire duodenum and proximal 15 cm of jejunum, the head of the pancreas, the gallbladder, and the distal bile duct. Alternatively, pylorus-preserving pancreatoduodenectomy (PPD) has similar long-term survival benefits and offers shorter operative times and decreased blood loss. Distal pancreatectomy has also been proposed for patients with resectable cancer in the body or tail of the pancreas. Surgical resection is the only treatment for IPMN.[23]

Chemotherapy

There is high local and distant recurrence of disease even in completely resected pancreatic cancers. Adjuvant chemotherapy, adjuvant radiotherapy, and adjuvant chemoradiation all have been shown to help decrease the recurrence rates and improve survival slightly, but this topic is very controversial. Most commonly, it is aimed at inhibition of tumor growth and spread in palliative attempt. Many different treatment protocols exist that make use of gemcitabine, folfirinox, and folfox 6. Many newer agents with specific pathway targets are being tested and include gene therapy agents, immunotherapy agents, and signal transduction inhibitors.[28]

Palliation

Treatment of non-resectable pancreatic cancer, which is majority of the cases, is focused around comfort and compassionate palliation. The most common issues are pain, weight loss, obstructive jaundice, pancreatic insufficiency, gastric outlet obstruction, depression, and fatigue.

- **Pain.** General principles of pain management should be followed. Specifically, the pain management of pancreatic cancer poses severe challenges as the tumor commonly invades the celiac and mesenteric plexi. Early care is focused around nonsteroidal anti-inflammatory agents with gradual shift to oral or transdermal narcotic agents. Regional anesthesia such as celiac blocks can be very helpful and avoid the adverse effects of narcotic pain medications. Radiation therapy and chemotherapy can be used as needed.
- **Obstructive jaundice.** The treatment of obstructive jaundice includes decompression of the gall bladder and biliary system by percutaneous ostomy tubes using interventional radiology, endoscopic ostomies, or surgical bypasses. Jaundice caused by deposition of bilirubin and its products in skin and subcutaneous tissue can cause severe pruritis. Bile acid sequestrants such as ursodeoxycholic acid and acid cholestyramine and neurodepressants like gabapentin or pregabalin could be used for intense pruritis in cases where biliary decompression is not possible.
- **Weight loss.** Weight loss is a common finding in any malignancy; however, very prominent in GI malignancies. There is complex interplay of molecules at biologic level, including tumor necrosis factor, interleukins, and many others leading to loss of appetite coupled with more caloric needs leading to cachexia and weight loss. This can in turn be associated with fatigue, weakness, and poor quality of life. Although the mainstay of treatment is supportive nutrition, certain agents such as megesterol acetate, medroxyprogesterone acetate, and dexamethasone can be used to improve appetite. Tricyclic antidepressant mirtazapine causes weight gain and sometimes be used. Metoclopramide and dronabinol are also potent appetite stimulants.
- **Pancreatic insufficiency.** Majority of the patients with pancreatic cancer will have some degree of fat malabsorption (about 65%) or/and protein malabsorption (50%). Replacement of pancreatic enzymes is helpful in such patients.
- **Gastric outlet obstruction.** Gastric outlet obstruction can be a challenge in patients who survive longer. It affects approximately 10% to 20% of patients who survive beyond 15 months of diagnosis. Prokinetic drugs such as metoclopramide, domperidone, and chlorpromazine are the mainstay of treatment; however, surgical bypass is an option for severe cases or anatomic obstruction.
- **Depression and fatigue.** A vast majority (up to 70%) of patients develop fatigue and depression that would require intervention, during the course of the disease. Patients who present with depressive symptoms should be evaluated for anemia and other causes of pseudodepression and treated accordingly. Depression in general can be treated typically with selective serotonin-reuptake inhibitors (SSRIs) and tricyclic antidepressants (TCAs), with SSRIs offering fewer side effects while TCAs offer additional analgesia benefit. Erythropoietin (EPO) can be used for anemia of chronic disease related to malignancy. Psychostimulants such as methylphenidate can be helpful in the treatment of fatigue.[29]

REFERENCES

1. Cartwright SL, Knudson MP. Evaluation of acute abdominal pain in adults. *Am Fam Physician* 2008;77(7):971–978.
2. Carrol JK, Herrick B, Gipson T, et al. Acute pancreatitis: diagnosis, prognosis, and treatment. *Am Fam Physician* 2007;75(10):1513–1520.
3. Steer ML, Waxman I, Freedman S. Chronic pancreatitis. *N Engl J Med* 1995;332(22):1482.
4. Pandol SJ. Acute pancreatitis. *Curr Opin Gastroenterol* 2005;21:538–543.
5. Fagenholz PJ, Castillo CF, Harris NS, et al. Increasing United States hospitalizations for acute pancreatitis 1988–2003. *Ann Epidemiol* 2007;17(7):491.
6. Stevens T, Conwell DL, Zuccaro G. Pathogenesis of chronic pancreatitis: an evidence-based review of past theories and recent developments. *Am J Gastroenterol* 2004;99(11):2256.
7. Forsmark CE, Baillie J, AGA Institute Clinical Practice and Economics Committee, AGA Institute Governing Board. AGA Institute technical review on acute pancreatitis. *Gastroenterology* 2007;132(5):2022.
8. Smotkin J, Tenner S. Laboratory diagnostic tests in acute pancreatitis. *J Clin Gastroenterol* 2002;34:459–462.
9. Fortson MR, Freedman SN, Webster PD IIIrd. Clinical assessment of hyperlipidemic pancreatitis. *Am J Gastroenterol* 1995;90:2134.
10. Takeda K, Ohtuki K, Kitagawa M, et al. Final draft of the diagnostic criteria for and criteria for severity assessment of acute pancreatitis 2005 report. Tokyo: The Intractable Pancreatic Disease Investigation and Research Group of the Japanese Ministry of Health, Labour and Welfare; 2006:27–34.
11. Banks PA, Freeman ML. Practice guidelines in acute pancreatitis. *Am J Gastroenterol* 2006;101(10):2379–2400.
12. Kiriyama S, Gabata T, Takada T, et al. New diagnostic criteria of pancreatitis. *J Hepatobiliary Pancreat Sci* 2010;17:24–36.
13. ACR Appropriateness Criteria° web page accessed at https://acsearch.acr.org/list
14. Ranson JH, Rifkin KM, Roses DF, et al. Prognostic signs and role of operative management in acute pancreatitis. *Surg Gynecol Obstet* 1974;139(1):69.
15. Larvin M. Assessment of clinical severity and prognosis. In: Beger HG, Warshaw AL, Buchler MW, et al., eds. *The Pancreas*. Oxford: Blackwell Science; 1998:489.
16. Buter A, Imrie CW, Carter CR, et al. Dynamic nature of early organ dysfunction determines outcome in acute pancreatitis. *Br J Surg* 2002;89(3):298.
17. Wu BU, Johannes RS, Sun X, et al. The early prediction of mortality in acute pancreatitis: a large population-based study. *Gut* 2008;57(12):1698.
18. Balthazar EJ, Robinson DL, Megibow AJ, et al. Acute pancreatitis: value of CT in establishing prognosis. *Radiology* 1990;174(2):331.
19. Williams M, Simms HH. Prognostic usefulness of scoring systems in critically ill patients with severe acute pancreatitis. *Crit Care Med* 1999;27(5):901.
20. Gardner TB, Vege SS, Chari ST, et al. Faster rate of initial fluid resuscitation in severe acute pancreatitis diminishes in-hospital mortality. *Pancreatology* 2009;9(6):770–776.
21. Tenner S. Initial management of acute pancreatitis: critical issues during the first 72 hours. *Am J Gastroenterol* 2004;99:2489–2494.
22. Thompson DR. Narcotic analgesic effects on the sphincter of Oddi: a review of the data and therapeutic implications in treating pancreatitis. *Am J Gastroenterol* 2001;96(4):1266–1272.
23. Freelove R, Walling AD. Pancreatic cancer: diagnosis and management. *Am Fam Physician* 2006;73(3):485–492.
24. McKenna S, Eatcock M. The medical management of pancreatic cancer: a review. *The Oncologist* 2003;8:149–160.
25. Michaud DS. The epidemiology of pancreatic, gallbladder, and other biliary tract cancers. *Gastrointestinal Endosc* 2002;56(6 Suppl):S195–S200.
26. Lomberk F, Fernandez-Zapico ME, Urrutia R. When developmental signaling pathways go wrong and their impact on pancreatic cancer development. *Curr Opin Gastroenterol* 2005;21:555–560.
27. Brune KA, Lau B, Palmisano E, et al. Importance of age of onset in pancreatic cancer kindreds. *J Natl Cancer Inst* 2010;102(2):119.
28. MacKenzie MJ. Molecular therapy in pancreatic adenocarcinoma. *Lancet Oncol* 2004;5:541–549.
29. El Kamar FG, Grossbard ML, Kozuch PS. Metastatic pancreatic cancer: emerging strategies in chemotherapy and palliative care. *Oncologist* 2003;8:18–34.

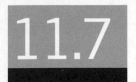

11.7 Diverticular Disease

Sean M. Oser, Parminder Nizran, Anne Walsh,
Tamara K. Oser

GENERAL PRINCIPLES

Diverticulosis is an acquired anatomic condition in which gastrointestinal (GI) mucosal tissue protrudes through weak areas of muscularis where feeding arteries penetrate. These outpouchings occur predominantly in the sigmoid colon but can be found in any portion of the GI tract. In westernized countries, the prevalence of colonic diverticulosis is high and increases with age, affecting about one-third of people by age 60 years and nearly two thirds by age 80.[1] Risk factors include low intake of dietary fiber, decreased tensile strength of the colon wall, abnormal colonic motility, visceral hypersensitivity, and genetic predisposition. In 80% of patients with diverticulosis, the condition is found incidentally and remains asymptomatic; such patients are therefore not considered to have a pathologic or disease process. However, 20% of patients with diverticulosis present with symptoms such as abdominal pain or hematochezia and are considered to have *diverticular disease*.[1,2]

SYMPTOMATIC DIVERTICULOSIS
Diagnosis

History

Patients with painful diverticulosis tend to be younger than those without symptoms and typically present with colicky or aching left lower quadrant abdominal pain of short duration. Pain is usually worse after meals and better after bowel movements. They may also complain of constipation.[2]

Physical Examination

The examination may be completely normal, or it may reveal some degree of left lower quadrant tenderness, but there should be no evidence of peritoneal irritation, inflammation, or mass.[2]

Laboratory and Imaging

Painful diverticulosis is a diagnosis of exclusion. All laboratory studies, including complete blood count (CBC), complete metabolic panel, erythrocyte sedimentation rate (ESR), C-reactive protein (CRP), and urinalysis, are typically normal. Diverticula are often found incidentally on barium enema or computed tomography (CT); colonoscopy is the "gold standard" diagnostic test to confirm the presence and location of diverticula, but their presence does not confirm the disease.[2]

Differential Diagnosis

Irritable bowel syndrome (IBS) may present similarly and often occurs concomitantly.[3] Diverticulitis, inflammatory bowel disease (IBD), gynecologic pathology, and other serious causes of acute abdominal pain should be ruled out, as symptomatic diverticulosis is a diagnosis of exclusion.

Treatment

Treatment has traditionally included increasing dietary fiber to the recommended 25 to 35 g per day along with increasing fluid intake in hopes of decreasing intraluminal pressure and improving stool caliber and consistency, thereby improving symptoms as well as decreasing the risk of diverticulitis.[2] However, recent studies have called into question fiber's efficacy in the management of diverticular disease, as data have been inconclusive.[1,4] If needed, an antispasmodic such as hyoscyamine can be used for relief of abdominal pain. Recent trials have shown benefit with newer regimens involving the use of mesalazine[5,6] and rifaximin with increased fiber,[7] but more studies are needed before off-label use of these expensive prescription medications can be recommended for long-term management. Probiotics have also shown recent promise in symptom management.[6,8]

DIVERTICULAR BLEEDING

Diagnosis

History

Diverticular bleeding occurs as a result of rupture of the vasa recta on the dome of a diverticulum, most commonly in the right colon. Bleeding is usually painless, and it may be occult or massive. Most patients are over age 60 and have comorbid health conditions.[9]

Physical Examination

Examination may reveal evidence of hypovolemia or anemia, depending on the extent of bleeding, but may also be normal. There is usually little or no abdominal tenderness. Rectal examination demonstrates hematochezia and/or stool that is positive for occult blood.[9]

Laboratory and Imaging

Laboratory studies may reveal anemia and/or iron deficiency, though with acute, new-onset bleeding, results may be normal. In patients with brisk bleeding and those who cannot tolerate colonoscopy, the site of bleeding may be identified first by radionuclide scan (tagged red blood cell scan) or arteriography (useful when the bleeding rate is at least 0.5 to 1 mL per minute), but colonoscopy is the preferred method of evaluation due to its higher diagnostic yield, low rate of complications, and availability for being performed immediately.[9]

Differential Diagnosis

Bleeding is not typically associated with diverticulitis. Angiodysplasia (of small bowel or colon, especially in patients over age 65), ischemic colitis, neoplasm, medication side effects, inflammatory conditions, and history of recent procedures such as colonoscopy with polypectomy should be considered. Hemorrhoidal bleeding is rarely massive. Variceal bleeding should be considered in patients with end-stage liver disease, alcoholism, or portal hypertension.[9]

Treatment

In up to 80% of patients, bleeding stops spontaneously with supportive therapy alone, though the risk of rebleeding is as high as 47%.[10] Endoscopic interventions include submucosal epinephrine injection, tamponade, and bipolar coagulation. Endoclips, banding, and laser photocoagulation may also be considered. Patients with severe bleeding may be treated with transcatheter embolization or intra-arterial vasopressin for up to 24 hours if the site of bleeding is known. Patients who are unable to tolerate continued bleeding or who fail medical management should be considered for surgery. Elective sigmoid resection should also be considered for the prevention of rebleeding in those who have experienced repeated bleeding episodes, as they are at especially higher risk of subsequent rebleeding. Other risk factors for rebleeding include older age at time of initial bleed, diverticulitis, peripheral vascular disease, and chronic kidney disease.[10]

DIVERTICULITIS

Diagnosis

History

This localized infection is a result of micro- or macroscopic perforation of a diverticulum due to erosion of its wall from increased intraluminal pressure and/or inspissated food particles. Patients present with abdominal pain (most often left-sided, but in Asian patients, right-sided disease is more common) and may have fever, chills, abdominal distention, nausea, anorexia, dysuria, and occasionally vomiting. Previous episodes of diverticulitis raise the risk of recurrence and should heighten clinical suspicion, though the risk of complicated diverticulitis declines with subsequent recurrences.[11] Peritonitis, bowel obstruction, abscess perforation, and fistula formation are possible complications.

Physical Examination

There may be relatively few findings if the inflammation is isolated to the pericolic fat, or findings of acute peritonitis may be evident. In early diverticulitis, temperature may be normal, or a low-grade fever may be present. On abdominal examination, there may be varying degrees of tenderness with or without rebound. In the presence of abscess or fistula, a mass may be palpable. Immunosuppressed patients may show few findings on initial physical examination, even in the presence of overt perforation.[1,12]

Laboratory and Imaging

CBC in uncomplicated disease is normal or may reveal leukocytosis. ESR and/or CRP may be elevated. Urinalysis may show microscopic hematuria and pyuria from irritation of the ureter or from vesicocolic fistula formation. Stool is positive for occult blood in up to 25% of patients. Plain film radiographs of the abdomen may reveal free intraperitoneal air if perforation occurs, and abdominal ultrasonography can show thickened bowel, but abdominal CT is the imaging test of choice. In addition to confirming the presence and location of bowel wall thickening and inflammation within the pericolic fat, CT can reveal any abscess, fistula, peritonitis, or obstruction, thereby readily distinguishing between complicated and uncomplicated disease. Water-soluble contrast enema is sensitive and specific for diverticulitis but less well tolerated and thus rarely utilized. Though previously recommended routinely, the role of colonoscopy after symptom resolution has become more controversial, with some supporting its continued use, and other recent studies finding no increased detection of advanced neoplasms.[11,13]

Differential Diagnosis

Ischemic colitis, colon cancer, obstruction, volvulus, IBD, nephrolithiasis, penetrating ulcer, and appendicitis, especially in patients with right-sided pain, should all be considered. In patients at risk, pelvic inflammatory disease, ectopic pregnancy, and ovarian cancer should also be ruled out.

Treatment

There has been a shift toward more outpatient management of *uncomplicated diverticulitis* for stable, reliable patients who can tolerate oral intake.[12] The patient should be started on a clear liquid diet. Antispasmodic medications and analgesics may be used judiciously for symptom relief. Supplemental fiber should not be given during acute episodes as it can exacerbate symptoms, but daily supplements after resolution may reduce risk of recurrence.[11] Antibiotic use has traditionally included a 7- to 10-day broad-spectrum course targeting anaerobes and Gram-negative aerobes; first-line regimens include oral courses of a quinolone with metronidazole, amoxicillin/clavulanate, or trimethoprim–sulfamethoxazole with metronidazole. However, recently mounting evidence has prompted a progressive reduction of use of oral antibiotics in uncomplicated diverticulitis.[11] As symptoms improve, diet may be advanced from clear liquids to low residue until the patient has recovered. Consumption of nuts, seeds, corn, and popcorn has not been shown to be associated with diverticulitis.[11,14] A dietary history should be reviewed, however, as some patients are able to pinpoint these or other foods as specific, consistent triggers, and identifiable triggers should be minimized or avoided.

Inpatient management is required for patients with complicated disease or for those who cannot tolerate oral intake, have significant comorbidities, or lack adequate support resources; such inpatient care consists of bowel rest, intravenous hydration, and intravenous antibiotics.[12] Coverage for Gram-negative aerobes and anaerobes may be achieved with clindamycin or metronidazole plus a quinolone or third-generation cephalosporin. An aminoglycoside can be added if there is concern about antibiotic resistance or if *Pseudomonas* infection is suspected. Effective single-agent treatment options include piperacillin/tazobactam and ticarcillin/clavulanate. Analgesics can be given as needed, but nonsteroidal anti-inflammatory drugs have been associated with a higher risk of complications (including perforation and bleeding), and their use is discouraged.[4,15,16]

Special Considerations

Patients with *complicated diverticulitis*, that is, those who develop perforation, abscess, fistula, or obstruction, and those who are septic, immunocompromised, or fail medical management are candidates for surgery.[17] In patients with abscesses, CT-guided needle drainage may delay the need for emergent surgery and allow the performance of an elective single-stage bowel resection. Previous guidelines recommended elective resection after two episodes of acute diverticulitis due to the high risk of recurrence and complications, but this has more recently come into question, as recurrences are usually uncomplicated, and as complication risk is highest with the first episode and lower with recurrent episodes.[11,18]

REFERENCES

1. Maconi G, Barbara G, Bosetti C, et al. Treatment of diverticular disease of the colon and prevention of acute diverticulitis: a systematic review. *Dis Colon Rectum* 2011;54:1326–1338.
2. Petruzziello L, Iacopini F, Bulajic M, et al. Review article: uncomplicated diverticular disease of the colon. *Aliment Pharmacol Ther* 2006;23:1379–1391.
3. Drossman D. The functional gastrointestinal disorders and the Rome III process. *Gastroenterology* 2006;130:1377–1390.

4. Strate LL, Modi R, Cohen E, et al. Diverticular disease as a chronic illness: evolving epidemiologic and clinical insights. *Am J Gastroenterol* 2012;107:1486–1493.
5. Kruis W, Meier E, Schumacher M, et al. Randomised clinical trial: mesalazine (Salofalk granules) for uncomplicated diverticular disease of the colon—a placebo-controlled study. *Aliment Pharmacol Ther* 2013;37:680–690.
6. Tursi A, Brandimarte G, Elisei W, et al. Randomised clinical trial: mesalazine and/or probiotics in maintaining remission of symptomatic uncomplicated diverticular disease—a double-blind, randomised, placebo-controlled study. *Aliment Pharmacol Ther* 2013;38:741–751.
7. Bianchi M, Festa V, Moretti A, et al. Meta-analysis: long-term therapy with rifaximin in the management of uncomplicated diverticular disease. *Aliment Pharmacol Ther* 2011;33:902–910.
8. Lamiki P, Tsuchiya J, Pathak S, et al. Probiotics in diverticular disease of the colon: an open label study. *J Gastrointestin Liver Dis* 2010;19:31–36.
9. Ghassemi KA, Jensen DM. Lower GI bleeding: epidemiology and management. *Curr Gastroenterol Rep* 2013;15:333.
10. Aytac E, Stocchi L, Gorgun E, et al. Risk of recurrence and long-term outcomes after colonic diverticular bleeding. *Int J Colorectal Dis* 2014;29:373–378.
11. Morris AM, Regenbogen SE, Hardiman KM, et al. Sigmoid diverticulitis: a systematic review. *JAMA* 2014;311:287–297.
12. Feingold D, Steele SR, Lee S, et al. Practice parameters for the treatment of sigmoid diverticulitis. *Dis Colon Rectum* 2014;57:284–294.
13. Sharma PV, Eglinton T, Hider P, et al. Systematic review and meta-analysis of the role of routine colonic evaluation after radiologically confirmed acute diverticulitis. *Ann Surg* 2014;259:263–272.
14. Strate LL, Liu YL, Syngal S, et al. Nut, corn, and popcorn consumption and the incidence of diverticular disease. *JAMA* 2008;300:907–914.
15. Strate LL, Liu YL, Huang ES, et al. Use of aspirin or nonsteroidal anti-inflammatory drugs increases risk for diverticulitis and diverticular bleeding. *Gastroenterology* 2011;140:1427–1433.
16. Lembcke B. The gastroenterologist's view. *Dig Dis* 2012;30:122–128.
17. Klarenbeek BR, Samuels M, van der Wal MA, et al. Indications for elective sigmoid resection in diverticular disease. *Ann Surg* 2010;251:670–674.
18. Chapman JR, Dozois EJ, Wolff BG, et al. Diverticulitis: a progressive disease? Do multiple recurrences predict less favorable outcomes? *Ann Surg* 2006;243:876–883.

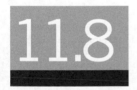

11.8 Irritable Bowel Syndrome

L. Peter Schwiebert

GENERAL PRINCIPLES

Definition

Irritable bowel syndrome (IBS) is abdominal discomfort or pain associated with abnormal bowel habits. Abnormal bowel habits include diarrhea-predominant, constipation-predominant, and alternating diarrhea and constipation. Current Rome III criteria for IBS include improvement with defecation, onset associated with a change in frequency of stools, and onset associated with a change in appearance of stools the previous 3 months, with symptoms beginning at least 6 months before diagnosis and not otherwise explained.

Epidemiology

Although up to 70% of patients with IBS do not consult a health care provider, **prevalence estimates** range between 3% and 25%; most studies suggest a 10% to 19% prevalence in the general population, with higher prevalence in females than in males. IBS and related functional bowel disorders account for >50% of gastroenterology consultations in the United States. IBS has **significant comorbidities**, including gastrointestinal (GI) and non-GI manifestations.

GI symptoms include lower GI symptoms consistent with Rome II criteria as well as associated nonspecific upper GI symptoms. For example, one large Japanese study found 34% of patients with IBS also had gastroesophageal reflux disease or functional dyspepsia. Non-GI comorbidities such as psychiatric disorders and sexual dysfunction are also common. Psychiatric diagnoses are present in up to two-third of patients with IBD, and severe IBS is associated with a history or physical or sexual abuse.[1]

Various estimates place the **annual cost of IBS** in physician visits, medications, and loss of productivity to sufferers in the United States at 20 billion dollars. This cost is comparable to or exceeds the cost of other common chronic conditions such as asthma, hypertension, and heart failure. Individuals with IBS also have significantly lower self-assessed health-related quality of life compared to controls.

DIAGNOSIS
History

Historical features (Rome III criteria) diagnose IBS, coupled with absence of "red flag" findings suggesting organic/structural disease. These "red flag" findings include the onset of symptoms after age 50, recent antibiotic use, nocturnal symptoms, unintended weight loss, hematochezia, anemia, or family history of inflammatory bowel disease/celiac sprue/malignancy. **Symptoms** of diarrhea, constipation, and remission in patients with IBS characteristically fluctuate, in fact, up to a third changing subtype diarrhea- versus constipation-predominant over a 12-week period.

The **Bristol Stool Scale** can assist both in characterizing stool type and in monitoring response to therapy. In this classification, stools have seven types, ranging from (a) hard lumps, like nuts, to (b) sausage-like but lumpy, to (c) snake-like with cracks on the surface, to (d) snake-like and smooth, to (e) soft blobs with clear-cut edges, to (f) mushy stool, to (g) watery stool without solid pieces. Types a and b are compatible with constipation, whereas types e to g are compatible with diarrhea. Other gastrointestinal symptoms in IBS may include a sensation of a lump in the throat, acid reflux, dysphagia, early satiety, intermittent dyspepsia, nausea, noncardiac chest pain, abdominal bloating, and flatulence.[2]

Diagnostic Testing

When there are "red flag" findings suggesting organic/structural disease, a colonoscopy is recommended. However, diagnostic testing may differ on the basis of clinical context, differential diagnoses, and specific "red flag" finding.

Laboratory Studies

In patients meeting IBS criteria, the American College of Gastroenterology Functional Disorders Task Force concluded that **routine diagnostic testing is not supported by the literature**, as the likelihood of an abnormal result is no different comparing those with IBS and controls. The only possible exception is to consider testing for celiac sprue in diarrhea-predominant or mixed presentation IBS (there is an approximate 4% incidence of sprue in these patients).

TREATMENT

Treatment for IBS is symptomatic and individualized, depending on the impact on the patient's quality of life. Evaluating efficacy of interventions is challenging, given a relatively high placebo response. Table 11.8-1 accounts for this by referencing, when available, randomized controlled trials.[3–7]

Referral

Possible referral to a gastroenterologist of individuals with IBS is appropriate if the diagnosis is in question or if the patient presents with findings of organic/structural disease.

Patient Education

Patient education in individuals with IBS is foundational to effective management. This includes **reassurance and a comprehensible explanation** of underlying physiology/pathophysiology of IBS, including discussion of the role of stressors and psychiatric influences. Scant evidence supports **dietary manipulation** in IBS; however, in some patients, a food diary may be beneficial in identifying particular foods (e.g., ethanol, caffeine, sorbitol, or fats) associated with symptoms.[2]

TABLE 11.8-1	Medications for IBS		
Class	**Examples**	**SOR**	**Comments**
Increased physical activity	–	A	Significant improvement in global symptoms
Probiotics	*Lactobacillus, Bifidobacterium, Streptococcus,* or combination	A	Significant improvement in abdominal pain and flatulence
Complementary alternative medication	Peppermint oil	A	Significant improvement in abdominal pain, global assessment, symptom score
Antispasmodics	Dicyclomine	A	Significant improvement in abdominal pain, global assessment, symptom score
Antidepressants	SSRIs (citalopram, paroxetine, fluoxetine) TCA (amitriptyline, desipramine, imipramine)	A	Significant improvement in global assessment, abdominal pain, symptom score
Antibiotics	Rifaximin[a]	A	Significant improvement in global assessment and bloating
Selective C-2 chloride channel activators	Lubiprostone	A	Significant improvement of global symptoms in constipation—predominant IBS
Antidiarrheals	Loperamide		Decreased stool frequency in diarrhea-predominant IBS
Laxatives	Polyethylene glycol		Improved bowel movement frequency, but not other symptoms in constipation-predominant IBS
Fiber	Psyllium		Ineffective

SOR, strength of recommendation (A = based on consistent, good quality, and patient-oriented evidence); SSRIs, selective serotonin reuptake inhibitors; TCA, tricyclic antidepressants.
[a]Dosed at 550 mg three times daily.

REFERENCES

1. Kaji M, Fujiwara Y, Shiba M, et al. Prevalence of overlaps between GERD, FD and IBS and impact on health-related quality of life. *J Gastroenterol Hepatol* 2010;25:1151–1156.
2. Wilkins T, Pepitone C, Biju A, et al. Diagnosis and management of IBS in adults. *Am Fam Physician* 2012;86(5):419–426.
3. Talley NJ, Herrick L, Locke GR. Antidepressants in functional dyspepsia. *Expert Rev Gastroenterol Hepatol* 2010;4(1):5–7.
4. Johannesson E, Simren M, Hans S, et al. Physical activity improves symptoms in irritable bowel syndrome: a randomized controlled trial. *Am J Gastroenterol* 2011;106:915–922.
5. Pimentel M, Lembo A, Chey W, et al. Rifaximin therapy for patients with irritable bowel syndrome without constipation. *N Engl J Med* 2011;364:22–32.
6. Moayyedi P, Ford AC, Talley NJ, et al. The efficacy of probiotics in the treatment of irritable bowel syndrome: a systematic review. *Gut* 2008;59:325–332.
7. Ruepert L, Quartero AO, de Wit NJ, et al. Bulking agents, antispasmodics and antidepressants for the treatment of irritable bowel syndrome. *Cochrane Database Syst Rev* 2011;(8):CD003460.

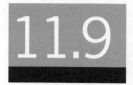

Inflammatory Bowel Disease

Michael A. Malone, Charis James, Neha Kaushik

GENERAL PRINCIPLES

The term inflammatory bowel disease (IBD) collectively includes the two major disorders, collectively known as Crohn disease (CD) and ulcerative colitis (UC), which are chronic, relapsing, and remitting inflammatory conditions of the gastrointestinal (GI) tract. Both have distinct pathologic and clinical characteristics, but their pathogenesis is poorly understood.

Epidemiology

The data that do exist suggest that the worldwide incidence of UC varies greatly between 0.5 and 24.5 per 100,000 persons, while that of CD varies between 0.1 and 16 per 100,000 persons worldwide, with the prevalence of IBD reaching up to 396 per 100,000 persons.[1] The most common age of presentation is from adolescence to 40 years, with a smaller increase in incidence in the 50- to 80-year age group. IBD is more common in developed countries. There is higher frequency in urban communities compared with rural areas.[2]

Pathology

- *Crohn disease:* CD is characterized by a granulomatous, transmural inflammatory infiltrate located at any level of the GI tract from mouth to anus, most commonly found in the ileocecal area. The transmural nature of the inflammatory process in CD results in fibrotic strictures. CD is a patchy, noncontinuous process.
- *Ulcerative colitis:* UC is characterized by recurring episodes of inflammation limited to the superficial mucosal layer of the colon and is continuous in nature. It is limited to the colon, commonly involves the rectum, and may extend in a proximal and continuous fashion to involve other parts of the colon.

Etiology

The pathogenesis of IBD remains obscure. The prevailing belief is that IBD is heterogeneous with several genetic and environmental factors playing a role. The final manifestation of the process is mucosal inflammation presenting with a wide variety of symptoms. Risk factors include being of Jewish ethnicity, while the incidence of IBD is lower in black and Hispanic populations compared to whites. Smoking may directly affect mucosal immune response. A western style diet is also associated with an increased risk of developing IBD.[2]

DIAGNOSIS

Accurate diagnosis rests with the analysis of the clinical presentation, the omission of infectious causes that may mimic IBD, and choosing the most appropriate study. The physician must obtain a complete history, including foreign travel, exposure to food-borne illness, and analgesic and antibiotic agents.[3]

- *Ulcerative colitis:* The diagnosis of UC is based on the presence of chronic diarrhea for more than 4 weeks and evidence of chronic colitis on endoscopy and biopsy. Since these features are not specific for UC, establishing the diagnosis also requires the exclusion of other causes of colitis by history, laboratory studies, and by biopsies of the colon obtained on endoscopy.
- *Crohn disease:* The diagnosis of CD is often made with endoscopic findings or imaging studies in a patient with a corresponding clinical history and examination. Colonoscopy is a conventional initial test for patients presenting with predominant diarrhea, whereas imaging studies are commonly used for those presenting with abdominal pain.

Clinical Presentation

Crohn Disease

CD can present acutely or chronically. The clinical manifestations of CD are more variable than those of UC.[4] Features of CD include abdominal pain, diarrhea that may be bloody, severe urgency, weight loss, loss of appetite, and fatigue. Symptoms manifest based on the site of involvement and disease pattern, fistulous versus obstructive. The terminal ileum is the most common site of involvement. The terminal ileum inflammation results in ileitis or ileocolitis and may manifest only as episodic right upper quadrant or periumbilical abdominal pain and diarrhea. This presentation can be mistakenly diagnosed as an acute appendicitis or diverticulitis.

Diarrhea is a common presentation of CD, but often fluctuates over a long period of time. CD, however, may also present as small bowel obstruction due to the decreased diameter of the inflamed colon. A history of prolonged diarrhea without bleeding, but with systemic features such as anorexia, fevers, weight loss, or anemia suggestive of IBD should suggest the diagnosis of CD. Although stools frequently reveal the presence of microscopic levels of blood, gross bleeding is less frequent in CD than in UC. An exception are patients with Crohn colitis, as bloody diarrhea usually indicates colonic involvement.

Less common GI presentations include refractory oral ulceration, perianal fistula or abscess, gastroduodenal disease (dyspepsia, anorexia, nausea and vomiting, epigastric pain), intra-abdominal abscess, or symptoms of enterovesical fistula (urinary tract infection, fecaluria). Extraintestinal manifestations are common in CD and include arthritis, uveitis, episcleritis, erythema nodosum, pyoderma gangrenosum, thromboembolism, renal stones, and renal failure.

Ulcerative Colitis

Patients with UC usually present with diarrhea often with gross rectal bleeding. The onset of symptoms is usually gradual, and symptoms are progressive over several weeks. Symptoms may be preceded by a self-limited episode of rectal bleeding that occurred weeks or months earlier. The severity of symptoms may range from mild disease with four or fewer stools per day with or without blood to severe disease with more than 10 stools per day with severe cramps and continuous bleeding.[5]

The majority of patients presenting with UC have proctitis, inflammation of the mucosal layer of the rectum. Proctitis manifests with rectal bleeding, rectal pain, urgency, tenesmus, and, sometimes, bowel incontinence.[5] Although the most common presentation in UC is bloody diarrhea, rectal disease may also cause constipation with hard, bloody, and mucus streaked stool. Abdominal pain is a frequent complaint and is described as crampy and colicky. Fever, anemia, nausea, vomiting, anorexia, and weight loss are common presenting signs and symptoms of UC.

Differential Diagnosis

The differential diagnosis for IBD includes lactose intolerance, appendicitis, cecal diverticulitis, ischemic or radiation colitis, ileocecal tuberculosis, giardiasis, small bowel lymphoma, the vasculitis associated with Behçet syndrome, HIV/AIDS, and cecal carcinoma. In women, gynecologic disease should be considered in the differential diagnosis. Irritable bowel syndrome (IBS) often mimics the presenting symptoms of UC and CD, but should never cause rectal bleeding or a positive fecal occult blood test.

Infections caused by *Shigella*, *Salmonella*, *Campylobacter*, *Escherichia coli* O157:H, *Yersinia*, and parasites (including amebiasis) should be considered. *Clostridium difficile* infection should also be included in the differential diagnosis, particularly in patients recently treated with antibiotics. In immunocompromised patients, cytomegalovirus infection can mimic CD.

Physical Examination

General inspection may reveal an individual with fever and pallor. Examination of the head may reveal conjunctivitis, iritis, or episcleritis. Ulcers may be seen in mouth. Joint arthralgias are seen, and erythema nodosum or pyoderma gangrenosum may affect the skin. An examination of the abdomen may reveal right lower quadrant tenderness or even a palpable mass in CD and left lower quadrant pain in UC. Abdominal distention and abnormal bowel sounds indicate bowel obstruction in CD. Rectal examination should be performed, to check for rectal tenderness and the presence of blood. The perianal region as up to one-third of patients with CD will develop perianal disease.

Laboratory Testing

Several laboratory studies are of value in assisting with the diagnosis and management of IBD and provide supporting information. However, no laboratory test is specific enough to adequately and definitively establish the diagnosis of IBD. Basic laboratory workup consists of complete blood count; liver function tests; electrolytes; renal function; albumin; vitamin B_{12}; and markers of inflammation such as erythrocyte sedimentation rate, C-reactive protein (CRP), and fecal calprotectin.[6] CRP levels are generally higher in CD than in UC. CRP determination may have a role in distinguishing between these diseases, as well as in differentiating patients with IBD from those with symptoms caused by other conditions.[7] Testing for fecal calprotectin may help identify patients with intestinal inflammation from IBD, but it is not routinely done in clinical practice.[8]

Before making a definitive diagnosis of IBD, it is recommended to perform a stool culture, ova and parasite studies, bacterial pathogens culture, and evaluation for *C. difficile* infection.[9] HIV testing should be considered, as opportunistic GI tract infections can present with diarrhea, weight loss, and abdominal pain.

Autoantibodies

Perinuclear antineutrophil cytoplasmic antibodies (pANCAs) have been identified in some patients with UC, and anti-*Saccharomyces cerevisiae* antibodies (ASCAs) have been found in patients with CD. The combination of positive pANCA and negative ASCA is highly suggestive of UC. Inversely, a combination of positive ASCA and negative pANCA is more specific for CD. However, at this time, serologic markers cannot be used to definitively rule in or exclude IBD. Therefore, these tests should be used only as an adjunct to conventional testing.[10–13]

Imaging

Radiologic imaging is generally needed to evaluate patients with probable small bowel disease, and therefore typically is not used in the evaluation of UC. They are most useful to evaluate the upper GI tract in CD and allow documentation of the length and location of strictures in areas not accessible by colonoscopy. Several imaging modalities are available, including conventional upper GI series with small bowel follow-through (SBFT), computed tomography (CT) and CT enterography, ultrasound, and magnetic resonance imaging (MRI).

Barium enemas may be useful to evaluate the lower GI tract in cases of limited or no access to endoscopy, in cases of incomplete colonoscopy, or to measure stricture length. **Barium enema should be avoided in patients who are severely ill since it may precipitate ileus with toxic megacolon.** CT and MRI have lower sensitivity than barium enema for the detection of subtle early mucosal disease but are equivalent in patients with established and severe disease.[14] CT and MRI may demonstrate marked thickening of the bowel wall, but this finding is nonspecific. Wall thickening may occur from smooth muscle contraction, but the presence of inflammatory changes such as mesenteric fat stranding, wall enhancement, and increased vascularity significantly increases the predictive value of the imaging. Ultrasonography, magnetic resonance imaging (MRI), and CT scanning have similar accuracy for the entire bowel and are reliable in identifying fistulas and stenosis, but ultrasound may lead to false positives for abscesses. Ultrasound and MRI are often preferred over CT scanning due to radiation exposure with CT.[15]

Ulcerative Colitis

Abdominal imaging is not required for the diagnosis of UC, but may be performed in patients who present with symptoms of colitis. If a radiological test is ordered for suspected UC, the most useful modality is the air-contrast barium enema. If severe colitis or obstruction is suspected, a three-position abdominal series can be obtained to rule out perforation, obstruction, or toxic megacolon. Abdominal radiography is usually normal in patients with mild to moderate disease, but in patients with severe or fulminant UC it may identify proximal constipation, mucosal thickening or "thumbprinting" secondary to edema, and colonic dilation.

Crohn Disease

Imaging has traditionally involved barium studies, such as barium enema or upper GI series with SBFT, but the use of CT and MR enterography is becoming the standard imaging for patients with CD. MRI can be useful for the detection of perianal fistulas in CD. Abdominal CT can be a useful modality when there is clinical suspicion for an intra-abdominal abcess.

Endoscopy

Sigmoidoscopy is a reasonable initial diagnostic test to perform for suspected UC. However, colonoscopy tends to be the preferred endoscopic procedure for IBD and is one of the most valuable tools available to the physician for the diagnosis of IBD. Colonoscopy can be used for the diagnosis of CD, especially if the ileocecal valve can be traversed and the terminal ileum examined. This is often the only method of diagnosing early ileal or colonic CD. Colonoscopy is also an effective method of assessing the extent of UC, which can be useful in determining if systemic or local therapy is appropriate.

Colonoscopy is almost never warranted during bouts of severe colitis or in the patient with toxic megacolon, although there is debate about the safety of the examination in this situation. Typically, there is a cobblestone appearance of the colon in CD, with areas of normal mucosa between involved areas. In UC, inflammation is continuous with erosions and friability apparent.

Barium enema is a less desirable alternative, but may be indicated when a complete colonoscopy cannot be performed for technical reasons. Esophagogastroduodenoscopy (EGD) is used for the evaluation of upper GI tract symptoms, particularly in patients with CD. Capsule enteroscopy may also aid in the diagnosis of small bowel CD when the standard diagnostic workup with a colonoscopy and upper endoscopy is negative.[10]

TREATMENT (TABLE 11.9-1)

The care of a patient with IBD can be either medical or surgical in nature or, in many patients, a combination of both. The management algorithm is also dependent on whether the diagnosis is CD or UC. The medical approach for patients with IBD is to improve symptoms and aid in mucosal healing. The main treatment goals are the achievement of disease remission and the prevention of flares. In mild to moderate IBD, a step-up approach with medication is typically done until a response is achieved. A typical step-up approach is listed below, with step 1 being the first treatment and step 3 being utilized only if needed.

- Step 1: Aminosalicylates and/or antibiotics
- Step 2: Corticosteroids
- Step 3: Immunomodulators/biologic therapies

The first step in medication therapy for IBD is usually aminosalicylates. There are several different aminosalicylates, but none has been consistently demonstrated to be superior to the others for all patients. There are five oral aminosalicylate preparations available in the United States. They are sulfasalazine, mesalamine, balsalazide, and olsalazine. Enema and suppository formulations are also available. All the aminosalicylates are derivatives of 5-aminosalicylic acid (5-ASA) with the major difference between them being the mechanism and site of delivery. The aminosalicylates appear to have greater efficacy for the treatment of UC than for CD, for which efficacy data are limited.

If the patient's condition fails to respond to an adequate dose of aminosalicylates, the second step is often corticosteroids.[16] Treatment options for the treatment of patients who do not respond to steroids, have frequent relapses, or become steroid dependent include azathioprine, 6-mercaptopurine, methotrexate, and biologic therapies. There are several studies with biologic therapies (antitumor necrosis factor therapies) that have shown a decrease in the rate of surgery, the use of corticosteroids, and the rate of hospitalization.[17-21]

Hospitalization

With severe symptoms, abnormal vital signs, severe colitis, intra-abdominal abscess, or other complications, management should occur in the hospital setting. The patient should be given intravenous (IV) rehydration, left nil per oral (NPO), and receive IV therapy (usually with high dose steroids) as soon as the diagnosis is made. In these cases, it is prudent to seek consultation from a gastroenterologist or surgeon. Consultation is also advised for patients who do not respond to initial outpatient management, or develop complications such as fistula, obstruction, or abscess.

Outpatient Treatment

Local therapy of proctitis and sigmoid disease (mild to moderate) should be attempted before using systemic treatment. Patients with CD should discontinue the use of oral contraceptives and smoking. IBD sufferers should avoid the use of nonsteroidal anti-inflammatory drugs. Systemic agents effective in IBD include 6-mercaptopurine, azathioprine, methotrexate, cyclosporin (in UC only), and antitumor necrosis factor therapies.

If the use of newer systemic agents is considered or complex therapy is necessary, this is best undertaken after consultation. Once remission occurs, maintenance therapy should be considered. However, a meta-analysis indicates that, despite multiple available therapies, remission rates remain high for IBD.[22] Symptomatic therapy for diarrhea (codeine, loperamide) is contraindicated in severe disease and megacolon.

TABLE 11.9-1 Inflammatory Bowel Disease: Management Options

Local agent	UC indications dose	CD indications dose	Contraindication	Side effects
Hydrocortisone (HCT) enema (cortenema) 100 mg	Enema (100 mg) Proctitis, sigmoid disease single agent in mild disease, supplement to systemic treatment 1 appl qhs × 21 d	For CD of lower colon/rectum, same doses as with UC	Obstruction, local abscess, perforation, peritonitis, recent anastamosis, fistulas Sensitivity to drug/class, infections	Local irritation, rectal bleeding, systemic absorption Serious side effects not reported
HCT foam (Cortifoam) 90 mg	As with HCT enema 1 appl PR qd–bid × 2–3 wk, then qod	For CD of lower colon/rectum, same doses as with UC	See HCT enema	See HCT enema
HCT Suppositories 100 mg	As with HCT enema	For CD of lower colon/rectum, same doses as with UC	See HCT enema	See HCT enema
Mesalamine suppositories (Rowasa) 500 mg	As with HCT but more effective 500 mg PR bid	As with HCT but more effective 500 mg PR bid	Sensitivity to drug/class, obstruction, local abscess, perforation, peritonitis, fistulas	Local irritation, rectal bleeding
Mesalamine enemas (4 g/60 mL)	As with HCT but more effective 1–4 g/d PR maintenance 1–4 g qod	As with HCT but more effective 1–4 g/d PR maintenance 1–4 g qod	See mesalamine suppositories	See mesalamine suppositories
Systemic agent				
IV steroids HCT (Solu-Cortef) Methylprednisolone (Solu-Medrol)	Effective for remission induction only HCT 300 mg/d Methylprednisolone 40–60 mg/d	Effective for remission induction only HCT 300 mg/d Methylprednisolone 40–60 mg/d	Drug sensitivity Relative with infections, caution if congestive heart failure, diabetes, tuberculosis, hypertension	Adrenal insufficiency, psychosis, immunosuppression, peptic ulcer, osteoporosis, and others
PO steroids Prednisone (Deltasone) CIR budesonide for CD of ileum	As with IV steroids Prednisone 40–60 mg/d	As with IV steroids Prednisone 0.25–0.75 mg/kg/d CIR budesonide 9 mg PO qam	See IV steroids	See IV steroids
PO sulfasalazine (Azulfidine 500 mg tabs)	Remission induction 2–6 g/d (1 g qid), maintenance 2–4 g/d; administer with folate 0.4–1 mg/d	Effective in ileocolonic disease only—induction 3–5 g/d (1 g qid) maintenance 3 g/d; administer with folate 0.4–1 mg/d	Hypersensitivity to drug/class/sulfa/salicylates, renal/hepatic dysfunction, porphyria, obstruction, caution G6PD deficiency	Poorly tolerated esp. at high doses (GI) rashes, Stevens–Johnson syndrome, hemolytic anemia, GI, headache, pancreatitis, hepatitis, sperm ab.

Local agent	UC indications dose	CD indications dose	Contraindication	Side effects
PO mesalamine 5-ASA (Asacol-ileocolonic release 400 mg, Pentasa 250 mg jejunum to colon)	Remission induction 4–4.8 g/d (Asacol 1200 mg qid) Maintenance 400–800 mg qid, prob. ineffective	Remission induction Asacol 1–1.2 g qid, Pentasa 1 g qid, better for proximal disease? maintenance same as remission effectiveness?	Hypersensitivity to drug/class, caution in impaired renal function	Anaphylaxis, confusion, headache, GI, pharyngitis, dizziness, asthenia, others
PO antibiotics Metronidazole (Flagyl) ± Ciprofloxacin (Cipro)	N/A	Effective in remission alone or in combination–first choice for perianal disease. Flagyl 250 mg qid ± Cipro 500 mg bid	Hypersensitivity to drug/class, pregnancy, caution with central nervous system disorder	GI, seizures, rash, photosensitivity, liver function test elevation, neuropathy and antabuse reaction with flagyl, tendonitis with Cipro
Methotrexate (intractable Crohn remission induction)	Role is unclear	25 mg IM weekly; effective in remission induction in refractory disease and reduction of steroid doses by 50%	Hypersensitivity to drug/class, pregnancy, breastfeeding, immunodeficiency alcohol abuse, caution with renal/ hepatic dysfunction	Ulcerative stomatitis, anemia, leucopenia thrombocytopenia Immune suppression
Infliximab	Varying doses and regimens, most often 5 mg/kg IV infusion	Varying doses and regimens; most often 5 mg/kg IV infusion; most effective Rx for fistulizing CD	Hypersensitivity to drug/class or murine proteins Active infection Congestive heart failure NYHA III, IV Caution with seizure, hematologic disorder, latent tuberculosis, multiple sclerosis, elderly	Fever, chills, myalgias, H/A, fatigue Sepsis, pneumonia, opportunistic infections, hepatotoxicity, serum sickness-like reaction, bone marrow suppression

COMPLICATIONS

Colon cancer is a complication of IBD. Colonic mucosa that is involved with IBD is more likely to develop dysplasia and carcinoma. With extensive colonic involvement by CD, the rate of malignant transformation is probably similar to that seen with UC.[23] The optimal frequency of screening for carcinoma in IBD is controversial, but colonoscopy and biopsy should be performed regularly.[24] Generally, surveillance colonoscopy beginning 8 years after diagnosis and every 1 to 3 years thereafter is recommended.[25]

Complications of IBD include acute hemorrhage, sepsis, gallstones, intestinal ischemia, osteoporosis, depression and anxiety, intra-abdominal abcess (CD), and colon perforation. Fistulas are also a common complication of CD and form in 15% of patients with this diagnosis. The fistulas can be perirectal, cutaneous, enterovaginal, and enterovesicular. Toxic megacolon is another possible complication of IBD characterized by colonic diameter ≥ 6 cm or cecal diameter > 9 cm and the presence of systemic toxicity.[26] Patients with severe IBD or toxic megacolon will appear acutely ill with abdominal tenderness, dehydration, tachycardia, hypotension, and fever.

Extraintestinal manifestations of IBD include ocular changes of episcleritis and uveitis, reactive arthropathy with ankylosing spondylitis, and the dermatologic manifestations of erythema nodosum and pyoderma gangrenosum. There is an increased incidence of nephrolithiasis, especially in CD. A serious complication, seen most often in UC, is sclerosing cholangitis.

REFERENCES

1. Lakatos PL. Recent trends in the epidemiology of inflammatory bowel diseases: up or down? *World J Gastroenterol* 2006;12(38):6102–6108.
2. Hanauer S. Inflammatory bowel disease: epidemiology, pathogenesis and therapeutic opportunities. *Inflamm Bowel Dis* 2006;12:S3–S9.
3. Bernstein CN, Fried M, Krabshuis JH, et al. World Gastroenterology Organization Practice Guidelines for the diagnosis and management of IBD in 2010. *Inflamm Bowel Dis* 2010;16(1):112–124.
4. Burgmann T, Clara I, Graff L, et al. The Manitoba Inflammatory Bowel Disease Cohort Study: prolonged symptoms before diagnosis—how much is irritable bowel syndrome? *Clin Gastroenterol Hepatol* 2006;4(5):614.
5. Silverberg MS, Satsangi J, Ahmad T, et al. Toward an integrated clinical, molecular and serological classification of inflammatory bowel disease: report of a Working Party of the 2005 Montreal World Congress of Gastroenterology. *Can J Gastroenterol* 2005;19(Suppl A):5A.
6. Prantera C, Davoli M, Lorenzetti R, et al. Clinical and laboratory indicators of extent of ulcerative colitis. Serum C-reactive protein helps the most. *J Clin Gastroenterol* 1988;10(1):41–45.
7. Schoepfer AM, Trummler M, Seeholzer P, et al. Discriminating IBD from IBS: comparison of the test performance of fecal markers, blood leukocytes, CRP, and IBD antibodies. *Inflamm Bowel Dis* 2008;14(1):32.
8. van Rheenen PF, Van de Vijver E, Fidler V. Faecal calprotectin for screening of patients with suspected inflammatory bowel disease: diagnostic meta-analysis. *BMJ* 2010;341:c3369.
9. Kornbluth A, Sachar DB. Ulcerative colitis practice guidelines in adults: American College of Gastroenterology, Practice Parameters Committee. *Am J Gastroenterol* 2010;105(3):501–523.
10. World Gastroenterology Organisation (WGO). *World Gastroenterology Organisation Global Guideline. Inflammatory bowel disease: a global perspective.* Munich, Germany: World Gastroenterology Organisation (WGO); 2009.
11. Peeters M, Joossens S, Vermeire S, et al. Diagnostic value of anti-Saccharomyces cerevisiae and antineutrophil cytoplasmic autoantibodies in inflammatory bowel disease. *Am J Gastroenterol* 2001;96(3):730.
12. Granito A, Zauli D, Muratori P, et al. Anti-Saccharomyces cerevisiae and perinuclear anti-neutrophil cytoplasmic antibodies in coeliac disease before and after gluten-free diet. *Aliment Pharmacol Ther* 2005;21(7):881.
13. Mow WS, Vasiliauskas EA, Lin YC, et al. Association of antibody responses to microbial antigens and complications of small bowel Crohn's disease. *Gastroenterology* 2004;126(2):414.
14. Mowat C, Cole A, Windsor A, et al; IBD Section of the British Society of Gastroenterology. Guidelines for the management of inflammatory bowel disease in adults. *Gut* 2011;60(5):571–607.
15. Panés J, Bouzas R, Chaparro M, et al. Systematic review: the use of ultrasonography, computed tomography and magnetic resonance imaging for the diagnosis, assessment of activity and abdominal complications of Crohn's disease. *Aliment Pharmacol Ther* 2011;34(2):125–145.
16. Ford AC, Bernstein CN, Khan KJ, et al. Glucocorticosteroid therapy in inflammatory bowel disease: systematic review and meta-analysis. *Am J Gastroenterol* 2011;106(4):590–599.

17. Schnitzler F, Fidder H, Ferrante M, et al. Mucosal healing predicts long-term outcome of maintenance therapy with infliximab in Crohn's disease. *Inflamm Bowel Dis* 2009;15(9):1295–1301.
18. Baert F, Moortgat L, Van Assche G, et al. Mucosal healing predicts sustained clinical remission in patients with early-stage Crohn's disease. *Gastroenterology* 2010;138(2):463–468.
19. Colombel JF, Sandborn WJ, Reinisch W, et al. Infliximab, azathioprine, or combination therapy for Crohn's disease. *N Engl J Med* 2010;362(15):1383–1395.
20. Ha C, Kornbluth A. Mucosal healing in inflammatory bowel disease: where do we stand? *Curr Gastroenterol Rep* 2010;12(6):471–478.
21. Feagan BG, Lémann M, Befrits R, et al. Recommendations for the treatment of Crohn's disease with tumor necrosis factor antagonists: an expert consensus report. *Inflamm Bowel Dis* 2012;18(1):152–160.
22. Akobeng AK, Gardener E. Oral 5-ASA for maintenance of medically-induced remission in Crohn's disease. *Cochrane Database Syst Rev* 2006:2.
23. Sharon R, Schoen RE. Cancer in inflammatory bowel disease. An evidence-based analysis and guide for physicians and patients. *Gastroenterol Clin North Am* 2002;31:237–254, 2002.
24. Collins PD, Mpofu C, Watson AJ, et al. Strategies for detecting colon cancer and/or dysplasia in patients with inflammatory bowel disease. *Cochrane Database Syst Rev* 2006;(2):CD000279.
25. Rubin DT, Kavitt RT. Surveillance for cancer and dysplasia in inflammatory bowel disease. *Gastroenterol Clin North Am* 2006;35:581–604.
26. Greenstein AJ, Sachar DB, Gibas A, et al. Outcome of toxic dilatation in ulcerative and Crohn's colitis. *J Clin Gastroenterol* 1985;7(2):137.

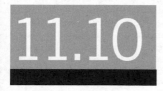

11.10 Anorectal Disease and Hemorrhoids

Munima Nasir, Nadine S. Hewamudalige, Paul A. Botros

GENERAL PRINCIPLES

Anorectal disease and hemorrhoids are commonly seen within primary care practice. Colon cancer is particularly important to diagnose as it is the cause of more than 50% of all gastrointestinal (GI) disease litigation against primary care providers.[1] Once cancer, which can coexist with benign conditions, has been excluded, more than 90% of anorectal complaints can be managed in the primary care office.[2]

ANAL FISSURES
General Principles

Definition

A fissure is a crack or linear tear in the anal mucosa in the distal anal canal from dentate line to anal verge. Anal fissures are usually found in the posterior midline of the skin, but in 10% to 20% of cases, they are located anteriorly.[3]

Pathophysiology

Fissure persistence is due to the repeated cycle of pain and reinjury of the tear from the passage of stools and subsequent spasm of the internal sphincter muscle, which leads to reduced anodermal perfusion and poor healing.

Etiology

Etiology is unknown. Primary anal fissures are commonly attributed to the passage of a hard stool or explosive diarrhea, and in some cases, anoreceptive intercourse and childbirth.[4]

Diagnosis

Clinical Presentation

Fissures generally produce tearing or burning pain and bright red bleeding associated with defecation.

History

The patient will often report a recent passage of a **hard stool or explosive diarrhea** with acute onset of severe **pain on defecation** as well as bright red blood on the toilet paper.[4] This pain can last several hours.

Physical Examination

Gentle lateral retraction of the buttocks allows for visualization of the fissure. Patients are often too uncomfortable to tolerate a digital rectal examination or anoscopy. These evaluations may be delayed until the fissure is healed or the pain has lessened; however, an examination under anesthesia, or endoscopic evaluation should be considered if the diagnosis is in doubt or the patient does not respond to treatment.[4]

Differential Diagnosis

Fissures **off the midline, laterally or present in multiples** should prompt consideration of other medical disorders such as inflammatory bowel disease, anal carcinoma, acquired immune deficiency syndrome (AIDS), tuberculosis, occult abscesses, leukemic infiltrates, herpes, or syphilis.[5] Screening laboratories may be helpful in these instances.

Treatment

The mainstay of anal fissure treatment (like that of hemorrhoids) begins with conservative treatment including increased **fluid** and **fiber** ingestion, the use of warm **sitz baths**, and the use of **stool softeners** such as docusate sodium. Roughly half of patients who are eligible for conservative management can expect healing, but recurrence is still likely among these patients without proper patient education and compliance.[4]

Medications

Topical steroids or topical anesthetics by creams, suppositories, or ointments can be used in the management of acute anal fissure pain, and are considered part of conservative management. Topical nitrates (isosorbide dinitrate, nitroglycerine, isosorbide-5-mononitrate or glyceryl trinitrate [GTN]) and topical calcium-channel blockers (such as diltiazem or nifedipine) can be used for 6 to 8 weeks in the medical management of refractory or chronic anal fissures. Botulinum toxin has inconsistent evidence for support of its use in medical management.[6] A recent Cochrane review concluded that in the treatment of acute and chronic fissure in children, these managements increase the chance of cure marginally compared to placebo, but topical nitrates, especially GTN may provide significant pain reduction[6,5] The addition of the oligoantigenic elimination diet (exclusion of foods associated with hypersensitivity, such as cow's milk, wheat, eggs, tomato, chocolate) to medical management in chronic fissures has been shown to reduce pain and may promote healing[6,7] Overall, for chronic fissures in adults, all medical management is less effective than surgery.[6]

Surgery

Surgical management is the treatment of choice for refractory and chronic anal fissures, and may be considered without a trial of medical management.[6] **Lateral internal sphincterotomy** is the procedure of choice. A small percutaneous incision is made into the internal sphincter, cutting muscle fibers without entering the anal canal. This technique is simple and effective, but the potential for permanent incontinence exists. Caution should be used in considering this management for high-risk patients such as the elderly, multiparous women, previous biliopancreatic bypass for obesity, or previous proctologic surgery.[5] Other surgical interventions do exist, such as anal fissurotomy, the conversion of a chronic fissure into an acute to promote healing, and the anal advancement flap (AAF), which has recently gained popularity as an alternative to lateral internal sphincterotomy (LIS).[8] The main advantage of the AAF technique is the reduction of risk of fecal incontinence.[8]

Referrals

Cancer can coexist with benign conditions such as hemorrhoids and so a complete assessment is needed for patients whose bleeding source is in doubt.

Follow-Up

Anal fissure pain may prevent a thorough examination on initial diagnosis; a complete examination to exclude cancer and assess source of bleeding is required in follow-up.

ANORECTAL ABSCESSES AND FISTULAS
General Principles

Definition

An anal fistula is an abnormal connection from an abscess to the anal canal or external skin. Abscesses and fistulas both begin as **infections in the glandular crypts of the anus** and progress to localized collections of pus.

TABLE 11.10-1	**Management Recommendations for Patients with Anorectal Abscesses**	
Type/classification	**Presentation/physical exam/tests**	**Treatment goals**
Perianal abscess— most abscesses track down toward the skin	Pain and swelling at the anal verge external to the dentate line	Incision and drainage with the aide of a drainage catheter, gauze, or seton in the office under local anesthesia
Ischiorectal abscess—grows through the external sphincter and into the fat of the ischiorectal fossa	1. May also be seen or produce pain overlying the buttocks away from the anal verge 2. **No abnormality may be appreciated on examination.** Intrarectal ultrasound should be considered	**Nontoxic appearing patient:** Incision and drainage as an outpatient if the abscess points to the perirectal skin area **Toxic appearing patient**: Incision and drainage should be performed in the **operating theater**
Submucosal abscess—tracks cephalad between the inner circular and outer longitudinal muscle layers of the anorectal wall	The patient complains of anal pain, and **a highly painful bulge can be palpated within the rectum**	Treatment options include surgical drainage into the rectum under general or spinal anesthesia
Supralevator abscess—abscess can arise from cryptoglandular anal disease or from an abdominal suppurative condition	Can arise from: 1. Anal disease or 2. An abdominal suppurative condition (pelvic inflammatory disease, diverticulitis, ruptured appendicitis) Consider imaging and **endoscopy or barium enema**, which may reveal a bulge in the rectal mucosa	Important to identify and treat the process leading to abscess formation as well as to relieve the abscess itself by surgical drainage Pelvirectal **abscesses** are **drained in the operating room** through an intra-anal incision rather than through the ischiorectal space

Clinical Course

As an abscess enlarges, its anatomic location determines its classification and eventual treatment need (Table 11.10-1). Fistulas form in up to 50% of all untreated perianal abscesses[9] and in 26% to 38% of treated abscesses.[9–11]

Anatomy

Most abscesses extend down toward the skin to become a **perianal abscess**. The lesser-encountered abscesses are **ischiorectal, submucosal**, and **supralevator** (Table 11.10-1).

Pathophysiology

Usually 8 to 10 anal glands are located circumferentially within the anal canal at the level of the dentate line;[12] blockage of anal glands permits the growth of bacteria, which may ultimately lead to the formation of an abscess.

Etiology

An acute **infection in the anal glands** can progress to an abscess and can lead to a chronic fistula-in-ano. Other causes include Crohn disease; trauma; tuberculosis; foreign bodies; and fissures that bore into the anal muscle, hematologic malignancy, actinomycosis, and anal surgery.

Clinical Presentation

Clinical presentation is dependent on the size and location of the abscess (Table 11.10-1).

Diagnosis

History

Swelling, throbbing, and severe continuous pain in the anal or rectal area are the most common symptoms. The pain may or may not be related to a bowel movement.

Physical Examination

Abscesses may cause pain, erythema, and swelling or no abnormal findings, if the abscess is in the intersphincteric or ischiorectal space.

Imaging

In elusive cases, intra-anal ultrasound examination under anesthesia may be needed. CT or MRI may be helpful if there is a high suspicion with nonpalpable rectal lesions or masses.[13]

Surgical Diagnostic Procedures

An examination under anesthesia may be required.

Pathologic Findings

An abscess may originate in the intersphincteric space because the anal glands terminate there. The abscess then can travel up, down, or circumferentially around the anus.

Classification

Abscesses are classified according to their location (Table 11.10-1).

Differential Diagnosis

The differential diagnosis also includes a pilonidal sinus, hidradenitis suppurativa, carcinoma, Bartholin gland abscess, and lymphoma.

Treatment

Anal abscesses should be drained in a timely manner. Lack of fluctuation should not be a reason to delay treatment. Antibiotics may have a role in special circumstances, including valvular heart disease, immunosuppression, extensive cellulitis, or diabetes.[14]

Medications

Antibiotics are an unnecessary addition to routine incision and drainage of uncomplicated perianal abscesses.[15] Antibiotics are reserved for patients who are immunocompromised or who have diabetes, or who have signs of systemic infection, such as high fever.

Surgical Management

Incision and drainage on discovery using a cruciate incision (in the shape of a plus sign) should be made as close to the anal orifice as possible. Direct compression of the tissues expresses the pus, and a gauze, seton, or mushroom catheter can be placed to drain the abscess cavity.

Referrals

Large or high abscesses require drainage in the operating room.

Complications

- **Fistula.** About 50% of abscesses that drain spontaneously or following surgery develop into a fistula,[9,15] and 26% to 38% of treated abscesses will develop into fistulas.[9] Fistulas often require complicated and extensive surgical procedures and are best referred to a specialist for treatment. Physicians should not probe fistulas in the office setting. Hospitalization and intravenous antibiotics are reserved for patients who are immunocompromised or diabetic or who have signs of systemic infection, such as high fever.
- **Protocol.** Flexible sigmoidoscopic examination is indicated to evaluate the mucosa of the distal colon for signs of inflammatory bowel disease. The index of suspicion for Crohn disease is increased by a history of episodes of diarrhea, abdominal cramping, and weight loss, and the appearance, location, and multiplicity of the fistulas.

ANAL WARTS, POLYPS, AND NEOPLASMS
Anal Condylomas

General Principles

- **Definition.** Warts are caused by the human papillomavirus (HPV), the most common sexually transmitted viral infection in the United States.[16]

- **Epidemiology.** About 1% of sexually active people have anal warts. Cases in women account for 67% of the total cases.[17]
- **Etiology.** About 35 HPV types primarily infect the squamous epithelium of the lower anogenital tracts.[18]
- **Pathophysiology.** *HPV* types 6 and *11* cause 90% of all genital warts. It is thought that most squamous cell cancers of the anal area are caused by HPV 16 and 18.[16]
- **History.** Anal intercourse is a causative factor in many (up to 80%) but not all patients. Symptoms of anal warts include pruritus, bleeding, anal wetness, and pain. Frequently, the warts are asymptomatic.

Diagnosis

- **Physical examination.** They can vary from small flat papules to many small raised points, in contrast to the flat *condylomata lata* of secondary syphilis.
- **Monitoring.** Infection with HPV has been associated with an increased risk of cervical and anal cancers.[19]
- **Differential diagnosis.** Secondary syphilis.

Treatment

- **Medications.** Treatments include topical podofilox, topical 5% 5-fluorouracil (5-FU), interferon injections, cryosurgical destruction, electrosurgical ablation, surgical excision, or laser ablation. Multiple treatment modalities exist, but even when bulky lesions have resolved, the virus remains.
- **Surgery.** Surgical excision and cautery yield the highest success rate. Laser seems to offer no advantage over cautery. Cure rates of 63% to 91% are reported. Disadvantages include the need for anesthesia and the presence of bioactive HPV in cautery-induced fumes.
- **Protocol.** Topical 5-FU cream and serial examinations, rather than extensive excision, have been advocated in HIV-positive patients with dysplasia.[20] Excision is reserved for patients with obvious lesions of the skin.
- **Risk management.** Clinical or latent infection with HPV may lead to the development of anal cancer.
- **Patient education.** Patients should be advised that condoms are very effective in preventing transmission of HPV but the risk of transmission still exists.
- **Follow-up.** Anal Pap smears can be performed to examine anal dysplasia associated with HPV. Anogenital warts infections in immunocompromised patients are more aggressive and more often dysplastic.
- **Special considerations.** In HIV-positive patients, dysplasia and histologic evidence of HPV can occur in the absence of gross warts.[20]

Management of Polyps and Neoplasms

Anal polyps are common benign growths that may represent residual from prior hemorrhoids or fistulas. Condylomas or tumors also can appear as a polyp, and so uncertain lesions in the anal canal should be biopsied.

Anal malignancies are less common, but basal cell carcinoma, squamous cell carcinoma, melanoma, or prolapsed rectal carcinoma all can occur. Anal cancer accounts for 1.5% of all gastrointestinal malignancies.[21] The incidence of anal malignancies are more common in adults over age 60 and in females. It is estimated that 90% of cases are caused by HPV.[22]

HIV is also an independent a risk factor and has caused anal malignancies to become an epidemic in the HIV-infected population. Smoking has also become an independent risk factor for anal cancer. Smoking cessation reduces this risk.[23]

Diagnosis can be difficult as there are no hallmark signs of malignancy. Any questionable lesion should be studied via imaging and biopsy. Imaging can include endoanal ultrasound, CT, or MRI; however, biopsy is the most reliable method of diagnosis.[24]

Treatment should be directed toward removal of the lesion and preservation of the anus. Chemoradiotherapy is the gold standard of treatment. Surgical management is necessary in 30% of cases due to unresponsiveness to chemoradiotherapy or recurrence. Tumor size is the most important factor regarding prognosis. T1–T2 lesions have a survival rate of 80% to 90%. T4 lesions have a survival rate of 50%.[25]

PRURITUS ANI
General Principles

- **Definition.** Pruritus ani is excessive and often intractable anal itching due to multiple causes.
- **Pathophysiology.** Pruritus ani may be idiopathic or secondary to an underlying disorder (infection, allergies, stool leakage), and specific treatment leads to resolution of symptoms. Complications may include bleeding and fissures.

- **Etiology.** 1% to 5% of the population is affected by this condition, and is the second most common anorectal condition, after hemorrhoids.[26] Although poor hygiene may lead to pruritus ani, vigorous cleansing and application of medications also can produce itching. Other causes include contact dermatitis, lichen sclerosus, seborrhea, lichen planus, psoriasis, infections due to pinworms (*Enterobius vermicularis*), most common among young children and institutionalized adults, and chronic *Candida* infection; parasites, systemic diseases (diabetes mellitus), anorectal disease (fissures, skin tags, proctitis, prolapsing hemorrhoids), irritants in stool (coffee, cola, chocolate, milk, beer, and others), and some medications. Scratching of the affected area causes an exacerbation in inflammation, which in turn triggers an increasing urge to continue to scratch. This scratch–itch cycle is at the core of the chronicity of this condition.[26]

Diagnosis

History

Patients often complain of anal pain and intense itching, burning, and soreness around the rectum.[27] Some complain of abdominal pain additionally.[28] It is important to review the aspects of past medical history for recent antibiotic use, skin disorders, rectal and/or vaginal discharge, as well as social history for anorectal intercourse, poor hygiene or exacerbation with caffeine use, which decreases resting anal canal pressure. Additionally, in elderly patients with chronic back pain, pruritus ani has been shown to be a manifestation of lumbosacral radiculopathy; therefore, obtaining a thorough history is paramount in excluding other causes for pruritus ani.[29]

Physical Examination

Patients are conventionally examined in the left lateral Sims position (on left side with left hip and left lower extremity straight, with right hip and knee bent), but the knee-chest position (patient rests on knees and upper chest with bottom in the air) may provide a much more broad field of view. The drawback to the knee-chest position is the risk of not visualizing hemorrhoids, since the large intestine is pulled down and the hemorrhoids are less likely to protrude.[27] Moistness of perianal skin and bleeding from excoriations may be present. A rectum and sigmoid colon examination should be performed noting the pattern of irritation (symmetrical vs. asymmetrical). Topical anesthetic cream can be used to alleviate patient discomfort.[30] Any abnormal skin should be biopsied.

Surgical Diagnostic Procedures

Surgical diagnostic procedures include anoscopy and endoscopy.

Pathologic Findings

On anoscopy, a symmetrical pattern of anal irritation is usually a diet-induced pruritus, whereas asymmetrical patterns of anal irritation are caused by infectious sources. Leakage of stool or mucus due to fecal incontinence, prolapse of the rectum, or hemorrhoids can cause irritation and itching.

Differential Diagnosis

Pruritus ani is poorly understood. Underlying premalignant lesion such as Bowen disease or Paget disease may cause similar symptoms and should be excluded.

Treatment

Behavioral

Any foods or beverages (such as teas, coffees, and chocolate) that appear to aggravate symptoms should be avoided. Use of or practices involving perianal irritants such as creams, ointments, care products, excessive cleansing with perfumed soaps, or rubbing with toilet paper or wash clothes should be discouraged. A program of gentle, but effective hygiene should be promoted. Wiping gently with wet facial tissue or baby wipes is recommended. Minimizing moisture with a wisp of absorbent cotton in the anal cleft changed several times a day can help prevent skin maceration and further itching. The patient should be instructed to use plain water and his or her hand to wash the perineum in the tub or shower. Creams or emulsifying ointments that do not cause irritation may be used instead of soap.[26] A diet high in fiber with plenty of fluids (similar to the diet for hemorrhoids) is recommended.

Medications

If the specific cause is known, then treatment should be optimized toward the specific disease process. A sedating antihistamine such as hydroxyzine may be used to alleviate nocturnal pruritus.[26] Some patients have been effectively treated with topical antifungals and low-potency steroids. A 2- to 4-week course of 1% hydrocortisone cream can be used.[31] Patients should be warned that chronic use of hydrocortisone will thin the anal skin and may lead to more problems.[26] Topical Capsaicin, Tacrolimus 0.1% ointment, and Intradermal methylene blue injections have demonstrated success in symptom reduction for patients with refractory idiopathic pruritus ani.[32–34]

Referrals

Often, the idiopathic form of pruritus ani can become a chronic condition with waxing and waning of symptoms. The physician should be aware that a previously overlooked underlying problem may be the cause of the pruritus. Assistance from a dermatologist may also be helpful and should be considered.

ANORECTAL INFECTIONS

General Principles

Definition

Anorectal infections are those causing the rectal and anal tissues to become inflamed.

Etiology

It is usually sexually transmitted with the highest risk from anal intercourse, either perianal contamination from cervical infection or direct infection from anal intercourse with men or women.[35] Among HIV-infected men who have sex with men, rectal gonorrhea was the most frequent infection, which is of grave concern due to the rise in drug-resistant gonococcal infections.[36,37] Other common pathogens include *Chlamydia trachomatis*, lymphogranuloma venereum (LGV) from *C. trachomatis* L1, L2, and L3, *Shigella, Escherichia coli, Clostridium difficile*, those causing syphilis, *Entamoeba histolytica*, herpes simplex virus, and cytomegalovirus. Infectious etiologies can often be confused with inflammatory bowel disease; thus, it is very important to distinguish one from another.[38]

Diagnosis

Clinical Presentation

Infectious proctitis can often be asymptomatic, but symptoms present as rectal discomfort, pruritus, rectal discharge, tenesmus, bleeding, genital or anorectal ulcers, other mucocutaneous lesions, lymphadenopathy, skin rash, or the continual urge to defecate.[35,38]

History

Patient may report anorectal pain, severe rectal pain after a bowel movement, rectal discharge, constipation, and/or anorectal itching/burning. A recent history of travel with fever and/or diarrhea, in addition to a detailed sexual history is vital, as proctitis occurs predominantly among persons who participate in receptive anal intercourse.[38]

Physical Examination

Rectal: Tenderness, mucopurulent discharge, ulcerations, warts or vesicular lesions, inguinal lymphadenopathy, and red skin rash may be noted on examination.[35]

Laboratory Studies

Swab, Gram stain in addition to culture for bacteria or viruses from anal canal, dark-field microscopy, Venereal Disease Research Laboratory or rapid plasma reagin blood tests, nucleic acid amplification tests, stool microscopy, rectal biopsy, urethral or cervical cultures can also be helpful in distinguishing the many causes of infectious proctitis. Positive tests should be confirmed with a fluorescent treponemal antibody-absorbed (FTA-Abs) test. There are no clear recommendations made for diagnosing gonococcal proctitis, but all patients under suspicion based on history and physical examination should be tested for chlamydia, syphilis, and HIV.[39]

Surgical Diagnostic Procedures

Anoscopy and endoscopy. Anoscopy should be performed on patients with history of tenesmus, rectal discharge, or anorectal pain with or without a history of receptive anal intercourse.[38]

Treatment

If an anorectal exudate is found on examination, or if polymorphonuclear leukocytes are found on a Gram-stained smear of anorectal secretions, the following therapy may be prescribed pending results of additional laboratory tests. Ceftriaxone 250 mg IM in a single dose PLUS either doxycycline 100 mg orally twice a day for 7 days or azithromycin 1 g orally in a single dose.[39] Alternatives to Ceftriaxone include Ceftizoxime 500 mg IM in a single dose, Cefoxitin 2 g IM in a single dose with Probenecid 1 g orally. Cefixime 400 mg orally in a single dose can also be used, but it is not a first-line therapy and requires a test-of-cure after 1 week.[39,40] Flouroquinolones are no longer recommended.[39] If syphilis is suspected, penicillin G (injection), tetracycline, or azithromycin should be considered. Patients with suspected or documented herpes proctitis should be managed in the same manner as those with genital herpes, for example, acyclovir, valacyclovir (Valtrex), and famciclovir (Famvir). If painful perianal ulcers are present or mucosal ulcers are seen on anoscopy, presumptive therapy should include a regimen for treating genital herpes and doxycycline 100 mg orally twice daily for 3 weeks for treatment of LGV. Appropriate diagnostic testing for LGV in accordance with state or federal guidelines should be executed.[39]

Risk Management
Partners of patients with sexually transmitted enteric infections should be tested for the index diseases.

Follow-Up
Follow-up should be based on specific etiology and severity of clinical symptoms. Reinfection may be difficult to distinguish from treatment failure.

HEMORRHOIDS
General Principles
Definition
Hemorrhoids can be divided into those below the dentate line in the greatly innervated anoderm, the external hemorrhoids, and those above the dentate line, the internal hemorrhoids.

History
A targeted history on the nature, duration, and severity of symptoms; dietary fiber intake; and bowel habits should be gathered. A history of rectal bleeding should prompt a family medical history to evaluate the possibility of familial colorectal neoplastic syndromes and the need for a more extensive colon evaluation.[41] Complete colon evaluation with colonoscopy or barium enema with flexible sigmoidoscopy is typically indicated for patients with rectal bleeding who meet the indications for colonic evaluation (Table 11.10-2).

Thrombosed External Hemorrhoids
- **Definition.** When external hemorrhoids become thrombosed, patients may experience extreme pain and bleeding with defecation.
- **Pathophysiology.** External hemorrhoids may thrombose spontaneously, possibly secondary to straining at stool or heavy lifting. The exact etiology remains unknown.

TABLE 11.10-2	Indications for Complete Colonic Evaluation	
Age	**Last normal endoscopy**	**Family history**
50 yr old	No complete colonic exam **within 10 yr**	N/A
40 yr old or older	**No complete colonic exam within 10 yr**	**Single first-degree relatives** with colorectal cancer or adenoma diagnosed at age >60
40 yr old or older	**No complete exam within 3–5 yr**	**Two or more first-degree relatives** with colorectal cancer or adenomas
Positive fecal occult blood Iron deficient anemia for screening people with possible genetic mutations	Use colonoscopy, instead of barium enema, for diagnostic evaluation of patients with positive findings on other screening tests	N/A

Adapted from Winawer S, Fletcher R, Rex D, et al. Colorectal cancer screening and surveillance: clinical guidelines and rationale—update based on new evidence. *Gastroenterology* 2003;124:544–560.

Diagnosis
- **History.** The patient often complains of a rapid onset of a palpable and painful perianal lump.
- **Physical examination.** On visual inspection, a tender mass at the external anal opening is appreciated.

Treatment
- **Surgery**
  - **Surgical management of thrombosis.** Acutely swollen and tender thrombosed external hemorrhoids may be surgically removed if the physician encounters the lesions in the first 72 hours after onset. An elliptic excision may be performed to unroof the hemorrhoid. Once the entire clot is excised, the physician can leave the wound open with gauze placed over the area to collect drainage or alternatively, the wound is closed with a buried subcuticular absorbable suture.
  - **Nonoperative.** After 72 hours, the discomfort of the procedure probably outweighs the relief provided from the surgery. In this circumstance, avoidance of constipation, patient analgesia, and ice or sitz baths to the perineum may result in more rapid symptom relief than will surgical excision.[42]
- **Patient education.** Instructions on high-fiber diet, stool softeners, warm sitz baths, and anal hygiene.

Internal Hemorrhoids

General Principles
- **Definition.** The anal cushions are blood-filled sacs that reduce the effects of stool passing through the anal canal. With the chronic passage of hard stool or straining, the anal cushions can lose their fibrocollagenous support. The cushions then dilate and prolapse into the anal canal, thus becoming hemorrhoids.
- **Classification.** See Table 11.10-3.

Diagnosis
- **Clinical presentation.** Internal hemorrhoids are painless and occur above the dentate line.
- **History.** The major symptoms of internal hemorrhoids are painless bleeding and protrusion. Patients may report the sensation of a lump or complain of bright red blood coloring the tissue or commode water. Hemorrhoids can prolapse and stain a patient's underwear, and increase anal moisture leading to itching.
- **Physical examination.** The diagnosis of internal hemorrhoids is made with the beveled anoscope. Internal hemorrhoids occur in three consistent positions in the anal canal. With the patient in the left lateral position, the physician usually examines the patient from the right side of the table with the patient's head to the left. The three locations for internal hemorrhoids are the right posterior position (10 o'clock position in the canal), right anterior position (2 o'clock position in the canal), and left lateral position (6 o'clock position in the canal).

TABLE 11.10-3	**Classification, Presentation, and Treatment of Internal Hemorrhoids**	
Grade	**Presentation**	**Treatment**
First degree	Internal hemorrhoids **do not** protrude through the anal orifice	Dietary management Fluid and fiber intake Avoid straining
Second degree	Internal hemorrhoids protrude through the anus but **spontaneously reduce**	Anal hygiene/sitz baths/moistened toilettes
Third degree	Internal hemorrhoids protrude and must be **manually replaced** into the rectum	Rubber band ligation Infrared coagulation Bipolar diathermy (electrosurgery) Hemorrhoidectomy
Fourth degree	Hemorrhoids **protrude permanently and cannot be replaced**	Hemorrhoidectomy is the surgical procedure of choice

TABLE 11.10-4	Management Recommendations for Patients with Fissures or Hemorrhoids

1. Take nonprescription ibuprofen (three 200-mg tablets three times a day with food) and acetaminophen (two tablets every 6 h) if needed for discomfort. Avoid taking narcotics (such as codeine), which can produce further constipation.
2. A sitz bath (soaking in a tub of warm water) for 20 min several times a day can reduce discomfort and promote healing of the tissues.
3. Use stool softeners for at least 2 wk to promote softer stools and to allow the tissues to heal. Start with nonprescription docusate sodium (two 100-mg capsules two times a day) and increase the dosage if you remain constipated.
4. Drink at least five to six full glasses of water or fluid daily.
5. A daily stool bulking agent will promote softer stools and improved colon health. Psyllium or methylcellulose powder (1 tablespoon) can be taken in a glass of orange juice daily to make these substances more palatable. Most patients experience bloating, gas, or cramping with the bulking agents initially, but generally this resolves after 2 wk. You can use simultaneous stool softeners when starting the bulking agents.
6. Do not use enemas or place anything in the rectum for the next 2 wk. Local application of ointments, creams, or pads to the anal tissues is permitted.
7. The National Institutes of Health recommends at least five servings of fresh fruits and fresh vegetables daily. A proper diet can promote soft stools and reduce the chances of recurrent anal disease.
8. Because stool in the rectum rapidly becomes dried out, do not delay going to the bathroom when you feel the rectum fill. Do not sit for long periods on the toilet or strain on the toilet. Please remove all reading materials from the bathroom.

Treatment

- **Medications.** When dietary manipulation does not work, more aggressive treatment is needed. These measures can apply to **grades 1, 2, and 3 internal hemorrhoids** (Table 11.10-4). Unless the patient has **fourth-degree internal hemorrhoids,** aggressive nonsurgical treatment is usually tried. (Most patients with **fourth-degree hemorrhoids** require surgical intervention.)
- **Surgery.** Internal hemorrhoids are most often managed medically (Table 11.10-3). Patients who fail conservative treatment can be considered for surgical intervention. Surgical excision of internal hemorrhoids often is painful and expensive. Surgical or laser excision of internal hemorrhoids has been largely replaced by other outpatient treatment modalities.
- **Nonoperative. Rubber band ligation** of internal hemorrhoids has been performed for many years. One or two small latex rings are placed at the base of the hemorrhoid, resulting in necrosis and sloughing of the hemorrhoid in the following week. The equipment for banding is inexpensive, but the procedure can produce moderate discomfort. Banding also rarely can produce pelvic sepsis, a life-threatening condition. In a meta-analysis of 18 prospective, randomized trials, rubber band ligation was found to be the most effective of the office procedures. It is associated with a lower recurrence rate, but more overall pain than sclerotherapy or infrared coagulation.[43,44]
- **Special therapy.** Infrared coagulation is an office technique for first-, second-, and third-degree internal hemorrhoids. Three to five exposures to each hemorrhoid generally reduce blood flow and shrink the lesion.
- **Other treatment modalities.** Bipolar diathermy (electrosurgery) produces a similar effect on the hemorrhoid as the infrared treatment. A low-voltage galvanic probe also is used for office treatment of hemorrhoids. These office treatments produce similar healing rates and are well tolerated. Cryotherapy and sclerotherapy generally have been abandoned for these newer, and safer, modalities.
- **Referrals.** Surgical evaluation is recommended for recalcitrant hemorrhoids or fourth-degree hemorrhoids.
- **Counseling.** A high-fiber diet with 25 to 30 g of daily fiber should be introduced gradually into the diet and accompanied by six to eight glasses of fluid daily. Patients are encouraged to read the package regarding the amount of fiber per serving.[44] Fiber supplementation with psyllium or hydrophilic colloid may be added to achieve the optimal amount of daily fiber.

REFERENCES

1. Gerstenberger PD, and Plumeri PA. Malpractice claims in gastrointestinal endoscopy: analysis of an insurance industry data base. *Gastrointest Endosc* 1993;39:132.

2. Pfenninger JL, Zainea GG. Common anorectal conditions: part II. Lesions. *Am Fam Physician* 2001;64(1):77. www.aafp.org/afp.

3. Cross KL, Massey EJ, Fowler AL, et al; ACPGBI. The management of anal fissure: ACPGBI position statement. *Colorectal Dis* 2008; 10(Suppl 3):1–7. http://onlinelibrary.wiley.com/doi/10.1111/j.1463-1318.2008.01681.x/abstract;jsessionid=950752F9BAB6CCF6A6580F21DFF4421E.f01t04. Accessed January 30, 2014.

4. Madoff RD, Fleshman JW. AGA technical review on the diagnosis and care of patients with anal fissure. *Gastroenterology* 2003;124(1):235–245. http://www.sciencedirect.com/science/article/pii/S001650850350035X. Accessed January 30, 2014.

5. Altomare DF, Binda GA, Canuti S, et al. The management of patients with primary chronic anal fissure: a position paper. *Tech Coloproctol* 2011;15(2):135–141. http://link.springer.com/article/10.1007%2Fs10151-011-0683-7/fulltext.html. Accessed January 30, 2014.

6. Nelson RL, Thomas K, Morgan J, et al. Non surgical therapy for anal fissure. *Cochrane Database Syst Rev* 2012;2:CD003431. http://onlinelibrary.wiley.com/doi/10.1002/14651858.CD003431.pub3/abstract;jsessionid=B81513B289D9B874736A2884A4403312.f03t01. Accessed January 30, 2014.

7. Carroccio A, Mansueto P, Morfino G, et al. Oligo-antigenic diet in the treatment of chronic anal fissures. Evidence for a relationship between food hypersensitivity and anal fissures. *Am J Gastroenterol* 2013;108(5):825–832. http://www.nature.com/ajg/journal/v108/n5/full/ajg201358a.html. Accessed January 30, 2014.

8. Patel SD, Oxenham T, Praveen BV. Medium-term results of anal advancement flap compared with lateral sphincterotomy for the treatment of anal fissure. *Int J Colorectal Dis* 2011;26(9):1211–1214. http://link.springer.com/article/10.1007%2Fs00384-011-1234-4/fulltext.html. Accessed January 30, 2014.

9. Abcarian H. Anorectal infection: Abscess-fistula. Clinics in colon and rectal surgery 2011. 24:14.

10. Piazza DJ, Radhakrishnan J. Perianal abscess and fistula-in-ano in children. *Dis Colon Rectum* 1990;33:1014.

11. Niyogi A, Agarwal T, Broadhurst J, et al. Management of perianal abscess and fistula-in-ano in children. *Eur J Pediatr Surg* 2010;20:35.

12. Rizzo JA, Naig AL, Johnson EK. Anorectal abscess and fistula-in-ano: evidence-based management. *Surg Clin North Am* 2010;90:45.

13. Glasgow SC, Dietz DW. Uncommon colorectal neoplasms. *Clin Colon Rectal Surg* 2006;12(2):61–68.

14. Breen E, Bleday R., Perianal abscess: clinical manifestations, diagnosis, treatment. UpToDate. In: Post TW, ed. Waltham, MA: UpToDate. http://www.uptodate.com/contents/perianal-abscess-clinical-manifestations-diagnosis-treatment? Accessed February 13, 2014.

15. Whiteford M. Perianal abscess/fistula disease. *Clin Colon Rectal Surg* 2007;20(2):102–109.

16. Pfister H. The role of human papillomavirus in anogenital cancer. *Obstet Gynecol Clin North Am* 1996; 23(3):579–595.

17. Burk RD, Kelly P, Feldman J, et al. Declining prevalence of cervicovaginal human papillomavirus infection with age is independent of other risk factors. *Sex Transm Dis* 1996;23(4):333–341.

18. Fleischer AB Jr, Parrish CA, Glenn R, et al. Condylomata acuminata (genital warts): patient demographics and treating physicians. *Sex Transm Dis* 2001;28(11):643.

19. Franco EL, Rohan TE, Villa, LL. Epidemiologic evidence and human papillomavirus infection as a necessary case of cervical cancer. *J Natl Cancer Inst* 1999;91:506–511.

20. Karamanoukian R, DeLaRosa J, Cosman B, et al. Conservative management of anal squamous dysplasia in patient with human immunodeficiency virus. *Dis Colon Rectum* 2000;43:A5.

21. Jemal A, Murray T, Samuels A, et al. Cancer statistics, 2003. *CA Cancer J Clin* 2003;53:5–26.

22. Parkin DM. The global health burden of infection-associated cancers in the year 2002. *Int J Cancer* 118(12):3030–3044.

23. Tseng HF, Morgenstern H, Mack TM, et al. Risk factors for anal cancer: results of a population-based case—control study. *Cancer Causes Control* 2003;14(9):837–846.

24. Glynne-Jones R, Northover JM, Cervantes A. Anal cancer: ESMO Clinical Practice Guidelines for diagnosis, treatment and follow-up. *Ann Oncol* 2010;21(Suppl 5):v87–v92.

25. Mirta S, Crane L, Diagnosis, treatment, and prevention of anal cancer. Curr Infect Dis Rep 2012;14(1):61–66.

26. Fargo MV, Latimer KM. Evaluation and management of common anorectal conditions. *Am Fam Physician* 2012;85(6):624–630. http://www.aafp.org/afp/2012/0315/p624.html. Accessed January 30, 2014.

27. Kuehn HG, Gebbensleben O, Hilger Y, et al. Relationship between anal symptoms and anal findings. *Int J Med Sci* 2009;6(2):77–84. http://www.ncbi.nlm.nih.gov/pmc/articles/PMC2653786/. Accessed January 30, 2014.

28. Heard S. Pruritus ani. *Aust Fam Physician* 2004;33(7):511–513. http://www.racgp.org.au/afp/200407/14491. Accessed January 30, 2014.

29. Cohen AD, Vander T, Medvendovsky E, et al. Neuropathic scrotal pruritus: anogenital pruritus is a symptom of lumbosacral radiculopathy. *J Am Acad Dermatol* 2005;52(1):61–66. http://www.sciencedirect.com/science/article/pii/S0190962204015543. Accessed January 30, 2014.

30. Billingham RP, Isler JT, Kimmins MH, et al. The diagnosis and management of common anorectal disorders. *Curr Probl Surg* 2004;41(7):586–645. http://www.sciencedirect.com/science/article/pii/S0011384004000255. Accessed January 30, 2014.

31. Al-Ghnaniem R, Short K, Pullen A, et al. 1% hydrocortisone ointment is an effective treatment of pruritus ani: a pilot randomized controlled crossover trial. *Int J Colorectal Dis* 2007;22(12):1463–1467. http://link.springer.com/article/10.1007%2Fs00384-007-0325-8/fulltext.html. Accessed January 30, 2014.

32. Lysy J, Sistiery-Ittah M, Israelit Y, et al. Topical capsaicin—a novel and effective treatment for idiopathic intractable pruritus ani: a randomised, placebo controlled, crossover study *Gut* 2003;52(9):1323–1326. http://gut.bmj.com/content/52/9/1323.long. Accessed January 30, 2014.

33. Sutherland AD, Faragher IG, Frizelle FA. Intradermal injection of methylene blue for the treatment of refractory pruritus ani. *Colorectal Dis* 2009;11(3):282–287. http://onlinelibrary.wiley.com/doi/10.1111/j.1463-1318.2008.01587.x/abstract;jsessionid=653C4A74742CE2F9B8C5D7D44F5D8AA3.f02t04. Accessed January 30, 2014.

34. Suys E. Randomized study of topical tacrolimus ointment as possible treatment for resistant idiopathic pruritus ani. *J Am Acad Dermatol* 2012;66(2):327–328. http://www.sciencedirect.com/science/article/pii/S0190962211005998. Accessed January 30, 2014.

35. Miller KE. Diagnosis and treatment of Neisseria gonorrhoeae infections. *Am Fam Physician* 2006;73(10):1779–1784. http://www.aafp.org/afp/2006/0515/p1779.html. Accessed January 30, 2014.

36. Mayer KH, Bush T, Henry K, et al. Ongoing sexually transmitted disease acquisition and risk-taking behavior among US HIV-infected patients in primary care: implications for prevention interventions. *Sex Transm Dis* 2012;39(1):1–7. http://www.ncbi.nlm.nih.gov/pmc/articles/PMC3740591/. Accessed January 30, 2014.

37. Bolan GA, Sparling PF, Wasserheit JN. The emerging threat of untreatable gonococcal infection. *N Engl J Med* 2012;366(6):485–487. http://www.nejm.org/doi/full/10.1056/NEJMp1112456. Accessed January 30, 2014.

38. Hoentjen F, Rubin DT. Infectious proctitis: when to suspect it is not inflammatory bowel disease. *Dig Dis Sci* 2012;57(2):269–273. http://link.springer.com/article/10.1007%2Fs10620-011-1935-0/fulltext.html. Accessed January 30, 2014.

39. Workowski KA, Berman S; Centers for Disease Control and Prevention (CDC). Sexually transmitted diseases treatment guidelines, 2010 [Erratum: 2011;60(01):18. http://www.cdc.gov/mmwr/preview/mmwrhtml/mm6001a8.htm. Accessed January 30, 2014]. *MMWR Recomm Rep* 2010;59(RR-12):1. http://www.cdc.gov/mmwr/preview/mmwrhtml/rr5912a1.htm. Accessed January 30, 2014.

40. Allen VG, Mitterni L, Seah C, et al. Neisseria gonorrhoeae treatment failure and susceptibility to cefixime in Toronto, Canada. *JAMA* 2013;309(2):163–170. http://jama.jamanetwork.com/article.aspx?articleid=1556149. Accessed January 30, 2014.

41. Church J, Simmang C. Practice parameters for the treatment of patients with dominantly inherited colorectal cancer (familial adenomatous polyposis and hereditary nonpolyposis colorectal cancer). *Dis Colon Rectum* 2003;46:1001–1012.

42. Cataldo P. Practice parameters for the management of hemorrhoids (revised). *Dis Colon Rectum* 2005;48:189–194.

43. MacRae HM, McLeod RS. Comparison of hemorrhoidal treatment modalities: a meta-analysis. *Dis Colon Rectum* 1995;38:687–694.

44. Orkin BA, Schwartz AM, Orkin M. Hemorrhoids: what the dermatologist should know. *J Am Acad Dermatol* 1999;41:449.

11.11 Colorectal Cancer

Eugene Orientale Jr., Nasser Mohamed,
Colton R. Redding

GENERAL PRINCIPLES

Colorectal cancer (CRC), one of the most prevalent cancers in the Western world, is the second most common cause of cancer-related death in the United States. For men and women in United States, CRC is the second leading cause of cancer-related deaths and the third most common cancer after prostate and lung cancer in men and breast and lung cancer in women.[1]

Epidemiology

In the most recent CDC statistical analysis in 2010, 131,607 people in the United States were diagnosed with colorectal cancer and 52,045 people had died of it. The disease has a high prevalence, passes through a long asymptomatic yet detectable phase, and has a high cure rate when detected at an early stage. In addition, CRC has a high mortality rate when advanced disease occurs. The incidence and mortality report from the CDC between 2002 and 2010 had shown that incidence of CRC decreased from 52.3 per 100,000 in 2003 to 45.5 per 100,000 in 2007. It also showed that the overall age-adjusted CRC death rate decreased from 19.0 per 100,000 in 2003 to 16.7 per 100,000 at that time. Approximately 50% of the improvement in mortality can be attributed to increased screening, with 35% attributed to reductions in risk factors such as smoking and obesity, and 12% to improved CRC treatment.[2] Thus, CRC is ideally suited to prevention and early detection programs, which are discussed at the end of this chapter.

Pathophysiology

Colonic polyps are of two general types.

- Hyperplastic polyps sometimes cannot be distinguished from other polyps solely on the basis of endoscopic appearance. They are sessile, are 10 mm or less, and tend to occur in the distal colon. A smooth and uniform appearance may uniquely distinguish these lesions. On gross inspection, small (less than 5 mm) hyperplastic polyps are often referred to as "diminutive" and need not be biopsied or ablated.
- Neoplastic polyps are mucosal outgrowths that may be broadly based or pedunculated. Although most polyps do not undergo neoplastic transformation, most CRCs originate from polyps through a 10- to 15-year process. Polyps undergo metaplastic transformation approximately 40% to 60% of the time. Three cell patterns are recognized.
  - Adenomatous polyps (tubular or glandular cell pattern) are histologically arranged in densely packed tubular glands and are the least malignant adenoma.
  - Villous (papillary cell pattern) polyps are arranged in fingerlike projections and are less common than tubular adenomas. A villous polyp has a higher malignant potential; if larger than 2 cm, it has a 50% chance of containing invasive cancer.
  - Mixed adenomatous–villous polyps have mixed-cell patterns and are common in large tumors. The risk for malignancy depends on the size and percentage of the villous cell pattern.
- Colorectal cancer
  - Histologic classification is of value for prognosis and treatment selection.
    - Adenomatous CRC is the most common neoplasm and is further differentiated by grade (poorly, moderately, and well differentiated). As with other neoplasms, poor differentiation in histologic specimens is associated with worse prognosis.
    - Mucinous CRC is an uncommon form that secretes abundant extracellular mucin and has a poor prognosis.
    - Signet ring CRC (linitis plastica) is composed of cells distorted by intracellular mucin into a signet ring shape. It is typically associated with metastasis at the time of diagnosis.
  - The Dukes classification, though somewhat less precise than the tumor–necrosis–metastasis (TNM) scheme, is commonly used because of its simplicity (Table 11.11-1). Prognosis is directly related to depth of invasion.[3]

TABLE 11.11-1	Dukes Classification Scheme for Colon Cancer	
Stage	Description	5-year survival (%)
A	Confined to the bowel wall	90
B	Through the wall and locally invasive (no lymph node involvement)	60–80
C	Metastasis to regional lymph nodes	20–50
D	Distant metastasis (peritoneum, liver)	5

DIAGNOSIS

- **Risk factors.** These include advancing age, race (African American), obesity, type 2 diabetes, personal history of CRC or polyps, family history, cigarette smoking, inflammatory bowel disease, and familial genetic syndromes (familial polyposis and hereditary nonpolyposis colorectal cancer).[4] Certain diets and alcohol consumption also correlate with increased risk for CRC.
- **Presentation.** There is a lack of correlation between duration of symptoms at diagnosis and survival. Early detection can be both elusive and challenging, with more than 65% of patients presenting with advanced disease.
  - Bleeding is most commonly occult, but patients can also present with melena or hematochezia.
  - Pain may be secondary to intestinal obstruction or metastasis.
  - Altered bowel movements range from diarrhea to obstipation. In elderly individuals, any change in bowel habits should prompt diagnostic consideration.
  - Constitutional complaints include fatigue, malaise, fever, and weight loss.
  - Metastatic disease may present with jaundice, pruritus, and ascites (liver); respiratory complaints (lung); or pathologic fracture (bone).
  - Weight loss, anemia, and a palpable mass comprise the triad often associated with a proximal lesion.
  - Asymptomatic presentation is not uncommon.

TREATMENT

- **Polyps.** Because polyps have malignant potential, they should be biopsied or removed at the time of colonoscopy. Larger sessile polyps sometimes require either surgical or piecemeal colonoscopic resection. Polypectomy is performed with the use of wire snare or biopsy forceps technique, both of which may be accomplished with concomitant electrocautery.
- **Cancer.** Management varies according to histology, location, and stage.
  - Colonoscopy with polypectomy may obviate the need for surgery. In some cases, even large biopsy-proven cancerous lesions can be removed in piecemeal fashion.
  - Surgery is the general treatment for cancers beyond Dukes stage A. The goal is complete removal or destruction of neoplastic tissue with maximal preservation of surrounding tissues.
  - Adjuvant chemotherapy with 5-fluorouracil plus leucovorin is used in selected stage II patients and in stage III patients. The American Society of Clinical Oncology (ASCO) recommends considering certain populations for the therapy, including patients with inadequately sampled nodes, T4 lesions, perforation, statistically significant survival benefit, or poorly differentiated histology.[5] The routine use of adjuvant chemotherapy for medically fit patients with stage II colon cancer is not recommended, as it is not supported with statistically significant survival benefit. The national comprehensive cancer network (NCCN) recommends adding oxaliplatin to the 5-fluorouracil plus leucovorin regimen (FOLFOX4) for patients with stage III disease. Oral capecitabine has also been shown to be effective in patients with stage III disease.[6]
  - Radiation can be of benefit in the management of rectal cancer and advanced CRC and in palliation for patients with unresectable disease.
  - Surveillance with cancer markers or colonoscopy has not demonstrated any improvement in survival rate. Carcinoembryonic antigen (CEA) is nonspecific and thus not useful for screening. For existing CRC, CEA may be used as a marker for disease recurrence every 3 months for the first year after resection, and then every 6 months for 2 more years. Colonoscopy is generally performed 12 months after resection and every 3 to 5 years after that. CT scan of chest and abdomen every 6 to

12 months for the first 3 years postresection can be considered in patients who are at higher risk for recurrence. Currently, other laboratory and radiological examinations are of unproven benefit, and it is recommended that they should be restricted to patients with suspicious symptoms.[6]

SPECIAL CONSIDERATIONS AND PREVENTION

- **Diet.** A diet high in red/processed meat correlates with higher incidence of colon cancer. Diets high in vegetables, fruits, and whole grains have been linked with a decreased risk of colorectal cancer. Fiber supplements themselves are ineffective at decreasing the risk of colorectal cancer. It is unclear if other dietary components (e.g., certain types of fats) affect colorectal cancer risk at this time.[4]
- **Aspirin.** The daily use of aspirin has been shown to decrease both the incidence of CRC and the occurrence of metastasis.[7]
- **Physical activity.** There is increasing evidence that physical activity and exercise contribute to decreasing the risk of colon cancer.[4,6]
- **Screening.** Screening for adenomatous polyps in an aggressive and systematic manner has proved effective in the prevention of CRC. Family physicians with full colonoscopic skills may play an integral role in the containment of this common cancer.
- **Screening modalities:**
  - **Digital rectal examination (DRE).** DRE is not considered a cost-effective means of detecting CRC. Less than 10% of CRCs arise within the reach of the examining finger. DRE should always precede a flexible sigmoidoscopy or colonoscopy. When performed solely with DRE, stool guaiac testing has a high false-positive rate and should not be considered part of routine screening for CRC.
  - **Fecal immunochemical testing (FIT) and fecal occult blood testing (FOBT).** Annual screening of asymptomatic individuals after age 50 is effective (sensitivity 72% to 88%, specificity 98%, and positive predictive value 10% to 17%) and decreases CRC mortality by up to 33%.[8] FIT and FOBT are usually performed on stool specimens acquired on each of the three consecutive bowel movements. Any positive test should prompt a further diagnostic workup with colonoscopy. False positives can be caused by consumption of red meat, turnips, horseradish, vitamin C, and certain medications (aspirin, nonsteroidal anti-inflammatory drugs), as well as benign conditions, such as diverticulosis or hemorrhoids. Some find FIT preferable because there are no dietary or drug restrictions required for testing.
  - **Flexible sigmoidoscopy.** This office procedure, performed with a 60-cm scope, is capable of screening from the rectum to the splenic flexure. It can diagnose up to two thirds of colonic lesions and has been shown to reduce CRC mortality by 60% to 80% at a fraction of the cost of colonoscopy.[8] Patient acceptability and compliance are significant issues. The procedure is embarrassing for some patients and requires an uncomfortable bowel preparation that might involve a liquid diet, laxative, electrolyte purge solution, or enema prior to the procedure. Conscious sedation is not required and complications are uncommon, with intestinal perforation occurring about once in 5,000 to 10,000 examinations. The U.S. Preventive Services Task Force (USPSTF) currently recommends routine screening every 5 years beginning at age 50. The combination of annual FOBT and periodic flexible sigmoidoscopy is a cost-effective means of CRC detection in the general population.[9]
  - **Air-contrast barium enema (ACBE).** This radiologic procedure allows visualization of the entire colon. Patient compliance and acceptability are comparable to that of flexible sigmoidoscopy. It has limitations in evaluation of the rectum and sigmoid colon but can be useful for proximal lesions. ACBE has a sensitivity of only 48% for large, 1-cm polyps and 41% for >6-mm polyps. Specificity ranges from 99% for large cancers to 90% for large polyps.[10] The American Cancer Society (ACS) recommends ACBE be repeated every 5 years. ACBE is over twice the cost of flexible sigmoidoscopy and has a similar complication profile, but can be useful in patients who refuse endoscopy.
  - **Colonoscopy.** This method remains the final common pathway of all other positive screening tests. With adequate bowel preparation, it is almost 100% specific and 95% sensitive for detection of neoplasm. Biopsy or polypectomy can be performed. A bowel preparation is always necessary, and conscious sedation improves patient acceptability. The current recommendation by the ACS for frequency of colonoscopy is at 10-year intervals starting at the age of 50, with increased frequency of surveillance based upon size, pathology, and number of polyps. Some family physicians are now acquiring skills in full colonoscopy, which ultimately may be a significant factor in the early detection of CRC.

- **Virtual colonoscopy.** This is also called computed tomographic colonography. This method uses x-rays and computers to produce two- and three-dimensional images from the rectum to the lower end of the small intestine and then displays them on a screen. However, if a polyp or growth is found using this method, a colonoscopy would need to be done for removal or biopsy of the lesion.[11] It is not yet considered a cost-effective means of screening for CRC, but if performed, is also recommended at 5-year intervals by the ACS.
- **Genetic testing of stool.** Studies are being done to find new ways to recognize DNA mutations in cells found in stool samples. New cells replace cells from the lining layer of the colon and rectum, which are constantly shed into the stool. Finding intact-appearing DNA that lacks the changes of apoptosis in stool samples may be useful in finding colorectal cancers.[12] Although stool DNA testing was performed in the past, it is no longer available in the United States, and thus, not recognized as part of routine screening by the ACS.

REFERENCES

1. U.S. Department of Health and Human Services, Centers for Disease Control and Prevention. Colorectal cancer, fast facts. www.cdc.gov/colorectalcancer/basic_info/fast_facts.htm. Accessed March 20, 2014.
2. Centers for Disease Control and Prevention. Vital signs: colorectal cancer screening, incidence, and mortality—United States, 2002—2010. http://www.cdc.gov/mmwr/preview/mmwrhtml/mm6026a4.htm. Accessed March 20, 2014.
3. Fry R, Fleshman J, Kodner I. Cancer of the colon and rectum. *Clin Symp* 1989;41:2.
4. American Cancer Society. Detailed guide, colon and rectum cancer. What are the risk factors for colorectal cancer? www.cancer.org. Accessed March 20, 2014.
5. Benson AB III, Schrag D, Somerfeld MR, et al. American Society of Clinical Oncology recommendations on adjuvant chemotherapy for stage II colon cancer. *J Clin Oncol* 2004;22(16)3408–3419.
6. Labianca R, Nordlinger B, Beretta GD, et al. Primary colon cancer: ESMO Clinical Practice Guidelines for diagnosis, adjuvant treatment and follow-up. Ann Oncol 2010;21(Suppl 5):v70–v77. doi:10.1093/annonc/mdq168.
7. Kahn MJ, Morrison DG. Chemoprevention for colorectal carcinoma. *Hematol Oncol Clin North Am* 1997;11(4):779.
8. Mandel JS, Bond JH, Church TR, et al. Reducing mortality from colorectal cancer by screening for fecal occult blood. *N Engl J Med* 1993;328:1365–1371.
9. Centers for Disease Control and Prevention. Colorectal Cancer Screening Tests. http://www.cdc.gov/cancer/colorectal/basic_info/screening/tests.htm. Accessed March 20, 2014.
10. Rockey D, Paulson E, Niedzwiecki D, et al. Analysis of air contrast barium enema, computed tomographic colonography, and colonoscopy: prospective comparison. *Lancet* 2005;365(9456):305–311.
11. Fenlon HM, Nunes DP, Schroy PC III, et al. A comparison of virtual and conventional colonoscopy for the detection of colorectal polyps. *N Engl J Med* 1999;341(20):1496–1503.
12. Dong SM, Traverso G, Johnson C, et al. Detecting colorectal cancer in stool with the use of multiple genetic targets. *J Natl Cancer Inst* 2001;93(11):858–865.

CHAPTER 12

Renal and Urologic Problems

Section Editor: Shawn P. Murdock

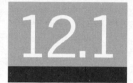

Cystitis
and Bacteriuria

Bridgette Pudwill

GENERAL PRINCIPLES
Definitions

Acute cystitis is an infection of the urinary bladder (the lower urinary tract) that does not involve the upper urinary tract (kidneys). Cystitis is commonly referred to as a urinary tract infection or a UTI. UTIs are a common complaint in the clinic, and are usually uncomplicated in nature.

Significant bacteriuria, which represents bacterial infection, is defined as growth of greater than 10^5 colony-forming units (CFU) per milliliter on a urine culture.[1]

Epidemiology

Most episodes of acute cystitis occur in young, sexually active women. The incidence is 0.7 UTIs per person year in this demographic. Conversely, the incidence of UTI in postmenopausal women is much lower at 0.07 UTIs per person year. The incidence of lower UTIs is much lower in men, infants, and children; in these patients evaluation for an underlying cause should be done.

Risk factors for a woman to develop acute cystitis include recent sexual activity, recent spermicide use, and a history of UTIs. Risk factors for uncomplicated UTIs in young men include insertive anal intercourse and lack of circumcision. Most episodes of acute cystitis in children or elderly males are associated with anatomical urologic abnormalities, bladder outlet obstruction (e.g., prostate enlargement), or recent instrumentation.[2]

Complications

While young women are at the highest risk of developing a UTI, they are also most likely to have an uncomplicated course of illness. Pregnant women are an exception to this, and are at risk for developing preterm labor, preterm delivery, and pyelonephritis in the setting of a UTI.

There are few reasons to screen for and treat asymptomatic bacteriuria in men. Screening for asymptomatic bacteriuria is warranted prior to transurethral resection of the prostate or other urologic procedures, for which mucosal bleeding is anticipated because of the risk of postprocedure bacteremia and sepsis.[3]

Anatomy and Pathophysiology

Acute cystitis is an infection of the bladder and may include infection of the distal ureters and urethra (the lower urinary tract), but by definition does not involve the proximal ureters or kidneys.

Men are much less likely to develop a UTI than women secondary to having a longer urethra, drier periurethral area, and the presence of antimicrobial substances in prostatic fluid.

Bacteriuria and acute cystitis occur when fecal flora colonize the vaginal introitus, and the bacteria then ascend to the bladder via the urethra.[2]

Microbiology

The large majority of uncomplicated UTIs (75% to 95%) are caused by *Escherichia coli*. Other less common pathogens include Enterobacteriaceae species (*Proteus mirabilis* and *Klebsiella pneumoniae*) and *Staphylococcus saprophyticus*. Rarely do other Gram-negative or Gram-positive organisms cause un-complicated acute cystitis.[4] In healthy, non-pregnant young women, isolates of Group B streptococci, enterococci, lactobacilli, and coagulase-negative staphylococcal species other than *S. saprophyticus* from a voided urine sample should be considered contaminant.[5]

DIAGNOSIS
Clinical Presentation

Although a definitive diagnosis of UTI requires a urine specimen with a culture, a good history can often identify patients with a likely diagnosis of cystitis. The history is also useful in distinguishing from other causes of dysuria, such as sexually transmitted disease (STD), gynecologic disorders, and mechanical or chemical irritation. History is helpful when trying to distinguish cystitis and lower UTIs from pyelonephritis and upper UTIs. Empiric antibiotics after the history can be a cost-effective method of treating cystitis.[2]

History

The history should include a complete description of the symptoms, including the onset and du-ration of dysuria; urinary urgency, hesitancy, and frequency; urinary incontinence; hematuria; and suprapubic pain. Systemic symptoms or their lack should be included such as fever, chills, nausea and vomiting, and costovertebral angle (CVA) discomfort. There should be a complete review of systems, with particular focus on gynecologic symptoms such as vaginal discharge, vaginal pain, or irregular menstrual bleeding.

The record should also include a medical history that encompasses a sexual history; a gynecologic and obstetrical history; a medication history; past infections and other relevant medical history; and a family history.

Patients should be asked to describe any personal history that includes activities that might cause mechanical or chemical irritations such as bubble baths, vaginal douching, or scented tampons or pads.[2]

Physical Examination

Patients with cystitis often have a normal physical examination. The examination should be used to help distinguish between upper and lower UTIs. Examination should include temperature, blood pressure, and pulse. Assessment for CVA tenderness should be done. A pelvic examination should be performed if indicated by the history.[2]

Laboratory Studies

The gold standard test is the urine culture and sensitivity. Significant bacteriuria has been defined as 10^5 CFU per mL. Lower colony counts may be used for patients with symptomatic infections, and treatment should not be delayed due to lower colony counts. Urine dipstick for leukocyte esterase, nitrites, protein, or occult blood may be used to aid in the diagnosis of UTI.[2]

Differential Diagnosis

- Pyelonephritis
- Chlamydia urethritis
- Gonococcal urethritis
- Candidal vulvovaginitis
- Trichomonal vaginitis
- Chemical urethritis from soaps, tampons, douches, or spermicides
- Atrophic vaginitis

TREATMENT
Medications

Many patients will respond to symptomatic treatment with phenazopyridine (100 to 200 mg PO TID). Antibiotic therapy can be divided into single-dose, short-term, long-term, and suppressive/pro-phylactic treatment. For most patients with uncomplicated cystitis, single-dose or short-term therapy is appropriate.[1]

Single-Dose Therapy[1,2]
- Fosfomycin, 3 g mixed in 4 oz of water

Short-Term Therapy (3-day)[1,2]
- Preferred:
  - Trimethoprim/sulfamethoxazole (160 mg/800 mg), 1 tab PO BID for 3 days
  - Trimethoprim (100 mg), 1 tab PO BID for 3 days
  - Nitrofurantoin SR (100 mg), 1 tab PO BID for 5 days
  - Pivmecillinam (400 mg), 1 tab BID for 5 days
- Alternative treatment regimens (to be used in cases of allergy or culture proven resistance):
  - Ciprofloxacin (250 mg), 1 tab PO BID for 3 days
  - Levaquin (250 or 500 mg), 1 tab PO daily for 3 days
  - Ofloxacin (200 mg), 1 tab PO BID for 3 to 7 days
  - Cephalexin (500 mg), 1 tab PO BID for 3 to 7 days
  - β-Lactam antibiotics for 3 to 7 days

A 3-day course of antibiotics is as effective as longer courses in patients with acute, uncomplicated cystitis. Longer-term treatment (7-day) is appropriate for patients who do not respond to a 3-day regimen. Treatment length of 7, 10, or even 21 days may be appropriate for patients with complicated infection, recurrent infection, or pyelonephritis. Prophylaxis or suppression should be considered in women with three or more infections in a year. Options include patient-initiated therapy, postcoital prophylaxis, or daily prophylactic therapy.[1,2]

Referrals

Patients with recurrent infections or those who do not respond to therapy should have further evaluation of their urinary tract. This may include cystoscopy, ultrasonography, intravenous pyelography, or retrograde ureterography. Referral to a urologist or urogynecologist is appropriate for these patients.[2]

Patient Education

Medication Instructions

All patients receiving drug treatment should receive instruction in proper use of antibiotics and potential adverse effects from the medication. These effects could include drug reactions or allergies, decreased effectiveness of birth control pills while taking antibiotics, and the risk of development of yeast vaginitis while on antibiotics.[1]

Follow-Up

Patients should return to the doctor if symptoms have not resolved or markedly improved within 48 hours of starting antibiotic treatment. Warning signs would include fever, chills, vomiting, or flank pain.[2]

Complications

The most common complication of untreated cystitis is the development of upper UTI such as pyelonephritis. Symptoms of pyelonephritis include fever, chills, nausea or vomiting, flank pain, and elevated white blood count. Other potential complications include renal abscess and peritonitis.[2]

SPECIAL CONSIDERATIONS

These recommendations are intended for uncomplicated cystitis and bacteriuria. Complicated UTIs require a different approach.[2]
- Immunocompromise (e.g., HIV, chemotherapy)
- Urinary tract obstruction, acute or chronic (e.g., nephrolithiasis)
- Neurogenic bladder
- Congenital anomalies
- Chronic catheterization
- Recent instrumentation of the urinary tract
- Age (<10 years or >65 years)
- Pregnancy

ACKNOWLEDGMENT

This author would like to acknowledge and thank the previous author, John E. Delzell, Jr., for his contributions to this chapter.

REFERENCES

1. Gupta K, Hooton TM, Naber KG, et al. International clinical practice guidelines for the treatment of acute uncomplicated cystitis and pyelonephritis in women: a 2010 update by the Infectious Diseases Society of America and the European Society for Microbiology and Infectious Diseases. *Clin Infect Dis* 2011;52(5):e103.
2. Hooton TM. Uncomplicated urinary tract infection. *N Engl J Med* 2012;366(11):1028.
3. Nicolle LE, Bradley S, Colgan R, et al; Infectious Diseases Society of America; American Society of Nephrology; American Geriatric Society. Infectious Diseases Society of America guidelines for the diagnosis and treatment of asymptomatic bacteriuria in adults. *Clin Infect Dis* 2005;40(5):643.
4. Czaja CA, Scholes D, Hooton TM, et al. Population-based epidemiologic analysis of acute pyelonephritis. *Clin Infect Dis* 2007;45(3):273.
5. Hooton TM. Clinical practice. Uncomplicated urinary tract infection. *N Engl J Med* 2012;366(11): 1028–1037.

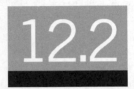

12.2 Hematuria

Anthony J. Strickland

GENERAL PRINCIPLES

Definition

Hematuria is simply detectable blood in the urine. A visible change in urine color caused by blood is called **gross** or **macroscopic** hematuria, whereas **microscopic** hematuria is detectable only under a microscope and defined as three or more red blood cells (RBCs) per high-powered field.[1]

Anatomy

Bleeding can originate at any point in the urinary tract. Potential sources include the kidney, renal vasculature, ureters, bladder, prostate, or urethra. The anatomic proximity of the female external urinary system with the reproductive system should not be overlooked as blood from the reproductive tract may contaminate an improperly collected sample.[1]

Epidemiology

Adults

Microscopic hematuria is found in 0.19% to 21% depending on the population. Malignancies are found in up to 5% of individuals with asymptomatic microscopic hematuria.[2]

Children

Gross hematuria occurs in 1.3 cases per 1,000 urgent care visits. Microscopic hematuria was present in 4% of children aged 8 to 15 in one study.[2]

Pathophysiology

The underlying cause of the hematuria is best determined by identifying the source. This is generally broken down into glomerular and nonglomerular bleeding. Damage to the glomerulus through inherited or acquired disease causes leaking of blood through the basement membrane. In this situation, the RBCs often become dysmorphic, or mix with mucoproteins in the glomerulus to form red cell casts. In contrast, urinary RBCs from nonglomerular bleeding have a normal appearance. Lack of RBC casts or dysmorphic RBCs does not rule out a glomerular source of bleeding. Significant proteinuria (>300 mg per 24 hours) may help support a glomerular source of blood loss.[2,3]

DIFFERENTIAL DIAGNOSIS

The *differential diagnosis* of hematuria is listed in Table 12.2-1.[2]

TABLE 12.2-1   Differential Diagnosis of Hematuria[2,3]

Glomerular

IgA nephropathy	Goodpasture syndrome
Idiopathic hypercalciuria	GPA aka Wegener granulomatosis
Idiopathic hyperuricosuria	Alport syndrome
HUS	Thin basement membrane nephropathy
HSP	aka benign familial hematuria
Glomerulonephritis	Mesangial proliferative
Lupus nephritis	Postinfectious (strep, viral)
Membranoproliferative glomerulonephritis	Loin pain-hematuria syndrome

Interstitial

Polycystic kidney disease	Acute tubular necrosis
Infection: pyelonephritis, tuberculosis,	Acute interstitial nephritis
schistosomiasis	Hyperuricosuria
Nephrolithiasis	Hypercalciuria

Neoplastic

Renal cell carcinoma	Wilms tumor
TCC	Rhabdoid tumor
Prostate cancer	Congenital mesoblastic tumor
Angiomyolipoma	

Vascular

Renal artery/vein thrombosis	Arteriovenous malformation
Sickle cell disease/trait	Coagulopathy, congenital or acquired
Platelet disorder	Hemophilia A or B
Malignant hypertension	

Lower urinary tract

Calculi (ureteral, bladder)	Trauma
Benign prostatic hypertrophy	Prostatitis
Cystitis (bacterial, viral, drug)	Endometriosis
Urethritis	Epididymitis
Foreign body	Urethral stricture
Posterior urethral valves	

Other causes

Exercise-induced	Sexual intercourse
Menstrual contamination	Nutcracker syndrome

DIAGNOSIS
Clinical Presentation

Gross Hematuria

Both adults and children will likely present for evaluation with symptoms of gross hematuria as it is usually quite distressing. Patients may note bright red blood in their urine, on the toilet paper, or perhaps a darkening of their urine to a "cola" or "tea" color. It is important to find out if the patient experienced pain with the hematuria. Abdominal or flank pain, dysuria, urinary frequency, and urgency may be seen with urolithiasis, a common cause of gross hematuria. Lower UTIs (i.e., cystitis, urethritis), neoplasm, and benign prostatic hypertrophy are the leading causes of gross hematuria in adults. Although UTIs are also common among children, painless gross hematuria in children is suspicious for glomerulonephritis, hypercalciuria, or IgA nephropathy.[3]

Microscopic Hematuria

Microscopic hematuria is generally discovered in one of two ways. Some patients may present with flank pain or irritative voiding symptoms, which prompt a urine dipstick to be performed in the office. Others may be asymptomatic and have a urine dipstick performed for screening reasons, such as preoperative exams, or at a well-child visit. A positive dipstick must always be confirmed with careful microscopic examination. Potential causes of false positives include menstruation, recent sexual

TABLE 12.2-2	Risk Factors for Urinary Tract Malignancy[2,3,6]

Male sex
Age >35 yr
Smoking history
Occupational exposure to dyes or chemical (aromatic amines, benzenes)
Prior/current treatment with cyclophosphamide
History of phenacetin use (banned in the United States in 1983 and associated with TCC)
History of pelvic irradiation
History of gross hematuria
Chronic indwelling foreign body
History of analgesic abuse (associated with carcinoma of the kidney)
Dietary nitrites/nitrates
Schistosomiasis
Chronic cystitis and bacterial infection associated with urinary calculi and obstruction of the upper urinary tract

activity, and vigorous exercise. These activities should be avoided at the time of subsequent confirmatory urinalysis. In a patient with a single positive urine microscopy with casts, significant proteinuria, or with risk factors for urinary tract malignancy (Table 12.2-2), further evaluation for the source of hematuria should proceed without requiring a confirmatory urinalysis.[1,2]

HISTORY

The following key points should be obtained in the history:[1,3]
- **Urine color.** Yellow or pink urine with red clots suggests collecting system disease, whereas dark, "cola" or "tea" color suggests glomerular source.
- **Timing.** Is the hematuria transient or persistent? When did the blood appear during urination? Early in void suggests urethritis, and end of void suggests trigonitis.
- **Review of symptoms**
  - Fever (infection, systemic disease, tumor)
  - Gastrointestinal symptoms (hemolytic uremic syndrome [HUS] and Henoch–Schonlein purpura [HSP])
  - Recent upper respiratory illness (IgA nephropathy, postinfectious nephritis)
  - Skin infection (poststreptococcal nephritis)
  - Cough (Goodpasture, granulomatosis with polyangiitis [GPA/WG])
  - Rash (vasculitis)
  - Edema or sudden weight gain (nephropathy)
  - Irritative voiding symptoms (calculi, cystitis, urethritis, bladder tumor)
  - Unexplained weight loss or night sweats (malignancy, tuberculosis)
  - Symptoms of prostatic obstruction (BPH)
  - Blood clots in the urine (almost always due to extraglomerular bleeding)
- **Medical history**
  - Prior instrumentation of the urinary tract
  - Prior genitourinary cancer
  - Prostatic disease
  - Prior history of hematuria
  - Prior history of nephrolithiasis
  - Menstrual history
  - Recent trauma or vigorous exercise
  - Use of anticoagulants (the use of anticoagulants is not sufficient to prevent further evaluation of hematuria)
  - Medications that may cause acute interstitial nephritis such as cyclophosphamide and NSAIDS.[2,3]
- **Social history**
  - Tobacco use
  - Occupational exposure to aromatic amines and benzenes (textiles, fuels)
  - Travel to areas endemic for tuberculosis or *Schistosoma haematobium*
  - Recent intercourse. (Trauma may cause bleeding, residual semen in urinalysis may cause false positives.)[1–4]

- **Family history**
  - Hearing loss (Alport syndrome)
  - Renal disease (Alport, IgA nephropathy, PCKD)
  - Renal stones
  - Blood disorders (sickle cell disease, hemophilia, platelet disorders).[3]

PHYSICAL EXAMINATION

Given the multitude of causes for hematuria, a thorough physical examination is warranted. In men, examining the urethra for lesions and a prostate examination for nodules or signs of prostatitis are essential. For women, a pelvic examination must be performed to inspect the periurethral area for lesions and to rule out a vaginal or uterine source. In children, growth should be assessed, as failure to thrive may be a symptom of chronic renal disease. Other key findings include fever, hypertension, rash, joint tenderness or swelling, and abdominal or flank tenderness or masses.[1]

LABORATORY

Urinalysis

- **Urine dipstick.** The initial laboratory study for suspected hematuria is a urinalysis. This test is highly sensitive, detecting as few as one to two RBCs per high-powered field. However, the specificity is low due to many false positives. The urine dipstick specifically detects reactivity with hemoglobin; therefore, hemoglobinuria, myoglobinuria, and some iodine compounds can cause false positives. False negatives may be caused by excessive vitamin C ingestion, urinary pH <5.1, or a urinary dipstick that has had prolonged exposure to air before use.[3]
- **Urine protein.** Proteinuria greater than 300 mg per 24 hours (roughly correlating to 3+ on dipstick) is highly suggestive of a glomerular source for the hematuria. Any proteinuria noted on dipstick should be further evaluated with a spot urine protein to creatinine ratio or a 24-hour urine collection for analysis of protein content.[3]
- **Microscopy.** Unless the patient clearly has symptoms of cystitis and the urinalysis suggests this by revealing pyuria, a positive urine dipstick should always be confirmed by microscopy. This more accurately quantifies the RBCs, as well as investigates the sample for evidence of dysmorphic RBCs and RBC casts which suggest renal or glomerular etiologies, respectively.[1,3]

Urine Cytology

Urine cytology may be helpful in detection of urinary tract malignancies. The sensitivity is increased for high-grade tumors, but is limited in its ability to detect low-grade tumors or renal cell carcinoma. Urine cytology has utility with patients at increased risk (Table 12.2-2)[1–3] or as part of the workup in adults with microscopic hematuria who will not undergo cystoscopy.

Urine Culture

Urine culture should be obtained in all patients with hematuria to exclude an infectious etiology. A positive urine culture should be treated for infection with urinalysis in 6 weeks to ensure resolution of the infection and hematuria.[1,2]

Other Urine Tests

Urine eosinophils can help evaluate for acute interstitial nephritis. If the patient has a travel history to areas that are endemic for tuberculosis or schistosomiasis, consideration of indicated cultures, serology, and microscopy are warranted.

Blood Tests

Any patient with suspected renal etiology should be evaluated with serum creatinine and CBC.[2] Other tests for underlying causes of glomerulonephritis may include antinuclear antibody (systemic lupus erythematosus), antistreptolysin antibody (poststreptococcal glomerulonephritis), complement levels, antiglomerular basement membrane antibody titers, and antineutrophilic cytoplasmic antibody titers (vasculitis). Serum IgA can be ordered if IgA nephropathy is suspected.

Imaging

- **Adults:** The preferred imaging modality to evaluate nonglomerular hematuria is now multiphasic CT urography, which has largely replaced intravenous pyelography (IVP) in adults.[4] Multiphasic CT urography combines the benefits of conventional CT scanning (with and without contrast) with the ability of an IVP to accurately visualize renal anatomy. CT without contrast may be necessary for patients with contraindications. Although less sensitive than CT, renal ultrasound may also be used to detect renal masses >3 cm, hydronephrosis, nephrolithiasis/nephrocalcinosis, and to some extent the renal parenchyma, particularly if significant cost, contrast, or other medical limitations exist.[5,6] However, a negative ultrasound does not rule out nephrolithiasis.[4] MR urography is also a potential modality being explored but has not yet found its place in current diagnostic algorithms.

- **Children:** Unlike adults, renal and bladder ultrasound is the recommended initial imaging study in children.[7] It can detect many urinary tract abnormalities, such as those listed above, while avoiding the relatively high radiation dose of contrast-enhanced CTU (7.7 mSv). If hematuria is secondary to blunt trauma, CT with and without contrast is justified as an initial investigatory modality.[5,6]

Diagnostic Procedures

- **Cystoscopy** is the ideal modality for evaluating the lower urinary tract as it is capable of both visualization and intervention (biopsy, etc.). It is also the only modality able to visualize the urethra and periurethral zone of the prostate. All patients with gross hematuria and no evidence of glomerular disease or infection should undergo cystoscopy as part of their evaluation. Those with microscopic hematuria should also undergo cystoscopy if they are over 35 years of age and benign causes have been ruled out.[1]
- **Renal biopsy** is often performed in the evaluation of a suspected glomerular source. It is rarely indicated in isolated microscopic hematuria, even if the differential diagnosis is IgA nephropathy or thin basement membrane disease, since the biopsy results would not change the management.[1]

TREATMENT

The treatments of hematuria are as numerous and varied as the differential diagnosis. In evaluations that identify a particular etiology, treatment is based on the diagnosis. If no serious etiology is readily identified, no treatment is indicated.

Follow-Up

The cause of hematuria is often elusive, and follow-up varies widely based on diagnosis and risk factors. Workup and treatment of hematuria often involves sensitive examinations and uncomfortable procedures such as cystoscopy. Therefore, it is not uncommon to get resistance from patients who minimalize their symptoms or incidental laboratory finding. Given that malignancies are found in up to 5% of individuals with asymptomatic microscopic hematuria, diligence with follow-up is of utmost importance. Annual follow-up for persistent hematuria is recommended.[1,2]

Patient Education

- Patients with isolated microscopic hematuria should be educated and encouraged to include this as part of their medical history, as some people may have undiagnosed disease such as early transitional cell carcinoma (TCC), IgA nephropathy, or thin basement membrane disease, which could progress to renal dysfunction.[2]
- Patients with gross hematuria should be reassured that it is uncommon to become anemic from urinary tract bleeding. In fact, very little blood will make urine red, about one-fifth of a teaspoon in 2 pints of urine.[2]

ACKNOWLEDGMENT

The author would like to acknowledge the previous authors for their work on the previous version of this chapter.

REFERENCES

1. Davis R, Jones JS, Barocas DA, et al. *Diagnosis, evaluation and follow-up of asymptomatic microhematuria (AMH) in adults: AUA guideline.* Linthicum, MD: American Urological Association Education and Research, Inc. (AUA); 2012:1–30.
2. Sharp VJ, Barenes KT, Erickson BA. Assessment of asymptomatic microscopic hematuria in adults. *Am Fam Physician* 2013;88(11):747–754.
3. Gerber GS, Brendler CB. Evaluation of the urologic patient: history, physical examination, and urinalysis. In: Wein AJ, Kavoussi LR, Novick AC, et al., eds. *Campbell-Walsh urology.* 10th ed. Philadelphia, PA: Saunders; 2011:86–87.
4. Mazouz B, Almagor M. False-positive microhematuria in dipsticks urinalysis caused by the presence of semen in urine. *Clin Biochem* 2003;36(3):229–231.

5. Lang EK, Thomas R, Davis R, et al. Multiphasic helical computerized tomography for the assessment of microscopic hematuria: a prospective study. *J Urol* 2004;171(1):237–243.
6. Eikefjord EN, Thorsen F, Rørvik J. Comparison of effective radiation doses in patients undergoing unenhanced MDCT and excretory urography for acute flank pain. *Am J Roentgenol* 2007;188(4):934.
7. Dillman JR, Coley BD, Karmazyn B, et al. *Expert panel on pediatric imaging. ACR Appropriateness Criteria* hematuria—child. Reston, VA: American College of Radiology (ACR); 2012.

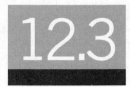

12.3

Pyelonephritis

Ayesha F. Chaudry

Pyelonephritis is characterized by bacterial invasion of the renal parenchyma. Presenting signs and symptoms may include the classic signs of cystitis, as well as flank pain, costovertebral angle tenderness, fever, general malaise, nausea, vomiting, or prostration. Pyelonephritis can have many complications if untreated, including bacteremia and sepsis (more often when there is underlying pathology or debilitation), which necessitates early diagnosis and presumptive therapy.

GENERAL PRINCIPLES
Definition

Pyelonephritis is defined as a **bacterial infection of the upper urinary tract** and, more specifically, the renal parenchyma and renal pelvis. This topic is often discussed in conjunction with other urinary tract infections (UTIs, i.e., cystitis, urethritis, and prostatitis) because they share similar pathophysiology and bacterial etiologies.[1]

Epidemiology

Although pyelonephritis is less common than other UTIs such as cystitis, acute cases occur roughly 250,000 times a year and are estimated to be responsible for roughly 100,000 hospitalizations each year. The incidence of pyelonephritis increases during pregnancy and occurs during 1% to 2% of all pregnancies.[2]

Classification

Pyelonephritis can be differentiated into two categories: uncomplicated and complicated. An **uncomplicated** case of pyelonephritis would be where the infection is caused by a known pathogen in an immunocompetent adult with a normal urinary tract and renal function. A **complicated** case of pyelonephritis would include one of the following: an unusual pathogen, an immunocompromised host, an elderly or very young patient, and an abnormality in the urinary tract or in renal function.[1,3]

Pathophysiology

Pyelonephritis is thought to be caused by the ascent of bacteria up through the urethra and bladder, finally reaching the kidney. Infection may reach the kidneys hematogenously, but this usually occurs in debilitated, chronically ill, and immunocompromised patients. In men, hypertrophy or infection of the prostate can predispose to UTIs. Metastatic staphylococcal or fungal infection may spread from distant foci in the bone or skin.[1,4,5]

Etiology

There are many different pathogens that can cause pyelonephritis. *E. coli* is the most common pathogen, causing more than 80% of infections. Because older patients are more likely to have catheter use or instrumentation, *E. coli* causes less than 60% of acute pyelonephritis cases in this population. These patients are more likely to end up with Gram-negative infections with bacteria such as *Klebsiella*, *Serratia*, *Pseudomonas*, and *Proteus*. Other common bacterial agents include *Enterobacter*, *Staphylococcus saprophyticus*, and *Enterococcus*.[2]

DIAGNOSIS

Clinical Presentation

Some combination of the following signs and symptoms is usually present, but in elderly or compromised patients, any or all may be absent: fever, flank pain, costovertebral angle tenderness, general malaise, nausea, vomiting, prostration, urinary frequency and/or urgency, dysuria, suprapubic pain, bacteriuria, pyuria, and hematuria.[1]

History

Adults typically present with fever, low back pain, costovertebral angle pain, and general malaise. They may also often present with nausea, vomiting, or diarrhea. A significant proportion of adults present only with lower tract symptoms: frequency, dysuria, urgency, and suprapubic discomfort. In infants, small children, and elderly people, the presentation may be vague, with irritability, lethargy, altered mentation, anorexia, and, eventually, dehydration. Onset may be insidious, or acute—as, for example, following traumatic removal of an indwelling catheter over a chronically infected prostate—and may be associated with sepsis. Again, keep in mind that in elderly or immunocompromised patients, fever may be the only presenting symptom, and there may be no localizing symptoms at all.[1,4]

Physical Examination

There are several key things to look for on physical examination. During the checking of vitals, look for fever and tachycardia. During the abdominal examination, palpate the mid- and lower abdomen, and percuss the flank of the patient to assess tenderness. Look for tenderness on deep pressure in one or both costovertebral angles, which is suggestive of upper tract disease. Suprapubic tenderness on examination tenders to suggest lower tract infection. With male patients you want to differentiate an upper tract infection from urethritis or prostatitis. The penis should be gently milked to look for urethral discharge, and a rectal examination should be performed to look for a boggy prostate. If a woman is also complaining of vaginal discharge, a vaginal examination would be appropriate.[1,6]

Laboratory and Imaging

- **Urinalysis.** You should perform a dipstick urine on every patient in whom you suspect pyelonephritis. Unless there is obstruction, urinalysis should show pyuria (positive leukocyte esterase and/or nitrites), usually bacteriuria—opinions vary on how many colony-forming units (CFU) per mL constitute a positive test—and often hematuria, white cell casts, and proteinuria. If a patient has lower counts of bacteria on microscopy, they may still have pyelonephritis, especially if they are pregnant or if they are male.
- **Urine cultures** are positive in 90% of patients with acute pyelonephritis and culture specimens should be obtained before initiating treatment, so that the culture can be used to guide or evaluate treatment. Cultures typically grow more than 10^{-5} organisms per mL, but, particularly with fastidious or nosocomial organisms, 10^{-3} organisms per mL may be consistent with renal infection (Ramakrishnan; Gupta). *E. coli*, other Enterobacteriaceae, *Staphylococcus saprophyticus*, and *Enterococcus* still account for more than 90% of cases. *Klebsiella*, *Enterobacter*, and *Proteus* are becoming more common. Sexually transmitted disease (STD) pathogens are common in at-risk populations. *Serratia*, *Pseudomonas*, and *Staphylococcus epidermidis*, as well as other unusual organisms, are primarily nosocomial.
- **Blood cultures** are not necessary unless you are uncertain of the diagnosis, the patient is immunosuppressed, or a hematogenous source is suspected.
- **Complete blood count** (CBC) usually shows leukocytosis with left shift but is not necessarily required in the initial workup.
- **Other laboratory findings.** Elevated blood urea nitrogen (BUN), creatinine, erythrocyte sedimentation rate (ESR), C-reactive protein (CRP), and electrolyte disturbances may be found in more severe disease.

Imaging

Ultrasonography (US) is indicated if obstruction, stones, or hydronephrosis is suspected. If US is nonspecific, consider computed tomography (CT). Intravenous pyelogram (IVP) is relatively contraindicated.[7]

Monitoring

With outpatient treatment, you should monitor patients within 72 hours after beginning therapy to see if they have defervesced or experienced an improvement in their symptoms. If there has been no improvement in symptoms, you should reassess the patient and consider admitting him or her to the hospital. If fever is still present after 96 hours, another urinalysis and urine culture would be appropriate to assess bacterial sensitivity and to guide a change in therapy.

Classification

When working up a patient with pyelonephritis, it is important to assess the severity of the infection, as this will determine whether the patient needs inpatient or outpatient management. An uncomplicated case would be where the patient is stable in the sense of being only moderately ill and still able to take fluids and medication by mouth. In this case, the patient may be treated with oral antibiotics on an outpatient basis, or given a loading dose of parenteral antibiotics initially, and sent home to finish the course with oral treatment.

When deciding whether to admit a patient or not, there are several indications for inpatient treatment. Absolute indications include persistent vomiting, progression of uncomplicated UTI, suspected sepsis, uncertain diagnosis, and urinary tract obstruction. Relative indications include a patient over age 60, poor social support, anatomic urinary tract abnormality, and immunocompromised (diabetes, sickle cell disease, malignancy, transplant patient).

Differential Diagnosis

Some of the conditions that may have a similar clinical picture include kidney stones, urinary tract obstruction, renal infarction, renal vein thrombosis, hemorrhage into a renal tumor or cyst, abdominal pathology (cholecystitis, empyema, peptic ulcer, pancreatitis, appendicitis), pelvic inflammatory disease, basal pneumonia, herpes zoster, and referred pain from a lesion of the vertebrae.[6]

TREATMENT
Behavioral

Patients should be advised to increase their fluid intake to at least 1,500 mL per day.

Medications

- **Outpatient treatment.** Seven to 14 days of an oral fluoroquinolone is the recommended treatment for outpatient therapy, given that these drugs have good absorption in the gastrointestinal tract and good kidney penetration. Studies have shown that oral fluoroquinolone use is nearly as effective as the intravenous (IV) preparation of fluoroquinolones. Other drugs that may be used as alternatives for susceptible bacteria are oral amoxicillin–clavulanate potassium (Augmentin), a cephalosporin, or trimethoprim–sulfamethoxazole (TMP–SMX). It should be noted that TMP–SMX is a fraction of the cost of the newer drugs.[5,8]
- **Inpatient treatment.** Three recommended treatments for initial inpatient treatment are (all parenteral): (a) a fluoroquinolone, (b) an aminoglycoside with or without ampicillin, and (c) an extended-spectrum cephalosporin with or without an aminoglycoside. If a urine culture shows Gram-positive cocci, ampicillin–sulbactam, with or without an aminoglycoside, is recommended. Once the patient is afebrile, clinically stable, and is tolerating medications and fluids by mouth, you may discharge the patient to home and finish with oral antibiotics. Patients who are immunosuppressed may require 21 days of antibiotic therapy.
- **Adjunctive therapy.** Hydration and pain relief are also key components of therapy for pyelonephritis. For pain relief, use oral or parenteral narcotics for the first 48 hours. For severe dysuria, give phenazophyridine (Pyridium), 200 mg tid PO. If severe pain persists after 48 hours, or fever after 96 hours, consider imaging. If nausea and vomiting are present, give PO or per rectum (PR) antiemetics. If fever is present, give acetaminophen PO or PR. Nonsteroidal anti-inflammatory drugs are best avoided as these drugs may impair renal function.
- If someone is advanced to the stage of **sepsis**, you want to aggressively rehydrate, administer parenteral antibiotics, and initiate anticipatory management of potential cardiorespiratory collapse (shock).
- **Cost considerations.** It should be noted that TMP–SMX is a fraction of the cost of the newer drugs. Oral therapy with any drug is invariably cheaper than parenteral therapy.
- **Surgery.** Obstructed pyelonephritis is a closed-space infection (abscess) and requires immediate urologic drainage.

Patient Education

Instruct patients in appropriate prophylactic measures. **Fluid intake should be at least 1,500 mL per day** to enhance recovery, avoid obstruction from urinary sediment, and reduce reinfection in patients with urinary tract abnormalities or catheters. Anticipate a preventive or suppressive program in the case of recurrence. For women, anticipate symptoms of candida infections.

Follow-Up

All patients should receive another urine culture following treatment with antibiotics to assess the success of treatment. Generally, this is done 1 to 2 weeks after finishing antibiotic therapy. If symptoms never abate, or if they return during treatment, another urine culture should be repeated promptly.[1]

Complications

- **Treatment failure.** Initial failure of a patient to defervesce in 96 hours should be evaluated for complicating factors. Diagnosis can usually be established by renal US and CT scan.

  If obstruction or perinephric abscess is present, surgical drainage and combination parenteral therapy with β-lactam antibiotic and aminoglycoside are indicated.
- **Failure of bacteriologic cure.** In the case of failure of bacteriologic cure or early relapse within 1 month, take the following actions: (a) diagnosis can be made via urinalysis, culture and sensitivity testing, and renal panel; (b) treat with a 14- to 30-day treatment course with a culture-determined antibiotic.
- **Multiple recurring infections:** Diagnosis can be made via US for anatomical abnormalities, by renal scan for differential function, or by IVP. Treat with 3- to 6-month suppression therapy with nitrofurantoin, 50 mg per day (more than 50 years of use has resulted in minimal resistance), or TMP–SMX, half a tablet per day, or norfloxacin (Noroxin), 400 mg per day. Suppression therapy often allows for restoration of normal defense mechanisms.

SPECIAL CONSIDERATIONS

- **Children with recurring infections.** Evaluate for reflux or structural abnormalities with US and renal scanning or voiding cystourethrography. Suppression therapy is appropriate if severe degree of reflux or anatomical anomaly is present, but more studies are needed to determine the effectiveness of long-term antibiotics for prevention in susceptible children. Surgery may be indicated but is usually unnecessary. The goal of treatment is prevention of symptoms, scarring, and stone formation.[2,9]
- **Pregnancy.** Pyelonephritis in pregnancy can cause many severe complications, including transient renal insufficiency (occurs in more than 25% of women), pre-eclampsia, gestational hypertension, preterm labor and delivery, respiratory insufficiency, septic shock, and disseminated intravascular coagulation. Pregnant women should be screened for asymptomatic bacteriuria during weeks 12 to 16 and, if positive, treated with 3 to 5 days with an oral cephalosporin, nitrofurantoin, or TMP–SMX to avoid pyelonephritis later in pregnancy. TMP–SMX should be avoided at term because of the possibility that sulfonamides increase risk of neonatal kernicterus. Hospitalize if the patient is not clearly stable. **Quinolones are not approved.** If infection is recurrent, suppress with nitrofurantoin 100 mg per day.[10]
- **Geriatric patients.** Evaluate for stones, prostatic obstruction, or incomplete bladder emptying with urinalysis, catheterization for residual, and imaging as indicated. Review hygiene. Consider estrogen deficiency if the patient is postmenopausal. Consider chronic bacteriuria. Expect multiple and resistant organisms. Consider *Candida* infection in debilitated patients. Consider other predisposing factors, such as malnutrition, incontinence, immobility, and drugs. The treatment should be specific to the problem. Address underlying factors, and consider suppression for chronic bacteriuria if the patient has had an episode of pyelonephritis with uremia or sepsis.
- **Nosocomial infections.** Therapy should cover *Pseudomonas aeruginosa, S. epidermidis, S. aureus,* and *Serratia marcescens.*
- **Sexually active patients.** For treatment, consider *Trichomonas vaginalis, Neisseria gonorrhoeae, Chlamydia trachomatis,* and *Ureaplasma.*
- **Indwelling catheters.** Treatment consists of removal of the catheter or suppression. Rotate suppression antibiotics every 6 months and expect resistant organisms. Sterile insertion of catheters is key, as are avoiding long-term catheterization if possible, using intermittent catheterization, closed drainage systems, and silver-alloy-coated catheters. Suppression prevents sepsis but not bacteriuria.[11]
- **Urosepsis.** Consider predisposing factors. Consider suppression if predisposing factors are not resolvable.
- **Prostatitis** (see Chapter 12.4). Diagnosis is based on physical examination findings or demonstration of high concentration of bacteria in prostatic secretions or post-massage urine sample. *Treatment:* Administer TMP–SMX or a quinolone for 1 to 3 months. If bacteria are not identified, treat with doxycycline, 100 mg bid, for 14 to 30 days.

- **Epididymitis.** Evaluate for STD. Treatment requires a 30-day course of medication.
- **Stones.** To diagnose, follow closely for persistence of urea-splitting organisms, such as *Proteus mirabilis.*
- **Women with frequent recurrences.** Treat with a single dose of nitrofurantoin, 50 mg, or a half-tablet of TMP–SMX, or 100 mg of TMP on mornings after sexual intercourse.[12]
- **Renal failure.** Use ceftriaxone, a quinolone, or aztreonam.

ACKNOWLEDGMENT

In the end I would like to thank for the great hard work and thorough contribution by Dr. Kathryn W. Hare to this book chapter, which helped me immensely in the revision process.

REFERENCES

1. Ramakrishnan K, Scheid DC. Diagnosis and management of acute pyelonephritis in adults. *Am Fam Physician* 2005;71(5),933–42.
2. White B. Diagnosis and treatment of urinary tract infections in children. *Am Fam Physician* 2011;83(4):409–415.
3. Nicolle LE. Complicated pyelonephritis: unresolved issues. *Curr Infect Dis Rep* 2007;9(6):501–507.
4. Longo DL, Fauci AS, Kasper DL, et al. Urinary tract infections and pyelonephritis. In: Harrison TR, Braunwald E, eds. *Harrison's principles of internal medicine*. 18th ed. New York, NY: McGraw-Hill; 2012.
5. Gupta K, Hooton TM, Naber KG, et al. International clinical practice guidelines for the treatment of acute uncomplicated cystitis and pyelonephritis in women: A 2010 update by the Infectious Diseases Society of America and the European Society for Microbiology and Infectious Diseases. *Clin Infect Dis* 2011;52(5):e103.
6. Shoff WH, Green-McKenzie J, Edwards C, et al. Acute pyelonephritis: the differential diagnosis and workup. http://emedicine.medscape.com/article/245559. Accessed March 29, 2014.
7. Kawashima A, Leroy AJ. Radiologic evaluation of patients with renal infections. *Infect Dis Clin North Am* 2003;17(2):433–456.
8. Peterson J, Kaul S, Khashab M, et al. A double-blind, randomized comparison of levofloxacin 750 mg once-daily for five days with ciprofloxacin 400/500 mg twice-daily for 10 days for the treatment of complicated urinary tract infections and acute pyelonephritis. *Urology* 2008;71(1):17.
9. Williams GJ, Craig JC. Long-term antibiotics for preventing recurrent urinary tract infection in children. *Cochrane Database Syst Rev* 2011;(3):CD001534.
10. Colgan R, Hyner S, Chu S. Uncomplicated urinary tract infections in adults. In: Grabe M, Bishop MC, Bjerklund-Johansen TE, et al., eds. *Guidelines on urological infections*. Arnhem, The Netherlands: European Association of Urology (EAU); 2009:11–38.
11. Hooton TM, Bradley SF, Cardenas DD, et al. Diagnosis, prevention, and treatment of catheter-associated urinary tract infection in adults: 2009 International Clinical Practice Guidelines from the Infectious Diseases Society of America. *Clin Infect Dis* 2010;50(5):625.
12. Kodner CM, Thomas-Gupton EK. Recurrent urinary tract infections in women: diagnosis and management. *Am Fam Physician* 2010;82(6):638–643.

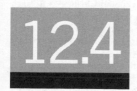

12.4 Epididymitis and Prostatitis

Emily J. Jones, Hina Anjum

Epididymitis and prostatitis are infections of the male urinary tract usually caused by extension of infection from the urethra or the bladder. Infections are typically caused by urinary tract and sexually transmitted infection (STI) pathogens. The most likely pathogen and empiric therapy are predicted based on the patient's age.[1–5]

EPIDIDYMITIS

Bacterial infection of the epididymis is usually caused by an ascending urethritis.[4]

General Principles

Epidemiology

In men >35 years old, the most common pathogens are enteric pathogens such as *E. coli*. In men <35 years old, sexually transmitted pathogens, such as *Neisseria gonorrhoeae* and *Chlamydia trachomatis* are more common. History of urethral instrumentation or unprotected insertive anal intercourse makes enteric bacteria more likely. History of STI in a sex partner makes STI pathogens more likely.[2,5]

Diagnosis

Clinical Presentation

The most common chief complaint is rapid onset unilateral scrotal pain, often radiating up the spermatic cord to the groin and possibly the flank. Pain is followed within 3 to 4 hours by unilateral scrotal swelling, redness, and induration. The testis then swells to twice normal size. Patient often has fever up to 40°C (104°F).[4,5]

History

Frequently, patients have a history of recent urethritis.[5]

Physical Examination

Physical examination reveals an exquisitely tender, swollen epididymis, which early on is adjacent to a normal testis. Within a few hours, the testis also swells, until it is not possible to differentiate between epididymis and testis by palpation. Reactive hydrocele may develop. Elevating the scrotum above the symphysis (Prehn sign) may reduce pain.[4]

Laboratory Studies

Laboratory tests should include clean-catch urine for culture if enteric organisms suspected or urethral swab or urine for testing for gonococci and *Chlamydia* if STI suspected.[4,5]

Differential Diagnosis

Testicular Torsion

If testicular torsion is missed, testis may be lost within 6 hours. Torsion is uncommon in men >25 years old. It has an abrupt onset and is frequently accompanied by nausea and vomiting. There may be a history of similar episodes with spontaneous resolution. On examination early, only the testis is tender. Swelling and edema develop quickly, making it difficult to differentiate torsion from epididymis. Prehn sign reveals increased pain in torsion.[4] If any question of torsion, prompt surgical consultation is indicated to prevent loss of testis. Ultrasonography may be useful to determine whether swelling is in testis or epididymis. Technetium scans show increased uptake in epididymitis and decrease in torsion.[4,6]

Treatment

- **Medications.** Empiric antibiotics should be started promptly after obtaining appropriate laboratory studies.[5] In patients at risk for enteric bacteria (>35), antibiotics appropriate for cystitis (such as trimethoprim–sulfamethoxazole, a cephalosporin, or a quinolone) should be administered until culture results are available. In those at risk for STIs (<35), an appropriate antibiotic (such as ceftriaxone, 250 mg IM, followed by doxycycline, 100 mg bid for 10 days, or ofloxacin, 300 mg bid for 10 days) should be started.[3,7]
- **Supportive care.** This includes bed rest, scrotal elevation, and pain control. Ice may help within first 48 hours.[4]
- **Follow-up.** Improvement should be noted in 3 days. Lack of improvement should be cause for re-evaluation of therapy. Any recent sexual partners of men with STI epididymitis should be evaluated and treated within 30 days if possible.[4]
- **Patient education.** Education on safe sexual practices to prevent STIs, use of condoms during insertive anal intercourse, avoiding urethral instrumentation.[4]

PROSTATITIS

It is inflammation of prostate gland. Prostatitis is a broad diagnosis that includes acute illness requiring immediate attention to chronic conditions and an incidental finding noted during evaluation and treatment of other urological conditions.

Epidemiology

The prevalence of prostatitis is approximately 8.2%. It accounts for 8% of visits to urologists, and up to 1% of visits to primary care physicians. Overall, prostatitis syndromes are a very common presentation in the clinical setting and tend to occur in young and middle-aged men.[8] However, acute bacterial prostatitis accounts for a minority of these cases.

Risk Factors

Acute prostatitis can occur in the setting of cystitis, urethritis, or other urogenital tract infections. Thus, underlying conditions such as functional or anatomical anomalies (e.g., urethral strictures) that predispose to other urogenital infections can increase the risk of prostatitis. Prostate infections following urogenital instrumentation, including chronic indwelling bladder catheterization, intermittent bladder catheterization, and prostate biopsy, are well documented.[9]

Anecdotally, trauma (e.g., bicycle or horseback riding), dehydration, and sexual abstinence have been thought to predispose to prostatitis. However, these factors have not been established by well-controlled studies.

Classification

- NIH classification system:
  - **Category I:** Acute bacterial prostatitis
  - **Category II:** Chronic bacterial prostatitis
  - **Category III:** Chronic pelvic pain syndrome that includes (**IIIA**) inflammatory (same as nonbacterial prostatitis in traditional scheme) and (**IIIB**) noninflammatory (same as prostatodynia)
  - **Category IV:** Asymptomatic inflammatory prostatitis, which refers to asymptomatic prostatitis found incidentally on biopsy[8]

Acute Bacterial Prostatitis

Acute bacterial prostatitis, NIH type I, is an acute bacterial infection of the prostate; patients are typically seen in the outpatient setting or emergency department. Left untreated, it can lead to overwhelming sepsis or the development of prostatic abscess.

E. coli is the most commonly isolated organism, but other Gram-negative organisms, such as *Klebsiella*, *Proteus*, and *Pseudomonas*, and Gram-positive *Enterococcus* species are often isolated as well.

Clinical Presentation

Urinary symptoms may be irritative (e.g., urinary frequency, urgency, dysuria) or obstructive (e.g., hesitancy, poor or interrupted stream, straining to void, incomplete emptying). Pain may be present in the suprapubic or perineal region, or in the external genitalia. Systemic symptoms of fever, chills, malaise, nausea, emesis, and signs of sepsis (tachycardia and hypotension) may be present as well.

Physical Examination

On physical examination, the prostate should be gently palpated. The prostate is tender, enlarged, and boggy; prostatic massage should not be performed and may be harmful. On abdominal examination, a palpable, distended bladder indicates urinary retention.[10,11]

Chronic Bacterial Prostatitis

Chronic bacterial prostatitis, NIH type II, is a persistent bacterial infection of the prostate lasting more than 3 months. *E. coli* is the most common cause, but other Gram-negative organisms are often isolated as well.[12]

Clinical Presentation

Patients may have irritative voiding symptoms and testicular, perineal, low back, and occasionally distal penile pain. They might present with recurrent or relapsing urinary tract infections, urethritis, or epididymitis with the same bacterial organisms.

Physical Examination

On physical examination, patients are usually afebrile, and on digital rectal examination the prostate may feel normal, tender, or boggy.

Chronic Pelvic Pain Syndrome

NIH type IIIA (inflammatory) and IIIB (noninflammatory). Differentiation between these groups has been made based on the presence of leukocytes in expressed and post-massage prostatic secretions, urine, or semen. One of the greatest challenges with the treatment of chronic prostatitis/chronic pelvic pain syndrome is that there is no clear understanding of the etiology; however, suggested explanations include infection, autoimmunity, and neuromuscular spasm.

Clinical Presentation and Physical Examination

Chronic pelvic pain syndrome is pain attributed to the prostate with no demonstrable evidence of infection. On examination, tenderness of the prostate, or less commonly the pelvis, is present in about one half of patients.

Asymptomatic Prostatitis

Asymptomatic prostatitis, NIH type IV, is diagnosed when inflammatory cells are identified on prostate biopsy or leukocytes are noted on semen analysis during urologic evaluation for other reasons. The clinical significance of this type of prostatitis is uncertain, and treatment is based on the primary reason for the urologic evaluation. When the indication for biopsy is an elevated prostate-specific antigen (PSA) level, it is important to remember that normalization of the PSA value after antibiotic or 5-α-reductase inhibitor therapy does not rule out the diagnosis of prostate cancer, and continued urologic evaluation is warranted.

Diagnosis

Category 1: Midstream urine culture should be obtained. The presence of more than 10 white blood cells per high-power field suggests a positive diagnosis. Other laboratory testing (e.g., CBC, electrolyte levels, blood culture) is determined by the severity of the presentation. Residual urine should be documented if a patient has a palpable bladder or symptoms consistent with incomplete emptying.[10]

In **Category II**, urinalysis may be negative. Urine culture may be negative, but expressed prostatic secretions or ejaculate may show >15 leukocytes per high-power field, and cultures usually positive.

Differential Cultures

First, 10 mL of urine in a void (VB$_1$), 10 mL from midstream (VB$_2$), expressed prostatic secretions (EPS) obtained by prostate massage, and 10 mL of urine following massage (VB$_3$) are obtained and examined microscopically and cultured. If VB$_1$ shows the highest numbers of white blood cells (WBCs) and colonies on culture, urethritis is diagnosed. If VB$_2$ is highest, cystitis is more likely. If EPS or VB$_3$ (or both) is highest, Category II is confirmed. Category IIB shows WBCs, but culture results are negative. Category IIIB shows neither WBCs nor positive culture results.

Differential diagnosis includes cystitis and urethritis as well as differentiating the categories of prostatitis. Differential cultures may be necessary. An alternate screen in patients with no evidence of urethritis is pre- and post-massage test. Urine specimens obtained before and after prostatic massage and then compared for the presence and amount of bacteria and leukocytes. This is the same as comparing VB$_2$ and VB$_3$ and is nearly as accurate.

Treatment

- **Medications**
  - **Category I.** Empiric therapy should be started at the time of evaluation, coverage can be tailored to the isolated organisms once urine culture results are available. Mildly to moderately ill patients may be treated in the outpatient setting; severely ill patients or those with possible urosepsis require hospitalization and parenteral antibiotics. Once patients have become afebrile, they may be transitioned to oral antibiotics based on the culture results. Minimal duration of treatment is 4 weeks; however, the optimal period has been shown to be 6 weeks, because of the possible persistence of bacteria, with repeat evaluation recommended at that time.[11]
  - **Category II.** An appropriate antibiotic with good tissue penetration in the prostate should be selected. Fluoroquinolones have demonstrated the best tissue concentration and are recommended as first-line agents. Second-line drugs include doxycycline, azithromycin, and clarithromycin (Biaxin). A 4- to 6-week course of therapy is usually recommended; however, a 6- to 12-week course is often needed to eradicate the causative organism and to prevent recurrence, especially if symptoms persist after completion of the initial therapy. For HIV patients, treatment for 4 to 6 weeks is recommended, followed by suppressive therapy for unspecified time.
  - **Category III.** There is no preferred first-line treatment for patients with chronic pelvic pain syndrome. It is reasonable to try antimicrobials, α-blockers, or anti-inflammatory medications first; however, if a patient does not respond to treatment, repeated trials are not warranted. In addition, it is important to consider multimodal therapy with a combination of medications or possible

adjunctive therapy with nonpharmacologic modalities. Men with chronic pelvic pain syndrome represent a highly complex group of patients, and urology referral is often necessary.
- **Nonoperative.** Supportive treatment includes rest, analgesics (nonsteroidal anti-inflammatory drugs often helpful), hydration, and stool softeners. Warm sitz baths may provide relief. For urinary retention, consider suprapubic bladder drainage. Foley catheter causes increased risk of sepsis. **Category III** may improve with avoidance of caffeine, alcohol, and spices.[11]

ACKNOWLEDGMENT

The author would like to acknowledge Douglas S. Parks for his work on the previous version of this chapter.

REFERENCES

1. Liang XL, Pang YR. Clinical features of chronic epididymitis: report of 63 cases. *Zhonghua Nan Ke Xue* 2012;18(3):257–259.
2. Ludwig M. Diagnosis and therapy of acute prostatitis, epididymitis and orchitis. *Andrologia* 2008;40(2):76–80.
3. Malhotra M, Sood S, Mukherjee A, et al. Genital chlamydia trachomatis: an update. *Indian J Med Res* 2013;138(3):303–316.
4. Trojian TH, Lishnak TS, Heiman D. Epididymitis and orchitis: an overview. *Am Fam Physician* 2009;79(7):583–587.
5. Walker NA, Challacombe B. Managing epididymo-orchitis in general practice. *Practitioner* 2013;257(1760):21–5, 2–3.
6. Srinath H. Acute scrotal pain. *Aust Fam Physician* 2013;42(11):790–792.
7. Raynor MC, Carson CC 3rd. Urinary infections in men. *Med Clin North Am* 2011;95(1):43–54.
8. Krieger JN, Nyberg L Jr, Nickel JC. NIH consensus definition and classification of prostatitis. *JAMA* 1999;282(3):236–237.
9. Mosharafa AA, Torky MH, El Said WM, et al. Rising incidence of acute prostatitis following prostate biopsy: fluoroquinolone resistance and exposure is a significant risk factor. *Urology* 2011;78(3):511–517.
10. Sharp VJ, Takacs EB, Powell CR. Prostatitis: diagnosis and treatment. *Am Fam Physician* 2010;82(4):397–406.
11. Meyrier A, Fekete T. Acute bacterial prostatitis. UpToDate. http://www.uptodate.com/home/index.html. Accessed March 10, 2014.
12. Zhao WP, Li YT, Chen J, et al. Prostatic calculi influence the antimicrobial efficacy in men with chronic bacterial prostatitis. *Asian J Androl* 2012;14:715–719.

12.5 Benign Prostatic Hyperplasia

Kathryn Helena Filutowski

GENERAL PRINCIPLES
General Knowledge

Benign prostatic hyperplasia (BPH) is a nonmalignant enlargement of the prostate gland. Histologically, it is characterized by the presence of discrete nodules in the periurethral zone of the prostate gland.[1] Cellular accumulation and gland enlargement may result from epithelial and stromal proliferation, impaired preprogrammed cell death (apoptosis), or both.[2] As the prostate enlarges, the layer of tissue surrounding it stops it from expanding, causing the gland to compress the urethra. The bladder wall becomes thicker and causes urinary incontinence and eventual overflow incontinence, which can impair a male's quality of life. The voiding dysfunction that results from prostate gland enlargement and bladder outlet obstruction (BOO) is termed lower urinary tract symptoms (LUTS).

Prevalence

The prevalence of histologically diagnosed prostatic hyperplasia increases from 8% in men aged 31 to 40, to 40% to 50% in men aged 51 to 60, to over 80% in men older than age 80.[3]

Potential Risk Factors

- Older age
- Black race have an increased risk of needing surgery related to BPH[3]
- Higher free prostate-specific antigen (PSA) levels, heart disease
- Higher levels of testosterone and estradiol
- Family history of bladder cancer
- Use of β-blockers

Negative factors: Asian race, cigarette use (1 to 20 cigarettes per day), exercise, drinking more than three drinks per day, cirrhosis (shown to decrease levels of androgens), and use of nonsteroidal anti-inflammatory drugs (NSAIDs).[3]

Pathogenesis and Pathophysiology

The enlarged gland has been proposed to contribute to the overall LUTS complex via at least two routes: (a) direct BOO from enlarged tissue (static component) and (b) from increased smooth muscle tone and resistance within the enlarged gland (dynamic component).[4] Other causes that can lead to BPH include:

- Age-related higher levels of the estrogen/androgen ratio
- Dysregulation of stromal growth factor as the tissue concentration of several growth factors is increased in hyperplastic tissue.[3]
- Inflammatory infiltrates are thought to play a role; however, this has not been fully identified. If there is a causal mechanism, it may explain why NSAIDs improve symptoms of BPH.[3]
- High immunoreactivity for interleukin-2 and bcl-2 is consistent with the decreased apoptotic rate of BPH.[3]

DIAGNOSIS (EVALUATION)

History

Symptoms may include urinary frequency, nocturia, hesitancy, urgency, and weak urinary stream are gradual and progress over time. A detailed history is important to rule out other causes of BPH. Questions to ask include history of type 2 diabetes, symptoms of neurologic disease, sexual dysfunction, general fitness level, hematuria, history of urethral trauma, urethritis, or urethral instrumentation that could lead to urethral stricture, family history of BPH or prostate cancer, or treatment with drugs that could impair bladder function.[5] The AUA/International prostate symptom score (IPSS) is useful in measuring treatment outcomes (Table 12.5-1).

Physical Examination

Examination should include an abdominal, genital, and digital rectal examination (DRE), and a focused neurologic examination (to exclude neurogenic bladder). Specifically, clinician should assess prostate size (normal is 7 to 16 g) and consistency and to detect nodules, induration, and asymmetry, all of which raise suspicion for malignancy.[6]

Laboratory and Imaging

The AUA 2010 guidelines recommend that:

- **Urinalysis** is useful in detecting proteinuria (renal disease), hematuria, infection (bacteriuria, nitrite, and esterase positive), casts (renal disease), and crystals (calculus). Hematuria may also indicate calculus, chronic renal disease, or malignancy in elderly patients.
- **Serum creatinine** is not recommended according to the AUA 2010 guidelines; however, the European Association of Urology (EAU) advises for its testing. They say it is a good baseline and a cost-effective choice.[4]
- **Serum PSA** may be used as a screening test for prostate cancer in these men with BPH, preferably in men between the ages of 50 and 69 years and before therapy for BPH is discussed. However, the following should be kept in mind with PSA:
  - The specificity of the serum PSA assay is lower in men with obstructive symptoms than in asymptomatic men.[6]
  - High values occur in men with prostatic diseases other than cancer, including BPH.
  - Some men with prostatic cancer have serum PSA concentrations of 4.0 ng per mL (a widely used cutoff value) or less.

TABLE 12.5-1　The American Urological Association Symptom Index for Benign Prostatic Hyperplasia

Questions to be answered	Not at all	Less than 1 time in 5	Less than half the time	About half the time	More than half the time	Almost always	Your score
Over the past month, how much have you had a sensation of emptying you bladder completely after urinating?	0	1	2	3	4	5	
Over the past month, how often have you had to urinate again less than 2 hr after you finished urinating?	0	1	2	3	4	5	
Over the past month, how often have you found you stopped and started again several times when you urinated?	0	1	2	3	4	5	
Over the past month, how often have you found it difficult to postpone urination?	0	1	2	3	4	5	
Over the past month, how often have you had a weak urinary stream?	0	1	2	3	4	5	
Over the past month, how often have you had to push or strain to begin urination?	0	1	2	3	4	5	
Over the past month, how many times did you most typically get up to urinate from the time you went to bed at night until the time you got up in the morning?	0	1	2	3	4	5	

Sum of numbers (AUA symptom score)

Total score
0–7: mild symptoms
9–19: moderate symptoms
20–35: severe symptoms

Quality of life due to urinary symptoms	Delighted	Pleased	Mostly satisfied	Mixed about equally satisfied and unsatisfied	Mostly dissatisfied	Unhappy	Terrible
If you were to spend the rest of your life with your urinary condition the way it is now, how would you feel about that?	0	1	2	3	4	5	6

Optional Tests
- **Maximal urinary flow rate.** It is tested if greater than 15 mL per second excludes clinically important BOO due to BPH.
- **Measurement of postvoid residual urine (PVR)** by in-and-out catheterization, ultrasound, or cystography. Large PVR correlates with severe BPH and chronic renal insufficiency, but does not predict need for surgery. Normal men have less than 12 mL of residual urine.[7]
- **Urine cytology.** Urine cytology may be helpful in men with predominantly irritative symptoms. It may be considered in men with a smoking history, since this is a risk factor for bladder cancer.[6]
- **Newer technologies.** It is also possible that newer imaging modalities, such as contrast-enhanced MRI and MR diffusion, will be able to differentiate glandular-ductal versus stromal-low ductal tissues.[8] Such information may aid in the detection of cancer and its grading. It is still unclear whether this information will prove to be cost-effective.

Differential Diagnosis

The differential includes urethral stricture (history of urethral trauma, urethritis, urethral instrumentation), bladder neck obstruction, carcinoma of the prostate or urinary bladder (hematuria, persisting LUTS not responding to treatment, hard nodular prostate on DRE, elevated PSA), and urolithiasis (pain, hematuria).
- Other considerations include lower urinary tract infections (UTIs), including prostatitis (frequency, urgency, abdominal pain, perirectal pain, constitutional symptoms, boggy and tender prostate) and neurogenic bladder (history of cerebral or spinal injury or tumor, stroke, degenerative joint disease of the spine, spinal or pelvic surgery; urinary retention or incontinence; focal neurologic deficits on examination; cystoscopy and pressure flow studies are useful).[6]

TREATMENT OPTIONS

Watchful Waiting (Active Surveillance)
- Appropriate for patients with mild symptoms (symptom score less than 7) and minimally enlarged prostate.[4]
- Medications exacerbating symptoms or inducing urinary retention (sedating antihistamines, decongestants) should be avoided.
- Voiding at regular intervals, pelvic floor exercises, and avoidance or treatment of constipation are recommended.
- Fluid intake should be minimized before bedtime; caffeine and alcohol intake are reduced.

Medication

Indicated when symptoms of BPH impact the patient's quality of life in spite of implementing the above treatment or AUA-SI score ≥ 8.[4] Two classes of drugs, α-adrenergic antagonists and 5-α-reductase inhibitors (5-ARIs), act upon the dynamic (tension of prostatic smooth muscle in the prostate, prostate capsule, and bladder neck) and fixed (the bulk of the enlarged prostate impinging upon the urethra) components of BOO, respectively.[9]
- α-Blockers
  - Smooth muscles in the prostate gland contract in response to α-adrenergic receptor stimulation, causing constriction of the prostatic urethra. α_1-Receptor antagonists improve LUTS by promoting smooth muscle relaxation.
  - FDA has approved terazosin, doxazosin, tamsulosin, alfuzosin, and silodosin for the treatment of the symptoms of BPH.[9]
    ∘ Dosage and adverse effects (Table 12.5-2).
  - These are considered the most effective monotherapy for improving LUTS in men with BPH.[4]
  - Symptom improvement is typically noted within 2 to 4 weeks of initiating α-blocker therapy.[1]
  - *Side effects:* Most important are orthostatic hypotension and dizziness. Terazosin and doxazosin need to be initiated at bedtime, and dose needs to be titrated up over several weeks.[9]
- 5-ARIs
  - These act upon the fixed component of prostate by reducing its size. 5-α-Reductase blockers inhibit the conversion of testosterone to dihydrotestosterone, suppressing prostate growth.[10]
  - FDA has approved finasteride and duasteride for the treatment of BPH.
  - For dosage and adverse effects, see Table 12.5-2.
  - These have been shown to affect the clinical course of BPH, reducing the risk of acute urinary retention (NNT = 26) and surgical intervention (NNT = 18) 4 years after therapy.[11]
  - It usually takes 6 to 12 months in order to see any symptom relief.

| TABLE 12.5-2 | Medical Therapies for Benign Prostatic Hyperplasia | | |

Medication	Dosage	Cost per month (generic)[a]	Comments
α-Blockers			
Doxazosin (Cardura)	Start at 1 mg daily; maximum 8 mg daily	$45 (26–28)	Risk of orthostatic hypotension
Prazosin (Minipress)	Start at 1 mg twice daily; maximum 5 mg three times daily	39 (18–24)	
Terazosin (Hytrin)	Start with 1 mg taken at bedtime; maximum 20 mg taken at bedtime	68 (18–20)	
Selective α-blockers			
Alfuzosin (Uroxatral)	10 mg daily	77 (—)	No effect on resting blood pressure; risk of orthostatic hypotension
Tamsulosin (Flomax)	0.4 mg daily	77 (—)	
5-α-Reductase inhibitors			
Dutasteride (Avodart)	0.5 mg daily	96 (—)	Six months of treatment is needed to achieve
Finasteride (Proscar)	5 mg daily	100 (94)	Symptom relief

[a]generic price listed first; brand price listed in parentheses.
Edwards JL. Diagnosis and management of benign prostate hypertrophy. *Am Fam Physician* 2008;77(10):1403–1410.

- Combination therapy
  - is an appropriate and effective treatment for patients with LUTS associated with demonstrable prostatic enlargement based on volume measurement, PSA level as a proxy for volume, and/or enlargement on DRE.[4]
- Alternative therapies
  - Saw Palmetto
  - Rye grass pollen extract (Cernilton)
  - Pygeum
    - AUA does not recommend for treatment of LUTS related to BPH[4]

Nonsurgical Treatment (Minimally Invasive Treatment)

Useful in those with significant comorbid disease, and in patients requiring chronic anticoagulation.[4]
- **Transurethral needle ablation of the prostate (TUNA).** Low-energy radiofrequency ablation performed under local anesthesia, which improves symptom scores and urinary flow rates in 50% to 60% of patients, with minimal complications.[4]
- **Transurethral microwave thermotherapy (TUMT).** It involves heating prostatic tissue using computer-regulated microwaves under local anesthesia. Higher energy TUMT is useful in patients with larger glands. It improves symptom scores and urinary flow. Serious thermal injuries may result.[4]

Surgical Treatment

The AUA recommends surgery in patients with renal insufficiency secondary to BPH, recurrent UTIs, bladder stones or gross hematuria due to BPH, acute urinary retention, or those who have LUTS refractory to other therapies.[4]
- **Laser therapies.** Transurethral holmium laser ablation of the prostate (HoLAP), transurethral holmium laser enucleation of the prostate (HoLEP), and holmium laser resection of the prostate (HoLRP) are effective treatment alternatives to transurethral resection of the prostate and open prostatectomy in men with moderate to severe LUTS and/or those who are significantly bothered by these symptoms.[4]
- **Transurethral incision of the prostate (TUIP).** Making two deep incisions distal to each ureteral orifice through the bladder neck and the prostatic adenoma toward the verumontanum, down to the capsule of the prostate. It is recommended for men with BOO and minimal prostate enlargement, especially those with comorbid illnesses.[4]
- **Open prostatectomy.** This procedure is performed infrequently (in under 5%) on patients with large prostates, who are good surgical candidates. Retropubic, transvesical, and perineal approaches exist.[4]

• **Newer treatment.** In September 2013, the FDA approved Urolift, the first permanent implant to relieve low or blocked urine flow in men aged 50 years and older with an enlarged prostate.[12] It relieves the urine flow by pulling back the prostate tissue that is pressing on the urethra.[12]

Special Considerations: Indications for Referral to a Urologist

• History of worsening LUTS, acute urinary retention, hematuria, urinary incontinence without response to conservative and medical treatment
• Palpable urinary bladder or high PVR
• Urolithiasis, recurrent UTIs
• Hard and irregular prostate, elevated PSA[9]

ACKNOWLEDGMENT

The author would like to acknowledge Kalyanakrishnan Ramakrishnan for his work on the previous version of this chapter.

REFERENCES

1. Edwards JL. Diagnosis and management of benign prostatic hyperplasia. *Am Fam Physician* 2008;77(10):1403–1410.
2. Deters LA, Kim ED. Benign prostatic hypertrophy. Medscape. http://emedicine.medscape.com/article/437359-overview#a0101. Accessed November 3, 2013.
3. Cunningam GR, Cadmon D. Epidemiology and pathogenesis of benign prostatic hyperplasia. UptoDate. www.uptodate.com. Accessed November 2, 2013.
4. American Urological Association. Guideline on the management of benign prostatic hyperplasia (BPH). http://www.auanet.org/common/pdf/education/clinical-guidance/Benign-Prostatic-Hyperplasia.pdf. Accessed November 3, 2013.
5. Parsons JK, Carter HB, Partin AW, et al. Metabolic factors associated with benign prostatic hyperplasia. *J Clin Endocrinol Metab* 2006;91:2562.
6. Cunningam GR, Cadmon D. Clinical manifestations and diagnostic evaluation of benign prostatic hyperplasia. UptoDate. www.uptodate.com. Accessed November 2, 2013.
7. DiMare JR, Fish SR, Harper JM, et al. Residual urine in normal male subjects. *J Urol* 1963;96:180.
8. Noworolski SM, Vigneron DB, Chen AP, et al. Dynamic contrast-enhanced MRI and MR diffusion Imaging to distinguish between glandular and stromal prostatic tissues. *Magn Reson Imaging* 2008;26:1071.
9. Cunningam GR, Cadmon D. Medical treatment of benign prostatic hyperplasia. UptoDate. www.uptodate.com. Accessed November 2, 2013.
10. McNaughton-Collins M, Barry MJ. Managing patients with lower urinary tract symptoms suggestive of benign prostatic hyperplasia. *Am J Med* 2005;118(12):1331–1339.
11. McConnell JD, Bruskewitz R, Walsh P, et al. The effect of finasteride on the risk of acute urinary retention and the need for surgical treatment among men with benign prostatic hyperplasia. Finasteride Long-Term Efficacy and Safety Study Group. *N Engl J Med* 1998;338(9):557–563.
12. Crane M. FDA OKs New Device to Treat BPH. Medscape. medscape.com/viewarticle/810981. Accessed November 3, 2013.

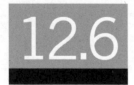

12.6 Prostate Cancer

Svetlana Moore

GENERAL PRINCIPLES

Prostate cancer is the most common noncutaneous cancer in men in the United States. An estimated one in six white men and one in five African American men will be diagnosed with prostate cancer in their lifetime, with the likelihood increasing with age. It is the second most common cause of cancer death in males.[1]

Anatomy

Prostate cancer usually arises in the peripheral zone of the gland, but it may also occur laterally or centrally and is often multifocal. If it grows, it may become locally invasive—penetrating the prostate capsule, invading the seminal vesicles, spreading to pelvic lymph nodes, and eventually reaching distant lymph nodes in the abdomen and beyond. Bone is usually the first site of metastasis beyond the lymph nodes, with liver and lung metastases occurring later.[2]

Epidemiology

The American Cancer Society estimates that there will be 238,590 new cases of prostate cancer diagnosed in 2013 and 29,700 deaths. Incidence increases after age 50, with more than two thirds of prostate cancers diagnosed after the age of 65.[3] Possessing certain genes increases the risk of prostate cancer. History of prostate cancer in a brother or father doubles the risk of the disease. African American men have a 60% higher incidence of prostate cancer compared to whites, whereas Asian and Hispanic Americans have lower rates than whites. African American men are also more often diagnosed with advanced disease and twice as likely as other American men to die of prostate cancer. Since the early 1990s, prostate cancer screening has dramatically increased the number of prostate cancers diagnosed in the United States, with a simultaneous shift toward earlier stage at diagnosis. Meanwhile, prostate cancer deaths declined. However, depending on the prostate-specific antigen (PSA) value, pathologic stage, and histologic grade of the tumor, approximately 30% of patients with clinically localized prostate cancer are estimated to progress despite initial treatment with intent to cure.[4]

Pathophysiology

Prostate cancer develops when the rates of cell division and cell death are unequal, leading to uncontrolled tumor growth. Further mutations of a multitude of genes, including the genes for p53 and retinoblastoma, can lead to tumor progression and metastasis. Most prostate cancers (95%) are adenocarcinomas.[2]

Etiology

Environmental risk factors include cigarette smoking, a diet high in fat or chromium, and obesity. Elevated levels of luteinizing hormone and of testosterone/dihydrotestosterone ratios are associated with mildly increased risk. Genetic changes associated with poor survival in prostate cancer include loss of one or both copies of the tumor suppressor gene *PTEN*, *TMPRSS2-ERG* chromosome fusion, *P53* mutations, and overexpression of *MYC*. Prospective trials are needed to assess these markers more thoroughly before their implementation in clinical management. Currently, none of them is measured in routine practice.[5]

DIAGNOSIS

Asymptomatic Men

Digital rectal examination and PSA evaluation are the two components necessary for a modern screening program. The indications for screening are controversial. In 2011, a USPSTF draft statement recommended against PSA screening of all ages who do not have symptoms considered highly suspicious for prostate cancer.[6] The American Cancer Society recommends that PSA evaluation and digital rectal examination (DRE) be offered annually, beginning at age 50 years to men who have at least a 10-year life expectancy, and that they should be offered as early as age 40 years to high-risk men. Information should be provided to patients regarding potential risks and benefits of intervention. Risks of screening include diagnosis and treatment of a clinically insignificant cancer, resulting in complications such as impotence or incontinence. A 2010 study concluded that in the 75- to 80-year age group discontinuation of PSA screening may be safe in African American men, with an initial PSA level of less than 6.0 ng per mL and in Caucasian men with an initial PSA of less than 3.0 ng per mL, because men in these groups are unlikely to develop high-risk prostate cancer.[7]

Symptomatic Men

Prostate cancer usually causes no symptoms in its early stages. When they occur, symptoms may include urinary frequency, urgency, hesitancy, or nocturia. If the cancer invades the neurovascular bundle, erectile dysfunction may result. Hematuria and hemospermia are relatively uncommon presenting symptoms. When metastatic, prostate cancer may cause bone pain or other symptoms due to distant lesions. When older men present with new symptoms of urinary obstruction or with symptoms that could be caused by bony metastases, the diagnosis of prostate cancer should be considered.[8]

Physical Examination

DRE is part of the diagnostic evaluation for prostate cancer for symptomatic men. On DRE, asymmetric areas of induration or frank nodules that are detected in the posterior and lateral aspects of the prostate gland are suggestive of prostate cancer. Tumors not detected by DRE include the 25% to 35% occurring in other parts of the gland and small, T1, cancers that are not palpable.[8]

Laboratory Studies

PSA is a protein made solely by prostate cells, so the antigen is highly specific for the prostate. However, it is not prostate cancer specific, and other prostate conditions, such as benign prostatic hyperplasia (BPH) or prostatitis, can affect PSA levels. The lack of specificity for prostate cancer has led to considerable controversy about the role of routine PSA testing. The controversy is compounded by the knowledge that not all cancers detected by routine screening require treatment. PSA levels generally increase with age and prostate size. The norm for a man less than age 50 years is <1 ng per mL, whereas it is >3 ng per mL for men over the age of 60 years. Some researchers advocate race-specific reference ranges.[9]

Monitoring

When PSA values are slightly elevated and DRE is normal, biopsy is sometimes deferred in favor of close monitoring of PSA values over time. In these cases, PSA may be initially repeated in a month or two and then again every 6 to 12 months. The change in PSA levels over time is referred to as PSA velocity. PSA exists in free and bound forms in the serum, with more bound PSA secreted by glands that have disrupted cellular architecture. As the proportion of free-to-total PSA drops below 20%, the likelihood of prostate cancer increases. Therefore, free PSA is often ordered to help decide whether to obtain a biopsy in borderline cases. Generally, PSA should be repeated before a biopsy is recommended since almost a third of patients will have a decrease to baseline levels if PSA is repeated a month or so later.[9]

Imaging

Transrectal ultrasound (TRUS) is not an accurate screening tool, but is used to guide needle biopsies that are done for diagnostic purposes. Pelvic and abdominal computed tomography (CT) and radionuclide bone scans are ordered when there is clinical suspicion of regional or distant metastases. Conventional endorectal magnetic resonance imaging (MRI) is helpful for localizing cancer within the prostate and seminal vesicles and for local staging. Dynamic, contrast-enhanced MRI and MR spectroscopic imaging are complementary in local staging, but their use is currently limited to a research setting.[10]

Surgical Diagnostic Procedures

Diagnosis of prostate cancer is typically made with the aid of a transrectal core needle biopsy. Biopsies focus on abnormal areas found on DRE and TRUS and also include multiple specimens covering all areas of the gland. Benign findings are often followed by repeat biopsy when the clinical diagnosis remains in doubt. The most common side effects of prostate biopsy are transient hemospermia and hematuria.[10]

Tumor Stage

The American Joint Committee on Cancer (AJCC) has developed a prostate cancer staging system based on the TNM (tumor, nodes, metastases) system. Stages 1 and 2 are defined, respectively, as nonpalpable and palpable tumors confined to the prostate. Stage 3 tumors extend through the prostate capsule and may involve the seminal vesicles but not the lymph nodes or other adjacent structures. Stage 4 tumors invade adjacent structures or have spread to regional lymph nodes or more distant sites.[11]

Gleason Score

Tumors may be well differentiated or poorly differentiated at any stage, and the level of tumor differentiation can be graded with a score of 1 to 5, with 5 being the most poorly differentiated. The Gleason score is the sum of grades for the two most prevalent patterns of differentiation seen on biopsy. A Gleason score of 4 or less is classified as a low-grade tumor. Scores of 5 to 7 are intermediate, and scores of 8 or above are high grade. The Gleason score adds prognostic information that can be used to guide treatment decisions, especially for Stage 1 and Stage 2 tumors.[10]

Clinical Staging

At present, approximately 90% of prostate cancers are localized at the time of diagnosis, and complete staging with bone scans, CT scans, and other imaging tests are usually reserved for patients who are clinically suspected to have a cancer that has spread beyond the prostate gland, such as in the case of a PSA >10 ng per mL or a high Gleason score. Seminal vesicle biopsy and pelvic lymph node dissection (PLND, which can now be done laparoscopically) are also sometimes used for more definitive clinical staging when needed to guide treatment.[12]

Differential Diagnosis

In asymptomatic men with a normal DRE, a mildly elevated PSA has a relatively low specificity and may be due to BPH, chronic prostatitis, or increased age. Local symptoms from prostate cancer can sometimes mimic BPH and include urinary frequency, hesitancy, nocturia, and weak stream. When these symptoms develop rapidly, they may be more indicative of cancer. When infection is suspected, an empiric trial of antibiotics with repeat PSA testing after treatment is sometimes tried before referring a patient for biopsy. Clinicians should consider the possibility of metastatic prostate cancer in older men presenting with new atypical back pain or other bone pain syndromes.[13]

TREATMENT
General Treatment Recommendations for Prostate Cancer

Selecting initial treatment requires assessing the risk of the disease spreading or progressing, which is based on evaluating life expectancy, comorbidities, biopsy grade (Gleason score), clinical stage, and PSA level.[14]

Treatment Recommendations for Clinically Localized Prostate Cancer

Very Low Risk of Recurrence
Patients with clinical stage T1c, Gleason score ≤6, PSA <10 ng per mL, fewer than three positive prostate cores, with a life expectancy <20 years, should be treated with active surveillance and observation.[14]

Low Risk of Recurrence
Patients with clinical stage T1–T2a, Gleason score of 2 to 6, PSA <10 ng per mL, with a life expectancy <10 years, should be treated with active surveillance.

Treatment of patients with a life expectancy ≥10 years includes active surveillance **OR** radical prostatectomy (RP) with or without PLND if predicted probability of lymph node metastases ≥2%. Patients with low-risk cancer are not candidates for pelvic lymph node irradiation or androgen deprivation therapy (ADT).[14]

Intermediate Risk of Recurrence
Patients with clinical stage T2b–T2c, Gleason score 7, and PSA 10 to 20 ng per mL, who have a life expectancy <10 years should be treated with active surveillance **OR** radiation therapy with daily image-guided radiotherapy (IGRT) with or without short-term ADT for 4 to 6 months with or without brachytherapy. Patients with a life expectancy ≥10 years should be treated with RP with PLND. Administering ADT before, during, and after radiation prolongs survival.[14]

High Risk of Recurrence
Patients with clinical stage T3a, Gleason score 8 to 10, and PSA >20 ng per mL should be treated with radiation therapy plus long-term ADT for 2 to 3 years or radiation therapy with daily IGRT plus brachytherapy.

Alternative treatment recommendations for localized prostate cancer include cryotherapy, high-intensity focused ultrasound, and particle beam therapy.[14]

Treatment Recommendations for Locally Advanced Prostate Cancer

Very High Risk
Clinical stage T3b–T4 treatment options include radiation therapy with IMRT plus long-term ADT for 2- to 3-year **OR** radiation therapy with IMRT with daily IGRT plus brachytherapy with or without short-term ADT.[14]

Metastatic Disease
Any T, N1 treatment includes ADT **OR** radiation therapy with IMRT with IGRT plus long-term ADT for 2 to 3 years. Any T, any N, M1 treatment should include only ADT.

Bisphosphonates are recommended for all men with hormone-refractory prostate cancer and bone metastases that have been shown to reduce pathologic bone fracture.[14]

Referrals

Treatment of prostate cancer often involves a variety of specialists, including a urologic oncologist and a radiation oncologist. Clear communication with the patient and treating physicians has the potential to help patients navigate complex diagnostic and treatment decisions.

Follow-Up

No randomized trials have yet defined the optimal surveillance strategy following treatment therapies for localized prostate cancer.

The standard follow-up for all patients is PSA testing and clinical evaluation. Current follow-up recommendations for patients who have undergone definitive therapy for localized disease are to monitor the serum PSA every 6 to 12 months for 5 years and then annually thereafter. Routine imaging procedures are not indicated in the absence of symptoms or a rising serum PSA.

The current recommendation for patients with metastatic prostate cancer is to monitor for disease progression and the side effects of long-term ADT. Patients should keep up with physician's appointments and measurements of serum PSA level every 3 to 6 months.[15]

REFERENCES

1. Cornelis F, Rigou G, Le Bras Y, et al. Real-time contrast-enhanced transrectal US-guided prostate biopsy: diagnostic accuracy in men with previously negative biopsy results and positive MR imaging findings. *Radiology* 2013;269(1):159–166.
2. Jamal A, Siegel R, Ward E, et al. Cancer statistics, 2006. *CA Cancer J Clin* 2006;56:106–130.
3. Siegel R, Naishadham D, Jemal A, Cancer statistics, 2013. *CA Cancer J Clin* 2013;63:11.
4. American Cancer Society. Cancer Facts and Figures 2010. http://www.cancer.org/research/cancer factsstatistics/cancerfactsfigures2010/index. Accessed November 20, 2013.
5. Markert EK, Mmizuno H, Vazquez A, et al. Molecular classification of prostate cancer using curated expression signatures. *Proc Natl Acad Sci USA* 2011:108(52):21276–21281.
6. Chou R, Croswell JM, Dana T, et al. Screening for prostate cancer: a review of the evidence for the U.S. Preventive Services Task Force. *Ann Intern Med* 2011;155(11):762–771.
7. Tang P, Sun L, Robertson CN, et al. Prostate specific antigen-based risk-adapted discontinuation of prostate cancer screening in elderly African American and Caucasian American men. *Urology* 2010;76(5):1058–1062.
8. Harris R, Lohr KN. Screening for prostate cancer: an update of the evidence for the U.S. Preventive Services Task Force. *Ann Intern Med* 2002;137:917–929.
9. Gann PH, Hennekens CH, Stampfer MJ. A prospective evaluation of plasma prostate-specific antigen for detection of prostate cancer. *JAMA* 1995;273:289–294.
10. Choi WW, Williams SB, Gu X, et al. Overuse of imaging for staging low risk prostate cancer. *J Urol* 2011;185(5):1645–1649.
11. Greene FL, Page DL, Fleming ID, et al, eds. *AJCC cancer staging handbook*. 6th ed. New York, NY: Springer; 2002:309–316.
12. Bostwick DG. Grading prostate cancer. *Am J Clin Pathol* 1994;102:S38–S56.
13. Smith DA, Catalona WJ. Rate of change in serum prostate specific antigen levels as a method for prostate cancer detection. *J Urol* 1994;152:1163–1167.
14. Ghavamian R. Prostate Cancer Treatment Protocols. http://emedicine.medscape.com/article/2007095-overview. Accessed November 20, 2013.
15. Penson DF, Vogelzang N, Lee WR, et al. Follow-up surveillance during and after treatment for prostate cancer. http://www.uptodate.com/contents/follow-up-surveillance-during-and-after-treatment-for-prostate-cancer. Accessed November 6, 2013.

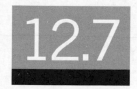

Chronic Kidney Disease

Jitendrakumar D. Sodvadiya, Kimberly J. Jarzynka

General Principles

Chronic kidney disease (CKD) is defined as "abnormalities of kidney structure of function, present for >3 months, with implications for health."

Criteria for CKD include either of the following for >3 months:
- Decreased glomerular filtration rate (GFR) <60 mL/min/1.73 m^2
- Markers of kidney damage (one or more):
  1. Albuminuria (albumin excretion rate [AER] ≥30 mg per 24 hours; albumin-to-creatinine ratio [ACR] ≥30 mg per g [≥3 mg per mmol])
  2. Urine sediment abnormalities
  3. Electrolyte and other abnormalities due to tubular disorders
  4. Abnormalities detected by histology
  5. Structural abnormalities detected by imaging
  6. History of kidney transplant.[1,2]

Epidemiology

It is estimated that greater than 10% of adults (greater than 20 million people) have CKD of varying severity. Prevalence increases after the age of 50 and is most common in adults greater than age 70. It is present in one-third of adults with diabetes and one-fifth of adults with hypertension. Diabetic and hypertensive patients make up approximately 70% of new cases of end-stage renal disease (ESRD) in the United States. African Americans are about 3.5 times more likely to develop ESRD than whites, and Hispanics are about 1.5 times more likely to develop ESRD than non-Hispanics.[3]

Risk Factors

Clinical Factors
- Diabetes
- Hypertension
- Autoimmune disease
- Systemic infections
- Urinary tract infections
- Urinary stones
- Lower urinary tract obstruction
- Neoplasia
- Family history of CKD
- Recovery from acute kidney injury (AKI)
- Reduction in kidney mass
- Exposure to certain drugs
- Low birth weight

Sociodemographic Factors
- Older age
- **U.S. ethnic minority status:** African American, American Indian, Hispanic, Asian or Pacific Islander
- Exposure to certain chemical and environmental conditions (lead, cadmium, arsenic, mercury, uranium)
- Low income or education[1,2,4]

Classification

See Tables 12.7-1 and 12.7-2.[1]

TABLE 12.7-1	GFR Categories in CKD[1]	
GFR category	Terms	GFR (mL/min/1.73 m^2)
G1[a]	Normal or high	≥90
G2[a]	Mildly decreased	60–89
G3a	Mildly to moderately decreased	45–59
G3b	Moderately to severely decreased	30–44
G4	Severely decreased	15–29
G5	Kidney failure	<15

GFR, glomerular filtration rate.
[a]In the absence of evidence of kidney damage, neither G1 nor G2 fulfills the criteria for CKD.

TABLE 12.7-2	Albuminuria Categories in CKD[1]			
Category	Terms	AER (mg/24 h)	ACR (mg/mmol)	ACR (mg/g)
A1	Normal to mildly increased	<30	<3	<30
A2	Moderately increased	30–300	3–30	30–300
A3	Severely increased[a]	>300	>30	>300

AER, albumin excretion rate; ACR, albumin-to-creatinine ratio; CKD, chronic kidney disease.
[a]Including nephrotic syndrome (albumin excretion usually >2,200/24 h [ACR >2,220 mg/g; >220 mg/mmol].

DIAGNOSIS
History
Many patients with CKD are asymptomatic and are found incidentally on routine laboratories or imaging studies performed for other reasons. Symptoms associated with CKD do not typically occur until the final stages (i.e., Stages 3 to 5) in the disease progression and more profoundly when kidney function deterioration is substantial enough to produce uremia (i.e., GFR less than 15 mL/min/1.73 m^2). These symptoms could include generalized fatigue, symptoms associated with anemia, volume depletion or volume excess, and symptoms consistent with uremia, including generalized weakness, anorexia, nausea, vomiting, or mental status change. Bone pain is also common late in the course of CKD. Many of the earlier historical findings are related to the initiating events, underlying disease, or other risk factors listed above. History to determine cardiovascular disease risk and smoking status should also be explored.[4–6]

Physical Examination
Abnormal physical findings associated with CKD occur late in the process (i.e., Stage 5), except those related to underlying disease processes. Late findings include edema; hypertension; decreased urine output; pallor; easy bruising; cardiac dysrhythmias induced by hyperkalemia; asterixis, seizures, mental status change; and other neurologic manifestations of uremia. Physical evidence of hypovolemia, heart failure, or other causes of kidney hypoperfusion would suggest the potential of acute renal failure in the setting of CKD. Hypertension and presence of an abdominal bruit, findings consistent with peripheral vascular disease or carotid artery disease could suggest renal vascular disease. Acute muscle tenderness and swelling may indicate muscle injury. Abdominal, pelvic, and prostate evaluation may reveal the source of postrenal obstruction. Musculoskeletal findings such as arthritis or synovitis, fever, skin rash, or pulmonary lesions could suggest an autoimmune disease or vasculitis as an etiology for CKD.[4,6]

Laboratory and Imaging
Initial evaluation of CKD should include serum creatinine with GFR estimation, serum electrolytes, glucose, urine sediment, urine ACR, and renal ultrasound. A fasting lipid panel and EKG should be included to assess cardiovascular disease risk.

Creatinine secretion increases with advancing CKD, but may be normal in the earliest stages of CKD. An initial doubling of baseline serum creatinine levels may represent as much as a 50% loss of kidney function even when the doubling of the serum creatinine results in levels still within normal ranges. Measurement of serum creatinine levels alone to assess renal function does not account for differences caused by age, ethnicity, gender, weight, muscle mass, protein intake, or protein loss. GFR estimate equations that take these variables into account will more accurately determine renal function. Serum creatinine levels and GFR estimates performed serially over time can help determine whether the renal damage is a chronic or acute process, and can approximate the rate of kidney function decline in later stages of CKD. Blood urea nitrogen (BUN) increase is at 10:1 relationship with creatinine for that portion of BUN related to declining GFR (nonrenal causes of BUN elevation include gastrointestinal bleeding, high protein diets, and enhanced tissue destruction).

The preferred method for evaluating proteinuria is a urine ACR. Other tests (in decreasing order of preference) include urine protein-to-creatinine ratio, reagent strip urinalysis for total protein with automated reading, and reagent strip urinalysis for total protein with manual reading. Confirmatory testing (repeating ACR on an early morning sample or albumin or total protein excretion rate in a timed urine sample) is indicated if factors that can affect protein excretion without kidney damage are present. These factors include menstrual blood contamination, UTI, exercise, upright posture in orthostatic proteinuria, septicemia, intrinsic biological or genetic variability, degradation of albumin before analysis due to freezing, age (lower in children and elderly), race (lower in Caucasian than black individuals); muscle mass (lower in people with amputations, paraplegia, muscular dystrophy, or other causes of muscle atrophy); gender (lower in females); AKI; and samples with very high albumin concentrations (may be falsely reported as low or normal using some assays).[3]

Diminished kidney capacity to concentrate urine and maximally acidify urine, as well as conserve sodium in response to decreased effective circulating volume, is an indicator of advanced CKD. Urine sediment examination may reveal red blood cells and casts in certain glomerulopathies and white blood cells and casts in kidney infections.

Renal ultrasound will reveal the presence of small echogenic kidneys in late CKD stages with normal or large kidneys in earlier stages and large kidneys caused by hyperfiltration in early disease. Ultrasound can also reveal the presence of urinary tract obstruction and abnormalities of kidney parenchyma (e.g., cysts). Plain imaging may reveal evidence of nephrocalcinosis. Computed tomography (CT) scan of the abdomen can provide better resolution of kidney structural changes. Contrasted imaging studies should be avoided. Captopril renal scans may be used in detecting the presence of renal artery stenosis at early stages of CKD.

Other tests to identify rare causes of CKD can include serum protein electrophoresis for plasma cell dyscrasias, antinuclear antibody (ANA), and dsDNA antibody for systemic lupus erythematosis and consumption of serum complement for certain autoimmune glomerulopathies and antiglomerular basement membrane for Goodpasture syndrome.

To identify progression of CKD, assessment of GFR and albuminuria should be obtained at least annually, but should occur more frequently in individuals at higher risk of progression and/or when measurement will impact therapeutic decisions. When GFR falls below 60 (CKD 3 to 5), the patient should also be evaluated for complications of CKD including anemia, malnutrition, mineral and bone disorders, neuropathy, and overall decreased level of functioning and well-being.[1,2,4,6]

Differential Diagnosis
See Table 12.7-3.[7,8]

TREATMENT

Management of chronic renal disease begins with the recognition of individuals who are at risk for this problem before the presence of markers that indicate early renal dysfunction. Interventions to control hypertension and diabetes and avoidance of renal-toxic agents should be perceived as kidney-protective strategies. Interventions aimed at slowing the progression of CKD included control of hypertension, hyperglycemia, and proteinuria; reducing protein intake; as well as implementing strategies for cardiovascular risk reduction to include appropriate exercise, weight loss, reduce sodium intake, control of dyslipidemias, and smoking cessation in both diabetic and nondiabetic nephropathy. Although the cardiovascular risk reduction activities have not been shown to be associated with slowing the progression of CKD, their impact on cardiovascular health is essential since patients with CKD have accelerated risk for cardiovascular disease events.[1,2,5–7]

Hypertension

Chronic and uncontrolled hypertension can accelerate the loss of kidney function. Strict blood pressure (BP) control is recommended for both diabetic and nondiabetic nephropathy since evidence

TABLE 12.7-3	Differential Diagnosis of CKD[7,8]
Acute kidney injury	Nephrosclerosis
Alport syndrome	Obstructive urinary tract disease
Amyloidal kidney	Polycystic kidney disease
Chronic glomerulonephritis	Rapidly progressive glomerulonephritis
Chronic pyelonephritis	Renal artery stenosis
Congenital abnormality of metabolism	Renal hypoplasia
Diabetic nephropathy	Renal/urinary tract tuberculosis
Drug induced nephropathy	Renal/urinary tract calculus
Goodpasture syndrome	Renal/urinary tract tumor
Gouty kidney	Systemic lupus erythematosus nephritis
Malignant hypertension	Wegener granulomatosis
Multiple myeloma	Other unclassifiable nephritis
Nephropathy of pregnancy/toxemia	

shows that these interventions slow progression of CKD. According to JNC 8 guideline, BP target for patients 18 years and older with CKD is less than 140/90. Treatment should be initiated if BP is greater than 140/90. There is no evidence to recommend a specific BP goal for people aged 70 years and older with GFR <60. Initial or add on antihypertensive treatment should include angiotensin-converting enzyme inhibitors or angiotensin II blocking agents to improve kidney outcomes regardless of race or diabetes status, but they should not be used together. Usually all agents can be employed to control hypertension in patients with CKD. Thiazide diuretics and, in advancing disease (GFR <30 to 40), loop diuretics may be required to lower BP, reduce sodium retention, and provide additional kaluresis in response to the associated hyperkalemia.[9–11]

Glycemic Control

Tight glycemic control to hemoglobin A1C HbA$_1$c to about 7.0% has been shown to slow the progression of microvascular complications and CKD. Target hemoglobin A1C should be extended above 7.0% in individuals with comorbidities, limited life expectancy, and risk of hypoglycemia.[1,2,12,13]

Microalbuminuria and Macroalbuminuria

Testing for microalbuminuria in diabetic patients should be performed annually as it allows detection of diabetic nephropathy at an earlier stage before a decline in GFR or an elevation in BUN and creatinine occurs. The use of ACE inhibitors and angiotensin II receptor blockers (ARBs) when microalbuminuria or macroalbuminuria is detected has been shown to slow the progression of diabetic and nondiabetic kidney disease independent of the presence of systemic hypertension. One must carefully monitor these agents to avoid hyperkalemia especially in advancing stages of CKD. ACE inhibitors and ARBs are not indicated for primary prevention of kidney disease diabetic patients without hypertension or albuminuria.[1,2,13,14]

Hyperlipidemia

Although the effect of the control of hypercholesterolemia on the progression of CKD is not known, the increase association of coronary artery disease (CAD) with patients who have CKD is a compelling reason to lower low-density lipoprotein (LDL) levels to decrease atherogenesis.

In patients age ≥50 years with CKD and GFR >60, Statin is recommended. In patients age ≥50 years and GFR <60 (not posttransplant), treat with a Statin or Statin/ezetimibe combination. In patients age 18 to 49 with CKD without dialysis or transplant, treat with Statin if one or more of the following risk factors are present: known CAD, diabetes, prior ischemic stroke, and estimated 10-year cardiovascular risk >10%. For patients on dialysis, do not initiate treatment for hypercholesterolemia, but it may be continued if patients are already receiving treatment. Statin treatment is recommended in adult renal transplant recipients. There is no evidence to suggest LDL target is beneficial. Therefore, the DKIGO work group suggests to not measure follow-up LDL unless the result would alter management.[1,2,13,15]

Dietary Restriction

Patients with CKD should receive a formal dietary assessment and advice tailored to the severity of CKD. Reasonable protein restriction that avoids protein malnutrition individualized to each patient should be employed although there is no evidence to suggest any impact on the progression of chronic CKD. The restriction of dietary protein to 0.6 to 0.8 g/kg/day in patients with GFR <50; and 0.3 to 0.5 g/kg/day in patients with GFR <20 who are not on dialysis is recommended. Caloric intake should be between 23 and 35 kcal/kg/day in patients with CKD. In patients with CKD Stages 3 to 5, sodium and potassium should be restricted to <2 g per day, phosphorus should be restricted to 800 to 1000 mg per day, and calcium to 2000 mg per day. Vitamin D should be replaced to maintain adequate serum levels.[1,2,16]

Mineral and Bone Disorders (Renal Osteodystrophy and Extraskeletal/ Vascular Calcification)

Phosphate retention occurs early in CKD and worsens as GFR decreases, which causes a fall in serum calcium levels. Hypocalcemia is exacerbated by decreased intestinal calcium absorption due to decrease renal synthesis of 1,25(OH)D. Hypocalcemia and hyperphosphatemia indirectly stimulate parathyroid hormone (PTH) release, which leads to bone disease, vascular calcification, cardiovascular disease, and increased mortality.

In patients with GFR less than 45 mL/min/1.73 m^2, testing should include serum calcium, phosphate, PTH, alkaline phosphatase, and vitamin D levels. Although fracture rates and fracture-related mortality are elevated in CKD, routine bone density testing is not recommended in patients with GFR less than 45 mL/min/1.73 m^2 as the information may be inaccurate and misleading. Monitoring phosphate levels, restricting phosphate intake, and using phosphate binders to maintain normal phosphorus levels will ameliorate some of the negative impact of PTH elevation and calcium lowering, and decrease the development of renal osteodystrophy and extracellular/vascular calcification. Vitamin D replacement is only recommended with documented deficiency, not solely to suppress PTH in non-dialysis patients. In vitamin D–deficient patients, replacement increases Bone Mineral Density (BMD) and muscle strength, reduces fracture risk and falls, and reduces PTH. Bisphosphonate therapy is recommended for treatment of osteoporosis and/or high fracture risk in CKD patients with GFR greater than 60 mL/min/1.73 m^2 and GFR 30 to 60 mL/min/1.73 m^2 with a normal PTH. Dose modification may be necessary.[1,2,5]

Hyperkalemia

When GFR falls below 20 mL per minute (i.e., Stages 4 and 5), hyperkalemia occurs because of diminished kidney potassium excretory capacity, especially with acute potassium loads. Potassium intake should be restricted as noted above. If hyperkalemia occurs, the source of excess potassium intake, decreased potassium excretion, or cellular extrusion of potassium should be eliminated. Further treatment of persistent and severe hyperkalemia is directed at antagonizing myocardial effects by using calcium gluconate, shifting potassium intracellularly with glucose and insulin or with sodium bicarbonate if metabolic acidosis is severe, removal of potassium-sparing diuretics, and use of ion-exchange resins, for example, sodium polystyrene sulfate and, in emergency settings, dialysis.[1,2,5]

Metabolic Acidosis and Sodium and Water Hemostasis

The acidosis, hypervolemia, and hyponatremia of CKD, which usually starts in Stage 4, require the use of sodium bicarbonate when pH is less than 7.3 and serum bicarbonate concentrate (HCO_3^-) is less than 22 mEq per L. Sodium chloride restriction should be implemented based on the clinical setting as noted above. Water restriction may be required in patients who develop hyponatremia when they consume free water at rates greater than the kidney water clearance rate.[1,2]

Hyperuricemia

Hyperuricemia (uric acid level greater than 7 mg per dL) is common in CKD patients, and there is a growing body of evidence to suggest an association with hyperuricemia in CKD and adverse cardiovascular outcomes. However, there is insufficient evidence to currently support or refute the use of uric acid–lowering agents in individuals with CKD and either symptomatic or asymptomatic hyperuricemia for the specific goal of delaying progression of CKD.[1,2]

Anemia

Anemia of CKD usually starts at Stage 3 and is due to declining erythropoietin production causing a decrease in red blood cell (RBC) production. Partial correction of the anemia of kidney disease improves the quality of life in predialysis and dialysis patients although there is no evidence it changes the progression of CKD.
• Evaluate for other causes with complete blood count, absolute reticulocyte count, serum ferritin, transferrin saturation, B$_{12}$, and folate. Search for source of blood loss.

- Oral or IV iron is recommended if serum ferritin <100 ng per mL and transferrin saturation <20%.
- Erythropoiesis-stimulating agents (ESAs) are recommended with Hgb <10 g per dl and when transfusion is anticipated due to rapid hemoglobin decline. Goal Hgb is between 9 and 11.5 g per dL with ESA treatment.
- Transfusion if iron and ESA are ineffective; risk if ESA outweighs benefit; acute hemorrhage; unstable CAD; rapid pre-op Hgb correction is required. No specific Hgb threshold is recommended. Treat if the patient is symptomatic.

Monitoring
- CKD with anemia not on ESA: every 3 months with CKD Stage 3 to 5 non-dialysis, or Stage 5 on peritoneal dialysis. Monthly for CKD Stage 5 on hemodialysis.
- CKD with anemia on ESA: monthly.[1,2,17,18]

Medication Management and Patient Safety

Prescribers should always take GFR into account when dosing medications for CKD patients. Consultation with a pharmacist is advantageous in this setting, and to provide counseling to patients regarding their prescribed and over-the-counter medications. Temporary discontinuation of potentially nephrotoxic and renally excreted drugs (including, but not limited to ACE-Is, ARBs, aldosterone inhibitors, direct renin inhibitors, diuretics, NSAIDs, metformin, lithium, and digoxin) is recommended in patients with GFR less than 60 mL/min/1.73 m^2 who have serious illness that increases the risk of AKI. Herbal agents should be avoided. Metformin should be discontinued once the GFR falls below 30 mL/min/1.73 m^2, but can be used with caution with GFR 30 to 44 mL/min/1.73 m^2. If the GFR is 45 mL/min/1.73 m^2 or higher, metformin should be continued. For all CKD patients on potentially nephrotoxic agents, GFR, electrolyte, and drug levels should be monitored regularly.[1,2]

Immunizations

All patients with CKD should receive a yearly influenza vaccine. Pneumococcal and hepatitis B vaccines are recommended in patients with a GFR less than 30 mL/min/1.73 m^2, and those at high risk. Immunologic response to hepatitis B should be confirmed with serologic testing. Consideration of live vaccines should include an appreciation of the patients' immune status and should follow CDC guidelines.[1,2]

Referrals

Patients with CKD should be referred to specialist for further evaluation in any of the following case.
- CKD Stages 4 and 5
- Unsure etiology
- Heavy proteinuria with ACR ≥70 mg per mmol unless it is due to diabetes or already treated
- Proteinuria with ACR ≥30 mg per mmol along with hematuria
- Active urine sediment
- Rapidly declining estimate of GFR (eGFR) (more than 5 mL/min/1.73 m^2 in 1 year or more than 10 mL/min/1.73 m^2 within 5 years).
- Patient with rare or genetic cause of disease.
- Resistant hypertension or suspected renal artery stenosis
- Difficult management issues: anemia, secondary hyperparathyroidism metabolic bone disease, and electrolyte disturbance.[1,2,14]

Kidney Replacement Therapy

Consultation with a kidney team should occur early in the predialysis period to promote transition of patients to kidney replacement therapy in a nonurgent setting. This early contact with the kidney team ensures that patients have an appropriate understanding of the types of kidney replacement therapies available to them. The kidney team can also affect the quality of life of the predialysis kidney patient by providing specific patient education and assessments concerning medical treatment of CKD as well as treatment of associated problems. Current kidney replacement therapies include hemodialysis, intermittent peritoneal dialysis, continuous ambulatory peritoneal dialysis, and kidney transplantation. The choice of kidney replacement therapy should be individualized based on the availability of a donor kidney, the patient's desire for independence, previous abdominal surgeries, underlying medical conditions, and patient's age. Initiation of dialysis (which usually occurs with GFR 5 to 10 mL/min/1.73 m^2) is indicated for one or more of the following: signs or symptoms due to kidney failure (uremia, serositis, acid–base or electrolyte abnormalities, pruritis); inability to control volume status or BP; progressive deterioration in nutritional status refractory to dietary interventions; or encephalopathy.[1,2]

REFERENCES

1. Kidney Disease: Improving Global Outcomes (KDIGO) CKD Work Group. KDIGO 2012 clinical practice guideline for the evaluation and management of chronic kidney disease. *Kidney Int Suppl* 2013;84(Suppl 3):1–150.
2. Inker LA, Astor BC, Fox CH, et al. KDOQI US commentary on the 2012 KDIGO clinical practice guideline for the evaluation and management of CKD. *Am J Kidney Dis* 2013;63(5):713–735.
3. Centers for Disease Control and Prevention (CDC). National Chronic Kidney Disease Fact Sheet: General Information and National Estimates on Chronic Kidney Disease in the United States, 2014. Atlanta, GA: US Department of Health and Human Services, Centers for Disease Control and Prevention. http://www.cdc.gov/diabetes/pubs/pdf/kidney_factsheet.pdf. Updated September 18, 2012. Accessed August 22, 2014.
4. Baumgarten M, Gehr T. Chronic kidney disease: detection and evaluation. *Am Fam Physician* 2011;84(10):1138–1148.
5. Rosenberg M. Overview of the Management of Chronic Kidney Disease in Adults. UpToDate. http://www.uptodate.com/contents/overview-of-the-management-of-chronic-kidney-disease-in-adults. Updated May 16, 2014. Accessed September 1, 2014.
6. Fatehi P, Hsu C. Diagnostic Approach to the Patient with Acute Kidney Injury (Acute Renal Failure) or Chronic Kidney Disease. UpToDate. http://www.uptodate.com/contents/diagnostic-approach-to-the-patient-with-acute-kidney-injury-acute-renal-failure-or-chronic-kidney-disease. Updated October 27, 2014. Accessed September 1, 2014.
7. Arora P. Chronic Kidney Disease. Medscape. http://emedicine.medscape.com/article/238798-overview. Updated September 9, 2014. Accessed September 15, 2014.
8. Uchida S. Differential Diagnosis of Chronic Kidney Disease (CKD): by primary diseases. *Japan Med Assn J* 2011;54(1):22–26.
9. National Kidney Foundation. KDOQI clinical practice guideline for diabetes and CKD: 2012 update. *Am J Kidney Dis* 2012;60(5):850–886.
10. James PA, Oparil S, Carter BL, et al. 2014 evidence-based guideline for the management of high blood pressure in adults: report from the panel members appointed to the Eighth Joint National Committee (JNC 8). *JAMA* 2014;311(5):507–520. doi:10.1001/jama.2013.284427.
11. KDIGO clinical practice guideline for the management of blood pressure in chronic kidney disease. *Kidney Int Suppl* 2012;2(5):337–414.
12. Taler SJ, Agarwal R, Bakris GL, et al. National Kidney Foundation KDOQI US commentary on the 2012 KDIGO clinical practice guideline for management of blood pressure in CKD. *Am J Kidney Dis* 2013;62(2):201–213. © 2013 by the National Kidney Foundation, Inc.
13. National Kidney Foundation. KDOQI clinical practice guideline for diabetes and CKD: 2012 update. *Am J Kidney Dis* 2012;60(5):850–886.
14. Standards of medical care in diabetes. VI. Prevention and management of diabetes complications. *Diabetes Care* 2013;36(Suppl 1):S28–S39.
15. KDIGO clinical practice guideline for lipid management in chronic kidney disease. *Kidney Int Suppl* 2013;3(3):259–305.
16. American Dietetic Association. Chronic kidney disease evidence-based nutrition practice guideline. Chicago (IL): American Dietetic Association; 2010 Jun. Accessed at http://www.guideline.gov/content. aspx?id=23924 on October 27, 2014.
17. U.S. Food and Drug Administration. FDA drug safety communication: modified dosing recommendations to improve the safe use of erythropoiesis-stimulating agents (ESAs) in chronic kidney disease. http://www.fda.gov/Drugs/DrugSafety/ucm259639.htm. Accessed September 1, 2011.
18. Kidney Disease: Improving Global Outcomes (KDIGO) Anemia Work Group. KDIGO clinical practice guideline for anemia in chronic kidney disease. *Kidney Int Suppl* 2012;2(4):279–335.

Urolithiasis

Nathan J. Timmer

GENERAL PRINCIPLES

- **Definition.** Urolithiasis refers to calculi (stones) in any part of the urinary tract.[1,2] Kidney stones, nephrolithiasis, or renal calculi are terms commonly used in place of urolithiasis.
- **Anatomy.** At the time of diagnosis, stones may be found in any part of the urinary tract, from the minor calyces in the kidney to the urethra.[2]
- **Classification.** Stones may be of any composition from calcium (calcium oxalate, the most common, and calcium phosphate), uric acid, struvite (magnesium ammonium phosphate), or cystine. It is possible one patient may produce more than one type or combination of stone.[3]
- **Epidemiology.** Kidney stones are relatively common, affecting approximately 1% of the population, with men being affected 2:1 over women.[1,2] Most renal calculi are found in the third through the fifth decade of life.[2] For patients affected, reoccurrence rates approach 50%.[1] Stones composed of calcium make up nearly 80% of all stones.[3] Calcium stones are more common in men than in women. Struvite stones, which represent 10% to 15% of all urinary calculi, are more common in women, as they are often the result of urinary tract infections (UTIs) from urease-producing bacteria.[1,2] Uric acid stones represent 5% to 8% of all urinary calculi and are more common in men as well; this may be because gout is more common in men and half of all patients with uric acid stones have gout.[1,2] Cystine stones are rare, representing 1% of all calculi, and occur in men and women with equal prevalence.[2] All stones are radiopaque except uric acid stones, which are radiolucent.[2]
- **Pathophysiology.** Kidney stones are thought to form secondary to any process that alters the kidney's delicate balance of prolithogenic factors and factors inhibiting the formation of stones, thus allowing a stone to precipitate out of solution in the urine. Stone-forming factors include the following: increased dietary oxalate, decreased fluid intake, increased dietary protein (specifically from animals), increased dietary sodium, and high-dose vitamin C.[1] In addition to these easily modifiable risk factors, there are other difficult-to-modify risk factors such as hypercalciuria, hyperoxaluria, primary hyperparathyroidism, hypocitraturia, and hyperuricosuria.[1,3] Major risk factors to developing a calcium oxalate stone in addition to the preceding include prior history of a stone and family history of stones. Uric acid stones are thought to arise from saturation of urate crystals in the urine. Fifty percent of people with uric acid stones also have gout.[2] Struvite stones are thought to form as the result of urease-producing bacteria, especially the *Proteus* species. These stones can become quite large and have the potential to become staghorn calculi, that is, calculi that fill and obstruct the entire renal pelvis.
- **Mechanism of injury.** Stones in the renal pelvis can be an incidental finding in asymptomatic patients.[4] Stones become painful when they become lodged in the urinary tract and the body attempts to move them along. Contraction of the ureter against the stone produces a severe, colicky pain. Often, there is some bleeding associated with this, found as gross or microscopic hematuria.

DIAGNOSIS

- **Clinical presentation.** Stones present with acute onset of severe colicky pain. The pain is often unilateral and its location depends on the location of the stone in the urinary tract. The pain is often referred to the cutaneous areas T11–L2 that supply the ureter and is variably described as flank pain that commonly radiates to the testicle or labia on the ipsilateral side.[3,5] The pain moves as the stone moves, and a person with previous stones may be able to tell if the stone is about to pass. Patients often find it difficult to find a comfortable position and may readjust frequently, trying to find stated position. Hematuria is present in up to 90% of stones, but its absence does not rule out a stone.[3] Nausea and vomiting often accompany the pain. If the stone is located in the distal ureter, dysuria, frequency, and urgency may also be present.[2]
- **Physical examination.** Patients have a lack of physical examination findings other than the pain. Tachycardia, diaphoresis, and hypertension as a result of the pain may be present. Fever is absent unless a concurrent urinary tract infection is also present. Flank pain is present, but not made worse by costovertebral angle percussion.

- **Differential diagnosis.** An acute onset of flank or abdominal pain has a broad differential diagnosis, including multiple organ systems. Renal cell carcinoma may bleed and clot off a ureter, thus producing renal colic.[3] Other illnesses that may present with vague abdominal pain but are not classically colicky in nature, such as acute appendicitis, diverticulitis, or abdominal aneurysm. Other colicky types of pain include biliary colic or an ectopic pregnancy. Last, renal colic may be faked by patients for secondary gain in those seeking narcotics.[3]
- **Laboratory studies.** Urinalysis looking for blood and the presence of infection are routinely obtained. No other abnormalities should be expected in a case of simple, first-time episode of nephrolithiasis in the acute setting. However, a metabolic panel is commonly obtained to check renal function and electrolytes like calcium.[2]
- **Imaging.** The current gold standard for diagnosis of a kidney stone is helical computed tomography (CT) scan without contrast. The specificity of a helical CT with 3- to 5-mm cuts is 98% and sensitivity 95% in one study, and specificity is consistently close to 100% in various studies.[3] CT imaging also allows the physician to see any obstruction caused by the stone and will aid in the differential diagnosis of the pain if a stone is not present. Kidney–ureter–bladder (KUB) radiography will not demonstrate radiolucent stones, such as uric acid stones.[3] Intravenous pyelogram (IVP) is the next best choice; however, it is neither as sensitive nor as specific, and it is often a slower test. Ultrasound may also be used to detect urinary tract obstruction and radiolucent stones. Ultrasound can be used safely during pregnancy. The combination of ultrasound with KUB may provide comparable results to CT alone.[3]
- **Monitoring.** It should be noted that the time for passage of each stone is variable and there is no set time limit.[4] Stones may pass in a little as a few hours, or it may take weeks. In a patient with a distal stone less than 5 mm with pain well controlled, the physician may well continue to observe for a month or more.
- **Pathologic findings.** After a stone has been diagnosed, patients should be asked to strain their urine for collection of the stone.[4] The stone should then be sent for stone analysis. The type of stone will guide treatment and strategies for prevention of reoccurrence.

TREATMENT

- **Medications.** Narcotics are often required to control the pain in the acute setting. Nonsteroidal anti-inflammatory drugs (NSAIDs) are also effective. Both indomethacin and ketorolac have been used in the acute setting alone and in combination with narcotics. Anti-emetics and IV fluids are also frequently used. If a stone is expected to pass, the patient may be sent home with either opiate and/or NSAIDs for pain control. To aid in the passage of the stone, α-blockers and calcium-channel blockers are thought to help decrease tone throughout the urinary tract and allow stones to pass more easily.[3,5] Meta-analysis shows that α-blockers are superior to calcium-channel blockers and are the preferred agents.[6] If infection or obstruction is present, an antibiotic like a fluoroquinolone should be started.
- **Surgery.** Urology consult is warranted if there is acute kidney injury, obstruction, urosepsis, stones larger than 5 mm, a patient fails outpatient therapy, or if the pain is uncontrollable.[3] Size is the single best predictor if a stone will pass, and a stone of 4 mm or less will most likely pass on its own.[3] In one study, stones 5 to 7 mm have a passage rate of 60%.[3]
- **Nonoperative.** Nonoperative treatments include shock wave lithotripsy and active surveillance.[2,4]
- **Operative.** Surgical treatment modalities include ureteroscopic lithotripsy, laparoscopy, and percutaneous nephrolithotomy.[4] Ureter stents may also be placed to facilitate stone passage.
- **Counseling.** Prevention of reoccurrence is based largely on the type of stone.[1] For nearly all stone types, increased daily water intake of approximately 2 to 3 L is the single best recommendation to prevent recurrence. Patients may also be counseled to modify their diet based on the type of stone found. Medications may be suggested to patients based on their metabolic profile and the type of stone, as discussed below.
- **Follow-up.** For patients with recurrent stones, a 24-hour urine should be collected preferably 1 to 2 months after acute even and tested for urine volume and pH, and excretion of calcium, uric acid, citrate, oxalate, creatinine, and sodium.[4] Serum calcium and parathyroid hormone are also helpful. Thiazide diuretic may reduce the amount of calcium present in the urine. Hypocitraturia may be treated with potassium citrate.[2,7] Hyperuricosuria may benefit from a low-purine diet and prevent the occurrence of calcium oxalate stones.[2] For patients with uric acid stones, allopurinol should be given.[2] For patients with struvite stones, antimicrobial therapy and surveillance may be beneficial.

SPECIAL CONSIDERATIONS

- **Pregnancy.** Kidney stones can occur during pregnancy. If the pregnancy is early on, an ectopic pregnancy must be ruled out. During pregnancy, there is an increase in calcium excretion in the urine relative to urine volume, so a simple increase in glomerular filtration rate cannot account for the increase.[8] Despite this, nephrolithiasis is a rare event. When reviewing imaging studies, it must be kept in mind that the normal pregnant patient will have a dilation of the ureters secondary to progesterone-mediated smooth muscle relaxation. Stones will often pass secondary to this relative dilation.[8] Opiates can be used for pain during pregnancy while NSAIDs are not recommended.
- **Children.** Management of stones in children is very similar to adults. Narcotics, NSAIDs, α-blockers, anti-emetics, and IV fluids are all used in children. Guidelines for stone passage and referral to urologist are also similar. Radiation exposure should be considered when ordering imaging. There has been some evidence of kidney stones in children treated long term with ceftriaxone.[3]

ACKNOWLEDGMENT

The author would like to acknowledge Michael A. Green for his work on the previous version of this chapter.

REFERENCES

1. Mount DB, Loscalzo J. Nephrolithiasis. In Dan L, Anthony F, Dennis K, Stephen H, Jameson J, Joseph L *Harrison's principles of internal medicine.* 18th ed. New York, NY: McGraw-Hill; 2013:998–1000.
2. Wesson J. Nephrolithiasis. In: Dario MT. *Kochar's Clinical Medicine for Students.* 5th ed. Philadelphia, PA: Wolters Kluwer/Lippincott Williams & Wilkins; 2009:535–538.
3. Curhan GC, Aronson MD, Preminger GM. Diagnosis and Acute Management of Suspected Nephrolithiasis in Adults. UpToDate. http://www.uptodate.com/contents/diagnosis-and-acute-management-of-suspected-nephrolithiasis-in-adults? Updated June 1, 2013. Accessed January 2, 2014.
4. Preminger GM, Curhan GC. The First Kidney Stone and Asymptomatic Nephrolithiasis in Adults. UpToDate. http://www.uptodate.com/contents/the-first-kidney-stone-and-asymptomatic-nephrolithiasis-in-adults? Updated 19 June 2013. Accessed January 2, 2014.
5. Lendvay TS, Smith J, Stapleton FB. Acute Management of Nephrolithiasis in Children. UpToDate. http://www.uptodate.com/contents/acute-management-of-nephrolithiasis-in-children? Updated June 18, 2013. Accessed January 2, 2014.
6. Preminger GM, Tiselius HG, Assimos DG, et al; EAU/AUA Nephrolithiasis Guideline Panel. 2007 guideline for the management of ureteral calculi. *J Urol* 2007;178:2418–2434.
7. Curhan GC. Prevention of Recurrent Calcium Stones. www.uptodate.com. Accessed January 2, 2014.
8. Rose B. Nephrolithiasis During Pregnancy. www.uptodate.com. Accessed January 2, 2014.

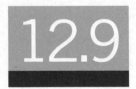

12.9 Urinary Incontinence

Robert Daro

BACKGROUND

Urinary incontinence (UI), an involuntary, unintended leakage of urine, is a common condition with prevalence reported at 16.2% to 81.9% affecting 20 million adults in the United States, with prevalence increasing with age. Although not a lethal condition, it is associated with great medical costs, increased risk of skin breakdown, falls, low self-esteem, social isolation, and depression. The average cost per individual in the United States with Stress UI is $5,624 per treatment.[1–5]

GENERAL PRINCIPLES

The cause of UI can typically be determined by the primary care provider through a thorough history and targeted physical examination. Diagnostic studies may be indicated for more complicated cases of UI, but imaging is not routinely recommended in the initial therapy. The detailed history, alone, is often telling enough to formulate a plan of care. However, the physician must remember to ask about this common condition as embarrassment associated with UI may interfere with patients volunteering this information.[4–6] Postvoid residuals (PVRs) are generally not useful in an initial evaluation. Specific factors including urinary retention, recent pelvic surgery, and neurologic disease warrant PVR testing. In addition, because of cost and difficulty of testing, urodynamic testing is not recommended for initial testing. Other imaging is generally not indicated. In addition to a UI for all cases, laboratory testing is not necessary unless a specific pathology is thought to be contributing.[7]

CLASSIFICATIONS

The classification of UI is based on the associated pathophysiologic abnormality, and patients may have features of any mixture of these types.

- **Transient UI** has abrupt onset and resolves when the underlying condition is treated. The causes of transient UI can be remembered by the mnemonic DIAPERS (delirium, infection, atrophic urethritis, pharmaceutical, excessive urinary output, restricted mobility, and stool impaction).[4]
- **Chronic UI** can be divided into four types: stress UI, urge UI, overflow UI, and functional UI.
  - **Stress UI** occurs when pressure within the bladder exceeds bladder sphincter pressures. These commonly occur during times of increased intra-abdominal pressure such as with sneezing, coughing, or changing sitting/standing positions.[8] Patients will describe loss of small volumes of urine and PVR volumes are usually normal (<50 mL). Stress UI is the most common type and affects approximately 35% of those with UI. This common urinary complaint is essentially a sphincter disorder caused by pelvic floor muscular relaxation or sphincter/bladder outlet incompetence from prior instrumentation (i.e., obstetrical repair) or prostate surgery.[4] The history alone is usually diagnostic and sufficient. A bladder stress test and PVR can confirm the diagnosis.[7]
    - **Behavioral therapy:** Along with weight loss, the initial treatment strategy for men and women with stress UI is the pelvic floor strengthening, or "Kegel" exercises. These exercises can produce positive results in up to 38% of stress UI. There are a number of exercise regimens and in general comprehensive, clinic based and longer training produces better results.[2,3]
    - **Pharmacologic therapy:** There are no FDA-approved medications for stress UI.[2] Although topical estrogen is widely used to increase urethral thickness and sensitive α-adrenergic receptors in the urethral sphincter, a meta-analysis of studies of estrogen effect on stress UI found no improvement in urine loss. This lack of evidence on efficacy and concerns about estrogen supplementation posed by the Women's Health Initiative make estrogen a poor choice for the treatment of stress UI.[9] Pseudoephedrine, phenylephrine, and duloxetine all have limited evidence and adverse effects in the treatment of stress UI.[2,8]
    - **Other modalities:** Stimulation of the pelvic floor with noninvasive electrical and magnetic stimulation along with a myriad of minimally invasive procedures has been met with varying success. Pessaries have few contraindications and remain a viable option for treatment.[2]
    - **Surgical options:** After conservative therapy has failed, surgical therapy including slings and urethroplexy as directed by a urogynecologist are further options for treatment of stress UI.[2,3]
  - **Urge incontinence** is the leakage of often large amounts of urine and the inability to delay voiding after the sensation of bladder fullness is detected. Like stress UI, urge UI typically involves normal PVR volumes. This type of UI is often associated with neurologic disorders, such as dementia or cerebrovascular disease. Most patients with UI, however, do not have a neurologic disease, and this type is the most common form of UI experienced by older adults. This disorder is due to detrusor hyperactivity.[4,8]
    - **Behavioral therapy:** Scheduled toileting at increasing intervals can aid in increasing compliance in the bladder over time. Bladder training with learning to control detrusor urge by learning to sit still and allow the bladder contraction to pass, typically less than 60 seconds, and only then move to the restroom to void along with Kegel exercises all remain first-line therapy.[2]
    - **Pharmacologic therapy:** Best used with behavioral therapy, medications focus on decreasing detrusor over activity. A number of anticholinergic drugs are available. Pharmacologic therapy is limited by anticholinergic side effects, such as dry mouth, delirium, and constipation. Mirabegron is a β-adrenergic agonist not to be used with uncontrolled hypertension. Botox to the detrusor can relieve symptoms for up to 6 months.[2,8,10]
    - **Electrical therapy:** Office based-tibial nerve stimulators have good results in three quarters of patients. Surgically implanted devices, most commonly a sacral nerve stimulator inserted into the tissue of the lower back or buttocks may improve UI by stimulating the S3 sacral nerve and decrease detrusor muscle contractility.[2]

- **Overflow UI** is the frequent or continuous leakage from mechanical forces over a distended/full bladder or from other effects of urinary retention on bladder or sphincter function. PVRs are usually high (>100 mL). This type of UI is often a consequence of bladder outlet obstruction from prostatic enlargement. Another cause of overflow UI is bladder hypoactivity, referred to as "neurogenic bladder." This is most commonly encountered in patients with spinal cord injury, longstanding diabetes mellitus, or vitamin B_{12} deficiency. Anticholinergic medications may induce a hypoactive bladder and medication review is crucial. Therapy is directed by the etiology.[4,5]
  - **Bladder outlet obstruction:** The target of medicinal therapy is relaxation of the internal urethral sphincter with α-adrenergic-blocking agents and bladder decompression as described below. Available α-blockers include terazosin (Hytrin), doxazosin (Cardura), and tamsulosin (Flomax). Orthostatic hypotension is the typical limiting side effect of the α-blockers and may be less problematic with the more selective tamsulosin than the other agents. Transurethral resection of the prostate may be warranted for patients who do not respond well to pharmacologic treatment or who are limited by orthostasis.[5,8]
  - **Medication side effect:** Removal of the offending agent and decompression with an indwelling Foley catheter for 7 to 14 days may allow the bladder to resume some contractile activity.
  - **Neurogenic bladder:** This type of overflow UI responds poorly to pharmacologic therapies. Patients may successfully manage their voids by being taught to do intermittent straight catheterization several times a day or placement of a chronic indwelling catheter may be considered.[5]
- **Functional UI** occurs in patients with normal bladder function from some extrinsic cause. Detrusor and sphincter function are intact, but the patient is either unable to recognize the urge to void or physically unable to get to the toilet on time. Debility, dementia, delirium, and cerebrovascular disease are common causes of functional UI.[4]
  - There is no available pharmacotherapy for functional UI. Treatment focuses on scheduled toileting and the use of incontinence supplies. Chronic indwelling catheterization is not suggested but may be warranted when perineal or sacral wounds are present.[4]

REFERRAL

In addition to the above indications, referral should be considered with uncertain diagnosis, suspected cancer, neurologic disease, pelvic pain or mass, hematuria, previous surgery, and cases that do not respond to initial therapy.[7]

ACKNOWLEDGMENT

This author would like to thank Mary McDonald and Sarah Parrott, the authors of the previous version of this chapter, for their contributions.

REFERENCES

1. Sensoy N, Dogan N, Ozek B, et al. Urinary incontinence in women: prevalence rates and impact on quality of life. *Pak J Med Sci* 2013;29(3):818–822.
2. Hersh L, Salzman B. Clinical management of urinary incontinence in women. *Am Fam Physician* 2013;87(9):634–640.
3. Carpenter D, Visovsky C. Stress urinary incontinence: a review of treatment options. *AORN J* 2010;91(4):471–478.
4. Weiss BD. Diagnostic evaluation of urinary incontinence in geriatric patients. *Am Fam Physician* 1998;57(11):2675–2684.
5. Moore KN, Gray M. Urinary incontinence in men: current status and future directions. *Nurs Res* 2004;53(6):S36–S41.
6. Artibani W, Cerruto M. The role of imaging in urinary incontinence. *BJU Int* 2005;95:699–703.
7. DuBeau CE. Approach to women with urinary incontinence. In: Falk S, ed. *UpToDate*. 2013. http://www.uptodate.com. Accessed March 12, 2014.
8. Moreland RB, Brioni JD, Sullivan JP. Emerging pharmacologic approaches for the treatment of lower urinary tract disorders. *J Pharmacol Exp Ther* 2004;308(3):797–804.
9. Rossouw JE, Anderson GL, Prentice RL, et al. Risks and benefits of estrogen plus progestin in healthy postmenopausal women: principal results from the Women's Health Initiative Randomized Controlled Trial. *JAMA* 2002;288:321–333.
10. Jayarajan J, Radomski S. Pharmacotherapy of overactive bladder in adults: a review of efficacy, tolerability, and quality of life. *Res Rep Urol* 2014;6:1–16.

12.10 Acute Kidney Injury

Dustin C. Carpenter, Shri Lalitha Rayavarapu

GENERAL PRINCIPLES

The term acute renal failure has now been replaced by acute kidney injury (AKI) to highlight the fact that even small decreases in renal function that do not result in significant organ damage are associated with increased morbidity and mortality.[1–5]

Definition

AKI is a sudden loss of kidney function resulting in increase in serum creatinine or decrease in urine output, leading to accumulation of waste products (usually <48 hours). The Kidney Disease/Improving Global Outcomes (KDIGO) AKI Workgroup defined the following criteria:

- Increase in SCr by ≥0.3 mg per dL (≥26.5 μmol per L) within 48 hours; or
- Increase in SCr to ≥1.5 times baseline, which is known or presumed to have occurred within the prior 7 days; or
- Urine volume <0.5 mL/kg/h for 6 hours.[5]

Epidemiology

There are limited data on overall epidemiology of AKI due to underreporting, regional disparities, and inconsistency of definition. Prevalence of AKI is on the rise worldwide. In the United States, prevalence ranges from 1% in the community up to approximately 7% of all hospital admissions. Five percent to 20% of critically ill patients experience an episode of AKI during the course of their illness, 4% to 9% of which require renal replacement therapy (RRT). Age plays a significant role in the epidemiology of AKI around the world. Although it is mostly seen in the elderly population in developed countries, younger adults and children are more affected in developing countries.[3,6–8]

Classification

See Table 12.10-1.

DIAGNOSIS

History

Obtaining a comprehensive history based on risk factors, noted in Table 12.10-2, is essential in the clinical assessment of the patient. Particular attention should be paid to assessing volume status, exposure to nephrotoxic substances, systemic illness, and underlying chronic conditions that could put the patient at risk for AKI. The clinical presentation varies with etiology and severity of renal injury, as well as any associated diseases. Patients with mild to moderate AKI are usually asymptomatic and

TABLE 12.10-1	Staging of Acute Kidney Injury	
Stage	**Serum creatinine**	**Urine output**
1	1.5–1.9 times baseline OR ≥ 0.3 mg/dL (≥26.5 μmol/L) increase	< 0.5 mL/kg/h for 6–12 h
2	2.0–2.9 times baseline	<0.5 mL/kg/h for ≥12 h
3	3.0 times baseline OR Increase in serum creat to ≥4.0 mg/dL (≥353.6 μmol/L) OR Requires renal replacement therapy OR Decrease in eGFR to <35 mL/min/1.73 m^2 in pts <18 yrs	0.3 mL/kg/h for ≥24 h OR anuria for ≥12 h

Creat, creatinine; eGFR, estimated glomerular filtration rate.

Adapted from International Society of Nephrology. KDIGO Clinical Practice Guideline for Acute Kidney Injury. *Kidney Int Suppl – J Int Soc Nephrol* 2012;2:89–115.

TABLE 12.10-2	Exposures and Susceptibilities for Nonspecific AKI
Exposures	**Susceptibles**
Sepsis	Dehydration or volume depletion
Critical illness	Advanced age
Circulatory shock	Female gender
Burns	Black race
Trauma	Chronic kidney disease
Cardiac surgery (especially cardiopulmonary bypass)	Chronic diseases (heart, lung, liver)
Major noncardiac surgery	Diabetes
Nephrotoxic drugs	Cancer
Radiocontrast agents	Anemia
Poisonous plants and animals	Human immunodeficiency virus

Adapted from International Society of Nephrology. KDIGO Clinical Practice Guideline for Acute Kidney Injury. *Kidney Int Suppl – J Int Soc Nephrol* 2012;2:89–115.

are incidentally found on routine laboratory testing. Patients with severe cases may be symptomatic and present with listlessness, confusion, fatigue, anorexia, nausea, vomiting, weight gain, or edema. Patients may present with oliguria (urine output less than 400 mL per day), anuria (urine output less than 100 mL per day), or normal volumes of urine (nonoliguric AKI). Anuria suggests AKI due to one of the three causes: urinary tract obstruction, a severe type of acute tubular necrosis (ATN) called cortical necrosis, or blood vessel blockage by clot or other obstruction.

Assessment of **prerenal AKI** should include awareness of any recent volume loss (e.g., history of vomiting, diarrhea, diuretic overuse, hemorrhages, or burns), or any underlying cardiac or liver disease.

In **intrinsic renal AKI**, certain findings may suggest the cause and portion of the kidney affected. Patients currently taking any nephrotoxic medications (over the counter, illicit, or herbal) may suggest ATN. History of hypotension, trauma, or myalgia can suggest rhabdomyolysis, also pointing to ATN, as well as recent radiographic studies that required contrast agents. A history of systemic diseases as mentioned in Table 12.10-3, may suggest a glomerular component. Indications of interstitial causes include medication use, rashes, arthralgia, fevers, and infectious illness. Nephrotic syndrome, trauma, flank pain, anticoagulation, vessel catheterization, or vascular surgery in the history should lead one to consider a vascular cause.

Postrenal findings include urinary urgency or hesitancy or polyuria. Any history of gross hematuria, history of stones, any cancers of urinary and reproductive systems, and any previous urological or gynecologic surgeries may suggest a postrenal cause of AKI.[2,9–11]

Physical Examination

For physical findings, see Table 12.10-3.

Laboratory and Imaging

Initial laboratory evaluation should include serum electrolytes, blood urea nitrogen (BUN) and creatinine level, fractional excretion of sodium (FE_{Na}), urinalysis, and complete blood count. If the patient is on a Na-wasting diuretic, a fractional excretion of urea (FE_{Urea}) should be ordered instead. Other laboratory indices helpful in a selected group of patients include BUN/serum creatinine ratio, rate of rise in serum creatinine concentration, urine osmolality, and urine volume.

Increased levels of BUN and creatinine are hallmarks of renal failure. Serum creatinine levels should be compared to previous values to determine duration and acuity of disease. AKI by definition is a rise in creatinine within 48 hours. In the outpatient setting, however, it may be difficult to be certain when the rise occurred. High serum creatinine level in a patient with previously normal levels suggests an acute process, whereas a rise over weeks to months represents subacute or chronic. As a general rule, if serum creatinine increases more than 1.5 mg/dL/day, rhabdomyolysis must be ruled out. Creatinine elevation is a late marker for renal dysfunction. Once creatinine is elevated, severe reduction in glomerular filtration rate has already occurred.

A ratio of BUN to creatinine can exceed 20:1 in conditions that favor enhanced reabsorption of urea, such as volume contraction (prerenal AKI). BUN can also be elevated with gastrointestinal and mucosal bleeding, steroid treatment, or protein loading.

TABLE 12.10-3	Physical Examination Findings and Common Associated Diseases	

System	Examination findings	Common disease complications
Skin	Livedo reticularis, digital ischemia, butterfly rash, palpable purpura	Systemic vasculitis
	Maculopapular rash	Allergic interstitial nephritis
	Track marks (IV drug abuse)	Endocarditis
Eyes	Keratitis, iritis, uveitis, dry conjunctivae	Autoimmune vasculitis
	Jaundice	Liver disease
	Band keratopathy	Multiple myeloma
	Signs of diabetes mellitus	Retinopathy
	Signs of hypertension	
	Atheroemboli	
Cardiovascular system	Irregular rhythms (atrial fibrillation)	Thromboemboli
	Murmurs	Endocarditis
	Pericardial friction rub	Uremic pericarditis
	Increased jugulovenous distention, rales, S_3 heart sound	Heart failure
Abdominal	Pulsatile mass or bruit	Atheroemboli
	Abdominal or costovertebral angle tenderness	Nephrolithiasis, papillary necrosis, renal artery thrombosis, renal vein thrombosis
	Pelvic, rectal masses; prostatic hypertrophy; distended bladder	Urinary obstruction
	Limb ischemia, edema	Rhabdomyolysis
Pulmonary	Rales	Goodpasture syndrome, Wegener granulomatosis
	Hemoptysis	Wegener granulomatosis

Modified from Workeneh BT, Agraharkar M, Gupta R. Acute Kidney Injury. Medscape. http://emedicine.medscape.com/article/243492-overview. Accessed November 25, 2013.

The measurement of FE_{Na} is helpful in distinguishing prerenal from intrinsic causes of AKI, especially in the setting of oliguria. A value of less than 1% indicates a prerenal cause of AKI. A value greater than 2% indicates an intrinsic renal cause. For patients currently on diuretic therapy, FE_{Na} is less reliable in prerenal states due to natriuresis caused by the diuretic. For these patients, fractional excretion of urea (FE_{Urea}) may help, with values less than 35% indicating a prerenal cause.

$$FE_{NA} = 100 \times \frac{(\text{urinary sodium} \times \text{serum creatinine})}{(\text{serum sodium} \times \text{urinary creatinine})}$$

$$FE_{Urea} = 100 \times \frac{(\text{urinary urea} \times \text{serum creatinine})}{(\text{serum urea} \times \text{urinary creatinine})}$$

A urinalysis with microscopy is an important noninvasive test in the initial workup. It can guide the differential diagnosis and direct further workup, especially in intrinsic renal disease. Renal tubular cells or casts, or pigmented casts suggest ATN. Eosinophils and white blood cell casts suggest allergic interstitial nephritis. Red blood cell casts and proteinuria greater than 3 g suggest multiple myeloma, glomerulonephritis, or vasculitis. Orthotolidine positive without red blood cells suggests myoglobinuria or hemoglobinuria.

Blood work including complete blood count (CBC) and serologic tests can help with the diagnosis of AKI. The presence of acute hemolytic anemia on CBC with differential and smear showing schistocytes suggests the possibility of hemolytic uremic syndrome (HUS) or thrombotic thrombocytopenic purpura (TTP). Serologic tests can be very informative, but cost prohibitive if not regularly ordered.

Such tests include complement levels, antinuclear antibody (ANA), antineutrophil cytoplasmic antibody (ANCA), anti-glomerular basement membrane (anti-GBM) antibody, hepatitis B and C viral studies, and antistreptolysin (ASO).

New biomarkers are being developed to help diagnose patients with AKI sooner and to identify those at risk. The most promising to date is urinary neutrophil gelatinase-associated lipocalin (NGAL), which has been shown to detect AKI in patients undergoing cardiopulmonary bypass. Plasma B-type natriuretic (BNP) and NGAL have been shown to be strong predictors of early AKI patients with lower respiratory tract infections. A BNP over 267 pg per mL or NGAL greater than 231 ng per mL has identified AKI in patients in some studies, with sensitivity of 94% and specificity of 61%.

Renal ultrasonography should be performed in most patients with AKI, especially in older men, to rule out obstruction. Presence of postvoid residual urine greater than 100 mL by bladder scan or urethral catheterization suggests postrenal AKI and requires renal ultrasonography to detect hydronephrosis or outlet obstruction. Small kidneys seen on images can suggest chronic renal failure. To diagnose extrarenal causes of AKI, computed tomography or magnetic resonance imaging may be required. Kidneys are typically of normal size on ultrasound with renal parenchymal disease.

Aortorenal angiography can identify renal vascular diseases such as renal artery stenosis, renal atheroembolic disease, atherosclerosis with occlusion, and necrotizing vasculitis.

Renal biopsy may be necessary for patients whose prerenal and postrenal causes have been excluded and the cause of intrinsic damage is unclear. It is particularly important when clinical assessment and laboratory findings suggest a diagnosis that requires confirmation prior to initiating therapy. Biopsy may need to be performed urgently in patients with oliguria with rapidly worsening AKI, hematuria, and RBC casts.[2,9-11]

Differential Diagnosis

See Table 12.10-4.

TREATMENT
Medications

After a diagnosis of AKI has been established, management is primarily supportive in nature and consists of adequate renal perfusion by achieving and maintaining hemodynamic stability and avoiding hypovolemia. Any nephrotoxic agents should be stopped, or renally dosed if stopping is not indicated. Correcting electrolyte imbalances in AKI is important. The primary electrolyte imbalances include hyperkalemia, hyperphosphatemia, hypermagnesemia, hyponatremia, hypernatremia, and metabolic acidosis. Contrast media should be avoided, so if images are required, noncontrast studies are recommended. Supportive therapies should be pursued on the basis of standard management practices.

If fluid resuscitation is required, isotonic solutions (normal saline) are preferred over hyperoncotic solutions (dextran, hydroxyethyl starch, and albumin). Reasonable goal is a mean arterial pressure greater than 65 mmHg, which may require the use of vasopressors in patients with persistent hypotension. Cardiac function can be optimized as needed with positive inotropes, or afterload and preload reduction.

Vasodilators do not have complete defined role in AKI. Dopamine has been used in the past because of its selective dilation of renal vasculature at small doses. Dopamine also reduces sodium absorption; this enhances urine flow, which may prevent tubular cast obstruction. Studies have failed to establish this beneficial role, and one study demonstrated that low-dose dopamine may worsen renal perfusion in patients with AKI. Therefore, it is no longer recommended for this purpose. The vasodilator fenoldopam may reduce the need for RRT and lowers mortality rate in patients with AKI, but larger trials are still needed before its use can be recommended.

Loop diuretics seem to have no effect on outcome of established AKI, but are recommended for treatment of volume overload in patients that can maintain urine output. Often high intravenous doses are required for greater diuretic effect. IV infusions are helpful in the ICU setting and promote a sustained natriuresis with reduced ototoxicity compared with conventional bolus dosing. Furosemide plays no role in converting an oliguric AKI to a nonoliguric AKI or in increasing urine output when the patient is not hypervolemic. However, response to furosemide can be a good prognostic sign.

Indications for emergent initiation of RRT (dialysis) in the setting of AKI include life-threatening changes in fluid, electrolyte, and acid–base balance that are refractory to medical management; uremic pericarditis or pleuritis; uremic encephalopathy; and certain poisonings and intoxications. There is no difference between the use of intermittent hemodialysis and continuous renal replacement therapy (CRRT). CRRT may have a role in patients who are hemodynamically unstable, and have prolonged renal failure after a stroke or liver failure. Peritoneal dialysis is not frequently used in AKI patients. It can be used in acute cases and can be better tolerated hemodynamically than conventional hemodialysis.[1,5,9-11]

TABLE 12.10-4 Causes of Acute Kidney Injury

Prerenal	Intrinsic	Postrenal
Hypovolemia (extrarenal loss) • Vomiting and diarrhea • Hemorrhage • Burns • Stevens–Johnson syndrome • Sweating • Pancreatitis (renal loss) • Diuretic overuse • Osmotic diuresis (DKA)	**Glomerular** • Glomerulonephritis (postinfectious or other) • Goodpasture syndrome • Wegner granulomatosis • Churg–Strauss syndrome • Cryoglobulinemia • Lupus	**Intrarenal obstruction** • Renal calculi • Clot • Tumor **Extrarenal obstruction** • Prostatic hypertrophy • Retroperitoneal fibrosis • Urethral stricture • Bladder, cervical, prostate or other pelvic/retroperitoneal mass • Obstructed Foley catheter • Neurogenic bladder
Systemic vasodilation • Sepsis • Anaphylaxis • Anesthetics • Drug overdose	**Tubular** • Ischemic (prolonged hypotension) • Exogenous nephrotoxins (radiocontrast agents, aminoglycosides, cisplatin, methotrexate, ethylene glycol, amphotericin B, acyclovir, indinavir) • Endogenous nephrotoxins (hemolysis, rhabdomyolysis, tumor lysis syndrome, myeloma)	
Intrarenal vasoconstriction • Drugs (NSAID, ACE-I, ARB, norepinephrine, cyclosporine, tacrolimus, radiocontrast agents) • Cardiorenal syndrome • Hepatorenal syndrome • Abdominal compartment syndrome • Hypercalcemia	**Interstitial** • Medications (PCN analogues, cephalosporins, sulfonamides, ciprofloxacin, acyclovir, rifampin, phenytoin, PPIs, NSAIDs, interferon) • Infections (pyelonephritis, viral or fungal nephritides) • Systemic diseases (sarcoidosis, lupus, Sjogren syndrome, lymphoma, leukemia, tubulonephritis, uveitis)	
	Vascular • Renal vein thrombosis • Renal artery obstruction (thrombosis, emboli, dissection, vasculitis) • Microangiopathy (TTP, HUS, DIC, preeclampsia) • Malignant hypertension • Renal infarction • Scleroderma renal crisis • Transplant rejection	

DKA, diabetic ketoacidosis; NSAID, nonsteroidal anti-inflammatory drug; ACE-I, angiotensin-converting enzyme inhibitor; ARB, angiotensin II receptor blockers; PCN, penicillin; PPI, proton pump inhibitor; TTP, thrombotic thrombocytopenic purpura; HUS, hemolytic uremic syndrome; DIC, disseminated intravascular coagulation.

Adapted from Workeneh BT, Agraharkar M, Gupta R. Acute Kidney Injury. Medscape. http://emedicine.medscape.com/article/243492-overview. Accessed November 25, 2013 and Rahman M, Shad F, Smith MC. Acute kidney injury: a guide to diagnosis and management. *Am Fam Physician* 2012;86(7):631–639.

Referrals

Optimal management of AKI requires close collaboration among primary care physicians, nephrologists, hospitalists, and other subspecialists participating in the care of the patient. Patients with AKI should be hospitalized unless the condition is mild and clearly resulting from an easily reversible cause. Nephrology consultation should be sought early in the course of AKI.[1,5,9–11]

Patient Education

Patients should be counseled to avoid medications that are nephrotoxic. Nonsteroidal anti-inflammatory drugs are one of the most commonly used, and most patients are unaware of their nephrotoxicity. Because of the electrolyte imbalances, diet may need to be addressed with patients as well. In cases with hyperkalemia, dietary potassium should be restricted. Restriction of salt and fluids are crucial in the management of oliguric AKI.

Prognosis

The prognosis of patients diagnosed with AKI varies from case to case. Patients with AKI are more likely to develop chronic kidney disease in the future. They are also at higher risk of end-stage renal disease and premature death. Those with an episode of AKI should be monitored for development of chronic kidney disease. Prognosis is directly related to the cause of AKI and the presence or absence of any preexisting kidney disease. It also depends on the duration of the dysfunction prior to therapeutic intervention.[8-10]

Inpatient mortality rate for AKI is 40% to 50%, with the rate for ICU patients higher than 50%. Variation depends on the type of AKI and patient comorbidities. ICU patients with sepsis-associated AKI have significantly higher mortality rates than nonseptic AKI patients. Survival rate is nearly 0% among those with AKI who have an Acute Physiology and Chronic Health Evaluation II (APACHE II) score higher than 40. Survival rate is 40% among those who have APACHE II score of 10 to 19. Most deaths are not due to AKI itself, but rather underlying comorbidities such as cardiopulmonary disease or infection. Half of the patients diagnosed with AKI recover renal function completely, with the majority of the rest having incomplete recovery. Only 5% to 10% require maintenance hemodialysis.[9,11]

Prevention

With the high morbidity and mortality associated with AKI, it is important for primary care physicians to identify patients who are at high risk and implement preventative strategies: Those over 75 years old; those with diabetes or chronic kidney disease; those with cardiac failure, liver failure, or sepsis; and those patients exposed to contrast agents or who undergo cardiac surgery are all at the highest risk.[10]

In the hospital setting, it is important to prevent AKI from developing, primarily by preventing hypotension, or correcting it rapidly if it does occur. It is also important to evaluate renal function prior to any surgeries. Avoid prescribing any neurotoxic medication, correcting any volume deficits or electrolyte imbalances, and treating oliguria and infections quickly are all additional steps in preventing AKI in the hospital setting. Incidence of contrast nephropathy can be reduced by hydrating patients before procedure, replacing traditional agents with nonionic contrast, and limiting the quantity of any contrast agent used.[5,11]

REFERENCES

1. Okusa MD, Rosner MH. Overview of the management of acute kidney injury (acute renal failure). UpToDate. 2013. http://www.uptodate.com/contents/overview-of-the-management-of-acute-kidney-injury-acute-renal-failure. Accessed November 25, 2013.
2. Fatehi P, Hsu C. Diagnostic approach to the patient with acute kidney injury (acute renal failure) or chronic kidney disease. UpToDate. 2013. http://www.uptodate.com/contents/diagnostic-approach-to-the-patient-with-acute-kidney-injury-acute-renal-failure-or-chronic-kidney-disease. Accessed November 25, 2013.
3. Lewington A, Kanagasundaram S. *Clinical practice guidelines: acute kidney injury.* 5th ed. UK Renal Association. 2011. http://www.renal.org/guidelines/modules#downloads. Accessed March 10, 2014.
4. Praught ML, Shlipak MG. Are small changes in serum creatinine an important risk factor? *Curr Opin Nephrol Hypertens* 2005;14:265–270.
5. KDIGO clinical practice guideline for acute kidney injury. *Kidney Int Suppl* 2012;2:89–115.
6. Lameire N, Van Biesen W, Vanholder R. The changing epidemiology of acute renal failure. *Nat Clin Pract Nephrol* 2006;2:364–377.
7. Cerdá J, Lameire N, Eggers P, et al. Epidemiology of acute kidney injury. *Clin J Am Soc Nephrol* 2008;3(3):881–886.
8. Kohli HS, Bhat A, Jairam A, et al. Predictors of mortality in acute renal failure in a developing country: a prospective study. *Ren Fail* 2007;29(4):463–469.
9. Workeneh BT, Agraharkar M, Gupta R. Acute Kidney Injury. Medscape. http://emedicine.medscape.com/article/243492-overview. Accessed November 25, 2013.
10. Rahman M, Shad F, Smith MC. Acute kidney injury: a guide to diagnosis and management. *Am Fam Physician* 2012;86(7):631–639.
11. Demirjian S, Nally J. Acute Kidney Injury. Cleveland Clinic Center for Continuing Education. https://www.clevelandclinicmeded.com/medicalpubs/diseasemanagement/nephrology/acute-kidney-injury/. Accessed November 25, 2013.

CHAPTER 13

Problems Related to the Female Reproductive System

Section Editor: Amber M. Tyler

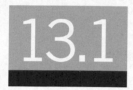

Vaginitis and Cervicitis

Heather L. Paladine, Urmi A. Desai

VAGINITIS
General Principles

Definition

Vaginitis is the general term for disorders of the vagina caused by infection, inflammation, or changes in the normal vaginal flora, and represents the most common gynecologic diagnosis seen in primary care. Symptoms commonly include vaginal discharge, odor, pruritus, or irritation. The majority of cases of vaginitis are caused by bacterial vaginosis (BV), *Candida*, and *Trichomonas*. A common antecedent of these symptoms is disruption of the normal vaginal flora, often due to douching, antibiotics, irritation (including vaginal intercourse), or sexually transmitted infections (STIs). Various physical examination and laboratory tests can help to determining the cause of vaginal complaints, though this remains challenging when typical microscopy findings are not present. Recent technology utilizing nucleic acid amplification to identify organisms associated with the major causes of vaginitis may provide more precise tools for diagnosis and treatment in the future, but are not yet widely available.[1]

Bacterial Vaginosis

BV, the most common cause of vaginitis symptoms, accounts for up to 30% of cases of vaginitis in women of childbearing age. BV is not sexually transmitted, but rather represents a disturbance of the normal vaginal flora from the usual *Lactobacillus* predominance to an increased growth of *Gardnerella vaginalis* and anaerobes.[1]

Diagnosis
Clinical Presentation
The classic presentation of BV is a thin, gray, homogeneous vaginal discharge. An unpleasant, fishy odor may be present. Symptoms often recur or are worse following menses or intercourse. In some women, BV may cause endometritis or pelvic inflammatory disease (PID).[1]

Physical Examination and Laboratory Studies
Amsel's criteria are used to confirm the diagnosis of BV.[2] Because the involved organisms are part of normal vaginal flora, culture is usually not helpful. Three of four positive criteria are consistent with a 90% chance of BV. The criteria include:

- Homogeneous, thin vaginal discharge
- pH >4.5
- Positive whiff test (fishy odor when 10% potassium hydroxide, KOH, is added to a sample of the vaginal discharge on a slide)
- Clue cells on wet mount microscopic examination (see Figure 13.1-2)

Treatment and Prevention of Recurrence

Many women with *Gardnerella* overgrowth (often reported on Pap tests) are asymptomatic. These women do not need treatment unless they are at risk for HIV infection (because BV can increase susceptibility to HIV) or undergoing a procedure such as hysterectomy or therapeutic abortion. Although previous studies have demonstrated an association between BV and pregnancy complications such as preterm labor in pregnant women, there is inconsistent evidence that treatment of asymptomatic BV in pregnant women is associated with lower preterm birth rates. However, oral treatment is preferred for symptomatic pregnant women due to the possibility of upper genital tract infections. Treatment of sexual partners is not indicated.[3]

Medications

First-line treatments include:

- Oral metronidazole (500 mg twice a day for 7 days).[1]
- Metronidazole gel 0.75% (5 g applied nightly to the vagina for 5 days)
- Clindamycin cream 2% (5 g applied nightly to the vagina for 7 days)

Recurrent Bacterial Vaginosis

Cure rates after treatment are 80% to 90% after 1 week, but recurrence rates can be up to 15% to 30% at 3 months. Three or more episodes within 1 year can be considered recurrent BV. Prevention of recurrent BV consists of avoiding triggers that may alter vaginal flora and pH, including douching. For treatment, consider:

- A longer course of oral metronidazole (500 mg twice a day for 14 days).
- Oral clindamycin (300 mg twice a day for 14 days).
- Consider offering suppressive therapy with topical clindamycin gel twice weekly for up to 6 months to reduce recurrences.[3]

Vaginal Candidiasis

Candida species may be identified in the vaginal flora of up to 10% to 20% of females of reproductive age and may not necessarily cause symptoms.[4] Candida vulvovaginitis represents the presence of *Candida* with associated vulvovaginal inflammation. It is usually is caused by *Candida albicans*, but occasionally is caused by other *Candida* species.

Diagnosis

Clinical Presentation

Candida vaginitis presents as a thick, white, "cottage cheese" vaginal discharge. Pruritus of the vagina or vulva is common; women may also experience vulvar swelling or dysuria.[1]

Laboratory Studies

- Microscopic examination with KOH (reveals hyphae or budding yeast forms). Gram stain can also be used but is more expensive and time-consuming (see Figure 13.1-1B).
- Fungal culture (should only be considered for resistant symptoms or recurrent candidiasis).
- pH 4 to 4.5 (normal).

Treatment and Prevention of Recurrence

Both topical and oral preparations of azoles are available for treatment of symptomatic infection. Topical preparations may be over-the-counter (OTC), and physicians should keep in mind that patients may self-treat with these regardless of the cause of vaginitis. Typical duration of treatment with topical azoles is 3 days, though a 7-day course may be preferable for severe infections and pregnant women. The safety of oral treatment in pregnant women has not been established, so topical treatment may be preferable.[1]

Medications

- *OTC treatments*: miconazole or clotrimazole for a 3- to 7-day course.
- *Prescription topical azoles*: terconazole, tioconazole, or butoconazole for a 3- to 7-day course.
- Oral treatment with one 150-mg tablet of fluconazole.

Recurrent Vulvovaginal Candidiasis

Recurrent infections are defined as four episodes within 1 year, and a vaginal culture should be considered in these cases to determine the presence of azole-resistant species. Combined

---

[1]Counsel patients that oral metronidazole may cause a disulfiram reaction if alcohol is concurrently consumed.

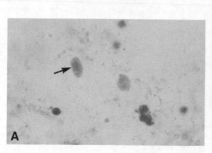
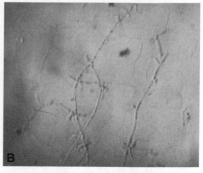

Figure 13.1-1. Vaginal smears of common vaginitis pathogens. **A:** *Trichomonas vaginalis.* **B:** *Candida albicans.* (A: Reproduced with permission from Sun T. *Parasitic disorders: pathology, diagnosis, and management.* 2nd ed. Baltimore, MD: Lippincott Williams & Wilkins; 1999; B: Reproduced with permission from Fleischer GR, Ludwig S. Baskin MN. *Atlas of pediatric emergency medicine.* Philadelphia, PA: Lippincott Williams & Wilkins; 2004.)

estrogen/progesterone oral contraceptives have been shown to be a risk factor for infection. Women with recurrent infections should also be considered for HIV and diabetes testing. In studies, there is variability in the percentage of women who develop symptomatic *Candida* vaginitis following antibiotic treatment; however, prevention includes avoiding unnecessary antibiotics. For women susceptible to *Candida* infections, consider prophylactic treatment concurrently with antibiotics when necessary. Probiotics have not been shown to be effective for prevention of *Candida*, but more studies are needed. Recurrent infections (especially non-*albicans Candida* species) may respond better to prescription rather than OTC treatments, or a longer duration of therapy or maintenance therapy.[5] Possible regimens include:

• 7 to 14 days topical therapy.
• Oral fluconazole (100, 150, or 200 mg dose) every third day for total three doses.

  AND

• One of the above initial doses plus oral fluconazole weekly for 6 months.

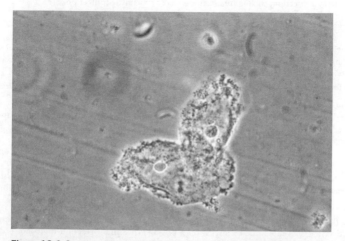

Figure 13.1-2. Clue cells. Clue cells are epithelial cells with clumps of bacteria clustered to their surface. These cells indicate the presence of bacterial vaginosis. (Courtesy M. Rein, Centers for Disease Control and Prevention Public Health Image Library.)

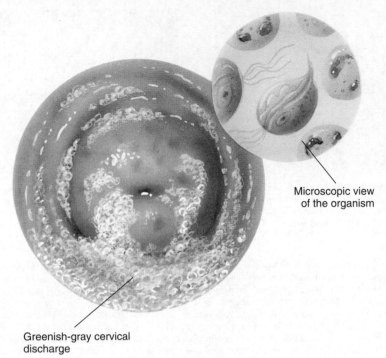

Microscopic view
of the organism

Greenish-gray cervical
discharge

Figure 13.1-3. Trichomonal vaginitis. (From Anatomical Chart Company. *Atlas of pathophysiology.* 3rd ed. Philadelphia, PA: Lippincott Williams & Wilkins; 2010:313.)

Trichomoniasis

Trichomoniasis is a protozoal infection caused by the organism *Trichomonas vaginalis*. In contrast to BV and *Candida* infection, trichomoniasis is a sexually transmitted infection.

Diagnosis

Clinical Presentation

Women with *T. vaginalis* infections typically have a profuse, yellow/green, frothy vaginal discharge with an unpleasant odor (see Figure 13.1-3). Vulvovaginal irritation can also be present. Examination of the cervix may reveal punctate hemorrhages on the cervix and vagina ("strawberry cervix"). Patients may complain of postcoital bleeding. Many of these infections are asymptomatic.[6]

Laboratory Studies

- Microscopic examination with the presence of mobile, flagellated trichomonads on wet mount (see Figure 13.1-1A).
- The vaginal pH is elevated (>4.5).
- Pap tests are specific but not sensitive for infections with *Trichomonas*. Infections based on Pap test results should be treated, but a normal Pap test does not rule out infection.[7]
- Cultures or nucleic acid amplification testing (NAAT) should be sent when there is a suspicion for *Trichomonas* infection despite a normal wet mount result due to high false negative rates for this test.

Treatment and Prevention of Recurrence

Standard treatment is a single oral dose of metronidazole, and topical therapy has been shown to be less effective. Patients should be counseled on a possible disulfiram reaction if alcohol is consumed concurrently. Patients should be counseled on prevention of future episodes through the use of male or female condoms.[7]

Medications

- A single 2-g dose of metronidazole.
- Tinidazole in a single oral 2-g dose is also likely as effective. Topical metronidazole has been shown to be less efficacious than oral metronidazole.
- Sexual partners should be treated as well. Resistant or recurrent infections may require a higher dose or longer duration of treatment with metronidazole (i.e., 500-mg orally twice daily for 7 days); no other medication is currently available in the United States to treat trichomoniasis. Patients with an allergy to metronidazole should undergo desensitization treatment.

Atrophic Vaginitis

Atrophic vaginitis is caused by estrogen deficiency and usually occurs in postmenopausal women.[1]

Diagnosis

Clinical Presentation

Like other forms of vaginitis, atrophic vaginitis is often asymptomatic. Symptoms include vaginal soreness, burning, dyspareunia, and occasionally bleeding or spotting.

Physical Examination

The vaginal mucosa is thin, friable, and pale or erythematous if inflammation is present. It can appear dry, or patients may have a thin, watery discharge.

Laboratory Studies

- Vaginal pH is increased (5 to 7).
- Wet mount reveals parabasal cells (small, round epithelial cells with large nuclei) and polymorphonuclear leukocytes if inflammation is present.

Treatment

Patients can be reassured that mild symptoms are normal and do not require treatment. Dryness can be treated with vaginal lubricants. Topical or oral estrogen replacement is used to treat more bothersome symptoms of atrophic vaginitis, though patients should be counseled on long-term risks of endometrial carcinoma, particularly with higher doses of estrogen. Consider use of oral progesterone along with estrogen for long-term treatment.[1]

CERVICITIS

General Principles

Definition

Cervicitis refers to inflammation of the uterine cervix and is characterized by a purulent cervical discharge or a friable cervix on examination. White blood cells on wet mount or Gram stain are also common, although there is no standard number of white blood cells that confirms the diagnosis.[8]

Epidemiology

Chlamydia trachomatis and *Neisseria gonorrhea* are the most common identified causes of cervicitis; however, these infections may account for only 20% to 50% of women with cervicitis.[5] Other common causes of cervicitis include infectious causes (*Mycoplasma, Ureaplasma*, bacterial vaginosis, herpes simplex, cytomegalovirus, *Trichomonas*, and adenovirus) and nonspecific inflammation.[9] In some women, a cause will not be identified after diagnostic evaluation.[8]

Diagnosis

History

Vaginal discharge, postcoital bleeding, dyspareunia, and irregular vaginal bleeding are common symptoms of cervicitis. Many women are asymptomatic, and cervicitis may be found on an examination done for other reasons, such as Pap smear collection.[3]

Physical Examination

Physical examination commonly reveals mucopurulent discharge, cervical ectropion, and a friable cervix that continues to bleed after passage of a cotton swab through the cervical os. Women with cervicitis should also be examined for cervical motion tenderness, as this can indicate the presence of pelvic inflammatory disease.

Laboratory and Imaging

Women who present with cervicitis should initially be tested for gonorrhea, *Chlamydia*, BV, and *Trichomonas*. Testing for *Chlamydia* and gonorrhea is done with a NAAT and can be performed on urine, vaginal, or cervical samples. The diagnosis of BV is made by Amsel's criteria (see Bacterial Vaginosis section). Trichomonal infection can be diagnosed on wet mount or through NAAT or culture.[8]

Differential Diagnosis

In addition to infectious causes, clinicians should consider the possibility of chemical irritants or cervical malignancy.[8]

Treatment

Medications

High-risk women, including younger women who are at risk due to their age, should receive empiric treatment for gonorrheal and chlamydial infections. When *Trichomonas* or BV is diagnosed in a woman with cervicitis, she should be treated. Empiric antibiotic treatment is not recommended for women who are at low risk or who have negative test results for specific infections.[8] Please see the chapters on Chlamydia and Gonorrhea for more details about the treatment of these infections.

Patient Education

Gonorrhea, *Chlamydia*, and *Trichomonas* infections are spread by intercourse with an infected partner.[3] Male and female condoms reduce the risk of transmission. It is important to recognize that a diagnosis of a sexually transmitted disease can be very stressful for a patient and her partner.

REFERENCES

1. Hainer B, Gibson M. Vaginitis: diagnosis and treatment. *Am Fam Physician* 2011;83:807–815.
2. Amsel R, Totten PA, Spiegel CA, et al. Nonspecific vaginitis: diagnostic criteria and microbial and epidemiologic associations. *Am J Med* 1983;74:14–22.
3. Centers for Disease Control and Prevention. Sexually transmitted disease treatment guidelines. *MMWR* 2010;59(No. RR-12):1–110.
4. Tibaldi C, Cappello N, Latino MA, et al. Vaginal and endocervical microorganisms in symptomatic and asymptomatic non-pregnant females: risk factors and rates of occurrence. *Clin Microbiol Infect* 2009;15:670–679.
5. Pappas PG, Kauffman CA, Andes D, et al. Clinical practice guidelines for the management of candidiasis: 2009 update by the Infectious Diseases Society of America. *Clinical Infect Dis* 2009;48(5):503–535.
6. Bachmann LH, Hobbs MM, Seña AC, et al. Trichomonas vaginalis genital infections: progress and challenges. *Clinical Infect Dis* 2011;53(Suppl 3):S160–S172.
7. Gülmezoglu AM, Azhar M. Interventions for treating trichomoniasis in women. *Cochrane Database Syst Rev* 2011;(5):CD000220. doi: 10.1002/14651858.CD000220.pub2.
8. Taylor SN, Lensing, S, Schwebke J, et al. Prevalence and treatment outcome of cervicitis of unknown etiology. *Sex Transm Dis* 2013;40:379–385.
9. Patel MA, Nyirjesy P. Role of mycoplasma and ureaplasma species in female lower genital tract infections. *Curr Infect Dis Rep* 2010;12:417–422.

13.2

Dysmenorrhea and Premenstrual Syndrome

Elizabeth K. Dayton

DYSMENORRHEA

General Principles

Definition/Pathophysiology

Dysmenorrhea is cramping pain associated with menstruation. Primary (functional) dysmenorrhea is a painful paroxysmal syndrome that precedes or may accompany menses. It is not associated with pelvic pathology. Secondary dysmenorrhea is painful menses caused by pelvic disease. The pain is thought to be due to elevated levels of prostaglandin $F_2\alpha$. Prior to the onset of menses, cyclic progesterone withdrawal leads to the degradation of endometrial cell membranes. The cellular debris is converted to arachidonic acid, which is further metabolized by cyclo-oxygenase (COX) enzymes to form prostaglandins.[1] The prostaglandins stimulate endometrial and uterine smooth muscle contractility and promote myometrial vasoconstriction. Ischemia develops, causing an angina equivalent in the uterus and results in pain. Other studies have also shown elevated leukotriene levels to be a contributing factor. Vasopressin was thought to be an aggravating agent, but vasopressin antagonists have shown no effect on the relief of menstrual pain.[2]

Epidemiology/Etiology

Primary dysmenorrhea is one of the most common gynecologic complaints, thought to affect from 50% to 90% of women of reproductive age. It is a leading cause of absenteeism for women under 30 years of age and the leading cause of school absences for adolescent women.[3] Secondary (acquired) dysmenorrhea is pain that results from a pelvic abnormality. Endometriosis is the most common cause of secondary dysmenorrhea.[4] Other possible etiologies include reproductive tract structural anomalies, adenomyosis, uterine tumors and leiomyomata, polyps, chronic salpingitis, pelvic inflammatory disease (PID), intrauterine device (IUD) use, cervical stenosis, irritable and inflammatory bowel syndromes, and urologic disorders. Several authors have correlated dysmenorrhea with smoking cigarettes, high intake of omega-6 fatty acids, nulliparity, depression, and stress. Causation has yet to be proved in rigorous controlled studies.

Diagnosis

Clinical Presentation

Primary dysmenorrhea usually appears within 12 months after menarche. It is characterized by symptom onset around the time of menses. Pain can be colicky or spasmodic and is usually felt in the lower abdomen, back, and thighs. Patients may also experience nausea, vomiting, diarrhea, headache, fatigue, and dizziness—prostaglandin-mediated symptoms. Menstrual flow may be heavier than normal. Symptoms are often worst on the first day of menses and then gradually resolves. Physical examination will be unrevealing. A pelvic examination is not initially required to make the diagnosis, especially in nonsexually active and virginal women. The diagnosis can generally be made on the basis of history alone. If an adolescent is sexually active, a pelvic examination should be performed due to the high risk of PID in this population.[4] If the history and physical examination are inconsistent, or initial therapies are unsuccessful, further evaluation for secondary causes of dysmenorrhea should be pursued.

In secondary dysmenorrhea, onset is typically more than 2 years after menarche. Pain is not limited to the menstrual cycle. Pelvic and rectovaginal examinations should be performed if endometriosis is suspected. Physical examination may reveal adnexal masses, fixed uterus or reduced uterine mobility, and uterosacral nodularity in patients with endometriosis; mucopurulent cervical discharge in those with PID; and uterine asymmetry or enlargement in those with adenomyosis.[4]

Treatment

First-line therapy is either a nonsteroidal anti-inflammatory drug (NSAID; e.g., naproxen, ibuprofen, mefenamic acid-nonspecific COX inhibitors) or a specific COX-2 inhibitor (e.g., celecoxib). These medications act to decrease prostaglandin production, thereby decreasing both menstrual flow and prostaglandin-mediated pain. Medications should be taken 1 to 2 days before the onset of menses and continued on a fixed regimen for about 3 days.[4] Because of the recent concerns about the safety of COX-2 inhibitors, the short duration of therapy for relieving primary dysmenorrhea, and the low cost of NSAIDs, it is prudent to recommend established NSAIDs with better long-term safety data as the preferred treatment.[5] Topical heat has been shown to be more effective than placebo and may be as effective as NSAIDs in small studies.[4] Other pharmacologic therapies for dysmenorrhea have included oral contraceptives (either traditional or extended cycle dosing), leuprolide, danazol, depot medroxy-progesterone, levonorgestrel-containing IUD, nifedipine, terbutaline, oral guaifenesin,[6] magnesium, thiamine, aspirin, B_{12}, vitamin E, fish oil supplements, and the Japanese herb Toki-shakayaku-san.[5]

Nontraditional modalities include acupuncture and acupressure, transcutaneous electrical nerve stimulation (TENS) unit therapy, and local application of unidirectional static magnets; however, there is limited and inconsistent evidence on their effectiveness.[7] Surgery is considered the intervention of last resort. Surgical interventions include laparoscopic uterosacral nerve ablation, presacral neurectomy, and hysterectomy. The first-line treatment for dysmenorrhea caused by endometriosis is combined oral contraceptives.[4] Treatment for secondary dysmenorrhea is directed to the specific underlying cause and referral to the appropriate specialist for further medical or surgical treatment should be made.[5]

Despite the great prevalence of dysmenorrhea, many patients will not report symptomatology unless the provider specifically inquires. Some chronic complications with inadequately treated primary dysmenorrhea include anxiety and depression. Infertility can become a complication with certain causes of secondary dysmenorrhea. Inquiry and intervention can result in significant improvement of quality of life for these women.

PREMENSTRUAL SYNDROME

General Principles

Definition

Premenstrual syndrome (PMS) is a poorly understood psychoendocrine condition characterized by an array of somatic, cognitive, affective, and behavioral disturbances that recur in cyclic fashion during the luteal phase of the menstrual cycle and resolve with the onset of menstruation. More than 150 symptoms have been documented, varying from mild to severe enough to disrupt normal activities and interpersonal relationships. Not all cycles are associated with PMS symptoms and not all premenstrual changes should be labeled PMS.

Pathophysiology/Etiology

PMS represents a biophysiologic, endocrine phenomenon. Altered levels of various hormones have been offered as the cause for premenstrual symptomatology, including estrogen, progesterone, pro-lactin, growth hormone, thyroid hormone, follicle-stimulating hormone, luteinizing hormone, antidiuretic hormone, insulin, prostaglandin, and cortisol. Studies have failed to confirm any of these as absolutely causative.[8] However, women with PMSs are thought to have an altered response to normal gonadal steroids during the luteal phase and their effect on neurotransmitters such as serotonin and GABA in the CNS.[9] Premenstrual symptomatology and behavior may also stem from social, psychologic, or cognitive dysfunction.

Diagnosis

Clinical Presentation

There is no typical presentation of PMS. Some of the more common physical symptoms include abdominal bloating and cramping, breast tenderness, fluid retention and weight gain, acne, cold sores, fatigue, and head and muscle aches. Emotional changes include anxiety, panic, depression, heightened aggressiveness, hostility, food craving, forgetfulness, insomnia, irritability, mood lability, poor concentration, tearfulness, and reduced coping skills. In 2000, the American College of Obstetrics and Gynecology (ACOG) published a practice bulletin of 10 PMS diagnostic criteria. According to ACOG, the diagnosis of PMS requires that a woman has one or more of the affective or somatic symptoms listed. Symptoms must occur during the 5 days before menses (late luteal phase) in each of the three prior menstrual cycles; be relieved within 4 days of the onset of menses; and not recur until at least cycle day 13. The symptoms must be bothersome to the patient. They must exist in the absence of any pharmacologic therapy, hormones, alcohol, or recreational drugs. Finally, all other psychiatric or medical disorders must be excluded.[10] The American Psychological Association (APA) included severe PMS in the *Diagnostic and Statistical Manual of Mental Disorders* 5th edition (DSM-5) as an axis I diagnosis called premenstrual dysphoric disorder (PMDD). The DSM-5 defines PMDD as a severe form of PMS in which symptoms of anger, irritability, and internal tension are prominent.[11] A woman must experience five or more from a list of 11 symptoms to fit PMDD criteria. As with the diagnosis of PMS, the symptoms must be experienced only in the luteal phase; all other diagnoses must be excluded; and the patient must have experienced them for the majority of cycles within the past year.[10]

History/Physical/Laboratory

A detailed history must be obtained, including menstrual history and inquiries about alcohol, tobacco, and recreational drugs. A complete physical examination must be performed. The need for in-depth neurologic or psychologic evaluation may become apparent. No specific diagnostic test is available for detecting PMS/PMDD. Laboratory investigation should be tailored to the individual patient. For example, complete blood count and thyroid studies should be considered in patients with menorrhagia or chronic fatigue. Charting the menstrual cycle and documenting symptomatology must be done for two to three cycles. Patients write down the symptoms that trouble them most and rate the severity throughout the entire menstrual cycle. The Daily Record of Severity of Problems (DRSP) form, a self-administered questionnaire, is the most commonly used tool.[11] Presence of luteal phase symptoms in at least two cycles, lack of follicular phase symptoms, and absence of other specific disease entities strongly suggest the diagnosis of PMS or PMDD.

Treatment

Nonpharmacologic

The clinician must individualize the treatment plan to maximize therapeutic response. Treatment should begin with a 2- to 3-month trial of lifestyle changes while the patient records symptoms. This is recommended in women with mild PMS that do not cause distress or socioeconomic dysfunction.[12] Stress management strategies should be taught. Sufficient rest should be advocated. Regular aerobic exercise has been demonstrated to alleviate some PMS symptomatology, probably due to endogenous endorphin release. A well-balanced diet with adequate protein, fiber, and complex carbohydrates is essential for everyone's good health. However, these recommendations have not been investigated in rigorous controlled studies. Caffeine, salt, excess sugar, tobacco, alcohol, and recreational drugs may worsen physical symptoms and emotional lability. Multivitamins, calcium, and magnesium supplements may be helpful. Pyridoxine (vitamin B_6) may reduce fatigue, depression, and irritability in selected women. However, there is no convincing evidence that any of these are more effective than placebo and carry a potential for harm such as peripheral neuropathy with high-dose B_6.[12]

Pharmacologic

If premenstrual complaints do not respond to the above and the presence of psychological disorders, substance abuse or hypothyroidism has been considered, medical therapy can be initiated. Symptom logs assist the clinician in tailoring treatment to individual needs. Prostaglandin inhibitors can relieve headaches, body aches, and dysmenorrhea. Spironolactone 25 to 50 mg bid during cycle days 14 to 28 may reduce fluid retention. Danazol and bromocriptine have been utilized in the past to reduce mastalgia. However, adverse side effects limit their usefulness.

Without menstrual cyclicity, PMS cannot occur. Oral contraceptives, depomedroxyprogesterone, levonorgestrel-containing IUDs, and gonadotropin-releasing hormone agonists have been tried with variable success. Oral contraceptive pills (OCPs) that contain the progestin drospirenone (an anti-mineralocorticoid and anti-androgen) are effective in reducing bloating and mood changes that accompany the placebo pill week. In 2012, the FDA stated the OCP-containing drospirenone may be associated with a higher risk of venous thromboembolism compared with levonorgestrel and other progestins.[12] The recommendation is to assess each individual's risk of Venous thromboembolism (VTE) prior to starting this medication in a new user. Multiple herbs have been utilized with variable success and safety in treating premenstrual symptoms. These include evening primrose oil, black currant oil, chaste tree extract, black cohosh, wild yam root, dong quai, kava kava, and St. John's wort. Interactions with other medications the patient might be taking must always be considered.[13]

Selective serotonin-reuptake inhibitors (SSRIs) are the first-line drugs for treating PMDD. Sertraline or fluoxetine are typically used first.[12] They can be administered daily or only during the luteal phase (starting on cycle day 14). Treatment only during the luteal phase has fewer adverse side effects and is less expensive; however, it is important to ensure the patient is asymptomatic during the follicular phase or else she will be undertreated.[12] If SSRIs are ineffective or patient still has residual symptoms despite SSRI therapy, one option is to augment treatment with low-dose alprazolam.[12] Alprazolam is an anxiolytic with proven effectiveness for symptoms of premenstrual tension, anxiety, irritability, and hostility. However, its addictive potential makes it a second-line treatment. Buspirone is an effective anxiolytic that is not addictive.

PMS is a complex disorder of reproductive-aged women. Successful management requires continued communication and collaboration between patient and clinician.

REFERENCES

1. Harel Z. Cyclooxygenase-2 specific inhibitors in the treatment of dysmenorrhea. *J Pediatr Adolesc Gynecol* 2004;17:75–79.
2. Shushan A. Complications of menstruation and abnormal uterine bleeding. In: DeCherney A, Nathan L, Goodwin TM, et al., eds. *Current diagnosis & treatment: obstetrics & gynecology.* 11th ed. New York, NY: McGraw-Hill; 2013:61–619.
3. Sultan C, Gaspari L, Paris F. Adolescent dysmenorrhea. In: Sultan C, ed. *Pediatric and adolescent gynecology. Evidence-based clinical practice.* 2nd ed. Basel: Karger; 2012:171–180.
4. Osayande A, Mehulic S. Diagnosis and initial management of dysmenorrhea. *Am Fam Physician* 2014;89:341–346.
5. Danakas G, Alvero R. Dysmenorrhea. In: Ferri FF, ed. *Ferri's clinical advisor 2014.* Philadelphia, PA: Mosby; 2014:352.
6. Marsden JS, Strickland CD, Clements TL. Guaifenesin as a treatment for primary dysmenorrhea. *J Am Board Fam Pract* 2004;17:240–246.
7. Eccles NK. A randomized double-blinded, placebo-controlled pilot study to investigate the effectiveness of a static magnet to relieve dysmenorrhea. *J Altern Complement Med* 2005;11:681–687.
8. Winer SA, Rapkin AJ. Premenstrual disorders: prevalence, etiology and impact. *J Reprod Med* 2006;51:339–347.
9. Rapkin AJ, Akopians AL. Premenstrual Syndrome. https://www.clinicalkey.com/. Updated January 7, 2014. Accessed January 16, 2014.
10. Futterman LA, Rapkin AJ. Diagnosis of premenstrual disorders. *J Reprod Med* 2006;51:349–358.
11. Yonkers KA, Casper RF. Clinical manifestations and diagnosis of premenstrual syndrome and premenstrual dysphoric disorder. *UpToDate.* www.uptodate.com/home/index.html. Updated November 8, 2013. Accessed January 16, 2014.
12. Kasper RF, Yonkers, KA. Treatment of premenstrual syndrome and premenstrual dysphoric disorder. *UpToDate.* www.uptodate.com/home/index.html. Updated March 17, 2014. Accessed March 28, 2014.
13. Kaur G, Gonsalves L, Thacker HL. Premenstrual dysphoric disorder: a review for the treating practitioner. *Cleve Clin J Med* 2004;71:303–321.

13.3 Abnormal Genital Bleeding in Women and Girls

Angela M. Riegel

GENERAL PRINCIPLES
Definition
Abnormal genital bleeding is any blood loss from the vaginal or perineal area other than the individual menstrual pattern of flow of a premenopausal girl or woman, or the expected cyclic hormonal bleeding in a postmenopausal woman taking hormones.

Terminology

A revised terminology system for abnormal uterine bleeding (AUB) in non–gravida-reproducing women was introduced in 2011 by the International Federation of Gynecology and Obstetrics. Within this system, the etiologies of the symptoms of AUB are classified as "related to uterine structural abnormalities" and "unrelated to uterine structural abnormalities" and categorized by the acronym PALM-COEIN (polyp, adenomyosis, leiomyoma, malignancy and hyperplasia, coagulopathy, ovulatory dysfunction, endometrial, iatrogenic, and not yet classified).[1]

Anatomy

Bleeding coming from structures surrounding the vagina, rectum, and perineum must be differentiated from uterine bleeding originating from the cervical os. Pregnancy, structural pelvic pathology such as fibroids or polyps, benign and malignant tumors, anovulation, and coagulopathies are the leading causes.

Epidemiology

The incidence of genital bleeding from all causes is unclear, but AUB accounts for nearly one-third of all gynecologic visits, mostly at menarche or perimenopause. In postmenopausal women, an estimate of uterine bleeding in the first 12 months is 409 per 1,000 person-years, but only 42 per 1,000 person-years 3 years postmenopause.

Classification

- **Nonuterine.** The actual source of the bleeding may not be obvious. A laceration of the cervix, or of the vagina, especially if high in a fornix, may appear to be uterine bleeding. Urinary, rectal, or vulvar bleeding may be mistaken for vaginal bleeding.
  - *Vulvar or vaginal*: infection, laceration, tumor, foreign body
  - *Extravaginal*: perineal, urinary, rectal
  - *Systemic/medical*: bleeding diathesis, thrombocytopenia; von Willebrand disease; liver, renal, endocrine disease
- **Uterine.** Age-grouping is important.
  - *Age*: premenarche—any bleeding is abnormal
  - *Age*: 13 to 40
    - The clinician should consider pregnancy-related causes, especially ectopic pregnancy, even when bleeding is light or moderate, and even in young and perimenopausal women. Once pregnancy is ruled out, the diagnosis of dysfunctional uterine bleeding (DUB), although one of exclusion, does not require total certainty before reasonable treatment for anovulation is implemented.
    - Anovulatory bleeding (DUB) is common and may be treated as such without an exhaustive search for all other causes initially, as long as there is a normal medical history, pregnancy test, complete blood count (CBC), Pap smear when appropriate and a normal bimanual pelvic examination. Although not all uterine bleeding in this group will prove to be DUB, serious pathology in the face of normal findings is unlikely. If hormonal manipulation fails, a more complete workup can follow. Over age 35, an endometrial biopsy should be done.[2]
  - *Age*: 40 and older—higher index of suspicion of neoplasm. A very different scenario pertains to the peri- and postmenopausal woman, in whom bleeding must be investigated before anovulation can be assumed.
  - *Age*: Postmenopausal—neoplasm until proven otherwise, unless known hormonal cause.

Etiology

- Pregnancy should be considered.
- Anovulation is a common cause (DUB, defined as uterine bleeding associated with anovulation, in the absence of other pathology):
  - *Physiologic*: Adolescence (although 4% to 20% of adolescents have a coagulopathy underlying their abnormal bleeding), perimenopause (although abnormal bleeding must be considered neoplastic or hyperplastic until proven otherwise), lactation, and pregnancy.
  - *Pathologic*: Hyperandrogenic anovulation (e.g., polycystic ovary syndrome, congenital adrenal hyperplasia, androgen-producing tumors), hypothalamic dysfunction (e.g., secondary to anorexia nervosa), hyperprolactinemia, hypothyroidism, primary pituitary disease, premature ovarian failure, and iatrogenic factors (e.g., secondary to radiation therapy or chemotherapy).

- Iatrogenic or treatment-induced:
  - Estrogen withdrawal occurs after removal or irradiation of ovaries, or after giving and then withdrawing estrogen to a person without ovaries. (Midcycle bleeding can be due to preovulation drop in estrogen.)
  - Estrogen breakthrough is due to stimulation of endometrium from unopposed low- or high-level estrogen. (Low-dose estrogen produces intermittent light spotting; high-dose estrogen yields amenorrhea followed by profuse bleeding. Cyclic progesterone corrects this.)
  - Progestin withdrawal occurs only if there has been prior estrogen priming.
  - Progestin breakthrough can occur when endometrium becomes so atrophic that lack of estrogen effect yields too little and too ragged a lining for synchronous cellular events. (Estrogen replacement therapy can restore responsiveness. This occurs after months on oral contraceptives (OCs) or depoprogesterone. Adding estrogen for a week usually corrects the problem.)
- Noncyclic uterine bleeding (non-DUB)
  - Uterine leiomyoma, leiomyosarcoma, endometrial polyp(s)
  - Endometrial hyperplasia or carcinoma
  - Cervical or vaginal neoplasia
  - Endometritis, adenomyosis
  - Bleeding associated with pregnancy (threatened or incomplete abortion, trophoblastic disease, ectopic pregnancy)
  - Bleeding associated with the puerperium (retained products of conception, placental polyps, subinvolution of the uterus)
  - Coagulopathies (von Willebrand disease, platelet abnormalities, thrombocytopenic purpura)
  - Iatrogenic causes, medications, and devices—intrauterine devices (IUDs), diaphragms, pessaries
  - Systemic diseases (liver, renal, thyroid, other endocrine)
- Infection, laceration or contusion, tumor, foreign body
- Perineal, rectal, urinary disease
- Systemic medical causes include bleeding diatheses, especially thrombocytopenia; von Willebrand disease; and liver, renal, endocrine disease
- Ovulatory excessive bleeding[2]

DIAGNOSIS/TREATMENT
Clinical Presentation
Abnormal genital bleeding can range from urgent or emergent bleeding to mild irregular bleeding in between menstrual cycle. Most common cause is pregnancy or its complications.

Assessment/History
When taking a detailed history, several questions must be answered, including pregnancy status, reproductive status, and the source of bleeding. This will help determine differential diagnosis and disposition of the patient. History should include relevant medical history, menstrual history, sexual history, contraceptive history, family history of bleeding disorders and thyroid diseases, and risk factors for endometrial cancer.

Severity
- **Rate of flow.** How heavy is the bleeding? Pad counts are unreliable because of differences of absorbency but may give a rough estimate. The patient's own opinion is probably more valid. When did it start? Is the blood bright red or dark, with or without clots? If it is heavier than she has ever seen it, if it is flowing, if brighter red than menstrual blood, and if there are clots or pieces of tissue, there might be significant hemorrhage and the patient should not wait even a short time. If she cannot get to the office immediately, she should go to the nearest emergency room, by ambulance or 911. She should be instructed to retrieve any tissue passed for the purpose of analysis.
- **Amount of flow.** A rough estimate of blood loss can be made by asking how much more bleeding than a usual period she has had since onset. (Normal menstrual blood loss is 20 to 80 cc.)[2]

Associated Symptoms
Has there been fever, dizziness, abdominal pain, and diarrhea? Any of these could signal associated pelvic infection or abscess, shock, severe loss of blood volume, dehydration, other intra-abdominal pathologic process, or bleeding tendency.

Physical Examination
Check vital signs; do abdominal, perineal, vaginal, pelvic, and rectal examination. The examination must meticulously pinpoint the exact source, which may not be obvious. A physical examination with

good exposure for the speculum examination, and optimal palpation of pelvic organs using bimanual and rectovaginal techniques, is crucial to finding serious and treatable pathology. Obesity and hirsutism should be noted. An estimate of prior hormonal influences should be made in an attempt to classify the type of anovulation.[2]

Basic Laboratory Tests

Initial tests should include pregnancy test (β-human chorionic gonadotropin) and CBC with platelets and differential. Additional testing based on history and physical examination may include endocrine, thyroid function tests, prolactin level, androgen level, follicle-stimulating hormone/luteinizing hormone, estrogen levels, and coagulation studies.[2,3]

Examination Findings

Examination findings may suggest other studies, such as endometrial biopsy or colposcopy, hysteroscopy, pelvic and/or endovaginal sonography (transvaginal scan [TVS]), hysterosalpingography, and saline infusion hysterosonography (saline infusion sonography [SIS]), usually performed by radiologists or gynecologists. Most procedures carry known risks, benefits, and advantages, and are chosen based on individual needs of the specific patient and circumstance.

Ultrasonography

Pelvic ultrasound is the first-line imaging study in women with AUB. Transvaginal examination should be performed, unless there is a reason not to do a vaginal examination. Ultrasound is effective at characterizing uterine and adnexal lesions. If it is performed in a postmenopausal woman, an endometrial biopsy is mandatory when the endometrial thickness is greater than 4 mm. In premenopausal women, endometrial findings on ultrasound is not a useful test since major variation during normal menstrual cycle.[4]

Endometrial Biopsy

After pregnancy has been excluded, endometrial biopsy should be performed to exclude endometrial neoplasia or endometritis. Endometrial biopsy should be performed in all women age 45 years or older with AUB, women below age 45 years with persistent AUB who failed medical management, those with a history of unopposed estrogen exposure, or those at high risk for endometrial cancers.[3]

Management

Treatment for specific pathology depends on the underlying cause and may be managed by the family doctor or may require referral to a gynecologist, endocrinologist, or gynecologic oncologist. Acute, heavy bleeding requires close observation, accurate determination of the source and likely cause, and immediate therapy. Hospitalization, hydration, and transfusion may be required.

Medical Management

In the hemodynamically unstable patient, fluid resuscitation and blood replacement are the first priority. Therapeutic options are intravenous high-dose estrogen, intrauterine tamponade, uterine curettage, uterine artery embolization, and hysterectomy. High-dose intravenous estrogen (Permarin) 25 mg is given every 4 to 6 hours for 24 hours. If bleeding does not subside after 8 hours, other treatments should be used.[5] Antiemetics should be given for nausea.

In patients that are hemodynamically stable with severe uterine bleeding patient, first-line therapy is high-dose oral estrogen (Premarin) 2.5 mg four times per day until the bleeding subsides or is minimal. After oral estrogen has been discontinued, oral progestin (medroxyprogesterone acetate) 10 mg per day for 10 days should be initiated.[6] Other options include high-dose oral monophasic contraceptives (containing 35 mcg ethinyl estradiol) three times a day for 7 days or medroxyprogesterone acetate 20 mg orally three times a day for 7 days.[6] Tranexamic acid, an antifibrinolytic drug, dosed at 1.3 g three times a day for 5 days is another option that may be used for women with contraindications to hormonal therapy.[7] For all patients, the contraindications to these therapies need to be considered before administration. In patients that are experiencing mild to moderate uterine bleeding, first-line therapy is usually oral estrogen–progestin contraceptives. Oral estrogen–progestin should contain 30 to 35 mcg ethinyl estradiol to reduce bleeding.[6] For women with contraindications to estrogen therapy, levonorgestrel-releasing IUD is a reasonable choice.

Once the acute episode of bleeding has been controlled, multiple treatment options are available for long-term treatment of chronic AUB. These included OCs, progestin therapy (oral or intramuscular), levonorgestrel intrauterine system, tranexamic acid, and nonsteroidal anti-inflammatory drugs. Duration of treatment depends on circumstances of bleeding, fertility or contraceptive needs, and the age of the patient. Anemic patients should receive iron supplementation.

Patients with known or suspected bleeding disorders may respond to hormonal and nonhormonal management. Consultation with hematologist is recommended. Patients with von Willebrand disease may respond to desmopressin. For severe bleeding, recombinant factor VIII and von Willebrand factor may be required to control bleeding. Avoid nonsteroidal anti-inflammatory drugs for patient with bleeding or platelet dysfunction.[8]

Surgical Management

The need for surgical treatment is based on the clinical stability of the patient, the severity of bleeding, contraindications to medical management, the patient's lack of response to medical management, and the underlying medical condition of the patient. Surgical options include dilation and curettage (D&C), endometrial ablation, uterine artery embolization, and hysterectomy. The choice of surgical modality is based on medical factors plus the patient's desire for future fertility.

Special Considerations

- **Structural or anatomical causes concurrent with DUB.** Fibroids, especially when large, can degenerate and be the primary source of bleeding. However, fibroids are common and their presence, especially if small, does not mean that they are the source of the bleeding. DUB may still be the primary diagnosis, as may cancer. DUB or infection can occur with an IUD in place, which may be retained if treatment of the underlying cause is successful.
- **Postmenopausal bleeding**
  - For the woman not on hormones, the decision is clear. She needs a thorough investigation of the cause of the bleeding, including endometrial sampling, to rule out endometrial cancer. Hysteroscopy, TVS, or SIS may be needed.
  - For the woman on hormones, an individual decision must be made based on her prior problems and her hormone regimen.
    - ○ Unopposed estrogen should not be used for long-term chronic AUB. If patients are identified as taking unopposed estrogen, they must have endometrial biopsy.
    - ○ Although continuous or monthly progesterone is protective, endometrial cancer risk is not entirely removed by its addition to the estrogen regimen. Cancer must be ruled out by endometrial biopsy in the face of persistent bleeding.
    - ○ Patients taking progesterone less than monthly should have endometrial sampling if bleeding is off schedule. It is reasonable to obtain an endometrial sample without prior ultrasonographic examination; the procedure is simple and yields definitive tissue, although it can also miss areas.
    - ○ Patients taking tamoxifen are at higher risk for endometrial cancer; those taking raloxifene are at lower risk.[9]
- **Perimenopause.** Although hormonal therapy remains controversial, it is now common in perimenopause. Decision-making must take into account the special circumstances of the bleeding. In some cases, one can treat the hormonal transition as DUB or hormonal bleeding, before doing more testing. In others, endometrial sampling and/or imaging is advised. It is better to err on the side of sampling/imaging.
- **Cervical stenosis.** If endometrial biopsy is impossible, an ultrasound scan with an acceptable endometrial stripe (less than 4 to 5 mm) may suggest that therapy for DUB is reasonable. If the endometrial stripe is greater than 8 mm, referral to a gynecologist (with probability of D&C) is indicated.

REFERENCES

1. Munro MG, Critchley HO, Broder MS, et al. FIGO classification system (PALM-COEIN) for causes of abnormal uterine bleeding in nongravida women of reproductive age. *Int J Gynaecol Obstet* 2011;113:3–13.
2. Sweet MG, Schmidt-Dalton TA, Weiss PM. Evaluation and management of abnormal uterine bleeding in premenopausal women. *Am Fam Physician* 2012;85(1):35–43.
3. Committee on Practice Bulletins—Gynecology. Practice bulletin no. 128: diagnosis of abnormal uterine bleeding in reproductive-aged women. *Obstet Gynecol* 2012;120:197–206.
4. American College of Obstetricians and Gynecologists. ACOG committee opinion no. 440. The role of transvaginal ultrasonography in the evaluation of postmenopausal bleeding. *Obstet Gynecol* 2009;114:409–411.
5. American College of Obstetricians and Gynecologists. ACOG committee opinion no. 557: management of acute abnormal uterine bleeding in nonpregnant reproductive-aged women. *Obstet Gynecol* 2013;121:891–896.
6. Munro MG, Mainor N, Basu R, et al. Oral medroxyprogesterone acetate and combination oral contraceptives for acute uterine bleeding: a randomized controlled trial. *Obstet Gynecol* 2006;108:924–929.

7. James AH, Kouides PA, Abdul-Kadir R, et al. Evaluation and management of acute menorrhagia in women with and without underlying bleeding disorders: consensus from an international expert panel. *Eur J Obstet Gynecol Reprod Biol* 2011;158:124–34.
8. American College of Obstetricians and Gynecologists Committee on Adolescent Health Care; American College of Obstetricians and Gynecologists Committee Gynecologic Practice. ACOG committee opinion no. 451. Von Willebrand disease in women. *Obstet Gynecol* 2009;114:1439–1443.
9. Speroff L, Fritz M. Postmenopausal hormone therapy. In: Fritz MD, Speroff L, eds. *Clinical gynecologic endocrinology and infertility*. 8th ed. Baltimore, MD: Lippincott Williams & Wilkins; 2011:749–854.

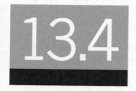

Pap Smear Evaluation for Cervical Cancer

Dena M. Jundt

GENERAL PRINCIPLES

Definition

The Pap smear is the primary detection tool for cervical cancer. Since its widespread acceptance following publication of Papanicolaou and Traut's paper in 1943,[1] developed countries using the Pap smear as screening have had dramatic drops in rates of cervical cancer. Cervical cancer resulted in 3,939 deaths in the United States in 2010.[2]

Pathophysiology

The cervix is the inferior extension of the uterus. The vaginal portion is covered by squamous epithelium peripherally and centrally to a point referred to as the squamocolumnar junction (SCJ), where columnar (glandular) epithelium progresses from that point inward through the cervical os and into the body of the uterus. At birth, the SCJ is effaced more laterally on the vaginal portion of the cervix compared to the finding in a nonpregnant adult. A process known as squamous metaplasia results in the change from columnar to squamous epithelium between the original SCJ and the "new" SCJ. This area is referred to as the transformation zone (TZ). Virtually all cervical dysplasia and cancer occurs within the limits of the TZ, as it is the most "mitotically active" region of the cervix.

Risk factors for development of cervical cancer include human papillomavirus (HPV) exposure, early age of initiation of sexual activity, multiple sexual partners, cigarette smoking, and *in utero* diethylstilbestrol (DES) exposure. There is a dramatic difference (approximately threefold) between more and less developed countries in the incidence of cancer, primarily due to the availability of screening via the Pap smear.[3]

It is now well established that HPV is the causative agent of cervical cancer. This sexually transmitted virus exists in over 100 "strains," most of which are not felt to be oncogenic. The known "high-risk" HPV subtypes are strains 16, 18, and approximately 10 others. Types 16 and 18 are responsible for approximately 70% of cervical cancers. Types 6, 11, and others are implicated as causes of condyloma. The other known risk factors for cervical cancer accelerate the oncogenicity of the high-risk subtypes; in addition, acquiring a new partner who exposes the patient to new low-risk strains accelerates the risk of cancer in a patient who already has high-risk strains of HPV.[3]

HPV is transmitted when infected genital epithelial cells desquamate during intercourse and bind to basal keratinocytes in areas of microtrauma on the sexual partner. The immune response of the host is usually inadequate to kill the virus because the virus does not kill the infected cells. It is believed that 20% of infections are handled through humoral immunity, and approximately 20% of infected patients have persistent infection despite therapy. The majority of patients, therefore, respond to therapy for warts or dysplasia with a lasting clinical remission. Patients with persistent infection may progress to low-grade disease, high-grade (cervical intraepithelial neoplasia, or CIN) disease, or invasive cancer. Severe dysplasia may still take up to 7 years to progress to invasive cervical cancer.[3]

DIAGNOSIS
Clinical Presentation

The great majority of patients who present with cervical cancer have had no screening for several years. The precursor conditions are imminently treatable when caught in any stage prior to invasive disease. Other than presenting for routine annual screening, patients may present with intermenstrual or post-coital bleeding, or have been referred for colposcopy because of a gross lesion.

History

Important aspects of the history, in addition to elucidation of risk factors mentioned above, include documentation of last menstrual period (LMP), any history of prior abnormal Pap or HPV testing, and history of prior treatment(s) for cervical disease. In older patients who may be menopausal, current or former hormone replacement therapy should be documented.[4]

Physical Examination

Screening should begin at age 21 with cytology alone every 3 years. Women less than age 21 should not be screened regardless of the time of first sexual intercourse. Women age 30 to 65 should be screened with cytology and HPV contesting every 5 years or with cytology alone every 3 years. It is not necessary to screen women after age 65 with prior negative screening. Direct visualization of the cervix with a speculum examination is necessary for collection of a sample for Pap smear. Patients should avoid douching or intercourse for 24 hours prior to the procedure. Metal speculums should be warmed with water; the new thin-layer preps do not require avoidance of lubrication for insertion of the speculum, but most pathologists still feel it should be avoided when possible. Note should be taken of any bleeding that is spontaneous or induced by contact with the instruments used to collect the sample. Any lesions, such as leukoplakia and Nabothian cysts, should be documented. A thorough bimanual examination is a standard part of an annual evaluation, with attention to size and position of the uterus and any nodularity or masses noted in the parauterine and adnexal regions.[4]

Laboratory Studies

Thin-layer ("thin-prep") cytology is now the standard collection technique for Pap smear. This specimen has the same sensitivity as older, conventional smears and also allows for detection of HPV in the same sample. The "broom" is centered over the cervical os and twirled with pressure against the cervix two full rotations, and then deposited into the collection medium. In patients whom have had hysterectomy for advanced cervical dysplasia/cancer, the vaginal cuff is sampled. It is standard care now to request reflex testing for high-risk HPV subtypes if "atypical squamous cells of undetermined significance" (ASCUS) is found in the sample (discussed further under Pathologic Findings).[4]

Pathologic Findings

Adequacy of the collection is noted on the pathologist's report; if endocervical cells are not detected in a patient who has a cervix, whether or not it should be recollected depends on age and HPV status. If the specimen is reported as inadequate, it should be recollected in 2 to 4 months. The Bethesda system adopted in 2001 includes the following:
- **Statement of adequacy of the sample**
- **A general categorization** of the findings, benign or malignant
- **Descriptive diagnoses** that may include benign changes (reactive, or secondary to infection). Epithelial changes may be squamous or glandular. The squamous components include ASCUS; HPV changes including "koilocytotic atypia," low-grade squamous intraepithelial lesion (LSIL), high-grade squamous intraepithelial lesion (HSIL), and squamous cell cancer (SCC). The glandular components include atypical glandular cells of undetermined significance (AGUS), adenocarcinoma *in situ* (AIS), and adenocarcinoma.[5]

TREATMENT
Nonoperative

Patients with Pap smears showing ASCUS with high-risk HPV subtypes present, and with LSIL, HSIL, or SCC need colposcopic evaluation. ASCUS without high-risk HPV present may repeat co-testing in 3 years. Those with cytology negative but HPV-positive test results can be followed with repeat co-testing in 12 months or HPV DNA typing may be done and those with HPV 16 or 18 should undergo colposcopy. Any other subtypes may repeat co-testing in 1 year. Patients with

AGUS should undergo colposcopy, and endometrial biopsy if appropriate. Adenocarcinoma, in situ or otherwise should be referred to a gynecologic oncologist, as the source of the abnormal cells could be endometrial, tubal, ovarian, or even from non-gynecological abdominal metastasis.[4]

Operative

After colposcopy with appropriate biopsies and endocervical curettage, patients are managed on the basis of American Society for Colposcopy and Cervical Pathology (ASCCP) guidelines. Recommendations may include a diagnostic excisional procedure.[4]

Counseling

With the ease and efficacy of modern techniques for the management of Pap smear abnormalities, virtually all patients can be assured that they will never develop cervical cancer if they maintain appropriate follow-up visits for any abnormalities. Counseling about the risk factors for accelerating their risk of cancer (new contacts, smoking) is appropriate.[4]

Follow-Up

Telephone follow-up with abnormal Pap smear results is usually appropriate. Normal results are often notified by mail. Patients should be specifically told when their next screening is due. Guidelines for follow-up Pap, HPV testing, and/or colposcopy are well established by the ASCCP.[4]

Complications

Other than transient discomfort and occasional mild spotting, collection of Pap smears is not associated with any complications.

REFERENCES

1. Papanicolaou GN, Traut HF. Diagnosis of uterine cancer by the vaginal smear. *Yale J Biol Med* 1943;15:924.
2. U.S. Cancer statistics Working Group. *United States cancer statistics: 1999–2010 incidence and mortality web-based report*. Atlanta, GA: U.S. Department of Health and Human Services, Center for Disease Control and Prevention and National Cancer Institute; 2013. www.cdc.gov/uscs. Accessed July 19, 2014.
3. Feldman S, Sirovich BE, Goodman A. Screening for cervical cancer: Rationale and recommendations. *Uptodate.* uptodate.com. Accessed July 19, 2014.
4. Saslow DS, Solomon D, Lawson HW, et al. American Cancer Society, American Society for Colposcopy and Cervical Pathology, and American Society for Clinical Pathology screening guidelines for the prevention and early detection of cervical cancer. *CA Cancer J Clin* 2012;62(3):147–172.
5. Solomon D, Davey D, Kurman R, et al. The 2001 Bethesda System terminology for reporting results of cervical cytology. *JAMA* 2002;287:2114–2119.

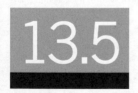

13.5 Pelvic Inflammatory Disease

Martin A. Quan

GENERAL PRINCIPLES

Definition

Acute pelvic inflammatory disease (PID) is an ascending infection of the female genital tract involving the uterus, fallopian tubes, ovaries, and adjacent pelvic structures.

Epidemiology

• More than 750,000 American women are diagnosed and treated for acute PID each year.[1]
• Direct medical costs of PID are estimated at $1.5 billion per year.[2]

Pathophysiology

- PID arises from the ascent of microorganisms from the vagina and cervix into the upper female genital tract.
- Although PID commonly stems from a cervicitis caused by *Neisseria gonorrhoeae* or *Chlamydia trachomatis*, there is evidence that an imbalance in the vaginal ecosystem, such as that seen in bacterial vaginosis, may also play a role in initiating the ascending infection.[3]

Etiology

- Microorganisms recovered from the upper genital tract of women with PID include *C. trachomatis*, *N. gonorrhoeae*, and anaerobic and aerobic bacteria of the endogenous vaginal flora, including *Prevotella* species, *Peptostreptococcus*, aerobic *Streptococcus*, *Gardnerella vaginalis*, *Haemophilus influenzae*, and enteric Gram-negative rods.[4]
- Epidemiologic risk factors that identify a patient at increased risk for acute PID include age less than 25 years, sexarche prior to age 16 years, multiple sexual partners, history of a sexually transmitted disease (including PID), the postinsertion period in intrauterine device (IUD) users, vaginal douching, and the presence of bacterial vaginosis.[2,5,6]

DIAGNOSIS

- As a result of the difficulty of diagnosis and its serious consequences if left untreated, guidelines for its diagnosis developed by the U.S. Centers for Disease Control and Prevention (CDC) reflect a lowering of the diagnostic threshold.[7]
- Once competing diagnoses are adequately excluded in a woman at risk for sexually transmitted diseases (STDs), the CDC recommends that a provisional diagnosis of PID be made and a therapeutic trial of antibiotics be initiated in patients who meet one or more of the following criteria on pelvic examination:
  - Cervical motion tenderness
  - Uterine tenderness
  - Adnexal tenderness
- Although not required, corroborating diagnostic laboratory, imaging, and surgical procedures should be sought in patients with an unclear diagnosis, no evidence of lower-genital-tract inflammation, and severe symptoms, or who fail to respond to therapy.[3,7]

Clinical Presentation

PID can present with a wide spectrum of nonspecific clinical symptoms and signs, ranging in degree from mild to severe.

History

- Lower abdominal pain, usually described as constant and dull, of less than 14-days duration is the most common complaint reported by patients with acute PID.
- Other manifestations include abnormal vaginal discharge, abnormal vaginal bleeding, gastrointestinal upset, and dysuria.
- Right upper quadrant pain secondary to perihepatitis (Fitz–Hugh–Curtis syndrome) is seen in up to 10% to 15% of patients.[8]

Physical Examination

- Cervical motion tenderness and adnexal tenderness (unilateral in up to 20% of cases) are the physical findings most frequently elicited in patients with PID.
- Rebound tenderness is present in two thirds of patients, and an adnexal mass or fullness in 16% to 49% of patients.
- Although a temperature of 38.3°C or higher supports the diagnosis, it is important to be aware that fever is a variable finding present in 24% to 60% of patients.[9]

Laboratory Studies

- *White blood count.* A leukocytosis is present only 60% of the time.
- *Erythrocyte sedimentation rate (ESR).* Although classically elevated in PID, the ESR is normal (less than 15 mm per hour) in 25% of patients.
- *C-reactive protein.* An elevated C-reactive protein (CRP) >10 mg per dL has been found in up to 93% of patients with PID.[10]
- Examination of the male partner for the presence of urethritis can be a source of confirmatory evidence for the diagnosis of PID.

- A sensitive pregnancy test should be routinely obtained in all patients with suspected PID because of the great difficulty encountered in clinically differentiating patients with PID from those with ectopic pregnancy.[11]
- The finding of mucopurulent cervicitis or evidence of white cells on microscopic examination of a saline preparation of vaginal fluid is seen in the great majority of patients with PID. If both are absent, the diagnosis of PID is unlikely and alternative causes of pain should be considered.[7,10,12]
- Laboratory documentation of a cervical infection with *N. gonorrhoeae* or *C. trachomatis* corroborates the diagnosis of PID.[7]
  - Cultures have traditionally been regarded as the gold standard.
  - Nucleic acid amplification tests for the detection of *C. trachomatis* and *N. gonorrhoeae* are preferred.

Imaging

- **Transvaginal pelvic ultrasonography.** Sonographic findings supportive of the diagnosis include:
  - Thickened, fluid-filled fallopian tubes
  - Fluid in the cul-de-sac
  - A complex, multiloculated adnexal mass
  - Hyperemia on power Doppler transvaginal sonography[3,13]
- **Magnetic resonance imaging (MRI).** MRI findings that support the diagnosis of PID include:
  - Fluid-filled tubes
  - Thickened tube walls with a dilated lumen
  - An ill-defined adnexal mass with thickened walls containing fluid[14,15]

Surgical Diagnostic Procedures

- **Endometrial biopsy.** The histopathologic finding of neutrophil and plasma cell infiltration in the endometrial stroma obtained on biopsy confirms the diagnosis of PID.[10]
- **Diagnostic laparoscopy**
  - Diagnostic laparoscopy is regarded by many authorities as the standard for the diagnosis of acute PID.
  - Criteria required for the diagnosis include abnormal erythema and edema of the fallopian tubes and sticky exudate on tubal surfaces and from fimbriated ends.[10]

TREATMENT

- Once the diagnosis of PID is made, 2010 CDC guidelines favor hospitalization under the following circumstances:
  - A surgical emergency, such as ectopic pregnancy or acute appendicitis, cannot be adequately excluded
  - A tubo-ovarian abscess is present
  - Pregnancy
  - Failure to respond clinically to oral antimicrobial therapy
  - Severe illness, nausea and vomiting, or high fever
  - Inability to follow or tolerate an outpatient oral regimen[7]

Medications

Antibiotic therapy is the cornerstone of treatment for acute PID. Empirical, broad-spectrum antimicrobial therapy targeting *N. gonorrhoeae*, *C. trachomatis*, enteric Gram-negative facultative bacteria (including *Escherichia coli*), and certain anaerobic bacteria is recommended.

- **Inpatient regimens.** Parenteral therapy can be discontinued as soon as 24 hours after the patient has improved clinically. Regimens recommended by the 2010 CDC guidelines are as follows:
  - Doxycycline 100 mg IV (or PO) q12h, plus cefoxitin 2 g IV q6h (or cefotetan 2 g IV q12h), followed by doxycycline 100 mg PO bid for a total of 14 days.
  - Clindamycin 900 mg IV q8h, plus gentamicin 2.0 mg per kg IV, followed by 1.5 mg per kg IV q8h, followed by either doxycycline 100 mg PO bid, or clindamycin 450 mg PO four times daily to complete 14 days of total therapy.[7]
- **Outpatient regimens.** Suggested regimens are as follows:
  - Cefoxitin 2 g IM plus probenecid 1 g PO concurrently, or ceftriaxone 250 mg IM, plus doxycycline 100 mg PO bid for 14 days with or without metronidazole 500 mg PO bid for 14 days.
  - Other parenteral third-generation cephalosporin (e.g., ceftizoxime or cefotaxime), plus doxycycline 100 mg PO bid for 14 days with or without metronidazole 500 mg PO bid for 14 days.[7]

Surgery

- Surgical treatment has a limited role in the management of PID.
- Possible indications include the confirmation of the diagnosis in a patient failing to respond to therapy, excision of chronically infected pelvic organs, and draining of pelvic abscesses.

Nonoperative

- General supportive measures, such as bed rest, sexual abstinence until cure is achieved, hydration, and provision of antipyretics and appropriate analgesia, are recommended in the management of PID.
- Although there is no evidence that IUDs have to be removed in women diagnosed with acute PID, if the IUD is not removed CDC guidelines mandate that close clinical follow-up be provided.

Follow-Up

- Patients should be seen within 3 days after initiation of therapy.
- Patients who fail to respond require careful reevaluation of both the diagnosis and therapy.
- Male sex partners who have had contact with the patient during the preceding 60 days should be evaluated and provided empiric treatment for *Chlamydia* and gonorrhea. If more than 60 days have elapsed since the patient's last sexual intercourse, the patient's most recent sexual partner should be treated.
- Patients should be provided counseling regarding safe sexual behavior, the use of condoms as a means for preventing the transmission of STDs, and the advisability of HIV testing.
- Periodic screening for *Chlamydia* is recommended in sexually active women at risk for this infection, such as unmarried women 25 years of age or younger.[16]

Complications

- Tubal factor infertility is seen in 8% to 12% of patients after one episode of PID, 20% to 25% after two episodes, and 40% to 50% after three episodes or more.
- Chronic pelvic pain has been reported in 15% to 20% of patients after PID.
- The risk of ectopic pregnancy is increased 3- to 10-fold in a patient with a history of PID.[6,8]

REFERENCES

1. Sutton MY, Sternberg M, Zaidi A, et al. Trends in pelvic inflammatory disease hospital discharges and ambulatory visits, United States, 1985–2001. *Sex Transm Dis* 2005;32:778–84.
2. Gradison M. Pelvic inflammatory disease. *Am Fam Physician* 2012;85:791–796.
3. Soper DE. Pelvic inflammatory disease. *Obstet Gynecol* 2010;116:419–428.
4. Sweet RL. Treatment of acute pelvic inflammatory disease. *Infect Dis Obstet Gynecol* 2011;2011:561909. doi: 10.1155/2011/561909.
5. Simms I, Stephenson JM, Mallinson H, et al. Risk factors associated with pelvic inflammatory disease. *Sex Transm Infect* 2006;82:452–457.
6. Taylor BD, Darville T, Haggerty CL. Does bacterial vaginosis cause pelvic inflammatory disease? *Sex Transm Dis* 2013;40:117–122.
7. Centers for Disease Control and Prevention. Sexually transmitted diseases treatment guidelines, 2010. *MMWR* 2010;59(No. RR-12):63–69.
8. Banikarim C, Chacko MR. Pelvic inflammatory disease in adolescents. *Semin Pediatr Infect Dis* 2005;16:175–180.
9. Quan M. Pelvic inflammatory disease: diagnosis and management. *J Am Board Fam Pract* 1994;7:110.
10. Jaiyeoba O, Soper DE. A practical approach to the diagnosis of pelvic inflammatory disease. *Infect Dis Obstet Gynecol* 2011;2010:753037. doi: 10.1155/2011/753037.
11. American College of Obstetricians and Gynecologists. ACOG practice bulletin no. 94. Medical management of ectopic pregnancy. *Obstet Gynecol* 2008;111:1479–1485.
12. Mitchell C, Prabhu M. Pelvic inflammatory disease: current concepts in pathogenesis, diagnosis and treatment. *Infect Dis Clin N Am* 2013;27:793–809.
13. Cicchiello LA, Hampe UM, Scoutt LM. Ultrasound evaluation of gynecologic causes of pelvic pain. *Obstet Gynecol Clin North Am* 2011;38:85–114.
14. Li W, Zhang Y, Cui Y, et al. Pelvic inflammatory disease: evaluation of diagnostic accuracy with conventional MR with added diffusion-weighted imaging. *Abdom Imaging* 2013;38:193–200.
15. Vandermeer FQ, Wong-You-Cheong JJ. Imaging of acute pelvic pain. *Clin Obstet Gynecol* 2009;52:2–20.
16. Gottlieb SL, Xu F, Brunham RC. Screening and treating chlamydia trachomatis genital infection to prevent pelvic inflammatory disease: interpretation of findings from randomized controlled trials. *Sex Trans Dis* 2011;40:97–102.

13.6 Menopause

Alisha E. O'Malley

GENERAL PRINCIPLES

Definition

Menopause is defined as the failure of ovarian follicle development in the presence of adequate gonadotropin stimulation, resulting in the cessation of spontaneous menstrual periods. A woman is considered to be postmenopausal after 12 months of amenorrhea without another physiologic or pathological cause.

Epidemiology

The average age for menopause is 51 years.[1] Factors that can lower the age of menopause include smoking, hysterectomy, oophorectomy, genetic disorders, autoimmune disorders, high altitude, and a history of chemotherapy or radiation.

Classification

Menopause may be secondary to surgical intervention or drug effect, particularly chemotherapeutic agents. Evidence of menopause before 40 years of age is considered premature ovarian failure and usually necessitates a workup.

Pathophysiology

Vasomotor symptoms are not fully understood but may relate to estrogen withdrawal and a narrowed thermoregulatory zone, resulting in increased sensitivity to temperature change. Symptoms are often worse in obese women, possibly due to the insulating effects or endocrine effects of adipose tissue. Vasomotor symptoms are also associated with depression, anxiety, smoking, and low socioeconomic status.[1] The vaginal epithelium is estrogen-dependent, and declining estrogen levels lead to thinning of the vaginal mucosa, loss of rugae, and narrowing and shortening of the vagina. There is also a loss of subcutaneous fat in the labia majora. Vaginal pH increases, altering vaginal flora, and vaginal secretions decrease. These changes may result in infection, fissures or tears, fusion of labia minora, and shrinking of the clitoris and urethra. Decreased libido may be secondary to dyspareunia, stress, depression, or hormonal changes. Estrogen deficiency leads to decreased osteoblastic activity with increased osteoclastic activity, resulting in osteoporosis and risk for fractures.

DIAGNOSIS

Clinical Presentation

Perimenopause, or the menopausal transition, often begins as early as 6 years before the last period.[1] During this time, women may experience signs or symptoms such as irregular periods, mood changes, insomnia, weight gain, bloating, vaginal dryness, decreased libido, headaches, or vasomotor instability (hot flashes). Hot flashes, which affect 80% of perimenopausal women, are described as intense warmth and profuse sweating, which may be accompanied by palpitations and redness of the skin. They last from seconds to minutes, rarely up to 1 hour, and may occur as often as 20 times per day. As ovarian response to gonadotropins declines in the postmenopausal years, associated symptoms decrease, also. After menopause, fibroids, endometriosis, and adenomyosis become less symptomatic. Prolapse of genitourinary organs may occur as loss of pelvic muscle tone occurs. Atrophic vaginitis may lead to insertional dyspareunia. Atrophic cystitis may mimic a urinary tract infection (UTI), and is also a risk factor for UTIs.

History

The history should focus on gynecologic and cardiovascular history, family history of breast or uterine cancer, and risk factors for osteoporosis and coronary artery disease. Note the frequency and severity of menopausal symptoms and their effect on the patient's overall function.

Physical Examination

The physical examination should be complete, including vital signs, thyroid, cardiovascular, breast, and pelvic examination. Pelvic examination at first reveals reddened vaginal epithelium as the skin thins and capillaries are more visible. After time, the number of capillaries decreases and the vaginal epithelium becomes pale. Rugation of the vaginal mucosa decreases, the uterus and ovaries diminish in size, and loss of pelvic tone may lead to prolapse. A palpable ovary on bimanual examination in a postmenopausal woman is abnormal and warrants a full evaluation. Pap smear should be completed if not up-to-date.

Laboratory Studies

A persistently elevated follicle-stimulating hormone (FSH) level confirms the diagnosis of menopause. Eventually FSH will increase 10- to 20-fold, while luteinizing hormone (LH) will increase to three times that of premenopausal levels. Conversely, estradiol and inhibin levels decline. Estradiol, inhibin, and LH values are not necessary to diagnose menopause. If the diagnosis is uncertain, repeat measurement of FSH and LH every 2 to 3 months may be helpful. Laboratory testing may include thyroid function tests or other tests as indicated by history and physical examination. Urine culture should be done for women complaining of UTI symptoms, even if they may be related to atrophic cystitis.

Imaging

Imaging is not necessary to diagnose menopause. Pelvic ultrasound to assess for endometrial hyperplasia is recommended in postmenopausal uterine bleeding. Bone densitometry testing should be done starting at 65 years of age or earlier for those with risk factors. Bone loss accelerates in the late perimenopausal years and continues after menopause. Mammograms are currently recommended for all women ages 50 to 74 and may be indicated for certain women at younger ages.

Surgical Diagnostic Procedures

Endometrial biopsy to rule out endometrial cancer should be performed on women with abnormal uterine bleeding and an endometrial stripe measuring more than 5 mm by ultrasound.

Differential Diagnosis

The differential diagnosis of vasomotor instability includes alcohol withdrawal, anxiety disorders, carcinoid tumor, epilepsy, insulin reaction, pheochromocytoma, thyrotoxicosis, and drug effects.

TREATMENT

Treatment of menopausal symptoms should be tailored to the severity of symptoms. Mild symptoms may be treated with behavioral modification, whereas more severe symptoms may require pharmacologic therapy. There is a significant placebo effect in the treatment of hot flashes, with up to 25% reduction in the number of hot flashes with placebo in controlled trials.[1]

Behavioral

Nonpharmacologic treatments for hot flashes include fans; cool drinks; lower ambient temperature; loose or layered clothing; and avoidance of alcohol, caffeine, and spicy foods. Risk of osteoporosis may be reduced by weight-bearing exercise and smoking cessation.

Medications

Estrogen has been used in the treatment of perimenopausal symptoms for more than 50 years. Selective serotonin reuptake inhibitors (SSRIs), serotonin–norepinephrine reuptake inhibitors (SNRIs), gabapentin, and clonidine can be useful alternatives to hormonal therapies for treatment of vasomotor symptoms. Paroxetine is the only nonhormonal treatment approved by the FDA for treatment of vasomotor symptoms. The FDA has approved ospemifene for treating moderate-to-severe dyspareunia in postmenopausal women. Estrogens, selective estrogen receptor modulators (SERMs), and bisphosphonates are approved for the prevention and treatment of osteoporosis.

- **Hormone replacement therapy (HRT)** is the most effective therapy for vasomotor symptoms of menopause. HRT may also improve mood symptoms, fatigue, incontinence, and vaginal dryness. Low-dose estrogen (0.3 to 0.45 mg per day conjugated estrogen, 0.5 mg per day micronized estradiol, 5 mcg per day ethinyl estradiol, or 0.025 to 0.0375 mg per week transdermal estradiol) or ultra-low-dose estrogen (0.25 mg per day micronized estradiol or 0.014 mg per week transdermal estradiol) regimens have a better side effect profile and may be effective. HRT may be administered orally or transdermally in the forms of patches, gels, or sprays. Contraindications to estrogen therapy include undiagnosed vaginal bleeding, liver disease, pregnancy, venous thromboembolism (VTE), and personal history of breast cancer. Well-differentiated early endometrial cancer after complete treatment is no longer an absolute contraindication.

- **Risks of HRT:** The Women's Health Initiative (WHI) study, a large randomized controlled trial (RCT) of healthy women 50 to 77 years old, demonstrated that after an average of 5 years of combined HRT, women had slightly increased risk of coronary artery disease, stroke, VTE, and breast cancer and a decreased risk of colon cancer and fractures.[2] For women receiving estrogen without progestin, there was an increased risk of VTE but not of cardiovascular disease or breast cancer.[3] It should be noted that these women were already past the menopausal transition, so it is difficult to extrapolate these data to general populations. Later analysis of the WHI data in women 55 to 60 years of age and within 10 years of menopause suggests a possible cardioprotective effect of HRT for these younger women. However, follow-up of these women at 13 years confirmed that the risks of combined HRT for primary prevention outweigh the benefits.[4] A Cochrane review of HRT completed in 2012 similarly showed that HRT should not be used for primary prevention because the risks outweigh the benefits. Different forms of HRT may have different risk profiles based on observational studies, and additional randomized trials are needed to further investigate this. Yearly mammograms are necessary for all women on HRT. An on-going discussion should be held at each healthcare maintenance visit regarding symptoms and treatment, with the goal of using the lowest possible dose of HRT for the shortest amount of time possible for each individual patient. Discontinuation may lead to return of vasomotor symptoms in up to half of women, regardless of age and duration of use. There are insufficient data to recommend tapering the dose versus abrupt cessation.
- **Estrogen/progestin combination therapy** is necessary in patients with an intact uterus or with endometriosis remaining after hysterectomy to avoid endometrial hyperplasia and development of endometrial cancer. Some studies suggest that addition of progestin to estrogen replacement leads to greater improvement of vasomotor symptoms. The progestin in combination therapy may be dosed in either a continuous or a cyclic manner.
- **Continuous progestin dosing** causes breakthrough bleeding in half of women in the first 6 months of therapy. Endometrial biopsy is indicated for breakthrough bleeding beyond this time frame. The progestin dose may be doubled if no pathology is found on biopsy.
- **Cyclic progestin dosing** causes less breakthrough bleeding but may worsen migraine headaches. Nonsmoking perimenopausal women may use low-dose oral contraceptive pills for regulation of menses, relief of vasomotor symptoms, and contraception.
- **Progestin-only therapy** has some evidence of relieving vasomotor symptoms. However, there are limited data on the safety of progestin alone. Furthermore, the rate of breast cancer was higher in the combined arm than in the estrogen-only arm of the WHI, indicating a possible correlation between progestin therapy and breast cancer risk.
- **Vaginal estrogen** in the form of cream, ring, or tablet may reverse vaginal atrophy if dosed daily for 1 to 2 weeks. This benefit is maintained with two to three treatments per week or a decreased daily dose. There is theoretical concern for endometrial hyperplasia or cancer in long-term vaginal estrogen therapy. However, a Cochrane meta-analysis showed no increase in either of these outcomes, so addition of progestin is not necessary for patients using vaginal estrogen.[1] Vaginal estrogen at low doses may be used indefinitely. The 3-month estradiol-releasing vaginal ring is often easier to use than daily tablets or creams.
- **SERMs** such as **tamoxifen** and **raloxifene** have not been shown to be beneficial in treating vasomotor or vaginal symptoms. **Ospemifene** (60 mg per day) is a novel SERM that has been shown to improve vaginal atrophy without stimulating the endometrium, and was recently approved by the FDA for treatment of moderate-to-severe dyspareunia in postmenopausal women. Side effects include hot flashes, vaginal discharge, muscle spasms, and excessive sweating.
- **Estrogen/SERM combination therapy** may be an alternative to estrogen plus progestin. A combination of **conjugated estrogen and bazedoxifene (Duavee)** has been approved by the FDA recently for treatment of vasomotor symptoms and to prevent osteoporosis in postmenopausal women with a uterus. This medication significantly reduces the number of vasomotor symptoms and increases bone mineral density compared to placebo.[5]
- **Plant-derived phytoestrogens** found in soy, wheat, cereals, nuts, and apples are converted to estrogens in the gut. These estrogens may have agonist and/or antagonist activity when bound to estrogen receptors. Controlled trials have not shown these to be efficacious for treatment of vasomotor symptoms.

- **Testosterone therapy** has not been shown to decrease vasomotor symptoms, and has adverse effects of acne, hirsutism, and dyslipidemia. A Cochrane review did show that addition of testosterone to HRT improves sexual function in postmenopausal women.[6]
- **SSRIs and SNRIs such as paroxetine, citalopram, fluoxetine,** and **venlafaxine** may reduce hot flashes. Side effects may include dry mouth, dizziness, nausea, constipation, sweating, and sexual dysfunction, but these often resolve with time or dose adjustment. Only paroxetine (7.5 mg per day) is FDA-approved for treatment of vasomotor symptoms.
- **Gabapentin** (900 mg per day) is associated with a 45% decrease in frequency and 54% decrease in severity of hot flashes.[7] Side effects include dizziness, somnolence, and peripheral edema.
- **Clonidine** (0.1 mg per day) may reduce hot flashes, although data are limited. Possible side effects include insomnia, dry mouth, and drowsiness.
- **Vitamin E** therapy (800 U per day) has had anecdotal reports of improvement in hot flashes. However, no significant benefit was noted over placebo during controlled trials.
- **Water-based or silicone-based lubricants** may help symptoms of vaginal dryness.
- Data do not support the use of **compounded bio-identical hormones; synthetic steroids; alternative therapies such as acupuncture and reflexology; or herbal remedies** such as **black cohosh, evening primrose,** or **red clover extract. Black cohosh** in particular should not be used for more than 6 months due to concern for liver toxicity.

Follow-Up

Follow-up in 3 to 6 months after initiation of therapy for menopausal symptoms is recommended to determine the adequacy of the regimen and review side effects. Once an appropriate regimen has been established, the patient should be evaluated yearly.

REFERENCES

1. ACOG practice bulletin 141: management of menopausal symptoms. *Obstet Gynecol* 2014;123:202–216.
2. Rossouw J, Anderson G, Prentice R, et al.; Writing Group for the Women's Health Initiative Investigators. Risks and benefits of estrogen plus progestin in healthy postmenopausal women: principal results From the Women's Health Initiative randomized controlled trial. *JAMA* 2002;288:321–333.
3. Anderson G, Limacher M, Assaf A, et al.; Women's Health Initiative Steering Committee. Effects of conjugated equine estrogen in postmenopausal women with hysterectomy: the Women's Health Initiative randomized controlled trial. *JAMA* 2004;291:1701–1712.
4. Manson J, Chlebowski R, Stefanick M, et al. Menopausal hormone therapy and health outcomes during the intervention and extended poststopping phases of the Women's Health Initiative randomized trials. *JAMA* 2013;310:1353–1368.
5. Tella SH, Gallagher JC. Bazedoxifene + conjugated estrogens in HT for the prevention of osteoporosis and treatment of vasomotor symptoms associated with the menopause. *Expert Opin Pharmacother* 2013;14:2407–2420.
6. Somboonporn W, Bell R, Davis S. Testosterone for peri and postmenopausal women. *Cochrane Database Syst Rev* 2005;(4):CD004509. doi: 10.1002/14651858.
7. Guttuso T Jr, Kurlan R, McDermott M, et al. Gabapentin's effects on hot flashes in postmenopausal women: a randomized controlled trial. *Obstet Gynecol* 2003;101:337–345.

Benign Breast Conditions and Disease

Brian P. Jundt

GENERAL PRINCIPLES

Definition

Benign breast conditions encompass a multitude of conditions united only in that cancer and precancerous lesions are excluded. Many women present to their physician for benign conditions of the breast that they perceive to be abnormal. Common complaints include pain, hypertrophy, breast lumps, breast infections, and nipple discharge. The health care provider must differentiate benign from malignant disease, reassure patients with benign conditions, manage common symptoms and conditions, and seek consultation when necessary. The provider must recognize the emotional distress common during this process and provide timely and effective communication.

Anatomy and Breast Development

The adult breast is a tear-shaped milk-producing gland supported and attached to the chest wall by the Cooper suspensory ligaments. The adult breast is located between the second and sixth ribs in the vertical axis, between the sternal edge and the midaxillary line in the horizontal axis, and extends into the axilla. Each breast is composed of 15 to 20 lobes, each composed of multiple lobules. Glandular milk-producing lobules drain through a series of branching ducts to the nipple, and are supported by fibrous tissue, or stroma. Typically, there are 6 to 10 pinhole openings on the areola, each draining a duct that leads to a single lobe. Because more lobes are present in the outer quadrants, especially the upper outer quadrants, many breast conditions (including breast cancer) occur more frequently in these regions.[1]

Breast development and change may be seen as a process of dynamic change beginning with embryonic development and continuing through the postmenopausal years. Newborns commonly have hypertrophied breast tissue caused by stimulation from maternal estrogen and progesterone. In most cases spontaneous regression occurs. Prepubertal children may develop unilateral or bilateral soft mobile subareolar nodules of uniform consistency that usually resolve spontaneously within a few months. Biopsy should be avoided as it may impair pubertal breast development. In girls, puberty marks the normal onset of glandular proliferation within the breast. For most girls, breast bud development (thelarche) is the first sign of puberty (typically between ages 10 and 12), while full breast development is usually the last sign. Thelarche is considered "premature" if it occurs earlier than age 8. Premature thelarche without other signs of pubertal development or accelerated growth is usually benign. No treatment is needed if medical evaluation excludes true precocious puberty, estrogen-producing tumors, ovarian cysts, or exogenous estrogen exposure. Other signs of puberty generally begin within 6 months of breast development and are completed within 4 years. Breast development may begin on one side and be asymmetrical. If there is a discrepancy in size, the left breast is usually larger. Breast development is considered "delayed" if stage 1 persists beyond 13.5 years; stage 2 persists more than 1 year; stage 3 greater than 2.2 years; or stage 4 more than 6 to 8 years.[1]

The normal breast changes in size and texture throughout the menstrual cycle as well. During the premenstrual phase, acinar cells, or the cells of the terminal duct-lobule unit, increase in number and size, the ductal lumens widen, and breast size and turgor increase. These changes reverse in the postmenstrual phase.[1]

Gynecomastia, or the proliferation of glandular breast tissue in a male, is common in the middle phases of pubertal development and in adulthood. In puberty, this may be attributed to serum estradiol levels rising to adult levels before serum testosterone levels. Although it can be psychologically disturbing, workup is indicated only if there is rapid progression, onset before puberty, or association with true precocious puberty. More than 90% of affected boys experience regression within 3 years.[2]

Classification of Conditions

Nipple Anomalies

The most common anomaly is polythelia, or, accessory nipple. Ectopic nipple tissue may occur at any point in the embryonic breast line, from the groin to the axilla. In many instances, an accessory nipple may be misdiagnosed as a nevus or dermatofibroma. Other nipple findings include discharge, Paget disease, and painful nipples.

Breast Infections

Infectious disease of the breast may include mastitis, abscess, or cellulitis. In evaluating and treating infections of the breast, it is important to determine whether the woman is lactating.

Structural/Functional Anomalies

These changes encompass many common complaints, including palpable masses as well as cyclical and noncyclical breast pain.

ASSESSMENT OF AN INDIVIDUAL WITH BREAST COMPLAINTS

History

In taking the history of the breast complaint, it is important that many areas of relevant history are obtained. Questions should focus on areas such as breast lump characteristics, diet and medications, family history, past medical and surgical history, social history, gynecological history, and context in which the breast lump was discovered.

In gathering history of breast lump characteristics, questions should be focused on changes in size of lump over time and in relation to menstrual cycle, how long the mass has been present, and if any pain, swelling, erythema, or discharge has been present. Past and current medications along with whether or not the patient has been on hormone therapy should be documented also. Important medical and surgical history should include questions about any personal history of breast cancer, previous lumps or biopsies, recent breast trauma, and any past or current radiation or chemotherapy. Family history should include information on any family member with a history of breast or ovarian cancer. Along with past medical, surgical, and family history, a social history should be obtained and include tobacco use, illicit substance use, and alcohol use. Finally, a gynecological history should be obtained and include age at first childbearing, age at menarche, age at menopause if applicable, current lactation status, history of breastfeeding, and number of children.[3–5]

Examination of the Breast

- Inspection is first followed by palpation. The examination should be performed in a well-lit room, and privacy is facilitated by draping parts of the body not being examined. Inspection occurs with the patient seated, arms at side; seated with hands on hips; seated with arms above the head; and supine with one arm raised at a time. Changes in size, shape, symmetry, or texture are noted. Palpation is performed with the patient supine, arms flexed at a 90-degree angle at the sides utilizing the "triple touch" technique of palpation of superficial, intermediate, and deep tissue planes. Palpation includes supraclavicular, infraclavicular, and axillary nodes. Compression may identify a mass and/or elicit a discharge. Nipples should be examined for deviation, retraction, skin changes, or discharge.[6]

Laboratory Evaluation

Currently, genetic screening is not part of the routine evaluation of individuals with breast-related complaints.

Diagnostic Tests

- **Imaging.** Mammography is discussed elsewhere in this manual. When mammography is indicated, a "diagnostic" rather than a "screening" mammogram is obtained to evaluate women with breast complaints. Important diagnostic information may be obtained regarding a known or undetected mass. However, a negative mammogram should never preclude biopsy of an appropriate palpable lesion. Since mammography is unable to visualize lesions well in younger women, ultrasonography may be preferable in women under 30 years of age to differentiate whether a mass is solid or cystic and as an adjunct to aspiration or biopsy. Magnetic resonance imaging is utilized in patients with silicone breast implants, women with a family history of breast cancer or known genetic susceptibility, and special circumstances. These circumstances include patients who have had breast conserving surgery, have known carcinoma needing further evaluation, have axillary metastasis and unknown primary tumor, have extensive postoperative scarring, or have extremely dense stroma.[6]

- **Aspiration.** A cystic lesion or lesion of uncertain nature may be aspirated both diagnostically and therapeutically.[6]
- **Fine-needle aspiration (FNA).** FNA involves cytologic aspirate of a mass using a 22- to 25-gauge needle usually with ultrasound or stereotactic guidance. Specimen must have adequate number of epithelial cells for interpretation (sensitivity 98% to 99% for malignancy).[6]
- **Fine-needle aspiration and biopsy (FNAB).** Indications for biopsy include any suspicious lesion; bloody nipple discharge or bloody fluid following cyst aspiration; persistent mass; suspicious skin changes; inflammatory changes unresponsive to antibiotic; suspicious axillary nodes; or suspicious microcalcifications on mammography. A 14- to 18-gauge needle is used to obtain six scores of the mass for histology.[6]
- **Triple test.** The "triple test" combines physical examination, mammography, and FNAB. The test utilizes a Triple Test Score. The three-point scale is used for each component of the test. A score of 1 is benign, 2 is suspicious, and 3 is malignant. A Triple Test Score of 3 to 4 is consistent with a benign lesion, a score of 5 indicates that further information should be obtained such as an excisional biopsy, and a score of greater than 6 indicates possible malignancy is present.[6]
- **Excisional biopsy.** The excisional biopsy is the gold standard for evaluating breast masses. The entire lesion is removed usually in an operating room. The biopsy can be both diagnostic and therapeutic if negative margins are present. Due to the increase in FNAB, excisional biopsies have declined.[6]

Pathologic Findings

Benign breast lesions diagnosed by the above methods may be subdivided based on the degree of risk they confer for the future development of malignancy. Such categorization is usually determined by proliferation and atypia. Lesions associated with an increased risk of developing breast cancer include any proliferative lesion, common benign lesions in patients older than 50 (such as cyst, adenosis, mammary duct ectasia fibrosis, metaplasia, fibroadenoma), mild/moderate or florid hyperplasia without atypia and simple papilloma. This risk is likely increased in patients with a strong family history of breast cancer. Findings with a small increase in relative risk include ductal hyperplasia without atypia, sclerosing adenosis, diffuse papillomas, complex fibroadenomas, and radial scars. Lesions conferring moderately increased risk include atypical ductal hyperplasia and atypical lobular hyperplasia. Both of the aforementioned lesions also confer an increased risk for development of breast cancer in the contralateral breast.

   Emotional well-being of the patient. The evaluation of a breast complaint is extremely stressful for many women. Most patients assume that their sign or symptom indicates cancer. The provider should anticipate the emotional responses typical in patients and family members. Timely assessment, diagnostic evaluation, and consultation when necessary should be provided. It may be useful to inquire how best to assist with the period of uncertainty and how the patient would like results conveyed to her. Realistic estimates of the likely time involved in diagnosis are beneficial. Adequate time should be made available to address questions and additional methods of contact (office visits, telephone calls, or e-mail) should be offered.[4]

BREAST PAIN

Mastalgia is an extremely common complaint among women accounting for 66% of physician visits for breast complaints, which may interfere significantly with quality of life. Pain without an associated mass is unlikely to be the presenting symptom of breast cancer, although evaluation may lead to the coincidental diagnosis of cancer. Mastalgia may be classed as cyclical or noncyclical, and may be acute or chronic.

- **Epidemiology.** Mastalgia is a more common complaint in premenopausal women than in postmenopausal women.
- **Classification/etiology.** Breast pain may be classified as cyclical (2/3) or noncyclical (1/3). Cyclical breast pain commonly occurs as a result of estrogen stimulation of ductal elements, and progesterone stimulation of the stromal such as during the normal menstrual cycle. Noncyclical causes of pain may include extramammary or chest wall pain, neuropathic pain, trauma, fat necrosis, infection, painful breast mass or cyst, and a multitude of other causes.
- **History.** Pertinent historical details include alleviating or aggravating factors, quality, radiation, severity, location, and laterality. It is important to illicit timing with regard to menstrual cycle, association with oral contraceptive pills or hormone replacement use, recent birth, pregnancy, loss of pregnancy, or termination. History of trauma, heavy muscular exertion, and constitutional symptoms should be sought.

- **Physical examination.** Physical examination should be used to evaluate for mass or nipple discharge; to localize areas of tenderness; and to assess for lymphadenopathy and changes in symmetry, contour, and overlying skin.
- **Laboratory studies and imaging.** Standard laboratory testing may be sought to assess for infection. Mammography or ultrasound may be useful in assessing for masses.[3,5]

Noncyclical Breast Pain

- **Trauma.** Trauma may produce a hematoma or rupture of a cyst and may also lead to fat necrosis. The patient will typically complain of pain and tenderness following an injury. Mild swelling and discoloration may be present. Unless a coagulopathy is suspected, no diagnostic tests are indicated. Fat necrosis is usually caused by preceding trauma and may be more likely if there is a history of fibrocystic breast disease. Physical examination reveals localized pain, swelling, and erythema. Evaluation should be performed to exclude malignancy if symptoms persist for more than a week, although fat necrosis commonly results in a residual calcified mass.
- **Ductal ectasia.** Distention of subareolar ducts due to inflammation may lead to pain of the breast. Typically fever with acute local pain and tenderness is associated. The degree of pain is correlated to the degree of inflammation.
- **Hormone replacement therapy.** Up to one-third of women receiving postmenopausal hormone therapy may experience breast pain. This typically will resolve over time.
- **Large pendulous breasts.** Large breasts may stretch Cooper's ligaments, which can cause pain. Typically the breasts will be pendulous in nature, and other myalgias such as the neck, back, or shoulder may be present.
- **Lactation-related pain.** Breast engorgement is a common cause of breast pain in new mothers. Breast engorgement usually occurs on the second or third postpartum day. Lactating women may also develop pain secondary to a galactocele or milk-filled cyst. These often resolve spontaneously.
- **Mastitis.** Both mastitis and breast abscesses almost always occur in lactating women or in women with a history of a bite or penetrating trauma. Mastitis commonly presents 1 week or more after delivery. Moderate to severe pain, tenderness, erythema, swelling, and warmth are usually localized to one breast, often to one quadrant or lobule. Axillary adenopathy may be present and there may be purulent drainage. The patient may be febrile and appear toxic. History and physical examination are diagnostic. Leukocytosis is common. Breast milk cultures are not useful, and *Staphylococcus aureus* is typically causative in breastfeeding women. Treatment for mild infection includes anti-inflammatory agents and cold compresses along with 10 to 14 days on oral antibiotics deemed safe for a nursing infant. Dicloxacillin 500 mg qid; cephalexin 500 mg qid; or clindamycin 300 mg qid for penicillin-allergic patients are recommended if a low suspicion for methicillin-resistant *S. aureus* (MRSA) is present. If a high suspicion for MRSA is present, clindamycin 300 mg qid, trimethoprim–sulfamethoxazole one to two tabs bid, or linezolid 600 mg bid is recommended. Patients should be reassessed in 48 to 72 hours. Breastfeeding should be continued on the affected breast to encourage drainage (the infant is not at risk for developing infection). Breast pumping is also appropriate.
- **Abscess.** Pitting edema over an area of inflammation and fluctuation is suggestive of abscess development. For patients with infections unresponsive to conservative management, severe infection, abscess, or deep infection, the wound should be drained and cultured. Breastfeeding should be continued and oral antibiotics should be started. Antibiotic regimens are the same as for mastitis listed above. If hemodynamic instability is present, hospitalization and initiation of vancomycin should be started. Nonpuerperal abscesses are usually caused by anaerobic bacteria if subareolar and by staphylococci in other locations. Nonpuerperal abscesses are treated with clindamycin or metronidazole. If the clinical setting is atypical, the woman is not breastfeeding, or she does not improve with antibiotics, a biopsy of indurated areas to exclude an underlying cancer should be considered. Presence of a periareolar inflammatory mass, breast abscess in a nonlactating woman, or a mammary duct fistula should raise suspicion of periductal mastitis.[5–7]

Cyclical Breast Pain

- **Etiology.** Most cyclical breast pain is associated with the menstrual cycle. Pain is usually worse in the luteal phase and abates following menstruation. Most women report some degree of cyclical breast pain at some point in their lives; 21% experience severe pain that interferes with function. Pain is typically bilateral and diffuse. Cyclical breast pain is not always associated with premenstrual syndrome (PMS), but 60% of women with PMS report breast pain as the predominant symptom. There is a high likelihood of spontaneous resolution of cyclical breast pain.

- **Treatment.** Watchful waiting and reassurance may be acceptable in up to 85% of patients. Breast support and analgesia with acetaminophen and anti-inflammatories may be beneficial. There is no evidence of benefit from dietary change. Progesterone and diuretics have also not been proved to be effective. Danazol has significant adverse effects (voice change, hirsutism, weight gain, acne), but 200 mg daily in the luteal phase (day 14 to 28) may be effective and minimize the total dose.[7] Tamoxifen 10 mg daily is efficacious as a continuous dose only during the luteal phase, but side effects limit its long-term use. Bromocriptine- and gonadotropin-releasing hormone agonists have also been successfully used for severe pain but are associated with a number of side effects. Additional therapies may include:
  - Evening primrose oil 500 mg, two tablets tid, has been demonstrated efficacious in a randomized controlled clinical trial with no apparent adverse effects.
  - Lowering the dose of estrogens in the treatment of postmenopausal women may be helpful, and the addition of an androgen to hormone replacement therapy may alleviate symptoms as well.
  - The use of oral contraceptives has not been well studied, but low-dose estrogen and 19-norprogesterone may be effective in relieving symptoms.[3,5]

Breast Mass

Benign breast masses are most commonly fibroadenomas or cysts, but must be differentiated from malignant disease. Benign breast masses will often change with the menstrual cycle, while worrisome masses are persistent throughout. Greater than 90% of palpable breast masses in women between 20 and 55 are benign. Masses may be discrete or poorly defined, but differ from the surrounding breast tissue and the corresponding area in the contralateral breast. Cancer should be excluded in a woman who presents with a solid mass. A woman with a clinically suspicious lesion should undergo mammography and/or ultrasound, and biopsy. Characteristics of a mass that are concerning for malignancy include single lesion, hard, fixed/immobile, irregular border, and size greater than 2 cm. Any asymmetry, skin dimpling, nipple discharge, and lymphadenopathy must also be assessed.[3,7]

- **Breast cysts.** Cysts may be solitary or multiple, and may be difficult to differentiate from solid masses on physical examination. Cystic disease peaks women 35 to 50 years of age. Ultrasound may be used to differentiate solid versus cystic masses and aspiration may be both diagnostic and therapeutic. Cysts should be surgically biopsied if they contain bloody fluid, fail to resolve completely after drainage, or recur after 4 to 6 weeks. It is not necessary to send aspirated fluid for cytologic examination. Nonpalpable cysts identified during routine mammography do not require further evaluation or treatment.
- **Fibrocystic breast changes.** Fibrocystic changes are the most common benign condition of the breast. Most experts consider such changes to be part of the natural history of the breast as histologic changes consistent with this diagnosis may be found in the majority of asymptomatic women. Changes are most common in women 35 to 45 years old and are rare in postmenopausal women. No treatment is necessary unless the woman is symptomatic (for example, from an enlarging cyst) or if physical findings are worrisome for possible cancer.
  - **Anatomy.** Fibrocystic changes consist of an increased number of cysts or fibrous tissue in an otherwise normal breast.
  - **Epidemiology.** Fibrocystic change may be divided into three subgroups with predominant histologic characteristics and age distributions. Hyperplasia commonly occurs in women in their 20s and presents as stromal proliferation and pain in the upper and outer quadrants. Adenosis is caused by proliferation of glandular cells and presents commonly as multiple 2- to 10-mm breast nodules in women in their 30s. Cystic disease occurs more commonly in women older than 40 with the painful enlargement of multiple or solitary cysts.
  - **History.** When symptoms are present, the most common symptom is cyclical pain (mastalgia). The pain is generally bilateral, located in the upper outer quadrants, begins a few days prior to menstruation, diminishes with the onset of menses, and may be associated with an increase in breast size. Family history is common.
  - **Physical examination.** Cysts are smooth, regular, rubbery, and easily movable lumps or areas of local tenderness without a discrete mass. Cysts can range in size from 1 mm to many centimeters. Compression causes tenderness. Larger cysts are more common as women age. To assess for possible menstrual changes, it may be helpful to repeat the examination with the patient at another

point in her cycle. It may be difficult to discern a cyst from a solid mass on physical examination. Pale green to brown nipple discharge may be noted in cystic disease.

- **Diagnostic evaluation.** Although fibrocystic symptoms typically differ from those associated with malignancy, if there is any doubt regarding the diagnosis or if a single mass is present, further evaluation for breast mass is needed. There is no increased risk of cancer in women with fibrocystic changes in a woman younger than 50 years unless proliferative or hyperplastic lesions with atypical epithelial cells are present on biopsy.
- **Management.** Most women do not require treatment. Treatment, if necessary, is focused on the predominant symptom or sign such as pain or a mass. A well-padded support bra and loose light clothing may relieve discomfort and weight reduction is recommended in women with a body mass index greater than 30 mm per kg. Calcium may be beneficial, but many other previously recommended therapies (dietary restriction of caffeine and methylxanthines in chocolate, tea, coffee, soda, and theophylline; use of vitamins, including A, E, and thiamine; and use of diuretics) have not proven efficacious in randomized controlled clinical trials. Additional management may include the following:
  - Low-estrogen/high-progesterone oral contraceptives may be used, but the patient may not notice significant change until 1 to 2 years of use.
  - Progesterone, such as medroxyprogesterone 5 to 10 mg daily for 10 days before menses, may be given for a trial of 4 to 6 months. Side effects may include weight gain, depression, breakthrough bleeding, and lipid alterations.
  - If thyroid-stimulating hormone (TSH) is elevated even when other thyroid hormones are normal, a trial of thyroid replacement may be helpful.
  - cis-Linoleic acid (evening primrose oil) at a dose of 1 g every 8 hours may be beneficial. However, the benefit may not be seen for 3 to 4 months.
  - Danazol is the only pharmacologic agent approved by the U.S. Food and Drug Administration for treatment of fibrocystic breast changes. Many women achieve the needed benefit, but significant side effects (hirsutism, amenorrhea, weight gain of 4 to 6 pounds, hot flashes, and acne) are common. Danazol is generally reserved for women with severe symptoms. Dose at 200 to 800 mg per day PO initially and then may decrease to 50 to 100 mg per day as maintenance once response is achieved. Some women benefit from 200 mg daily, given on days 14 to 28 of the menstrual cycle. Duration of treatment is usually limited to 3 to 6 months. Once danazol is discontinued, the treatment response may persist for months to years.
  - Tamoxifen, an antiestrogen, reduced breast pain in approximately 70% of patients within 3 to 6 months in several studies. In premenopausal women younger than 49 years, 20 mg per day was found to cause no increase in the incidence of deep venous thrombus, pulmonary embolism, stroke, transient ischemic attack (TIA), or endometrial cancer. Tamoxifen 10 mg per day may be effective when used only during the luteal phase (days 15 to 25), but its use should be restricted to fewer than 6 months. Side effects may include hot flashes, gastrointestinal (GI) symptoms, and vaginal discharge.
  - Surgery (subcutaneous mastectomy; oophorectomy) should be considered only after medical management has failed for women with recalcitrant symptoms. Surgery may be useful for patients with one large dominant cyst.
  - Bromocriptine- and luteinizing hormone–releasing agents have also been used but have significant side effects.[3,5]
- **Fibroadenoma.** Fibroadenoma, the most common solid tumor, contains both fibrous and glandular elements. These tumors occur in young women, most commonly ages 15 to 35. Multiple lesions may develop. Growth may be rapid especially at the end of a menstrual cycle and in pregnancy. Older women characteristically have a single, solitary, more slowly growing lesion. Fibroadenomas frequently calcify and may involute after menopause. Occasionally they may develop in a postmenopausal woman after administration of estrogen.
  - **History.** A painless mass is generally discovered by the patient and reported to the physician.
  - **Physical examination.** A well-defined, rubbery, mobile, nontender, 1 to 5 cm mass can generally be palpated. The usual location is in an upper quadrant.
  - **Diagnostic procedures.** A FNAB should be performed or have the patient return in 3 to 6 months for repeat ultrasound and breast examination. Cyroablation may be another option for fibroadenomas confirmed by biopsy. Mammography is not usually helpful, especially in young patients.

- **Breast cancer risk.** Fibroadenomas are neither cancerous nor premalignant but may require excisional biopsy to confirm the diagnosis.
- **Management.** Excisional biopsy is both diagnostic and curative.[5]
- **Cystosarcoma phyllodes** is a rapidly growing fibroadenoma that recurs if not completely excised. This tumor is rarely malignant, but, because of its extreme size, simple mastectomy may be necessary to achieve complete removal.

NIPPLE ANOMALIES
Nipple Discharge

Nipple discharge is an extremely common concern in young women and most isolated complaints of discharge are of a benign origin. It is practical to divide nipple discharge into two categories based on the presence or absence of galactorrhea. Normal, healthy women commonly have some degree of clear or milky nipple discharge following pregnancy and lactation that can either spontaneously drain from the breast or be produced by palpation. This discharge may be more frequently noted just before menses or with breast stimulation as part of sexual activity. This benign discharge has a small volume, and the amount does not change over time. However, characteristics of pathologic discharge include unilaterality; presence from a single duct; association with an underlying mass; spontaneous, intermittent, and persistent occurrence in a postmenopausal woman; and bloody to serosanguinous color.

- **History.** History should elicit the nature of discharge, underlying mass, laterality, single- or multiple-duct involvement, relation to menses, color of discharge, the menopausal status of the patient, association with hormonal therapy, and whether the discharge appears spontaneously or must be expressed. The amount and type of nipple stimulation should also be explored. Nipple discharge in a postmenopausal woman is more ominous and is more likely to be caused by cancer.
- **Physical examination.** A complete breast examination should be performed, with attention to identifying masses, underlying induration, and lymphadenopathy as well as characterizing the discharge. Warm compresses placed on the breast may enhance the ability to detect a discharge. It is important to note whether the discharge originates from one or more ducts. A "pseudo-discharge" is a stain on clothes originating from outside the breast (such as from an abrasion, eczema, or viral condition like herpes). If nipple crusting is present, Paget disease should be excluded by a skin biopsy.
- **Fluid characteristics.** The characteristics of the fluid may aid in diagnosis. Green, black, creamy, or mucoid discharge is characteristic of fibrocystic breast disease. Straw-colored discharge is most commonly due to a papilloma (which is benign histologically and has only a slight potential for malignant degeneration). Bloody or serosanguinous discharge is associated with malignancy, but may also represent bleeding papilloma or fibrocystic change with an intraductal component. Bloody discharge, or brown-green discharge suggesting old blood, should be investigated further. Cheesy discharge often results from duct ectasia, a chronic inflammatory reaction resulting in permanent distention of the major ducts. The typical patient with duct ectasia is a multiparous woman 40 years or older who notes thick, white, or discolored cheesy material draining from the nipple and noncyclical, burning breast pain. Purulent discharge could indicate an underlying mastitis.
- **Diagnostic procedures**
  - **Mammography.** A mammogram should be performed in women with abnormal discharge older than 30 years of age and may reveal abnormalities such as the presence of an associated mass.
  - **Ultrasound.** Ultrasound should be performed in conjunction with mammography. It should be directed at the periareolar area to visualize any dilated ducts. Visualization of ductal pathology as small as 0.5 mm can be seen.
  - **Galactography.** The role of galactography and/or ductography requires that iodine be injected into the duct with discharge. Intraductal filling defects, complete ductal obstruction, or an abnormality in the ductal wall may be seen. A negative galactogram does not replace the need for terminal duct excision.
  - **Magnetic resonance imaging (MRI) and MR ductography.** MRI and MR ductography have the ability to provide three-dimensional images of the ducts that are dilated. The role of this technology continues to evolve and is not completely understood yet.

- **Fluid analysis.** The discharge can be tested for the presence of blood (with a heme occult slide). Gram staining can be performed to identify white blood cells if there is a concern for infection. Fat stain can demonstrate fat globules indicative of milk if galactorrhea is suspected. Cytologic examination of the nipple discharge has no definite benefits.
- **Management.** Management includes surgical exploration of the duct and removal of the papilloma, if present.[3-5]

Galactorrhea

Galactorrhea consists of a milky discharge from the breast beyond 6 months postpartum in a non-breastfeeding woman. Although galactorrhea can have many causes, it is usually benign. It has been described in women who jog because friction between the nipple and clothing can stimulate prolactin. Athletic activities may also trigger endorphin release from the hypothalamus, which stimulates prolactin secretion. Correlation is poor between the presence of lactation and serum prolactin level. Galactorrhea is not associated with an increased risk of breast cancer.

- **History.** History should include recent childbirth, excessive breast stimulation, and medication use. Additionally, it should be determined whether galactorrhea is present from both nipples and from multiple ducts. Galactorrhea from multiple ducts in a nonlactating woman may occur in certain syndromes (Chiari–Frommel, Argonz–Del Castillo). Processes that inflame or irritate the chest wall such as thoracotomy, herpes zoster infection, radiation to the chest wall, burn, may also cause galactorrhea (presumably from a stimulatory increase in prolactin secretion) and should be investigated. Any associated change in menstrual pattern, such as amenorrhea or oligomenorrhea, is suggestive of a central nervous system lesion and approximately 20% of patients with galactorrhea will have a prolactin-secreting pituitary tumor. Headache or visual change may indicate the presence of an intracranial process. Conditions that affect the pituitary and/or the hypothalamus (tuberculosis and multiple sclerosis) and other chronic medical conditions (chronic renal failure, hypothyroidism, Cushing disease) may cause galactorrhea and should be explored in the past medical history.
- **Medication history.** Medications may be the cause of galactorrhea in up to 20% of patients. Drugs associated with galactorrhea include digitalis, marijuana, heroin, dopamine receptor blockers, phenothiazine, haloperidol, metoclopramide, isoniazid, antidepressants, reserpine, methyldopa, atenolol, cimetidine, benzodiazepines, amphetamines, verapamil, cocaine, progesterones, oral contraceptives, copper-containing intrauterine devices (IUDs), and others. Herbal products that can cause galactorrhea include fenugreek seed, fennel, and red clover. Post–oral contraceptive galactorrhea may occur as well where the milk production is triggered by the withdrawal of estrogen and progesterone. This usually resolves spontaneously. Some patients eventually develop radiologically evident pituitary adenomas.
- **Diagnostic evaluation.** Serum prolactin level, TSH, and renal function tests can be useful. Further endocrine workup may be indicated. If serum prolactin is greater than 100 ng per mL, brain computed tomography (CT) or MRI is necessary to rule out pituitary adenoma. Non-pituitary prolactin-producing malignancies are less common but include bronchogenic carcinomas, renal adenocarcinomas, Hodgkin disease, and T-cell lymphoma. A CT or MRI scan is necessary if serum prolactin is elevated; if serum prolactin is normal but the patient has an aberration in her menstrual pattern; or if any central nervous system symptoms or signs are present.
- **Management.** Any medication associated with galactorrhea should be withdrawn. Any thyroid abnormalities detected on workup should be treated. If serum prolactin is elevated, a workup for pituitary adenoma is indicated. If elevated serum prolactin but no pituitary adenoma is demonstrable, treatment may still be indicated to decrease the risk of hyperprolactin-associated osteoporosis. If a microadenoma is present but fertility is not desired, and the risk of osteoporosis does not warrant treatment, patients can be followed without therapy. Microadenomas may regress spontaneously and do not typically transform into macroadenomas. Serum prolactin levels can be followed every 6 months, with repeat CT or MRI every 2 to 5 years. If a macroadenoma is present, therapy is indicated to prevent further growth. Medical management consists of bromocriptine, 2.5 mg per day for 1 week, increased to 2.5 mg bid–tid, or pergolide and cabergoline. Side effects may include nausea, nasal congestion, and postural hypotension. Tumor regrowth may occur following withdrawal of the medication. Bromocriptine can be used to lower prolactin levels to normal to allow fertility and to shrink tumor size preoperatively. Transsphenoidal surgery is an option for large tumors and in patients with macroadenomas who wish to become pregnant. However, surgical success is limited as these tumors frequently recur. Radiation may be an option for patients who are not surgical candidates.[5,7]

Painful Nipples

Breastfeeding Women

Tenderness of the nipples is a common symptom when breastfeeding is initiated. Proper positioning of the baby is necessary, so that the most cracked or tender portion of the breast is at the corner of baby's mouth and not aligned with the roof of the mouth or tongue, and correct techniques to "break suction" are essential. Nursing position may be changed. Any engorgement should be treated. Alternate which breast is presented first and begin with the less sore one. Warm or cold compresses and crushed ice applied to nipples before nursing may be beneficial. Milk should be expressed until "let-down" occurs. Avoid petrolatum and zinc oxide. The area can be washed with warm water and can air dry with colostrum applied.

Nipples should be examined for the presence of fissures or local infection. If candidal disease is suspected, treat with topical nystatin or antifungals. Thrush or *Candida* diaper rash in the newborn or maternal *Candida* vaginitis should be treated concurrently.

A plugged milk duct can present as a white blister on the nipple following breastfeeding and a hardened area in the breast. Soak the nipple in warm water before next nursing. Gently rub a clean washcloth across the tip of the nipple. As baby nurses, massage behind the hard area to encourage milk expression.

Non-Breastfeeding Women

Nipples can develop painful localized irritation and bleeding in joggers. Small elastic bandages can be applied to the nipple before running or other athletic activities. Emollients or low-dose hydrocortisone cream may ameliorate symptoms.

A unilateral, weeping, ulcerated, irritated nipple is suggestive of Paget disease, especially in middle-aged or older women, and may be associated with an underlying ductal carcinoma. Further evaluation is necessary.[1,5,7]

Gynecomastia

Gynecomastia has a bimodal distribution. Most boys at puberty develop bilateral gynecomastia, which resolves without treatment within 3 years. It is also common for men in their 50s and 60s to experience breast enlargement. Gynecomastia associated with pain, asymmetry, rapid onset or progression, galactorrhea, and/or erectile dysfunction requires further workup. Association with precocious puberty is also a concerning sign.

Drugs and medications that can cause gynecomastia include an extensive list. Many categories of medications, including antiandrogens, antibiotics, antiulcer drugs, chemotherapeutic drugs, cardiovascular drugs, drugs of abuse, hormones, psychoactive drugs, and some miscellaneous drugs. It is recommended that if a patient has gynecomastia, this list of medications be reviewed and the patient's medication list removed of potential causative agents if able.

Medical conditions that cause gynecomastia include cancer (testes, liver, bronchiole, stomach, or pancreas, especially the human chorionic gonadotropin (hCG)–producing neoplasms), hyperthyroidism, hypogonadism, cirrhosis, renal failure, severe pulmonary disease, Klinefelter syndrome, testicular feminization, and refeeding after starvation.

Laboratory evaluation includes thyroid function tests, renal and liver function studies; if these are normal, luteinizing hormone, hCG, estradiol, and testosterone should be obtained. If hCG is elevated, testicular ultrasonography and search for other hCG-secreting tumors should be undertaken. If estradiol is elevated, a search for an estrogen-secreting tumor should be undertaken.

Older men develop gynecomastia at an age close to that at which male breast cancer occurs. If a breast mass is felt, a combination of physical examination and FNA can establish the correct diagnosis in the majority of patients. Mammography may add little additional information.[1,2,5,7]

REFERENCES

1. Andolsek KM, Copeland JA. Benign breast conditions and disease. In: Taylor RB, ed. *Family medicine: principles and practice.* 6th ed. New York, NY: Springer-Verlag; 2003:895–902.
2. Dickson G. Gynecomastia. *Am Fam Physician* 2012;85:716–722.
3. Onstad M, Stuckey A. Benign breast disorders. *Obstet Gynecol Clin N Am* 2013;40:459–473.
4. Amin A, Purdy A, Mattingly JD, et al. Benign breast disease. *Surg Clin N Am* 2013;93:299–308.
5. Salzman B, Fleegle S, Tully AS. Common breast problems. *Am Fam Physician* 2012;86:343–349.
6. Klein S. Evaluation of palpable breast masses. *Am Fam Physician* 2005;71:1731–1738.
7. Santen RJ, Mansel R. Current concepts: benign breast disorders. *N Engl J Med* 2005;353:275–285.

GENERAL PRINCIPLES

Definition

Breast cancer is formed in the tissue of the breast. Ductal carcinoma develops in the lining of the milk ducts and lobular carcinoma develops from the lobules. Cancer confined to the primary tissue is defined as "in situ" and may become invasive in an estimated one-third of cases.[1] Lobular carcinoma in situ (LCIS) is not a true cancer or precancer, but an indicator for increased risk.[1] The majority of invasive carcinomas are ductal adenocarcinomas (80%), while infiltrating lobular carcinomas are a minority (up to 15%).[2] Inflammatory cancers and Paget disease often have an atypical presentation and are less common (1% to 4%).[2]

Epidemiology

The global incidence of invasive breast cancer is 22.9%, making it one of the most common invasive cancers in all women, and a leading cause of cancer death worldwide.[3]

Current estimates in the United States are a lifetime risk of 12.3% or one in eight for women with 40,000 deaths occurring annually. Approximately 79% of new cases and 88% of breast cancer deaths will have occurred in women aged 50 and older. About 1 in 3,000 of all breast cancers occurs in pregnant women, the most common cancer detected in pregnancy which does not change the prognosis.[1]

Risk factors with a relative risk of >4.0 for breast cancer include (a) female sex (>99% of breast cancer cases), (b) increasing age (65+), (c) biopsy-confirmed atypical hyperplasia, (d) certain genetic mutations such as BRCA1 and/or BRCA2, (e) two or more first-degree relatives with breast cancer diagnosed premenopausally, (f) increasing breast density, and (g) personal history of breast cancer. Risk factors with a relative risk of 2.1 to <4.0 include (a) personal history of breast cancer, (b) one first-degree relative with breast cancer, (c) high-dose radiation to the chest, and (d) high endogenous estrogen or testosterone levels. Other risk factors with lower relative risks (1.1 to 2.0) include (a) age at first delivery (>30); (b) early menarche (<12 years); (c) late menopause (>55 years); (d) nulliparity; (e) no history of breastfeeding; (f) height (tall) ; (g) recent and long-term use of hormone replacement therapy with estrogen and progestin; (h) obesity (postmenopausal), (i) personal history of endometrial, ovary, or colon cancer; (j) alcohol consumption; (k) higher socioeconomic status; (l) Ashkenazi (Eastern European) Jewish heritage; and (m) diethylstilbestrol (DES) exposure.[1]

Risk models to predict the relative or the absolute risk of breast cancer consist of BRCA probability tools and Breast Cancer Risk Assessment Models (Gail model). The Gail model of risk assessment is the most validated to predict risk and to direct screening guidelines. While risk factors are important, breast cancer can occur in the absence of known risk factors in nearly 60% of women.[4]

Breast cancer is a predominantly females disease, with less than 1% seen in males. Risk factors include family history, a higher incidence of genetic mutations involving the BRCA genes, and obesity. Worse prognosis is seen in male breast cancers.[1]

Classification

The concept of breast cancer as a homogenous disease has evolved into a complex disease state based on molecular subtypes, risk factors, clinical behavior, and response to treatment.[5] In addition to the tissue of origin, and the histopathology, breast cancer is classified by grade into low, intermediate, and high, based on the loss of breast cancer cell differentiation using the Nottingham scheme.[5] The clinical method of classification is based on tumor size, spread to regional lymph nodes, and the presence or absence of distant metastases known as the TNM staging system.[4] Whether the cancer stage is early (stage I, IIA, or T2N1), advanced (T3NO), or metastatic (stage 1V) determines the treatment modalities, prognosis, and risk of recurrence.[4] Molecular subtypes are based on the receptor status.[2] The presence or absence of estrogen receptors (ERs), progesterone receptors (PRs), or human epidermal growth factor receptor 2 (HER2) defines the immunohistochemistry.[2] If all the receptors are absent, the tumor is determined to be triple negative.

DIAGNOSIS

Clinical Presentation

The typical presentation is an asymptomatic mass detected by screening mammography or by breast examination found by the patient or clinician.[2] Less common symptoms include breast pain; skin irritation or distortion; and nipple abnormalities such as spontaneous discharge, erosion, or inversion particularly with Paget disease.[1] Rarely does a metastatic breast cancer present with signs of secondary spreads such as skin changes and nodules, bone or joint pain, hepatomegaly, or axillary node enlargement, occasionally even prior to a detectable lump in the breast.[2]

History

The history should include date the lump was found, prior breast problems and biopsies, and risk factor assessment. A detailed family history is essential.[1]

Physical Examination

The breasts should be examined in the upright and supine positions and inspected for differences in size, retraction or eczematous changes of the skin or nipple, and signs of inflammation and lymphedema. The flat surface of the fingertips should be used to palpate the breast tissue using the vertical strip, three-pressure methods. Characteristics, size, and location of a mass should be noted and constitute the clinical breast examination (CBE). The contralateral breast should be similarly examined. The axillary and supraclavicular areas should be checked for adenopathy. Suspicious masses are generally solitary, discrete, hard, fixed, nontender, and unilateral; however, cancer cannot be excluded based solely on physical examination findings.[6]

Concerning findings include axillary lymphadenopathy, nipple inversion, or skin changes such as retraction. Rarely if advanced, signs of spread can be evident. A complete physical examination should include a pelvic examination if indicated.[5]

Imaging

Screening mammography of an asymptomatic woman provides two views of each breast using x-ray and will detect 78% of breast cancers in women with an 83% sensitivity for women over 50. About 17% breast cancers will be missed on routine breast imaging. Breast density is a major confounding factor.[7] See Table 13.8-1 for screening guidelines.

Diagnostic mammography is used to evaluate women with signs or symptoms of breast cancer and may include additional views or ultrasonographic imaging. Digital mammography utilizes computer-aided diagnosis and interpretation of mammography. Magnetic resonance imaging (MRI) of the breasts may be used in very high-risk patients, particularly in those with gene mutations. In women with breast implants, a special technique called implant displacement views can assure that breast tissue is not hidden; an MRI may be preferred.[8]

Tomosynthesis, a three-dimensional x-ray imaging with digital reconstruction, has been approved by the FDA in 2013, and somo-v Automated Breast Ultrasound System (ABUS) was approved in 2012 as an adjunct to mammography.[9] To evaluate for metastatic disease, PET, CT, and bone scans are used to detect spread. Clinical and self-breast examinations, along with screening mammograms, have been the mainstay of population screening. Despite the improvement in detection and reduction of breast cancer mortality, routine screening has been recently reviewed to have contributed to over diagnosis and overtreatment leading to several national organizations to revise previous recommendations.[10]

Currently, the onset and cessation as well as the intervals of screening in all age groups, are increasingly controversial and under review. A consensus has not been reached. In general, women are encouraged to use breast self-awareness and enter an individualized decision based on risk and preference. The use of risk models and decision aids can be helpful but have not been validated for use in the general population.[11]

Surgical Diagnostic Procedures

Definitive diagnosis of a suspicious mass depends on tissue sampling. Breast imaging should be performed prior to biopsy to avoid possible distortion from hemorrhage. Fine-needle aspiration (FNA) is done to obtain samples from a solid mass for cytology. Core biopsy collects a larger sample size, requires a small skin incision, and, however, has the benefits of higher specificity and the use of immunohistopathology, but slightly lower sensitivity. Stereotactic biopsies utilize imaging for accurate localization and are indicated for deeper masses or for suspicious calcifications seen on a screening mammogram. Lumpectomy or an open excisional biopsy may be indicated when needle biopsies are negative, but the mass is clinically suspicious. Axillary node or the sentinel node biopsies are critical for staging and may be undertaken prior to surgery or more commonly intraoperative.[2]

Pathologic Findings

Pathology reports from breast biopsies include tumor type, in situ or invasive pathology, and immunohistopathology status. With tumor resection, surgical margins are evaluated and if lymph node sampling was conducted, presence of cancer cells is determined. Nonmalignant conditions comprised the bulk of breast disease and include fibrocystic breast disease, fibroadenomas, hamartomas, and other benign tumors and can often have similar presentation and features.

TREATMENT

Breast cancer requires a variety of treatment options depending on the presenting stage and pathology, the patient's age and preferences. Early stage breast cancer is treated conservatively in a majority of cases.[1] LCIS following a diagnosis with biopsy can be followed with observation alone. Locally advanced and metastatic breast cancer requires a multimodal treatment plan.[2]

Surgery

The primary treatment for the majority of all breast cancers is surgical resection. Types of surgery consist of varying amounts of removal of involved breast and adnexal tissue and include lumpectomy, quadrantectomy, simple mastectomy, and the modified radical mastectomy.[1] The type of surgery is determined by the stage of the tumor and must include the patient's preference for breast conservation surgery.[2]

Modified radical mastectomy has replaced the classical radical mastectomy as the most common type of surgery. Axillary and sentinel node biopsies are performed for advanced breast cancer at the time of breast surgery. Sentinel node biopsy has replaced the standard axillary surgery due to reduced morbidity and sequelae. After surgical treatment for breast cancer, the patient may elect to undergo breast reconstruction.[1]

Radiation

Radiation therapy consists of external beam or brachytherapy and is used after surgical excision and on occasion intraoperatively.[1] Radiation is indicated most often with invasive disease to provide locoregional benefits and reduce microscopic spread.[12]

Breast conserving therapy is a combination of breast conserving surgery, with mandatory moderate dose of radiation therapy in an attempt to provide better cosmesis in appropriate patients. No change has been found for prognosis.[1]

Systemic Therapy

Chemotherapy, hormonal therapy, and biologic options in various combinations (depending on the tumor size, histology, hormone receptor status, and stage) are considered systemic therapy. These therapies have contributed significantly to the improved outcomes in breast cancer. Neoadjuvant therapy is used prior to surgery and has been associated with improved outcomes, particularly with late-stage cancers by initiating tumor regression and reducing spread. Surgery is always indicated after completing the therapy independent of the initial outcome or regression. Adjuvant therapy is used following surgery and continued for varying periods of times.[1]

Chemotherapy consists of combinations of cyclophosphamide, methotrexate, 5-fluorouracil, doxorubicin, epirubicin, and paclitaxel. Multidrug therapy is more effective than single-drug therapy for breast cancer treatment.[13] Chemotherapy is indicated generally for stage 2 to 4 cancers and may be the only option in receptor negative disease. Chemotherapy can be withheld in low risk early stage ER+ breast cancer. However, it is superior to hormonal therapy even in receptor positive tumors with advanced disease.[14]

Adjuvant hormonal therapy is particularly significant in estrogen receptor–positive cancers[1] and is determined by the menopausal status.[14] Tamoxifen blocks the estrogen receptor and can even be used prior to a diagnosis of cancer in high-risk women as preventative therapy. In postmenopausal women, the aromatase inhibitors (letrozole, anastrozole, and exemastane) are indicated due to ineffectively of tamoxifen, and may be the only neoadjunctive therapy if chemotherapy is contraindicated.[14]

Trastuzumab (Herceptin) is a targeted monoclonal antibody and offers survival benefit for women with HER2-positive advanced breast cancer, when combined with chemotherapy as adjuvant therapy. Everolimimus suppresses tumor growth and can support hormone therapy.

TABLE 13.8-1	Recommendations for Breast Cancer Screening for Women with Average Risk	

Organization	Routine mammography	Clinical breast examination
U.S. Preventative Services Task Force (USPSTF)	Biennial screening mammography women 50–74 (B)[a]	Evidence of CBE's additional benefit, beyond mammography is inadequate (I)
American Cancer Society	Once a year age 40 and older	Every 3 yr women in their 20s and 30s. Once a year starting age 40.
American Academy of Family Medicine	Routine biennial screening for women 50–74 yr of age	Insufficient evidence
American College of Obstetrics and Gynecology	Once a year age 40 and older	Every 3 yr women in their 20s and 30s. Once a year starting age 40.
National Cancer Institute	Every 1–2 yr starting age 40	No specific recommendation

[a]USPSTF grade evidence: B, Inconsistent or fair evidence; benefits of screening are only moderately greater than the harm. I, evidence that the intervention is effective is lacking, of poor quality or conflicting and the balance of benefits, harms, and costs cannot be determined.

Surgery is the safest treatment, especially early in pregnancy. Radiation and chemotherapy have greater adverse effects intrapartum and postpartum. Third-trimester patients can be observed until delivery and then receive prompt therapy.[1]

Prognosis and Follow-Up

Prognosis for breast cancer has improved over the past 30 years with a 34% reduction of breast cancer mortality. Prognosis is largely determined by the stage. Developed countries report higher survival rates.[3] Early stage offers the best results and the 10-year survival for early stage lesions is 75% to 85%. Death can occur 15 to 20 years later, making posttreatment surveillance imperative for primary breast cancer and secondary cancer. Cancer survivorship is becoming important as mortality due to cancer is decreasing and the increased risk of death due to cardiovascular disease is increasingly being recognized. A multidisciplinary approach is recommended.[2]

Primary Prevention

Although many of the risk factors are not modifiable, a number of modifiable lifestyle risk factors—smoking, postmenopausal obesity, physical inactivity, and possibly diabetes—have been associated with increased risk. Avoiding weight gain, exercising, smoking cessation, breast feeding, and reducing alcohol have been promoted to reduce up to 20% to 42% of breast cancer.[1]

Secondary Prevention

Between 3% and 5% of all women who have breast cancer have mutations in the BRCA 1 and 2 genes with a lifetime risk of 50% to 80% of breast cancer. Bilateral prophylactic surgery may be indicated for select women at the highest risk for breast cancer, and appropriate counseling is essential. Prophylactic ovarian and uterine removal is occasionally indicated in for the highest risk cohort. Treatment with tamoxifen or raloxifene can be used as chemoprevention for very select subtypes.[1]

REFERENCES

1. American Cancer Society. Breast cancer facts and figures 2013–12014. http://www.cancer.org/acs/groups/content/@research/documents/document/acspc-042725.pdf. Accessed February 28, 2014.
2. Brufsky A, McGuire K, Leone J. Breast Cancer. First Consult, MD Consult. Web site. http://www.mdconsult.com/das/pdxmd/body/442859946-2/0?type=med&eid=9-u1.0-_1_mt_1014646. Accessed April 8, 2014.

3. Ferlay J, Soerjomataram I, Ervik M, et al. GLOBOCAN 2012 v1.0, Cancer Incidence and Mortality Worldwide: IARC Cancer Base No. 11. Lyon, France: International Agency for Research on Cancer; 2013. http://globocan.iarc.fr. Accessed April 8, 2014.
4. Stopeck AT, Chalasani P, Thompson PA. Breast Cancer. Medscape website. http://emedicine.medscape.com/article/1947145-overview. Accessed April 7, 2014.
5. Elston CW, Ellis IO. Pathological prognostic factors in breast cancer. I. The value of histological grade in breast cancer: experience from a large study with long-term follow-up. *Histopathology* 1991;19:403–410.
6. Apantaku LM. Breast cancer diagnosis and screening. *Am Fam Physician* 2000;62:596–602.
7. Oestreicher N, Lehman CD, Seger DJ, et al. The incremental contribution of clinical breast examination to invasive cancer detection in a mammography screening program. *Am J Roentgenol* 2005;184: 428–432.
8. National Cancer Institute. Fact Sheet. http://www.cancer.gov/cancertopics/factsheet/detection/mammograms. Accessed April 7, 2014.
9. National Cancer Institute. FDA approves Ultrasound imaging system for dense breast tissue. http://www.cancer.gov/ncicancerbulletin/100212/page11. Accessed April 8, 2014.
10. Gøtzsche PC, Jørgensen KJ. Screening for breast cancer with mammograph. *Cochrane Database Syst Rev* 6: CD001877. doi:10.1002/14651858.CD001877.
11. Pace LE, Keating NL. A systematic assessment of benefits and risks to guide breast cancer screening decisions. *JAMA* 2014;311:1327–1335.
12. Breastcancer.org. Radiation therapy. http://www.breastcancer.org/treatment/radiation. Accessed April 4, 2014.
13. Taghian A, El-Ghamry MN, Merajver SD. Overview of the treatment of newly diagnosed, non-metastatic breast cancer. http://www.uptodate.com/contents/overview-of-the-treatment-of-newly-diagnosed-non-metastatic-breast-cancer?source=search_result&search=newly+diagnosed+breast+cancer&selected Title=2%7E150. Accessed February 28, 2014.
14. Smith IE, Chua S. ABC of breast diseases: medical treatment of early breast cancer. III: chemotherapy. *BMJ* 2006;332:161–162.

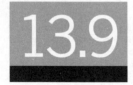

13.9 Colposcopy

Jennifer G. Chang

GENERAL PRINCIPLES

Diagnosis and management of genital epithelial dysplasia requires mastery of colposcopy, punch biopsy, and endocervical curettage (ECC). The colposcope is essentially a stereoscopic operating microscope combined with a bright-light source. Colposcopy with biopsy seeks to identify patients who may have invasive genital malignancy requiring advanced cancer therapies and women who have premalignant changes, which frequently can be managed with outpatient procedures, such as cryotherapy or loop electrosurgical excision procedure (LEEP). The ultimate challenge for the colposcopist is to distinguish normal from abnormal areas and direct biopsy to allow for histologic interpretation of abnormal areas.[1] Recent studies have questioned the diagnostic accuracy of colposcopic punch biopsy,[2] and suggest that a liberal approach to biopsy be taken to improve diagnostic yield.

INDICATIONS FOR COLPOSCOPY[1]

1. Abnormal cervical cancer screening (see Chapter 13.4)
   - Cytology (Papanicolaou [Pap] smear) with dysplasia or cancer
   - Evidence of high-risk (oncogenic) human papillomavirus (HPV) infection
   - Persistent unexplained atypia
   - Persistent unsatisfactory cytology[3]
2. Suspicious visible lesion of the cervix, vagina, or vulva
3. Follow-up of previously treated patients
4. History of diethylstilbestrol exposure

5. Colposcopy highly recommended
   • Patients with visible persistent condylomata
   • Unexplained vaginal discharge, itching, or bleeding
   • HIV-infected women
   • Intravenous drug abusers

CONTRAINDICATIONS FOR COLPOSCOPY[1]

Contraindications usually delay rather than prevent the examination, and include:
• Active gonococcal, chlamydial, or trichomonal infections
• Uncooperative patient
• Heavy, active menses

BASIC CERVICAL COLPOSCOPIC FINDINGS[1]

• Normal cervical findings
   • Squamous epithelium
   • Columnar epithelium
   • Squamous metaplasia
   • Squamocolumnar junction (SCJ)
   • Transformation zone (TZ)
• Variants of normal
   • Nabothian cysts
   • Atrophy
   • Pregnancy changes
   • Inflammatory or infectious process
   • Traumatic changes, clefts, or prior therapy
• Abnormal cervical mucosal patterns, indicating the need for biopsy
   • Leukoplakia (a white area prior to application of acetic acid)
   • Acetowhite change (a whitening following acetic acid application)
   • Punctation (a vessel pattern of small red dots usually within an acetowhite area)
   • Mosaic (a vessel pattern with the appearance of chicken wire)
   • Atypical vessel pattern (abnormal branching, hairpins, corkscrew patterns)

PATIENT PREPARATION FOR COLPOSCOPY

• Providing informational leaflets may improve patient knowledge and reduce psychosexual dysfunction associated with colposcopy.[4]
• Playing music during the procedure has been shown to reduce anxiety levels and pain.[4]

BASIC PROCEDURAL STEPS FOR COLPOSCOPY OF THE CERVIX[1]

   1. Perform a bimanual examination.
   2. Insert speculum. Gently blot off excess mucus.
   3. Adjust and focus colposcope initially on low power.
   4. Apply normal saline to clean the cervix; assess for leukoplakia or other gross lesions.
   5. Apply a solution of 3% to 5% acetic acid (i.e., vinegar) to allow for acetowhite changes within areas of dysplasia. Reapply acetic acid every 5 minutes as needed.
   6. Colposcopically examine the cervix:
      a. Determine whether or not the entire SCJ is visible.
      b. View with a green light filter to assess for abnormal vasculature
      c. Identify areas of abnormality that will require biopsy
   7. Lugol iodine solution may be applied to enhance one's impression of the presence or absence of lesions. Lack of black staining on *squamous* epithelium implies dysplasia.
   8. Perform ECC to evaluate for occult cervical canal disease, particularly when no lesions are visible on the ectocervix or when the examination is inadequate (entire TZ is not visible). ECC is **contraindicated** in pregnancy.
   9. Perform punch biopsies of abnormal areas, starting inferiorly.
   10. Apply Monsel's solution or silver nitrate for local hemostasis.
   11. Carefully examine the vagina and vulva, and biopsy abnormal areas.

TABLE 13.9-1	Summary of Recommendations for Management and Follow-Up of Cervical Dysplasia[3,5,6]		
Patient demographic	**Colposcopy result**	**Preceding cytology**	**Recommended follow-up**
Age 21–24 yr	No lesion or CIN 1	ASC-US or LSIL	Cytology 12 and 24 mo; routine screening if both normal
		ASC-H or HSIL	Inadequate colposcopy: excision Adequate colposcopy: cytology with colposcopy at 6 and 12 mo, or excision, or review pathologic findings
	CIN 2 (adequate colposcopy)		Observation preferred: cytology with colposcopy 6 and 12 mo
	CIN 3 (or CIN 2 with inadequate colposcopy)		Definitive therapy preferred
Age >24 yr	No lesion or CIN 1	ASC-US, LSIL, persistent HPV	Co-test at 12 mo • Normal: retest in 3 yr[a] • Either abnormal: colposcopy
		ASC-H or HSIL	Co-test at 12 and 24 mo: • Normal: retest in 3 yr[a] • Abnormal (low-grade): colposcopy • HSIL: diagnostic excisional procedure
	CIN 2 or greater		Definitive therapy
Pregnant	Normal or only low-grade lesions[b]	Any	6 wk postpartum colposcopy
	CIN 2–3[c]	Any	Surveillance colposcopy no sooner than every 12 wk; repeat biopsy only if lesion appears to progress or if referring cytology suggested cancer

CIN, cervical intraepithelial neoplasia; ASC-US, atypical squamous cells of undetermined significance; LSIL, low-grade squamous intraepithelial lesion; ASC-H, atypical squamous cells cannot rule out high-grade; HSIL, high-grade squamous intraepithelial lesion.
[a]Age-appropriate testing: cytology for <30 years, co-testing ≥30 years.
[b]Based on histology or colposcopic impression at initial colposcopy.
[c]Biopsy recommended at initial colposcopy for suspected high-grade lesions.

INTERPRETATION AND MANAGEMENT OF BIOPSY RESULTS

- The American Society for Colposcopy and Cervical Pathology (ASCCP) updated 2012 guidelines for management of cervical dysplasia incorporate HPV testing in postcolposcopy follow-up and emphasize less invasive management strategies, particularly for younger women who desire to preserve fertility.[3] See Table 13.9-1.
- A positive ECC result or colposcopic evidence of significant endocervical canal involvement requires further tissue biopsy with LEEP or cold knife conization, *except*:
  - An ECC with low-grade dysplasia in a patient with NO high-grade dysplasia on colposcopic-directed biopsies, whose prior cytology findings were considered low-grade (ASC-US or low-grade squamous intraepithelial lesion), may be managed with co-testing at 12 and 24 months, including endocervical sampling at 12 months.[3,5]
- Definitive therapy consists of excisional (LEEP, laser excision, cold knife cone) or ablative (cryotherapy) procedures. Ablative therapies are not acceptable in the setting of a positive ECC or an inadequate colposcopy.

- Cryotherapy, LEEP, and laser ablation (for large lesions) can be considered for persistent low-grade lesions (present longer than 2 years).
- Limited ectocervical dysplasia that does not involve the canal is rarely a sole indication for hysterectomy.
- Adenomatous or glandular dysplasia on biopsy or ECC usually requires cold cone biopsy to evaluate for possible adenocarcinoma of the canal. Endometrial biopsy may also be necessary if there is suspicion of endometrial sources of adenodysplasia.
- Histologic diagnosis of cervical cancer requires definitive staging and advanced therapy, such as radical hysterectomy and radiation therapy.

COMPLICATIONS AND MORBIDITY OF COLPOSCOPY[1]

- Bleeding from biopsy sites is usually minimal and readily controlled with Monsel's.
- Infection is extremely rare.
- Failure to biopsy abnormal areas may result in missing or underestimating the degree of dysplasia, and ultimately cause delayed or inadequate therapy.

REFERENCES

1. Newkirk GR. Colposcopic examination. In: Pfenninger JL, Fowler GC, eds. *Procedures for primary care.* 3rd ed. Philadelphia, PA: Mosby; 2011.
2. Underwood M, Arbyn M, Parry-Smith W, et al. Accuracy of colposcopy-directed punch biopsies: a systematic review and meta-analysis. *BJOG* 2012;119:1293–1301.
3. Massad LS, Einstein MH, Huh WK, et al. 2012 Updated consensus guidelines for the management of abnormal cervical cancer screening tests and cancer precursors. *Obstet Gynecol* 2013;121:829–846.
4. Galaal K, Bryant A, Deane KH, et al. Interventions for reducing anxiety in women undergoing colposcopy. *Cochrane Database Syst Rev* 2011;(12):CD006013 doi: 10.1002/14651858.CD006013.pub3.
5. American College of Obstetricians and Gynecologists. ACOG practice bulletin no. 140. Management of abnormal cervical cancer screening test results and cervical cancer precursors. *Obstet Gynecol* 2013;122(6):1338–1367.
6. Massad LS, Einstein MH, Huh WK, et al. *ASCCP Algorithms: Updated consensus guidelines for managing abnormal cervical cancer screening tests and cancer precursors.* Frederick, MD: American Society for Colposcopy and Cervical Pathology; 2013.

CHAPTER 14

Family Planning and Maternity Care

Section Editor: Ashley J. Falk

14.1 Contraception

Carey Christiansen Ford

Many forms of contraception exist, each of which has unique benefits and disadvantages. Counseling a patient regarding birth-control options should include discussion of many factors, including efficacy, convenience, duration of action, reversibility and return to fertility, effects on uterine bleeding, side effects, cost, and sexually transmitted disease (STD) protection (See Table 14.1-1 for a comparative summary of available contraceptive methods). Additionally, contraception has moral implications for some individuals that should not be overlooked. A patient's individual characteristics and medical history may also limit or influence the selection of an appropriate form of contraception, and a thorough medical history and review of systems should be taken. Attention should be given to cardiovascular, gynecologic, and reproductive conditions, as well as psychologic or psychiatric conditions that might affect adherence.

NATURAL FAMILY PLANNING

This includes several methods described below of calculating the fertile time of a woman's cycle and maintaining complete abstinence during that period. Estimates of reliability vary, and for maximal effectiveness strict adherence must be followed. Advantages are lack of hormonal manipulation, cost, availability, and avoidance of artificial interventions that may contradict the beliefs of some religious and cultural groups. Disadvantages include the low rate of effectiveness compared to other methods, and the need for education to be provided in order to use it effectively.[1]

The calendar method is based on three assumptions: (a) a human ovum is capable of fertilization only for approximately 24 hours after ovulation; (b) sperm can only fertilize an ovum for about 48 hours after intercourse; and (c) ovulation usually occurs 12 to 16 days before the next menses begins. After recording six menstrual cycles, the fertile period can be estimated. The earliest day of the fertile period is determined by the number of days in the shortest menstrual cycle subtracted by 18. The latest day of the fertile period is calculated by the number of days in the longest cycle subtracted by 11. Abstinence is maintained during that interval.[1]

Cervical Mucus Method

The woman attempts to predict her fertile period by examining the cervical mucus with her fingers. Under the influence of estrogen, the mucus increases in quantity and becomes progressively more elastic. After a peak day, the mucus becomes scant and dry secondary to the influence of progesterone and remains this way until the onset of the next menses. Intercourse is allowed 4 days after the cervical mucus peaks until menses begins.[1]

Symptothermal Method

This method predicts the first day of abstinence by either using the calendar method or the detection of mucus, whichever is noted first. The end of the fertile period is predicted by measuring basal body temperature. The basal body temperature is lowest during the follicular phase and rises in the luteal (postovulatory) phase of the menstrual cycle in response to progesterone. The rise in temperature can vary from 0.2°C to 0.5°C. The elevated temperatures begin 1 to 2 days after ovulation and correspond to the rising level of progesterone. Intercourse is allowed 3 days after the temperature rise.[1]

Lactational Amenorrhea Method

While breastfeeding, a woman's fertility is typically reduced. The lactational amenorrhea method (LAM) can be relied on when three criteria are met: (a) It has been 6 months or less since delivery; (b) the woman's menstrual cycle has not returned; and (c) the infant's nutritional needs are at least 90% met at the breast. This method relies on frequent breastfeeding, both day and night, to be effective. Mechanism of action is inhibition of ovulation by elevated prolactin level. Disadvantages to this method include variability and unpredictability of the return of menses, and uncertainty of some women of the anticipated duration of breastfeeding.[2]

Abstinence

Abstinence is the complete avoidance of sexual intercourse. Mechanism of action is exclusion of sperm from the female reproductive tract. Advantages include STD prevention or reduction, although skin-to-skin contact without intercourse can transmit some infections. Disadvantages include lack of preparation for unanticipated intercourse, as well as difficulty maintaining the degree of willpower and self-control required.

BARRIER METHODS

These methods physically prevent the union of ovum and sperm.

Male Condoms

Sheaths made of latex, polyurethane, or natural materials worn over the penis during intercourse. Effectively reduces the risk of STDs. Disadvantages include short shelf life, possibility of failure if used with oil-based lubricants, problems with correct usage, and decreased sensation.[3] Many people are allergic to latex, in which case polyurethane condoms, which are somewhat less effective, may be used.

Female Condoms

A polyurethane sheath inserted into the vagina up to 8 hours before intercourse. Provides some protection from STDs. Inner surface coated with lubricant but does not contain spermicide. May be cumbersome or uncomfortable to use, and may contribute to the development of a urinary tract infection if left in place for too long.[2]

Diaphragms and Cervical Caps

Diaphragms and cervical caps are cervical barriers inserted vaginally to prevent sperm from reaching the cervical canal. These barriers should be used in conjunction with spermicide to increase efficacy. Advantages include the absence of hormone exposure and reduced likelihood of sexually transmitted infection, but are not recommended in women at high risk for HIV exposure. Disadvantages include lower efficacy than other methods, vaginal irritation, and discomfort in some women.[1]

Intrauterine Device

T-shaped device is placed in the uterus through the cervix during a simple office procedure; prevent pregnancy primarily through prevention of fertilization by several mechanisms. Two general types are approved for use in the United States, the copper-releasing type (ParaGard) and hormone-releasing type (Mirena and Skyla). This device is very effective, with a duration of use from 3 to 10 years. Both types of IUD have excellent continuation rates, and may be safely used by adolescents, nulliparous women, and multiparous women.[4]

Progesterone-Releasing Device

Levonorgestrel coating releases progesterone at 14 to 20 µg per day. This device can remain in the uterus for 3 to 5 years depending on the formulation. Advantages include improvement in menorrhagia and dysmenorrhea.[5,6] This device may have other noncontraceptive benefits, including treatment of endometrial hyperplasia, protection from pelvic inflammatory disease (PID), and reduction in symptoms of endometriosis.[4]

Copper-Releasing Device

Copper coating releases ions that interfere with sperm mobility and create a spermicidal environment. The device may be in place for up to 10 years.[5] Bleeding and dysmenorrhea may temporarily increase after insertion.[3] This device may be inserted postcoitally as emergency contraception, then left in place for ongoing birth control. Initially, users may experience heavier menstrual bleeding with increased dysmenorrhea for the first several months, decreasing over the first year. Additionally, the risk of PID is slightly higher than with a progesterone-containing device, with exposure to a sexually transmitted infection.[4]

COMBINED CONTRACEPTIVES

- **Oral combined contraceptive pills.** Oral contraceptive pills (OCPs) are daily tablet containing a progestin and a synthetic estrogen. Many users rely on OCPs for their noncontraceptive benefits, including improvement in menstrual cycle regulation, acne, hyperandrogenism, dysmenorrhea, breast and ovarian cysts, premenstrual syndrome, endometriosis, and others.[7] Newer formulations exist that allow less frequent menses, with 84 active pill days and 7 placebo, rather than the standard "21 + 7" schedule. These pills prevent midcycle gonadotropin release and thus inhibit ovulation. Combined OCPs may be started at any time during the menstrual cycle; a barrier method is typically recommended for the first week after starting, unless started on the first day of menstrual bleeding.[8]
- **Contraindications** include uncontrolled hypertension, venous thromboembolism, coronary heart disease, cerebrovascular disease, postpartum <21 days, age >25 years and smoke >15 to 20 cigarettes per day, headaches with focal neurologic symptoms, diabetes with vascular complications, lactation (<6 weeks), breast cancer, pregnancy, liver disease, inherited thrombophilias, anticonvulsant drug use, and undiagnosed abnormal uterine bleeding.[1,7]
- **Ortho Evra patch.** It is worn on the torso, buttocks, or upper arm, and changed weekly for 3 weeks followed by a patch-free week of bleeding similar to placebo-pill week of OCPs. Its mechanism of action, benefits, risks, and contraindications to use of the patch are similar to those of combined OCPs. Conflicting data exist regarding possible increased risk of thromboembolism. This method may be started on first day of menses or on Sunday following first day of menses, and requires 1 week of backup barrier method.[1]
- **NuvaRing.** It is a flexible plastic ring worn intravaginally for 3 weeks and removed for a 1-week interval before a new ring is inserted. Its mechanism of action, benefits, risks, and contraindications to use are similar to those of combined OCPs. This method should be started within the first 5 days of menses with a backup barrier method used for the first week.[1]

PROGESTIN-ONLY CONTRACEPTIVES

Ovulation is prevented by inhibiting the midcycle release of gonadotropins. Atrophic endometrium and thickened cervical mucus also protect against pregnancy by minimizing ability of a fertilized ovum to implant and decreasing sperm penetration through endocervical canal, respectively.[9]

- Progestin-only pills include Micronor and Ovrette. To maintain efficacy, these pills must be taken within 3-hour window regularly. These are often prescribed to women who are breastfeeding. Unlike estrogen-containing contraceptives, there is no increased risk of thromboembolism.[9]
- **Etonogestrel.** A single-rod progestin implant (originally marketed as Implanon, subsequently as Nexplanon) is available in the United States. Excellent contraception is provided for 3 years after placement subdermally in the inner upper arm. Protection from pregnancy, typically by prevention of fertilization and ovulation, occurs within 24 hours of insertion and fertility returns rapidly after removal. Training sponsored by the manufacturer is required before implant can be purchased or inserted. There are few contraindications, but unscheduled bleeding, headache, acne, weight gain, breast tenderness, emotional lability, and abdominal pain are the most common side effects.[10]
- **Depo-Provera.** Medroxyprogesterone acetate is given intramuscularly every 3 months. This medication is highly effective and can be started any time, as long as pregnancy is ruled out. A backup barrier method is needed the first week. Typically, a grace period of up to 2 weeks may be offered to patients returning late for an injection, although after 1 week late (or 14 weeks from last injection), many physicians will perform a urine pregnancy test and have the patient use a backup method (such as condoms) for 1 week. This method is beneficial for those wishing to avoid an estrogen-containing method of contraception or in those patients whose lifestyles or comorbid conditions make having a menstrual period difficult, such as military personnel or those who are wheelchair-bound or institutionalized. Depo-Provera reduces the risk of PID in users, protects the endometrium, and reduces both dysmenorrhea related to endometriosis and menorrhagia and dysmenorrhea in general.[11] Data indicate that bone density decreases while using this medication; however, this is largely regained and there has not been any evidence of increased fracture risk while using or later in life.[11] Irregular bleeding, amenorrhea, and delayed return to fertility (up to 18 months) are common side effects, as are a possible increase in mood symptoms and headaches for some users prone to these.[11]

TABLE 14.1-1   A Comparative Summary of Available Contraceptive Methods

Method	Women who had an unintended pregnancy within the first year (%)		Women who continued use at 1 yr (%)	Risks and side effects
	Typical use	Perfect use		
No method	85	85	—	—
Spermicides	29	15	42	Allergy to spermicide
Withdrawal	27	4	43	None known
Periodic abstinence	Unknown	1–9	—	None known
Cervical cap with spermicide: parous/ nulliparous	32/16	26/9	46/57	Vaginal and bladder infections, allergy to spermicide
Diaphragm with spermicide	16	6	57	Vaginal and bladder infections, allergy to spermicide
Female condom	21	5	49	Difficult to use, vaginal and bladder infections
Male condom	15	2	53	Decrease in spontaneity, allergic reactions
Combined OC	8	0.3	68	Nausea, vomiting, headaches, dizziness, mood changes, breast tenderness, spotting, breakthrough bleeding
Patch (Ortho Evra)	0.8	0.6	68	Same as OC, application site reactions
Vaginal contraceptive ring (Nuva-ring)	0.65	0.3	68	Vaginitis, breast tenderness, spotting, bleeding
Depo-Provera injection	3	0.3	56	Menstrual changes, weight gain, headaches, mood changes
Copper IUD (Paragard)	0.8	0.6	78	Increase in menstrual flow and cramping, risk of perforation and PID after insertion
Levonorgestrel-releasing IUD (Mirena)	0.1	0.1	81	Irregular bleeding, releasing amenorrhea, risk of perforation and PID after insertion
Female sterilization	0.5	0.5	100	—
Male sterilization	0.15	0.1	100	—

OC, oral contraceptive; IUD, intrauterine device; PID, pelvic inflammatory disease.

Adapted from Hatcher RA, Zieman M, Cwiak C, eds. *A pocket guide to managing contraception 2004–2005.* Tiger, GA: Bridging the Gap Communications; 2005.

STERILIZATION

Tubal Sterilization

This is a surgical method of preventing the ovum from being fertilized or reaching the uterine cavity by occluding or otherwise interrupting the fallopian tubes. This method is effective and permanent. There is an associated decreased risk of PID and ovarian cancer in women who have undergone sterilization procedures.[12] Drawbacks to this method include the risks inherent to any surgical procedure as well as the permanence of the procedure. Sterilization regret is highly correlated with age younger than 30 and unpredictable life events such as change in marital status or death of a child.[12] Reversal is costly and unpredictable. Also, there is an increased risk for ectopic pregnancy, should pregnancy occur.

Vasectomy

Vasectomy is a surgical method of preventing the release of sperm in the ejaculate by disrupting the vas deferens typically with ligation and cautery. This method is less expensive than tubal ligation; restoring fertility after vasectomy is unreliable and expensive. Another method should be used until documentation of azoospermia, which may be about 10 weeks. Bleeding and infection are rare complications.[13]

EMERGENCY CONTRACEPTION

This term often refers to high-dose progestin in pill form used postcoitally to prevent pregnancy by preventing ovulation, altering cervical mucus, or preventing implantation of fertilized ovum. Progestin pills do not interrupt an already-implanted pregnancy, and is not teratogenic.[3] The copper IUD may also be used as emergency contraception, as well as the antiprogestin drug ulipristal. The copper IUD is the most effective form of postcoital contraception, with the additional benefit of remaining in place to provide ongoing protection.[14]

- **Ella.** 30 mg ulipristal is taken as soon as possible, but within 120 hours of intercourse.[14]
- **Plan B.** 75 µg levonorgestrel is taken within 72 hours of intercourse, with second 75 µg tablet taken 12 hours later.[3,13] Some sources say the first tablet may actually be given within 120 hours of intercourse.[3] Plan B is now readily available over the counter.
- Alternatively, combined OCPs may be used. The first dose should be given within the first 72 hours after unprotected intercourse, and the second dose given 12 hours after the first dose. Many brand name OCPs can be used for emergency contraception including:
  - *Preven Kit.* Two pills per dose (0.5 mg of levonorgestrel and 100 µg of ethinyl estradiol per dose)
  - *Ovral.* Two pills per dose (0.5 mg of levonorgestrel and 100 µg of ethinyl estradiol per dose)
  - *Lo/Ovral.* Four pills per dose (0.6 mg of levonorgestrel and 120 µg of ethinyl estradiol per dose)
  - *Nordette.* Four pills per dose (0.6 mg of levonorgestrel and 120 µg of ethinyl estradiol per dose)
  - *Triphasil.* Four pills per dose (0.5 mg of levonorgestrel and 120 µg of ethinyl estradiol per dose)
  - *Ovrette.* 20 pills per dose (1.5 mg of levonorgestrel per dose)
  - *Seasonale.* Four pills per dose (0.6 mg of levonorgestrel and 120 µg of ethinyl estradiol per dose)
  - *Alesse.* Five pills per dose (0.5 mg of levonorgestrel and 100 µg of ethinyl estradiol per dose)[3,13]

REFERENCES

1. Samra O. Contraception (online). http://www.emedicine.com. Accessed on April 4, 2014.
2. Zieman M, Hatcher R. *Managing contraception.* New York, NY: Ardent Media; 2012.
3. Steiner MJ, Dominik R, Rountree RW, et al. Contraceptive effectiveness of a polyurethane condom and a latex condom: a randomized controlled trial. *Obstet Gynecol* 2003;101:539–547.
4. Dean G, Goldberg A. *Intrauterine contraception (IUD): Overview.* www.uptodate.com. Accessed on April 4, 2014.
5. Johnson BA. Insertion and removal of intrauterine devices. *Am Fam Physician* 2005;71:95–102.
6. Herndon EJ. New contraceptive options. *Am Fam Physician* 2004;69:853–860.
7. CerelSuhl SL, Yeager BF. Update on oral contraceptives. *Am Fam Physician* 1999;60(7):2073–2084.
8. Martin KA, Barbieri AR. Overview of the use of estrogen progestin contraceptives. http://www.uptodate.com. Accessed on April 4, 2014.
9. Apgar BA, Greenberg G. Using progestins in clinical practice. *Am Fam Physician* 2000;62(8)1839–1846, 1849–1850.
10. Darney P, Patel A, Rosen K, et al. Safety and efficacy of a single-rod etonogestrel implant (Implanon): results from 11 international clinical trials. *Fertil Steril* 2009;91:1646.
11. Kaunitz A. *Depot medroxyprogesterone acetate for contraception.* www.uptodate.com. Accessed on April 4, 2014.
12. Baill IC, Cullins VE, Sangeeta P. Counseling issues in tubal sterilization. *Am Fam Physician* 2003;67:1287–1294, 1301–1302.
13. Dassow P, Bennett J. Vasectomy: an update. *Am Fam Physician* 2006;74:2069–2074.
14. Bosworth MC, Okesola PL, Low SB. An update on emergency contraception. *Am Fam Physician* 2014;89:545–550.

14.2 Infertility

Hilary B. Miller

GENERAL PRINCIPLES

The diagnosis of infertility is established after 1 year of regular unprotected intercourse in which a pregnancy has not been achieved. In women older than 35, infertility is diagnosed after 6 months of regular unprotected intercourse. **Fecundity** is the probability of achieving pregnancy in one menstrual cycle; approximately 50% of couples are able to conceive after 3 months, 75% after 6 months, and 90% after 1 year. In the Unites States, 12% of reproductive age women are affected by infertility; this proportion increases with the age of the female partner.[1–4]

There are many causes of infertility, including abnormalities of any portion of the male or female reproductive system. Infertility is due to a single cause in the majority of couples, but more than one factor may contribute to infertility. Therefore, a comprehensive history, physical examination, and diagnostic evaluation are recommended for all couples.[5]

Common Etiology and Pathophysiology

- **Male factors.** Male cause for infertility occurs in 25% of couples. The most common male etiologic factor is a varicocele. Other causative factors include low or absent sperm count, oligospermia or azoospermia, disorders of sperm function or motility, asthenospermia, and abnormalities of sperm morphology, teratospermia. Autoimmunity as a cause of male infertility is rare.[4]
- **Ovulatory dysfunction.** Disorders of ovulation account for approximately 27% of cases of infertility.[6] The possible causes may be grouped into four major categories:
  - **Hypothalamic anovulation** includes anatomical defects, congenital defects, psychologic trauma, anorexia nervosa, and pharmacologic agents.
  - **Ovarian anovulation** includes ovarian tumors, premature ovarian failure, ovarian dysgenesis, thyroid disease, and adrenal disease.
  - **Pituitary anovulation** includes pituitary tumors and ischemia.
  - **Integrative anovulation** includes nonpsychogenic weight disturbances and polycystic ovarian syndrome (PCOS).
- **Tubal.** Infertility due to tubal structural damage or adnexal adhesions accounts for approximately 22% of cases of infertility.[6] Tubal obstruction may result from previous episodes of salpingitis, although many cases of tubal occlusion are encountered in which no episodes of salpingitis are recalled by the patient. Endometriosis may result in the anatomical distortion of adnexal structures.
- **Endometriosis.** The chronic inflammation associated with endometriosis may disrupt normal conception by interfering with ovum capture and gamete and embryo transport, or by causing tubal damage. Endometriosis is the cause of approximately 5% of infertility cases.[6]
- **Unexplained infertility.** No specific etiologic factor is identified in approximately 17% of infertile couples after an initial diagnostic survey.[6]

DIAGNOSTIC EVALUATION

A thorough diagnostic survey of both partners is necessary to evaluate all areas of the reproductive system. The workup is begun for women under 35 years old after 12 months of infertility and after 6 months of infertility in women over 35 years old. A meeting with the couple early in the evaluation provides an opportunity to review reproductive biology, discuss the rationale for subsequent tests, and assess the couple's coping skills.

History

The initial assessment of the couple consists of a thorough history of each partner, taken individually, to assess current and past contributing symptoms, illness, medication, or surgery. The key elements of such a history are outlined in Table 14.2-1.[4]

Physical Examination

As with the history, a thorough physical examination of each partner is essential. Areas of special attention for each physical are listed in Table 14.2-2.[4]

TABLE 14.2-1	Key Areas of Infertility History

Marriage
Duration of infertility
Fertility in previous relationship
Sexual techniques
Frequency of intercourse (optimal is daily around time of ovulation)
Use of coital lubricants (often spermicidal)

Adult illness
Acute viral or febrile illness in past 3 mo
Orchitis
Renal disease
Sexually transmitted diseases
Tuberculosis

Occupation and habits
Exposure to radiation, chemicals, excessive heat (e.g., hot tub)

Childhood
Cryptorchidism
Age at puberty

Surgery
Herniorrhaphy
Retroperitoneal surgery
Vasectomy

Past medical history
Focus on endocrine conditions
Gynecologic history (Pap smear testing result, treatment)
Contraceptive use
Diethylstilbestrol (DES) use by mother
Douches and lubricant use
Menarche
Menses (regularity and flow)
Mittelschmerz

Drug use
Alcohol, tobacco, excessive caffeine, and other drugs
Anabolic steroids, nitrofurantoin, cimetidine

TABLE 14.2-2	Physical Examination in Infertility: Areas of Special Attention

Male	**Female**
Hair pattern	Breast formation and galactorrhea
Genitalia	Distribution of body fat
Meatus size and location	Hair pattern (virilization)
Prostate and seminal vesicles	Neurologic
Scrotum	Anosmia
Testicular size (>4 cm in long axis)	Visual fields
Varicocele (standing and with Valsalva maneuver)	Pelvis
Neurologic	External genitalia
Anosmia	Retrovaginal area (endometriosis)
Visual fields	Uterus and adnexa
	Vagina and cervix

TABLE 14.2-3	Laboratory and Diagnostic Testing in Infertility

Routine laboratory tests
Male
  CBC
  Semen analysis (at least 2, 4 wk apart)
  Urinalysis
Female
  CBC
  Pap smear
  Urinalysis
Special circumstances
Anovulation: serum prolactin and TSH
Galactorrhea: serum prolactin and TSH
Hyperandrogenism: serum prolactin, TSH, LH, FSH, DHEA-S, 17-OH progesterone
Advanced maternal age >35 yr/o: cycle day 2 FSH and estradiol. Indicates decreased ovarian reserve if FSH >10–20 mIU/mL. If estradiol elevated, >70 pg/mL cannot accurately interpret FSH results.

Laboratory Studies

Each couple is evaluated with a few routine laboratory and appropriately timed studies to assess every major reproductive factor that may contribute to infertility. This comprehensive diagnostic survey can and should be completed for the majority of couples in 3 to 6 months. The evaluation should be individualized on the basis of findings of the history and physical examination, but an initial survey of all major reproductive factors is necessary in all couples and can be coordinated by the family physician. The specifically timed diagnostic tests required for an infertility survey are outlined in Table 14.2-3.[4]

- **Male factors.** The male is evaluated with a complete blood count, urinalysis, and at least two semen analyses 4 weeks apart. Each semen analysis is performed on a fresh (within 2 hours), warm specimen obtained by masturbation after at least 2 days of abstinence. Normal results vary between laboratories, but in general include a volume (2 to 5 mL), complete liquefaction within 30 minutes, sperm count (>20 million per mL), sperm motility (>50%), and morphology (WHO >30% normal forms, Kruger Strict Criteria >14%). Evidence of oligospermia after two or more semen analyses requires further evaluation, including blood levels for luteinizing hormone, follicle-stimulating hormone (FSH), and testosterone. Etiology of semen abnormalities is outlined in Table 14.2-4.[4,7,8]
- **Ovulatory dysfunction.** Anovulation or inconsistent ovulation may be suggested by history (irregular menses, amenorrhea), and confirmed by an abnormally low-serum progesterone levels in the midluteal phase, or persistently negative home luteinizing hormone (LH) testing. If the patient is not ovulating, further laboratory evaluation is needed (see Table 14.2-3, Special circumstances). Those patients with a diminished ovarian reserve (FSH >10 mIU per mL) should be referred to an infertility specialist.[4]
- **Tubal factors.** The female partner must undergo an evaluation for tubal patency. A hysterosalpingogram is obtained if the history and physical examination show no evidence of tubal damage. Otherwise, the patient is referred for laparoscopy.[4]

TREATMENT

Treatment should not be initiated until the diagnostic survey is complete and the infertility cause or causes identified. The diagnosis should be shared with the couple together and the treatment options outlined. The workup, diagnosis, and treatment of infertility can precipitate intense emotional reactions. The physician should assist the couple in the development of mutual support. Periodic meetings with the couple to review diagnostic or treatment progress provide further opportunity to reinforce coping skills. Referral to self-help groups, such as RESOLVE, Inc. (www.resolve.org), assists the couple in broadening their support systems.

- **Male factors.** Consultation with urology is necessary to coordinate treatment for a varicocele or other causes of sperm dysfunction.
- **Ovulatory dysfunction.** Treatment with clomiphene should be considered for women diagnosed with anovulation. Amenorrheic and oligomenorrheic women attempting to conceive are among the most suitable patients for clomiphene. Patients with other cause for their anovulation respond

TABLE 14.2-4	Etiologies of Semen Abnormalities

Count abnormality

Oligozoospermia	Endocrinopathies (androgen receptor defect)
	Varicocele
	Maturation arrest
	Hypospermatogenesis
Azoospermia	Klinefelter syndrome
	Sertoli-cell–only syndrome
	Seminiferous tubule or Leydig cell failure
	Hypogonadotropic hypogonadism
	Ductal obstruction (Young syndrome)
	Varicocele

Volume abnormality

No ejaculate	Ductal obstruction
	Retrograde ejaculation
	Ejaculatory failure
	Hypogonadism
Low volume	Ductal obstruction
	Absence of seminal vesicles and vas deferens
	Retrograde ejaculation
	Infection

Motility/morphology dysfunction

Abnormal motility	Autoimmunity
	Infection
	Varicocele
	Sperm structural defects
	Metabolic abnormalities of sperm
	Abnormal viscosity
	Poor liquefaction of semen
Abnormal morphology	Varicocele
	Stress
	Infection

best to specific therapy, such as surgery for a pituitary tumor or medical therapy for thyroid disease. Obese women with insulin insensitivity and/or PCOS may benefit from metformin therapy initiated at 500 mg PO daily and titrated up over several weeks, with typical dosing of 1,500 mg daily. It is generally a preliminary option to clomiphene in women with obesity and insulin insensitivity.[7]

Clomiphene citrate is first-line pharmacotherapy for women with anovulatory causes of infertility. The starting dose for clomiphene citrate is 50 mg PO daily on menstrual cycle days 3 to 7. Ovulation should be expected 3 to 8 days after the treatment ends and should be confirmed by LH home detection kit and an elevated serum progesterone on day 21 (approximately 2 weeks after the last clomiphene dose). If midluteal progesterone is greater than 10 pg per mL, continue the same clomiphene dose on subsequent cycles. If the midluteal progesterone level is less than 10 pg per mL, the dose of clomiphene can be increased by 50 mg on subsequent cycles until the patient is ovulating. Most women should begin ovulation at 50 mg dosing. It is unusual to require more than 150 mg, maximum dose 250 mg, to achieve ovulation. At this point, adjunctive therapy with metformin or switching therapy may be considered. The patient should be aware of the common side effects of clomiphene therapy: ovarian enlargement (13.9% of cases), vasomotor flushes (10.7%), abdominal or pelvic discomfort (7.4%), and multiple gestation (<5% and usually twinning). If ovulation does not occur despite clomiphene therapy, consultation with an infertility specialist is recommended.[3,7]

- **Tubal damage, uterine anomaly.** Tubal deformity or blockage, intrauterine congenital anomalies, intrauterine adhesions, and leiomyomas are uncommon causes of infertility and can be diagnosed with ultrasound or hysterosalpingogram. These conditions may require surgical correction via laparoscopy or laparotomy with tubal microsurgery, although pregnancy outcomes may be more cost effectively achieved via in vitro fertilization (IVF).[7]

- **Endometriosis.** The treatment of infertile women with endometriosis depends on the degree and location of the endometrial deposits. Conservative surgical treatment may enhance fertility by destroying endometrial implants and endometriomas. The laparoscopic cauterization of early-stage endometriosis has been shown to improve pregnancy rates. Ovulation suppression by danazol, progestins, and gonadotropin-releasing hormone analogues has been shown not to be effective in the treatment of endometriosis-associated infertility. Superovulation with clomiphene or human menopausal gonadotropins has been shown to be effective in such patients.[3,7]

Prognosis, Referral

The specific prognosis of infertility is difficult to determine due to the multiple etiologies. For most causes of infertility, conception will not occur without specific treatment. However, favorable pregnancy rates are reported when specific therapy is instituted. If the comprehensive diagnostic workup fails to establish a diagnosis or if appropriate treatment is unsuccessful, the physician should consider referring the couple to an infertility specialist for additional treatment and consideration of intrauterine insemination or IVF. The options for adoption should also be discussed.[3]

REFERENCES

1. Fritz MA, Speroff L. *Clinical gynecologic endocrinology and infertility*. 8th ed. Baltimore, MD: Williams & Wilkins; 2010.
2. Kaplan JL, Porter RS, eds. 2011. *Merck manual of diagnosis and therapy*. 19th ed. Whitehouse Station, NJ: Merck Sharp & Dohme Corp; 2011.
3. Hull MG, Glazener CM, Kelly NJ, et al. Population study of causes, treatment, and outcome of infertility. *Br Med J* 1985;14(291):1693–1697.
4. Ghadir S, Ambartsumyan G, DeCherney AH. Infertility. In: DeCherney AH, Nathan L, Laufer N, et al., eds. *CURRENT diagnosis & treatment: obstetrics & gynecology*. 11th ed. New York, NY: McGraw-Hill; 2013:chap 53.
5. Mohan SK, Siladitya B. Demographics of infertility and management of unexplained infertility. *Best Pract Res Clin Obstet Gynecol* 2012;26(6):729–378.
6. Collins JA, Burrows EA, Willan AR, et al. The prognosis for live birth among untreated infertile couples. *Fertil Steril* 1995;64(1):22–28.
7. Lentz GM, Lobo RA, Gershenson DM, et al. *Comprehensive gynecology*. 6th ed. Philadelphia, PA: Elsevier Mosby; 2012.
8. Mishell DR, Davajan V, Lobo RA, eds. *Infertility, contraception and reproductive endocrinology*. 3rd ed. Cambridge, MA: Blackwell Scientific; 1991.

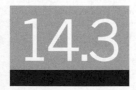

14.3 Genetic Disorders and Pregnancy

Lei Yu, Ashley J. Falk

GENERAL PRINCIPLES

Genetic disorders in pregnancy is a complex topic for patients and providers. For most genetic conditions, the benefits of prenatal diagnosis have not been scientifically evaluated, other than the option for a patient to terminate a pregnancy affected by a genetic disorder. Patients may be concerned about possible discrimination against themselves or future offspring. Genetic counseling is recommended to clarify these issues and discuss the implications of testing for patients who are at risk. This chapter reviews the most common genetic disorders found during pregnancy, specifically the ones for which screening tests are available.

Types of Genetic Disorders

- **Chromosome disorders** are caused by the loss, gain, or abnormal arrangement of one or more chromosomes. The incidence of these disorders in the population is about 0.2%. Down syndrome (trisomy 21) is discussed below.

- **Mendelian disorders** are single-gene disorders caused by a mutant allele at a single genetic locus. The transmission pattern is further divided into autosomal dominant, autosomal recessive, X-linked dominant, and X-linked recessive. The incidence of these disorders is about 0.35%. Screening for cystic fibrosis, hemoglobinopathies, and Tay–Sachs disease is discussed below.
- **Multifactorial disorders** involve interactions between genes and environmental factors. The nature of these interactions is poorly understood. Screening for cardiac defects and neural tube defects (NTDs) is described below.

CHROMOSOME DISORDERS: DOWN SYNDROME

Down syndrome (trisomy 21) occurs in 1 in 700 live births. The risk of having a fetus with Down syndrome increases with maternal age. Affected children have variable degrees of intellectual disability (mean IQ 50). About 40% to 50% of those children will have congenital heart defects, and there is an increased risk of duodenal atresia and tracheoesophageal fistula. Affected children also have increased problems with hearing, vision, hypothyroidism, leukemia, cervical spine instability, and Alzheimer disease.

Noninvasive Prenatal Screening for Down Syndrome

Various tests can be done though serum detection or ultrasound during the first and second trimester, including combined test, quadruple test, integrated test, and serum integrated test. The American College of Obstetrics and Gynecology (ACOG) recommends that all women be offered serum screening during their pregnancy,[1] Both the first and second trimester serum screening are simple to perform and have high rates of sensitivity with small false positive rates. Second trimester ultrasound is readily available but has a lower sensitivity for detection of Down syndrome.

- Early testing allows women who would choose termination of the pregnancy to do so at an earlier gestational age (when termination is safer). For women who would not choose termination, determination of the fetal abnormality allows patients to prepare for the baby and its added needs. It also allows providers to do further testing on the fetus (i.e., cardiac echo). Identification of pregnancies that have a fetus affected by Down syndrome will also assist physicians in management of the pregnancy. These pregnancies often have higher rates of pre-eclampsia, postdates pregnancy, and dysfunctional labor.
- **First trimester screening.** Serum and ultrasound markers that can be evaluated during weeks 10 to 13 of gestation. The serum markers are pregnancy-associated plasma protein A (PAPP-A) and the free unit of β-human chorionic gonadotropin (hCG). PAPP-A levels are 2.5 times lower in fetuses with Down syndrome and levels of the free unit of β-hCG are two times higher.
  - Increased nuchal translucency (NT) seen on ultrasound during weeks 11 to 13 of gestation is associated with Down syndrome, trisomy 18, and other aneuploidies. The combined test (serum markers and ultrasound for NT, together with maternal age) is recommended as an effective screening test in the general population with an approximate sensitivity of 85% and a false-positive rate (FPR) of 5%. It also can be used to detect trisomy 18.[2] However NT measurement requires specialized training and thus is not available in some regions. Women who have first trimester screening for Down syndrome still need to have an α-fetoprotein (AFP) level done in the second trimester for evaluation of NTDs.
  - The cost-effectiveness of combined screening in the first trimester is debatable. Compared to second trimester screening, performing fewer amniocenteses decreases the cost, while measuring NT with its high FPR increases the cost.
- **Second trimester screening.** The quadruple test is a serum study that evaluates AFP, β-hCG, inhibin A, and estriol levels. The test can be performed from 15 to 22 weeks of gestation and has a sensitivity of 85% with FPR of 5% to 6%.[3] Calculation of the serum marker levels combined with maternal age provides a personal risk score for each woman for her risk of having a fetus with Down syndrome. The screening test is considered positive if the calculated risk is greater than 1/270. This is the risk of a 35-year-old woman having a fetus with Down syndrome and is also the risk of a procedure-related loss from invasive testing for Down syndrome.
  - Incorrect gestational age is the most common reason for a false-positive result. Gestational age should always be first confirmed with an ultrasound prior to proceeding to invasive testing for an evaluation of a positive screen.
  - **Ultrasound.** Second trimester ultrasound can be used to identify major and minor structural abnormalities of the fetus that are associated with Down syndrome. Major structural abnormalities include heart defects and duodenal atresia. Minor ultrasound markers include increased nuchal fold, echogenic bowel, pyelectasis, echogenic cardiac focus, choroids plexus cysts, two-vessel cord, and absent nasal bone. Sensitivity for detection of Down syndrome with one or more makers is 79% with a FPR of 12%.

- **Integrated test.** The test integrates both first and second trimester measurements into a single test result. It typically includes NT and PAPP-A in the first trimester and quadruple test in the second trimester. Compared to combined test or quadruple test alone, it achieves an equivalent sensitivity (85%) with a much lower FPR of 1%. When measurement of NT is not available, serum integrated test can be used as an alternative (sensitivity 85% and FPR 4.4%).

Invasive Diagnostic Test

This test is available both to evaluate a positive screen for Down syndrome and also as primary screening for women over the age of 35.

- **Chorionic villus sampling (CVS)** can be performed from 10 to 13 weeks of gestation. A cannula is used to obtain a small amount of placental tissue via a transcervical (TC-CVS) or transabdominal (TA-CVS) approach. This provides a large amount of genetic material and karyotype results are often available in 48 hours.
  - Risks of the procedure include spontaneous fetal loss. The relative risk of fetal loss compared to amniocentesis is 1.3 (CI 1.2 to 1.5). However, when rates of TC-CVS are removed, the rate of loss is similar to amniocentesis. Other risks include bleeding, infection, and fetomaternal hemorrhage.
- **Amniocentesis** can be performed as early as 13 weeks gestation, but is more commonly done after 15 weeks. A needle is introduced into the amniotic cavity and amniotic fluid is removed. Sloughed fetal cells are cultured and DNA is extracted for karyotyping. Results can take up to 2 weeks.
  - Total fetal loss after amniocentesis is 6.1% with a procedure-related loss of 0.6%. Membrane rupture occurs 1.7% of the time, but most of the leaks are small, resolve spontaneously, and reaccumulate within a week. Other risks include indirect fetal injury, infection, and fetomaternal hemorrhage.

MENDELIAN DISORDERS
Cystic Fibrosis

Cystic fibrosis (CF) is the most common autosomal recessive disorder of Caucasians of Northern European descent. The carrier rate for a mutation is 1 in 25. Carrier rates are also high in Ashkenazi Jews (1 in 24). CF can cause abnormal pulmonary function, pancreatic insufficiency, or congenital absence of the vas deferens. The average age of survival is about 37 years and continues to increase.

- Serum screening can be done at any time, but ideally is best done prior to pregnancy. Because most screening tests detect only 90% of the mutations that cause CF, screening can decrease risk but not eliminate it.[4]
- The ACOG recommends that preconception and prenatal CF carrier screening be offered to all women of reproductive age.[5] Women who are not in high-risk groups (family history of CF, reproductive partner with CF, Caucasian of European descent, or Ashkenazi Jews) should be offered the test, but the decreased detectability of mutations should be discussed. If the patient is a carrier, screening should be offered to her partner. It is recommended to offer genetic counseling to couples in which both partners are carriers.
- The fetus can be tested for CF with amniocentesis, CVS, or fetal blood sample. Issues that need to be considered include the related fetal loss associated with invasive testing. Knowledge of the diagnosis for the fetus will most likely not change the neonatal course (except for monitoring/treatment of meconium ileus). In addition, parents need to be reminded that the same genotypes often have different phenotypic presentations, which makes prediction of morbidity and mortality from CF problematic.

Hemoglobinopathies

Hemoglobinopathies have an autosomal recessive inheritance pattern. High-risk groups are people of African, Southeast Asian, and Mediterranean descent. Complete blood count (CBC) is an appropriate first-line screening test for most at-risk women. Additionally, ACOG recommends that all women of African descent have hemoglobin electrophoresis at the same time.[6]

Women of Southeast Asian or Mediterranean descent with a low mean corpuscular volume (MCV) on CBC testing (less than 80 μ^3) should have hemoglobin electrophoresis to determine whether they are hemoglobinopathy carriers.

Prenatal genetic testing by CVS or amniocentesis is available for sickle cell disease, and for α- and β-thalassemia when the mutations have previously been identified in the parents.

Sickle Cell Disease

Sickle cell disease is the most common hemoglobinopathy; 1 out of 12 African Americans has sickle cell trait. Sickle cell trait can be detected by hemoglobin electrophoresis. If a woman who is pregnant or contemplating pregnancy tests positive, the next step is testing of the male partner. If both partners test positive, the couple should be referred for genetic counseling. Despite the relatively high prevalence of sickle cell disease, surveys have shown that most African American women of childbearing age do not understand the inheritance pattern or implications of the carrier state.

Thalassemia

α-Thalassemia trait (α-thalassemia minor) has two variants. In individuals of Southeast Asian descent, both α-globin genes on the same chromosome are deleted. They are at higher risk for a child with hemoglobin H disease (deletion of three of the four α-globin genes) and hemoglobin Bart (or α-thalassemia major, deletion of all four α-globin genes). Hemoglobin H results in mild to moderate hemolytic anemia. Hemoglobin Bart can lead to hydrops fetalis, intrauterine fetal demise, and pre-eclampsia.

In individuals of African descent with α-thalassemia trait, one α-globin gene is deleted on each copy of chromosome 16. They are not typically at risk for offspring with hemoglobin H or hemoglobin Bart. However, mild anemia is often present.

α-Thalassemia trait will not be detected on hemoglobin electrophoresis. DNA-based testing is needed for women with low MCV, no iron-deficiency anemia, and a normal hemoglobin electrophoresis.

Tay–Sachs Disease

The carrier rate for Tay–Sachs disease is 1 of 30 for people of Eastern European Jewish descent (Ashkenazi); people of French–Canadian and Cajun descent also have higher rates. Inheritance is autosomal recessive.

In this disorder, accumulation of gangliosides in the central nervous system results in progressive neurologic disease and death in early childhood.

In nonpregnant women, carrier screening can be performed by molecular or biochemical analysis.[7] Biochemical analysis has a higher carrier detection rate, especially in low-risk populations. However, in women who are pregnant or taking oral contraceptives, serum biochemical testing may yield a false-positive result. These women should have biochemical testing on peripheral leukocytes or molecular testing. Genetic counseling is recommended for high-risk patients to determine the correct type of testing and to interpret the test results.

MULTIFACTORIAL DISORDERS

Congenital Heart Disease

Congenital heart disease (CHD) is the most common congenital anomaly, occurring in 8 of 1,000 live births. Risk factors include family history of CHD, maternal diabetes, exposure to cardiac teratogens, noncardiac fetal anomalies detected on ultrasound, chromosomal abnormalities, single umbilical artery, fetal arrhythmias, nonimmune fetal hydrops, and increased NT.

The majority of CHD will occur in a low-risk population. In the United States, although routine ultrasound screening is not mandated, most women do undergo ultrasound screening during pregnancy. The International Society of Ultrasound in Obstetrics and Gynecology (ISUOG) recommends routine cardiac screening should include both four-chamber view and outflow tract views. The detection rate of CHD on routine 18- to 22-week ultrasound is very variable, ranging from 23% to 77%.[8] However, women with risk factors should be referred for fetal echocardiography.[9]

The advantages of early detection of CHD fall into three categories: offering patients the choice of pregnancy termination, prenatal intervention, and postnatal management. Prenatal intervention is still in the experimental stages. Although postnatal management, such as delivery at a tertiary care center and preparation for early surgery, would appear to have logical benefits, the advantages of this have been difficult to demonstrate in studies.

Neural Tube Defects

NTDs are the second most prevalent congenital anomaly. In the United States, NTDs occur in 1 in 1,000 pregnancies. The defects either appear in the spine (spina bifida, meningomyelocele, meningocele) or the cranium (anencephaly, which accounts for 50% of NTDs). Some NTDs are associated with genetic syndromes, but the majority are isolated defects.

NTDs most likely result from a combination of genetic and environmental influences. In a family with a child with a previous NTD, the relative risk of having another child with an NTD is 2% to 4%. Exposure to drugs that interfere with folic acid metabolism (carbamazepine, valproic acid) can cause NTDs. Maternal hyperthermia, diabetes, and obesity also increase the risk of having a fetus with an NTD. Finally, folic acid deficiency is known to increase the risk of NTDs. Preconception and early gestation (prior to 6 weeks) supplementation decrease the risk of NTDs.

Screening

Since 90% of NTDs occur in women with no prior history of having an affected fetus, it is recommended that all pregnant women be offered screening during weeks 15 to 20 of gestation.[10]

- **Maternal serum α-fetoprotein (MSAFP)** is elevated in 89% to 100% of pregnancies with a fetal NTD. An MSAFP greater than 2.0 to 2.5 multiples of the mean is 75% to 90% sensitive (5% FPR) for detection of all NTDs and greater than 95% sensitive (2% to 5% FPR) for detection of anencephaly.[11] Some factors such as gestational age, maternal weight, diabetes mellitus, fetal abnormality, and multiple gestations will affect the test results. Follow-up ultrasound examination should be offered to patients with positive MSAFP results.
- **Ultrasound** is used as both a screening and diagnostic examination, especially in high-risk pregnancies. It is 97% to 100% sensitive for the detection of NTDs and should be offered to all women with an abnormal MSAFP or women who are at high risk for a fetus with NTD during 18 to 20 weeks of gestation.
- **Amniocentesis** allows for removal of amniotic fluid and evaluation of amniotic fluid AFP (AFAFP) and acetylcholinesterase. Amniocentesis should be considered if the ultrasound is equivocal or normal with positive MSAFP result, or if the patient wishes to have karyotype determination of the fetus. If both AFAFP and amniotic acetylcholinesterase levels are abnormal, the fetus most likely has an open NTD (96% sensitivity, 0.14% false positive).
- Fetal magnetic resonance imaging (MRI) can be considered in cases where ultrasound failed to obtain ideal visualization. However, the diagnostic capability and efficacy needs further investigation.

OTHER CONGENITAL ANOMALIES

The rates of ultrasound detection of anomalies vary from over 90% for major defects such as hydrocephalus and anencephaly, to just over 17% for cleft lip and palate and foot deformities.[12] Because of this wide variability, the value of ultrasound screening for congenital anomalies is still unproven. Pregnant women should be informed about the detection rates of anomalies on ultrasound, and that many anomalies may be missed on ultrasound testing.

REFERENCES

1. ACOG Committee on Practice Bulletins. ACOG practice bulletin No. 77: screening for fetal chromosomal abnormalities. *Obstet Gynecol* 2007;109(1):217–227.
2. Messerlian GM, Farina A, Palomaki GE. First trimester combined test and integrated tests for screening for down syndrome and trisomy 18. www.uptodate.com. Accessed January 15, 2014.
3. Messerlian GM, Farina A, Palomaki GE. Second trimester maternal serum screening for Down syndrome. www.uptodate.com. Accessed January 15, 2014.
4. Wenstrom KD. Cystic fibrosis: prenatal genetic screening. www.uptodate.com. Accessed on December 30, 2013.
5. American College of Obstetricians and Gynecologists Committee on Genetics. ACOG committee opinion No. 486: update on carrier screening for cystic fibrosis. *Obstet Gynecol* 2011;117(4);1028–1031.
6. ACOG Committee on Obstetrics. ACOG practice bulletin No. 78: hemoglobinopathies in pregnancy. *Obstet Gynecol* 2007;109(1):229–237.
7. ACOG Committee on Genetics. ACOG committee opinion. Number 318, October 2005. Screening for Tay–Sachs disease. *Obstet Gynecol* 2005;106(4):893–894.
8. Copel J. Prenatal sonographic diagnosis of fetal cardiac anomalies. www.uptodate.com. Accessed January 15, 2014.
9. Carvalho JS, Allan LD, Chaoui R, et al.; International Society of Ultrasound in Obstetrics and Gynecology. ISUOG Practice Guidelines (updated): sonographic screening examination of the fetal heart. *Ultrasound Obstet Gynecol* 2013;41:348–359.
10. Driscoll DA, Gross SJ; Professional Practice Guidelines Committee. Screening for fetal aneuploidy and neural tube defect. *Genet Med* 2009;11(11):818–821.
11. Hochberg L, Stone J. Prenatal screening and diagnosis of neural tube defects. www.uptodate.com. Accessed January 15, 2014.
12. American College of Obstetricians and Gynecologists. ACOG practice bulletin No. 101: ultrasonography in pregnancy. *Obstet Gynecol* 2009;113(2):451–461.

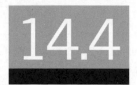

Prenatal Care
Irina Rozin

GENERAL PRINCIPLES

Family-centered prenatal care is the delivery of effective, efficient, accessible, safe, and economical quality care for the psychosocial, spiritual, and physical needs of the mother, child, father, and family unit. Family physicians with this philosophy view childbirth as a vital life event in the family and a foundational event in the formation of community and society. The family physician is ideally suited to provide this care, whether the family physician will deliver the baby or provide "shared prenatal care" with a delivering midwife or physician. An in-depth review of routine prenatal care is beyond the scope of this chapter; however, basic information that is frequently needed during prenatal care is provided, and Figure 14.4-1 illustrates important considerations and decision points in prenatal care.

DIAGNOSIS
History

A comprehensive history is required to provide appropriate prenatal care and distinguish between uncomplicated and higher risk obstetrical patients. Ideally, prenatal care begins before conception and includes preventive, health-maintenance care, counseling, and screening for risks to maternal and fetal health.[1] The following components should be included:

- **Medical/surgical history.** History of diabetes, hypertension, asthma, seizure disorder, mental illness, hematologic disorders, cancer, HIV, recurrent urinary tract infections. Past surgeries. Previous history of varicella.
- **Maternal care history.** Past history of complicated pregnancy or delivery. History of preterm delivery; prior cervical or uterine surgery. History of fetal anatomic abnormality or intrauterine fetal demise.
- **Psychosocial history.** History of eating disorder, substance use, mood disorder, psychosis, or postpartum depression.
- Family history of medical and genetic disorders; prescription and over-the-counter medication use; substance use; history of domestic violence; history of transfusions; and immunization status. Ascertain risk for tuberculosis as well as sexually transmitted infections (STIs) or diseases (STDs) caused by HPV, HIV, hepatitis B or C, gonorrhea, *Chlamydia,* herpes, or syphilis.[1]

Physical Examination

- **Initial visit.** The estimated date of delivery (EDD) is ascertained based on the patient's last menstrual period (LMP). Early ultrasound is indicated to determine the EDD whether there is uncertainty about the LMP.
- Examination should include height, weight, and body mass index (BMI); blood pressure; screening Pap smear for women who have not been recently screened and meet criteria. Obtain cervical cultures for gonorrhea (GC) and *Chlamydia* (Chl) in high-risk women (age <25 years; unmarried; Black, a history of STIs or STDs, new or multiple sexual partners, inconsistent use of barrier contraception; and living in communities with high infection rates).[1]
- Initial lab includes blood type and Rh, HIV, rubella, hepatitis B surface antigen (HBsAg), urine culture; varicella titer if unsure of history; and urine dipstick to determine baseline renal function.[1]
- All subsequent visits should include interval history and address any patient concerns or symptoms suggestive of preeclampsia or preterm labor, along with assessment of blood pressure, weight gain, fundal height, and fetal heart tones.
- Beginning with the start of the third trimester, visits should also include an assessment of fetal movement and abdominal palpation to assess fetal presentation at 36 weeks gestation.[1]
- There is no benefit in performing routine urine dipstick to check for proteinuria or glycosuria in low-risk women.[2]

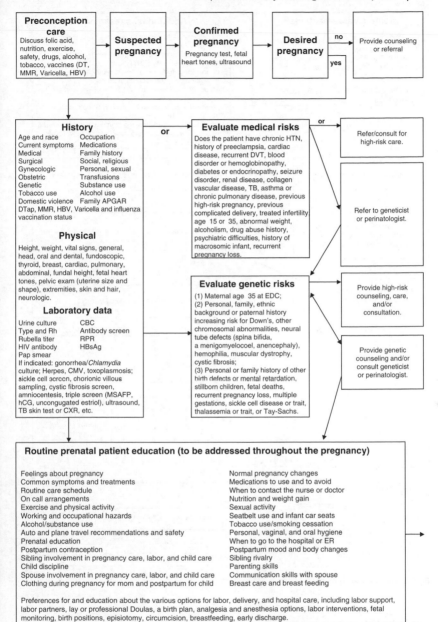

Figure 14.4-1. Important considerations and decision points in prenatal care. TB, tuberculosis; UTI, urinary tract infection; C&S, culture and sensitivity; CBC, complete blood count; CMV, cytomegalovirus; c/o, complains of; CXR, chest x-ray; DTap, diphtheria, tetanus, acellular pertussis vaccine; DVT, deep venous thrombosis; EDC, estimated date of confinement (due date); EGA, estimated gestational age; ER, emergency room; GDM, gestational diabetes mellitus; HBsAg, hepatitis B surface antigen; HBV, hepatitis B vaccine; hCG, human chorionic gonadotropin; HIV, human immunodeficiency virus; h/o, history of; HTN, hypertension; L&D, labor and delivery; MMR 5, measles, mumps, rubella vaccine; MSAFP, maternal serum α-fetoprotein; Rh, Rhesus factor; RPR, rapid plasma regain.

(continued)

Routine care—each visit	Additional assessments

Routine care—each visit

Interval history—maternal well-being (symptoms pain); signs and symptoms of preterm labor (contractions, cramping, or bleeding); symptoms of hypertensive disorders (headache, visual c/o); or any other new problems.

Exam—weight, blood pressure, fundal height, fetal heart tones.

Additional assessments

Offer multiple marker maternal serum analyte screen at 15–18 wk EGA.
Urine C&S with urinary complaints or every trimester if history of recurrent UTI or UTI this pregnancy.
Fetal anatomy ultrasound at 16–20 wk EGA.
If Rh-negative, antibody screen at 28 wk.
One-hour glucose tolerance test at 24–28 wk (earlier for prior h/o GDM).
Perform rectovaginal swab for group B Streptococcus (GBS) screen at 36 wk.
Hemoglobin or hematocrit at the start of the third trimester.
Consider 36 wk syphilis, gonorrhea, or chlamydia screen in high-risk patients.

Figure 14.4-1. (*continued*)

TREATMENT, INTERVENTIONS/RECOMMENDATIONS
Behavioral Counseling

- **Nutrition and weight gain.** Most pregnant women require an increase of 300 to 400 calories per day above nonpregnant levels throughout pregnancy.[3] For most patients, a well-balanced diet provides adequate nutrition during pregnancy. In general, special diets, skipping meals, and food avoidance may lead to nutritional deficiencies and inadequate weight gain during pregnancy. Recommendations for weight gain are based on a pre-pregnancy ideal body weight (IBW) or BMI.[3] The average weight gain in women with a normal BMI (18.5 to 24.9) is 25 to 35 pounds. Women who enter pregnancy substantially below their IBW (BMI less than 18.5) should gain a greater amount of weight during pregnancy (e.g., 28 to 40 pounds). Overweight (BMI 25 to 29.9) women should gain 15 to 25 pounds, and obese (BMI >30) women should be advised to gain less weight during pregnancy 11 to 20 pounds during pregnancy.[4]

- **Iron** is necessary to expand maternal red cell mass and for fetal–placental development. Iron consumption should be increased to **27 mg per day,** the amount found in most prenatal vitamins. **Dietary sources** include red meat, poultry, fish, whole grains, dried fruits, green leafy vegetables, and legumes, seeds, and nuts. **Vitamin C** enhances iron absorption from plant foods when taken with a meal. Women with **iron deficiency anemia** should receive an additional iron supplement of 30 to 120 mg per day until the anemia is corrected.[5] There is no evidence for routine iron supplementation as opposed to selective iron supplementation in populations with a low prevalence of iron deficiency.
- **Folate** supplementation is recommended to reduce the risk of neural tube defects (NTDs). Supplemental folate is ideally recommended in the pre-conceptual period, as the neural tube closes between 18 and 26 days after conception. The Centers for Disease Control and Prevention (CDC) recommend all low-risk fertile women to take **400 µg of folic acid daily, and increase to 600 µg daily during and throughout pregnancy.**[5] Women at increased risk for offspring with NTDs should take higher pre-pregnancy doses (4 mg per day). This includes personal or family history of NTD, maternal insulin-dependent diabetes, and women who are taking anticonvulsants.[5]
- **Calcium** is required for fetal skeletal development, particularly in the last trimester. Calcium absorption is increased during pregnancy and, if necessary, is easily mobilized from maternal stores. During pregnancy and lactation, elemental calcium intake should include at least **1,000 mg per day** in women 19 to 50 years old; for women and girls 14 to 18 years old, **1,300 mg** of calcium is recommended daily.[5]
- **Proteins** are a critical part in the fetus's proper brain development. As such, pregnant women are advised to ingest an **additional 5 to 6 g of protein** daily above the nonpregnant state.[3]
- **Vegetarian diets** may not provide adequate amounts of essential amino acids, iron, vitamin B_{12}, or complex lipids for normal embryonic development. Minor dietary alterations, such as increasing soy, legumes, and dairy products, may correct these deficiencies. Consultation with a registered dietician for further recommendations is advised.[5]
- **Mega-vitamins and natural medications (herbs, vitamins, and supplements).** Inquire about consumption of these substances. Excessive intake of these substances may prove toxic and possibly teratogenic.
- **Foods to limit or avoid** due to potentially adverse effects: high caffeine intake (more than 200 mg daily), unwashed produce, unpasteurized dairy products, undercooked meats, and fish potentially containing high levels of mercury.[5]
- **Exercise.** At least 30 minutes of moderate exercise on most days of the week is reasonable for most pregnant women. Pregnant women should avoid activities that put them at risk for falls or abdominal injuries.
- **Immunizations.** Live-virus vaccines are generally contraindicated for pregnant women because of the theoretical risk of transmission of the vaccine virus to the fetus. If a live-virus vaccine is inadvertently given to a pregnant woman, or if a woman becomes pregnant within 4 weeks after vaccination, she should be counseled about the potential effects on the fetus; however, it is not typically an indication to terminate the pregnancy.[6]
- Inactivated influenza vaccine is **recommended** for all women who are or will be pregnant during flu season.[6]
- **Tetanus/diphtheria/pertussis (Tdap)** is recommended during each pregnancy, regardless of the last time vaccination occurred. Vaccination may be given at any time during pregnancy, but administration between 27 and 36 weeks provides optimal timing for antibody transfer to the fetus to occur.[7]
- **Live** vaccines are contraindicated during pregnancy: **influenza (live-attenuated), measles, mumps, rubella, varicella.**
- The following vaccines can be safely administered if clinically indicated: **Hepatitis A, Hepatitis B.**
  - Recommendations for travel and other circumstances are published at the CDC Web site.[6]
- **Medications.** Few medications have been proven to be completely safe for use in pregnant women, especially in the first trimester. Benefits and risks must be carefully weighed before initiating prescription, over-the-counter, or natural medications.[1]

Patient Education

- **Breastfeeding education.** Breastfeeding education should be offered to all pregnant women at their first visit with the provider and should be encouraged throughout the pregnancy.[1]

- **Preterm labor precautions.** Pregnant women should be educated about the most common symptoms of preterm labor: low, dull backache; four or more uterine contractions per hour; increased pelvic pressure; change in vaginal discharge.[1]
- **Labor and delivery.** Pregnant women should be counseled about signs of labor, ruptured membranes, pain management, and what to expect in labor.[1]
- **Injury prevention.** Seat belts should be properly worn.[1]

Screening

- **Substance abuse.** All pregnant women should be screened for tobacco, alcohol, and illicit substance use.[1]
- **Domestic violence.** Domestic violence affects a significant number of pregnant women and may put both the woman and her fetus at risk. Patients generally accept screening questions about domestic violence.[8]
- **Asymptomatic bacteriuria.** Routine urine culture is recommended due to increased risk of pyelonephritis among pregnant women with asymptomatic bacteriuria.[9] Perform screening urine culture and sensitivity (C&S) at the initial visit. For patients with history of recurrent urinary tract infections (UTIs), UTI during pregnancy, or symptomatic infections, urine culture should be repeated each trimester.[9]

Genetic Screening

- **Chorionic villi sampling** may be offered between 10 and 12 weeks estimated gestational age (EGA). It is associated with 1% to 1.5% risk of spontaneous abortion (SAB) and may be associated with transverse limb defects. Amniocentesis may be offered after 15 weeks EGA and is associated with a 0.5% risk of SAB.[10]
- **Maternal serum analyte screen** should be offered at 15 to 20 weeks EGA to screen for NTDs and trisomies 21 and 18. Optimal timing is 15 to 18 weeks EGA to maximize accuracy and allow time for adequate follow-up counseling and testing.[11]
- **Fetal anatomy ultrasound** can be offered at 16 to 20 weeks EGA to evaluate for structural anomalies.[12]
- **Antibody screen** for Rh-negative women at the first prenatal visit, and again at 28 weeks EGA.
  - Administer Rho(D) immune globulin antepartum at 28 weeks and postpartum (if the baby is Rh-positive) to prevent hemolytic disease of the newborn in subsequent pregnancies.[13]
  - Rho(D) immune globulin is also indicated for spontaneous or induced abortion, ectopic pregnancy, chorionic villus sampling, amniocentesis, vaginal bleeding, significant abdominal trauma, external cephalic version, and transfusion of unmatched Rh-positive blood or any platelet transfusion.[13] For a more detailed discussion, see Chapter 14.8.
- **Gestational diabetes mellitus (GDM) screening** at 24 to 28 weeks (earlier if at increased risk).
- **Risk factors** include obesity, history of miscarriage or fetal death, age 40 or older, history of premature infant, family history of diabetes, polyhydramnios, history of infant with macrosomia (>4,000 g) or congenital malformation, pre-eclampsia, excessive weight gain, and glycosuria.[14]
  - **Screening** is based on risk factors. The American Diabetes Association recommends that all pregnant women be screened with a **50-g nonfasting glucose** challenge at **24 to 28 weeks**. Women at high risk of GDM should be screened at the first antepartum visit using the same 50-g nonfasting glucose challenge.[14] Women with a plasma glucose **exceeding 140 mg per dL** during a 1-hour glucose tolerance test (GTT) need a 3-hour GTT. Because of poor specificity, the use of random or fasting glucose values is not recommended as a screening tool for GDM.[14]
  - **Diagnosis.** Administer a 3-hour fasting GTT with a **100-g glucose** load. **Two or more** of these plasma values (*not* fingerstick values) must be met or exceeded for diagnosis of GDM: fasting, 95 mg per dL; 1 hour, 180 mg per dL; 2 hours, 155 mg per dL; and 3 hours, 140 mg per dL.[14]
- **Group B Streptococcus (GBS) screening.** Perform a rectovaginal swab at 35 to 37 weeks EGA. Colonized women, women with GBS bacteriuria, and women with a previous child with early-onset GBS infection should be treated with intravenous antibiotics at the time of labor or ruptured membranes.[15]
- **Screening for STIs.** Consider **syphilis, gonorrhea, or *Chlamydia*** screening in the third trimester in high-risk patients.
- **Bacterial vaginosis.** The United States Preventative Services Task Force (USPSTF) recommends against screening for bacterial vaginosis in asymptomatic women at low risk for preterm delivery. In women with a history of a previous preterm birth, there is insufficient evidence to assess whether the benefits outweigh the harms of screening asymptomatic women.[16]

SPECIAL CONSIDERATIONS

- **Nausea and vomiting of pregnancy (NVP), also called morning sickness,** is experienced by more than 70% of pregnant women.
  - **Lifestyle modifications should** encourage small frequent protein meals and increased rest. Avoidance of fried and heavily seasoned food, noxious odors, and environmental stimuli should also be recommended.
  - **Nonpharmacologic treatments** include biofeedback and self-hypnosis. Ginger suppresses gastric contractions and increases gastrointestinal motility. Ginger (250 mg oral capsules taken four times daily) significantly reduced nausea and vomiting compared with placebo in women who were <17 weeks pregnant.[17]
  - **Oral pharmacologic treatments**
    - **Pyridoxine (vitamin B₆)** is considered first-line treatment for NVP: 12.5 to 25 mg TID, or pyridoxine, 25 to 50 mg PO TID–QID used in combination with doxylamine, 10 to 12.5 mg PO QD–BID.[18] **Doxylamine** is available over the counter in 12.5-mg (Decapryn) and 25-mg tablets (Unisom Nighttime Sleep-Aid Tablets). The latter combination is contained in the prescription drug Diclegis.[19]
    - **Antiemetics**, antihistamines, phenothiazines, and benzamides are common prescription oral medications for NVP. An algorithm for the suggested evaluation and treatment with NVP is available.[18]
  - Newer data indicate that **hyperemesis gravidarum** may be associated with *Helicobacter pylori* infection. *H. pylori* infection may be safely and effectively treated with triple therapy (amoxicillin, metronidazole, and an H2-receptor blocker) after the first trimester of pregnancy.[20]
- **Vaginal bleeding** is common in early pregnancy, occurring in approximately **20% to 40%** of all pregnant patients. Any report of bleeding deserves further investigation to delineate between potentially serious and less worrisome causes.[21]
  - Evaluation should include a physical examination, laboratory studies (quantitative β-hCG and progesterone, blood type and Rh, serology, and cultures when indicated), and ultrasound. First trimester etiologies include threatened or spontaneous abortion, ectopic pregnancy, trophoblastic disease, cervical polyps, friable cervix, trauma, or malignancy. Bleeding that occurs in the second and third trimesters warrants immediate investigation for abnormally implanted placenta, placental abruption, or other potentially serious conditions[21] (see Chapter 14.10).
- **Vaginal discharge** is common in pregnancy, with many women noting increased vaginal discharge during pregnancy. If this becomes symptomatic, further investigation is warranted using culture and microscopic techniques. Optimal treatment for symptomatic vulvovaginal candidiasis consists of a topical imidazole (clomitrazole or miconazole) for 7 days.[22]
  - Treatment of symptomatic bacterial vaginosis may be achieved with a topical or oral agent. Whether treatment of bacterial vaginosis with oral metronidazole reduces the risk of preterm delivery remains unclear.[22] Increased vaginal discharge or secretions in the second or third trimester may signal preterm cervical changes or labor and may warrant sterile vaginal examination.
- **Back pain and pelvic pain** is common in pregnancy and aggravated by mechanical and hormonal factors. It occurs in more than two-thirds of pregnancies, and often interferes with daily activities and sleep.[23] Usual recommendations include stretching and strengthening exercise, oral or topical analgesics, massage, heat therapy, or ice therapy. Acupuncture has been demonstrated to be more effective in reducing pain than physiotherapy.[24]
  - Evidence for the use of specially shaped pillows instead of regular pillows to reduce nighttime back pain has been shown to be very low.[23]
  - Osteopathic manipulation therapy (OMT) conducted during the third trimester of pregnancy, when combined with conventional obstetric care, has been shown to decrease back pain and slow the progression of problems involving back function.[25] OMT intervention in the first and second trimesters has not been adequately studied.
- **Leg cramps** affect almost half of all pregnant women, particularly in the second and third trimesters of pregnancy; they mostly occur at night. Their cause is unknown, but may be associated with increased levels of lactic and pyruvic acids.[26] Stretching, taking a hot shower, and walking may alleviate leg cramps. Regular exercise and increased hydration may also help.[27] Evidence supporting the use of magnesium prophylaxis of pregnancy-associated leg cramps is conflicting and unclear at this time.[27]
- **Heartburn and gastroesophageal reflux disease (GERD)** may occur in the second to third trimesters and can be a source of significant discomfort.
  - **Nonpharmacologic interventions** include eating small, frequent meals; avoiding fried, greasy, and spicy foods; and eating slowly and chewing food well. Like nonpregnant patients with these

symptoms, it is helpful to avoid lying down immediately after eating, to take walks after meals, and to drink fluids between meals.

- **Pharmacologic agents** used to treat heartburn include:
  - **Antacids** (calcium carbonate, magnesium hydroxide and oxide, and aluminum hydroxide and carbonate). Systemic absorption of antacids is negligible; recommended doses are safe in pregnancy and lactation.[28] Antacids containing sodium bicarbonate or magnesium trisilicate should be avoided.
  - **Antisecretory agents** used for heartburn and GERD include the histamine H2-antagonists and proton pump inhibitors. **The histamine antagonists**, cimetidine (Tagamet) and ranitidine (Zantac), are the most well studied; they have generally shown significant symptom improvement with minimal side effects. Nizatidine (Axid) should be avoided due to the potential risk for fetal death and spontaneous abortion, as seen in animal studies.[28] Because of a lack of evidence regarding safety in the first trimester, histamine antagonists are not recommended during the first trimester. Of the **proton pump inhibitors**—lansoprazole (Prevacid), omeprazole (Prilosec), and pantoprazole (Protonix)—these have been most widely studied in pregnancy.[29] Omeprazole and lansoprazole are available without a prescription.

REFERENCES

1. American Academy of Pediatrics and the American College of Obstetricians and Gynecologists. *Guidelines for perinatal care.* 7th ed. Elk Grove Village, Illinois: AAP; 2012.
2. Alto WA. No need for glycosuria/proteinuria screen in pregnant women. *J Fam Pract* 2005;54:978–983.
3. Zolotor AJ, Carlough MC. Update on prenatal care. *Am Fam Physician* 2014;89(3):199–208.
4. American College of Obstetricians and Gynecologists. Committee opinion no. 548: weight gain during pregnancy. *Obstet Gynecol* 2013;121:210–212.
5. American College of Obstetrics and Gynecology Website. Nutrition during pregnancy educational pamphlet FAQ001. September 2013. http://www.acog.org/-/media/For-Patients/faq001.pdf?dmc=1&ts=20150108T1656382578
6. Guidelines for Vaccinating Pregnant Women. Abstracted from recommendations of the Advisory Committee on Immunization Practices (ACIP). April 2013. http://www.cdc.gov/vaccines/pubs/downloads/b_preg_guide.pdf
7. Centers for Disease Control and Prevention (CDC). Updated recommendations for use of tetanus toxoid, reduced diphtheria toxoid, and acellular pertussis vaccine (Tdap) in pregnant women—Advisory Committee on Immunization Practices (ACIP), 2012. *MMWR Morb Mortal Wkly Rep* 2013;62(7):131–135.
8. U.S. Preventive Services Task Force. Screening for intimate partner violence and abuse of elderly and vulnerable adults. January 2013. http://www.uspreventiveservicestaskforce.org/uspstf/uspsipv.htm. Accessed January 9, 2014.
9. Schnarr J, Smaill F. Asymptomatic bacteriuria and symptomatic urinary tract infections in pregnancy. *Eur J Clin Invest* 2008;38(Suppl 2):50–57.
10. American College of Obstetricians and Gynecologists. ACOG practice bulletin no. 88, December 2007. Invasive prenatal testing for aneuploidy. *Obstet Gynecol* 2007;110:1459–1467.
11. American College of Obstetricians and Gynecologists Committee on Genetics. Committee opinion no. 545: noninvasive prenatal testing for fetal aneuploidy. *Obstet Gynecol* 2012;120:1532–1534.
12. American College of Obstetricians and Gynecologists. ACOG practice bulletin no. 101: ultrasonography in pregnancy. *Obstet Gynecol* 2009;113:451.
13. Crowther CA, Middleton P, McBain RD. Anti-D administration in pregnancy for preventing Rhesus alloimmunisation. *Cochrane Database Syst Rev* 2013;2:CD000020.
14. American College of Obstetricians and Gynecologists. Practice bulletin no. 137: gestational diabetes mellitus. *Obstet Gynecol* 2013;122:406–416.
15. Verani JR, McGee L, Schrag SJ; Division of Bacterial Diseases, National Center for Immunization and Respiratory Diseases, Centers for Disease Control and Prevention (CDC). Prevention of perinatal group B streptococcal disease—revised guidelines from CDC, 2010. *MMWR Recomm Rep* 2010;59(RR-10):1–32.
16. U.S. Preventive Services Task Force. Screening for Bacterial Vaginosis in Pregnancy to Prevent Preterm Delivery, Topic Page. February 2008. http://www.uspreventiveservicestaskforce.org/uspstf/uspsbvag.htm
17. Ozgoli G, Goli M, Simbar M. Effects of ginger capsules on pregnancy, nausea, and vomiting. *J Altern Complement Med* 2009;15(3):243–246.
18. American College of Obstetrics and Gynecology. ACOG (American College of Obstetrics and Gynecologists) Practice bulletin: nausea and vomiting of pregnancy. *Obstet Gynecol* 2004;103(4):803–814.
19. Lexi-Comp Online. *Doxylamine and pyridoxine drug information.* Hudson, OH: Lexi-Comp Inc. https://online.lexi.com/crlsql/servlet/crlonline. Accessed March 9, 2014.
20. Mansour GM, Nashaat EH. Role of helicobacter pylori in the pathogenesis of hyperemesis gravidarum. *Arch Gynecol Obstet* 2011;284(4):843–847.

21. Norwitz ER, Park JS. Overview of the etiology and evaluation of vaginal bleeding in pregnant women. In: Barss VA, ed. *UpToDate*. Waltham, MA: UpToDate. Accessed March 8, 2014.

22. American College of Obstetricians and Gynecologists. ACOG practice bulletin clinical management guidelines for obstetrician-gynecologists, number 72, May 2006: vaginitis. *Obstet Gynecol* 2006;107:1195–1206.

23. Pennick V, Liddle SD. Interventions for preventing and treating pelvic and back pain in pregnancy. *Cochrane Database Syst Rev* 2013;8:CD001139.

24. Ee CC, Manheimer E, Pirotta MV, et al. Acupuncture for pelvic and back pain in pregnancy: a systematic review. *Am J Obstet Gynecol* 2008;198:254.

25. Licciardone JC, Buchanan S, Hensel KL, et al. Osteopathic manipulative treatment of back pain and related symptoms during pregnancy: a randomized controlled trial. *Am J Obstet Gynecol* 2010; 202:43.e1.

26. Young GL, Jewell D. Interventions for leg cramps in pregnancy. *Cochrane Database Syst Rev* 2002;(1):CD000121.

27. Bermas BL. Musculoskeletal changes and pain during pregnancy and postpartum. In: Barss VA, ed. *UpToDate*. Waltham, MA: UpToDate. Accessed March 8, 2014.

28. Law R, Maltepe C, Bozzo P, et al. Treatment of heartburn and acid reflux associated with nausea and vomiting during pregnancy. *Can Fam Physician* 2010;56(2):143–144.

29. Gill SK, O'Brien L, Einarson TR, et al. The safety of proton pump inhibitors (PPIs) in pregnancy: a meta-analysis. *Am J Gastroenterol* 2009;104:1541.

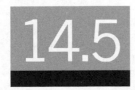

14.5 Ectopic Pregnancy

Elizabeth S. Pietralczyk

GENERAL PRINCIPLES

Ectopic pregnancy presents a major health problem to women of childbearing age. This condition is considered a medical emergency, and hemorrhage from ruptured ectopic pregnancy is still the leading cause of pregnancy-related maternal death in the first trimester.[1] Prompt diagnosis and treatment is a must in all patients presenting with signs or symptoms of ectopic pregnancy.

Definition

Ectopic pregnancy occurs when a fertilized ovum implants anywhere outside the endometrial lining of the uterine cavity. The most common location is the fallopian tube, which accounts for 97% of all ectopic gestations.[2] Other, less common, sites of implantation include the abdomen, peritoneum, cervix, ovary, and uterine cornua.

Etiology

Risk factors for ectopic pregnancy can be classified into high, intermediate, and low. High degrees of risk of ectopic pregnancy occur in patients with previous ectopic pregnancy, previous tubal surgery, known tubal pathology, and *in utero* diethylstilbestrol (DES) exposure. Intermediate risk is attributed to patients who are smokers and have a history of pelvic inflammatory disease (PID). Low risk is seen in patients who have had previous (nontubal) abdominal surgery or in patients who become pregnant at a young age (<18).[3,4] Women who are currently using an intrauterine device for contraception or who have had tubal ligation performed are much more likely to have an ectopic pregnancy if conception occurs. However, the risk of conception is obviously much lower with these contraceptive methods in place. All the aforementioned risk factors increase the chance of tubal pathology and thus tubal pregnancy.

Epidemiology

Ectopic pregnancy occurs in nearly 2 per 100 pregnancies. The incidence has increased sixfold between 1970 and 1992,[2] largely due to a rise in PID. The prevalence is reported to be as high as 18% of women presenting to the emergency department with first trimester bleeding and abdominal pain.[5]

DIAGNOSIS
History

Pelvic/abdominal pain, amenorrhea, and vaginal bleeding are the classic symptoms of ectopic pregnancy. Pain is almost always present before rupture, but is highly variable in location, character, and severity. The onset of pain is usually at 6 to 8 weeks gestational age. Often, there is amenorrhea followed by irregular vaginal bleeding. More than 50% may be asymptomatic before tubal rupture and have no identifiable risk factor for ectopic pregnancy, making the diagnosis difficult.[4]

Physical Examination

Signs may include localized lower quadrant tenderness with or without a palpable mass, peritoneal irritation, guarding and rebound tenderness (suggesting tubal rupture with hemoperitoneum), and cervical motion tenderness. Signs of shock, including pallor, diaphoresis, weakness, and orthostatic pulse and blood pressure changes, may be present.[4]

Laboratory Tests

An initial workup should include a complete blood count (CBC), quantitative β-human chorionic gonadotropin (β-hCG), and Rh determination. The β-hCG concentration in a normal intrauterine pregnancy (IUP) rises until 41 days of gestation at which time it plateaus at approximately 100,000 IU per L and the mean doubling time for the hormone is from 1.4 to 2.1 days. In ectopic pregnancy, the doubling time is 3 or more days. A falling value signals non-viability. A single value is not interpretable and serial testing should only be used if the patient remains hemodynamically stable.[5]

Imaging

Transvaginal ultrasound should be the initial diagnostic test in women known to be pregnant who present with first trimester vaginal bleeding and/or pelvic pain. If the imaging study is non-diagnostic, transvaginal ultrasound findings in conjunction with serial serum β-hCG concentrations facilitate a diagnosis of ectopic pregnancy. When β-hCG levels are higher than 1,500 IU per L (the so-called "discriminatory zone") with no visualized IUP, there should be a high suspicion for ectopic pregnancy regardless of symptoms.[5]

Differential Diagnosis

This includes appendicitis, PID, ruptured corpus luteum cyst, ovarian torsion, urinary tract disease, and threatened or incomplete intrauterine abortion. Consider concurrent problems, such as IUP and appendicitis, or IUP and ectopic pregnancy (rare, except in patients who have undergone fertility treatment). Also, rare types of ectopic pregnancy, including interstitial, abdominal, cervical, ovarian, or multiple, should be considered.

TREATMENT
Emergent Presentation

Emergency laparotomy or laparoscopy is indicated if signs of intraperitoneal bleeding or shock are present. Fluids and blood transfusions are given as required. Ultrasonographic examination may waste critical time.

Nonemergent Presentation

- **Surgery.** Surgical management is favored if pain is prolonged for more than 24 hours, quantitative β-HCG is more than 10,000 IU per L, when fetal cardiac activity is noted, or in ectopics larger than 3.5 cm on ultrasound. Laparoscopy or laparotomy is performed to remove the ectopic pregnancy.[5,6]
- **Methotrexate.** Eligible patients for this treatment have a gestational sac diameter less than 3.5 cm, with no fetal cardiac activity, and no evidence of rupture on ultrasound. There is no absolute cutoff for the level of β-HCG in medical management; however, higher β-HCG levels (greater than 5 to 10,000 IU per L) have a higher risk of subsequent rupture.[4–6] The current recommended regimen is a single intramuscular injection of the drug at 50 mg per m². Absolute contraindications include immunodeficiency, liver disease, blood dyscrasia, pulmonary disease, renal dysfunction, or peptic ulcer disease (PUD). The β-HCG level may rise for 3 to 4 days, but should then fall 15% between days 4 and 7. If this does not occur, a second dose of methotrexate or surgical treatment is considered.[5]
- **Expectant.** Nearly 47% of ectopic pregnancies can undergo expectant management. Expectant management should be undertaken only in hemodynamically stable patients with β-HCG levels less than 1,000 IU per L and declining. Ectopic mass must be less than 3 cm with no fetal heart rate.

Patients electing for expectant management need to be highly reliable, have close follow-up, and be counseled of the risk of ectopic rupture and hemorrhage.

Monitoring of Treatment

β-HCG should be followed weekly until undetectable, regardless of the method of treatment. Rho (D) immune globulin should be given to Rh-negative women.[1]

SPECIAL CONSIDERATIONS

The mortality rate for ectopic pregnancy in the United States has decreased from 1.15 to 0.50 deaths per 100,000 live births from 1980 to 2007 and continues to decline, largely due to improved detection and timely treatment.[7] Medical treatment has been shown to be as efficacious as surgical management in appropriate candidates. Complications from surgery include anesthesia risks, routine surgical risks, postoperative pain, and discomfort. Methotrexate side effects are minimal and self-limiting. The most common are stomatitis and conjunctivitis.

In patients with an ectopic pregnancy, another ectopic pregnancy occurs in 6% to 12% of patients. Patients should be counseled to practice "safe sex" to avoid pelvic infections. Finally, patients should be encouraged to discuss their feelings about the loss of the pregnancy and the possibility of compromised fertility in the future.

REFERENCES

1. Lozeau AM, Potter B. Diagnosis and management of ectopic pregnancy. *Am Fam Physician* 2005;72:1710–1714.
2. Seeber BE, Barnhart KT. Suspected ectopic pregnancy. *Obstet Gynecol* 2006;107(2):399–413.
3. Ankum WM, Mol BW, Van der Veen F, et al. Risk factors for ectopic pregnancy: a meta-analysis. *Fertil Steril* 1996;65(6):1093–1099.
4. Bickell NA, Bodian C, Anderson RM, et al. Time and ruptured tubal pregnancy. *Obstet Gynecol* 2004;104(4):789–794.
5. American College of Obstetricians and Gynecologists. ACOG practice bulletin no. 94: medical management of ectopic pregnancy. *Obstet Gynecol* 2008;111:1479–1485.
6. Goksedef BP, Kef S, Akca A, et al. Risk factors for rupture in tubal ectopic pregnancy. *Eur J Obstet Gynecol Reprod Biol* 2011;154:96–99.
7. Creanga AA, Shapiro-Mendoza CK, Bish CL, et al. Trends in ectopic pregnancy mortality in the United States 1980–2007. *Obstet Gynecol* 2011;117(4):837–843.

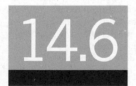

14.6 Medical Problems During Pregnancy

Ashley J. Falk

NAUSEA AND VOMITING OF PREGNANCY
General Principles

One of the most common complaints in pregnancy is nausea, affecting almost 85% of women. Another 50% will suffer from vomiting as well. Hyperemesis gravidarum is a severe form of this condition affecting about 1% of pregnant women.[1] Nausea and vomiting of pregnancy is most often managed conservatively, but may require hospitalization if symptoms are severe.

Nausea of pregnancy usually starts around 4 to 6 weeks, peaks at 8 to 12 weeks, and subsides by 20 weeks.

Pathophysiology

The mechanism of nausea and vomiting in pregnancy remains unclear, but the clinical course closely follows the waxing and waning levels of human chorionic gonadotropin. A newer hypothesis is that it may be related to *Helicobacter pylori*.[2]

Diagnosis

The most important part of the diagnosis of nausea and vomiting of pregnancy is history. Frequency and volume of vomiting as well as any weight loss is important. Migraine headaches and other gastrointestinal disorders should be considered in the differential diagnosis.

Physical examination to assess fluid status is also essential. Important signs are dry mucous membranes, tachycardia, orthostatic hypotension, and poor skin turgor. Weight loss greater than 5% of prepregnant weight, ketonuria, electrolyte abnormalities (hypokalemia), or dehydration (high urine specific gravity) may signify the development of hyperemesis gravidarum. Vomiting of this severity increases the risk of poor fetal outcome.

If hyperemesis gravidarum is suspected, laboratory evaluation should include blood levels of blood urea nitrogen, creatinine, alanine aminotransferase, aspartate aminotransferase, electrolytes, and lipase.

Treatment

Most nausea of pregnancy can be managed conservatively with dietary modifications. Eating small amounts of food several times may be helpful as well as avoiding odors, foods, and supplements that might serve as triggers such as fatty or spicy foods or iron supplements. Randomized controlled trials have not compared different types of diets to control nausea and vomiting in pregnancy.[1] About 10% of women with nausea and vomiting in pregnancy require medication therapy. Randomized trials support the use of vitamin B_6 (pyridoxine), 10 to 25 mg every 8 hours, and doxylamine, 25 mg at bedtime and 12.5 mg in the morning and afternoon. If symptoms persist, other treatment options include metoclopramide, promethazine, and ondansetron. A randomized controlled trial suggests that metoclopramide give in a dosage of 10 mg every 8 hours is as effective and better tolerated than promethazine for hyperemesis gravidarum.[3]

APPENDICITIS IN PREGNANCY
General Principles

The most common general surgical problem encountered during pregnancy is acute appendicitis.[4] Appendicitis in pregnancy may have an alternative presentation in pregnancy with right upper quadrant pain due to displacement of abdominal contents.

Appendicitis occurs in approximately 1 in 1,500 pregnancies. In one series, 30% of cases occurred in the first trimester, 48% in the second trimester, and 25% in the third trimester.[5]

Diagnosis

Diagnosis of acute appendicitis can be quite challenging in pregnancy, likely leading to the increased rates of appendiceal rupture. Factors confounding the diagnosis during pregnancy include the relatively high prevalence of abdominal/gastrointestinal discomfort, anatomic changes related to the enlarged uterus, and the physiologic leukocytosis of pregnancy. Pregnant women are less likely to have a classic presentation of appendicitis, especially in the third trimester. Although right lower quadrant pain at McBurney's point is the most common symptom at any point in pregnancy, pain may also localize to the mid- or upper right quadrant as the uterus enlarges and displaces the bowel.

Compression-graded ultrasonography is the preferred method of imaging the appendix during pregnancy.[6] Computed tomography has greater specificity and sensitivity for the diagnosis of appendicitis, but concerns of fetal radiation exposure limit its use to situations in which the clinical findings and ultrasound are inconclusive.

Treatment

Treatment of acute appendicitis is appendectomy. Maternal morbidity following appendectomy is comparable to that in nonpregnant women. The exception is in the case of appendiceal rupture, which significantly increases the rate of fetal loss.[7]

HYPERTENSION
General Principles

Hypertension is the most common medical problem in pregnancy affecting between 6% and 8% of gestations. There are four categories of hypertension in pregnancy as described by the National High Blood Pressure Education Program Working Group on High Blood Pressure in Pregnancy: chronic hypertension, gestational hypertension, preeclampsia, and preeclampsia superimposed on chronic hypertension.[8]

Hypertension in pregnant women is defined as blood pressure greater than 140/90 measured on more than one occasion. As many women are becoming pregnant at older ages, chronic hypertension now plays a larger role in management issues in pregnant women. Patients should be screened for hypertension at every visit.

Pathophysiology

Most cases of chronic hypertension in pregnancy are caused by essential, or primary, hypertension. This process involves complex hemodynamics and often is associated with obesity. Preeclampsia is associated with abnormal immunologically mediated invasion of the trophoblast into the endometrium. This leads to altered development of placental vasculature. Because the blood flow to the placenta is altered, it releases vasoactive hormones, which cause endothelial dysfunction. In addition, the clotting cascade is triggered by the activated endothelium. These hemodynamic changes lead to hypertension and end-organ damage seen in preeclampsia.

Diagnosis and Treatment

Chronic hypertension is defined as hypertension presenting before 20 weeks gestation or persisting beyond 12-week postpartum. Treatment is not required unless the patient's blood pressure is persistently greater than 150–180/100 to 110. In this case, treatment with methyldopa, labetalol, or nifedipine should be considered to prevent maternal end-organ damage. Intrauterine growth retardation is of concern in chronic hypertension and should be monitored for accordingly.[9]

Gestational hypertension, previously termed pregnancy-induced hypertension, describes the development of hypertension after 20 weeks gestation without proteinuria. Management should include close monitoring as 50% of patients will go on to develop preeclampsia. Treatment remains similar to that of chronic hypertension where medications are reserved for severe elevations in blood pressure.

Preeclampsia is a multiorgan disease process of unknown etiology defined as the development of hypertension and proteinuria (greater than 300 mg in a 24-hour urine specimen) after 20 weeks gestation.[10] Risk factors for the development of preeclampsia include chronic hypertension, chronic renal disease, obesity, maternal age greater than 40 years, multiple gestation, nulliparity, preeclampsia in a previous pregnancy, and pregestational diabetes mellitus. In cases of mild preeclampsia, expectant management is indicated. This constitutes maternal and fetal monitoring, including blood pressure measurement, laboratory evaluation, nonstress tests, and biophysical profiles along with ultrasound to assess fetal growth. Diagnostic criteria for severe preeclampsia include one or more of the following: resting blood pressure greater than 160 mmHg systolic or 110 mmHg diastolic on two or more occasions, proteinuria greater than 5 g in a 24-hour urine specimen, or any of the associated signs or symptoms (cerebral or visual disturbance, right upper quadrant pain, fetal growth restriction, oliguria, pulmonary edema, thrombocytopenia). Management of severe preeclampsia includes admission to the hospital for complete evaluation of maternal and fetal status. Treatment with magnesium sulfate, antihypertensives, and corticosteroids maybe indicated. Timing of delivery is based on fetal maturity and evaluation of fetal and maternal well-being.

Preeclampsia may progress to eclampsia (preeclampsia with seizure) or HELLP syndrome (hemolysis, elevated liver enzymes, low platelet count). Both of these are immediately life-threatening conditions, which require medical intervention, and plans should be made for prompt delivery.

URINARY TRACT INFECTIONS AND ASYMPTOMATIC BACTERIURIA
General Principles

Urinary tract infections are common in pregnant women. They can be defined as either lower tract (acute cystitis) or upper tract (acute pyelonephritis). Likewise, asymptomatic bacteriuria, the presence of a positive urine culture in a patient without symptoms, is also fairly common in pregnancy, affecting between 2% and 5% of pregnant women. While benign in the nonpregnant woman, asymptomatic bacteriuria in pregnancy does pose a threat to the well-being of mother and fetus. The most common causative agents are *Escherichia coli*, *Klebsiella*, *Proteus*, and *Streptococcus* group B.

Many physiologic changes lead to an increased tendency for pregnant women to harbor bacteria in their urine. Progesterone can cause smooth muscle relaxation, leading to less ureteral peristalsis and urine stasis. Hormones also cause the bladder to increase its capacity. In addition, mechanical changes such as compression of the ureters by the enlarging uterus and a positional change of the bladder due to shifting of the abdominal organs can also cause urinary stasis. Any stasis of the urine provides a good culture medium for bacteria.[11]

Diagnosis

Screening for asymptomatic bacteriuria should be performed at 12 to 16 weeks gestation (or at the first prenatal visit).[12] Rescreening is generally not performed in low-risk women. Acute cystitis is the presence of bacteriuria of the lower urinary tract with associated signs and symptoms such as dysuria, frequency, hematuria, and lower abdominal discomfort. Patients with acute pyelonephritis generally present with fever, flank pain, and nausea/vomiting, which may occur in the presence or absence of cystitis symptoms.[13] Laboratory evaluation should include a complete blood count (CBC) with differential, electrolytes, blood urea nitrogen, creatinine, urine analysis, and urine and blood cultures.

Treatment

For asymptomatic bacteriuria and acute cystitis, treatment options include nitrofurantoin 100 mg BID for 5 days at bedtime for 10 days; amoxicillin 500 mg BID for 5 days; or cephalexin 500 mg BID for 5 days. Urine culture should be repeated after treatment to ensure successful eradication. If the culture remains positive, antibiotic therapy should be adjusted to resistance patterns and duration of therapy increased to 7 to 10 days. Patients with a history of asymptomatic bacteriuria or acute cystitis should continue to be screened for recurrence on a monthly basis for the remainder of their pregnancy. If the patient continues to have recurrences, prophylactic treatment should be given for the remainder of the pregnancy using nitrofurantoin 50 to 100 mg PO at bedtime. Regular repeat urine cultures should be done throughout the pregnancy.

Because of the higher risk of complications, acute pyelonephritis in pregnancy is generally treated with hospital admission and intravenous antibiotics until the patient is afebrile or asymptomatic for at least 48 hours at which point a transition to oral antibiotics can be considered. Preferred antibiotic therapy is parenteral β-lactams. If symptoms and fever persist beyond the first 24 to 48 hours of treatment, imaging should be considered to further evaluate the urinary tract for obstruction or abscess.

Complications

About 30% of women with asymptomatic bacteriuria go on to develop pyelonephritis. Eradication of the bacteriuria reduces the risk of pyelonephritis to about 5%. In addition, treatment of asymptomatic bacteriuria has been shown to reduce the incidence of preterm labor, which is four times higher if untreated, as well as reduce the incidence of low-birth-weight infants. A case-control study of over 15,000 pregnant women found an increased risk of preeclampsia in association with either asymptomatic bacteriuria or symptomatic urinary tract infection.[14] Preterm birth is also more common in pregnant women with acute pyelonephritis during pregnancy.[15]

DIABETES MELLITUS
General Principles

Diabetes mellitus is a serious chronic illness that can have major effects on the outcome of pregnancy. Tight glycemic control is key to avoiding complications. Like hypertension, diabetes in pregnancy can be either pregnancy-induced or pre-existing. Gestational diabetes is defined as diabetes that is first recognized during pregnancy. This means that a patient could have pre-existing type 2 diabetes that is first recognized during routine prenatal laboratory tests. In this case, during the pregnancy, the disorder would be called gestational diabetes and if it continued after the pregnancy it would be reclassified as type 2 diabetes. Gestational diabetes is common (affecting 5% to 9% of pregnancies in the United States and growing in prevalence) and signals patients who are at increased risk of developing type 2 diabetes later in life even if they were euglycemic prior to pregnancy.

Gestational diabetes most often develops in the second or third trimesters, when the placenta begins to secrete hormones that cause increased insulin resistance. It is believed that patients with new-onset diabetes during pregnancy are likely predisposed to insulin resistance and that pregnancy simply pushes them over the edge into insulin resistance and hyperglycemia.

Diagnosis

Screening for gestational diabetes is important, but risk stratification is necessary. Patients who are obese, have a family history of diabetes mellitus, have a personal history of insulin resistance or delivery of a macrosomic infant, or have glucosuria are considered at high risk for developing gestational diabetes. Average-risk patients require screening for gestational diabetes between 24 and 28 weeks, whereas high-risk patients should be screened at the first prenatal visit and again at 24 to 28 weeks.[16]

Screening starts with a 50-g 1-hour oral glucose challenge. A positive test is a serum glucose measurement of >140 mg per dL after 1 hour. This test does not require fasting. A positive glucose challenge is followed up by a 100-g 3-hour oral glucose tolerance test. First, a fasting glucose level is measured (normal <95). Sequential serum glucose measurements are then taken 1 hour (normal <180), 2 hours (normal <155), and 3 hours (normal <140) after the 100-g dose of glucose. A positive test is determined if two or more of these measurements are above the normal range.

Treatment

First-line treatment for gestational diabetes should begin with dietary medication, often in consultation with an experienced nutritionist. If fasting blood sugars remain greater than 95, or 2-hour postprandial blood sugars remain above 120, pharmacologic therapy should be instituted. Insulin is often considered first-line; however, glyburide has been proven to be safe and effective for use in management of gestational diabetes, and there is increasing evidence to support the use of metformin.

Fetal surveillance is also an important part of the management of gestational diabetes. This may include screening for congenital abnormalities and twice weekly nonstress testing and weekly amniotic fluid index beginning in the third trimester. Timing of delivery remains somewhat controversial and should be based on glycemic control and other risk factors, but there is little evidence to support elective delivery prior to 39 weeks.

All patients with gestational diabetes should be rescreened at 6 to 12 weeks postpartum for persistent diabetes.

Complications

Hyperglycemia early in pregnancy has been shown to cause defects in organogenesis. During the first few weeks of gestation, when organogenesis occurs, the embryo cannot make its own insulin and maternal insulin does not cross the placenta. Thus, maternal hyperglycemia directly leads to hyperglycemia in the developing baby. For this reason, preconception glycemic control is important in diabetic women of childbearing age. Second, maternal hyperglycemia often leads to fetal macrosomia and problems with delivery as well as neonatal hypoglycemia and increased risk of neonatal death.

REFERENCES

1. Barclay L. ACOG guidelines for treating nausea and vomiting in pregnant women reviewed. *N Engl J Med* 2010;363:1544–1550.
2. Quinlan JD, Hill DA. Nausea and vomiting of pregnancy. *Am Fam Physician* 2003;68:121.
3. Tan PC, Khine PP, Vallikkannu N, et al. Promethazine compared with metoclopramide for hyperemesis gravidarum: a randomized controlled trial. *Obstet Gynecol* 2010;115(5):975–981.
4. Tamir IL, Bongard FS, Klein SR. Acute appendicitis in the pregnant patient. *Am J Surg* 1990;160:571.
5. Mahmoodian S. Appendicitis complicating pregnancy. *South Med J* 1992;85:19.
6. Wand PI, Chong ST, Kielar AZ, et al. Imaging of the pregnant and lactating patients: part 2, evidence based review and recommendations. *Am J Roentgenol* 2012;198:785.
7. Silvestri MT, Pettker CM, Brousseau EC, et al. Morbidity of appendectomy and cholecystectomy in pregnant and nonpregnant women. *Obstet Gynecol* 2011;118:1261.
8. Report of the National High Blood Pressure Education Program Working Group on High Blood Pressure in Pregnancy. *Am J Obstet Gynecol* 2000;183(1):S1–S22.
9. ACOG Committee on Practice Bulletin. Chronic hypertension in pregnancy. *Obstet Gynecol* 2001;98(1 Suppl):177–185.
10. Davison JM, Homuth V, Jeyabalan A, et al. New aspects in the pathophysiology of preeclampsia. *J Am Soc Nephrol* 2004;15(9):2440–2448.
11. Cunningham FG, Lucas MJ. Urinary tract infections complicating pregnancy. *Bailliere's Clin Obstet Gynecol* 1994;8:353.
12. Lin K, Fajardo K; U.S. Preventative Services Task Force. Screening for asymptomatic bacteriuria in adults: evidence for the U.S. Preventive Services Task Force reaffirmation recommendation statement. *Ann Intern Med* 2008;149:W20.
13. Hooton TM, Gupta K. Urinary tract infections and asymptomatic bacteriuria in pregnancy. www.uptodate.com. Accessed July 30, 2014.
14. Minassian C, Thomas SL, Williams DJ, et al. Acute maternal infection and risk of preeclampsia: a population-based case-control study. *PLoS One* 2013;8:e73047.
15. Wing DA, Fassett MJ, Getahun D. Acute pyelonephritis in pregnancy: an 18-year retrospective analysis. *Am J Obstet Gynecol* 2014;210:219.e1.
16. Metzger BE, Buchanan TA, Coustan DR, et al. Summary and recommendations of the Fifth international Workshop-Conference on Gestational Diabetes Mellitus. *Diabetes Care* 2007;30(Suppl 2):S251–S260.

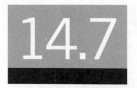

Postdate Pregnancy
Sean P. Wherry

GENERAL PRINCIPLES

Post-term or postdate pregnancy (PDP) is pregnancy lasting beyond 42 weeks, or 294 days measured from the first day of the last menstrual period.[1] The incidence of PDP ranges from 0.4% to 8.1%.[2]

An accurate estimate of gestational age based on early pregnancy ultrasound with measurement of the crown–rump length has been shown to decrease the incidence of postdate pregnancies when compared with other dating modalities (last menstrual period, and known date of conception).[2]

DIAGNOSIS

The most common cause of PDP is the inaccurate dating of the pregnancy. Other causes are unclear, but risk factures include previous PDP (50% recurrence rate); family history of PDP; primigravity; excessive maternal weight gain; maternal obesity; male fetal gender; lower socioeconomic status; and fetal abnormalities such as anencephaly, adrenal insufficiency, and placental sulfatase deficiency.[2]

TREATMENT

Treatment of PDP remains controversial. Expectant as opposed to active management between 41 and 42 weeks yields no statistically significant difference in perinatal or neonatal morbidity. Despite this, expectant management is associated with a statistically significant increased risk for cesarean delivery and meconium aspiration syndrome.[2,3] Births after completion of the 42nd week are associated with a slightly increased risk to the infant and are associated with greater number of deaths.[3,4]

Expectant Management

It is recommended that routine fetal surveillance for PDP begins between 40 and 42 weeks gestation. Despite this, there are no randomized controlled trials (RCTs) demonstrating the efficacy of such monitoring in the reduction of fetal mortality or morbidity. This fetal assessment can take the form of a biophysical profile (BPP), a modified BPP consisting of a non-stress test (NST) with an ultrasound for amniotic fluid index (AFI), or a contraction stress test. Abnormalities in any of these tests may indicate the need for induction. By convention, antenatal testing is started at $41+0$ with biweekly NSTs and weekly AFI. By 43 weeks gestation, all patients should be delivered due to the fact that fetal morbidity and mortality generally increase beyond that gestational age.[3]

Active Management

Active management of the PDP advocates for the induction of labor to reduce perinatal complications. The timing of the induction remains controversial. There are no RCTs comparing induction at 41 versus 42 weeks. The relative risk of perinatal mortality increases between 41 and 42 weeks (0.25 and 0.32, respectively). Resulting from this, it is generally recommended that labor be induced in women without signs of ensuing labor prior to the completion of the 41st week.[2] Elective induction of labor is associated with a nonsignificant difference in perinatal mortality compared with expectant management for PDP (relative risk 0.33, 95% CI: 0.10 to 1.09, $p = 0.07$; 11 RCTs). Elective induction of labor is associated with a significant reduction in meconium aspiration syndrome (relative risk 0.43, 95% CI: 0.23 to 0.79, $p = 0.007$; seven RCTs), a significantly lower mean birth weight (weighted mean difference -44.41, 95% CI: -79.37 to -9.45, $p = 0.01$; eight RCTs), and a significant reduction in cesarean section (relative risk 0.87, 95% CI: 0.80 to 0.96; $p = 0.004$; 13 RCTs). There were no statistical differences in other outcomes for the two groups.[5] Women should be informed that number of inductions needed to treat is 500 in order to prevent a single perinatal death and that women who opt for expectant management of PDP may have a higher rate of cesarean delivery than their active management counterparts.

- **Cervical ripening agents.** Dinoprostone, a prostaglandin E_2 (PGE$_2$) analogue, has been shown to improve induction outcome as well as decrease the length of induction time in patients with an unfavorable cervix. Prepidil (gel) in a standard dose of 0.5 mg administered intracervically can be used every 6 hours as needed to a maximum dose of 1.5 mg PGE$_2$ or 7.5 mL PGE$_2$ gel.[6] Cervidil (10 mg vaginal insert) is introduced into the posterior fornix of the vagina for 12 hours. Continuous fetal monitoring is recommended during use of either agent. Both agents require refrigeration and are extremely expensive. Misoprostol (Cytotec), a PGE_1 analogue, is also used for cervical ripening and labor induction (not Food and Drug Administration approved). Cytotec 25 to 50 μg inserted intravaginally into the posterior fornix used every 3 to 4 hours significantly reduces labor time. Uterine tachysystole and hyperstimulation can occur; therefore, continuous fetal monitoring is recommended. Misoprostol is temperature stable and inexpensive.[7]

- Membrane stripping or sweeping has also been used as a method for inducing labor. Sweeping membranes somewhere between every other day and once weekly starting at 39 weeks can reduce the number of women who reach 41 weeks gestation. Risks of the procedure include membrane rupture, infection, and bleeding.[8]

- Amniotomy, with or without oxytocin, is widely used to induce labor. Early amniotomy shortens the duration of labor and reduces the incidence of dystocia but does not reduce the need for anesthesia or cesarean section. Timing of the amniotomy is important because once it is done the patient is committed to delivery. Amniotomy is best performed in conjunction with the administration of some agent to induce contractions, when there are regular uterine contractions and the head is well applied to the cervix.[9]

- Oxytocin administration remains the most common form of labor induction. Various protocols exist. The use of the low-dose infusion (starting at 1.0 to 2.0 mU per minute and increasing the dose every 15 to 30 minutes with a maximum of 20 mU per minute) is associated with less uterine hyperstimulation, water intoxication, and antidiuretic effect than high-dose protocols. Misoprostol is also being used for labor inductions and has been shown to shorten times to delivery and a significant decrease in cesarean when compared with pitocin but has higher rates of tachysystole and hyperstimulation.[10] Fetal monitoring should be continuous during induction to ensure fetal well-being.[11]

COMPLICATIONS
Expectant Management

Neonatal complications include stillbirth, birth asphyxia, placental insufficiency, umbilical cord complications, bone fracture, pneumonia, septicemia, and meconium aspiration.[12] Macrosomia occurs more often (3% to 7% in PDP) and is associated with an increased risk for shoulder dystocia, neurologic injuries to the shoulder girdle, and cephalohematoma. Hypoglycemia is often seen during the neonatal period in the macrosomic infant. Post-maturity syndrome, characterized by peeling skin, calcified skull, and thin body due to wasting of subcutaneous fat, complicates up to 10% of pregnancies between 41 and 42 weeks, and increases to 33% of pregnancies at 43 weeks.[2] Maternal complications include an increased incidence of cephalopelvic disproportion, labor dystocia, anxiety, chorioamnionitis, postpartum hemorrhage, vaginal and rectal lacerations, endometritis, and double the rate of cesarean section.[2]

Active Management

See Chapter 14.10 for complications during induction of labor.

REFERENCES

1. ACOG Committee Opinion No. 579: definition of term pregnancy. *Obstet Gynecol* 2013;122(5):1139.
2. Simpson PD, Stanley KP. Prolonged pregnancy. *Obstet Gyneacol Reprod Med* 2011;21:257.
3. Clinical Practice Obstetrics Committee, Maternal Fetal Medicine Committee, Delaney M, Roggensack A, Leduc DC, et al. Guidelines for the management of pregnancy at 41+0 to 42+0 weeks. *J Obstet Gynaecol Can* 2008;30:800.
4. Gülmezoglu AM, Crowther CA, Middleton P, et al. Induction of labour for improving birth outcomes for women at or beyond term. *Cochrane Database Syst Rev* 2012;6:CD004945.
5. Wennerholm UB, Hagberg H, Brorsson B, et al. Induction of labor versus expectant management for post-date pregnancy: is there sufficient evidence for a change in clinical practice? *Acta Obstet Gynecol Scand* 2009;88(1):6–17.
6. Sawai SK, Williams MC, O'Brien WF, et al. Sequential outpatient application of intravaginal prostaglandin E2 gel in the management of postdate pregnancies. *Obstet Gynecol* 1991;78:19.
7. Wing D. Labor induction with misoprostol. *Am J Obstet Gynecol* 1999;181:339.
8. Cammu H, Haitsma V. Sweeping of the membranes at 39 weeks in nulliparous women: a randomized controlled trial. *Br J Obstet Gynecol* 1998;105:41.
9. Fraser WD, Turcot L, Krauss I, et al. Amniotomy for shortening spontaneous labour (Cochrane review). In: *The Cochrane Library*, Issue 2:2000. Oxford: Update Software.
10. Induction and augmentation of labor. ACOG Technical Bulletin Number 157—July 1991. *Int J Gynaecol Obstet* 1992;39(2):139–142.
11. Sulik SM. Postdate pregnancy. In: Taylor RB, ed. *Manual of family practice*. 2nd ed. Philadelphia, PA: Lippincott Williams & Wilkins; 2002.
12. Olsen AW, Westergaard JG, Olsen J. Perinatal and maternal complications related to post-term delivery: a national register-based study, 1978–1993. *Am J Obstet Gynecol* 2003;189:222.

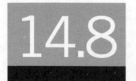 **Obstetric Problems During Pregnancy**
S. Lindsey Clarke, James W. Jarvis,
Daphne J. Karel

PREECLAMPSIA AND ECLAMPSIA

Preeclampsia is potentially life-threatening complication of late pregnancy characterized by hypertension, proteinuria, and multiorgan dysfunction. Preeclampsia is a progressive syndrome that requires frequent reevaluation of both maternal and fetal health. In severe cases, patients may develop abnormalities of the central nervous, hepatic, and hematologic systems, including generalized seizures known as eclampsia.

General Principles

Definitions

Preeclampsia is the new onset of systolic blood pressure (SBP) 140 mmHg or higher and/or diastolic blood pressure (DBP) 90 mmHg or higher after 20 weeks of gestation plus any of the following:[1]

- Proteinuria (300 mg or more in 24 hours or protein/creatinine ratio 0.3 or higher)
- Thrombocytopenia (platelet count less than 100,000 per μL)
- Impaired kidney function (creatinine more than 1.1 mg per dL or a doubling from baseline creatinine)
- Impaired liver function (transaminases more than twice normal values)
- Pulmonary edema
- Cerebral or visual symptoms

Eclampsia is the occurrence of generalized seizures in a preeclamptic woman; this is one of several severe features of preeclampsia. Other severe features of preeclampsia are shown in Table 14.8-1. Hypertension should be confirmed with two measurements at least 4 hours apart. Severely elevated BP readings may be verified after shorter intervals in order to facilitate timely intervention.

Epidemiology

Preeclampsia complicates 3.1% to 3.4% of pregnancies in the United States. With appropriate treatment, eclampsia occurs in less than 1% of preeclamptic patients. The incidence of eclampsia in the United States and Canada is approximately 5.6 to 5.9 per 10,000 deliveries. Risk factors for preeclampsia include nulliparity, age less than 20 years or greater than 35 years, African American ethnicity, preeclampsia in a previous pregnancy, prolonged interval since previous pregnancy, chronic hypertension, multiple gestation, diabetes mellitus, chronic kidney disease, connective tissue disease, antiphospholipid antibody syndrome, obesity, and family history of preeclampsia.

Classification

Preeclampsia is classified as a hypertensive disorder of pregnancy. However, hypertension is thought to be a sign rather than the cause of the underlying disease process.

Diagnosis

History

At the initial prenatal visit, screen patients for risk factors for preeclampsia, and note complications of previous pregnancies. Beginning at 20 weeks of gestation, assess patients routinely for headache, visual disturbances, abdominal pain, and edema. Preeclampsia usually presents in the third trimester of pregnancy but can occur any time after 20 weeks of gestation, during labor, or even after delivery. Postpartum cases are most likely to occur within 48 hours of delivery.

Symptoms, if present, indicate more severe disease. Neurologic symptoms include headache, visual changes, confusion, coma, hyperreflexia, stroke, and seizures (eclampsia). Visual changes consist of scotomata, diplopia, blurred vision, blind spots, and transient cortical blindness. Gastrointestinal symptoms include nausea, vomiting, and epigastric or right upper quadrant abdominal pain resembling heartburn. Edema of the legs, hands, and face may persist after bed rest. Dyspnea due to pulmonary edema may occur. Preeclampsia can progress rapidly.

Physical Examination

Measure BP at every prenatal visit and monitor weight regularly. Patients with preeclampsia may gain a pound of fluid or more daily. Lower extremity edema is a common finding in normal pregnancy, but edema of the face and upper extremities is more closely associated with preeclampsia. Fundal height measurements that do not match dates may indicate fetal growth restriction (FGR). Assess deep tendon reflexes in patients with preeclampsia.

Laboratory and Imaging

In patients who develop SBP 140 mmHg or higher and/or DBP 90 mmHg or higher after 20 weeks of gestation, measure urine protein excretion by one of the following methods:

- **24-hour urine protein (preferred):** 300 mg or more is diagnostic of preeclampsia
- **Protein/creatinine ratio on a random urine sample:** less than 0.15 is normal, 0.3 or higher is suggestive of preeclampsia
- **Urine dipstick protein:** 1+ or more (should be verified by quantitative testing)

Measure platelet count, serum creatinine, and liver enzymes both for diagnosis and for assessment of severity. Once a diagnosis of preeclampsia has been established, recheck platelets, creatinine, and liver enzymes at least weekly until delivery to monitor for worsening of disease. Preeclampsia with severe features may require more frequent testing.

Obtain peripheral blood smear and lactate dehydrogenase (LDH) to evaluate for hemolysis. The constellation of hemolysis, elevated liver enzymes (aspartate aminotransferase >70 IU per L), and low platelets (<100,000 per µL), known as HELLP syndrome, is a marker of severe disease. Hemolysis is evidenced by schistocytes on blood smear, LDH >600 IU per L, total bilirubin ≥1.2 mg per dL, or serum haptoglobin ≤25 mg per dL.

Careful monitoring for signs of maternal and fetal compromise is critical for timing of delivery. Fetal surveillance should be performed on the following schedule in preeclamptic women:

- Fetal movement counts daily (more than 10 kicks daily is considered normal)
- Non-stress test (NST) weekly
- Biophysical profile weekly, usually alternated with NST for total of two tests weekly; repeat more frequently for suspected FGR or oligohydramnios or as indicated by severity of maternal condition
- Ultrasound assessment of fetal growth every 3 weeks
- Umbilical artery Doppler velocimetry if pregnancy is complicated by FGR

Differential Diagnosis

Distinguishing preeclampsia from chronic hypertension and gestational hypertension may prove challenging. Preeclampsia can also be superimposed on chronic hypertension. Depending on the presentation, the differential diagnosis for preeclampsia and eclampsia may include hepatitis, acute fatty liver of pregnancy, migraine, stroke, epilepsy, pulmonary embolism, systemic lupus erythematosus, and thrombotic thrombocytopenic purpura–hemolytic uremic syndrome.

Treatment

Behavioral

Ambulatory management is appropriate until 37 weeks for patients with preeclampsia without severe features. Indications for hospitalization include preeclampsia with severe features, disease progression, uncertainty about diagnosis or severity, non-reassuring maternal or fetal condition, and barriers to treatment and follow-up. Bed rest has no proven benefit for preeclamptic patients and may increase the risk of venous thromboembolism. Sodium restriction is not recommended during pregnancy, because it may cause volume depletion.[1] Smoking during the third trimester greatly increases the risk of FGR and should be discontinued.

Medications

- **Anticonvulsants.** Magnesium sulfate should be given to prevent seizures in women who have preeclampsia with severe features (see Table 14.8-1).[2] Magnesium also is the drug of choice for eclampsia.[1] Start with a 6-g intravenous (IV) bolus followed by a 2-g per hour IV infusion. Check serum magnesium 4 hours later; therapeutic levels are 4.8 to 8.4 mg per dL. Monitor reflexes, respirations, mental status, and urine output. Continue the magnesium infusion for 24 to 48 hours postpartum until the patient is stable and diuresing well. Somnolence, muscle weakness, loss of deep tendon reflexes, bradycardia, and hypotension may herald magnesium toxicity. Toxicity is uncommon in women with normal renal function but can be reversed with IV calcium gluconate.

TABLE 14.8-1   Severe Features of Preeclampsia

- Systolic blood pressure ≥160 mmHg and/or diastolic blood pressure ≥110 mmHg on two measurements at least 4 h apart while at rest
- Thrombocytopenia (platelet count <100,000/μL)
- Impaired liver function (transaminases more than twice normal values, severe persistent right upper quadrant or epigastric pain)
- Progressive renal insufficiency (creatinine >1.1 mg/dL or a doubling from baseline creatinine)
- Pulmonary edema
- New-onset cerebral or visual symptoms

Data from American College of Obstetricians and Gynecologists; Task Force on Hypertension in Pregnancy. Hypertension in pregnancy. Report of the American College of Obstetricians and Gynecologists' Task Force on Hypertension in Pregnancy. *Obstet Gynecol* 2013; 122:1122–1131.

Some physicians administer magnesium sulfate to all women with preeclampsia during labor and the immediate postpartum period. However, the American College of Obstetricians and Gynecologists' (ACOG) Task Force on Hypertension in Pregnancy does not recommend the routine use of magnesium sulfate for preeclampsia without severe features.[1]

- **Antihypertensives.** Initiate antihypertensive therapy for sustained SBP 160 mmHg or higher or DBP 105 to 110 mmHg or higher. Lower BP gradually to a goal of 130 to 150 mmHg systolic and 80 to 100 mmHg diastolic. Avoid reducing mean arterial BP by more than 25% acutely.[1,3]
  Preferred antihypertensive agents for acute treatment include:[4]
  - Labetalol 20 mg IV over 2 minutes, then escalating doses of 20 to 80 mg IV every 10 minutes as needed up to a maximum cumulative dose of 300 mg. Labetalol may also be given as an IV infusion at a rate of 1 to 2 mg per minute.
  - Hydralazine 5 mg IV over 1 to 2 minutes, then 5 to 10 mg IV every 20 minutes as needed up to a maximum cumulative dose of 30 mg.
  Preferred drugs for ambulatory treatment include:
  - Methyldopa 250 mg by mouth two or three times daily up to 3 g daily.
  - Labetalol 100 mg by mouth twice daily; it is increased by 100 mg twice daily every 2 or 3 days as needed up to maximum 2,400 mg per day.
  - Nifedipine extended release 30 to 60 mg orally daily, maximum 120 mg daily.
  Angiotensin-converting enzyme inhibitors, angiotensin receptor blockers, direct renin inhibitors, atenolol, spironolactone, and other diuretics are contraindicated in pregnancy.[1,3]
- **Corticosteroids.** Corticosteroids, such as betamethasone 12 mg IM every 24 hours for two doses, should be given to enhance fetal lung maturity if delivery before 34 weeks of gestation is considered.[1]

Referrals

Patients with severe preeclampsia who are remote from term are best managed in tertiary care settings or in consultation with physicians who are experienced in the management of high-risk pregnancy. Delivery is curative. The vaginal route is preferred if feasible after consideration of gestational age, fetal presentation, cervical status, and maternal and fetal conditions. Timing of delivery should be individualized but typically is recommended as follows:[1,5]

- Preeclampsia without severe features, with stable maternal and fetal conditions: 37 weeks
- Preeclampsia with severe features but stable maternal and fetal conditions: 34 weeks
- Preeclampsia with unstable maternal or fetal conditions (e.g., uncontrollable severe hypertension, eclampsia, pulmonary edema, placental abruption, HELLP syndrome, disseminated intravascular coagulation, non-reassuring fetal status): soon after maternal stabilization regardless of gestational age

Counseling

Preeclampsia usually resolves spontaneously by 1 to 2 weeks postpartum; some cases may take up to 12 weeks. Eclampsia has been reported as late as 23 days postpartum. Women with preeclampsia have an increased risk of preeclampsia in subsequent pregnancies. The risk is highest in women with early-onset preeclampsia and preeclampsia with severe features. Aspirin 60 to 80 mg by mouth daily starting at 12 weeks of gestation has been shown to reduce the risk of recurrence. Preeclampsia confers an increased risk of hypertension and cardiovascular disease later in life. Hypertension that persists beyond the postpartum period should be managed as in nonpregnant adults.

Patient Education
Prior to hospital discharge, all women, including those without preeclampsia, should be instructed about the importance of prompt medical attention for signs and symptoms of postpartum preeclampsia.[1]

ALLOIMMUNIZATION OF ERYTHROCYTES IN PREGNANCY

Erythrocyte (red blood cell, RBC) alloimmunization in pregnancy has drastically diminished since 1968 but has not disappeared. The decreased incidence is due in part to smaller family sizes, but mostly due to the introduction of anti-D immune globulin, formerly referred to as $Rh_o(D)$ immune globulin. Careful attention to maternal blood typing, prior obstetric history of RBC immunization, and careful prophylaxis of the nonimmune gravida for all potential risks of fetal–maternal transfusion are critical elements of managing this potentially lethal complication of pregnancy.[6]

General Principles

Definition
Alloimmunization is the development of maternal antibodies that may result in adverse consequences for the fetus or newborn, and may occur in women who are Rh(D) negative, and rarely from an anti-ABO or other antigen.

Epidemiology
- **Major blood type antigens**
  - D or Rhesus D (formerly Rh) is the most clinically significant.
  - Other Rhesus (C, c, E, e).
  - ABO (usually not hemolytic, but 98% of all hemolytic disease is Rhesus or ABO).
  - Kell, Duffy, Kidd, and Diego are other rare hemolytic antigens.
- **Population distribution.** 15% of whites are D-negative, and 8% of blacks are D-negative; 1% of Asians and Native Americans are D-negative.
- **Incidence.** 6.8 per 1,000 births, with 25 per 10,000 with clinical significance.

Etiology
If an Rh-negative woman is exposed to a Rhesus antigen, she may develop IgG antibodies that can cross the placenta and sensitize fetal erythrocytes of an Rh-positive fetus. This may result in erythrocyte destruction, causing fetal or newborn complications.

- **Causes of alloimmunization**
  - Major antigens D or Rhesus D (formerly Rh) are the most clinically significant.
  - Incompatible blood transfusion is mostly seen with non-Rh and non-ABO sensitization.
  - Possible clinical settings of incompatible transplacental hemorrhage are as follows:
    - **Procedures:** Amniocentesis, cesarean section, and, to a lesser extent, external version
    - Any antepartum bleeding
    - Abortion, spontaneous and elective
    - Molar pregnancies
    - Fetal–maternal hemorrhage. In 75% of pregnancies, there is some evidence of fetal blood in the maternal circulation, most frequently less than 0.1 mL.
- **Fetal and perinatal complications** include immune hydrops fetalis (severe), anemia (mild to severe), heart failure, hyperbilirubinemia leading to kernicterus, extramedullary hematopoiesis, and fetal demise.

Diagnosis

Identify antibodies against fetal erythrocytes in the maternal circulation. Once the antibody is specifically identified, the hemolytic potential of these erythrocytes is determined.

Laboratory Studies
- **Rh/ABO typing.** Every pregnant patient should have Rh/ABO typing at the first prenatal visit.
- **Antibody screening.** Every patient must have an antibody screening; if positive, identification and titration of the antibody is essential. An indirect Coombs test is usually done to determine titers. The majority of maternal antibodies identified are nonhemolytic.

Management

- Prevention by screening and treating those at risk for alloimmunization is the key.
- D-positive (Rh-positive), O-type blood requires no therapy.

- D-negative gravidas should:
  - Receive anti-D immune globulin (Rh Ig, RhoGAM) 300 μg as a single dose at 28 to 32 weeks gestation. Consider repeat antibody screening at 28 to 32 weeks gestation to identify alloimmunization earlier in pregnancy.[6,7]
  - Receive anti-D immune globulin (Rh Ig, RhoGAM) 300 μg as a single dose within 72 hours of delivery when susceptible to alloimmunization (delivery of D-positive or Rh-unknown infant).[6,7]
  - Receive 300 μg anti-D (Rh Ig) within 72 hours of a potential transfusion (see Causes of Alloimmunization above). Some physicians still use minidose (50 μg) anti-D before 12 weeks of gestation.[6]
- Postpartum management should include any deliveries at risk for increased fetal–maternal transfusion (cesarean section, increased blood loss, pregnancy-induced hypertension, manual removal of the placenta). Consider quantifying the fetal–maternal transfusion if the baby's blood type is D-positive. The Kleihauer–Betke test assesses the amount of fetal blood in the maternal circulation. If less than 15 mL of blood is transfused, give the routine 300 μg of anti-D (Rh Ig); if more than 15 mL of blood is transfused, 300 μg per 15-mL transfusion should be given.
- The patient with a positive antibody screen and an identified antigen (D, C, c, E, or e) should be treated as follows:
  - If the antibody titer is 1:8 or higher or is elevated four times baseline in monthly measurement, the following should be considered looking for evidence of fetal anemia:
    - Ultrasound, including Doppler velocimetry of the middle cerebral artery
    - Amniocentesis for optical density
    - Fetal blood sampling[6]
- Treatment of suspected fetal complications is usually carried out in a perinatal center.
  - Intraperitoneal fetal transfusions are effective.
  - Intravascular fetal transfusion into the umbilical vein or intrahepatic vein is also effective.
  - Plasmapheresis, corticosteroids, and promethazine have no proven benefit.
  - Delivery decisions are based on the fetal risk of immaturity versus rising hemolysis risks with continued pregnancy.
  - Fetal distress may be present, with the characteristic sinusoidal heart rate indicating repetitive decelerations. The severely distressed fetus should be delivered.

    Delivery where a level II or III neonatal intensive care unit is available is essential in the sensitized mother. Fetal exchange transfusion should be readily available.[6,8]

PRETERM LABOR

Preterm labor (PTL) is a leading cause of neonatal morbidity and mortality in the United States. Early, accurate diagnosis of PTL provides for secondary prevention of premature births. Primary prevention attempts to reduce risk factors for prematurity and may include progesterone supplementation or cervical cerclage when indicated. Once the patient is in PTL, a comprehensive management plan is essential.

General Principles

Definition

PTL is defined as contractions occurring between 20 and 36 6/7 weeks gestation and producing cervical change, or alternatively, as regular contractions with cervical dilation ≥2 cm at presentation.[9]

Epidemiology

Twelve percent of births are complicated by prematurity, and half of these preterm births result from PTL. The other half results from medical indications for early delivery, such as preeclampsia. Large societal costs result from neonatal intensive care and long-term treatment for complications. Seventy percent of neonatal mortality, 36% of infant deaths, and more than 25% of persistent neurological impairment are attributable to preterm birth.[9]

Etiology

The etiology is multifactorial. See History and Risk Management below for details.

Diagnosis of Preterm Labor

Clinical Presentation

Detecting PTL early enough for effective intervention has proven to be a challenge in practice. The patient presents between 20 and 36 6/7 weeks of gestation with uterine contractions or irritability producing cervical dilatation and/or effacement.

History

The most significant risk factor for preterm birth is a prior preterm birth. Other risk factors include short cervical length, maternal substance abuse (tobacco, cocaine), low prepregnancy weight, uterine overdistension, abruption, bacterial infections, periodontal disease, bleeding in the current pregnancy, and short interpregnancy interval.[10] Menstrual history, outpatient records, and early ultrasounds should be reviewed to confirm dates. Usually, the patient will give a history of recent or intermittent contractions with or without other signs of labor, such as pelvic pressure or bloody show.

Physical Examination

- **PTL signs.** Contractions can be palpated. A single observer should document cervical change (such as effacement or dilation) over time. Uterine measurement and ultrasound can provide an estimate of gestational age.
- **Cervical examinations.** Cervical examination for dilation, effacement, and station may prove useful in women with a history suggestive of incompetent cervix and should be performed in women with a complaint of preterm contractions to evaluate for cervical change. In suspected premature rupture of membranes (PROM), digital cervical examination has been associated with an increased risk of infection and should be avoided unless the patient is in labor or delivery is imminent.[11]

Laboratory

Fetal fibronectin is an extracellular protein that is believed to act as an adhesive between the developing embryo and the uterine surface. A negative fetal fibronectin assay has an excellent negative predictive value for preterm delivery, and women with normal cervical length and negative fetal fibronectin have a very low risk of imminent delivery.[12] Preterm PROM has typically been diagnosed by amniotic fluid leakage (observing cervical canal for pooling during valsalva), pH testing using nitrazine (normal vaginal pH is 4.5 to 6.0 and amniotic fluid pH is 7.1 to 7.3), and microscopic identification of ferning on dried vaginal fluid. Newer tests for amniotic proteins such as placental alpha microglobulin-1 appear to have better diagnostic accuracy than the combined use of pooling, nitrazine, and ferning.[12]

Imaging

Short cervical length (<25 mm) on transvaginal ultrasound is associated with an increased risk of preterm delivery. Measurement of cervical length by transvaginal ultrasound before 24 weeks can be considered in women who do not have a prior history of preterm birth to select women who may benefit from prophylactic treatment. Women with a prior history of preterm birth of a singleton pregnancy are already considered high risk.[10]

Monitoring

Home uterine monitoring is ineffective for the prevention of PTL.[9] Hospital- or office-based monitoring can be helpful in the presence of symptoms.

Differential Diagnosis

The differential includes false labor, Braxton–Hicks contractions, incompetent cervix, and uterine irritability secondary to infection or dehydration.

Treatment

Behavioral

Bed rest and pelvic rest do not prolong pregnancy and may have adverse maternal effects.[10]

Conservative Management

- Treat underlying causes (urinary tract infection, cervicitis, dehydration, substance use).
- Routine hydration has not been proved effective in the prevention of preterm birth.[9]

Medications

- **Tocolytic therapy**
  - **Efficacy.** Tocolytics have successfully lengthened pregnancy by an average of 48 hours, which may provide enough time to administer corticosteroids and magnesium sulfate, or to transfer to a tertiary care center. The decision to use tocolytics should be influenced by maternal condition, fetal size and maturity, and fetal condition.
  - **Contraindications.** Contraindications include advanced labor, severe preeclampsia or eclampsia, chorioamnionitis, dead or distressed fetus, anomalies incompatible with life, fetal maturity, and maternal bleeding with hemodynamic instability. In preterm PROM, tocolytics may be considered for 48 hours only to allow time for corticosteroid administration or transfer to a higher level of care.[9]

- **Drug dosage and comparison.** Based on efficacy, β-adrenergic receptor agonists, calcium-channel blockers, or nonsteroidal anti-inflammatory drugs (NSAIDs) are first-line agents for tocolysis. However, β-agonists have a higher incidence of adverse drug reactions than the other two agents.[9] Combining tocolytics increases maternal morbidity and should be avoided. Maintenance therapy with tocolytics is not recommended. Table 14.8-2 presents a list of tocolytics, dosages, and potential complications.

TABLE 14.8-2	Tocolytics for Management of Preterm Labor		
	Dosage	Precautions/complications	Contraindications
First-line agents			
Nifedipine (calcium-channel blocker)	10–20 mg PO q4–6h; Alt: load 30 mg PO x1, then 20 mg PO after 90 min	Transient hypotension, dizziness, flushing, elevated liver transaminases	Maternal liver disease, hypotension, aortic insufficiency, and other preload-dependent heart diseases
Indomethacin (NSAID)	50–100 mg PR; and/or 25–50 mg PO q6h	Renal failure, hepatitis, oligohydramnios, GI symptoms, platelet dysfunction, in utero constriction of ductus arteriosus Possible risk of necrotizing enterocolitis and intraventricular hemorrhage in neonates and patent ductus arteriosus in newborn	Aspirin-sensitive asthma, coronary artery disease, GI bleed, renal or hepatic failure, platelet dysfunction or bleeding disorder, oligohydramnios, fetal cardiac, or renal anomalies
Sulindac (NSAID)	200 mg PO q12 (up to six doses)	Same as indomethacin	Same as indomethacin
Second-line agents			
Magnesium sulfate	**Tocolysis dose** 4–6 g IV load, then 2–4 g/h drip Therapeutic level 4.8–8.4 mg/dL **Neuroprotection** Consider 4 g load and 1 g/h (optimum dose not yet defined)	Dizziness, flushing, Pulmonary edema Toxic levels may cause profound hypotension, paralysis, tetany, cardiac arrest, respiratory depression, and renal failure Areflexia at 8–10 mg/dL, respiratory suppression at >10 mg/dL Neonatal depression	Hypocalcemia, myasthenia gravis, renal failure
Terbutaline (β$_2$-agonist)	0.25–0.5 mg SC q3–4h	Hypokalemia, tremor, hyperglycemia, hypotension, pulmonary edema, tachycardia and palpitations, cardiac insufficiency, chest pain, fetal tachycardia	Maternal arrhythmias, uncontrolled diabetes mellitus, hypertension, or thyrotoxicosis

GI, gastrointestinal; NSAID, nonsteroidal anti-inflammatory drug.
Data from American College of Obstetricians and Gynecologists. ACOG practice bulletin no. 127: management of preterm labor. *Obstet Gynecol* 2012;119:1308–1317; Hyagrive NS, Caritis SN. Prevention of preterm delivery. *N Engl J Med* 2007;357:477–487; American College of Obstetricians and Gynecologists. Magnesium sulfate before anticipated preterm birth for neuroprotection. Committee Opinion No. 455. *Obstet Gynecol* 2010;115:669–671.

- **Adverse effects.** Magnesium sulfate has been associated with serious maternal complications and neonatal depression when used at tocolytic doses, and should not be considered first line. If magnesium sulfate is being given for neuroprotection prior to 32 weeks of gestation, indomethacin may be the safest tocolytic to use in combination. Magnesium sulfate given in combination with either calcium-channel blockers or β-adrenergic receptor agonists has been associated with significant maternal complications. The NSAIDs can cause constriction of the ductus arteriosus in the fetus and a decreased amniotic fluid index. These effects are reversible if use is restricted to a short period (24 to 48 hours). Nifedipine has few adverse effects, with hypotension being the most significant. β-Adrenergic receptor agonists have been associated with maternal tachycardia, pulmonary edema, hypokalemia, and hypoglycemia.[9] See Table 14.8-2 for additional complications and precautions.
- **Corticosteroids**
  - **Efficacy.** Antenatal steroids given between 24 and 34 weeks estimated gestational age (EGA) to women at risk of preterm delivery within 7 days have been proved to reduce the incidence and severity of respiratory distress syndrome, intraventricular hemorrhage, necrotizing enterocolitis, and death.[9]
  - **Complications.** The benefit of antenatal corticosteroids outweighs any potential risk. As expected, closer monitoring of gestational diabetes may be necessary after steroid administration, and steroids may mask maternal fever. Antenatal corticosteroids are not associated with increased infection risk.[11]
  - **Dosage and comparison.** Corticosteroids result in significant benefits, starting within 24 hours and persisting for a week. Corticosteroids are indicated in PTL between 24 and 34 weeks EGA. A single repeat course of steroids may be considered if more than a week has passed since the initial course, and delivery is expected prior to 34 weeks.[13] There are two accepted steroid courses, chosen for their ability to cross the placenta, their longer duration of action, and their proven efficacy in clinical trials. Higher or more frequent doses than those listed below do not provide any additional benefit.[9]
    - Betamethasone: two 12-mg doses given IM 24 hours apart.
    - Dexamethasone: four 6-mg doses given IM 12 hours apart.
- **Antibiotics**
  - In preterm PROM before 34 weeks gestation, a 7-day course of antibiotics has been shown to prolong latency, reduce maternal infections, and improve neonatal outcome. Combination treatment with ampicillin and erythromycin is preferred in preterm PROM. Studies indicate that empiric antibiotics with intact membranes do not prolong the pregnancy in PTL. Treatment of group B *Streptococcus*–positive mothers prior to delivery has been proved to decrease the incidence of neonatal sepsis.[11] Maternal infections including bacterial vaginosis, urinary tract infections, and sexually transmitted infections should be treated.
- **Magnesium sulfate**
  - Intravenous magnesium sulfate has been shown to reduce the risk and severity of cerebral palsy when delivery is expected to occur prior to 32 weeks of gestation. Optimum treatment guidelines have not been established, and ACOG recommends hospitals develop protocols in accordance with one of the larger trials.[9]

Operative

Cerclage has been associated with a 30% reduction in the risk of preterm birth in singleton pregnancies with prior preterm birth and a very short cervix (<25 mm before 24 weeks). Cerclage increases the risk of preterm birth in women with twin gestations and a short cervix, and should be avoided. The role of cerclage in addition to progesterone supplementation has not been defined.[10]

Risk Management

Women with a prior spontaneous preterm singleton birth should be offered progesterone supplementation starting at 16 to 24 weeks of gestation for all subsequent singleton pregnancies to prevent PTL. Women without a prior preterm birth and with a short cervical length (≤20 mm) before 24 weeks of gestation should also be offered vaginal progesterone. Progesterone supplementation is not recommended for women carrying multiple gestations.[10]

Patient Education

All pregnant patients with signs or symptoms of labor should seek immediate medical attention. Counsel risk reduction, such as smoking cessation, proper nutrition, avoiding contact sports, and treating infections promptly.

Complications

Preterm infants have significant risk of pulmonary, neurologic, and enteral complications that require specialized medical care. Whenever possible, preterm delivery should occur in a hospital with specialized newborn care available.

REFERENCES

1. American College of Obstetricians and Gynecologists; Task Force on Hypertension in Pregnancy. Hypertension in pregnancy. Report of the American College of Obstetricians and Gynecologists' Task Force on Hypertension in Pregnancy. *Obstet Gynecol* 2013;122:1122–1131.
2. Duley L, Gülmezoglu AM, Henderson-Smart DJ, et al. Magnesium sulphate and other anticonvulsants for women with pre-eclampsia. *Cochrane Database Syst Rev* 2010;11:CD000025.
3. Bushnell C, McCullough LD, Awad IA, et al. Guidelines for the prevention of stroke in women: a statement for healthcare professionals from the American Heart Association/American Stroke Association. *Stroke* 2014;45(5):1545–1588.
4. Al Khaja KA, Sequeira RP, Alkhaja AK, et al. Drug treatment of hypertension in pregnancy: a critical review of adult guideline recommendations. *J Hypertens* 2014;32:454–463.
5. American College of Obstetricians and Gynecologists. ACOG committee opinion no. 560: Medically indicated late-preterm and early-term deliveries. *Obstet Gynecol* 2013;121:908–910.
6. American College of Obstetricians and Gynecologists. ACOG practice bulletin no. 75: management of alloimmunization during pregnancy. *Obstet Gynecol* 2006;108:457–464.
7. Crowther CA, Middleton P, McBain RD. Anti-D administration in pregnancy for preventing Rhesus alloimmunisation. *Cochrane Database Syst Rev* 2013;2:CD000020.
8. MacKenzie IZ, Bowell P, Gregory H, et al. Routine antenatal Rhesus D immunoglobulin prophylaxis: the results of a prospective 10 year study. *Br J Obstet Gynaecol* 1999;106:492–497.
9. American College of Obstetricians and Gynecologists. Practice bulletin no. 127: management of preterm labor. *Obstet Gynecol* 2012;119:1308–1317.
10. American College of Obstetricians and Gynecologists. Practice bulletin no. 130: prediction and prevention of preterm birth. *Obstet Gynecol* 2012;120:964–973.
11. American College of Obstetricians and Gynecologists. Practice bulletin no. 139: premature rupture of membranes. *Obstet Gynecol* 2013;122:918–930.
12. Di Renzo GC, Roura LC, Facchinetti F, et al. Guidelines for the management of spontaneous preterm labor: identification of spontaneous preterm labor, diagnosis of preterm premature rupture of membranes, and preventive tools for preterm birth. *J Matern Fetal Neonatal Med* 2011;24:659–667.
13. Crowther CA, McKinlay CJ, Middleton P, et al. Repeat doses of prenatal corticosteroids for women at risk of preterm birth for improving neonatal health outcomes. *Cochrane Database Syst Rev* 2011;6:CD003935.

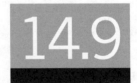

Intrapartum Care
Lyrad K. Riley

GENERAL PRINCIPLES

Intrapartum care of the healthy term pregnant woman is the subject of this chapter, beginning with her arrival at the labor ward with symptoms of labor.

DIAGNOSIS AND ADMISSION
History

The woman in labor typically gives a history of regularly occurring contractions of increasing frequency and intensity, associated with pain in the abdomen and/or back. Establish her estimated gestational age, gravidity, and parity. Ask whether she has had, and the time of, suspected rupture of the membranes. Ask whether it was clear, green (meconium), or bloody. Determine whether there has been abnormal bleeding and whether the fetus has been moving normally. Review her antenatal history for any significant problems during this pregnancy. Review her past obstetric history, medical history, and psychosocial history, identifying problems that are active or relevant to her current labor (e.g., diabetes or history of cesarean section) (see Chapters 14.6 and 14.8).

Physical Examination

Perform a focused physical examination at the time of admission, giving attention to the areas identified in the history as being of concern. Confirm the uterine size and presentation (with ultrasound if necessary). Inspect the vulva for herpes under bright light. Confirm a history of suspected rupture of the membranes with a combination of the following clues: sterile speculum examination looking for pooled fluid in the vagina, pH test, microscopic evidence of "ferning" when vaginal fluid is air dried on a slide, or use of a swab designed to detect the presence of placental α-microglobulin-1 in amniotic fluid. Digitally examine the cervix for dilatation (in centimeters), softness, effacement, and position, which allows calculation of the Bishop's score. Confirm a vertex presentation and ascertain its station relative to the ischial spines. Note the fetal heart rate (FHR) and the frequency and duration of contractions. To diagnose true labor, one should note the presence of cervical change in the setting of regular, painful contractions.

Investigations

In many facilities, it is routine to draw blood for a complete blood count and blood type and screen at the time of initiation of intravenous access, and to send urine for urinalysis. Verify the mother's group B Streptococcus screen results to determine whether intrapartum antibiotics should be used.

LABOR MANAGEMENT

The well-being of the maternal–fetal pair is dynamic throughout the labor process, which merits close observation. One should assess the plan on an ongoing basis and adjust management appropriately.

- **First stage,** from onset of labor to full dilatation at 10 cm, is divided into latent and active phases. The latent phase is marked by slow cervical dilation until 4 to 6 cm. The active phase is characterized by more rapid dilation.
  - **Monitoring and care**
    - **Maternal nutrition and position.** Allow clear liquid intake (water, ice chips, juice without pulp, soda, sports drinks) during labor.[1] Consider restricting intake of thicker liquids and solid foods during active labor to reduce risk of emesis and surgical complications. Allow women to ambulate or assume sitting or squatting postures as preferred.
  - **Fetal surveillance**
    - **Amniotic fluid.** When the membranes are ruptured, assess the fluid for the presence of meconium and blood. Meconium has been associated with increased perinatal morbidity, both as an indicator of fetal stress and a risk factor for aspiration. Blood may signify abruption.
    - **FHR monitoring.** Benefits are controversial, and can be either intermittent or continuous. With intermittent monitoring, the FHR is checked every 15 to 30 minutes, immediately following a contraction. This can be done by simple auscultation or by Doppler ultrasonography. Continuous FHR monitoring can be accomplished with either an external Doppler transducer or an internal fetal scalp electrode.
    - **Baseline FHR pattern.** Assess the FHR pattern for baseline rate and variability. The baseline FHR (i.e., the rate between contractions at term) is normally 110 to 160 beats per minute (BPM). Variability (the beat-to-beat variation in the FHR) is considered moderate (normal) from 6 to 25 BPM. Variability may be diminished or absent in the premature or "sleeping" fetus, or after parenteral analgesics. However, absence of variability may indicate fetal problems such as hypoxia or congenital anomalies. Tachycardia (>160 BPM) can be caused by maternal fever, drugs, or fetal hypoxia. Other less common causes of fetal tachycardia include fetal hyperthyroidism, fetal anemia, fetal heart failure, and fetal tachyarrhythmias. Bradycardia (<110 BPM) can be normal in the post-term infant or indicative of severe hypoxia, maternal systemic lupus erythematosus, or fetal heart block.[2]
    - **Periodic heart rate changes.** Document accelerations and decelerations. Accelerations are defined as increases in FHR peaking at least 15 BPM above baseline lasting at least 15 seconds. Decelerations are of three patterns: early, late, and variable. In early decelerations, the heart rate decreases with the start of the contraction and recovers as the contraction diminishes. This type of deceleration is associated with fetal head compression. Late decelerations begin as the contraction peaks. The lowest FHR is reached well after the peak of the contraction and recovery does not take place until after the end of the contraction. These may

be associated with uteroplacental insufficiency and resultant hypoxia. Variable decelerations usually have abrupt decreases in FHR (less than 30 seconds from onset to nadir) and begin at no fixed time in relation to the contraction, and may be the result of cord compression.

- Given the high false-positive rate of potentially concerning FHR tracings, there has been some effort to categorize them by a combination of baseline rate, variability, and the presence or absence of accelerations and decelerations as category I, II, or III. In the case of prolonged or recurrent late decelerations or fetal bradycardia, consider interventions such as a change in maternal position, supplemental oxygen by face mask, and IV fluid bolus, and check for cord prolapse. An abnormal FHR pattern unresponsive to these measures may indicate the need for immediate consultation with a cesarean capable provider.

- **Progress.** Periodically assess the cervix for further dilation, effacement, and descent of the head. These examinations should not be done more often than necessary to minimize discomfort and, when the membranes have already ruptured, the risk of infection. An acceptable rate of dilatation in the active phase may be 0.5 to 1.5 cm per hour, with primiparas generally progressing more slowly than multiparas. Slow progress may be, but is not necessarily, a sign of abnormal labor. Interpret the rate of progress in the context of both fetal and maternal well-being.[3]

- **Pain control can be nonpharmacologic or pharmacologic.** Anything that relaxes and distracts the woman from her pain is beneficial. Maternal movement and position changes help with pain tolerance. Encourage the use of hot and cold compresses, showers, massage, or music as desired by the patient. The presence of trained nonmedical birth attendants (doulas) increases both the rate of successful vaginal birth and patient satisfaction.[4]
  - **Systemic drugs.** Narcotics provide reasonable analgesia but are also associated with dose-related maternal sedation, hypotension, nausea, vomiting, and neonatal respiratory depression. Options include fentanyl, butorphanol, and nalbuphine.
  - **Regional anesthesia** options include the epidural, spinal, and pudendal anesthetics. Epidurals generally provide more effective pain relief than do intravenous narcotics. However, epidurals may lengthen labor and increase the rates of operative vaginal delivery, maternal fever, and hypotension.[5] Epidural placement does not need to be delayed until active labor.[6]

- **Second stage** comprises the time from 10 cm dilatation to delivery of the infant. Confirm full dilatation before pushing. Allow the unanesthetized woman to push in the position of her choice and according to her own urges. For women with an epidural, delayed pushing up to 2 hours (laboring down), unless there is an irresistible urge, visibility of head, or medical indication to shorten the second stage, may reduce the need for obstetric interventions. Give the patient guidance and feedback on her propulsive efforts. As long as there is progress, intervention is generally required only if there is a concern about maternal or fetal well-being.

  - **Care of the perineum.** Consider application of a warm washcloth to the perineum. Episiotomy should not be done unless indicated, as it does not reduce the risk of severe perineal trauma or urinary incontinence, nor does it improve perineal healing or prevent fetal trauma. Indications include relief of maternal or fetal distress or to provide room for maneuvers in case of an operative vaginal delivery or shoulder dystocia. Time episiotomies at the last possible moment to reduce blood loss. Local anesthetic is injected into the perineum along the anticipated line of the incision if required.

  - **Spontaneous delivery of the occiput-anterior infant**
    - **Delivery of the head.** Minimize perineal trauma by conducting a *controlled* delivery of the head. At crowning, guide the woman to give small, short pushes of submaximal power, to allow gradual stretching of the perineum. Allow the head to restitute spontaneously based on which way the shoulders are facing.
    - **Shoulders.** Check for the presence of a nuchal cord. Try to slip it over the head or shoulders; if too tight it may be necessary to double clamp and cut between the clamps. Deliver the anterior shoulder first by gentle downward traction on the head, then the posterior shoulder by upward traction. Watch and support the posterior perineum to control for lacerations and extensions. The rest of the infant easily follows. The cord is then clamped and cut. If the infant has good color, tone, and cry, consider waiting 30 to 60 seconds before clamping the cord, holding the infant below the level of the placenta.[7] The vigorous infant can then be placed directly on the maternal abdomen, where it should be warmed and dried. In the presence of meconium and a nonvigorous infant, try to minimize stimulation of the fetus until the infant's attendant determines whether there should be endotracheal suction to decrease the risk of meconium aspiration.

- **Third stage**
  - **Delivery of the placenta.** Spontaneous delivery of the placenta usually occurs within minutes. Maintain firm gentle traction on the cord while the abdominal hand pushes upward on the anterior wall of the uterus to reduce the risk of uterine inversion. Routine administration of oxytocics may shorten the third stage and reduce the risk of postpartum hemorrhage. **Dosage:** Oxytocin (Oxytocin injection, USP) 10 to 30 units IM or IV should be given after delivery of the anterior shoulder. Manual removal of the placenta is considered if the placenta is not delivered within 30 minutes.
  - **Vaginal repair.** Inspect the vagina, periurethral tissues, and cervix for tears. Confirm the presence or absence of a third (involving external anal sphincter) or fourth-degree (involving rectal mucosa) tear, and repair these first. Repair vaginal mucosa and perineum with 2–0 absorbable suture, ensuring hemostasis and anatomical restoration, with the minimal amount of suture required.
- **The postpartum transition period.** For the first few hours, monitor the woman closely for any evidence of bleeding and abnormal vital signs. Check her fundus frequently, and massage if not firm. If her flow seems too fast or heavy, then treat for postpartum hemorrhage (see Section 14.10) with uterotonic agents such as oxytocin, methylergonovine, carboprost, or misopropstol while evaluating for other potential causes of hemorrhage. Encourage and assist with early breastfeeding.

REFERENCES

1. Committee on Obstetric Practice, American College of Obstetricians and Gynecologists. ACOG committee opinion no. 441: oral intake during labor. Sep 2009, reaffirmed 2013.
2. American College of Obstetricians and Gynecologists. ACOG practice bulletin no. 116: management of intrapartum fetal heart rate tracings. *Obstet Gynecol* 2010;116(5):1232–40.
3. Caughey AB, Cahill AG, Guise JM, et al. Safe prevention of the primary cesarean delivery (joint ACOG/SMFM Consensus). *Am J Obstet Gynecol* 2014;210:179–199.
4. Berghella V, Baxter JK, Chauhan SP. Evidence-based labor and delivery management. *Am J Obstet Gynecol* 2008;199:445–454.
5. Anim-Somuah M, Smyth RM, Jones L. Epidural versus non-epidural or no analgesia in labour. *Cochrane Database Syst Rev* 2011;(12):CD000331 doi: 10.1002/14651858.
6. American College of Obstetricians and Gynecologists Committee on Obstetric Practice. ACOG committee opinion no. 339: analgesia and cesarean delivery rates. *Obstet Gynecol* 2006;107(6):1487–1488.
7. McAdams RM. Time to implement delayed cord clamping. *Obstet Gynecol* 2014;123:549–552.

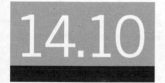

14.10 Complications During Labor and Delivery

Kevin C. Sisk

Bleeding in the third trimester, or antepartum hemorrhage, occurs in 2% to 5% of pregnancies. Nearly half of the identifiable cases of bleeding are attributable to either placental abruption or placenta previa.[1] Premature rupture of the membranes (PROM) and shoulder dystocia are more common than the hemorrhagic complications of labor and delivery, but are less likely to result in as significant maternal or neonatal morbidity or mortality.

PLACENTAL ABRUPTION
General Principles

Definition

Placental abruption, or abruptio placentae, is defined as premature separation of a normally inserted placenta from the endometrium.

Anatomy

Hemorrhage occurs at the decidual–placental interface and usually, but not always, dissects through to the cervix. It can occur in any trimester. Early in pregnancy, abruption can manifest clinically as threatened or spontaneous abortion, and on ultrasound as a subchorionic hemorrhage. Unless the abruption occurs traumatically as in an auto accident or as the consequence of uterine rupture, the bleeding derives from maternal vessels.

Epidemiology
Abruption is seen clinically in about 0.48% to 1.8% of all pregnancies with variation attributable to diagnostic technique.[2,3]

Classification
Abruption can be marginal, partial, or total. In the case where blood does not dissect through to the vagina, abruption is designated as concealed or occult.

Etiology
Risk factors include prior abruption, smoking, trauma, cocaine use, multifetal gestation, hypertension, preeclampsia, thrombophilias, advanced maternal age, preterm PROM, intrauterine infections, and hydramnios.[4] Abruption increases somewhat with increasing maternal age. Cocaine abuse is particularly important, causing at least a threefold increase in the rate of abruption. The increase in the use of this drug may in part be responsible for the increased national incidence of abruption.[5]

Pathophysiology
The exact mechanism of placental abruption is unknown despite a large body of clinical research, although the majority of the time it is considered the end result of a chronic process begun at an earlier gestation.[6] There is no doubt, however, that acute placental separation may result from traumatic shearing forces such as those experienced in an automotive accident.[4,7]

Mechanisms of Injury
- **Maternal.** Maternal mortality is rare with modern obstetrical management, but morbidity can occur due to blood loss, disseminated intravascular coagulation (DIC) and subsequent renal damage, or anemia. Most of the blood loss is maternal, but some fetal–maternal transfusions may occur, leading to isoimmunization.
- **Fetal.** Despite a majority of perinatal deaths being related to extreme prematurity, intrauterine fetal demise is possible even at term related to disruption of placental function, although usually with greater than 50% disruption of the placental interface.[8] Abruption is associated with poorer neurodevelopmental outcome in low-birth-weight infants but not in normal-weight infants.[9]

Diagnosis

History
Abruption is often an obstetrical emergency and the clinician must be looking for symptoms that may be subtle. The classical presentation consists of vaginal bleeding, contractions, and abdominal or back pain. Bleeding-related events including abruption should additionally be suspected in patients presenting with preterm labor.[8]

Physical Examination
Uterine tenderness, back pain, vaginal bleeding, and fetal distress may each be seen in more than half of cases. Less common but still occurring in more than 10% are hypertonic contractions, rapid progress of labor, preterm labor, and in 15% of cases, fetal demise.[5] Abruption may rarely present as shock.

Laboratory
Blood tests occasionally demonstrate renal failure and coagulation defects that are associated with increased maternal and fetal complications. Hypofibrinogenemia is found in 30% of patients with abruption and associated fetal demise. Proteinuria is also a common accompaniment of DIC. Other maternal serum markers may be elevated such as α-fetoprotein and human chorionic gonadotropin. In Rh-negative mothers, a Kleihauer Betke test may be done, which would indicate the presence of fetal cells in the maternal circulation. It may be helpful in diagnosing a concealed abruption as well as useful for dosing RhoGam if a larger than normal fetal maternal transfusion has occurred.

Imaging
- **Ultrasound.** An ultrasound examination should be performed as soon as possible when abruption is suspected. Although a clot may not be seen in as many as 50% of cases, the study is still useful in excluding placenta previa. A hemorrhage greater than 60 cc or 50% of the surface that attaches to the uterus is associated with a 50% mortality.[10]

- **Magnetic resonance imaging (MRI)** may detect a higher percentage of suspected cases of abruption where the diagnosis is not obvious clinically. However, lack of portability renders MRI less useful in an emergency situation.

Staging

The Sher classification lists three grades that can be used to help direct management.[11]

- **Grade I mild abruption.** Clot is often minimally symptomatic and discovered retrospectively, at the time of delivery after unexplained bleeding.
- **Grade II symptomatic abruption** (tender abdomen) with live fetus.
- **Grade III abruption with fetal demise.**
  - IIIA without coagulopathy
  - IIIB with coagulopathy

Treatment

Nonoperative

Labor may be allowed to progress if no fetal distress is noted, although rapid deterioration may be seen. Continuous electronic fetal monitoring is essential if the patient is allowed to labor. If contractions do occur, they are often hypertonic and accompanied by rapid cervical dilation secondary to prostaglandin release caused by uterine separation. This progression often precludes the additional need for labor augmentation.

Operative

A cesarean section is performed if there are signs of fetal distress or in the case of Stage III abruption. About half of symptomatic abruptions receive a cesarean section.[5]

Special Treatment

Coagulopathy may require replacement of blood products while waiting for the effects of the placental inflammation to reverse. Any significant bleeding in pregnancies where the mother is at risk for anti-D isoimmunization should prompt treatment with Rh immune globulin.

Patient Education and Prevention

In spite of the high incidence of recurrence (12%), preventive measures are not available to lower the increased incidence of fetal demise (7%) in pregnancies with a history of abruption.

PLACENTA PREVIA
General Principles

Definition

Placenta previa is defined as placental implantation overlying or in close proximity to the internal cervical os.[12]

Anatomy

Bleeding from separation of the placenta in the presence of previa is a common cause of bleeding in the second and third trimesters.[11]

Epidemiology

Placenta previa causes bleeding in about 0.5% of late pregnancies. A higher than normal rate of placenta previa is associated with previous cesarean section, previous induced or spontaneous abortion, advanced maternal age, and smoking.[10] The recurrence rate can be up to 7%.

Classification

Depending on the precise location of the placenta, the previa may be qualified as being total (completely covering the internal os), partial (partially covering), or marginal (edge of placenta touching the os). Vasa previa, where the fetal vessels divide before implanting on the margin and protrude through the os during labor, is a rare and often fatal variant.

Pathophysiology

Placenta previa, although it may be due to a random faulty localization of the placenta, is also associated with factors that cause damage to the vascular function or continuity of the endometrium. Up to 7% of patients with placenta previa may have an abnormal placental attachment (placenta accreta, increta, or percreta). This is noted especially in patients with repeated cesarean sections, indicating that both conditions may be related to endometrial defects. The rate of accreta may be as high as 65% after multiple cesarean sections.[5]

Etiology

Advanced maternal age, multiparity, prior cesarean section, history of uterine curettage, chronic hypertension, and smoking all increase the rate of placenta previa.[13]

Mechanisms of Injury

- **Fetal.** Perinatal fetal mortality is less than 5%, primarily due to increased premature births by cesarean section.[10] In addition to the common forms of morbidity associated with prematurity, neonatal anemia is common and related to the degree of maternal hemorrhage. Respiratory distress syndrome occurs more commonly than would be predicted by the rate of prematurity. Other effects, such as an increased incidence of congenital anomalies, may be associated with the causes of abnormal implantation. It is likely that a number of spontaneous abortions occur due to a low insertion of the placenta.
- **Maternal.** Women with placenta previa have a mortality of 0.03%, or about three times the overall U.S. rate of mortality in childbirth. Death may be due to hemorrhage from a digital examination in labor or postpartum hemorrhage from placenta accreta, increta, or percreta. These can cause exsanguination and must be anticipated, especially when previa occurs with a prior cesarean section. Other complications include an increase in cesarean birth, postpartum hemorrhage, blood transfusion, and hysterectomy.[14]

Diagnosis

Clinical Presentation

Placenta previa may present as painless bleeding in the second or third trimester or as heavy bleeding after an examiner unwittingly damages the presenting placenta or vessels.

History

The ubiquitous use of ultrasound has allowed most cases of placenta previa to be diagnosed in the antepartum period. Previa is frequently diagnosed prior to any bleeding and commonly overdiagnosed. One study of 267 patients having placenta previa diagnosed on ultrasound performed between 14 and 20 weeks gestation showed that the previa persisted to the time of delivery in only 2.5% of patients with partial or marginal previa, although it persisted in 26% of patients with total previa.[10] Placenta accreta may present as excessive bleeding in the third stage of labor due to incomplete separation. Placenta percreta and increta may also be associated with difficulty in delivering the placenta.

Physical Examination

Vaginal examination should be avoided if placenta previa is suspected before performing an ultrasound examination, due to the risk of perforating the portion of placenta that is palpable through the os. If the localization of a low-lying placenta is not clear from ultrasound a "double setup" examination may be performed in the operating room after the patient is prepared for cesarean delivery and the operative team is assembled.

Laboratory Studies

Blood tests are generally normal in the absence of anemia due to massive hemorrhage.

Imaging

- **Ultrasound.** An ultrasound should be performed with the onset of painless bleeding in pregnancy. False-positive and false-negative rates may each approach 5%. Bladder overdistention is associated with false positives, and consideration should be made to catheterize the bladder before performing an ultrasound. Clinical judgment is important. Heavy bleeding, especially when coexisting with signs of fetal distress, should lead to an immediate delivery without taking time to perform studies.
- **MRI** can clearly outline the location of a placenta previa, but it is much more expensive and less readily available.

Monitoring

- **Antepartum.** Monthly ultrasound can be performed to document whether, as the lower uterine segment grows, the placenta will no longer be low-lying, allowing for normal labor.
- **Preterm.** Patients with transient minor bleeding who are not in labor may be managed in consultation with a perinatologist. Avoiding vaginal examinations may increase the latent period. In preterm placenta previa prior to 36 weeks gestation without evident fetal jeopardy, authorities recommend attempting delay in delivery by avoiding vaginal examination. Reliable patients with minor degrees of bleeding who have been adequately observed for premature delivery and fetal distress may be managed at home without increased maternal or infant morbidity or mortality. In practice, few patients with symptomatic placenta previa meet these criteria.[5]

• **Term and intrapartum.** Prompt delivery should be the goal in term placenta previa. Hemorrhage and shock must be managed aggressively, and the delivering physician should be prepared to perform an emergency cesarean section or hysterectomy if bleeding from placenta accreta cannot be controlled. Continuous electronic fetal monitoring is needed when labor is allowed. Maternal hypotension should be managed with two large-bore intravenous lines, type and cross match, consideration of transfusion, and prompt delivery.

Differential Diagnosis

Physical examination and history are usually sufficient to help differentiate abruptio and previa from normal bleeding. Bleeding may also be due to trauma upon a friable cervix and the normal bloody show in early labor. DIC caused by sepsis or infection and clotting disorders are rare and may be anticipated with a prior history or signs of shock.

Treatment

Behavioral

Women who are managed expectantly are restricted from vaginal intercourse or use of tampons.

Medications

In preterm placenta previa prior to 36 weeks gestation without evident fetal jeopardy, authorities recommend attempting delay in delivery by tocolysis (see below).

Surgery

Cesarean section is performed if fetal distress or significant hemorrhage is evident.

Special Considerations

Regional anesthesia is less likely to exacerbate heavy bleeding than general anesthesia and is preferred for cesarean sections in patients with symptomatic previa.

PREMATURE RUPTURE OF MEMBRANES
General Principles

Definition

PROM is a loss of integrity of the fetal membranes with leakage of amniotic fluid that occurs more than 1 hour before the onset of active labor. The duration between membrane rupture and the onset of active labor contractions is defined as the latent period.

Epidemiology

PROM occurs in 5% to 10% of term and 30% of preterm deliveries.[5]

Classification

PROM may be subdivided into PROM at term or preterm (PPROM), which occurs prior to 37 weeks of gestation.

Pathophysiology

Many cases of PROM are thought to be due to inflammation from subclinical infections of the genital tract. The bacterial enzymes that facilitate colonization as well as local release of inflammatory cytokines are thought to weaken fetal membranes.[15] Vascular damage may be a cause, as in diabetes or hypertension.

Etiology

Positive cultures of amniotic fluid are present in 30% of pregnancies with PPROM. Smoking and vaginal bleeding are associated but it is not known how. Previous PROM is a risk factor. Other risk factors include vaginal group B streptococcal (GBS) colonization, cigarette smoking, hypertension, diabetes, amniocentesis, and cervical surgery during pregnancy.

Mechanisms of Injury

• **Maternal.** Most complications are related to infection. The rate of postpartum endometritis historically approached 30%, but the widespread use of antibiotics has greatly reduced this. Abruption occurs to a larger degree than that in the total birth population but at less a rate than seen in other preterm deliveries.[16]

• **Fetal.** Subclinical infection is common, but less than 10% of neonates actually develop sepsis after PROM. Most complications are related to prematurity. Although PPROM poses a significant risk of morbidity and mortality to the neonate, 75% of cases of PROM occur at term and generally run a benign course. PROM increases the frequency of neonatal sepsis from 0.1% to 1.4%. Fatalities are common in neonatal sepsis, especially in low-birth-weight infants (20% in very low-birth-weight infants vs. 12% in normal-weight infants) and those with GBS sepsis. Although an increase in the latency period in term pregnancy increases the incidence of sepsis, the neonatal mortality is unaffected. Even the presence of acute chorioamnionitis for up to 24 hours does not increase neonatal mortality in term births.[5]

Diagnosis

Clinical Presentation
Patients will notice a gush of fluid or leaking fluid prior to the onset of labor.

History
If the flow does not persist, the physician should ask the patient to examine the clothing for an odor of urine.

Physical Examination
- On examination of the vagina with a sterile speculum, a flow of fluid, sometimes containing vernix caseosa or meconium, is diagnostic, as is seeing or palpating the fetal scalp.
- Signs of acute chorioamnionitis, or acute infection complicating premature rupture, include fever and foul or cloudy amniotic fluid.
- Readiness of the cervix for labor is determined by direct observation and digital examination. Engagement of the presenting part, cervical softness, forward position of the os, dilatation, and effacement all indicate impending labor and are features which are more likely to result in successful induction of labor with oxytocin.

Laboratory
- **Ferning.** Amniotic fluid dries with a characteristic arborization pattern, called *ferning*, seen on microscopic examination. False-positive fern test results may rarely be seen in the presence of scant fluid due to the presence of cervical mucus.
- **Nitrazine test.** This test checks for elevation of the normally acidic vaginal pH due to the presence of amniotic fluid. False-positive results are more common than with the fern test and may be caused by bacterial vaginosis or by contamination of the vaginal sample with blood, lubricant jelly, or povidone–iodine.
- **Fetal fibronectin** can be detected in a vaginal fluid sample not otherwise contaminated by blood, semen, or lubricant gel. If negative, this test is useful in ruling out a premature delivery in the next 2 weeks.[17]
- **Chorioamnionitis** may be associated with DIC. Chorioamnionitis occurs in 3% to 25% of PROM cases. When this condition is suspected, clotting studies and measurement of renal and hepatic function should be done.
- **Amniocentesis** to evaluate pulmonary maturity may be performed in preterm PROM before 35 weeks. A decreased level of amniotic fluid glucose provides rapid confirmation of chorioamnionitis.
- **GBS colonization** can increase morbidity and mortality. Those who have no prior testing or a negative GBS screen should have a single swab of the vagina and rectum sent for testing.
- **Coagulation** studies and studies of renal function should be performed if signs of chorioamnionitis develop.

Monitoring
- **Fever.** In addition to frequent fetal monitoring, those with PROM need routine measures of temperature to help anticipate chorioamnionitis.
- **Hyperstimulation.** The use of prostaglandin analogues may cause hyperstimulation of the uterus. This is defined as the presence of prolonged (≥2 minutes) contractions, excessively frequent contractions, or tachysystole (≥6 in 10 minutes) and fetal distress (late decelerations or fetal bradycardia).

Treatment

Medication
- **Preterm PROM**
  - **Tocolysis.** Tocolysis is often used in preterm PROM before 35 weeks, but little evidence exists for its effectiveness in improving fetal outcomes. Indomethacin and parenteral terbutaline have the best evidence supporting their use in prolonging the latent period, although parenteral magnesium sulfate and ritodrine are also commonly used.[18]
  - **Corticosteroid administration** has been extensively utilized to induce the production of mature lung surfactant. There is good evidence that they are effective in reducing neonatal mortality and

morbidity due to respiratory distress syndrome and intraventricular hemorrhage.[19] A typical dose of corticosteroids is betamethasone 12 mg IM in two doses 24 hours apart.

- **Antibiotic prophylaxis** is designed to lengthen latency through a reduction of amnionitis when given to women with PROM before 37 weeks gestation. It has additionally been shown to reduce neonatal infection as well as use of supplemental oxygen and surfactant. Co-amox-iclav, however, should be avoided, as it has been shown to increase the risk for necrotizing enterocolitis.[20]
- **Term PROM**
  - **Ripening the cervix.** Digital examination is performed. If the cervix is not dilated more than 2 cm, vaginal application of a prostaglandin can cut the latency period by at least half, as was shown in several studies. Cervidil, an insert impregnated with 10 mg dinoprostone (prostaglandin E), may be the preferred preparation because it can be removed in the case of hyperstimulation. Administration of misoprostol (25 to 50 μg vaginally every 3 to 6 hours to a maximum of 100 μg) is a much less expensive alternative that frequently has the advantage of resulting in regular contractions in addition to ripening the cervix. Prostaglandins are also safe and effective in the induction of labor if the cervix is ripened and not dilated beyond 5 cm.[21]
  - **Oxytocin.** Induction of labor with an intravenous infusion of oxytocin decreases latency significantly but seems not to affect the low rate of maternal or neonatal mortality in term pregnancy. A Cochrane Database systemic review indicates that induction does offer reduction in chorioamnionitis and endometritis without increasing operative deliveries in comparison with expectant management.[22]
  - **Antibiotic prophylaxis.** The CDC and American Academy of Pediatrics recommend treating a mother with prophylactic antibiotics if she is GBS-positive within the previous 5 weeks or GBS-unknown and: (a) delivery is likely to occur after 18 hours of ruptured membranes, (b) current gestation is <37 weeks, or (c) there is a fever greater than 38°C. Additional indications for GBS prophylaxis include prior infant with GBS disease and GBS bacteriuria during the current pregnancy.[23]

Counseling

The benefits—a lower risk of maternal and neonatal infection and increased maternal satisfaction—and risks—increased epidural anesthesia and internal monitoring—must be presented to the patient when oxytocin or prostaglandin is offered.[24]

Special Considerations in PPROM

- **Digital examination.** In preterm PROM, digital examination shortened the latent period from 11 to 2 days in one study. This may be avoided by assessing cervical dilatation and effacement by sterile speculum examination, vaginal or transperineal ultrasound.[5]
- **Transport.** In hospitals without neonatal intensive care units, transport of the mother if delivery is not imminent may improve neonatal mortality by 60%.[18]

SHOULDER DYSTOCIA
General Principles
Definition

Shoulder dystocia is defined as an impaction of the fetal shoulder girdle behind the maternal pubis symphysis during vaginal delivery such that additional maneuvers beyond gentle traction are required to enact delivery of the shoulders.[25]

Epidemiology

Shoulder dystocia is reported to occur from 0.2% to 3% of all vaginal deliveries with variability dependent on the subjective assessment of the practitioner.[25] Shoulder dystocia is much more common in larger babies, with a rate of 5% seen in those weighing 4,000 to 4,250 g, 9% with weight 4,250 to 4,500 g, 14% with weight 4,500 to 4,750 g, and 21% in infants weighing greater than 4,500 g.[26] However, more than half the cases of shoulder dystocia occur in infants with weights in the normal range and are unanticipated.[10]

Mechanisms of Injury

- **Maternal**
  - There is an increased rate of trauma to the birth canal, including lacerations and symphysis separation. Transient lateral femoral cutaneous neuropathy can be seen.[27] These are related to the size of the fetus as well as the maneuvers performed to permit delivery.

- **Neonatal**
  - Neonatal brachial plexus injuries are the most common neurologic sequelae of shoulder dystocia, with varying occurrence reported from 4% to 40%.[28] An Erb palsy affects C5 and C6 nerve roots and typically presents as unilateral arm weakness and an asymmetrical Moro response, with impaired active abduction of the ipsilateral arm with preserved hand movements. A Klumpke palsy affects palmar strength resulting from damage to C8 and T1 nerve roots.[18] Clavicular and humeral fractures are also reported, though less common. Death or brain damage may also ensue as a result of hypoxemia from umbilical cord impaction by the fetus.

Diagnosis

Clinical Presentation

A positive "turtle sign," or retraction of the fetal head against the perineum following its delivery, may contribute to diagnosis. No consensus yet exists on objective measures, including time thresholds that accurately define a shoulder dystocia. This subjectivity largely contributes to the variability in incidence reported in the literature.[29]

Monitoring

Umbilical cord pH monitoring in cases of shoulder dystocia has been shown to be unpredictable with statistically significant, yet clinically insignificant, decrease in umbilical pH.[30]

Treatment

Management of shoulder dystocia is facilitated by use of the HELPERR mnemonic.[18] The maneuvers are performed in a rapid sequence, although not necessarily in this order.

- **H.** Call for **H**elp.
- **E. E**pisiotomy may help facilitate the maneuvers, although data have recently put this practice in to question. Several studies have demonstrated an increase in severity (degree), frequency, and length of perineal lacerations without reduction in maternal or fetal morbidity.[31]
- **L.** The McRoberts maneuver consists of actively flexing the maternal **L**egs against her abdomen from the dorsal lithotomy position. Though this position does not increase the pelvic volume, it does straighten the sacrum in line with the lumbar spine and allow the pubic symphysis to move in the cephalic position.[31] Buhimschi et al.[32] additionally showed an increase in maternal expulsion forces in this position.
- **P. P**uprapubic **P**ressure may help disengage the shoulder and is commonly done in junction with McRoberts maneuvering early on in the course. Fundal pressure increases the impaction and must be avoided. Pressure may be applied to the fetal shoulders in a side-to-side, rocking motion (Rubin maneuver I).
- **E. "E**nter" the pelvis for internal maneuvers. Push the fetus's anterior shoulder toward the fetal chest (Rubin maneuver II). Push the posterior shoulder from the pectoral region toward the fetus's back (Wood screw maneuver). The Wood and Rubin II maneuvers push the fetus in the same direction and can be performed simultaneously. The Wood screw can also be performed in reverse if these motions fail.
- **R.** Next try to **R**emove the posterior arm by pushing behind the humerus, sweeping the arm across the chest.
- **R. R**olling the patient onto all fours, the Gaskin maneuver, may disimpact the shoulder by increasing the pelvic width.

Other methods, which are rarely necessary, include deliberate fractures of the fetal clavicle, cephalic replacement (the Zavanelli maneuver), and symphysiotomy.

REFERENCES

1. Navti OB, Konje JC. Bleeding in late pregnancy. In: James D, Steer PJ, Weiner CP, et al. *High risk pregnancy*. 4th ed. St. Louis, MO: Elsevier Saunders; 2011:1037–1051.
2. Rasmussen S, Irgens LM, Bergsjo P, et al. The occurrence of placental abruption in Norway 1967–1991. *Acta Obstet Gynecol Scand* 1996;75(3):222–228.
3. Ananth CV, Oyelese Y, Yeo L, et al. Placental abruption in the United States, 1979 through 2001: temporal trends and potential determinants. *Am J Obstet Gynecol* 2005;192(1):191–198.
4. Oyelese Y, Ananth CV. Placental abruption. *Obstet Gynecol* 2006;108(4):1005–1016.
5. Scott JR, Gibbs RS, Karlan BY, et al., eds. *Danforth's obstetrics and gynecology*. 9th ed. Philadelphia, PA: Lippincott Williams & Wilkins; 2003.

6. Ananth CV, Oyelese Y, Prasad V, et al. Evidence of placental abruption as a chronic process: associations with vaginal bleeding early in pregnancy and placental lesions. *Eur J Obstet Gynecol Reprod Biol* 2006;128(1–2):15–21.

7. Vladutiu CJ, Weiss HB. Motor vehicle safety during pregnancy. *Am J Lifestyle Med* 2012;6(3):241–249.

8. Ananth CV, Berkowitz GS, Savitz DA, et al. Placental abruption and adverse perinatal outcomes. *JAMA* 1999;282(17):1646–1651.

9. Spinillo A, Fazzi E, Stronati M, et al. Severity of abruptio placentae and neurodevelopmental outcome in low birth weight infants. *Early Hum Dev* 1993;35(1):45–54.

10. Gabbe SG, Niebyl JR, Simpson JL, et al., eds. *Obstetrics: normal and problem pregnancies.* 6th ed. New York, NY: Churchill Livingstone; 2012.

11. Dutta DK. *Dutta's obstetrics haemorrhage made easy.* New Delhi, India: Jaypee Brothers Medical; 2007.

12. Vergani P, Ornaghi S, Pozzi I, et al. Placenta previa: distance to internal os and mode of delivery. *Am J Obstet Gynecol* 2009;201(3):266.e1–266.e5.

13. Faiz AS, Ananth CV. Etiology and risk factors for placenta previa: an overview and meta-analysis of observational studies. *J Matern Fetal Neonatal Med* 2003;13(3):175–190.

14. Onwere C, Gurol-Urganci I, Cromwell DA, et al. Maternal morbidity associated with placenta praevia among women who had elective caesarean section. *Eur J Obstet Gynecol Reprod Biol* 2011;159(1):62–66.

15. Mercer B. Antibiotics in the management of PROM and preterm labor. *Obstet Gynecol Clin North Am* 2012;39(1):65–76.

16. Markhus VH, Rasmussen S, Lie SA, et al. Placental abruption and premature rupture of membranes. *Acta Obstet Gynecol Scand* 2011;90(9):1024–1029.

17. American College of Obstetricians and Gynecologists. ACOG Practice Bulletin. Assessment of risk factors for preterm birth. Clinical management guidelines for obstetrician-gynecologists. Number 31, October 2001. (Replaces Technical Bulletin number 206, June 1995; Committee Opinion number 172, May 1996; Committee Opinion number 187, September 1997; Committee Opinion number 198, February 1998; and Committee Opinion number 251, January 2001). *Obstet Gynecol* 2001;98(4):709–716.

18. Atwood L, Deutchman M, Bailey E, et al. *ALSO course syllabus.* 4th ed. Leawood, KS: American Academy of Family Physicians; 2000.

19. Miracle X, Di Renzo GC, Stark A, et al; Coordinators Of World Association of Perinatal Medicine Prematurity Working Group. Guideline for the use of antenatal corticosteroids for fetal maturation. *J Perinat Med* 2008;36(3):191–196.

20. Kenyon S, Boulvain M, Neilson JP. Antibiotics for preterm rupture of membranes. *Cochrane Database Syst Rev* 2013;12:CD000246.

21. Cunningham FG, Leveno KJ, Bloom SL, et al., eds. *Williams' obstetrics.* 22nd ed. Norwalk, CT: Appleton & Lange; 2005.

22. Dare MR, Middleton P, Crowther CA, et al. Planned early birth versus expectant management (waiting) for prelabour rupture of membranes at term (37 weeks or more) [Review]. *Cochrane Database Syst Rev* 2006;(1):CD005302 doi: 10.1002/14651858.

23. Committee on Infectious Diseases; Committee on Fetus and Newborn, Baker CJ, Byington CL, Polin RA. Policy statement—recommendations for the prevention of perinatal group B streptococcal (GBS) disease. *Pediatrics* 2011;128(3):611–616.

24. MORE[OB] Risk management comprehensive programs such as ALSO[4] and MORE[OB] are available to professionals. Ottawa, Canada: Society of Obstetricians and Gynaecologists of Canada. www.moreob.com version 2.9.3. Accessed August 1, 2006.

25. American College of Obstetrician and Gynecologists. Shoulder dystocia. ACOG practice bulletin no. 40. *Obstet Gynecol* 2002;100:1045–1050.

26. Nesbitt TS, Gilbert WM, Herrchen B. Shoulder dystocia and associated risk factors with macrosomic infants born in California. *Am J Obstet Gynecol* 1998;179(2):476–480.

27. Heath T, Gherman RB. Symphyseal separation, sacroiliac joint dislocation and transient lateral femoral cutaneous neuropathy associated with McRoberts' maneuver. A case report. *J Reprod Med* 1999;44(10):902–904.

28. Doumouchtsis SK, Arulkumaran S. Are all brachial plexus injuries caused by shoulder dystocia? *Obstet Gynecol Surv* 2009;64(9):615–623.

29. Grobman W. Shoulder dystocia [Review]. *Obstet Gynecol Clin North Am* 2013;40(1):59–67.

30. Stallings SP, Edwards RK, Johnson JW. Correlation of head-to-body delivery intervals in shoulder dystocia and umbilical artery acidosis. *Am J Obstet Gynecol* 2001;185(2):268–274.

31. Gottlieb AG, Galan HL. Shoulder dystocia: an update [Review]. *Obstet Gynecol Clin North Am* 2007;34(3):501–531, xii.

32. Buhimschi CS, Buhimschi IA, Malinow A, et al. Use of McRoberts' position during delivery and increase in pushing efficiency. *Lancet* 2001;358(9280):470–471.

Postpartum Care
Katrina N. Wherry

EARLY POSTPARTUM PROBLEMS (0 TO 2 WEEKS)
Pain

General Principles
Classification. Commonly women can experience breast pain, pelvic or perineal pain, headaches, backaches, or surgical site pain.

Diagnosis
Evaluation. Observe for mastitis, wound dehiscence, or evidence of wound infection.

Treatment
- **Medications for mild to moderate pain**
  - Ibuprofen 600 mg PO q6h
  - Acetaminophen 500 to 1000 mg PO q6h
  - Acetaminophen with codeine 30 mg (Tylenol No. 3) PO q4–6h (caution in breastfeeding patients)[1]
- **Medications for severe pain**
  - Morphine and hydromorphone are unlikely to reach the infant in clinically significant levels, so they can be safely used in the breastfeeding patient.[2]

Special Therapy
- **Perineal pain:** Use local cooling agents.[3]
- **Breast engorgement:** On demand nurse with at least eight episodes in 24 hours in the first 1 to 2 weeks after delivery.

Primary Postpartum Hemorrhage

General Principles
Classification. Postpartum hemorrhage is defined as blood loss of more than 500 mL after delivery. Causes of postpartum hemorrhage include uterine atony most commonly, retained placenta, genital tract lacerations, uterine rupture, and coagulation disorders.[4]

Diagnosis
Evaluation. Look for signs of shock; examine uterus for tone; and examine cervix, vagina, and labia for lacerations. Obtain complete blood count, type and cross, and coagulation studies.

Treatment
Volume replacement with IV fluids or blood products as needed. Perform uterine massage with removal of blood clots, retained placenta, or correction of inversion. Repair lacerations and use uterine tamponade if indicated.

Medications
- Oxytocin 10 to 40 units in 1,000 cc IV fluids, titrate rate
- Methylergonovine maleate (Methergine) 0.2 mg IM q2–4h (use cautiously if hypertensive)
- Carboprost tromethamine (Hemabate) 250 μg IM q 90 to 120 minutes
- Misoprostol 200 μg PO plus 400 μg SL, or 800 μg per rectum

Surgery
Perform hypogastric or uterine artery ligation, uterine compression sutures, or hysterectomy.

Anemia

General Principles
Classification. Anemia is seen in a majority of women in the early postpartum period, and is usually secondary to blood loss from delivery. Most women with mild anemia are asymptomatic.

Diagnosis
Evaluation. Look for skin pallor, postural hypotension, tachycardia, fatigue, and weakness. Check hemoglobin 24 hours after delivery, or sooner if indicated.

Treatment
For severe or symptomatic anemia, transfuse with packed red blood cells.
Medications. For mild to moderate anemia, give ferrous sulfate 325 mg daily-bid, until hemoglobin normalizes.

Endometritis
General Principles
Classification. Postpartum endometritis is defined as an infection of the endometrial lining, the myometrium, and the parametrium. Endometritis develops in approximately 10% of women who have delivered by cesarean section, and 5% who have delivered vaginally. Causal organisms include Group B *Streptococcus, Enterococcus faecalis, Staphylococcus epidermidis, Staphylococcus aureus, Prevotella bivia, Peptostreptococci* spp., *Clostridium* spp., *Gardnerella vaginalis, Escherichia coli*, and *Bacteroides* spp.[5]

Diagnosis
Evaluation. Physical findings include elevated temperature, tachycardia, uterine tenderness, and purulent vaginal discharge. Obtain white blood cell count with differential, urinalysis, electrolytes, and creatinine (also, if indicated, endometrial/vaginal cultures, blood cultures, and pelvic imaging).

Treatment
Medications. Give intravenous antibiotics until patient is afebrile for 24 to 48 hours. If symptoms have completely resolved, the patient can be discharged without oral antibiotics. Antibiotics choices include:

- Piperacillin/tazobactam 3.375 g IV q6h
- Ampicillin/sulbactam 1.5 to 3 g IV q6h plus gentamicin 5 mg per kg IV q24h
- Clindamycin 900 mg IV q8h plus gentamicin 5 mg per kg IV q24h
- Metronidazole 500 mg IV q8h plus gentamicin 5 mg per kg IV q24h
- If initial antibiotics fail, evaluate for resistant bacteria, pelvic abscess, or septic pelvic thrombosis.[5]

Risk management. Preventive strategies include limiting the number of intrapartum vaginal examinations, limiting duration of labor and ruptured membranes, and using prophylactic antibiotics at the time of cesarean section.
Complications. Complications include peritonitis, pelvic abscess, dynamic ileus, bowel obstruction, and necrosis of the lower uterine segment.[5]

The "Blues"
General Principles
Classification. The postpartum "blues" is defined as a transient, self-limited mood disturbance occurring within the first 2 weeks after delivery. These episodes affect a majority of mothers, and last hours to days.

Diagnosis
Evaluation. Interview and examination are based on the clinical presentation. Symptoms can include sadness, mood lability, crying, anxiety, insomnia, poor appetite, and irritability.

Treatment
Behavioral
Treatment consists of support and reassurance.

DELAYED POSTPARTUM PROBLEMS (>2 WEEKS)
Fatigue
General Principles
Classification. Fatigue is seen in a majority of women after childbirth, and may last for weeks to months. Causes include the physical sequelae of childbirth (general recovery, anemia, infections), parenting demands, postpartum hypothyroidism, or postpartum depression.

Diagnosis

Evaluation. Physical examination should include a depression screening questionnaire and a search for evidence of anemia or hypothyroid disease. Laboratory analysis can include complete blood count and thyroid-stimulating hormone level.

Treatment

Behavioral. Treat the cause, encourage use of social supports, and curtail work and other obligations, if possible.

Medications. Use iron replacement for anemia or treat hypothyroid disease if appropriate.

Postpartum Thyroiditis

General Principles

Classification. Postpartum thyroiditis is an autoimmune disorder that classically consists of a hyperthyroid phase at 2 to 6 months postpartum, followed by a hypothyroid phase at 3 to 12 months postpartum. Usually, women return to a euthyroid state by 12 months postpartum, but a minority will continue to be hypothyroid indefinitely. Prevalence ranges from 1.1% to 16.7%, with a mean prevalence of 7.5%.[6]

Diagnosis

Evaluation. A thorough history should be obtained. Symptoms of hyperthyroidism can include fatigue, palpitations, heat intolerance, and nervousness. Symptoms of hypothyroidism can include fatigue, dry hair and skin, impaired concentration, and depression. A focused thyroid examination should be performed to assess for palpable thyroid nodules. Laboratory studies should include thyroid-stimulating hormone, which will be low in the hyperthyroid phase, and elevated in the hypothyroid phase. Thyroid imaging is usually unnecessary. Thyroid ultrasound should be included if a nodule or nodules are palpated.

Treatment

Medications. If symptomatic in hyperthyroid phase, give propranolol 10 to 20 mg PO qid. If symptomatic in hypothyroid phase, give levothyroxine, and continue treatment either until 1 year postpartum or until mother has finished childbearing.[6]

Mastitis, Breast Abscess

General Principles

Classification. Approximately 1% to 5% of nursing mothers experience mastitis and/or breast abscesses. Causal organisms include *Staphylococcus aureus* (most common), *E. coli*, *Klebsiella pneumoniae*, and *Streptococcus* species. Predisposing factors include a decrease in nursing frequency or irregular nursing, inadequate drainage, cracked nipples, and fatigue.[7]

Diagnosis

Evaluation. The patient can present with several clinical manifestations to include fever, chills, body aches, malaise, and an inflamed breast. A careful breast examination should be performed to assess for localized edema or fluctuance that could be consistent with an abscess. Laboratory analysis should include white blood cell count and differential. If abscess is present, obtain cultures and sensitivities on aspirate. An ultrasound should be performed if an abscess is suspected.[8]

Treatment

Behavioral

Frequent nursing is recommended as part of the treatment of mastitis. If an abscess is present, nursing with the opposite breast is recommended. Warm and cold compresses can provide relief, as well as gentle massage to the affected area. The patient should be advised to drink sufficient fluids.

Medications

- **Antibiotics:** Choices include cephalexin 500 mg PO qid or cefazolin 0.5 to 1.5 g IV q6–8h; or amoxicillin–clavulanate 500/125 mg PO tid.[8]
- **Analgesics:** Acetaminophen 1 g PO q6h or ibuprofen 600 mg PO q6h.

Surgery. If abscess is present, incise and drain. Alternatively, use ultrasound guidance to aspirate small abscesses (<3 cm) or to place a drainage catheter for larger abscesses (3 cm or greater).[8]

Risk management. To prevent mastitis, the nursing patient should be advised to nurse frequently and to take measures to avoid fatigue.

Marital/Partner and Sexual Changes

General Principles
Classification. Most couples do not resume intercourse until about 2 months or longer after delivery. Thereafter, sexual interest and activity may be reduced for several months, and sexual problems occur fairly often. In addition, marital/partner satisfaction tends to decline after the birth of a first child, and this decline may persist until children reach school age. The declination in marital/partner satisfaction may be related to changing roles, increased work responsibilities, and fatigue. Factors associated with postpartum sexual dysfunction include assisted vaginal delivery, vaginal or perineal lacerations, mediolateral episiotomy, depression, and vaginal atrophy secondary to estrogen withdrawal, which may be exacerbated by breastfeeding.[9]

Diagnosis
Evaluation. A thorough interview should include inquiry about partner relationship and sexual concerns at mother's postpartum visit. A vaginal/perineal examination should be conducted if any sexual complaints are related to physiologic changes.

Treatment
Behavioral. Inform partners of anticipated postpartum sexual changes, reassure them that problems often resolve, and encourage partners to continue to affirm and support one another.
Medications. For dyspareunia due to vaginal atrophy and dryness, consider vaginal lubricants or short-term use of estrogen cream.
Risk management. To reduce the risk of perineal trauma, limit episiotomies.[9]

Postpartum Depression

General Principles
Classification. The incidence of postpartum depression is 5% to 7% in the first 3 months of postpartum, which is similar to the rates of major depression in the general population. A risk factor of previous history of postpartum depression strongly increases the patient's risk of depression with subsequent deliveries. Some studies suggest that up to 50% of women with a history of postpartum depression will experience it again. Other risk factors include depressive symptoms during pregnancy, history of major depressive disorder, poor social support, major life events during pregnancy, family history of postpartum depression, gestational diabetes, and delivery of multiples.[10]

Diagnosis
Evaluation. The presence of at least five of the following symptoms (two of them must be the first two listed) over a 2-week period (and is impairing normal functioning) is necessary for the diagnosis of postpartum depression: depressed mood, anhedonia, decreased energy, changes in sleep pattern, weight change, decreased concentrating ability, guilt, psychomotor retardation, and suicidal ideation. Screening should take place during the postpartum visit (or the infant's pediatric exams) using a validated tool such as the Edinburgh Postnatal Depression Scale (EPDS). Thyroid-stimulating hormone should be measured to rule out a hypothyroid state that can contribute to the patient's depressive symptoms.[10]

Treatment
Nonpharmacologic. Individual or group psychotherapy has been demonstrated to be an effective treatment for postpartum depression. Interpersonal therapy and cognitive behavioral therapy are the most commonly used types of therapies.[10]
Medications. Selective serotonin reuptake inhibitors (SSRIs) are the first-line medication therapy of choice for postpartum depression given their effectiveness and favorable adverse effects profile. There is no evidence to support that one SSRI is more effective in treating postpartum depression in women who are not nursing. An approach to initiating therapy can include beginning with a starting dose for 4 days and then increasing to the lowest usual effective treatment dose with follow-up planned at 2 weeks. If the EPDS score does not improve by four points at the time of reassessment and the patient is not experiencing adverse effects, then the dose should be increased to the next effective treatment dose and follow-up should be arranged in another 2 weeks. If the patient continues not to respond despite appropriate treatment doses, psychotherapy, and adequate follow-up (usually every 2 to 4 weeks), then the patient should be referred for psychiatric evaluation. Nursing mothers may be hesitant to begin treatment. A thorough discussion about the risks and benefits of treatment should be held. Risks of persistent depressive symptoms can include infant sleep problems, poor mother–infant bonding, delays in infant growth and development, and increased risk of anxiety or depression for the infant later on.[10]

REFERENCES

1. Chou D, Abalos E, Gyte GM, et al. Paracetamol/acetaminophen (single administration) for perineal pain in the early postpartum period. *Cochrane Database Syst Rev* 2013;1:CD008407.
2. Deussen AR, Ashwood P, Martis R. Analgesia for relief of pain due to uterine cramping/involution after birth. *Cochrane Database Syst Rev* 2011;(5):CD004908 doi: 10.1002/14651858.CD004908.pub2.
3. East CE, Begg L, Henshall NE, et al. Local cooling for relieving pain from perineal trauma sustained during childbirth. *Cochrane Database Syst Rev* 2012;5:CD006304.
4. Anderson J, Etches D. Prevention and management of postpartum hemorrhage. *Am Fam Physician* 2007;75(6):875–882.
5. Faro S. Postpartum endometritis. *Clin Perinatol* 2005;32:803–814.
6. Stagnaro-Green A. Postpartum thyroiditis. *Best Pract Res Clin Endocrinol Metab* 2004;18(2):303–316.
7. Leung AKC, Sauve RS. Breast is best for babies. *J Natl Med Assoc* 2005;97(7):1010–1019.
8. Ulitzsch D, Nyman MKG, Carlson RA. Breast abscess in lactating women: US-guided treatment. *Radiology* 2004;232:904–909.
9. Flynn P, Franiek J, Janssen P, et al. How can second-stage management prevent perineal trauma? *Can Fam Physician* 1997;43:73–84.
10. Hirst K, Moutier C. Postpartum major depression. *Am Fam Physician* 2010;82(8):926–933.

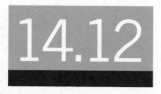

14.12 Diagnostic Ultrasound in Obstetrics

Zackary J. Kent

GENERAL PRINCIPLES

Once a rudimentary imaging procedure is used to assess basic features, diagnostic ultrasound in obstetrics now involves a vast array of capabilities, including high-frequency transvaginal probes, three- and four-dimensional imaging, and sophisticated digital workstations (to name a few). Although this technology has increased the clinician's ability to gather data about a pregnancy, its method, utility, and application continue to be debated. The focus in this chapter will be limited to three types of ultrasound examinations, as defined by the American Institute of Ultrasound in Medicine (AIUM): first trimester ultrasound examination, the standard second- or third-trimester ultrasound examination, and a limited ultrasound examination.

SAFETY

The primary concerns regarding negative bioeffects of ultrasonography in pregnancy have been involved the potential for thermal injury and microbubble formation, which has been demonstrated in animal studies under conditions that are not typical of routine obstetrical ultrasound. Pulsed doppler (spectral, power, and color flow) should not be used in the first trimester.[1] The AIUM advocates prudent use of the procedure and adherence to the "As Low As Reasonably Achievable" principle, namely ultrasound should be considered only when it is indicated, minimizing exposure time and exposure intensity.[2] According to the available evidence, exposure to diagnostic ultrasonography during pregnancy appears to be safe.[3]

FIRST TRIMESTER ULTRASOUND EXAMINATION (1 WEEK TO 13 WEEKS + 6 DAYS)

- **Typical indications (not all inclusive)** include confirmation of the presence of intrauterine pregnancy, evaluation of suspected ectopic pregnancy, evaluating the cause of vaginal bleeding, estimating gestational age, diagnosis or evaluation of multiple gestations, confirmation of cardiac activity, and aneuploidy screening or assessment for fetal anomaly.
- **Study parameters:** A standard first trimester ultrasound should confirm the presence (or absence) of an intrauterine pregnancy, assess the number of gestations, estimate the gestational age of the pregnancy, evaluate fetal cardiac activity, and evaluate adnexal structures when possible.

- **Intrauterine pregnancy:** When the maternal serum β-human chorionic gonadotropin (β-hCG) level is between 1,000 and 2,000 mIU per mL (by first international reference preparation), a gestational sac is normally visible by transvaginal ultrasound. This range is also referred to as the discriminatory zone. If the gestational sac is not seen by 2,000 mIU per mL, an ectopic pregnancy must be excluded.[4]
- **Number of gestations:** The uterus should be scanned in both horizontal and vertical planes to assess the number of gestations. Decreased perinatal mortality has been demonstrated when twins were identified before 20 weeks gestation.[5]
- **Estimation of gestational age:** The mean gestational sac diameter (MSD) and crown–rump length (CRL) are used to estimate the gestational age of the pregnancy, with the CRL providing greater accuracy over the MSD and is preferred when a fetal pole is present. The MSD is evaluated by measuring the gestational sac at its greatest dimension in three orthogonal planes (height, width, and depth). The CRL is the maximum visible length of the embryo. Care must be taken not to include the umbilical cord or yolk sac in the crown–rump measurement. The 95% confidence interval (by Hadlock) is ±8% of the predicted gestational age; therefore, earlier ultrasound measurements will have a smaller margin of error for dating purposes. For example, a fetus measuring 7 weeks will be ±4 days, where a fetus measuring 13 weeks will be ±7 days.
- **Evaluation of fetal cardiac activity:** The presence of cardiac activity should be documented by M-mode or through two-dimensional video capture. Normal fetal heart rates (FHRs) vary by gestational age. At 6 weeks, normal FHR is 95 to 127 BPM, at 7 weeks normal FHR is 117 to 153, at 8 weeks normal FHR is 140 to 179 BPM, at 9 weeks normal FHR is 154 to 194 BPM, and at 10 weeks normal FHR is 147 to 187 BPM.[6] Thereafter, a normal FHR will progress to 120 to 160 BPM.
- **Evaluation of adnexal structures:** When possible, the cervix, uterus, ovaries, and cul-de-sac should be evaluated.

SECOND- AND THIRD-TRIMESTER ULTRASOUND EXAMINATION

- **Typical indications (list not all inclusive)** include screening for fetal anomalies, evaluation of fetal anatomy, estimation of gestational age, evaluation of fetal growth, evaluation of vaginal bleeding, evaluation of cervical insufficiency, determination of fetal position, evaluation of fetal well-being, and suspected amniotic fluid abnormalities.
- **Study parameters:** A standard second- or third-trimester ultrasound should evaluate fetal cardiac activity, fetal number, fetal presentation, a qualitative or semiquantitative estimate of amniotic fluid volume, placental location and relationship to the internal os, the number of umbilical cord vessels, placental cord insertion site, a gestational age estimate through fetal biometry, a fetal weight estimation, maternal anatomy, and fetal anatomic survey.
- **Fetal anatomy**
  - Second trimester screening anatomy examinations are typically done between 18 and 22 weeks gestation. The ability of routine ultrasound to detect fetal anomalies in an otherwise low-risk unselected population remains highly controversial, as there is conflicting evidence regarding the benefit routine ultrasound screening for fetal anomalies.[5]
  - The experience of the sonographic examiner, the specific defect, the gestational age, and overall population risk are cornerstones to detection. Baseline detection rate of any type of anomaly is about 50% with central nervous system, and urinary tract anomalies detection rates are higher (~80%) than that of cardiac and musculoskeletal anomalies (~30% to 40%).[7]
- **Placental location, fetal presentation, and amniotic fluid index**
  - The placenta typically adheres to the anterior or posterior wall of the uterus. Placenta location is of concern when it approaches or covers the internal os. This is called placenta previa and it occurs in about 5% of pregnancies. Abnormal placentation in the form of placenta accreta, percreta, and increta can, at times, be diagnosed by ultrasound. Sonographically, they appear as multiple placental lakes and give a "Swiss cheese" appearance. These abnormal attachments of the placenta to the uterine myometrium are a significant source of maternal hemorrhage and rarely death. Even more rarely, a vasa previa can be detected if the ultrasound protocol includes examination of the cord insertion.[8]
  - The amniotic fluid index (AFI) is a quantitative assessment of the amount of amniotic fluid surrounding the fetus. Various techniques including a four-quadrant approach and single deepest vertical pocket approach have been described. Normal amount is typically 8 to 18 cm. A normal AFI infers a level of reassurance of fetal well-being secondary to an adequate urine output and thus renal perfusion. Although definitions vary, oligohydramnios is typically identified with an

AFI <5 cm or maximal vertical pocket <2 cm, and polyhydramnios is typically identified with an AFI >25 cm.[9]
- **Fetal biometry for assessment of gestational age and growth and weight**
  - During the second and third trimesters, fetal biometry is used for gestational age assessment and growth evaluation. Measurements of the fetal biparietal diameter, abdominal circumference, and femoral diaphysis length are combined and compared to published nomograms to predict growth percentile. The variability of gestational age estimations, however, increases with advancing pregnancy.
  - **Intrauterine growth restriction (IUGR)** can be diagnosed if interval growth is abnormal or if the ratio of abdominal circumference to other parameters is abnormal. Definitions vary regarding what constitutes IUGR, with some authors citing <10 percentile, whereas others use <3 percentile. When IUGR is identified, umbilical artery doppler velocimetry (systolic and diastolic flow) is helpful in assessing the nature and prognosis of the fetal growth restriction, and has been shown to reduce morbidity and mortality.
- **Assessment of fetal well-being**
  - In the latter half of pregnancy, it often becomes necessary to assess fetal well-being. This can be due to acute issues like decreased fetal movement and vaginal bleeding. The most severe causes of vaginal bleeding in the third trimester include placental abruption, placenta previa, uterine rupture, vasa previa, and the previously described placental attachment abnormalities (placenta accreta, increta, percreta). Ultrasound is of significant use in diagnosing these conditions, with the exception of placental abruption where less than a quarter of cases are identified sonographically.[10]
  - Complications of pregnancy such as gestational diabetes, chronic or gestational hypertension, or pre-eclampsia may infer a greater risk to the fetus. The basic evaluation, a modified biophysical profile, includes the AFI (described above) and the nonstress test. The role of ultrasound is in the more in-depth biophysical profile that sonographically looks at four fetal parameters: fetal breathing motion, fetal activity, fetal muscular tone, and AFI. A score of either 0 or 2 points is given to each category. A score of 8 of 8 is considered reassuring.

Limited Ultrasound Examination

A limited ultrasound examination is performed when a specific question requires investigation. This examination does not replace a standard (or complete) ultrasound evaluation, and is most commonly performed when a standard evaluation has been previously performed, or when a standard evaluation will be performed later. For example, determination of the fetal presentation prior to vaginal delivery is performed by Leopold maneuvers and cervical examination. If the presenting part is uncertain, a limited ultrasound is performed to make the determination.

SPECIAL CONSIDERATIONS
- **Assessment of fetal viability in the first trimester**
  - A pregnancy is considered viable if it can potentially result in a liveborn baby, while ectopic pregnancies and failed intrauterine pregnancies are considered nonviable.[11] The embryo is the second structure to appear in the gestational sac after the yolk sac. Fetal cardiac activity can generally be detected by transvaginal ultrasound during week 6 or when the embryo is 5 mm in length. From a practical management standpoint, it is most helpful to identify nonviable pregnancies and pregnancy failures, while pregnancies of uncertain viability are typically followed with subsequent ultrasound evaluations at an appropriate interval. Findings diagnostic of pregnancy failure include a CRL ≥7 mm an no heartbeat, a mean sac diameter ≥25 mm and no embryo (a blighted ovum or anembryonic gestation), the absence of an embryo with a heartbeat ≥2 weeks after an ultrasound showing a gestational sac without a yolk sac, and the absence of an embryo with a heartbeat ≥11 days after an ultrasound showing a gestational sac with a yolk sac.[12]
- **Cervical length measurements**
  - The value of routine cervical length measurement in otherwise low-risk pregnancies has not been established in population-based studies, though studies have found that a cervical length <25 mm before 24 weeks gestation is associated with an increased risk for preterm delivery. Women identified with a cervix <15 mm prior to 24 weeks should be treated with vaginal progesterone.[13] Women with a history of preterm birth <34 weeks and a cervical length <25 mm prior to 24 weeks gestation should be offered a cervical cerclage.[14] Transvaginal cervical length is a useful

screening tool for women with preterm contractions, as a cervical length >25 mm prior to 34 weeks has a negative predictive value of 99% for delivery within 7 days, and 94% for delivery prior to 35 weeks.[15] Finally, there is little correlation between transabdominal cervical length and transvaginal cervical length; therefore, a transvaginal evaluation should be obtained if there is an indication for an ultrasound measurement of cervical length.[15] Numerous studies have looked at the role of cervical length as a predictor for preterm delivery. Mixed results were found on the basis of study designs and populations studied. The cervix is described as "funneled" or "funneling" when the internal os is opened and forms a funnel or beak-shaped appearance on ultrasound. Funneling is most concerning when it is persistent and occurs before 32 weeks. The appearance of funneling combined with an overall cervical length of 3 cm or less are features consistently associated with preterm delivery. Who should be scanned? High-risk women with previous preterm birth and symptomatic women with preterm contractions seemed to benefit from cervical length monitoring. The predictive value of scanning a woman with no risk factors is very low. Studies showed that most low-risk women with a shortened cervix (less than 2.5 cm) went on to deliver after 35 weeks. American College of Obstetricians and Gynecologists recommends against routine ultrasound screening of the cervix in low-risk women but states that offering screening after 16 to 18 weeks in high-risk women is reasonable.[10]

ACKNOWLEDGMENT

The author acknowledges Stephanie L. Werner for her authorship of a previous version of this chapter.

REFERENCES

1. AIUM Statement on the Safe Use of Doppler Ultrasound During 11–14 week scans (or earlier in pregnancy). Approved April 18, 2011. http://www.aium.org/officialStatements/42
2. Kremkau FW. *Diagnostic ultrasound, principles and instruments.* 7th ed. Philadelphia, PA: WB Saunders; 2006.
3. Torloni MR, Vedmedovska N, Merialdi M, et al; ISUOG-WHO Fetal Growth Study Group. Safety of ultrasonography in pregnancy: WHO systematic review of the literature and meta-analysis. *Ultrasound Obstet Gynecol* 2009;33(5):599–608.
4. Sohaey R. First trimester ultrasounds. http://medlib.med.utah.edu/kw/human_reprod/lectures/clin_radiology/. Accessed July 28, 2014.
5. Ewigman BG, Crane JP, Frigoletto FD, et al. Effect of prenatal ultrasound screening on perinatal outcome. RADIUS Study Group. *N Engl J Med* 1993;329:821.
6. Papiaoannou G. Normal ranges of embryonic length, embryonic heart rate, gestational sac diameter and yolk sac diameter at 6–10 weeks. *Fetal Diagn Ther* 2010;28:207–219.
7. Levi S. Ultrasound in prenatal diagnosis: polemics around routine ultrasound screening for second trimester fetal malformations. *Prenat Diagn* 2002;22:285.
8. Munim S, Nadeem S, Khuwaja NA. The accuracy of ultrasound in the diagnosis of congenital abnormalities. *J Pak Med Assoc* 2006;56(1):16–18.
9. Lazebnik N, Lazebnick R. The role of ultrasound in pregnancy-related emergencies. *Radiol Clin North Am* 2004;42:315–327.
10. American College of Obstetricians and Gynecologists. ACOG practice bulletin no. 101: ultrasonography in pregnancy. *Obstet Gynecol* 2009;113:451–461.
11. Doubilet PM, Benson CB, Bourne T, et al; Society of Radiologists in Ultrasound Multispecialty Panel on Early First Trimester Diagnosis of Miscarriage and Exclusion of a Viable Intrauterine Pregnancy. Diagnostic criteria for nonviable pregnancy early in the first trimester. *N Engl J Med* 2013;369:1443–1451.
12. Fonseca E. Progesterone and the risk of preterm birth among women with a short cervix. *N Engl J Med* 2007;357:462–469.
13. American College of Obstetricians and Gynecologists. ACOG practice bulletin no. 142: cerclage for the management of cervical insufficiency. *Obstet Gynecol* 2014;123:372–379.
14. Schmitz T. Selective use of fetal fibronectin detection after cervical length measurement to predict spontaneous preterm delivery in women with preterm labor. *Am J Obstet Gynecol* 2006;194:138–143.
15. Friedman AM, Srinivas SK, Parry S, et al. Can transabdominal ultrasound be used as a screening test for short cervical length? *Am J Obstet Gynecol* 2013;208:190.e1–190.e7.

Pregnancy Loss and Stillbirth

Ryan Frank

GENERAL PRINCIPLES

Couples with pregnancy loss require empathy and understanding as pregnancy loss is an emotionally traumatic experience. In addition, if pregnancy loss is recurrent, evaluation can be frustrating and difficult because the etiology of their recurrent pregnancy loss may not be determined and there are few evidence-based diagnostic and treatment strategies. Observational studies describe psychological sequelae, such as depression, post-traumatic stress disorder, and anxiety, as well as deleterious effects on maternal–child attachment, in pregnancies subsequent to a stillbirth (even if expected). As a result, it is important for all care providers to be knowledgeable about these issues when they approach parents facing a pregnancy loss and stillbirth.

Definition

- **Spontaneous abortion:** Spontaneous abortion, or miscarriage, is defined as a clinically recognized pregnancy loss before the 20 week of gestation.
- **Stillbirth:** Stillbirth is defined as pregnancy loss after 20 weeks gestation. If the gestational age is not known, fetal weight may be used to distinguish a stillbirth from a miscarriage. Early stillbirths are typically defined as 20 to 27 weeks of gestation, whereas late stillbirths occur at or after 28 weeks of gestation.

Epidemiology

Spontaneous abortion is most commonly caused by chromosomal abnormalities in the embryo or exposure to teratogens. Chromosomal abnormalities account for approximately 50% of all miscarriages. Most such abnormalities are aneuploidies; structural abnormalities and mosaicism are responsible for a small proportion. Congenital anomalies may be caused by chromosomal or other genetic abnormalities, by extrinsic factors (e.g., amniotic bands), or by exposure to teratogens. Trauma and invasive intrauterine procedures such as chorionic villus sampling and amniocentesis increase the risk of abortion.

The etiology of stillbirths includes obstetric complications (abruption, multiple gestation, preterm birth), placental disease, fetal genetic/structural abnormalities, maternal or fetal infection, umbilical cord abnormalities, hypertensive disorders, and other maternal medical conditions.[1]

Obstetrical History and Risk Factors

- **Maternal age at the time of conception.** There is an increased incidence of pregnancy loss with increasing maternal age, which is due to an increased incidence of aneuploidy, resulting in a decreased implantation rate. Data show a pregnancy loss incidence of 9% to 17% among patients under the age of 30, which increases to 40% in patients over age 40[2] (Figure 14.13-1).
- **Previous spontaneous abortion.** There is an approximately 20% risk of abortion after a previous spontaneous abortion (up from 11% to 13%). This risk increases to 28% and 33% after two and three cases of spontaneous abortion, respectively.[3] There are many other risk factors for spontaneous abortion and recurrent spontaneous abortion (SAB) (see Table 14.13-1).

Classification

- Threatened abortion presents as vaginal bleeding in the presence of a viable pregnancy with a closed cervix.
- Inevitable abortion occurs when the cervix has dilated and the membranes have ruptured, but the products of conception remain in utero.
- Missed abortion is characterized by intrauterine fetal death and retention of the products of conception.
- Complete abortion refers to the spontaneous passage of all the products of conception and does not require medical treatment.
- Recurrent abortion refers to a history of three or more spontaneous abortions.
- Empty sac (blighted ovum) is characterized by the nondevelopment of gestational sac associated with mild symptoms.

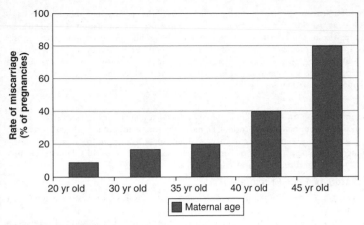

Figure 14.13-1. Maternal age effect on rate of miscarriage.

TABLE 14.13-1	Other Risks for Spontaneous Abortion[1,3]
Hypothyroidism	**Maternal infections**
Diabetes mellitus	Bacterial vaginosis
Polycystic ovary syndrome	*Listeria monocytogenes*
Thrombophilia	Measles
Antiphospholipid antibodies	Mumps
Systemic lupus erythematosus	Coxsackie virus
Intrauterine causes	Toxoplasmosis
Asherman syndrome	*Ureaplasma* and *Mycoplasma*
Fibroids	**Diet and lifestyle**
Uterine malformations	Coffee consumption
Substance abuse	Obesity
CNS stimulants	Smoking
Cocaine	

- Incomplete abortion refers to incomplete passage of products of conception often with persistence of symptoms.
- Septic abortion is spontaneous abortion accompanied by intrauterine infection.

DIAGNOSIS
History
- **Clinical signs and symptoms** that may be associated with fetal death include cessation of previously perceived fetal movements, a decrease in pregnancy-related symptoms (e.g., nausea, breast tenderness), and uterine bleeding/passage of fetal contents or contractions.
- The gestational age should be calculated on the basis of menstrual history or ultrasound assessment. Obstetrical and previous pregnancy history is important to obtain, especially in the case of possible recurrent pregnancy loss. The history should focus on the presence and characteristics of any vaginal bleeding and pelvic pain, and on the passage of fetal tissue.

Physical Examination
- **Hand-held Doppler device.** A hand-held Doppler ultrasound can be used to detect fetal heart rate in the late first trimester. Loss of a previously detected fetal cardiac activity raises suspicion for a missed abortion. However, further evaluation with ultrasonography is required.
- **Pelvic examination.** A complete pelvic examination should be performed to evaluate site of bleeding and whether the cervix is dilated and whether products of conception are visible at the cervix

or in the vagina. These features are used to classify the status of the spontaneous abortion (see Classification section), which impacts management. A bimanual pelvic examination is performed to determine uterine size; an abdominal examination may also be useful when gestational age is greater than 12 weeks. In normal pregnancy, the size of the uterus should be consistent with gestational age. A small for gestational age uterus raises suspicion of a spontaneous abortion. A purulent cervical discharge or uterine tenderness suggests a possible septic abortion, which should also be suspected in women who appear ill or are febrile.

Imaging

- **Pelvic ultrasound.** Pelvic ultrasonography is the most useful test in the diagnostic evaluation of women with suspected spontaneous abortion. The most important finding is fetal cardiac activity, but fetal size, gestational sac, and presence of yoke sac should all be evaluated. In general, these early pregnancy sonograms are performed transvaginally, as the gestational sac and its contents are best evaluated in early gestation through a transvaginal approach.

Potential Predictors of Failed Pregnancy

- **Gestational sac.** A gestational sac ≥25 mm with the absence of a yolk sac or embryo suggested an abnormal pregnancy.
- **Fetal cardiac activity.** Fetal cardiac activity confirms a live pregnancy. The absence of cardiac activity in an embryo of any crown–rump length (CRL) raises suspicion of an abnormal pregnancy. However, the finding of fetal cardiac activity does not exclude the possibility of a subsequent miscarriage.
- **Abnormal gestational sac.** A gestational sac that is abnormally small or large in relation to the embryo within is associated with an increased risk of spontaneous abortion. Other findings suggesting a poor pregnancy outcome include a gestational sac with an irregular contour, a decidual reaction <2 mm in thickness, absence of the double decidual sac sign, decreased echodensity of the choriodecidual reaction, and low sac position in the uterus.
- **Subchorionic hematoma.** A subchorionic hemorrhage or hematoma is a risk factor for spontaneous abortion, particularly when it amounts to 25% or more of the volume of the gestational sac. Pregnancy outcome associated with subchorionic hematoma also relates to location, with worse outcomes observed for retroplacental hematomas, compared with marginal hematomas. The only management option for subchorionic hematoma is expectant.
- **Abnormal yolk sac.** An abnormal yolk sac may be large for gestational age, irregular, free floating in the gestational sac rather than at the periphery, or calcified.
- **Slow fetal heart rate.** Embryonic heart rate below 100 beats per minute (BPM) at 6 to 7 weeks raises suspicion of an abnormal pregnancy.

Laboratory Evaluation

- **Human chorionic gonadotropin.** A serum human chorionic gonadotropin (hCG) should be drawn. A single hCG concentration is used as a baseline is if the ultrasound findings are nondiagnostic or if ectopic pregnancy is suspected. In such cases, serial hCG measurements should be done. In failed pregnancies, a decline in serum hCG is usually apparent based upon two measurements at least 48 hours apart (as hCG should almost double in that time).[4]
- **Blood type and antibody screen.** An Rh(D) typing and antibody screen should be drawn if not previously performed during the current pregnancy. Women with bleeding in pregnancy who are Rh(D) negative should be given anti-D immune globulin.

A hemoglobin and hematocrit should be drawn if significant blood loss is suspected. A white blood cell count should be drawn only if septic abortion is suspected.

TABLE 14.13-2 Counseling[7,8]

Bereaved parents should be provided with:
  Medical care, as appropriate
  Support in viewing, holding, and then separating from the baby
  Emotional support in what may be a chaotic environment
  Grief assessment and counseling
  An opportunity to obtain as complete information as possible about the course of events, cause of death, risk of recurrence in a future pregnancy, and potential interventions, such as prenatal diagnosis or therapy

TREATMENT

Threatened Abortion

Women with threatened abortion have traditionally been managed expectantly until their symptoms resolve; a definitive diagnosis of nonviable pregnancy can be made; or there is progression to an inevitable, incomplete, or complete abortion. The use of progestin to reduce the risk of miscarriage among women with threatened abortion is controversial.

Septic Abortion

Suspected septic abortion with retained products of conception should be managed by stabilizing the patient, obtaining blood and endometrial cultures, promptly administering parenteral broad-spectrum antibiotics, and surgically evacuating the uterine contents.

Complete Abortion

Tissue that is passed should be examined to confirm that it is (or is not) the product of conception. This should be confirmed with ultrasound.

Incomplete, Inevitable, and Missed Abortion

- **Expectant management:** For women with early pregnancy loss at less than 13 weeks of gestation who have stable vital signs and no evidence of infection expectant management is an option with close observation.
- **Medical management:** Medical management can be used to for those that want to avoid surgery. Misoprostol is the drug of choice. The advantages of misoprostol over other drugs are its low cost and low incidence of side effects when given intravaginally. The risk of a major complication is rare. Misoprostol can be used either vaginally or orally. Mifepristone can be added or oxytocin (in the case of stillbirth).[5]
- **Surgical management:** The conventional treatment of first or early second trimester failed pregnancy is dilatation and curettage (D&C) or dilatation and evacuation (D&E) to prevent potential hemorrhagic and infectious complications from the retained products of conception.[6]
- **Stillbirth:** Patients should be offered induction of labor soon after diagnosis of fetal death. Commonly using misoprostol for cervical ripening and oxytocin to induce labor. Some couples may choose to delay induction or even wait for spontaneous labor; prompt induction is not medically necessary. C-section may be needed in patients with previous C-section.
- **Alloimmunization prevention:** Women who are Rh(D) negative should be given anti-D immune globulin (Rhogam).
- **Resolution of positive hCG:** Serum hCG values typically return to normal within 2 to 4 weeks after a completed abortion and should be followed to zero.
- **Counseling:** Grief counseling is important to acknowledge the patient's (and partner's) grief and provide empathy and support. If reversible risk factors for spontaneous abortion are present, these can be addressed, as appropriate, in a nonjudgmental way.[7,8] There are many times when the etiology may be unknown (see Table 14.13-2).

Referrals

For patients who need surgical intervention referral to OB/GYN or MFM may be needed. Also, in couples with recurrent pregnancy loss, referrals to OB/GYN or Genetic Counseling may also be indicated following initial workup or evaluation.

REFERENCES

1. Stillbirth Collaborative Research Network Writing Group. Causes of death among stillbirths. *JAMA* 2011;306:2459.
2. Nybo Andersen AM, Wohlfahrt J, Christens P, et al. Maternal age and fetal loss: population based register linkage study. *BMJ* 2000;320:1708.
3. Stirrat GM. Recurrent miscarriage. *Lancet* 1990;336:673.
4. Prine LW, MacNaughton H. Management of early pregnancy loss. *Am Fam Physician* 2011;84(1):75–82.
5. Neilson JP, Gyte GM, Hickey M, et al. Medical treatments for incomplete miscarriage (less than 24 weeks). *Cochrane Database Syst Rev* 2010;(1):CD007223.
6. Forna F, Gülmezoglu AM. Surgical procedures to evacuate incomplete abortion. *Cochrane Database Syst Rev* 2001;(1):CD001993.
7. Hughes P, Turton P, Hopper E, et al. Assessment of guidelines for good practice in psychosocial care of mothers after stillbirth: a cohort study. *Lancet* 2002;360:114.
8. Säflund K, Sjögren B, Wredling R. The role of caregivers after a stillbirth: views and experiences of parents. *Birth* 2004;31:132.

CHAPTER 15

Musculoskeletal Problems and Arthritis

Section Editor: Christopher W. Bunt

15.1 Osteoarthritis

John R. Gimpel

EPIDEMIOLOGY AND PATHOPHYSIOLOGY

Osteoarthritis (OA) is the most common arthritic disorder.[1–3] Most healthy asymptomatic people will have developed some evidence of this degenerative process by the age of 55. Risk factors include age older than 50, previous joint injury, obesity, prolonged occupational or sports stress (especially competitive contact sports), female gender, and heredity.[1–3] OA is considered to be more degenerative than inflammatory, resulting from failure of chondrocytes to maintain the homeostatic balance between degradation and synthesis of the extracellular matrix. This results in biomechanical and immune thinning of the articular cartilage and bone, and thickening of the synovium.[2] Bony spurs (osteophytes) form at the articular edges, with local (and generally mild) inflammation involving the joint capsule and adjacent ligaments.

DIAGNOSIS
Clinical Presentation

OA usually presents in a middle-aged or older person as mild, dull, aching pain in one or more joints. Pain typically worsens with activity, improves with rest, and can be aggravated by damp, cold weather. There are no systemic symptoms or signs. Stiffness occurs with inactivity but commonly improves after about 15 minutes of exercise. Morning stiffness lasts less than 30 minutes. Patients may report joint instability or "buckling." The patient often complains of pain and reduced function and, in the case of knee and hip disease, difficulty walking and climbing stairs. Usually, the symptoms will wax and wane, with increasing involvement of more joints over time. However, the patterns and trajectory of the disease are highly variable and often cannot be predicted.[2,3]

Physical Examination

The distribution of joints affected—distal interphalangeal (DIP) and proximal interphalangeal (PIP) in the hands and feet—in OA is different from that in rheumatoid arthritis (RA), and it is more likely than other arthritides to preferentially affect weight-bearing joints such as the hips, knees, and cervical and lumbar spine. The affected joints will likely be enlarged and cool to the touch, with limited range of motion. Crepitus is both a sensitive and a specific criterion for the disease. There may be effusions in large joints. OA of the wrists, ankles, and shoulders is often the result of trauma or other secondary causes. Most commonly affected joints are the DIP and PIP joints of the hands, the thumb carpometacarpal joint (first CMC), the big toe (first MTP), DIP joints of the feet, the knees and hips, and the spine. Degenerative change in the spine is common, with formation of osteophytes (bony spurs) at the facet joints that can produce local pain as well as compression of spinal nerve roots, causing neuropathy (weakness and sensory loss). When disc degeneration and osteophyte formation are severe, subsequent spinal canal stenosis can cause direct injury to the spinal cord in the neck or lumbar spine areas. Spinal stenosis can present with symptoms that mimic claudication.[2,3]

Laboratory Findings

Synovial fluid analysis is useful in ruling out possible inflammatory or crystal-induced arthritis, but is not often necessary in patients with OA. The erythrocyte sedimentation rate (ESR) is normal except in the rare case of erosive OA or primary generalized OA, which may have an inflammatory presentation much like RA.

Radiologic Findings

Imaging is useful for monitoring disease progression rather than making a diagnosis since osteoarthritic changes are routinely found in asymptomatic patients. These findings include asymmetric joint space narrowing (vs. symmetric narrowing in RA), osteophyte formation, calcification of cartilage, cyst formation, and subchondral sclerosis. Computed tomography and magnetic resonance imaging can be helpful to evaluate possible cervical or lumbar spinal stenosis or other causes of nerve impingement.[2,3]

TREATMENT

General and Nonpharmacologic

The aim of treatment is to decrease pain and improve function. Nonpharmacologic treatment is generally considered first-line. Obese patients should be encouraged to lose weight, especially before orthopedic surgery for joint replacement, and weight loss improves long-term progression of OA.[2,3]

Physical, Structural, and Manual Therapies

Exercise programs are a proven mainstay for OA treatment. Twice-daily exercise programs and low-impact aerobic conditioning produce increased strength and pain reduction. Aquatic exercise can be considered the first part of a longer exercise program for OA patients. Activity that causes pain lasting longer than 90 minutes should be avoided. Exercise directed at the muscle group or groups that support affected joints (e.g., quadriceps for the knees) can be beneficial to reduce the wear and tear on the affected joints. The use of braces, supportive shoes, and other orthotics can relieve pain from asymmetric walking patterns.[3–9]

Acupuncture may lead to small but clinically relevant benefits for peripheral joint OA. Balneotherapy (spa therapy/mineral baths), electromagnetic field treatment, osteopathic manipulative treatment, and other manual therapies may improve pain and quality of life, but further controlled studies are warranted.[4,10,11] Therapeutic ultrasound and also thermotherapy with ice massage or cold packs may likewise provide clinically relevant benefit in patients with knee OA.

Dietary Supplements and Pharmacologic Treatment

Glucosamine sulfate, which is derived from oyster and crab shells, may provide substrate for proteoglycan synthesis and may have mild anti-inflammatory effects. Patients treated with glucosamine (Rottapharm) 1,500 mg daily in three divided doses, may show mild to moderate efficacy compared with placebo in relieving painful symptoms. Short-term use of glucosamine seems to be well-tolerated, with the most common adverse effect of gastrointestinal discomfort occurring less than with nonsteroidal anti-inflammatory drugs (NSAIDs).

Chondroitin sulfate, made from shark and cow cartilage, may provide some anti-inflammatory effects, and, like glucosamine, may be superior to placebo in reducing pain of OA. Likewise, chondroitin sulfate, 1,200 mg daily in three divided doses, is also well-tolerated by patients, and has a somewhat slower onset of action but possibly a longer duration than NSAIDs for OA. Therefore, chondroitin sulfate or glucosamine should be taken for at least 1 month before any symptom relief would be expected. There is little evidence that the combination of glucosamine and chondroitin sulfate is any better than either used alone.

Nonrandomized and small trials have shown potential clinically relevant benefits in patients with OA with the following dietary supplements: S-adenosyl methionine (SAMe) and avocado–soybean unsaponifiables.

Prescription pharmacologic treatment can be recommended for pain relief and for faster onset than glucosamine and chondroitin. Acetaminophen, up to 3,000 mg per day, is superior to placebo and has a similar safety profile, so it is generally considered first-line pharmacological therapy for pain relief in OA. At higher doses, acetaminophen can cause some gastrointestinal symptoms, and overdoses or use with excessive alcohol has been associated with hepatotoxicity. Acetaminophen is likely not as efficacious as NSAIDs for pain reduction in people with knee or hip OA, but may be equivalent in functional improvements. If there is an unacceptable response to acetaminophen, NSAIDs can be added and titrated to effect. The use of topical capsaicin (0.025% cream applied four times daily) for OA affecting the knee, ankle, finger, wrist, or shoulder may be beneficial with the minor side effects of a local burning sensation. It is postulated to act as an irritant–counterirritant. Care is needed to avoid contact with the eyes. In the same fashion, topical analgesic creams (e.g., salicylate cream, diclofenac sodium topical gel) may be effective for focal joint pain, and can be applied four times daily. Arnica gel may be as effective as a gel containing NSAIDs, but side effects may be slightly worse. Tramadol, a non-opioid centrally acting analgesic, can be added to NSAID therapy for short-term use to help with severe pain, and duloxetine has been approved for use in chronic musculoskeletal pain including that from OA. The minimal to moderate beneficial effects of oral or transdermal opioids for OA patients are likely outweighed by the substantial risk of adverse events.[3,12–17]

Intra-Articular Therapy

Intra-articular steroid injections have a well-established role in providing short-term benefit for patients with knee OA pain flare-ups and effusion. Joint lavage does not appear to provide relevant benefit for pain or functional improvement for patients with knee OA.

Viscosupplementation is now being utilized widely—particularly for OA of the knees, with relatively low risks of adverse reactions. These viscous agents are injected into the joint space to (theoretically) replace depleted hyaluronic acid (a natural substance essential for maintaining joint fluid viscosity). Sodium hyaluronate (Hyalgan) and Hylan G-F20 (Synvisc) are generally given in two to five injections (2 mL) over 2 to 4 weeks, whereas Synvisc-One can be given in a single injection that may provide relief for 6 months. Adverse effects (e.g., pain, swelling, allergic reaction) generally occur in 5% of cases. Studies have confirmed short-term relief of pain, more prolonged effects than intra-articular steroids, and good patient-oriented evidence with viscosupplementation for OA of the knee. However, costs of the injection series are significant. Prolotherapy, with injection of 10% dextrose solutions, has also shown some efficacy for pain and stiffness in knee OA.[2,3,18–23]

Surgical Treatment

Patients with severe OA not responding to medication and those with intractable pain or serious functional impairment should be referred to an orthopedic surgeon for osteotomy or arthroplasty. Fewer than one half of patients with OA who undergo arthroscopic debridement (simple lavage or abrasion arthroplasty) will have sustained pain reduction. Long-term outcomes for joint replacement/arthroplasty are good.[2,3,24]

Prevention

In both primary and secondary prevention of OA, the most important factor in protecting the weight-bearing joints is maintenance of an appropriate body weight. Exercise, especially for supporting joints (quadriceps for knees, abdominal muscles for lumbar spine), plays an important role, and adaptive equipment and mobility aides can reduce disability. Patients should also be advised to maintain an adequate vitamin D intake.[2,3]

ACKNOWLEDGMENT

The author would like to acknowledge the contributions of Richard Pascucci, DO, and J. Michael Finley, DO, in the review of this chapter.

REFERENCES

1. Rice D. Musculoskeletal conditions: impact and importance. United States Bone and Joint Decade. 2000. www.usbji.org. Accessed December 1, 2005.
2. Klippel JH, Stone JH, Crofford LeJ, et al. *Primer on the rheumatic diseases.* 13th ed. Atlanta, GA: Arthritis Foundation; 2008.
3. Van Manen MD, Nace J, Mont MA. Management of primary knee osteoarthritis and indications for total knee arthroplasty for general practitioners. *J Am Osteopath Assoc* 2012;112(11):709–715.
4. Verhagen AP, Bierma-Zeinstra SM, Boers M, et al. Balneotherapy for osteoarthritis. *Cochrane Database Syst Rev* 2007;(4):CD006864 doi: 10.1155/2013/638050.
5. Rutjes AW, Nuesch E, Sterchi R, et al. Therapeutic ultrasound for osteoarthritis of the knee or hip. *Cochrane Database Syst Rev* 2010;(1):CD003132 doi: 10.1002/14651858.
6. Brosseau L, Yonge KA, Robinson V, et al. Thermotherapy for treatment of osteoarthritis. *Cochrane Database Syst Rev* 2003;(4):CD004522 doi: 10.1002/14651858.

7. Bartels EM, Lund H, Hagen KB, et al. Aquatic exercise for the treatment of knee and hip osteoarthritis. *Cochrane Database Syst Rev* 2007;(4):CD005523 doi: 10.1002/14651858.
8. Li S, Yu B, Zhou D, et al. Electromagnetic fields for treating osteoarthritis. *Cochrane Database Syst Rev* 2013;12:CD003523 doi: 10.1002/14651858.
9. Fransen M, McConnell S. Exercise for osteoarthritis of the knee. *Cochrane Database Syst Rev* 2008;(4):CD004376 doi: 10.1002/14651858.
10. Manheimer E, Cheng K, Linde K, et al. Acupuncture for peripheral joint osteoarthritis. *Cochrane Database Syst Rev* 2010;(1):CD001977 doi: 10.1002/14651858.
11. Rutjes AW, Nuesch E, Sterchi R, et al. Transcutaneous electrostimulation for osteoarthritis of the knee. *Cochrane Database Syst Rev* 2009;(4):CD002823 doi: 10.1002/14651858.
12. Towheed TE, Maxwell L, Anastassiades TP, et al. Glucosamine therapy for treating osteoarthritis. *Cochrane Database Syst Rev* 2005;(2):CD002946 doi: 10.1002/14651858.
13. Towheed TE, Maxwell, L, Judd MG, et al. Acetaminophen for osteoarthritis. *Cochrane Database Syst Rev* 2006;(1):CD004257 doi: 10.1002/14651858.
14. Cameron M, Chrubasik S. Topical herbal therapies for treating osteoarthritis. *Cochrane Database Syst Rev* 2013;5:CD010538 doi: 10.1002/14651858.
15. Rutjes AW, Nuesch E, Reichenbach S, et al. S-Adenosylmethionine for osteoarthritis of the knee or hip. *Cochrane Database Syst Rev* 2009;(4):CD007321 doi: 10.1002/14651858.
16. Cepeda MS, Camargo F, Zea C, et al. Tramadol for osteoarthritis. *Cochrane Database Syst Rev* 2006;(3):CD005522 doi: 10.1002/14651858.
17. Nuesch E, Rutjes AW, Husni E, et al. Oral or transdermal opioids for osteoarthritis of the knee or hip. *Cochrane Database Syst Rev* 2009;(4):CD003115 doi: 10.1002/14651858.
18. Laupattarakasem W, Laopaiboon M, Laupattarakasem P, et al. Arthroscopic debridement for knee osteoarthritis [Review]. *Cochrane Database Syst Rev* 2008;(1):CD005118 doi: 10.1002/14651858.
19. Reichenbach S, Rutjes AW, Nuesch E, et al. Joint lavage for osteoarthritis of the knee. *Cochrane Database Syst Rev* 2010;(5):CD007320 doi: 10.1002/14651858.
20. Bellamy N, Campbell J, Robinson V, et al. Intraarticular corticosteroid for treatment of osteoarthritis of the knee. *Cochrane Database Syst Rev* 2006;(2):CD005328 doi: 10.1002/14651858.
21. Bellamy N, Campbell J, Robinson V, et al. Viscosupplementation for the treatment of osteoarthritis of the knee. *Cochrane Database Syst Rev* 2006;(2):CD005321 doi: 10.1002/14651858.
22. Rabago D, Patterson JJ, Mundt M, et al. Dextrose prolotherapy for knee osteoarthritis: a randomized controlled trial. *Ann Fam Med* 2013;11(3):229–237.
23. Rabago D, Patterson JJ. Prolotherapy: an effective adjunctive therapy for knee osteoarthritis. *J Am Osteopath Assoc* 2013;113(2):122–123.
24. Brouwer RW, Raaij van TM, Bierma-Zeinstra SM, et al. Osteotomy for treating knee osteoarthritis. *Cochrane Database Syst Rev* 2007;(3):CD004019 doi: 10.1002/14651858.

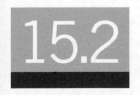

15.2 Rheumatoid Arthritis and Related Disorders

John J. Olshefski

The rheumatic diseases include more than 100 diagnoses. In this chapter, we focus on four commonly seen connective tissue diseases: rheumatoid arthritis (RA), juvenile idiopathic arthritis, systemic lupus erythematosus (SLE), and systemic sclerosis.

RHEUMATOID ARTHRITIS
Definition
RA is a chronic, systemic inflammatory synovitis that can affect many different joints.

Anatomy
Typically involves wrist, metacarpophalangeal (MCP) or proximal interphalangeal (PIP) joints.

Epidemiology

Prevalence: 1% lifetime prevalence worldwide; peaks between 30 and 50 but can occur at any age.[1]

Pathophysiology

RA signs and symptoms are secondary to the activation of proinflammatory cells that infiltrate the synovium. These cells increase the production of proinflammatory cytokines, including tumor necrosis factor alpha (TNF-α) and interleukin-6 (IL-6), which cause bone and cartilage damage.

Etiology

Unknown. Risk factors include cigarette smoking, female gender, and family history of RA.[1]

Mechanisms of Injury

As described above in Pathophysiology.

Diagnosis

- 2010 American College of Rheumatology/European League Against Rheumatism Classification system aims at earlier recognition and diagnosis of RA.
- **Patients to be tested:** Those with at least one joint with definite clinical synovitis or patients with synovitis that cannot be better explained by another disease.
- **Score-based system:** At least six points needed for definitive diagnosis.[1]
    - **A.** Joint involvement
        - **a.** 0 points for 1 large joint
        - **b.** 1 point for 2 to 10 large joints
        - **c.** 2 points for 1 to 3 small joints
        - **d.** 3 points for 4 to 10 small joints
        - **e.** 5 points for more than 10 joints, at least one of which is a small joint
    - **B.** Serology
        - **a.** 0 points for negative rheumatoid factor (RF) and negative anti-citrullinated protein antibody (ACPA)
        - **b.** Two points for low-positive RF or low-positive ACPA (higher than upper limit of normal for lab or assay but less than three times the upper limit of normal)
        - **c.** Three points for high-positive RF or high-positive ACPA (greater than three times the upper limit of normal for laboratory or assay)
    - **C.** Acute phase reactants
        - **a.** 0 points for normal erythrocyte sedimentation rate (ESR) and normal C-reactive protein (CRP)
        - **b.** 1 point for elevated ESR or elevated CRP
    - **D.** Duration of symptoms
        - **a.** 0 points for less than 6 weeks of symptoms
        - **b.** 1 point for 6 weeks or more of symptoms

Clinical Presentation

Patients often present with stiffness and pain in multiple joints. Morning stiffness that lasts greater than 1 hour is suggestive of the diagnosis.[1]

History

Gradual onset of joint pain with systemic symptoms (weakness, fatigue, anorexia).

Physical Examination

Symmetric joint involvement; most often hands, sometimes feet; with effusions, tenderness, and restricted range of motion.

Laboratory Studies

RF (up to 30% false-negative early in disease course); ACPA in combination with RF improves both sensitivity and specificity.

Imaging

Earliest radiographic findings include soft tissue swelling, periarticular osteopenia, and erosions (present in up to 25% at first visit); later findings include joint space narrowing and visible deformity.

Monitoring

At each visit, evaluate for subjective and objective evidence of active disease.

- Degree of joint pain (by visual analog scale [VAS])
- Duration of morning stiffness
- Duration of fatigue
- Presence of actively inflamed joints on examination (tender and swollen joint)

Differential Diagnosis

Systemic lupus erythematosus, seronegative spondyloarthropathies, polymyalgia rheumatica, acute rheumatic fever, systemic sclerosis, and sarcoidosis.

Treatment

Behavioral

The patient's recognition of the chronic, progressive nature of the disease is central to healthy adjustment to the diagnosis and optimal participation in therapy. Providers should educate the patient and family about the disease and provide longitudinal care. The Arthritis Foundation also has valuable educational materials and programs (http://www.arthritis.org/resources).

Medications

Early aggressive therapy with disease-modifying antirheumatic drugs (DMARDs) is advocated to prevent or delay joint destruction. Although nonsteroidal anti-inflammatory drugs (NSAIDs) may initially control symptoms, the opportunity to control the disease may be lost if more potent therapies are not initiated early.

NSAIDs. Although all NSAIDs are associated with gastrointestinal (GI) side effects, selective cyclo-oxygenase-2 (COX-2) inhibitors produce equivalent pain relief with somewhat reduced GI complications compared with nonselective NSAIDs. However, placebo-controlled trials suggest increased risk of thrombotic cardiovascular events with COX-2 selective NSAIDs. The American College of Rheumatology Guidelines for the Management of Rheumatoid Arthritis recommends that physicians weigh the potential risks and benefits of treatment with these medications.

DMARDs. DMARDs should be initiated within 3 months of diagnosis. They are usually used in combination with NSAIDs and often with other DMARDs if control cannot be obtained with a single DMARD. They are broken into two groups: nonbiologic and biologic.

- **Nonbiologic DMARDs**
  - Methotrexate (Rheumatrex) inhibits dihydrofolate reductase. Temporarily discontinue with development of any pulmonary symptoms. Avoid alcohol. Ensure non-pregnant state and adequate birth control. Monitor complete blood count (CBC) and liver-associated enzymes. Supplement with folic acid. The most commonly used and most studied DMARD.[1]
  - Leflunomide (Arava) inhibits pyrimidine synthesis. Possible side effects include GI and liver effects.
  - Antimalarials: Hydroxychloroquine (Plaquenil) blocks toll-like receptors. Because of rare ocular toxicity, perform a baseline retinal examination, and repeat this every 6 months while on medication.
  - Less commonly used nonbiologic DMARDs are gold sodium thiomalate (Myochrysine) and aurothioglucose (Solganal), penicillamine, and cyclophosphamide.
- **Biologic DMARDs**
  - TNF-α inhibitors may dramatically suppress disease activity. Etanercept (Enbrel), infliximab (Remicade), and adalimumab (Humira) have been effective in reducing signs and symptoms of RA in patients refractory to methotrexate. Other DMARDs target additional anti-inflammatory mediators (IL-1, T cells, and B cells). Biologic DMARDs have significant safety considerations, contraindications, and costs and should be used in consultation with a rheumatologist. Generally, patients on biologic DMARDs are more susceptible to tuberculosis and other opportunistic infections.[1]

Glucocorticoids. Low-dose oral glucocorticoids and local injections of glucocorticoids are highly effective for relieving symptoms in patients with active RA. Individual joint steroid injections should be given no more often than every 3 months.

Surgery

Patients with unacceptable levels of pain and/or limitation of function because of structural joint damage should be considered for surgical treatment.[1]

Referrals

Instruction in joint protection techniques, energy conservation, range of motion, muscle strengthening, and aerobic exercise are all important in achieving the goal of maintaining function. Physical and occupational therapists may be needed to assist with this teaching. Patients with RA should also be referred to a rheumatologist to help determine the ideal treatment regimen.

JUVENILE IDIOPATHIC ARTHRITIS

Definition

Juvenile idiopathic arthritis (JIA) is a persistent arthritis present for at least 6 weeks with an onset less than 16 years of age, after excluding other known conditions. Seven subtypes have been identified; see "Classification" below.

Anatomy

Knees, ankles, wrists, and elbows are most frequently involved, but all joints can be affected.

Epidemiology

More common in girls than in boys; prevalence approximately 1 per 1,000.[2]

Classification

See Table 15.2-1.

Pathophysiology

Inflammatory mediators in joints produce joint injury and eventual destruction.

Etiology

Unknown, thought to be a complex of genetic traits related to immunity and inflammation.

Diagnosis

See Table 15.2-1 for classification.

Clinical Presentation

As noted in classification.

History

Many patients complain little of joint pain, but limit or modify motion due to pain. Decreased activity and morning stiffness are common.

TABLE 15.2-1	International League of Associations for Rheumatology (ILAR) Classification of JIA
Category	**Criteria for diagnosis**
Systemic onset arthritis	Fever and at least one of erythematous rash, generalized lymph node enlargement, hepatosplenomegaly, or serositis
Oligoarthritis	One to four joints involved in first 6 mo of disease
Polyarthritis w/ negative RF	At least five joints involved and negative RF
Polyarthritis w/ positive RF	At least five joints involved and positive RF
Enthesitis-related arthritis	Arthritis and enthesitis, or arthritis or enthesitis with at least two of the following: sacroiliac joint tenderness, positive HLA B-27 antigen, symptomatic anterior uveitis, or arthritis onset after age 6 yr in males
Psoriatic arthritis	Arthritis and psoriasis, or arthritis and at least two of the following: dactylitis, nail pitting, or psoriasis in first-degree relative
Unclassified	Fits none or more than one of the other categories

Data from Kim KH, Kim DS. Juvenile idiopathic arthritis: diagnosis and differential diagnosis. *Korean J Pediatr* 2010;53(11):931–935.

Physical Examination
- **Systemic onset disease:** Spiking fevers, an evanescent centripetal salmon-pink rash, generalized lymphadenopathy, and hepatosplenomegaly may occur.
- **Oligoarticular disease:** Lacks systemic features except iridocyclitis.
- **Polyarticular disease:** Multiple joints are involved without systemic symptoms, but malaise, growth retardation, weight loss, mild adenopathy, and low-grade fevers are sometimes present.

Laboratory Studies
RF and antinuclear antibody (ANA) are rarely positive in systemic disease. RF-positive children with polyarticular onset have a worse prognosis and more vasculitis than those with polyarthritis who are RF negative. In oligoarticular disease of early onset (before 6 years), most are ANA positive and RF negative.

Imaging
Radiologic joint damage occurs in most patients with systemic arthritis and polyarthritis within 2 years of onset and in oligoarthritis within 5 years.

Differential Diagnosis
Trauma; malignancy; sarcoidosis; SLE; progressive systemic sclerosis; infections (viral, rickettsial, and other bacterial); and serum sickness.

Treatment

Behavioral
Patients and families should be encouraged to seek supportive counseling to assist in dealing with a chronic illness in a child.

Medications
Systemic onset: NSAIDs (ibuprofen and naproxen are available as elixirs; tolmetin and naproxen are approved in patients as young as 2 years; ibuprofen as young as 6 months) and systemic corticosteroids.

- **Oligoarthritis.** NSAIDs are the mainstay of treatment. If unresponsive to 4 to 6 weeks of NSAIDs or in patients with flexion contractures then intra-articular corticosteroids (triamcinolone hexacetonide) should be considered. Treat as polyarthritis if the patient is unresponsive to therapies or has small joint involvement.[3] Methotrexate can be used as initial therapy if disease activity is high or if the patient has poor prognostic features (i.e., arthritis of hip or cervical spine or radiographic evidence of joint damage).[2]
- **Polyarthritis, RF negative.** NSAIDs for symptom control; methotrexate started early, may increase dose if initially ineffective.
- **Polyarthritis, RF positive.** Treated per protocols for RA in adults.
- **Enthesitis-related arthritis.** Sulfasalazine may be most effective, particularly for boys over age nine, although evidence is lacking.
- **Psoriatic arthritis.** Can present as oligo-, poly-, or enthesitis-related arthritis and should be treated as the parallel JIA subset, since evidence is limited for psoriatic arthritis in children.[3]

Special Therapy
Early consultation with physical and occupational therapy to maintain or regain muscle and joint strength, range of motion, and function.

Referrals
Early involvement of an ophthalmologist to identify and treat iridocyclitis is mandatory to prevent disability. Early involvement of a rheumatologist is essential.

SYSTEMIC LUPUS ERYTHEMATOSUS

Definition

SLE is a multisystem inflammatory disease.

The presence of four or more of the American Rheumatological Association Preliminary Criteria for SLE is a reliable indicator of the diagnosis:[4]

- **Malar rash,** tending to spare the nasolabial folds
- **Discoid rash,** follicular plugging with alopecia and atrophic scarring in older lesions
- **Photosensitivity**
- **Oral ulcers,** classically painless

- **Nonerosive arthritis** involving two or more peripheral joints
- **Serositis,** pleuritis or pericarditis
- **Renal disorder** manifested by persistent proteinuria >0.5 g per day or cellular casts on urine microscopy
- **Neurologic disorder** manifested by seizures or psychosis
- **Hematologic disorder,** hemolytic anemia with reticulocytosis, leukopenia (<4,000 cells per μL on two or more occasions), lymphopenia (<1,500 cells per μL on two or more occasions), or thrombocytopenia (<100,000 cells per μL)
- **Immunologic disorder,** antibody to double-stranded DNA or Smith antigen
- **ANA** positive (in the absence of any drugs known to be associated with "drug-induced lupus" syndrome)

Epidemiology
- 90% of patients are women of child-bearing age.
- Prevalence ranges from 20 to 150 cases per 100,000; more common in African Americans.
- In United States, more than 250,000 people have been diagnosed with SLE.[4]

Etiology
Unknown. Autoantibodies are typically present for years before the diagnosis of SLE.

Mechanisms of Injury
Autoantibodies produce multisystem inflammatory damage.

Diagnosis
Clinical Presentation
Arthritis or arthralgia is usually the earliest symptom.

History
Almost all patients are fatigued and feel general malaise.[5] Pleuritis, pericarditis, or a combination of both may produce chest pain. Central nervous system changes may result in subtle changes in cognitive function, depression, or seizure disorder.

Physical Examination
Approximately 85% of patients have skin, hair, and mucous membrane involvement, ranging from mild malar rash to ulcerations, patchy to diffuse alopecia, and mucosal ulceration. Symmetrical arthritis is usually present, and most commonly involves the PIP joints (80%), followed by wrists, knees, ankles, elbows, and shoulders. Little objective joint inflammation is appreciated on physical examination.

Laboratory Studies
Anemia, elevated ESR or CRP, and polyclonal gammopathy reflect systemic inflammation. ANA is positive in more than 99% of patients with SLE (titer greater than 1:40) but is nonspecific. Antibodies to double-stranded DNA (anti-ds DNA) or the Smith nuclear antigen (Anti-Sm) are highly specific for SLE.[5]

Imaging
A chest radiograph should be performed to evaluate pulmonary involvement; an echocardiogram can evaluate for valvular heart disease.

Differential Diagnosis
Other connective tissue disorders (e.g., progressive systemic sclerosis, RA), neoplasm, and infection.

Treatment
Behavioral
Patients with photosensitivity should avoid sunlight and use higher sun protection factor sunscreens.

Medications
Therapy should be individualized based on disease severity.

- Joint pain and mild serositis are generally well controlled with NSAIDs; antimalarials are also effective.
- Cutaneous manifestations are treated with topical corticosteroids.
- Intradermal corticosteroids are helpful for individual discoid lesions, particularly on the scalp.

Referrals

Rheumatology referral is recommended for initial consultation regarding therapy and for patients poorly responsive to first-line therapy.

Patient Education

Education should be provided regarding recognition of disease flares and anticipated course of the illness.

Complications

The leading cause of death in patients with SLE is infection (one-third of all deaths).[4] Serum creatinine levels >3 mg per dL or evidence of diffuse proliferative involvement on renal biopsy are poor prognostic factors.

SYSTEMIC SCLEROSIS/SCLERODERMA

Definition

Systemic sclerosis (SSc) is a chronic connective tissue disease that causes extensive microvascular damage and collagen deposition in skin and internal organs.

Epidemiology

Annual incidence is estimated at 10 to 20 cases per million; females are affected more often than men.[6]

Etiology

Unknown.

Mechanisms of Injury

Fibrotic changes occur in the skin and visceral organs, primarily in the lung, kidney, and esophagus.

Diagnosis

Based on clinical findings.

Clinical Presentation

- **Limited scleroderma (lSSc) or CREST syndrome**—calcinosis, Raynaud phenomenon, esophageal dysmotility, sclerodactyly, and telangiectasia
  - Skin involvement occurs mostly in distal extremities, but may affect the face
  - Lung involvement is common—typically pulmonary hypertension
  - Raynaud phenomenon and severe gastroesophageal reflux disease are characteristic
- **Diffuse scleroderma (dSSc)** has more widespread skin involvement—affecting areas proximal or distal to the elbows and knees as well as the face
  - Greater than 90% have Raynaud phenomenon
  - Interstitial lung disease is common
  - Renal crisis—present in 3% to 10% of all patients with systemic sclerosis—greatest risk within first 3 years after diagnosis[6]
    - Often presents with acute hypertension and progressive renal failure and proteinuria as well as microscopic hematuria
    - Possible to be normotensive but actually is hypertensive compared with baseline
    - Important to monitor baseline blood pressures

History

Most patients present with Raynaud phenomenon and edema of fingers; arthralgias may be present.[4] Rarely, esophageal symptoms occur first.

Physical Examination

1. Early in disease—edema of hands and feet
2. Later in disease course—thickening of skin of fingers (sclerodactyly)
3. Digital pits secondary to Raynaud phenomenon and other findings as outlined in CREST syndrome above

Laboratory Studies

- Greater than 90% of patients have positive ANA; nucleolar pattern associated with dSSc and centromere pattern with lSSc. ESR is often normal.[6]

- Anticentromere antibody testing is positive in 60% to 80% with limited disease (good prognosis if positive).[6]
- Antitopoisomerase-1 antibody (anti-Scl-70) can be positive in 20% to 40% with diffuse disease.
- Screen for visceral involvement with CBC, urinalysis, creatinine, pulmonary function tests, and diffusion capacity of carbon monoxide.

Imaging
Perform a chest radiograph to evaluate for pulmonary fibrosis; and perform esophageal motility studies.

Surgical Diagnostic Procedures
Skin biopsy.

Differential Diagnosis
- **Limited diseases:** mycosis fungoides, amyloidosis, porphyria cutanea tarda, reflex sympathetic dystrophy
- **Diffuse diseases:** idiopathic pulmonary fibrosis, primary biliary cirrhosis, GI dysmotility problems, SLE and overlapping syndromes

Treatment

Behavioral
Because of the sometimes disfiguring nature of the disease, counseling is recommended for supportive care. Protect extremities from cold temperatures.

Medications
- Raynaud disease should be managed with calcium-channel blockers (long-acting) or peripheral α-blockers. May also try pentoxifylline and stellate ganglion block.[6]
- Penicillamine for skin changes, in addition to moisturizing agents.
- Proton pump inhibitors and H2-receptor blockers for esophageal reflux symptoms. Promotility agents may be helpful.
- Monitor blood pressure and make early use of angiotensin-converting enzyme inhibitors.

Surgery
Progression of disease may eventually require lung and renal transplantation.

Referrals
Physical and occupational therapy should be involved early to prevent and treat functional loss secondary to skin changes. Rheumatology can help with confirmation of initial diagnosis and comanagement. Pulmonary and renal consults as needed with disease progression.

REFERENCES

1. Wasserman AM. Diagnosis and management of rheumatoid arthritis. *Am Fam Physician* 2011;84(11):1245–1252.
2. Beukelman T, Patkar NM, Saag KG, et al. 2011 American college of rheumatology recommendations for the treatment of juvenile idiopathic arthritis: initiation and safety monitoring of therapeutic agents for the treatment of arthritis and systemic features. *Arthritis Care Res* 2011;63(4):465–482.
3. Hashkes PJ, Laxer RM. Medical treatment of juvenile idiopathic arthritis. *JAMA* 2005;294(13):1671–1684.
4. Gill JM, Quisel AM, Rocca PV, et al. Diagnosis of systemic lupus erythematosus. *Am Fam Physician* 2003;68(11):2179–2187.
5. Rahman A, Isenberg D. Systemic lupus erythematosus. *N Engl J Med* 2008;358:929–939.
6. Hinchcliffe M, Varga J. Systemic sclerosis/scleroderma: a treatable multisystem disease. *Am Fam Physician* 2008;78(8):961–969.

15.3 Fibromyalgia

Jimmy H. Hara

Fibromyalgia is a nonarticular rheumatic pain syndrome characterized by widespread musculoskeletal pain and tenderness on palpation at characteristic sites, called tender points. It is considered to be a disorder of pain regulation and classified as a central sensitization or pain amplification syndrome.[1] Non-musculoskeletal symptoms often accompany the nonarticular musculoskeletal pain. Fatigue, sleep disturbance, anxiety or depression, headache, irritable bowel syndrome, dysmenorrhea, and paresthesias are among the more common non-musculoskeletal features. In 2010, preliminary criteria were recommended to capture these non-musculoskeletal symptoms, add additional regions of pain other than the tender points described in 1990, and suggest a symptom severity scoring system.[2]

DIAGNOSIS

History

Fibromyalgia occurs predominantly in Caucasian women (80% to 95%), who are 40 to 50 years old. The prevalence in the general population is 4% to 10%. Pain is the cardinal symptom and is widespread. According to the American College of Rheumatology, the pain must be above and below the waist, on both sides of the body, and along the axial skeleton.[2] Non-musculoskeletal symptoms, especially anxiety and depression, are commonly found, and frequently overlap with chronic fatigue syndrome.

Physical Examination

According to the American College of Rheumatology Fibromyalgia Classification criteria, there must be tenderness on digital palpation (using 4 kg of force, or enough to blanch the nail bed of the thumb) in at least 11 of the following 18 (nine pairs) tender point sites:

- **Occipital:** bilaterally at the suboccipital muscle insertions a few centimeters below the nuchal ridge.
- **Low cervical:** bilaterally at the anterior aspects of the intertransverse spaces at C5–C7.
- **Supraspinatus:** bilaterally above the medial border of the scapular spine.
- **Second rib:** bilaterally at the second costochondral junction.
- **Lateral epicondyle:** bilaterally 2 cm distal to the epicondyle.
- **Gluteal:** bilaterally in the upper outer quadrants of the buttocks in the anterior fold of gluteus minimus.
- **Greater trochanter:** bilaterally just posterior to the trochanteric prominence.
- **Knee:** bilaterally at the medial fat pad proximal to the joint line.

Laboratory Studies

There are no routine laboratory markers for fibromyalgia. Specifically, the complete blood count and erythrocyte sedimentation rate are usually normal. Rheumatologic serologies are not diagnostic. Although abnormalities in T-cell subsets have been described, these tests are not currently recommended for routine use.[3]

TREATMENT

Injection

The tendinitis, bursitis, and costochondral tender points (lateral epicondyle, trapezius, greater trochanter, knee, and second rib) may be injected with lidocaine (Xylocaine) and/or corticosteroid.

Stretch and Spray

The myofascial trigger points of Travell (occiput, low cervical, supraspinatus, and gluteal tender points) may be stretched and have a vapo-coolant applied; alternatively, these may be injected with 0.5% procaine.[3]

Pharmacotherapy

Low-dose tricyclic antidepressants, such as amitriptyline (Elavil), 10 to 50 mg per day, or cyclobenzaprine (Flexeril) 10 to 30 mg per day, are recommended. Likewise, selective serotonin reuptake inhibitors, such as fluoxetine, 10 to 20 mg per day or paroxetine (Paxil) 5 to 10 mg per day, or low-dose dual (serotonin and norepinephrine) reuptake inhibitors such as duloxetine (Cymbalta) 60 mg per day, or venlafaxine (Effexor) 75 to 150 mg per day may be tried. The anticonvulsant pregabalin (Lyrica) was the first drug to attain FDA approval for the treatment of fibromyalgia and the dual reuptake inhibitor milnacipran (Savella) was the second to achieve approval.[4] Nonsteroidal anti-inflammatory drugs and tramadol (Ultram) may also prove useful for the treatment of myofascial pain.[4]

Non-Pharmacologic Therapy

Exercise can be of significant benefit; low-impact aerobic activities such as walking, biking, swimming, or water aerobics are especially helpful.[5] A 2008 systematic review of 34 studies of aerobic exercise and fibromyalgia found beneficial effects on aerobic performance, pain amelioration, and global well-being.[6] Physical therapists and exercise physiologists familiar with fibromyalgia can provide helpful assistance and monitoring of progress. "Mind-body" interventions such as tai chi and yoga have demonstrated benefit in global well-being in a number of studies.[6] Electromyographic biofeedback training and cognitive behavioral therapy also have proven benefit in patients with chronic fibromyalgia symptomatology.[5-7]

REFERENCES

1. Sarzi-Puttini P, Atzeni F, Mease PJ. Chronic widespread pain: from peripheral to central evolution. *Best Pract Res Clin Rheumatol* 2011;25(2):133–139.
2. Wolfe F, Clauw DJ, Fitzcharles MA, et al. The American College of Rheumatology preliminary diagnostic criteria for fibromyalgia and measurement of symptom severity. *Arthritis Care Res* 2010;62(5):600–610.
3. Hara J. Myofascial syndromes (fibromyalgia and myofascial trigger points). In: Rakel R, ed. *Saunders manual of medical practice*. Philadelphia, PA: WB Saunders; 2006.
4. Goldenberg DL, Burckhardt C, Crofford L. Management of fibromyalgia syndrome. *JAMA* 2004;292(19):2388–2395.
5. Busch AJ, Schachter CI, Overend TJ, et al. Exercise for fibromyalgia: a systematic review. *J Rheumatol* 2008;35(6):1130–1144.
6. Hadhazy VA, Ezzo J, Creamer P, et al. Mind-body therapies for the treatment of fibromyalgia. A systematic review. *J Rheumatol* 2000;27(12):2911–2918.
7. Miller FL, O'Connor DP, Herring MP, et al. Exercise dose, exercise adherence, and associated health outcomes in the TIGER Study. *Med Sci Sports Exerc* 2014;46(1):69–75.

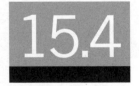

15.4 Gout

Kristen H. Goodell, Joseph W. Gravel Jr

GENERAL PRINCIPLES

Definition

Gout is an inflammatory disease caused by the deposition of uric acid crystals in and around joints, subcutaneous tissues (tophi), and kidneys.

Epidemiology

Gout primarily affects middle-aged men (ages 40 to 60) and postmenopausal women. The prevalence of gout has been increasing over the last two to three decades with self-reported prevalence of 3.9% of adults in the United States.[1] Increasing rates of obesity, hypertension, type 2 diabetes mellitus, and chronic kidney disease may be contributing to the increase.[2] Acute attacks of gout are less common in elderly people, in whom it may present insidiously or develop into chronic polyarticular arthritis.

Pathophysiology

Painful gouty attacks occur when uric acid crystals, a product of purine oxidation, are deposited in joints and subcutaneous tissues. Hyperuricemia is a marker for gout, but each can exist without the other. Defined as uric acid levels greater than 6.8 mg per dL,[3] hyperuricemia is present in about 5% of the U.S. male population, of whom only a small minority will develop gout. Approximately 40% of patients have normal uric acid levels during an acute episode of gout;[4] however, the risk of gout is proportional to the degree and duration of hyperuricemia. Levels normally rise during puberty in men and in postmenopausal women. It normally takes 20 to 30 years of hyperuricemia before a patient has a first episode of gouty arthritis. Primary hyperuricemia results from inborn errors of metabolism, either reduced excretion (90% of patients) or increased production (10%) of uric acid. Secondary hyperuricemia associated with gout can result from the use of thiazide diuretics, a high-purine diet (red meat and seafood), increased alcohol consumption, and obesity.[5,6]

Etiology

Risk of gout increases with increasing body mass index (BMI) and with weight gain over time. Weight loss, on the other hand, is protective against gouty attacks. Presence of hypertension is strongly associated with gout independent of renal failure and diuretic use.[5] High levels of purine-rich seafood and red meat consumption may increase uric acid levels, whereas consumption of dairy products is protective. Increased consumption of purine-rich foods has no effect on clinical gout.[6] Consumption of alcohol, in particular beer and spirits, increases the risk of gout. Ethanol metabolism increases serum lactate, which blocks renal uric acid excretion, leading to gouty attacks. Other factors provoking gouty attacks include rapid changes (either up or down) in serum uric acid levels, infection, surgery, renal failure, diuretic use, and emotional stress.

DIAGNOSIS

Clinical Presentation

Acute gout typically presents as an acutely painful monoarticular arthritis that may progress to chronic arthritis after years of progressively more severe and frequent episodes interspersed with variable symptom-free periods. The first metatarsophalangeal (MTP) joint is involved in 50% of initial acute gouty attacks (podagra), and 75% to 90% of patients with gout have first MTP involvement eventually. This is probably due to the microtrauma propensity of the first MTP and its relative coolness compared with the rest of the body. Gout severity ranges from vague aches and pains of low-grade polyarticular gout to dramatic attacks of extreme monoarticular pain to chronic polyarticular arthritis. Even in untreated gout, acute attacks resolve within several days to weeks. Presumptive diagnosis of acute gout can be made based on clinical signs and symptoms and a significant response to colchicine or nonsteroidal anti-inflammatory drugs (NSAIDs).

Timing of gouty attacks is quite variable and unpredictable, with the second and subsequent gouty attacks occurring weeks or decades later. However, gout recurs within 1 year in more than half of patients. As time passes, gouty attacks tend to occur more frequently, with greater severity, and with polyarticular involvement that is often refractory or poorly responsive to therapy. For unknown reasons, gouty attacks may be slightly more common in spring.

Gout in elderly people is often polyarticular and involves upper extremity joints (especially proximal interphalangeal joints and distal interphalangeal joints) and is associated with subcutaneous tophaceous deposits in the fingers, toes, and elbows. This may be misdiagnosed as rheumatoid arthritis.[7]

Women present 70% of the time with polyarticular disease rather than the classic monoarticular arthritis seen in men.[8]

Physical Examination

During acute gouty attacks, pain, swelling, redness, and exquisite tenderness develop suddenly in the joint and surrounding area, peaking within 24 to 48 hours. The heel, ankle, knee, midtarsal joints, and olecranon bursa can all be initially involved but less frequently than the first MTP. Acute polyarticular gout is less common but has a more dramatic presentation. Acute polyarticular gout can cause a high fever and leukocytosis, making it difficult to distinguish from septic arthritis.

Frequent, recurrent acute gouty attacks can lead to chronic gout, in which, joint swelling, deformity, and disability may be present. Deformity is caused by tophi, deposits of monosodium urate crystals in the soft tissue overlying joints.

Laboratory Studies

The presence of monosodium urate crystals in synovial fluid or tophi is diagnostic of gout. Negative joint cultures and hyperuricemia contribute to the presumptive diagnosis.

Pathologic Findings

In acute gout, needle-shaped urate crystals are found inside synovial fluid phagocytes or free within tophaceous deposits. These are strongly negatively birefringent under a polarized microscope lens. The calcium pyrophosphate crystals of pseudogout are, on the other hand, weakly positively birefringent and rhomboid-shaped.

Imaging

There are no imaging studies that are diagnostic of acute gouty arthritis. The classic radiographic finding of chronic gout is sharply marginated erosions proximal to the joint space with an overlying rim of cortical bone. Uric acid calculi can be seen as filling defects on intravenous pyelograms.

Classification

- **Acute gout** describes acute painful attacks of arthritis induced by urate crystal deposition. During the intervals between acute gouty attacks, patients with early gout are virtually asymptomatic.
- **Intercritical gout** describes these asymptomatic periods. Urate crystals can be aspirated from quiescent joints during these interval periods; therefore, the finding of urate crystals during an acute episode provides little reassurance of a nonseptic cause; antibiotic therapy should be based on clinical presentation, Gram stain, and culture.[9] Crystals remain present in joints as long as hyperuricemia persists; when serum uric acid levels are reduced to normal, urate crystals slowly dissolve and finally disappear from the joint.
- **Chronic tophaceous gout** has become increasingly rare due to more widespread drug treatment of hyperuricemia and gout. Tophi without prior episodes of gouty arthritis are unusual because they normally occur after gout has been present for more than 10 years. Tophi can occur anywhere but tend to occur in the helix of the ear, proximal ulnar surface of the forearm, olecranon, Achilles tendon, prepatellar bursa, or near active joints. **Secondary gout** is caused by overproduction or underexcretion of uric acid due to drugs or other disease processes. Overproduction of uric acid occurs in myeloproliferative and lymphoproliferative disorders, polycythemia, hemolytic anemia, multiple myeloma, and other malignancies. Renal disease, diuretics, low doses of salicylates, chronic lead intoxication ("saturnine gout"), nicotinic acid, alcohol, ethambutol, and pyrazinamide all cause underexcretion of uric acid. Acute uric acid nephropathy occurs primarily in patients undergoing chemotherapy for hematologic or myeloproliferative disorders and can be prevented by several days of allopurinol administration and adequate hydration before initiation of chemotherapy.

Differential Diagnosis

Gout can be misdiagnosed as inflammatory osteoarthritis, particularly given that erosions on radiographs are seen in both conditions. Gout may be mistaken for rheumatoid arthritis because tophi may resemble rheumatoid nodules, and rheumatoid factor often becomes weakly positive as people age. It may be difficult to differentiate cellulitis or septic arthritis from gout, particularly when a low-grade fever, leukocytosis, redness, or desquamation is present. The term pseudogout, for calcium pyrophosphate deposition disease, belies the difficulty in clinically differentiating it from gout. For definitive diagnosis, joint fluid must be aspirated for culture and a search for urate crystals.

Treatment Approach

All patients with an established gout diagnosis should receive patient education on the role of uric acid, risk factors, and the natural course of the disease. Counseling should include diet and lifestyle recommendations. A comorbidity checklist should be used to consider secondary causes of hyperuricemia, and nonessential medications, which induce hyperuricemia, should be considered for elimination.[2] Acute gouty arthritis attacks should be treated with pharmacologic therapy, preferably initiated within

24 to 48 hours of symptom onset. The choice of pharmacologic agent should depend largely on the severity of pain and the number of joints involved, acknowledging that combination therapy may be an appropriate option if pain is severe or one to two large joints are involved.[10]

Medications

NSAIDs, colchicine, and systemic corticosteroids are all considered appropriate first-line options for an acute gouty attack. Specific medication choice should be based upon patient preference, prior response to treatment, and associated comorbidities.[10]

- **NSAIDs** are recommended for use in acute gout and three (indomethacin, naproxen, and sulindac) have specific FDA approval for gout treatment. There is no evidence that one specific NSAID is superior to the others, but all NSAIDs should be prescribed at anti-inflammatory dosing levels and continued at that level until symptoms are completely resolved. Dosing may be tapered in patients with renal failure. COX-2 inhibitors are an option in patients with gastrointestinal (GI) contraindications or NSAID intolerance; celecoxib 800 mg one time followed by 400 mg on day 1 then 400 mg bid for 1 week was shown to be equal to indomethacin in acute gout.[10] NSAIDs can cause GI toxicity (nausea, abdominal discomfort, GI bleeding, peptic ulcer disease), nephrotoxicity, and central nervous system side effects (headache, dizziness, confusion). Therefore, they must be used with caution, especially in the elderly or in patients with underlying disease. **Colchicine** terminates most acute gouty attacks within 6 to 12 hours; however, it is limited by its GI side effects and is often poorly tolerated by the elderly. Colchicine is much more effective if given within the first 12 to 24 hours of an acute attack. Its mechanism of action is not entirely known but apparently reduces the inflammatory response to urate crystals and diminishes phagocytosis. Recommended dosing has changed, with the most recent guidelines now suggesting a loading dose of 1.2 mg of colchicine followed by 0.6 mg orally 1 hour later, and then 0.6 mg up to three times daily thereafter.[10] Possible bone marrow toxicity limits the total dose for a single day to 4.8 mg (less if the patient has hepatic or renal disease). Colchicine should be used prophylactically when initiating uric acid–lowering therapy to prevent precipitating an acute gouty attack. The optimal duration of prophylaxis is unknown, but it can usually be stopped after the uric acid level is brought down to a normal range for 2 months. Colchicine, 0.6 mg bid, is usually started several days before the urate-lowering therapy is started. **Corticosteroids** are an additional first-line treatment option. Prednisone or prednisolone at 5 to 10 mg per kg per day for 5 to 10 days can be given followed by discontinuation, or 2 to 5 days at the full dose may be followed by a 7- to 10-day taper. Rebound can be avoided by using colchicine prophylactically, 0.6 mg PO bid, which should then be discontinued 6 to 8 weeks later. In patients with gout involving one or two large joints (ankle, knee, wrist, elbow, hip, or shoulder) or who are unable to tolerate oral therapy, intra-articular corticosteroid injections are useful. These usually result in resolution of an acute gouty episode within 12 to 24 hours.
- **Combination therapy** may be appropriate for patients with severe acute gout (pain >7 on a 10-point pain scale) and for patients with an acute polyarthritis or involvement of more than one large joint, full doses of two of the pharmacologic modalities recommended above may be used in combination. The exception to this is a combination of corticosteroids and NSAIDs, which would pose an unacceptably high risk of GI side effects.[10]
- **Allopurinol** (Zyloprim) is a xanthine oxidase inhibitor that decreases the production of uric acid. For patients with recurrent gouty attacks (more than one per year), renal stones, renal damage, or uric acid–lowering therapy should be initiated. Allopurinol is effective in most patients regardless of the source of hyperuricemia (overproduction or underexcretion) because it produces a more soluble metabolite. A 24-hour urinary uric acid determination to differentiate urate overproduction from underexcretion is therefore unnecessary in most patients. Allopurinol is also better tolerated than uricosuric agents, has fewer drug–drug interactions, is effective in patients with renal failure or nephrolithiasis, and is used in a single daily dose. In patients receiving chemotherapy, allopurinol should be used when daily uric acid excretion exceeds 800 mg per 24 hours in male patients and 750 mg per 24 hours in female patients. Allopurinol may be started at 100 mg daily with food and increased at weekly intervals by 100 mg until a serum uric acid level of 6 mg per dL or less is attained. The average effective dose for mild gout is 200 to 300 mg per day, although some patients need 400 to 600 mg per day, particularly those with tophaceous gout or those on cancer chemotherapy. Enough fluids should be taken to keep daily urine output greater than 2 L. If an acute attack occurs while taking allopurinol, the dose should be maintained as is and the attack treated as usual (e.g., NSAIDs, colchicine). In elderly patients, a starting dose of 50 to 100 mg on alternate days, to a

maximum daily dose of 100 to 300 mg based on the patient's creatinine clearance and serum urate level, decreases the risk of hypersensitivity reactions.[8] Life-threatening hypersensitivity reactions to allopurinol involving skin, kidney, and liver occur rarely but are being recognized with increasing frequency. The most frequent adverse reactions to allopurinol are skin rash, GI reactions (diarrhea, nausea, and alkaline phosphatase, aspartate aminotransferase, and alanine aminotransferase elevations), and acute attacks of gout, which can be minimized by proper use. Renal function must be monitored in patients taking thiazide diuretics. Allopurinol may also cause a rash in patients taking ampicillin or amoxicillin, and it may potentiate anticoagulants.[8]

- **Febuxostat (Adenuric)**, a newer xanthine oxidase inhibitor, is also considered a first-line urate-lowering therapy, with no evidence of clear superiority between febuxostat and allopurinol. Febuxostat has been shown to be effective at reducing urate levels to <6 mg per dL. Some evidence indicates that it is slightly more effective at reducing uric acid levels, but with a slightly higher risk of precipitating an acute gout attack. The increased rate of acute attacks does not persist over time, and can be managed by prophylaxis with anti-inflammatory agents or colchicine.[11]

- **Uricosuric drugs** are indicated for patients who need urate-lowering therapy but are intolerant or unresponsive to xanthine oxidase inhibitors. These medications block renal tubular reabsorption of uric acid. As with allopurinol, they should never be started during an acute attack but should be maintained if started previously. Before using these agents, a 24-hour urine for creatinine clearance and urine uric acid should be performed, as uricosuric drugs are ineffective for a glomerular filtration rate less than 50 mL per minute and can increase the risk of urate stones if the urinary uric acid is already elevated (>800 mg per 24 hours). Urate stone formation can be minimized if patients maintain a high fluid intake and alkalinize the urine. These medications include probenecid and sulfinpyrazone.

- **Probenecid** (Benemid) is started at 250 mg bid for 1 week and then 500 mg bid after that. The dose is increased by 500 mg every 1 to 2 weeks until the serum urate level is normal or the 24-hour uric acid excretion is at or below 800 mg. The usual effective dose is 500 mg twice daily. Probenecid is well tolerated but is not effective in even mild renal insufficiency, and should not be used in patients with creatinine >2. It also should not be used with salicylates, as they antagonize its action. It can also raise plasma levels of penicillin, sulfonylureas, and NSAIDs. In patients with glucose-6-phosphate dehydrogenase deficiency, it can cause hemolytic anemia.

Special Therapy

Arthroscopic Removal of Urate Crystals

A small cohort study demonstrated that surgical removal of urate crystals from the first MTP joint reduced gout flares and improved function compared with standard therapy in patients followed for 4 years.[12]

Counseling

Although no randomized controlled trials have proved the effectiveness of counseling patients on decreasing the frequency of gouty attacks, it is prudent for the physician to counsel patients with a gout history about factors known to worsen the course of the disease. Counseling should suggest dietary decrease in meat and seafood, and a corresponding increase in dairy product consumption. Advice on weight loss may also be beneficial. The American College of Rheumatology advises a thorough patient education effort that includes a basic explanation of the disease, treatment options, and objectives of treatment, including the reduction of uric acid.[2]

Risk Management

Although there are multiple disease states that increase risk of gouty attacks, the presence of gout generally does not increase risks for other diseases or have multiple complications. One exception to this is in the kidney, namely, interstitial renal disease and nephrolithiasis. Men with gout have a twofold increased risk for developing kidney stones compared with men without gout. Therefore, it may be prudent to counsel men to increase fluid intake and decrease salt consumption to modify this risk factor.[13]

REFERENCES

1. Zhu YM, Pandya BJ, Choi HK. Prevalence of goat and hyperuricemia in the US general population: the National Health and Nutrition Examination Survey 2007–2008. *Arthritis Rheum* 2011;63(10):3136–3141.

2. Khanna D, Fitzgerald JD, Khanna PP, et al. 2012 American college of Rheumatology guidelines for management of gout. Part I: systematic nonpharmacologic and pharmacologic therapeutic approaches to hyperuricemia. *Arthritis Care Res* 2012;64(10):1431–1446.
3. Neogi T. Clinical practice. Gout. *N Engl J Med* 2011;364(5):443–452.
4. Schlesinger N, Baker DG, Schumacher HR. Serum urate during bouts of acute gouty arthritis. *J Rheumatol* 1997;24(11):2265–2266.
5. Choi HK, Atkinson K, Karlson E, et al. Obesity, weight change, hypertension, diuretic use, and risk of gout in men: the health professionals follow-up study. *Arch Intern Med* 2005;165(7):742–748.
6. Choi HK, Atkinson K, Karlson E, et al. Purine-rich foods, dairy and protein intake, and the risk of gout in men. *N Engl J Med* 2004;350(11):1093–1103.
7. Sturrock RD. Gout: easy to misdiagnose. *BMJ* 2000;320(7228):132–133.
8. Lally EV, Ho G, Kaplan SR. The clinical spectrum of gouty arthritis in women. *Arch Intern Med* 1986;146(11):2221–2225.
9. Johnson JR. Diagnosis of intercritical gout. *Ann Intern Med* 2000;132(10):843.
10. Khanna D, Khanna PP, Fitzgerald JD, et al. 2012 American college of Rheumatology guidelines for management of gout. Part II: therapy and anti-inflammatory prophylaxis of acute gouty arthritis. *Arthritis Care Res* 2012;64(10):1447–1461.
11. Tayar JH, Lopez-Olivo MA, Suarez-Almazor ME. Febuxostat for treating chronic gout. *Cochrane Database Syst Rev* 2012;11:CD008653. doi: 10.1002/14651858.CD008653.pub2
12. Wang CC, Lien SB, Huang GS, et al. Arthroscopic elimination of monosodium urate deposition of the first metatarsophalangeal joint reduces the recurrence of gout. *Arthroscopy* 2009;25(2):153–158.
13. Kramer HJ, Choi HK, Atkinson K, et al. The association between gout and nephrolithiasis in men: the health professionals' follow-up study. *Kidney Int* 2003;64(3):1022–1026.

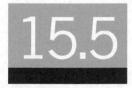

15.5 Overuse Injuries

Matthew C. Schaffer, Ted C. Schaffer

GENERAL PRINCIPLES

Definition

Overuse injuries occur when forces applied over time to a bone, muscle, tendon, or ligament exceed the ability of those tissues to adapt to the forces. Repetitive microtrauma leads to local tissue damage in the form of cellular and extracellular degeneration, and most likely occurs more often with a sudden change in mode, intensity, or duration of activity.

Epidemiology

More than 50% of pediatric sports injuries are overuse injuries.[1] More than 50% of occupational illnesses involve overuse from repetitive motion injuries.

Pathophysiology

The muscle-tendon unit is the most common site of injury, but other structures such as bone, cartilage, ligament, bursa, and fascia may be involved. In children, the growth plates are also vulnerable to the stress of repetitive injury.

Etiology

The etiology is multifactorial, involving a pathway of repetitive microtrauma and local tissue injury. Modification of both intrinsic and extrinsic risk factors is essential for injury treatment and prevention.
- **Intrinsic risk factors** are inherent characteristics of an individual's body. These include muscle inflexibility, muscle weakness, joint laxity, previous injury, anatomic malalignment, and lower extremity asymmetry. Frequently a deficit in one body area may affect function in another region.
- **Extrinsic risk factors** include equipment malfunction, training errors, environmental conditions, biomechanical errors, and ergonomic problems.[1]

TREATMENT APPROACH

- **Initial treatment** aims to reduce the inflammatory process with relative rest and ice.
  - **Ice.** Applied for 15 to 30 minutes every 2 to 6 hours over the first 24 to 48 hours as necessary.
  - **Nonsteroidal anti-inflammatory drugs (NSAIDs).** Controversial in acute and chronic injury—may reduce inflammation, but may also slow inflammatory-mediated healing.
  - **Modalities** such as ultrasound, electrical stimulation, or iontophoresis may reduce initial inflammation.
  - **Corticosteroid** injection may reduce inflammation for certain injuries (e.g., subacromial bursitis and de Quervain tenosynovitis). Side effects may include subcutaneous fat atrophy or necrosis, depigmentation, hyperpigmentation, tendon rupture, accelerated joint destruction, or infection. Diagnostic information may be obtained if injection of local anesthetic (1% lidocaine or 0.5% bupivacaine) reduces local pain.
- **Definitive treatment** includes identification and modification of predisposing risk factors. Exercises, especially eccentric exercises, address deficits in strength, flexibility, and proprioception. Rehabilitation efforts include correcting biomechanical abnormalities, such as poor throwing motion, as well as addressing poor ergonomics, such as chair height or computer screen adaptation. Incomplete rehabilitation of any previous injury is also addressed.

ROTATOR CUFF TENDINOPATHY

Diagnosis

Clinical Presentation

Rotator cuff tendinopathy is a common cause of nontraumatic shoulder pain in both children and adults. Pain is frequently insidious, and there is often a nocturnal component. In adults, impingement of the supraspinatus tendon as it runs beneath the subacromial arch is the most common cause of tendinopathy.

Physical Examination

Pain with shoulder abduction is the most common finding. Provocative maneuvers with forward flexion and internal rotation (Neer or Hawkins signs), which force the humerus into the subacromial space, will often reproduce symptoms.

Imaging

Radiographs are helpful in excluding other causes of persistent (greater than 6 weeks) shoulder pain, including calcific tendonitis, glenohumeral arthrosis, and bone tumors. A supraspinatus outlet view is helpful to evaluate the bony morphology of the anterior acromion. For diagnostic uncertainty coupled with persistent pain or for treatment nonresponders, magnetic resonance imaging (MRI), potentially with gadolinium contrast, is useful to help guide treatment.

Treatment

Nonoperative

Initial treatment includes ice, a limited course of NSAIDs, and avoiding aggravating factors. A subacromial corticosteroid injection combined with local anesthetic may confirm symptom source and reduce pain. More definitive therapy involves maximizing glenohumeral motion, stabilizing the scapulothoracic articulation, strengthening the rotator cuff, and addressing biomechanical or ergonomic errors.[2]

Operative

For adults with persistent impingement symptoms, MRI completion and referral for surgery to relieve bony impingement may be necessary.

EPICONDYLITIS

Diagnosis

Clinical Presentation

Epicondylitis is the most common overuse problem in the elbow. Pain, often insidious, is present over the affected epicondylar region. Excessive wrist extension precedes lateral epicondylitis, whereas excessive wrist flexion precedes medial epicondylitis. Lateral epicondylitis is more common than medial epicondylitis.

Physical Examination

With lateral epicondylitis, "tennis elbow," pain radiates distally along the extensor forearm muscles. Symptoms are reproduced with resisted wrist extension while the forearm is pronated and with resisted supination. With medial epicondylitis, "golfer's elbow," pain is commonly elicited with resistance to wrist flexion and forearm pronation. Reduced grip strength may be noted with either condition.

Imaging
For treatment nonresponders, MRI can help to identify tendon tears that may warrant surgical intervention.

Treatment

Nonoperative
Initial treatment includes ice with friction massage, relative rest, and a short course of NSAIDs. Avoiding pronation activities may be useful in lateral epicondylitis. A counterforce brace distal to the affected epicondyle may be useful, as may a short period of wrist splint immobilization to reduce the aggravating motion. When pain persists, a corticosteroid injection at the site of maximal tenderness may improve symptoms. Care should be exercised in a medial epicondyle injection to avoid infiltrating the ulnar nerve. Rehabilitation should include stretching and strengthening, especially eccentric strengthening of the forearm musculature, and biomechanical or ergonomic modifications.[3]

Operative
Rarely, treatment nonresponders may require surgical debridement for relief of symptoms.

CARPAL TUNNEL SYNDROME
Diagnosis

Clinical Presentation
Carpal tunnel syndrome is an entrapment neuropathy caused by compression of the median nerve between the transverse carpal ligament and the flexor tendons of the wrist. Symptoms of pain, paresthesias, and/or numbness occur in the sensory distribution of the median nerve, especially the index finger. Presentation occurs bilaterally in up to 50% of cases. Commonly affected groups include middle-aged women and workers with repetitive manual labor. Tasks requiring a strong grip with wrist flexion and extension or that have vibration exposure are at greatest risk. The majority of patients experience pain that is strong enough to awaken them from sleep, with relief obtained by shaking their wrist ("flick sign"). The syndrome affects up to 3% of the population, and is three times more common in women.[4]

Physical Examination
Pain in the distribution of the median nerve often can be elicited with percussion over the median nerve (Tinel sign), hyperflexion of the wrist (Phalen test), or compression of the median nerve (Durkan test). Severe cases often result in thenar atrophy. Diagnostic confirmation can be made with electromyography (EMG) and nerve conduction study (NCS) testing.

Imaging
Wrist radiographs are rarely of help, although a special carpal tunnel view can rule out other anomalies, such as a fracture of the hook of the hamate.

Treatment

Nonoperative
Initial identification of aggravating causes, including work modification, may be all that is needed for mild cases. Other early interventions may include nocturnal or job-specific splinting, while NSAID use is less certain to provide benefit.[5] Direct injection of corticosteroid into the carpal tunnel often alleviates symptoms initially, but a majority still progress to surgery.[5,6]

Operative
For refractory cases, or when EMG/NCS reveals moderate to severe nerve compression, median nerve decompression by incision of the transverse carpal ligament is recommended.

DE QUERVAIN TENOSYNOVITIS
Diagnosis

Clinical Presentation
De Quervain disease is characterized by inflammation of the first dorsal compartment of the wrist (containing the extensor pollicis brevis and abductor pollicis longus) as it passes over the radial styloid.

Excessive repetitive hand motion, especially involving radial and ulnar wrist deviation, is a frequent cause.

Physical Examination
Pain is exquisitely reproduced by sharp ulnar deviation of the hand with the thumb flexed (Finkelstein test).

Imaging
Imaging is rarely of help in making the diagnosis. Degenerative arthritis of the first carpal–metacarpal joint may be seen, but this problem manifests pain in a different location.

Treatment

Nonoperative
First-line treatment is local corticosteroid injection into the tendon sheath. Recent evidence suggests little to no added benefit from NSAIDs and/or thumb spica splinting versus injection alone. Iontophoresis may also be useful as an early modality.[7]

Operative
When nonoperative treatments fail to alleviate symptoms, surgical release of the compartment may be necessary.

TRIGGER FINGER
Diagnosis

Clinical Presentation
Trigger finger involves a stenosing tenosynovitis of the flexor tendons of the hand. Although the complaint may be of pain at the proximal interphalangeal (PIP) joint, the problem is actually located at the palmar surface of the metacarpophalangeal (MCP) joint.

Physical Examination
Most commonly, inflammation involves the A1 pulley, the first of five pulleys that guide the flexor tendon into the finger. Locking or triggering may occur as the stenosed tendon becomes trapped in the pulley.

Treatment

Nonoperative
Treatment is focused on a corticosteroid tendon sheath injection. For persistent or recurrent symptoms, a second injection several months later with application of a trigger-finger splint may be helpful, provided that the first injection yielded some symptomatic relief.

Operative
For patients who do not respond after a first injection, or whose symptoms recur after a second injection, surgical release of the pulley will be necessary.

PATELLOFEMORAL PAIN SYNDROME
Diagnosis

Clinical Presentation
Patellofemoral pain syndrome (PFPS) or patellofemoral dysfunction refers to anterior knee pain arising from the patellofemoral joint. Symptoms can range from mild activity-related knee pain to severe pain limiting ordinary activities. Pain typically worsens after prolonged sitting with the knees flexed ("theater sign") or with activities that require repetitive knee flexion, such as stair climbing/descending or running.

Physical Examination
Palpation often elicits tenderness of the medial or lateral patellar facets. Pain increases with downward pressure applied to the superior pole of the patella during isometric quadriceps contraction (patellar grind/compression test). Provocative maneuvers of the ligaments or menisci will be negative.

Imaging
Radiographs are most helpful in excluding other diagnoses, such as osteochondritis dissecans. A patellar "sunrise" or "merchant" view, which can reveal patella tilting, most commonly to the lateral side, is suggestive but not diagnostic of PFPS.

Treatment

Nonoperative

Treatment should be aimed at reducing pain and eliminating predisposing risk factors. Activities with significant quadriceps loading, such as stair climbing, should be minimized. After a brief period of relative rest, ice, and NSAIDs, a rehabilitation program should focus on correcting lower extremity deficits in flexibility, strength, and proprioception. Abnormal foot biomechanics, such as excessive pronation, should be addressed. Patellar taping techniques or bracing to correct malalignment may reduce symptoms.[8]

Operative

Surgery is rarely needed for PFPS. In refractory conditions, release of the lateral retinaculum can be considered.

ILIOTIBIAL BAND SYNDROME

Diagnosis

Clinical Presentation

Iliotibial (IT) band syndrome refers to lateral hip or lateral knee pain due to chronic friction of the IT band over the greater tuberosity of the femur and/or the lateral femoral condyle. Pain, usually achy in quality, is worsened by activities with repetitive knee and hip flexion, such as distance running and cycling.

Physical Examination

Palpation often elicits tenderness of the inflamed IT band over the lateral femoral condyle or greater trochanter, particularly if an associated bursitis has developed. Tightness of the IT band is usually demonstrated through a positive Ober test.[8]

Imaging

Although IT band syndrome is usually a clinical diagnosis, occasionally an MRI is obtained to exclude other potential surgical findings that may present similarly with knee lateral joint line tenderness, such as lateral meniscus injuries.

Treatment

Nonoperative

Treatment should be aimed at reducing pain and eliminating predisposing risk factors. After a brief period of relative rest, ice, and NSAIDs, a rehabilitation program should focus on stretching the IT band and hamstrings and strengthening the hip abductors, along with correcting training errors, such as excessive downhill running. Friction massage, such as with foam rolling, may help to break up the areas of thickening and scarring. Localized corticosteroid injection may be offered when pain and swelling persist despite more conservative measures.

Operative

In cases that are unresponsive to nonoperative management, surgical release may be considered.

PREPATELLAR BURSITIS–"HOUSEMAID'S KNEE"

Diagnosis

Clinical Presentation

Chronic inflammation of the prepatellar bursa results from recurrent trauma, such as repetitive kneeling.

Physical Examination

Acute trauma may also lead to immediate swelling of the prepatellar bursa, as can underlying infection. If infection is suspected, aspiration for Gram stain and culture should be performed.

Treatment

Nonoperative

Protective padding is an essential part of treatment in recurrent cases. When infection is suspected, antibiotics should be instituted after cultures are obtained. Chronic inflammation may respond to a corticosteroid injection.

Operative

For refractory cases, surgical excision of the bursa may be necessary.

MEDIAL TIBIAL STRESS SYNDROME—"SHIN SPLINTS"
Diagnosis
Clinical Presentation
Both the name and exact cause of this entity, which is common among runners, dancers, and other athletes, continue to generate controversy. Pain typically increases at the onset of activity, improves with continued activity, and resolves with rest; however, symptoms often intensify with higher activity levels. Contributing intrinsic factors include anatomic malalignment and deficits in flexibility and strength of the lower extremity. Extrinsic factors include inadequate or worn-down footwear, insufficient warm-up, uneven or hard running surfaces, and rapid advancement of a training regimen.

Physical Examination
The diagnosis is based on diffuse pain and tenderness at the posteromedial aspect of the tibia.

Imaging
Radiographs are useful primarily to rule out other disorders, such as tibial or fibular stress fractures.

Treatment
Nonoperative
Initial treatment includes relative rest, ice massage, and NSAIDs. Occasionally symptoms can persist for weeks, especially if the athlete continues at high levels of activity. Total rest, including cessation of all athletic activities, may be necessary to resolve symptoms. Definitive treatment also includes identification and correction of modifiable risk factors, along with a gradual increase to premorbid activity levels.[9]

PLANTAR FASCIITIS/FASCIOSIS
Diagnosis
Clinical Presentation
Heel pain from plantar fasciitis is caused by degenerative thickening (and potentially inflammation) of the aponeurosis that arises from the calcaneus and inserts distally on the proximal phalanges. The pain is typically most intense upon arising in the morning, with symptom improvement during activity. Risk factors include obesity, excessive foot pronation, poor lower extremity flexibility, planus or cavus foot type, and calf weakness. Patients may be active or sedentary.

Physical Examination
Frequently, severe pain and tenderness localize to a single plantar area slightly anterior to the medial calcaneal tubercle.

Imaging
Radiographs are of little diagnostic help. Although 50% of patients with plantar fasciitis show heel spurs on the anterior calcaneus, this finding is also present in up to 25% of asymptomatic individuals.

Treatment
Nonoperative
Initial measures should include relative rest, appropriate shoe support including shoe inserts, and calf stretching. As a second step, custom-made night splints, physical therapy, and corticosteroid injection may be helpful. Extracorporeal shock wave therapy may be effective in select populations, such as runners with chronic heel pain.[10]

Operative
In rare cases, surgical intervention is needed to relieve symptoms.

ACHILLES TENDINOPATHY
Diagnosis
Clinical Presentation
Patients complain of pain and swelling in the Achilles tendon, usually 4 to 7 cm proximal to the calcaneal insertion. Activity will exacerbate the pain.

Physical Examination
Dorsiflexion of the foot or local palpation reproduces the symptoms, and the patient may have an antalgic gait.

Treatment

Nonoperative

Ice, NSAIDs, relative rest, and gentle calf stretching should be the first treatments. Early referral for physical therapy should be added to address flexibility, resolve strength deficits (eccentric strengthening exercises are key), and correct biomechanical abnormalities. Recently, topical nitroglycerine has been demonstrated as a useful adjunct in promoting healing.[3]

STRESS FRACTURES

Diagnosis

Clinical Presentation

When repetitive weight-bearing activity causes the bony architecture to exceed a given threshold, a stress injury can occur. The process begins as a stress reaction; however, if allowed to progress unabated, a stress fracture will result. Risk factors include sudden increases in training regimen or activity level, osteopenia, poor biomechanics, and hormonal factors. In general, women are more susceptible than men.

History

Symptoms begin with progressive localized pain with activity that resolves with rest. If untreated, pain will occur with lower levels of activity, and eventually with rest. Approximately 90% to 95% of stress fractures involve the lower extremity, although specific sports can be associated with upper body injuries (rowing: rib fractures; throwing: humerus/ulnar fractures).

Physical Examination

Palpation usually elicits point tenderness over the bone with distal lower extremity involvement. In proximal lower extremity fractures, the pain may be more ill-defined. The most common sites for injury are the tibia, metatarsals, and fibula.

Imaging

Radiographs are often normal until 2 to 4 weeks from symptom onset, when reactive sclerosis of the bone appears. Bone scans may provide diagnostic confirmation as early as 72 hours from symptom onset, but early findings may be inconclusive. MRI is an expensive but very accurate diagnostic tool, with detection as early as 24 to 48 hours from symptom onset.

Classification

Stress fractures can be divided into high-risk and low-risk fractures based on their potential for long-term morbidity (Table 15.5-1). High-risk fractures have greater potential for complications such as

TABLE 15.5-1	Stress Fracture Identification			
Location	**Frequency**	**At risk for long-term morbidity?**	**Physical finding**	**Immediate treatment**
Second and third metatarsals	Common	No	Localized tenderness	Rest; symptomatic
Proximal fifth metatarsal	Occasional	Yes	Localized tenderness	NWB, casting vs. surgery
Tarsal navicular	Occasional in track and field	Yes	Midfoot pain	NWB, casting
Posterior-medial tibial shaft	Common	No	Localized tenderness	Rest; symptomatic
Mid-tibial anterior cortex	Rare	Yes	Anterior shin pain	Prolonged rest; occasionally surgery
Fibula	Common	No	Localized tenderness	Rest; symptomatic
Femoral shaft	Occasional	No	Thigh pain	Rest; symptomatic
Femoral neck	Rare	Yes	Groin pain	NWB, orthopedic referral

NWB, non-weight-bearing.

delayed union, nonunion, bony displacement, or completed fracture. Orthopedic consultation is advisable for these injuries, which require individualized and prolonged management.

Treatment

Nonoperative

Immediate treatment for low-risk stress fractures includes relative rest, ice, and analgesics. Pain relief should be expected within 1 to 2 weeks. Non-weight-bearing activities, such as swimming or stationary biking, and muscle stretching should be encouraged until pain resolution indicates healing; then a gradual increase in activity level can be resumed along with appropriate counseling and review of the training regimen to prevent injury recurrence. Return to full activity after low-risk stress fractures typically is expected within 3 weeks to 3 months.[11]

Operative

Once a high-risk stress fracture is suspected, activity should be very limited (often includes non-weight-bearing) until an accurate diagnosis is made and orthopedic consultation is obtained. Occasionally surgery may be indicated (Table 15.5-1).

SPECIAL CONSIDERATIONS—OVERUSE SYNDROMES IN CHILDREN

Osgood–Schlatter Disease

Diagnosis

- **Clinical presentation.** This traction apophysitis at the patellar insertion on the tibial tuberosity is a common complaint among peripubertal adolescents. Caused in part by longitudinal forces created by rapidly growing bones, Osgood–Schlatter disease is associated with increased physical activity.
- **Physical examination.** Palpation reveals localized edema and tenderness over the tibial tuberosity.
- **Imaging.** Imaging is needed only in refractory cases, primarily to rule out other problems such as bone tumors.

Treatment

- **Nonoperative.** Several days or weeks of relative rest, along with analgesics, reduce symptoms to a manageable level. A bony prominence may remain due to residual fragmentation of the upper tibial epiphysis. Improvement in lower extremity flexibility and reduction of quadriceps loading, especially with stair walking, will help to reduce symptoms. For refractory cases, several weeks of prolonged rest may be necessary.

Sever Disease

Diagnosis

- **Clinical presentation.** This is a calcaneal apophysitis, similar to Osgood–Schlatter disease, which occurs primarily in adolescent male soccer players.
- **Physical examination.** Inflammation at the insertion of the calcaneal apophysis leads to localized pain, tenderness, and swelling, which may be aggravated by activity.

Treatment

- **Nonoperative.** Treatment includes ice, relative rest, calf stretching, and often a temporary heel lift.[8,12]

Little League Elbow

Diagnosis

- **Clinical presentation.** This phrase is often used broadly to describe medial elbow pain due to repetitive valgus stresses in the skeletally immature thrower, most commonly involving baseball pitchers. Although other related abnormalities can result from a similar mechanism, the phrase "little league elbow" specifically implies medial epicondyle apophysitis. Contributing factors include improper warm-up, poor throwing mechanics, elevated pitch counts, and throwing curveballs.[9]
- **Physical examination.** Pain is reproduced with the throwing motion, and palpation usually reveals localized tenderness over the medial epicondyle.
- **Imaging.** Radiographs are important to exclude other bony abnormalities associated with little league elbow, such as osteochondral defects, loose foreign bodies, or growth plate irregularities.[8]

Treatment

- **Nonoperative.** Rest, ice, and occasionally a short course of NSAIDs are the first therapies. When symptoms subside, the patient may play a less-demanding position (e.g., first base) as long as he or she is pain-free while throwing. Stretching and strengthening of the muscles of the forearm, shoulder, and scapulothoracic region are the mainstays of rehabilitation. Return to pitching should be in months, not days or weeks.

Spondylolysis

Diagnosis

- **Clinical presentation.** Up to 50% of back pain in adolescent athletes may be caused by a vertebral defect in the pars interarticularis. The defect can be unilateral or bilateral, and is thought to be due to repetitive hyperextension of the posterior spine in gymnasts, ballet dancers, offensive linemen, and volleyball and soccer players. The problem most commonly affects the fourth and fifth lumbar vertebrae. Patients present with activity-related back pain exacerbated by hyperextension.
- **Physical examination.** The best test is pain reproduced with ipsilateral single leg hyperextension ("stork test"). Other findings may include hyperlordotic posture, decreased range of motion, and hamstring tightness.
- **Imaging.** Initial studies should include a full lumbar series with anteroposterior (AP), lateral, and oblique films. On the oblique view, spondylolysis manifests as a "Scotty dog sign," which is a complete fracture through the pars interarticularis. Radiographs may also demonstrate spondylolisthesis, which is the anterior or posterior displacement of a vertebral body on another. When spondylolysis is suspected but initial x-rays are negative, other more sensitive tests can be ordered, including a single photon emission computed tomography (SPECT) scan, MRI scan, or CT scan.

Treatment

- **Nonoperative.** Accepted treatment includes relative rest, analgesics, and often bracing to limit hyperextension. When bracing is used, it should be continued until the patient is completely asymptomatic or there is radiographic evidence of complete healing. In some cases, this may take up to 9–12 months. Physical therapy should focus on lumbar flexion, hamstring stretching, and core strengthening. The goal with prolonged treatment is to prevent nonunion and subsequent spondylolisthesis.[1,8]
- **Operative.** While treatment for low-grade (up to 50%) spondylolisthesis is similar to spondylolysis, more severe grades typically require surgical spine stabilization.

REFERENCES

1. DiFiori JP, Benjamin HJ, Brenner JS, et al. Overuse injuries and burnout in youth sports: a position statement from the American Medical Society for Sports Medicine. *Br J Sports Med* 2014;48:287–288.
2. St Pierre P. Rotator cuff pathology. In: O'Connor FG, Casa DJ, Davis BA, et al., eds. *ACSM's sports medicine: a comprehensive review.* Philadelphia, PA: Lippincott Williams & Wilkins; 2013:317–322.
3. Rodenberg RE, Bowman E, Ravindran R. Overuse injuries. *Prim Care Clin Office Pract* 2013;40:453–473.
4. Wipperman J, Potter L. Carpal tunnel syndrome—try these diagnostic maneuvers. *J Fam Pract* 2012;61:726–732.
5. Ashworth NL. Carpal tunnel syndrome. *Clin Evid* 2011;10:1114.
6. Atroshi I, Flondell M, Hofer M, et al. Methylprednisolone injections for the carpal tunnel syndrome: a randomized, placebo-controlled trial. *Ann Intern Med* 2013;159:309–317.
7. Crop JA, Bunt CW. Doctor, my thumb hurts. *J Fam Pract* 2011;60(6):329–332.
8. Hoang QB, Mortazavi M. Pediatric overuse injuries in sports. *Adv Pediatr* 2012;59:359–383.
9. Rodriguez CR, Fountain LB, Mularoni PP, et al. *Sports medicine in children. FP essentials*, Edition No. 417. Leawood, KS: American Academy of Family Physicians; February 2014.
10. Teh J, Suppiah R, Sharp R, et al. Imaging in the assessment and management of overuse injuries in the foot and ankle. *Semin Musculoskelet Radiol* 2011;15:101–114.
11. Liem BC, Truswell HJ, Harrast MA. Rehabilitation and return to running after lower limb stress fractures. *Curr Sports Med Rep* 2013;12:200–207.
12. Chang GH, Paz DA, Dwek JR, et al. Lower extremity overuse injuries in pediatric athletes: clinical presentation, imaging findings, and treatment. *Clin Imaging* 2013;37:836–846.

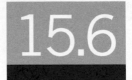

Arthrocentesis and Joint and Soft-Tissue Injections

Michael J. Henehan, Amy White Hockenbrock

The removal of joint fluid (arthrocentesis) and intra-articular (joint) or soft-tissue injection of medication are common primary care procedures. The indications and techniques for these procedures are outlined here.[1,2]

INDICATIONS
Arthrocentesis (Figure 15.6-1)

Diagnostic

Arthrocentesis is helpful to evaluate a joint effusion of uncertain etiology. The differential diagnosis includes septic arthritis, aseptic inflammation (rheumatologic process), degenerative changes, and traumatic effusion (hemarthrosis).

Therapeutic

In rare instances, repetitive joint aspiration is indicated to relieve pain and restore range of motion. In general, treatment of the underlying problem is preferred because the joint fluid will often reaccumulate rapidly, and repeated arthrocentesis may increase the risk of infection.

Intra-Articular and Soft-Tissue Injection (Figure 15.6-2)

Diagnostic

Intra-articular and soft-tissue injection can be helpful in definitively locating and differentiating the pain etiology.

Therapeutic

- Therapeutic injections relieve inflammation in tendon sheaths, bursae, muscles, and joints in inflammatory, noninfectious arthropathies.
- Therapeutic injections provide adjunctive therapy for joint and soft-tissue inflammation not responsive to systemic therapy.[1,2]

Risks and Risk Management

- **Intravascular injection.** Always aspirate back into your syringe before injecting any contents. If blood is aspirated, slightly withdraw and redirect the needle, and proceed again.

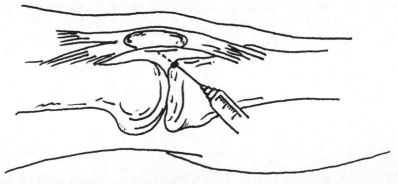

Figure 15.6-1. Arthrocentesis of the knee.

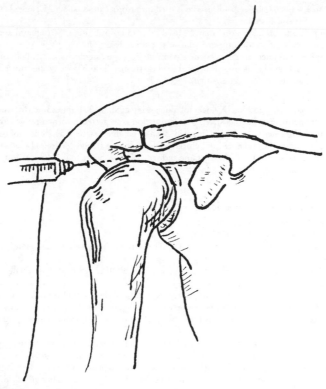

Figure 15.6-2. Injecting the subacromial space: lateral approach.

- **Tendon rupture.** Avoid injecting directly into a tendon. Ideally, the medication should be injected into the surrounding bursa or tendon sheath. Allow 2 weeks before re-injecting or permitting significant load-bearing activities when injecting around large tendons.
- **Hypersensitivity.** Ask about allergies to medication options before injecting.
- **Infection.** Use sterile technique and avoid multiple injections.
- **Anatomical hazards.** Review the anatomy to avoid nerves, large blood vessels, and organs.
- **Hematoma.** Apply a pressure dressing upon completion of the procedure.
- **Postinjection pain.** Pain occurs in about 5% of patients. It is thought to be a local inflammatory response. The pain usually lasts 24 to 36 hours and occurs within hours of the injection.
- **Tissue atrophy.** Fat degeneration and subsequent tissue atrophy can occur due to the catabolic properties of corticosteroids. The more superficial the injection, the more likely atrophy is to occur.
- **Skin discoloration.** This is usually a postinflammatory reaction hypopigmentation due to the corticosteroid. The change is most pronounced in dark-skinned individuals and is most likely to occur with superficial injections.[2]

Contraindications to Joint Injection
- Suspicion of septic arthritis or bacteremia.
- Known or suspected coagulopathy.
- Cellulitis overlying the proposed injection site.
- More than three steroid injections in a weight-bearing joint during a 12-month period (relative contraindication).[1,2]

Supplies
Antiseptic solution (e.g., povidone–iodine, alcohol swabs)

- **Syringes.** A 10- to 30-mL syringe is used for arthrocentesis, and a 3- to 10-mL syringe for joint or soft-tissue injection.

- **Needles.** An 18- to 20-gauge 1.5-in. needle is used for arthrocentesis, and a 25-gauge 1.5-in. needle for joint or soft-tissue injection.
- **Medication.** Local anesthetic alone may be used prior to arthrocentesis. Steroid and anesthetic are often used in combination for intra-articular or soft-tissue injection.
- **Other supplies.** Specimen containers, gauze pads, sterile gloves, sterile drapes, and plastic strip bandages are needed. A sterile hemostat is helpful to grasp the needle hub if the syringe must be removed to empty the aspirate or to switch syringes.[1,2]

Selecting Medications

For diagnostic trials, 1% lidocaine (Xylocaine) alone is injected; 0.5% bupivacaine (Marcaine) can be used if a longer anesthetic effect is desired. If inflammation is suspected, a corticosteroid can be added. Typically, either a long-acting steroid is injected, such as betamethasone (Celestone, Soluspan), or an intermediate-acting steroid, such as methylprednisolone acetate (Depo-Medrol). Lidocaine, bupivacaine, and the steroid can be mixed in the same syringe. All appropriate multidose vial and medication combination policies should be followed.[1,2]

TECHNIQUE
Arthrocentesis and Joint Injection

- Obtain and document informed consent.
- Use sterile technique, including sterile skin preparation.
- Decide what equipment and medication you will need and have it available before you start the procedure.
- Synovial fluid can be very viscous, so a large-bore needle (i.e., 18-gauge) is usually needed for aspiration.
- When using a large-bore needle for your procedure, local anesthetics can help relieve needle discomfort; 1% lidocaine superficially injected using a 27- or 30-gauge needle (i.e., a tuberculin needle and syringe) usually provides adequate anesthesia. Ethyl chloride sprayed on the skin immediately before inserting the needle can also be helpful.
- During aspiration of a joint, the fluid generally flows easily. If fluid is not immediately aspirated on entering the joint, the needle can be gently repositioned while suction is maintained.
- If the joint is to be injected after aspiration, leave the needle in place and change the syringe to inject the medication. This ensures that you are injecting into the joint. A sterile hemostat can be used to replace the needle.
- The total volume of fluid (anesthetic and steroid) as well as the corticosteroid dose depends on the joint size. In general, smaller joints require less steroid and a smaller injection volume (Table 15.6-1).
- If there is no joint effusion to aspirate and only a corticosteroid/lidocaine preparation is to be used, joint injection can be completed using the technique described above with the exception that a smaller bore needle (typically 25 gauge 1.5 in. for larger joints or a 27-gauge 0.5 in. for small joints) can be used. Preinjection local anesthetic is usually not necessary when using a small-gauge needle.[1,2]

TABLE 15.6-1	Volume of Injections and Steroid Dosages	
Anatomic area	**Total volume of injection (lidocaine + steroid)**	**Dose of steroid (examples)**
Small joints (e.g., digits, acromioclavicular joint)	0.5–1.0 mL	Betamethasone 0.5–2 mg; methylprednisolone 4–10 mg
Soft-tissue structures (e.g., tendon sheaths, carpal tunnel)	1–5 mL	Betamethasone 2–4 mg; methylprednisolone 20–40 mg
Medium joints (e.g., ankle, elbow) Soft-tissue structures (e.g., subacromial space, trigger points, bursae, epicondylitis)		
Large joints (e.g., knee)	3–10 mL	Betamethasone 4–6 mg; methylprednisolone 30–80 mg

Soft-Tissue Injection

- Obtain and document informed consent.
- Use sterile technique, including sterile skin preparation.
- Decide what equipment and medication you will need and have it available before you start the procedure.
- Local anesthetic is generally not needed for soft-tissue injections.
- During soft-tissue injections, the fluid should flow easily. If it does not gently reposition the needle and attempt to inject again. Always aspirate before injecting to avoid undesired intravascular injection.
- Soft-tissue injections work best when the fluid is infiltrated into several parts of the inflamed area. This can be done by fanning out the injection (Figure 15.6-3). With this technique, the needle is repositioned by withdrawing the needle tip back to just below the skin surface and then passing it back into a different location within the inflamed tissue. Part of the steroid preparation is injected with each repositioning.[1,2]

Synovial Fluid Analysis

Typical laboratory results include appearance, characteristic of mucin clot, cell count, glucose, Gram stain, culture, and crystal studies (Table 15.6-2). Additional studies that may be helpful in some situations include fungal culture as well as measurement of lactate dehydrogenase, complement, rheumatoid factor, and antinuclear antibodies.[1,2]

Additional Injection Options

Platelet-Rich Plasma Injection

Definition, Uses, and Indications

Platelet-rich plasma (PRP) injection is the process whereby a concentrated (defined as at least fourfold concentration) platelet-rich layer of the patient's centrifuged blood is injected into injured tendons,

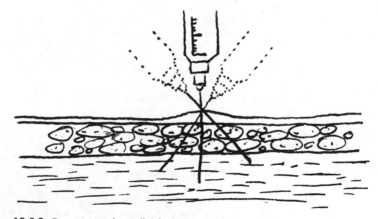

Figure 15.6-3. Repositioning the needle when injecting soft-tissue structures.

TABLE 15.6-2	Synovial Fluid Analysis		
Characteristic	**Normal**	**Inflammatory**	**Septic**
Color	Clear	Yellow	Cloudy
Viscosity	High	Low	Low
White blood cell count (mm^3)	0–200	2,000–50,000	>50,000
Neutrophils (%)	<25	Variable	>65

ligaments, muscles, or joints.[3] The technique was first developed in dentistry and veterinary medicine and has been more recently applied to orthopedics and sports medicine. Platelets contain higher concentrations of growth factors, including platelet derived growth factor, vascular endothelial growth factor, insulin-like growth factor, and basic fibroblast growth factor. It is believed that they accelerate the healing process in tendons, ligaments, and articular cartilage.

Technique

There is no standardized technique for PRP. All preparations involve phlebotomy, centrifuging the patient's blood, extracting the platelet concentrated layer, and injecting it in or around the damaged tissue. Currently, there is no standard concentration, additive mixture, or frequency of injections.

The actual injection technique is similar to that described earlier in this chapter, with the exception that a larger bore needle (18 to 20 gauge) is needed due to the viscosity of the PRP material. The injection should be performed under ultrasound guidance. Most clinicians advocate limited activities for a period of 1 to 2 weeks after the injection or injection series.

Risks

Risks are similar to those outlined in the corticosteroid section with the exception of tissue atrophy and skin discoloration, which are corticosteroid-specific. The incidence of infection appears to be very low, but the injections can be painful due to the inflammatory response that they generate. There is a theoretical risk that higher concentrations of PRP could predispose to malignancy or increase the risk of heterotopic bone formation.

Scientific Evidence

The medical literature lacks well-designed clinical studies that document definitive benefits for PRP, but the literature that does exist points to at least moderate benefit for lateral epicondylosis.[4] A recent study on the use of PRP for knee osteoarthritis showed mild benefit in moderate disease compared with hyaluronic acid injection.[5] At this time, most insurance companies still view PRP injections as experimental and do not cover the cost.

Viscosupplementation

Definition, Uses, and Indications

Viscosupplementation is an injection of synthetic hyaluronic acid or hyaluronan into arthritic synovial joints (knee, hip, and ankle). Studies in vitro were promising, but clinical effectiveness has been limited and controversial.[6] The mechanism of action is currently unclear. There are various manufacturers, which market viscosupplementation products that vary based on molecular weight and cost. Controversy exists regarding whether the different molecular weights contribute to the efficacy and side effects.[6]

Technique

Intra-articular injections are typically given in a series depending on the product used. Injections are given anywhere from a single dose to a series of five weekly injections.[7]

Preparations typically come in pre-filled syringes, and the injection technique is similar to that used with the injection of corticosteroids as outlined previously. Since the material is very viscous, a large-bore needle (18 to 20 gauge) is needed for the injection. Cost of a course of treatment typically ranges from $200 to $800 for the medication. Because of the conflicting data, some insurance companies will not cover the costs for this procedure.

Risks

Overall, viscosupplementation has been shown to be very safe. There is a about a 3% to 7% incidence of reactive synovitis resulting in pain and joint effusion.[6] Otherwise, the risks are similar to those outlined in the corticosteroid section, with the exception of tissue atrophy and skin discoloration, which are corticosteroid-specific.

Scientific Evidence

Recent studies show a modest beneficial effect for viscosupplementation in mild to moderate knee osteoarthritis. The magnitude and duration of the effect vary with different studies, but 5 to 13 weeks postinjection has the greatest symptom relief with a downgraded result of "minimal improvement" by 6 months.[7] Most of the literature show some symptom relief, but the threshold for significance is debated.

Prolotherapy

Definition, Uses, and Indications

Prolotherapy, also known as sclerotherapy, refers to the injection of an irritant into a joint space, ligament or tendon insertion site in order to reduce pain through the subsequent inflammatory reaction and immune response. Although various substances have been utilized,[8] the most commonly injected substance is 7% to 20% hyperosmolar dextrose. Prolotherapy's mechanism of action is not well-defined. The prevailing theory is that the injection will strengthen connective tissue and decrease ligament laxity through an inflammatory response within the tendon while destroying any neovascularization that has occurred.[9] While it has been utilized as an adjunct for chronic low back pain, arthropathies, and osteoarthritis, the most promising use of prolotherapy is in chronic tendinopathies.[10]

Technique

The injection technique is similar to that described previously with corticosteroids, with the difference being the substance injected. Using standard injection technique, half volume 50% dextrose can be combined with half volume 1% lidocaine for intra-articular injections. Tendinopathies typically require a peppering and fanning technique with a greater volume and multiple skin punctures. Tendinopathies require typically half volume normal saline, with a quarter volume 50% dextrose and a quarter volume 1% lidocaine.[11]

Risks

The risks and contraindications are similar to those detailed in the corticosteroid injection. Tissue atrophy and skin discoloration are less likely, but the prolotherapy solution will often produce a significant inflammatory response and associated pain.[11]

Scientific Evidence

The evidence for prolotherapy is continuing to grow but remains limited and controversial. The most evidence for prolotherapy involves the patellar, achilles, and hip adductor tendinopathies, along with plantar fasciitis and lateral epicondylosis.[8,9,12] While few studies lack even moderate grades for level of evidence, significant decreases in pain have been demonstrated in treatment for chronic tendinopathies.[8] Low back pain prolotherapy injections have shown improvement only when combined with other modalities or interventions. Sacroiliac injections have shown some promise, but the randomized control trials are lacking. Randomized controlled trials for both knee and finger osteoarthritis have shown positive trends toward decreasing pain and increasing range of motion.[8-10] Given the emerging evidence, many insurance companies do not cover prolotherapy.

REFERENCES

1. Fye KH, Imboden JB. Joint aspiration & injection. In: Imboden J, Hellman D, Stone J, eds. *Current diagnosis & treatment: rheumatology*. 3rd ed. New York, NY: McGraw-Hill; 2013:7–14.
2. Stitik T, Kim J, Gazillo G. Basic principles of joint and soft tissue injection procedures. In: Stitik TP, ed. *Injection procedures: osteoarthritis and related conditions*. New York, NY: Springer; 2011:3–32.
3. Hsu WK, Mishra A, Rodeo SR, et al. Platelet-rich plasma in orthopaedic applications: evidenced-based recommendations for treatment. *J Am Acad Orthop Surg* 2013;21(12):739–748.
4. Peerbooms JC, Sluimer J, Bruijn DJ, et al. Positive effect of an autologous platelet concentrate in lateral epicondylitis in a double-blind randomized controlled trial: platelet-rich plasma versus corticosteroid injection with a 1-year follow-up. *Am J Sports Med* 2010;38(2):255–262.
5. Cerza F, Carnì S, Carcangiu A, et al. Comparison between hyaluronic acid and platelet-rich plasma, intra-articular infiltration in the treatment of gonarthrosis. *Am J Sports Med* 2012;40(12):2822–2827.
6. Bellamy N, Campbell J, Welch V, et al. Viscosupplementation for the treatment of osteoarthritis of the knee. *Cochrane Database Syst Rev* 2006;(2):CD005321 doi: 0.1002/14651858.CD005321.pub2.
7. Trigkilidas D, Anand A. The effectiveness of hyaluronic acid intra-articular injections in managing osteoarthritic knee pain. *Ann R Coll Surg Engl* 2013;95(8):545–551.
8. Coombes BK, Bisset L, Vicenzino B. Efficacy and safety of corticosteroid injections and other injections for management of tendinopathy: a systematic review of randomised controlled trials. *Lancet* 2010;376(9754):1751–1767.
9. Childress MA, Beutler A. Management of chronic tendon injuries. *Am Fam Physician* 2013;87(7):486–490.
10. Distel LM, Best TM. Prolotherapy: a clinical review of its role in treating chronic musculoskeletal pain. *PM R* 2011;3(6 Suppl 1):S78–S81.
11. Rabago D, Patterson JJ, Mundt M, et al. Dextrose prolotherapy for knee osteoarthritis: a randomized controlled trial. *Ann Fam Med* 2013;11(3):229–237.
12. Rabago D, Best TM, Zgierska AE, et al. A systematic review of four injection therapies for lateral epicondylosis: prolotherapy, polidocanol, whole blood and platelet-rich plasma. *Br J Sports Med* 2009;43(7):471–481.

CHAPTER 16

Dermatologic Problems

Section Editor: Elisabeth L. Backer

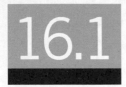

Pyoderma and Cellulitis

Michael L. O'Dell

Pustular skin infections are common complaints in family physicians' offices. Such illnesses are often related to a break in the skin and may have minor or life-threatening implications. Methicillin-resistant *Staphylococcus aureus* (MRSA) now causes most suppurative skin infections in many U.S. communities. Community-acquired MRSA is best treated with oral trimethoprim/sulfamethoxazole, clindamycin, or a tetracycline. More serious cases may require IV vancomycin, oral linezolid, or IV daptomycin.[1]

I. IMPETIGO

A. Clinical presentation of small-vesicle impetigo begins with small, reddened macules progressing to water-filled vesicles surrounded by a band of erythema. A honey-colored crust follows rupture of the vesicle. *Streptococcus* infection is often the cause of small-vesicle impetigo and, sporadically, impetigo predates poststreptococcal nephritis. *S. aureus* infection may cause small-vesicle impetigo as well.

B. Clinical presentation of bullous impetigo begins as a large flaccid blister or blisters. The blister quickly becomes filled with cloudy, purulent-appearing fluid. Occasionally, staphylococcal scalded skin syndrome accompanies bullous impetigo.

C. Treatment. Good hygiene speeds healing and helps prevent spread of the illness to others. Systemic therapy is needed in immunosuppressed patients, those with extensive disease, patients with eczema, or those who live in communities that are experiencing an outbreak of poststreptococcal nephritis. Systemic therapy should provide for coverage of MRSA in most communities.

II. ECTHYMA

A. Clinical presentation. Ecthyma occurs on the legs of the debilitated as small bullae, followed by an adherent crust and then by a slowly healing, ulcerated lesion. It should be differentiated from pseudomonas sepsis-related pyoderma gangrenosum, a life-threatening illness.

B. Ecthyma is caused by Group A streptococcus and is generally adequately treated with erythromycin, azithromycin, dicloxacillin, or cephalexin and attention to nutrition.

III. FOLLICULITIS, FURUNCLES (BOILS), CARBUNCLES, AND HIDRADENITIS SUPPURATIVA

A. Folliculitis

1. **Clinical presentation.** Lesions appear as yellowish pustules, with an encircling thin band of erythema around hair follicles, generally in the intertriginous areas. Often, patients have diabetes. Hot-tub folliculitis occurs in users of poorly maintained hot tubs.

2. Treatment includes improved hygiene and application of topical agents, such as mupirocin or bacitracin. Presence of extensive lesions warrants systemic therapy with coverage of MRSA. Hot-tub cellulitis is a self-limited illness, but immunocompromised patients should receive ciprofloxacin or other antipseudomonal medication.

B. Furuncle

1. **Clinical presentation.** A tender, fluctuant lesion, with surrounding erythema extending into the subcuticular space, is present. Furuncles more commonly occur in adolescents and in those with poor hygiene, seborrhea, diabetes, or immunodeficiency. Facial furuncles may result in cavernous sinus thrombosis.

2. Treatment for furuncles is drainage. Following drainage, antibiotics are generally not needed.[2] Systemic therapy should provide for coverage of MRSA in most communities.

C. **Carbuncle**
  1. **Clinical presentation.** Carbuncles appear as a collection of furuncles, generally on the back of the neck in men older than 40 years.
  2. **Treatment.** Drainage or debridement (or both) is required, and systemic antibiotics with MRSA coverage are often required. Surgical consultation is useful.

D. **Hidradenitis suppurativa**
  1. **Clinical presentation.** Furunculoid lesions are present in the axillae, inguinal area, scrotum, labia, or mons pubis. They usually occur in males or individuals with acne conglobata.
  2. **Treatment.** Drainage is necessary. Twice-daily use of an oral tetracycline or application of topical clindamycin 2% is useful.[3] Isotretinoin is also useful. Surgical excision is often necessary.

IV. ERYSIPELAS

A. **Clinical presentation.** Erysipelas is an acute illness marked by redness, pain, and swelling in the area of rash, which has a spreading, irregular, but sharply defined border. Lymphatic involvement is prominent. Erysipelas affects all age groups. Patients are often febrile and have an elevated white cell count. Sepsis may occur in the elderly, young children, persons with diabetes, or immunosuppressed individuals.

B. Oral penicillin, erythromycin plus rifampin, or ciprofloxacin can be used for treatment. Facial involvement should be managed with intravenous therapy to prevent cavernous sinus thrombosis.

V. CELLULITIS

A. **Clinical presentation.** Cellulitis is a spreading infection of the epidermis and subcutaneous tissue that generally begins following a break in the skin. The affected skin is warm, reddened, and painful without a sharply demarcated border. Source, location, immunocompetency, and rapidity of spread dictate treatment.
  1. Patients with uncomplicated cellulitis generally have a *Streptococcus* infection, although *S. aureus* infection is common as well.
  2. Injury in brackish water may result in halophilic *Vibrio* infection.
  3. Cellulitis near the eye may involve the orbit or be superficial to the septum of the orbit. It is often difficult to distinguish between the two infections. Infections of the orbital space (orbital cellulitis) often present with proptosis, chemosis, and pain with motion of the eye. Sinusitis is often present and is the source of the infection. Orbital cellulitis threatens life and vision and may quickly spread to the central nervous system or cause cavernous sinus thrombosis. Infections of the preseptal space (periorbital cellulitis) often result from superficial trauma; they lack signs of proptosis, chemosis, or pain with eye movement and are generally not life threatening.
  4. Infections of the face or neck may result from trauma but are often the result of poor dental hygiene. Odontogenic infections may quickly spread to the submental and retropharyngeal spaces, resulting in airway compromise and collapse.
  5. Diabetics and immunocompromised patients may harbor unusual organisms (see Chapters 17.2 and 19.4).

B. **Treatment.** The affected body part should be elevated.
  1. **Patients with uncomplicated disease.** Systemic therapy should provide for coverage of MRSA in most communities, with IV administration desirable if the patient has systemic signs or symptoms. In patients with lower extremity cellulitis, good household support is necessary to ensure elevation of the extremity, and hospital admission should be considered if home support is lacking.
  2. **Brackish water injury.** Antibiotic should cover halophilic *Vibrio*, such as doxycycline (200 mg immediately, 100 mg bid for 10 days), and an antipseudomonal aminoglycoside should also be given.
  3. Infection involving the orbit requires inpatient treatment with ophthalmologic or ear–nose–throat consultation for potential drainage. Systemic therapy should provide for coverage of MRSA in most communities and vancomycin is generally required.
  4. Infections of face or neck associated with trauma-induced infections require MRSA coverage in most communities. Infections of the face or neck resulting from poor dentition are managed with amoxicillin/clavulanate or clindamycin.

5. Management of cellulitis in immunocompromised patients and those with diabetes is best dictated by culture from the leading edge of infection. Empirical therapy should consist of MRSA coverage, or, if the patient appears significantly ill, vancomycin, linezolid, or daptomycin.

REFERENCES

1. Liu C, Bayer A, Cosgrove SE, et al. Clinical practice guidelines by the infectious Diseases Society of America for the treatment of methicillin-resistant *Staphylococcus aureus* infections in adults and children: executive summary. *Clin Infect Dis* 2011;52(3):285–292.
2. Drugs for bacterial infections. *Treat Guidel Med Lett* 2013;11(131):65–74.
3. Jemec GB. Clinical practice. Hidradenitis suppurativa. *N Engl J Med* 2012;366(2):158–164.

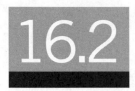

16.2 Fungal Infections of the Skin

Lars C. Larsen, Valerie B. Laing, Jonathon M. Firnhaber

TINEA INFECTIONS

Tinea infections are caused by the dermatophytes: *Trichophyton*, *Microsporum*, and *Epidermophyton*.[1] Infections may be subacute or chronic and are usually not invasive. These fungi selectively inhabit the keratin in the skin, hair, and nails. Tinea infections are not highly contagious.

Clinical Presentation

Infections commonly involve the scalp (*tinea capitis*), body (*tinea corporis*), groin (*tinea cruris*), feet (*tinea pedis*), hands (*tinea manuum*), face (*tinea faciei*), and nails (*tinea unguium*; onychomycosis). Annular erythema with scaling is characteristic. Edema, plaques, pustules, and vesicles may be present in varying degrees. Onychomycosis is characterized by elevation of the distal nail, with subungual thickening and crumbling.

Diagnosis

Diagnosis is based on the clinical presentation of lesions and confirmed by examination of a potassium hydroxide preparation of skin scrapings, nail debris, or broken hair. Scrapings from a leading edge of inflammation yield the highest results. Scalp infections caused by *Microsporum* species (less than 5% of cases in the United States; can be most common elsewhere) may fluoresce brilliant green with Wood light examination.[2] Fungal cultures are reserved for cases in which the diagnosis is in doubt. Documentation of cure in scalp infections and justification for prolonged systemic therapy in tinea capitis and onychomycosis are additional indications for cultures.

Management

Oral antifungal medications are necessary for the management of tinea capitis and most cases of onychomycosis. Topical agents are usually adequate for most other tinea infections, with oral medications occasionally required for extensive involvement or after failure of topical agents. Ancillary measures to avoid heat and moisture and increase exposure to air are beneficial.

• **Tinea capitis.** Oral treatment with griseofulvin for 4 to 6 weeks in adults (or until culture is negative; ultramicrosize tablets, 375 mg per day); children older than 2 years: microsize suspension for 6 to 12 weeks (or 2 weeks after signs and symptoms have resolved), 20 to 25 mg/kg/day (maximum dose 1,000 mg per day). Other effective treatments include terbinafine for 4 weeks (children: 10 to 20 kg, 62.5 mg per day; 21 to 40 kg, 125 mg per day; more than 40 kg, 250 mg per day; adults: 250 mg per day); itraconazole (Sporanox) for 2 to 4 weeks (children: 5 mg/kg/day; adults: 200 to 300 mg per day; or fluconazole (Diflucan) for 3 weeks (children: 6 mg/kg/day).

Concurrent twice-weekly shampooing (Head & Shoulders, Selsun Blue, or Nizoral) may reduce spore shedding.

• **Tinea corporis, tinea cruris, tinea pedis, tinea manuum, and tinea faciei.** Topical medication until 2 weeks after the rash clears is curative for most infections. Tinea pedis typically requires a longer course of treatment (up to 4 weeks). Oral therapy may be necessary for extensive, refractory, or recurrent disease. First-line medications effective against tinea include the following over-the-counter (OTC) medications: those containing terbinafine (e.g., Lamisil; 1% cream, spray, solution; daily; bid for tinea pedis) and butenafine (e.g., Lotrimin Ultra, Mentax; 1% cream daily for 14 days; bid for 7 days for tinea pedis). Naftifine (e.g., Naftin; 1%, 2% cream [daily], 1% gel [twice daily], 2% gel [daily for tinea pedis]; for 2 to 4 weeks) and luliconazole (Luzu; 1% cream daily for 1 to 2 weeks) are prescription medications. Other OTC and prescription medications that are slightly less effective include those containing clotrimazole (Lotrimin, clotrimazole; 1% cream, solution; Fungicure solution, spray; bid for 2 to 4 weeks), econazole (1% cream; daily for 2 to 4 weeks), miconazole (Lotrimin AF spray or powder, Micatin, Monistat-Derm, miconazole; 2% cream, Desenex 2% spray, powder; Neosporin AF 2% cream, spray; Zeasorb-AF 2% powder; bid for 2 to 4 weeks), oxiconazole (Oxistat; 1% cream, lotion; bid for 2 to 4 weeks), sulconazole (Exelderm; 1% cream, solution; bid for 3 to 4 weeks), ketoconazole (2% cream; daily for 2 to 6 weeks), and ciclopirox (Loprox, ciclopirox; 0.77% cream, gel, suspension; bid for 1 to 4 weeks). Sertaconazole (Ertaczo; 2% cream; bid for 4 weeks) is used to treat tinea pedis. Medications containing undecylenic acid and tolnaftate are inexpensive, but are significantly less effective. Oral medication regimens for adults: tinea corporis/cruris—terbinafine (Lamisil) (250 mg per day × 2 to 4 weeks), itraconazole (200 mg per day × 2 weeks or 200 mg twice daily × 1 week), fluconazole (150 mg once weekly × 2 to 3 weeks), or ultramicrosize griseofulvin (375 mg per day × 2 to 4 weeks); tinea pedis/manuum/faciei—terbinafine (250 mg per day × 2 weeks), itraconazole (100 mg per day × 4 weeks or 400 mg per day × 1 week), fluconazole (150 mg once weekly × 4 weeks), or ultramicrosize griseofulvin (375 mg twice daily × 4 to 8 weeks).

• **Onychomycosis.** Oral treatment regimens include terbinafine (highest mycotic cure rate)[3] (adults, single daily dose, 250 mg per day for 6 weeks for fingernails, 12 weeks for toenail infections), itraconazole (Sporanox; adults, 200 mg daily for 6 weeks for fingernails, 12 weeks for toenail infections or 200 mg bid for 1 week each month for 2 months for fingernails, 3 months for toenail infections), or fluconazole (adults, 150 mg once weekly for 6 to 12 months, until the abnormal nail has grown out). Topical medications for control of infection contain ciclopirox (Penlac nail lacquer, applied daily at bedtime up to 48 weeks).

Prevention

Preventive measures include wearing of loose undergarments, wearing of cotton socks or sandals, avoidance of other occlusive clothes, and tight control of blood sugar in persons with diabetes. Sharing of contaminated combs and hairbrushes should be discouraged.

CANDIDAL INFECTIONS

Superficial candidal infections of the skin and mucous membranes may be acute or chronic and are most often caused by the *Candida albicans* species. Infection is often associated with abnormalities of the epithelium or host immunologic system. Predisposing factors include antibiotic therapy, systemic conditions such as diabetes mellitus and HIV infection, and other skin conditions that cause maceration or a warm, moist environment. More significant systemic infections are typically associated with severe immunodeficiency, as may be seen in AIDS, cancer, and transplant patients. Cutaneous candidiasis is not highly contagious.

Clinical Presentation

Common sites of *Candida* infection include oral mucosa (thrush), angles of the mouth (angular cheilitis, perlèche), vaginal/perineal area (vulvovaginitis), on the glans and prepuce of the penis (balanitis), between moist skin folds (intertrigo), and in diaper areas of infants and adults (diaper dermatitis). Nail folds (paronychia), nails (onychomycosis), and the esophagus (esophagitis) are less common sites of infection. Skin infections typically present as beefy red plaques with satellite papules or pustules, or both; maceration, fissures, and exudate may be present. Lesions involving the mucous membranes appear as erythematous plaques and superficial erosions with adherent white exudate.

Diagnosis

Diagnosis is based on the typical clinical appearance of lesions and is confirmed by microscopic examination of a potassium hydroxide preparation of exudate, skin, or mucosal scrapings. Fungal pseudohyphae and budding yeast are frequently identified. Culture for the presence of *Candida* species is rarely needed.

Management

Topical antifungal agents are first-line therapy for candidal infections of the skin and mucous membrane; a short course of a systemic antifungal drug is also appropriate. Patients should be counseled to avoid heat and moisture, and unnecessary antibiotic or corticosteroid therapy. Diabetics should aim for optimum blood sugar control. Longer term systemic antifungal therapy is generally reserved for chronic and resistant infections, systemic infections, and for prophylaxis in immunocompromised hosts.

- **Thrush.** Most patients can be successfully treated with nystatin oral suspension used for 10 to 14 days or for 2 days after lesions clear. The dosage for infants is 1 mL in each side of the mouth qid; adult dosage is 4 to 6 mL in each side of the mouth qid, held as long as possible. Clotrimazole oral troches (10 mg five times per day for 14 days) and miconazole buccal tablets (50 mg daily for 14 days) are also effective. Treatment of adults with fluconazole (200 mg PO single dose or 100 mg PO daily for 5 days) or itraconazole (200 mg PO as a single dose) and treatment of children with fluconazole (3 mg per kg PO daily for 7 days) are alternatives.
- **Intertrigo, perlèche, diaper dermatitis, balanitis, paronychia.** Effective OTC topical medications include miconazole (Micatin, Monistat) and clotrimazole (Lotrimin AF; Mycelex); these are available in multiple vehicles, including cream, ointment, solution, and spray. Prescription topical medications include ciclopirox (Loprox 0.77% cream and gel, 8% solution; applied bid), miconazole (Monistat-Derm 2% cream; applied bid), ketoconazole (Nizoral 2% cream, applied daily), and econazole (1% cream; applied daily). Vusion is an ointment for *Candida* diaper dermatitis that provides an effective barrier protection to the skin of zinc oxide and petrolatum while delivering an anticandidal agent of 0.25% miconazole. If maceration is present in intertrigo or diaper dermatitis, soaks or compresses with Burow solution (aluminum acetate) for 15 to 20 minutes up to three times daily can be helpful. If a systemic agent is required for more extensive candidal infection, fluconazole or itraconazole (100 mg PO daily for 7 to 14 days) is effective.

Prevention

Preventive measures include wearing loose cotton undergarments, frequent diaper changes, conservative use of antibiotics and corticosteroids, tight control of diabetes, exposure of moist areas to air (including blow drying with cool air after bathing), and use of well-fitted dentures to prevent drooling. Prompt and aggressive treatment of oral, penile, vaginal, and perirectal infections may prevent transmission to sexual partners.

TINEA VERSICOLOR (PITYRIASIS VERSICOLOR)

Tinea versicolor results from infection of sebum-producing skin follicles by yeasts in the genus *Malassezia*.[4] Infection is common and is often chronic and recurrent. It is exacerbated by warm humid weather and use of oils on the skin. Tinea versicolor is not highly contagious.

Clinical Presentation

A fine scale covering lighter-colored skin is characteristic, with small circular lesions coalescing to involve large areas. It often becomes noticeable in the summers when the surrounding skin tans. Macules, plaques, and erythema may be present. Lesions vary in color and can be hypopigmented (white) or hyperpigmented (pink, tan, brown, or black). Although the upper chest, arms, and back are commonly affected, lesions may also be found on the face and intertriginous areas.

Diagnosis

Diagnosis is based on the clinical presentation of skin lesions and is confirmed by microscopic examination of a potassium hydroxide preparation of skin scrapings, which yields characteristic "spaghetti and meatballs" hyphae and spores. Culture for *Malassezia* is rarely needed.

Management

- **Topical regimens:** Selenium sulfide 2.5% lotion applied qhs and washed off in am for 7 days or prescription ketoconazole cream, oxiconazole lotion or cream, ciclopirox cream or suspension, OTC clotrimazole cream, or miconazole cream applied bid for 2 to 4 weeks.
- **Oral regimens (for widespread for recalcitrant disease):** Ketoconazole 200 mg qd × 10 days, alternative ketoconazole 400 mg × 1 (work up sweat and do not shower for 8 hours) repeat in 7 days. Note in July 2013 the FDA requested ketoconazole not be used for tinea versicolor and instead be reserved for serious systemic fungal infections. Itraconazole 200 mg qd × 7 days. Fluconazole 300 mg taken twice 1 week apart or 400 mg as single dose.
- **Prophylaxis for frequent recurrences:** Any of the topicals can be used weekly for several months.

Prevention

Skin oils should be avoided. Prophylactic therapy with selenium sulfide suspension usually prevents clinically significant recurrences in susceptible individuals.

REFERENCES

1. Moriarty B, Hay R, Morris-Jones R. The diagnosis and management of tinea. *BMJ* 2012;345:e4380. doi: 10.1136/bmj.e4380.
2. Kelly BP. Superficial fungal infections. *Pediatr Rev* 2012;33:e22. doi: 10.1542/pir.33-4-e22.
3. Westerberg DP, Voyack MJ. Onychomycosis: current trends in diagnosis and treatment. *Am Fam Physician* 2013;88(11):762–770.
4. Crespo-Erchigo V, Florenzio VD. Malassezia yeasts and pityriasis versicolor. *Curr Opin Infect Dis* 2006; 19:139–147.

16.3 Pediculosis and Mite Infestations

Jeffrey G. Jones

Pediculosis is an infestation with head lice (*Pediculus humanus* var. *capitis*), body lice (*P. humanus* var. *corporis*), or crab lice (*Phthirus pubis*). Hundreds of types of mites can cause symptoms in humans, the most common of which is scabies, an infestation with *Arcoptes scabiei* var. *hominis*. Mites or their products may be an important source of allergic reactions in people or they may cause symptoms by feeding and causing a pruritic dermatitis, as in the case of chiggers (Trombiculid mites), among many others.

CLINICAL MANIFESTATIONS

- **Pediculosis**
  - **Pediculosis capitis.** Head lice infest millions of children. The infestation is transmissible by close contact or fomites, and small epidemics in schools are common. Secondary infection with pustules, crusting, and cervical adenopathy are common. The infestation is found most commonly on the back of the head, the neck, and behind the ears.
  - **Pediculosis corporis.** Body lice infestation is seen primarily in homeless adults. The lice live on clothing, where they are generally found, along with eggs. Patients complain of itching and often have red pustules, 2 to 4 mm in diameter on an erythematous base. Chronic infestation leads to skin thickening and diffuse pigmentation. They may be a vector for the diseases of epidemic typhus, relapsing, and trench fever.[1]
  - **Pediculosis pubis.** Crab lice is a sexually transmitted infestation, with at least 30% of affected persons having at least one other sexually transmitted disease.[2] The majority of patients complain of pruritus. The infestation may spread to other thick hair, including eye lashes and axillary hair.

- **Scabies and chiggers**
  - **Scabies.** Mite infestation results from direct skin contact with an infected person or fomites. Scabies is ubiquitous, and pruritis is the most common symptom. On examination, burrows in the web spaces between the fingers, wrists, hands, feet, genitals, and waistline area are seen. The mite almost never affects the head and neck region in adults. Discrete vesicles and papules are frequently seen in similar locations. Secondary infection with pustules, nodules, and regional adenopathy may develop. **Crusted scabies** refers to the hyperkeratotic lesions found in immunosuppressed people, and is highly contagious because of the high number of mites.
  - **Chiggers.** The larval Trombiculid mite feeds on many hosts, including humans. The bites present as intensely pruritic, grouped erythematous papules, usually on the lower extremities. They may mimic scabies nodules, and can spread rickettsial infections in Asia.[3]

DIAGNOSIS
Pediculosis

- Head and pubic lice can be seen on the individual hairs by careful visual examination or under the microscope. The use of a fine-toothed comb (nit comb) aids in their detection.
- Nits, the eggs attached to hairs, are indicative of infestation by head and pubic lice.
- Examination of seams of clothing may reveal body lice and their eggs.

Scabies

The diagnosis is suspected when burrows are found or when dermatologic features in the characteristic locations are present. The definitive diagnosis is made with identification of the mite, egg, egg casing, or feces. The diagnosis can be aided by the following techniques.

- With a magnifying lens, the burrows can be seen in the typical locations. The dark spot at the end of the burrow is the mite. It can be removed with a needle and examined under the microscope.
- By adding a drop of potassium hydroxide to a slide with a skin scraping, better visualization of the mite, egg, egg casing, and feces is often possible.
- Apply mineral oil to a suspicious lesion to improve the yield. After the application of the mineral oil, scrape the lesion and look for mites, eggs, egg casings, or feces with and without potassium hydroxide.
- If burrows are not obvious, apply ink to a suspicious area of rash. After washing off the ink with alcohol, any area that remains stained represents a burrow. This area can be scraped with a scalpel and the material examined.

Chiggers

This condition is diagnosed by the characteristic history of being in grassy areas and location of lesions at areas of clothing constriction, such as the panty line.

TREATMENT (TABLE 16.3-1)

Drug resistance is becoming a problem for several classes of topical pediculicides, especially pyrethroids. Occluding oils and plant oils may prove to be important treatment modalities as resistance increases. Ivermectin, a broad-spectrum antihelmintic, is useful as an off-label treatment against lice and scabies. Topical or systemic antibiotics may be necessary for secondary infections. Topical steroids and antihistamines may be used to help control itching. Retreatment of nonresponsive patients after 1 to 2 weeks with an alternative regimen is recommended.[7]

PREVENTION

- All close contacts of individuals infected with pediculosis or scabies should be treated concomitantly.
- All clothing, bed linens, and towels should be washed and dried in a hot cycle or dry cleaned.
- Education regarding institution of adequate hygiene is important.

TABLE 16.3-1	Treatment of Pediculosis* and Scabies**		
Drug	**Lowest age/weight**	**Dosage and technique**	**Cost**[4]
Ivermectin lotion 0.5% (Sklice)*[5]	6 mo	Apply to dry hair and scalp for 10 min, then rinse	$$$$
Spinosad 0.9% susp (Natroba)*[5]	4 yr	Apply to dry hair for 10 min then rinse, repeat in 7–10 d prn	$$$$$
Benzyl alcohol 5% lotion (Ulesfia)*[5]	6 mo	Same as Spinosad	$$$$
Pyrethrins with piperonyl butoxide shampoo (Rid)*[5]	2 yr	Same as Spinosad	$
Permethrin 1% crème rinse (Nix)*[5]	2 mo	Apply to shampooed, towel-dried hair for 10 min, then rinse; repeat in 7–10 d	$$
Malathion 0.5% lotion (Ovide)*[5]	6 yr	Apply to dry hair for 8–12 h, then shampoo. Repeat in 7–9 d	$$$$
Ivermectin tablets Stromectol*/**[5,6]	15 kg	200–400 mcg/kg PO once; repeat 7–10 d later	$$
Permethrin 5% cream (Elimite)**[6]	2 mo	Massage cream into entire body, wash off after 8–14 h	$$
Crotamiton 10% (Eurax)**[6]	Not approved in children	Massage cream/lotion into entire body from chin down, on days 1, 2, 3, and 8	$$

*denotes drugs indicated for treatment of pediculosis
**denotes drugs indicated for treatment of scabies

REFERENCES

1. Sturchler DA. Exposure—a guide to sources of infection. Chapter 4. *Invertebrates*. Herndon, VA: ASM Press; 2006:85.
2. Chapel TA, Katta R, Kuszmar T. Pediculosis pubis in clinic for treatment of sexually transmitted disease. *Sex Transm Dis* 1979;6:257.
3. Jones JG. Chiggers. *Am Fam Physician* 1987;36(2):149.
4. Dermatology: Antiparasitics (Topical), In: *Tarascon Pocket Pharmacopoeia 2013 Edition*. 14th ed. Burlington, MA: Jones & Bartlett; 2013:149–150.
5. Ivermectin (Sklice) topical lotion for head lice. *Med Lett Drugs Ther* 2012;54:61–63.
6. The Medical Letter. *Drugs for parasitic infections*. 3rd ed. New York: The Medical Letter; 2013:55.
7. Currie BJ, McCarthy JS. Permethrin and ivermectin for scabies. *N Engl J Med* 2010;362(8):717.

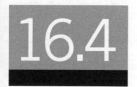

16.4 Acne Vulgaris

Daniel J. Van Durme, Lisa M. Johnson

GENERAL PRINCIPLES

Definition

A very common follicular disorder, particularly in adolescents.

Anatomy

Blocked pilosebaceous unit that leads to retained sebum and distention (comedones), inflammation (papules and pustules), or hypertrophy of sebum glands (nodules and cysts).[1]

Epidemiology

Extremely common—found in about 85% of patients between 15 and 24 years old.

Classification

Mild (noninflammatory): primarily comedones; moderate (inflammatory): primarily papules and pustules; severe (nodulo-cystic): primarily nodules and cysts.[1]

Pathophysiology and Etiology

Hypercohesive keratinocytes block follicular opening of pilosebaceous unit. This may be idiopathic or aggravated by androgens. The organism *Propionibacterium acnes* may proliferate and lead to inflammation.[2]

DIAGNOSIS
Clinical Presentation

Patients may present with a wide range of severity, sometimes very distressed over minimally visible lesions and at other times with minimal distress over marked physical findings.

Physical Examination

Most commonly found on the face, but may include the back, shoulders, and anterior chest wall; these areas should be examined to determine the extent of the disorder.

Differential Diagnosis

Acne vulgaris starts with microcomedones that then develop into comedones, papules, and pustules. In the absence of comedones, one should consider acne mechanica, steroid acne, or rosacea. Pustules and/or nodules in the perioral and nasal area that are unresponsive to typical antibiotic treatment for acne should lead to the consideration of Gram-negative folliculitis. Bacterial cultures may be used in establishing this diagnosis.[1]

TREATMENT
Behavioral

Avoid excess scrubbing of the skin, which can aggravate the condition; acne is not due to poor hygiene. There is no good evidence that diet affects acne. Avoid "picking" or "popping" as these can increase the likelihood of scarring. There is also an association between smoking and acne severity.[1]

Medications

Choice of medication is based on several factors: (a) the predominant lesion and skin type, (b) the distribution of lesions, (c) the patient's preferences that will affect compliance, and (d) some degree of trial and error.

- **Benzoyl peroxide** preparations (soaps, lotions, gels) used once or twice a day are an excellent starting point for all types of acne. There are many preparations available over the counter or as a prescription. The strengths range from 2.5% to 10%, with increased drying of the skin associated with higher concentrations (there is no increase in efficacy). The water-based preparations are also less drying. Benzoyl peroxide may also be used in conjunction with topical or oral antibiotics as it decreases bacterial resistance.[1–3]
- **Mild or comedonal acne.** This is best treated with a topical retinoid, such as tretinoin, adapalene, or tazarotene applied thinly at bedtime. Always start with the lowest dose and increase strength over several weeks or months as needed and as tolerated. Erythema and irritation are common at first and can be minimized by decreasing frequency to every other day or every third day as needed. The gel and alcohol forms are more dry, and stronger. They are best used in patients with relatively oily skin or when creams fail. Azelaic acid has keratolytic, antibacterial, and anti-inflammatory properties and has shown efficacy with both mild and moderate acne. It may lead to hypopigmentation, which can be advantageous in those prone to postinflammatory hyperpigmentation, but can be a problem in ethnic groups with more skin pigment. Azelaic acid is pregnancy category B and may be considered for selected use in pregnant women.[2–5]
- **Moderate or inflammatory (papular and pustular) acne.** This calls for the addition of antibiotics. Oral and topical agents can be used, depending on how widespread the lesions are and whether the patient prefers oral or topical therapy. Topical antibiotics are applied thinly bid after washing

(with benzoyl peroxide agent) and drying the skin. Common preparations are available as solutions, gels, lotions, ointments, and creams, including erythromycin, clindamycin, and sulfacetamide. Choice of the vehicle should depend on the patient's skin type. Those with oily skin may do better with the drying effects of gels and solutions, whereas those with dry skin may do better with the moisturizing effects of lotions, creams, and ointments. Topical erythromycin and clindamycin are most effective when used with benzoyl peroxide and there are commercial preparations that combine these into one. Topical dapsone has also been approved for use in acne; it has antimicrobial and anti-inflammatory effects.[2-5]

- Oral antibiotics are indicated when lesions are widespread (making topical application impractical) or severe. First-line agents include tetracycline or erythromycin at 1 g per day in divided doses. Tetracycline may cause photosensitivity, and qid dosing on an empty stomach makes compliance difficult. Gastrointestinal (GI) upset can be common with erythromycin, and increasing resistance is noted with this agent. Minocycline 50 to 100 mg qd-bid, or doxycycline 50 mg (occasionally 100 mg) qd-bid, and less commonly trimethoprim–sulfamethoxazole 160/800 mg bid can be helpful. Oral agents are generally stronger than topical agents and can be used when topicals fail.[2,3,5]
- **Nodulocystic acne,** the most severe form of acne vulgaris, can cause emotional and physical scarring. Treatment starts with judicious use of the agents above, but the condition can often be resistant to these therapies. When this happens, oral isotretinoin may be indicated; see special considerations below.
- **Oral contraceptives (OCs) and other hormonal agents.** Several combined OCs are FDA-approved for use in acne. These have low doses of estrogen and nonandrogenic progestins, such as norgestimate, levonorgestrel, or desogestrel. (Progestin only contraceptives may worsen acne.) Therapy must be used for 2 to 4 months to see effects.

The diuretic spironolactone has antiandrogenic properties and has been found to be useful in the treatment of acne as well.[1,2,5]

Counseling

The potential physical disfigurement from acne, whether temporary from the current lesions or from scarring, can be extremely distressing for the adolescent who is developing a self-image and who may be very self-conscious. The psychological trauma from acne for a developing adolescent should not be underestimated and general supportive counseling can be very helpful. This is also a valuable time to teach adolescents about self-care and responsibility for their own health.

Patient Education

Acne is controlled (not cured) with medications. The patient will need to continue to use treatments to prevent new lesions even after the current lesions have resolved. Treatments are designed to prevent new lesions far more than clearing existing lesions. Thus, topical treatments should be applied all over the affected area, not just on the lesions themselves. Some patients notice an initial worsening with treatment before it improves. They need to be warned of this, so they do not stop medications prematurely.

Follow-Up

Expect 4 to 8 weeks to see significant improvement with most treatments. Recommend follow-up about every 6 weeks until the optimal regimen has been determined, then every 2 to 3 months for maintenance and adjustments.

Results

Most acne can be well controlled with some combination of medications as listed above. It may take time to determine the ideal regimen, but patients should be reassured that there are extremely effective treatments to control this condition. Nevertheless, optimal treatment may never make the skin look "completely normal."

Complications

Complications include scarring from deep lesions or from self-inflicted picking at lesions.

SPECIAL CONSIDERATIONS

Isotretinoin can be *tremendously effective* in cases of severe, recalcitrant, nodulocystic acne. This agent is also *highly* teratogenic, and has numerous side effects, including myalgias, arthralgias, epistaxis, xerosis, liver function elevation, hyperlipidemia, and leukopenia. Frequent monitoring of bloodwork is advised. In order to obtain isotretinoin, the prescriber, pharmacy, and patient must receive specific information through an FDA risk management program called iPLEDGE and become registered (www.ipledgeprogram.com). The numerous administrative burdens and potential complications with this medicine have led many family physicians to stop prescribing this medicine and refer these patients to a dermatologist.

REFERENCES

1. Strauss J, Kowchuk D. Guidelines of care for acne vulgaris management. *J Am Acad Dermatol* 2007; 56:651–663.
2. Dawson A, Dellavale R. Acne vulgaris. *BMJ* 2013;346:f2634.
3. Williams H, Dellavalle R, Garner S. Acne vulgaris. *Lancet* 2012;379:361–372.
4. Titus S, Hodge J. Diagnosis and treatment of acne. *Am Fam Physician* 2012;86(8):734–740.
5. Olutunmbi Y, Paley K, English J. Adolescent female acne: etiology and management. *J Pediatr Adolesc Gynecol* 2008;21:171–176.

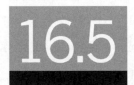

16.5 Common Dermatoses

Rhonda A. Sparks, Kalyanakrishnan Ramakrishnan, Brian R. Coleman

Dermatologic problems are commonly encountered in the primary care setting. This chapter reviews the diagnosis and management of seven of the most common dermatoses encountered in clinical practice.

PSORIASIS
General Principles

Definition
Psoriasis is a life-long papulosquamous dermatologic disorder that is transmitted genetically and characterized by chronic recurrent bouts of characteristic erythematous papules and scaling plaques.

Anatomy
Psoriasis can develop at sites of trauma (the so-called Koebner phenomenon) although it can affect any cutaneous surface. Areas that are common for psoriatic involvement include elbows, knees, scalp, gluteal cleft, and nails. In children under age 2, it may present as a diaper rash.[1](pp264–334)

Epidemiology
Psoriasis affects between 1% and 3% of the population. It is found equally in men and women, and usually presents in the second or third decade of life, but may be seen initially in infants and elderly people. Psoriasis is much less common in African Americans, Native Americans, and Asians than in whites. Patients with psoriasis are at an increased risk for atherosclerotic cardiovascular disease and metabolic syndrome.[2]

Classification
Several forms of psoriasis are defined by morphology and area of cutaneous involvement.

- **Chronic plaque psoriasis** is the most common morphologic presentation typically involving the elbows, knees, and sometimes the scalp.
- **Guttate psoriasis** (multiple, small, droplike) usually develops prior to age 20, and is usually preceded by a streptococcal or viral upper respiratory tract infection.
- **Generalized pustular psoriasis** is a rare, serious, and sometimes fatal variant. Patients develop fever, malaise, diarrhea, and leukocytosis. This form of psoriasis may be precipitated by withdrawal from systemic steroids.

- **Erythrodermic psoriasis** is another rare and potentially fatal form of psoriasis, occurring in patients with previously stable, chronic psoriasis. Light-sensitive psoriasis is usually precipitated by solar exposure (in some patients hypersensitive to ultraviolet light).
- **Psoriasis of the scalp** presents with characteristic plaques and is more difficult to treat as plaques are anchored to the scalp by hair.
- **Psoriasis of the palms and soles** may be a distinct entity marked by exclusive involvement of the palms and soles or involvement (though uncommon) as part of a generalized eruption.
- **Pustular psoriasis** of the palms and soles cause deep pustules of the central palm and central sole of the foot.
- **Keratoderma blennorrhagicum** is a form of psoriasis that develops in patients with Reiter syndrome.
- **Psoriasis inversus** affects less common areas, including the axillae, groin, sub-mammary folds, and other intertriginous areas.
- **HIV-induced psoriasis** may have an atypical clinical presentation, and an unusually severe course.[1(pp267–275)]

Pathophysiology

Typical psoriatic plaques show characteristic changes, including hyperproliferation of epidermal keratinocytes and hyperkeratosis, and infiltration of immunocytes along with angiogenesis, with resultant thickening and scaling of the erythematous skin. Mitotic activity of keratinocytes is greatly increased.

Etiology

A genetic predisposition to psoriasis is postulated, although the exact pattern of inheritance is unclear. It appears that genetic predilection in combination with environmental factors precipitates the disease. Symptoms of psoriasis usually improve during summer, which may reflect the presumed positive effect of sunlight. Of patients with childhood psoriasis, 71% have a positive family history.[3]

Diagnosis

Clinical Presentation

Characteristic dermatologic lesions of psoriasis are red, scaling papules that coalesce into larger plaques. The classic scale of psoriasis is silvery white. There may be small, pinpoint areas of bleeding known as Auspitz sign. The plaques of psoriasis may become thick, especially on the scalp. Psoriasis without scaling is most common in the intertriginous areas, where it can appear as smooth, red, or macerated plaques. Psoriasis affects the extensor surfaces more commonly than the flexures and, in its most common form, spares the palm, soles, and face. Severe psoriasis may be a presenting finding in HIV infection. Psoriatic nail changes and psoriatic arthritis are the most common extracutaneous manifestations of psoriasis, and occur in 5% to 20% of patients with psoriasis.[3] Scalp lesions are seen in approximately 50% of patients with psoriasis.

History

Approximately 30% of patients with psoriasis have their first episode before age 20.[1(pp264–334)] In many cases, the initial presentation is that of guttate psoriasis—psoriatic rash developing after a streptococcal or viral upper respiratory infection. Guttate psoriasis may resolve spontaneously, with recurrence of chronic plaque psoriasis being common. Pruritis is variable. Response to treatment is often temporary. Exacerbations and remissions are usual. Psoriatic arthritis is more common in patients with severe dermatologic disease. Medications may also precipitate or exacerbate the disease. These include lithium, quinidine, clonidine, iodine, indomethacin, some β-blockers, terfenadine, nonsteroidal antiinflammatory drugs, angiotensin-converting enzyme inhibitors, interferon-α, interleukin-2, isotretinoin, and antimalarial agents.

Physical Examination

Psoriasis most commonly presents with noninflammatory, well-defined, localized plaques involving the extensor surfaces of the elbows, the scalp, the gluteal cleft, and the nails of both the hands and feet. If these occur in intertriginous areas, they may appear inflamed (i.e., bright red and shiny). If a plaque resolves, the skin demonstrates a temporary brown or white macule. The joints may exhibit asymmetric arthritis of one or more joints of the fingers and toes, most often the proximal interphalangeal, distal interphalangeal, metatarsophalangeal, or metacarpophalangeal joints. The joint may be red, warm, painful, and exhibit soft tissue swelling known as "sausage finger." Range of motion may be decreased. Nail changes, including pitting, yellowing, and severe nail dystrophy, are most commonly seen among patients with joint involvement. Ocular involvement occurs in some patients with psoriatic arthritis. Uveitis, which is the most common manifestation, may present with insidious visual impairment or with acute, painful red eye.

Laboratory Studies

Laboratory tests are of limited value in this disease. If guttate psoriasis is suspected, throat cultures may be obtained to rule out streptococcal infection. There is a high incidence of positive, antistreptolysin O (ASO) titers in this group.[1(pp264–334)] If psoriatic arthritis is suspected, other rheumatologic causes of arthritis should be ruled out. Rheumatoid factor levels are usually normal, although a small percentage of patients with psoriatic arthritis will have mild elevations.[1(pp264–334)] Erythrocyte sedimentation rate (ESR), white blood cell counts, and uric acid levels may show mild elevation but have limited predictive value in the diagnosis of psoriatic arthritis.

Imaging

The most severe form of psoriatic arthritis is arthritis mutilans, which classically presents with marked deformity and destruction of the digits on radiograph.

Monitoring

The ESR is the best laboratory test to monitor disease activity.

Surgical Diagnostic Procedures

In rare instances, when the diagnosis is not apparent on clinical presentation, punch biopsy of skin lesions may be diagnostic.

Classification

Diagnostic classification is based on morphology and location of psoriatic lesions (see above). For treatment options, patients are classified according to percentage of body surface affected by psoriasis. Patients with less than 20% of body surface involvement can be managed with topical therapy. Patients with greater cutaneous involvement require more aggressive therapy.

Differential Diagnosis

Seborrheic dermatitis (SD) is commonly confused with psoriasis. Chronic eczema with lichenification may present with thickened plaques, and should be included in the differential diagnosis. Other considerations include superficial fungal infections, lichen planus, pityriasis rosea, squamous cell carcinoma, and cutaneous T-cell lymphoma.

Treatment

Behavioral

A positive correlation between the severity of psoriatic symptoms and psychologic stress has been demonstrated. Stress reduction techniques are therefore useful in some patients.

Medications

Treatment occurs via four basic modalities: topical applications, phototherapy, systemic treatments, and immunobiologics. Other experimental approaches will also be briefly discussed. Disease control, including decreasing frequency of exacerbations, should be the goal of therapy. The mainstay of treatment in mild and localized psoriasis (75% of patients) is topical therapy, with or without phototherapy.[4] The second group (25%) with moderate to severe psoriasis is usually treated with systemic treatment. Most common topical treatments include emollients, topical corticosteroids, vitamin D analogs (calcipotriene), vitamin A analog (tazarotene), anthralin, and tars. Topical steroids provide rapid response and control itching and inflammation. Disadvantages include tolerance and skin atrophy. Efficacy may be increased by using occlusive dressings. Calcipotriene produces long remissions but may cause severe irritation and burning. Tazarotene (a retinoid) can also be very irritating to the skin. Efficacy of these medications may be enhanced, and irritation decreased, by concomitant topical steroid use. Anthralin can be used in short bursts, and is effective for scalp psoriasis. It is most effective on chronic, noninflamed plaques, and when used with ultraviolet light (UVB) therapy. Tar solutions are effective in only a small percentage of patients and are best combined with UVB light.[4] Regimens including ultraviolet therapy require major commitment of time and money, making them less accessible.

Therapeutic options for severe psoriasis (involving greater than 20% of the cutaneous surface) include ultraviolet light (UVB), the use of psoralens, along with exposure to long-wave ultraviolet light (PUVA). PUVA therapy is effective for symptomatic control of severe and disabling plaque psoriasis, but requires significant time commitment, and is not effective for scalp lesions. Because of concerns with long-term exposure and toxicity, PUVA is most appropriate for patients older than 50 years. Other treatment options for severe psoriasis include methotrexate, acitretin, and cyclosporin. Methotrexate and cyclosporin are effective in psoriatic arthritis but are of limited value secondary to hepatotoxicity and nephrotoxicity, respectively.[1(pp264–334)] Combining PUVA with UVB, calcipotriene, tazarotene, acitretin, or methotrexate improves efficacy, and decreases cost and adverse effects of treatment. Frequent monitoring of renal, hepatic, and hematologic function is required with several of these agents.

Recent advances in psoriasis research have provided biologic agents that target key mechanisms in the pathogenesis of psoriasis. TNT-α inhibitors are the most commonly prescribed biologic agents and include adalimumab and atanercept.[1(pp264–334)]

Referrals
Treatment of severe psoriasis and frequent exacerbations and medications used in their management require frequent monitoring, best accomplished through specialized dermatologic care. If psoriatic arthritis is suspected, rheumatologic referral is recommended.

Patient Education
Patients should be informed of the chronic nature of this disease. Environmental factors, medications, and stress exacerbating psoriasis should be avoided.

Follow-Up
Frequent follow-up is important to determine effectiveness of treatment. Some systemic therapeutic agents require special testing to avoid medication side effects.

ACNE ROSACEA
General Principles
Definition
Rosacea is a chronic acneiform dermatologic disorder characterized by erythema, edema, papules and pustules, and telangiectasia, usually affecting middle-aged individuals. It is characterized by periods of remission and exacerbation.[5]

Anatomy
Rosacea commonly involves the central face, including the nose, forehead, cheeks, and periorbital and eyelid areas. Hyperplasia of the soft tissue of the nose (rhinophyma) may occur in long-standing rosacea.

Epidemiology
Rosacea most commonly occurs between the ages of 30 and 60 years, although it has rarely been reported in younger individuals. It is relatively common among individuals with light hair and eye color, fair skin, and those with a history of blushing or flushing.

Classification
Rosacea disorders are divided into four broad subtypes to guide diagnosis and treatment:

1. Erythematotelangiectatic (vascular) characterized by flushing, telangiectasia, and possibly edema
2. Inflammatory characterized by a spectrum from small papules and pustules to deep nodules
3. Phymatous characterized by marked skin thickening and surface nodularities
4. Ocular characterized by blepharitis and conjunctivitis

Other variants include granulomatous, pyoderma faciale, and perioral dermatitis.[6]

Pathophysiology
The cardinal features include erythema, edema, papules and pustules, and telangiectasia.[3]

Etiology
The cause of rosacea is unknown. It is clear that individuals with rosacea have a defective skin barrier and are hyperirritable. Infection with the hair mites *Demodex folliculorum* has historically been linked to rosacea, but without evidence. One study found an increased frequency of *Helicobacter pylori* infection, but current literature does not support this to be a causative factor.[6]

Diagnosis

Clinical Presentation
The earliest manifestations include facial erythema and fine telangiectasia typically involving the cheek. This may progress to a papular or cystic rash involving the cheeks, nose, or forehead. Patients may also present with ocular symptoms.

History
Patients with rosacea usually have a history of recurrent flushing, precipitated by hot or spicy foods, alcohol consumption, temperature changes (including ingested liquids) and extremes, or

emotional stimulus. Symptoms may also be brought on or aggravated by sun exposure, but solar skin damage is not a prerequisite for the development of rosacea.[5] Later in the disease process, patients may develop hyperplasia of sebaceous glands with accompanying papules, pustules, and nodules resembling acne vulgaris. Ocular symptoms may develop alone or in association with skin lesions, and may include burning, foreign body sensation, meibomian gland dysfunction, blepharitis, conjunctivitis, or episcleritis. Cystic lesions of the nose can occur late in the disease, mostly in middle-aged men.

Physical Examination
Classic skin findings include **erythema** of the forehead, cheeks, and nose. Close inspection may reveal telangiectasias. These may be accompanied by papules, pustules, nodules, and cysts. Comedones are not characteristic of rosacea. Granuloma formation, characterized by hard papules or nodules, may be severe and most apparent on the nose, representing rhinophyma. Ocular involvement may present with mild conjunctivitis, conjunctival hyperemia, telangiectasia of the lid, blepharitis, and chalazion. The National Rosacea Society Expert Committee recommends the presence of one or more of the following primary features for diagnosis:

- Flushing (transient erythema)
- Nontransient erythema
- Papules and pustules
- Telangiectasia

The following secondary features may appear with primary features:

- Burning or stinging
- Plaque
- Dry appearance
- Edema
- Ocular manifestations
- Peripheral location
- Phymatous changes[7]

Laboratory Studies
Laboratory studies are not helpful in diagnosis.

Surgical Diagnostic Procedures
Diagnosis of rosacea is clinical. Punch biopsy may be helpful if diagnostic uncertainty is present.

Differential Diagnosis
Differential diagnosis includes acne vulgaris, keratosis pilaris, SD, basal cell carcinoma, systemic lupus erythematosus (SLE), and chronic topical steroid use.[6] Rosacea is differentiated from acne vulgaris by the absence of comedones, and from SLE by the presence of papules and pustules. SD usually has prominent scales. Carcinoid syndrome is rare and may cause brief flushing. The cutaneous effects of chronic topical steroids can be indistinguishable from rosacea but resolves with its discontinuation.

Treatment

Behavioral
Control of symptoms is the goal of therapy.

Medications
The three topical medications approved by the Food and Drug Administration for rosacea include topical solutions of **metronidazole,** several brands of **sodium sulfacetamide with sulfur,** and **azelaic acid gel.** Metronidazole, either alone or combined with oral antibiotics, is frequently used for initial therapy to decrease inflammation and erythema. The azelaic acid gel is as effective as metronidazole, although its use is limited by skin irritation. Sodium sulfacetamide is less effective than metronidazole and azelaic acid gel. Topical agents should be used for at least 4 weeks before assessing effectiveness. If symptoms persist after initial topical therapy, tretinoin cream may be useful in papular or pustular lesions, and may be combined with topical antibiotics. Oral antibiotics may be necessary for nodular rosacea or in patients with ocular involvement. Oral antibiotics that have been shown to be effective include **tetracycline, metronidazole, erythromycin,** and **azithromycin.** Maintaining remission with **topical metronidazole** is required after initial therapy. **Isotretinoin** has been used effectively in the treatment of rosacea, including rhinophyma.[8]

Surgery
Vascular laser therapy and light therapy may be useful in telangiectasias.

Special Therapy
Minimizing sun exposure is important. Broad-spectrum sunscreen should be applied daily. Some sunscreens can cause irritation and trigger rosacea. Silicon-based preparations are the best. Cosmetic sensitivity is a common feature of rosacea and therefore cosmetic use should be minimized. Astringents and camphor-containing products should also be avoided.

Referrals
Referral to a dermatologist is indicated if response to topical and oral therapy is inadequate. Referral to an ophthalmologist is recommended if ocular rosacea is suspected.

Patient Education
See Special Therapy.

Follow-Up
After initial treatment, follow-up is required in 6 to 8 weeks to determine treatment efficacy.

Complications
Patients with rosacea can develop ocular symptoms that include subnormal tear production, corneal vascularization, and infiltration. Visual acuity may be affected.

ATOPIC DERMATITIS
General Principles

Definition
Atopic dermatitis (AD) is a chronic, inflammatory skin condition commonly seen in people with a personal or family history of allergic rhinitis or asthma. It is commonly referred to as "eczema." In modern usage, AD and atopic eczema are used interchangeably, and both are acceptable.

Anatomy
AD occurring in infants usually involves the cheeks and spares the perioral and perinasal areas. In childhood (2 to 12 years), it most commonly affects the flexure surfaces including the antecubital fossae, neck, wrists, and ankles. In adults (older than 12 years), AD involves the flexures but also may involve the hands and periorbital area.[9]

Epidemiology
The prevalence of AD has steadily increased over the past 50 years, and now affects more than 10% of children and 17.8 million people in the United States. More than 60% of patients present before the first year of life. It is rare in adults.[10]

Classification
Classification is based on age—infant phase (0 to 2 years), childhood phase (2 to 12 years), and adult phase (12 years and older).

Pathophysiology
Two models exist for possible causes of AD. First is thought to be a defect in filaggrin protein, which disrupts the epidermis. This leads to contact between the immune cells and antigens in the external environment. This process effectively modulates an inflammatory response to outside environmental factors.[10] The other mechanism thought to cause AD is an impaired epidermal function secondary to abnormalities in the skin.

Etiology
The precise immunologic mechanism involved in the development of AD is unclear. Allergic triggers such as some foods, dust mites, and animal dander have been implicated. AD-associated food allergies are more common in childhood, while airborne allergens are more commonly associated with AD in adults. Other triggers may include temperature change and sweating, excessive washing, contact with irritating substances, and decreased humidity.[11]

Diagnosis

Clinical Presentation
In infants, typical skin lesions include scaling on erythematous papules involving cheeks. These lesions may also affect the extremities or trunk, sparing the diaper area. In children, intensely pruritic patches

more commonly affect the flexure surfaces of the arms and legs. Adults present with a distribution of lesions similar to children but may also have lesions on the hands and eyelids.

History

Patients with AD usually have symptoms from childhood. Many patients with AD also exhibit symptoms of allergic rhinitis and/or asthma. Lesions are intensely pruritic. Patients may have history of recurrent bacterial, fungal, and viral skin infections. Food allergies in children and airborne allergens in adults may trigger AD flares.

Physical Examination

Acute lesions of AD are usually vesicles and may have exudate. More chronic lesions usually demonstrate thickened skin, increased skin markings (lichenification), and excoriated papules and plaques. The flexure areas most commonly involved include antecubital and popliteal fossae, wrists, and forearms. Severe cases may affect any skin surface, although lesions of the axillae, gluteal, or groin area are uncommon. Scratching, leading to destruction of melanocytes, results in areas of hypopigmentation. Associated clinical findings may include severe xerosis, development of ichthyosis, keratosis pilaris, hyperlinear palmar creases, and atopic pleats (appearance of an extra line on the lower eyelid, also known as Dennie–Morgan infraorbital fold).[12]

Laboratory Studies

Allergy testing may be of benefit to identify triggers causing AD flares.

Surgical Diagnostic Procedures

Punch biopsy may be indicated if clinical diagnosis is unclear.

Differential Diagnosis

Differential diagnosis of AD includes contact dermatitis, SD, drug reactions, psoriasis, and scabies. In infants, the rare disorders Wiskott–Aldrich syndrome and hyperimmunoglobulin E syndrome should be considered.

Treatment

Behavioral

Management of AD requires a comprehensive approach that addresses skin inflammation as well as elimination of exacerbating factors. Contact with wool, excessive heat, and other irritants should be minimized. Airborne allergens and allergenic foods must be identified and avoided. Skin hydration is key and skin must be moisturized by the application of nonirritating, hydrophobic lubricating agents.[13]

Medications

Acute flares of AD may require potent **topical corticosteroid** preparations for 7 to 10 days. **Tar preparations** can help control pruritus and resolve inflammation, decreasing the need for topical corticosteroids. Nonsedating antihistamines may have some anti-inflammatory effects but have not been shown to reduce pruritis significantly. Immunomodulators such as topical calcineurin inhibitors are now considered second-line therapy. The immunomodulators are recommended for short time periods due to potential side effects.[13] **Oral immunosuppressants** such as methotrexate or azathioprine may be considered in severe AD but should be avoided in children. Phototherapy (UVA + UVB) and oral immunosuppressants may be used for severe or resistant AD.[13]

Referrals

Referral to a dermatologist is appropriate if the diagnosis is uncertain, in patients failing to respond to conventional therapy, or if systemic immunosuppressive agents are considered necessary.

Protocol

Disease management should be considered in three phases: (a) induction of remission, (b) maintenance, and (c) rescue from flares. Induction of remission usually requires steroids while emollients are critical for maintenance therapy. Rescue from flares may involve treatment of secondary infections with oral antibiotics and avoiding exposure to triggers.

Follow-Up

Patients should be followed regularly to assess treatment efficacy.

Complications

Complications of chronic steroid use include skin atrophy, telangiectasia, striae, steroid rosacea, acne, hypopigmentation, and delayed wound healing.[13]

Special Considerations

Dealing with this chronic disease may result in emotional sequelae, but AD is not an emotional disorder as previously thought.

ALLERGIC AND IRRITANT CONTACT DERMATITIS
General Principles

Definition

Allergic contact dermatitis (ACD) is an inflammatory skin reaction that follows absorption of some antigen applied to the skin and recruitment of previously sensitized antigen-specific T lymphocytes. Irritant contact dermatitis (ICD) is an inflammatory skin reaction that results from direct epidermal damage produced by contact with an irritant and is not immunologic. ICD can affect any person at any time if the irritant and exposure are sufficient, while ACD requires a susceptible individual with prior sensitization by the allergen. Systemic contact dermatitis (SCD) is an inflammatory skin reaction that occurs in a previously sensitized person, following exposure to the allergen by ingestion, inhalation, or injection (e.g., patients allergic to poison ivy may develop a diffuse inflammatory skin reaction following ingestion of raw cashew nuts, which are chemically related to the specific allergen of poison ivy).[14,15]

Anatomy

Site of exposure of the suspected allergen is usually congruent with the distribution of the rash (under a watchband, elastic waistband, or shoe). Plants usually produce linear lesions at the site of contact. Half of all ACD involves the hands.[12] ACD usually affects the dorsum of the hand, where the skin is thinner. ACD secondary to allergens applied to the head will usually involve the hairline or ears, and spares the scalp, where the skin is thick. Airborne allergens, which can be transferred from the hands to the eyes and face, and cosmetics may cause facial involvement. The torso and groin are affected in the area of application of the allergen. Involvement of the oral mucosa is rare, but may occur with dental implants. Genitalia is commonly involved secondary to transfer of the allergens from hands.[16]

Epidemiology

ICD constitutes 80% of contact dermatitis. Industrial workers are at high risk for occupational skin exposure. The hands are the most commonly affected areas.[15]

Classification

Contact dermatitis is classified as ICD (irritant), ACD (allergic), or SCD (systemic) (see definition).

Pathophysiology

Unlike most clinical allergic diseases, which involve an immediate hypersensitivity response, ACD is a delayed (cell-mediated) hypersensitivity reaction that depends on previous sensitization in susceptible individuals. ICD results from direct epidermal damage. SCD involves systemic reexposure following previous sensitization to an allergen applied topically.

Etiology

ACD is caused by exposure to common contact allergens, including poison ivy, poison oak, poison sumac, nickel (the most common metal allergen), topical medications (neomycin and bacitracin), latex and rubber chemicals, formaldehyde, and fragrances.[17]

Diagnosis

Clinical Presentation

ACD presents as an acute pruritic eruption.

History

History should be directed at uncovering contact allergens—specifically work-related exposure, plant exposure, household products, jewelry, clothing, and cosmetics. The timing of an eruption may be as brief as 8 hours (common with plant exposure) and as remote as 1 week after exposure. Pruritus is uniformly present in CD.[16]

Physical Examination

The acute phase of ACD involves erythema, edema, and vesicles. Vesicles may coalesce to form bullae. Vesicles contain clear fluid and rupture spontaneously during the subacute stage (most common presentation). Vesicles are then replaced by papules, which develop crusting and scaling. Secondary bacterial infection may occur. As the papulovesicular lesions resolve, the chronic stage involving lichenification and scaling occurs.[14]

Laboratory Studies

Laboratory testing is not routinely recommended; however, patch testing may be used for patients with persistent eruptions and may be helpful to identify allergens.[15]

Staging

Lesions may present in acute, subacute, or chronic stages (see Physical Examination).

Differential Diagnosis

The differential diagnosis includes AD, SD, nummular eczema, dishydrotic eczema, photocontact dermatitis, psoriasis, T-cell lymphoma, scabies, tinea pedis, and bacterial, fungal, or viral skin infections.

Treatment

Behavioral

Central to ACD prevention and treatment is identifying specific allergens and avoiding contact with them. If the allergen cannot be avoided, wearing a protective barrier is recommended.

Medications

Initial treatment of vesicles and erythema includes cold compresses, which should be used for 15 to 30 minutes initially during the acute stage. Erythema may respond to topical corticosteroids. Hydroxyzine and diphenhydramine control itching. If dermatitis is severe or widespread, involves mucous membranes, or is unresponsive to initial therapy, **systemic corticosteroids** should be used. ACD due to plant allergens requires 10 to 21 days of treatment with **topical or oral corticosteroids** to prevent rebound dermatitis.[18]

Referrals

Referral to a dermatologist is warranted if the diagnosis is unclear or if the patient is unresponsive to conventional therapy.

Patient Education

See Behavioral.

Follow-Up

Patients should be instructed to follow up if rash does not resolve or worsens, as rebound dermatitis is possible and may be more severe than the initial eruption.

Special Considerations

The appearance of new lesions remote from the initial eruption, seen in plant contact dermatitis (Rhus dermatitis), may be confused with active spread of the disease. Contrary to popular belief, vesicle fluid does not contain allergen and cannot spread the inflammation.

SEBORRHEIC DERMATITIS
General Principles

Definition

SD is a chronic, inflammatory papulosquamous skin disease, characterized by erythema and scaling.

Anatomy

The term "seborrhea" suggests the anatomic distribution of this disorder, which is predominant in areas where sebaceous glands are abundant—the scalp, face, upper trunk, and intertriginous areas. Seborrhea also tends to present under areas of facial hair (mustache, beard, eyebrow), and nasolabial folds. In infants, seborrhea commonly affects the scalp and is termed "cradle cap."[19]

Epidemiology

In infants, seborrhea usually presents in the first 3 months of life. In adults, seborrhea is most commonly seen between 30 and 60 years of age.

Classification

Seborrhea is classified by age as **adolescent and adult SD** and **infant SD.** Infant SD may have a classic scalp distribution, or may be generalized.

Etiology

The etiology of SD is unknown. *Malassezia furfur* (formerly *Pityrosporum ovale*) has been implicated, but both genetic and environmental factors seem to influence the onset and course of the disease.[1(pp312–315)] Other possible stimulants include hormones, nutritional deficiencies, and a neurogenic cause (based on its association with parkinsonism and other neurologic syndromes).[20] It also appears to be triggered by stress and is both more prevalent and more intense in patients with the HIV syndrome.[19]

Diagnosis

Clinical Presentation

Patients with SD typically present with erythema and mild epidermal hyperproliferation leading to scaliness. SD in infants is not usually pruritic, whereas adult SD has varying degrees of pruritus.

History

The onset of seborrhea in infants is usually in the first 3 months of life with scalp involvement. Adults present with an itchy red rash. Patients may have a history of "dandruff" (mild seborrhea), with progression and worsening of symptoms. Symptoms may be worse in winter because of dry indoor environments. Sunlight may cause some patients to flare while promoting improvement in others. SD may have a chronic course in adults, with periods of remissions and exacerbations.

Physical Examination

SD of the scalp presents as mildly greasy scaling and erythema. Blepharoconjunctivitis may coexist. On the chest, SD presents with follicular and para-follicular papules with scales. In infants, SD presents with thick scales and erythema over the vertex of the scalp.[20] Application of lotions or oils to the scalp may cause SD to appear intensely erythematous without scaliness.

Laboratory Studies

Fungal cultures and potassium hydroxide (KOH) preparations may be indicated in resistant cases of SD.

Pathologic Findings

Histologically, SD reveals focal parakeratosis, with few neutrophils, moderate acanthosis, spongiosis, and nonspecific inflammation of the dermis. The most characteristic histological finding is neutrophils at the tips of dilated follicular openings.

Differential Diagnosis

SD of the scalp and face should be differentiated from tinea capitis, psoriasis, AD, contact dermatitis, erythrasma, and rosacea.[19] SD involving the trunk should be differentiated from pityriasis versicolor and pityriasis rosea. Underlying immunodeficiency should be suspected in generalized SD in infants, especially if associated with diarrhea and weight loss.[20] Immunodeficiency should also be suspected in adults who present with severe, recalcitrant cases of SD.

Treatment

Behavioral

Emotional stress has been linked to SD flares.

Medications

Effective treatment options include keratolytics, antifungals, and anti-inflammatory agents. Keratolytics induce sloughing of cornified epithelium. Salicylic acid, zinc pyrithione, and tar shampoos are effective for lesions involving the scalp and face. Treatment of infantile SD requires milder formulations. Shampoos may be used two to three times per week. Anti-inflammatory topical agents and shampoos such as fluocinolone shampoo and cream are also effective, especially in patients with SD involving the scalp. Patients may apply a topical steroid once or twice a day with a shampoo. Topical calcineurin inhibitors (Tacrolimus, Pimecrolimus) have anti-inflammatory and antifungal properties and are recommended for SD over facial skin.[20] Most antifungal agents are effective against *Malassezia* species associated with SD. Ketoconazole and selenium sulfide shampoos are commonly used. Ketoconazole preparations should be avoided in infants.[20] Phototherapy utilizing ultraviolet B light is an alternative in patients with extensive SD unresponsive to other measures.[19]

Special Therapy

Seborrheic blepharitis may respond to cleansing of the eyelashes with baby shampoo and cotton-tipped applicators. The use of ketoconazole in this area is controversial.

Referrals

Referral to dermatology is typically required only in recalcitrant or very severe cases.

Patient Education

Patients should be educated that this is a chronic disorder that may require continued maintenance therapy.

Special Considerations

SD is the most common cutaneous manifestation of AIDS.[1(pp312–315)] Severe intractable or extensive seborrhea should prompt evaluation for HIV infection. Infants with widespread SD, diarrhea, and inadequate weight gain and physical growth (failure to thrive) should be evaluated for immunodeficiency states.[20]

PITYRIASIS ROSEA
General Principles

Definition

Pityriasis rosea (PR) is an acute, self-limiting papulosquamous skin eruption, preceded by a viral illness in nearly three-fourths of patients.[1(pp316–318)]

Anatomy

PR typically involves the trunk and proximal extremities, but in rare cases may involve the arms, legs, and face. A reverse presentation, involving the extremities, is rarely seen.

Epidemiology

The average age of patients affected with PR is 23, with most cases occurring between 10 and 35 years of age. PR occurs most often in the spring and fall.

Classification

The initial phase involves appearance of the "herald patch," followed 7 to 14 days later by a generalized eruption—the "eruptive phase."

Etiology

The etiology of PR is unclear, although an infectious agent (Human Herpes Virus 6 and 7) is likely.[21] This is supported by the fact that PR occurs in clusters, rarely recurs (2%), and is preceded commonly by a prodromal illness.

Diagnosis

Clinical Presentation

Typical presentation is a prodromal viral illness (headache, malaise, pharyngitis), followed by the herald patch and subsequent smaller salmon-colored lesions during the eruptive phase.

History

Many patients will report an upper respiratory illness a few weeks prior to the rash. The herald patch is typically seen on the torso or proximal arm. Then, 7 to 14 days later, similar smaller oval lesions appear on the trunk and proximal extremities. The majority of patients (over 75%) will also report pruritus. The rash of PR resolves spontaneously in 5 to 8 weeks.[22]

Physical Examination

The herald patch is a 2- to 10-cm ovoid erythematous, raised patch with a peripheral collarette of fine scales. Subsequent eruption involves similar 5- to 10-mm salmon-colored lesions (hyperpigmented in African Americans) with a characteristic distribution following lines of cleavage (Christmas tree pattern). Lesions may show excoriation.

Laboratory Studies

Physicians may perform KOH testing to rule out tinea. Serologic testing for syphilis is a consideration in appropriate clinical settings.

Pathologic Findings

Histologically, PR demonstrates parakeratosis with or without acanthosis, spongiosis, and a perivascular infiltrate of lymphocytes and histiocytes.

Differential Diagnosis

Psoriasis, secondary syphilis, tinea corporis, Lyme disease, HIV seroconversion illness, and drug eruptions (e.g., hepatitis B vaccine, interferon, captopril, and clonidine) should all be considered.[16] Pityriasis Lichenoides Chronica is a variant of PR with similar morphology and distribution but has no herald patch and lasts longer than PR.[21]

Treatment

Behavioral

Patients should be counseled that PR is a self-limited illness.

Medications

PR, being self-limited, requires only symptomatic treatment in most patients. Oral antihistamines and topical agents (steroids and calamine lotion) may be used for relief of pruritus. Systemic steroids may be used in extensive lesions with severe pruritus, but may lengthen the course of the illness. Some studies show efficacy of antiviral agents (acyclovir, ganciclovir, foscarnet) in hastening resolution of lesions, especially if treated soon after their expression.[1(pp316–318)]

Special Therapy

PR may be alleviated by UVB phototherapy or natural sunlight exposure if started in the first week of symptoms.

Referrals

Consider referral to dermatology for variable lesion morphology, or if lesions are more extensive or last longer than expected.

Patient Education

Educate patients about etiology (unknown), infectivity (very low), relapse (uncommon), and complications (rare).

Follow-Up

Patients should be instructed to follow up if rash persists longer than 3 months.

Complications

Complications are rare, but postinflammatory hyperpigmentation or hypopigmentation may occur.[20] PD during pregnancy may result in miscarriage, preterm labor, and fetal demise; these patients should be counseled and referred for high-risk maternity care.[21]

REFERENCES

1. Habif TH. Psoriasis and other papulosquamous diseases. In: Habif TP, ed. *Clinical dermatology*. 5th ed. Philadelphia, PA: Mosby; 2010.
2. Armstrong AM, Harskamp CT, Armstrong EJ. Psoriasis and metabolic syndrome: a systematic review and meta-analysis of observational studies. *J Am Acad Dermatol* 2013;68(4):654–662.
3. Schon MP, Boehncke W-H. Medical progress: psoriasis. *N Engl J Med* 2005;18:1899–1912.
4. Levine D, Gottlieb A. Evaluation and management of psoriasis: an internist's guide. *Med Clin North Am* 2009;93:108–114.
5. Habif TH. Acne rosacea. In: Habif TH, ed. *Clinical dermatology*. 5th ed. Philadelphia, PA: Mosby; 2010:256–259.
6. Webster GF. Rosacea. *Med Clin North Am* 2009;93:1016–1027.
7. Wilkins J, Dahl M, Detmar M, et al. Standard grading system for rosacea: report of the National Rosacea Society Expert Committee on the classification and staging of rosacea. *J Am Acad Dermatol* 2004;50:907–912.
8. Goldgar C, Keahey D, Houchins J. Treatment options for acne rosacea. *Am Fam Physician* 2009;80: 461–468.
9. Weston WL, Howe W. Epidemiology, clinical manifestations, and diagnosis of atopic dermatitis (eczema). In: Dellavalle RP, ed. *UpToDate*. Waltham, MA: UpToDate. http://www.uptodate.com/contents/epidemiology-clinical-manifestations-and-diagnosis-of-atopic-dermatitis-eczema Accessed March 31, 2014.
10. Berke R, Singh A, Guralnick M. Atopic dermatitis: an overview. *Am Fam Physician* 2012;86(1):35–42.
11. Spergel JM. Role of allergy in atopic dermatitis (eczema). In: Sicherer SH, ed. *UpToDate*. Waltham, MA: UpToDate. http://www.uptodate.com/contents/role-of-allergy-in-atopic-dermatitis-eczema?source =search_result&search=Role+of+allergy+in+atopic+dermatitis+%28eczema&selectedTitle=1%7E150. Accessed March 31, 2014.
12. Habif TH. Atopic dermatitis. In: Habif TH, ed. *Clinical dermatology*. 5th ed. Philadelphia, PA: Mosby; 2010:154–180.
13. Weston WL, Howe W. Treatment of atopic dermatitis (eczema). In: Dellavalle RP, ed. *UpToDate*. Waltham, MA: UpToDate. http://www.uptodate.com/contents/treatment-of-atopic-dermatitis-eczema? source=search_result&search=Treatment+of+atopic+dermatitis+%28eczema%29.&selectedTitle= 1%7E150. Accessed March 31, 2014.
14. Habif TH. Contact dermatitis and patch testing. In: Habif TH, ed. *Clinical dermatology*. 5th ed. Philadelphia, PA: Mosby; 2010:130–153.

15. Usatine RP, Riojas M. Diagnosis and management of contact dermatitis. *Am Fam Physician* 2010;82(3):249–255.
16. Yiannias J. Clinical features and diagnosis of allergic contact dermatitis. In: Fowler J, ed. *UpToDate*. Waltham, MA: UpToDate. http://www.uptodate.com/contents/clinical-features-and-diagnosis-of-allergic-contact-dermatitis?source=search_result&search=Clinical+features+and+diagnosis+of+allergic+contact+dermatitis&selectedTitle=1%7E136. Accessed March 31, 2014.
17. Goldner R, Tuchinda P. Irritant contact dermatitis in adults. In: Fowler J, ed. *UpToDate*. Waltham, MA: UpToDate. http://www.uptodate.com/contents/irritant-contact-dermatitis-in-adults?source=search_result&search=Irritant+contact+dermatitis+in+adults&selectedTitle=1%7E33. Accessed March 31, 2014.
18. Brod B. Management of allergic contact dermatitis. In: Fowler J, ed. *UpToDate*. Waltham, MA: UpToDate. http://www.uptodate.com/contents/management-of-allergic-contact-dermatitis?source=search_result&search=Management+of+allergic+contact+dermatitis.&selectedTitle=1%7E136. Accessed March 31, 2014.
19. Naldi L, Rebora A. Seborrheic dermatitis. *N Engl J Med* 2009;360:387–396.
20. Schwartz RA, Janusz CA, Janniger CK. Seborrheic dermatitis: an overview. *Am Fam Physician* 2006;74:125–130.
21. Browning JC. An update on pityriasis rosea and other similar childhood exanthems. *Curr Opin Pediatr* 2009;21:481–485.
22. Stulberg DL, Wolfrey J. Pityriasis rosea. *Am Fam Physician* 2004;69:87–91.

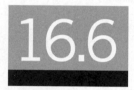

16.6 Urticaria

William A. Alto, Louis Paul Gianutsos

GENERAL PRINCIPLES
Definitions
- **Urticaria** is a common and reversible skin eruption characterized by multiple, palpable, circumscribed, erythematous, blanchable, pruritic papules (wheals) and plaques ranging in size from 2 mm to 30 cm.
- **Angioedema** occurs abruptly on the skin and mucous membranes, may or may not be erythematous, is seldom pruritic but may be painful.
- They are classified by their time course as acute or chronic (lasting more than 6 weeks) and by the presumed inciting agent or mechanism.

Pathophysiology
- **Urticaria** involves the superficial dermis.
- **Angioedema** involves the deep dermis and subcutaneous tissue.
- They result from **vasodilation and increased vascular permeability** caused by the release of mast cell mediators of inflammation, such as histamine and other vasoactive substances.
- Mechanisms are autoimmune, immune complement, and nonimmune mediated.

Epidemiology
- Acute urticaria affects up to 20% of individuals at some point during their life. Chronic urticaria has a prevalence of less than 1%, while angioedema affects about 40% of those with chronic urticaria.[1]

DIAGNOSIS
Clinical Presentation
- **Acute urticaria** (urticarial wheals) develop rapidly over 15 minutes and dissipate within 60 minutes to 24 hours. As lesions resolve new crops appear, and the patient may mistakenly report that the individual "hives" have been present for days or weeks.

- **Physical urticarias** are provoked by skin stimulation resulting in mast cell degranulation. Duration is brief, lasting only 30 to 60 minutes.
- **Angioedema** has indistinct borders, typically involves the mouth, lips, larynx, tongue, the genitalia, and mucosa of the gastrointestinal tract, and lasts 2 to 3 days.
- **Angiotensin-converting enzyme (ACE) inhibitor angioedema** does not have associated urticaria.

History

- **A careful history** often identifies the cause.
- **Gastrointestinal angioedema** causes abdominal pain.
- **Oral angioedema** may result in airway obstruction.

Physical Examination

- **Physical urticarias** can be identified by application of the offending agent or force.
- **Urticarial vasculitis** is an indicator of underlying disease and must be differentiated from the acute and chronic urticarial wheals. Urticarial vasculitis is suggested by the presence of painful wheals lasting more than 24 hours, wheals with underlying purpura, or those with residual hyperpigmentation.
- **Angioedema** frequently accompanies the urticarial wheals of chronic, cold, or solar urticaria.

Laboratory Studies

- The American Academy of Allergy, Asthma and Immunology recommends against routine diagnostic testing of patients with chronic urticaria.[2]
- **Antithyroid antibodies** may be found in chronic urticaria with an associated thyroiditis.
- **Complement assays** are used to diagnose hereditary angioedema.
- **Surgical diagnostic procedures:** Suspected urticarial vasculitis merits a biopsy.

Classification

- **Allergic urticaria** is immunoglobulin E (IgE) mediated (type 1 hypersensitivity).
- Direct contact, ingestion, or inhalation of an allergen causes hives.
- **Typical allergens** include grasses, pollens, insect toxins, drugs, foods, or simultaneous infections.
- **Medications** commonly associated with urticaria include penicillin, cephalosporins, sulfonamides, aspirin, nonsteroidal anti-inflammatory drugs, and vaccines.
- **Foods** frequently linked with transient urticaria are eggs, nuts, shellfish, strawberries, chocolate, and tomatoes.
- **Infectious agents** include hepatitis and Epstein–Barr virus, bacteria, and intestinal parasites.
- **Children with atopic dermatitis** are more likely to have urticaria.
- **Physical urticarias** comprise 20% to 30% of chronic urticarias.
- **Dermatographism** is the most common physical urticaria.
- **Cholinergic urticaria** is characterized by small (1 to 3 mm) pruritic papules with blanched centers. Physical exercise, hot showers, fever, and anxiety are antecedent stimuli.
- **Uncommon** (cold) and rare (solar, localized heat, delayed pressure, vibratory, and aquagenic) causes of urticaria can be identified by application of the offending agent or force.
- **Delayed-pressure urticaria** has a 4- to 6-hour lag time between the stimulus and the appearance of a wheal, which may last several hours.
- **Chemical or contact urticarias** do not involve IgE release.
- **Drugs** can cause the direct release of histamine in susceptible individuals: aspirin, amphotericin B, dextromethorphan, opiates, buproprion, selective serotonin-reuptake inhibitors (SSRIs), polymyxin B, scopolamine, and radiographic contrast-containing iodine.
- Nonimmunologic urticaria does not require prior exposure to the offending agent. It has a gradual onset over hours and makes up 90% of drug-associated urticaria.
- Certain foods, including spoiled mackerel and tuna, may cause urticaria because of their high histamine content (scombroid poisoning).
- **Chronic urticaria** is often attributed to an autoimmune etiology, but this remains unproven.
- **Focal infections,** candidiasis, and undiagnosed malignancy are rarely, if ever, the causes of chronic urticaria.
- **Angioedema is** most commonly an adverse reaction to drug therapy.
- ACE inhibitors cause angioedema without hives (Kinin pathway). One half of patients present during the first week on the medication.

- **Hereditary autosomal dominant angioedema is rare** (less than 0.4%). Penetrance is variable, and acquired cases occur, so that a family history may not be helpful. If the fourth component of complement (C4) is low, then the diagnosis should be confirmed with an assay of C1 esterase inhibitor, which is also low.

Differential Diagnosis

- **Erythema multiforme (EM)** may be confused with large urticarial wheals. EM has an acute onset and typically evolving target lesions that last at least 7 days and fade by 4 weeks.
- **Insect bites** may occasionally resemble urticaria. The patient's history and location of the lesions will help clarify the etiology.
- **Mastocytosis** (urticaria pigmentosa, solitary mastocytoma, systemic disease, and mastocytosis with associated hematologic disorders) is characterized by histamine and other vasoactive substances released from overabundant mast cells. Urticaria and flushing are common symptoms.
- **Dermatitis herpetiformis and bullous pemphigoid** can occasionally resemble urticaria. They are longer lasting.
- **Pruritic urticarial papules and plaques of pregnancy** is a fixed rash.
- **Angioedema** could be confused with facial cellulitis or the edema of superior vena cava syndrome.

TREATMENT

- A thorough **history** coupled with knowledge of frequently-implicated triggers can help prevent further attacks.
- **Local therapies** such as topical anti-pruritics, doxepin cream, and 1% menthol in aqueous cream are not very effective.[3]
- **Antihistamine therapy** with H_1 receptor blockers is more effective for acute urticarias. Regular dosing around the clock offers better control. Nonsedating antihistamines are first-line therapy.[3] Desloratadine and levocetirizine at up to four times normal dosing are effective in children and non-pregnant adults.[4,5] Loratadine is pregnancy category B at standard doses. Drug interactions should be considered at higher dosages.
- Older antihistamines are effective but not well tolerated at higher doses except at bedtime. They should be avoided in children less than 2 years of age.
- **Histamine H_2 blockers** have been used in conjunction with H_1 blockers, but there is insufficient evidence as to their effectiveness.[6]
- **Leukotriene antagonists** can be added for symptoms persisting beyond 6 weeks.[5]
- **Corticosteroids** given orally for 3 to 7 days can be used as a third-line agent.
- **Severe or refractory chronic urticaria** must be individualized and may ultimately necessitate immunosuppressive therapy with corticosteroids, cyclosporine, methotrexate, or tacrolimus. There is less evidence to support intravenous immunoglobulins, azathioprine, mycophenolate mofetil, cyclophosphamide, and anti-IgE. Evaluation and treatment are usually coordinated by dermatologists and allergists.
- Patients should be advised to avoid aspirin, other nonsteroidal anti-inflammatory agents, and opioid narcotics.
- Angioedema patients may require intubation. Epinephrine, first-generation antihistamines, and corticosteroids are used.

REFERENCES

1. Sánchez-Borges M, Asero R, Ansotequi IJ, et al. Diagnosis and treatment of urticaria and angioedema: a worldwide perspective. *World Allergy Organ J* 2012;11:125–147.
2. American Academy of Allergy, Asthma & Immunology. Choosing Wisely. http://www.choosingwisely .org/doctor-patient-lists/american-academy-of-allergy-asthma-immunology/. Accessed March 15, 2014.
3. Zuberbier T, Asero R, Bindslev-Jensen C, et al. EAACI/GA2LEN/EDF/WAO Guideline: management of urticaria. *Allergy* 2009;64:1427–1443.
4. Zuberbier T, Asero R, Bindslev-Jensen C, et al. EAACI/GA2LEN/EDF/WAO Guideline: definition, classification and diagnosis of urticaria. *Allergy* 2009;64:1417–1426.
5. Kavosh ER, Khan DA. Second-generation H1-antihistamines in chronic urticaria: an evidence-based review. *Am J Clin Dermatol* 2011;6:361–376.
6. Fedorowicz Z, van Zuuren EJ. Histamine H2-receptor blockers for urticaria. The Cochrane Library http://www.ncbi.nlm.nih.gov/pubmed/22419335. Accessed March 15, 2014.

Stasis Dermatitis, Venous (Stasis) Ulcers, and Pressure Ulcers

Ryan C. Petering

STASIS DERMATITIS
General

Definition

Stasis dermatitis (SD) is an eczematous skin condition associated with erythema hyperpigmentation, pruritis, erosions, edema, and lipodermatosclerosis.[1]

Classification

SD is a clinical indicator of chronic venous insufficiency (CVI). CVI is graded by CEAP (Clinical, Etiologic, Anatomic, Pathologic) classification system. The clinical classes are C0: no signs or symptoms of venous disease; C1: telangiectasias; C2: varicose veins; C3: edema; C4: SD changes (pigmentation, eczema, etc.); C5: healed venous stasis ulcer; and C6: active venous stasis ulcer. Etiology is categorized as primary (degeneration of veins and valves), secondary (damage to vein from deep vein thrombosis (DVT) or inflammatory conditions), or congenital. The anatomic classes are superficial or deep. The Pathologic category is divided into reflux or obstruction.[2]

Pathophysiology

The venous system of the lower extremity is composed of superficial, perforating, and deep veins. All veins have one-way valves that allow one-way flow of blood from the superficial veins to the deep veins. The valves prevent reflux of blood. Dysfunction of the venous system causes pooling of blood. This triggers a cascade of inflammatory changes and capillary damage that develops CVI. Older age, family history of venous insufficiency, standing occupation, injury, and history of phlebitis or clot are recognized risk factors for CVI.[3]

Diagnosis

History

SD typically has acute, subacute, chronic, and recurrent presentations. Common complaints are skin color changes, edema, itching, and drainage.

Physical Examination

SD is found on the lower extremities. Acute changes include red, itchy plaques that develop abruptly. Subacute and chronic eczematous changes (dry, flaking, peeling, or erythematous skin) may be seen. Hemosiderin deposition results in reddish brown pigmentation and fibrosis of the subcutaneous tissue. Lipodermatosclerosis refers to necrosis of fat with advanced SD that leads to narrowing of legs distally with an "inverted champagne bottle" appearance.[4] SD is first diagnosed with a presentation of a stasis ulcer.

Laboratory/Imaging

Venous duplex ultrasonography and ankle/brachial index (ABI) testing commonly may be ordered to rule out other conditions.

Differential Diagnosis

Cellulitis, contact dermatitis, and tinea corporis are common conditions that may mimic SD. The chronic nature of this condition will help in the diagnosis. Venous ulcers often coexist with SD.

Treatment

Behavioral

Treatment of SD requires significant lifestyle changes. Control of the edema associated with SD is essential. Elevation of the legs whenever possible and avoidance of prolonged standing can improve dependent edema. Compression stockings can be used to treat underlying venous insufficiency. Gradient compression stocking provide the greatest pressure (20 to 40 mmHg) around the ankle and gradually decrease proximally. Multilayered compression bandages are more expensive than single-layer bandages, but they provide faster healing. In severe cases, intermittent pneumatic compression pumps may be considered.[5]

Medications and Immunizations
The acute eczematous changes should be managed with topical steroids and lubricating creams. Oral antibiotics may be required if secondary cellulitis is suspected.

Patient Education
Patients should be educated on importance of regular exercise, avoidance of prolonged periods of sitting or standing, and need for frequent elevation of the legs.

VENOUS (STASIS) ULCER
General

Definition
A venous (stasis) ulcer (VU) is an ulcer commonly located on the lower leg and is associated with CVI.

Epidemiology
Older age, obesity, previous leg injuries, tobacco use, deep venous thrombosis, and phlebitis are risk factors for VU.[6,7]

Classification
See the CEAP classification above.

Diagnosis

History
Venous ulcers are often chronic and recurrent. Swelling and aching of lower legs are common. Mild trauma may precede VU development.

Physical Examination
Venous ulcers are shallow, painful, irregular shape, below the knee, and commonly on the medial aspect of the leg. VUs are commonly located in the "gaiter area" from mid-calf to the ankle. Dependent edema, varicose veins, purpura, and changes associated with SD may be present. It is important to assess pulses, sensation, and capillary refill time during the clinical examination.

Laboratory/Imaging
Venous ulcers are typically diagnosed clinically. Venous duplex ultrasonography and ABI testing are commonly ordered to rule out other conditions. Nonhealing ulcers may require tissue culture or biopsy if not responding to therapy.

Differential Diagnosis
Ulcers of the lower leg are typically arterial, venous, diabetic/neuropathic, or pressure related. Ulcers of the lower extremity are often caused by more than one etiology. Arterial ulcers are associated with pain, decreased pulses, and cool extremities. Neuropathic ulcers are often associated with diabetes and loss of sensation in the lower extremities. Pressure ulcers occur over pressure points and are surrounded by a thick callous. Infection, neoplasm, and vasculitis are less common causes of lower extremity ulceration.[5]

Treatment

Behavioral
Leg elevation and compression therapy is crucial for healing of VU.

Medications and Immunizations
Medium to high potency topical steroids should be used for surrounding eczema/dermatitis. Wet compresses with saline or silver nitrate can aid in the control of the inflammation. Systemic antibiotics should be used only in VUs that have a suspected secondary bacterial infection.

Referral
Vascular or general surgery referral is needed for ulcer debridement if necrosis is present or if the ulcer is not responding to medical therapy. A multidisciplinary team, which includes a dermatologist, vascular surgeon, and wound care expert, may be needed for difficult cases.

Patient Education
Patients should be educated on the importance of regular exercise, avoidance of prolonged periods of sitting or standing, and the need for frequent elevation of the legs.

PRESSURE ULCER
General

Definition
Pressure ulcers (PUs) are localized areas of tissue destruction caused by prolonged pressure usually over a bony prominence. Decubitus ulcers (DUs) are a type of pressure ulcer that occurs in bed-bound patients.

Epidemiology
PUs typically occur in elderly individuals, but can occur in any patient with known risk factors. Immobility, incontinence, poor nutrition, poor circulation, smoking, alcoholism, and diabetes have been found to increase the risk of PU.[6] Major contributing factors resulting in DUs are pressure, shear, friction, and moisture.

Classification
PUs are classified using a staging system. They are staged as follows:

- Stage 1: Nonblanchable erythema seen over intact skin
- Stage 2: Ulceration of epidermis, dermis, or both
- Stage 3: Ulceration extending to the subcutaneous layer
- Stage 4: Ulceration extending to muscle, bone, and/or supporting tissues[7]

Diagnosis

Physical Examination
PUs typically occur over bony prominences such as sacrum, ischial tuberosity, greater trochanter, medial and lateral malleoli, and calcaneous. Callus tissue may surround ulcers due to chronic pressure.

Laboratory/Imaging
PUs are typically diagnosed clinically. Venous duplex ultrasonography and ABI testing are commonly ordered to rule out other conditions. Nonhealing ulcers may require tissue culture or biopsy if not responding to therapy.

Differential Diagnosis
- Venous, arterial, and neuropathic ulcers are at times difficult to differentiate from PU.
- Neoplasm, vasculitis, or infection may present similar to PU.

Treatment

Behavioral
Frequent position changes are a cornerstone of management of PU. Many patients cannot control their immobility or other risk factors. Care takers need to implement positioning and protective care for PU. Good nutrition is also key for adequate protein and other nutrient to ensure healing. A dietician is often incorporated to assist in guiding nutrition therapy plan.

Medication/Immunizations
Topical cleansers and saline wound rinses may be beneficial.

Referral
Assessing and correcting risk factors is the goal of treatment in stage 1 ulcers. Stage 2 ulcers are typically treated using an occlusive dressing and avoiding all pressure to the area. Stage 3 and 4 ulcers are treated based on the degree and severity of the ulcer. Negative pressure therapy (wound vacuum) is a common modality for encouraging wound healing. Presence of necrotic tissue, exudates, or evidence of infection usually requires debridement. This can be performed using enzymatic, mechanical, or surgical techniques. Surgical referral and wound care consult may be necessary for stage 3 and stage 4 ulcers. Complicated reconstruction may be needed for wounds that require significant debridement.[8]

Prevention
Prevention is the key for high-risk patients. Patients with known risk factors should be identified to allow early initiation of preventive measures. Minimizing pressure with pressure-relieving devices and repositioning schedules as well as maintaining good nutrition and decreasing moisture can help prevent DU.

REFERENCES

1. Habif TP. Stasis dermatitis and venous ulceration: postphlebitic syndromes. In: Habif TP, ed. *Clinical dermatology.* 5th ed. 2009; Philadelphia, PA: Mosby, Elsevier.
2. Rabe E, Pannier F. Clinical, aetiological, anatomical and pathological classification (CEAP): gold standard and limits. *Phlebology* 2012;27 (Suppl 1):114–118.
3. Beebe-Dimmer JL, Pfeifer JR, Engle JS, et al. The epidemiology of chronic venous insufficiency and varicose veins. *Ann Epidemiol* 2005;15:175–184.
4. Kirsner RS, Pardes JB, Eaglestein WH, et al. The clinical spectrum of lipodermatosclerosis. *J Am Acad Dermatol* 1993;28:623–627.
5. deAraujo T, Valencia I, Federman DG, et al. Managing the patient with venous ulcers. *Ann Intern Med* 2003;138:326–334.
6. Cakmak S, Gul U. Risk factors for pressure ulcers. *Adv Skin Wound Care* 2009;22:412–415.
7. Resnick NM. Geriatric medicine. In: Fauci AS, Kasper DL, Longo DL, et al., eds. *Principles of internal medicine.* New York, NY: McGraw-Hill; 1998:42–43.
8. Levine SM, Sinno S, Levine JP, et al. An evidence-based approach to the surgical management of pressure ulcers. *Ann Plast Surg* 2012;69(4):482–484.

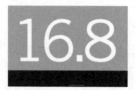

16.8 Common Skin Cancers

Stephanie T. Carter-Henry, Jeremy Golding

INTRODUCTION

Non-melanoma skin cancers are the most commonly diagnosed cancer in the United States—more than 1 million cases are diagnosed annually. Basal cell carcinoma (BCC) accounts for 80% of cases, and squamous cell carcinoma (SCC) accounts for 20%. Malignant melanoma (MM) was diagnosed in >76,000 people in the United States in 2012 and is an important cause of morbidity and mortality.[1] Prevention, early diagnosis, definitive treatment, and surveillance for recurrence are mainstays of treatment for each of these cancers and provide an opportunity for those in primary care settings to improve outcomes. Most definitive treatment is well within the scope of practice for general family medicine and office-based primary care. Familiarity with common presentations, differential diagnosis, risk stratification, and treatment options for BCC, SCC, and MM will be reviewed subsequently. This chapter provides the tools to approach diagnosis and treatment of skin cancer with confidence and evidence-based practice. In the event of diagnostic uncertainty, simple office biopsy can be invaluable for definitive diagnosis and treatment discussions.

Patient education should include methods to reduce the risk of skin cancer. Minimizing cumulative and high-intensity sun exposure is important for skin cancer prevention. Preventive measures include educating patients about use of sunscreen, use of protective clothing, and reduction of exposure to UVA and UVB rays. Following a diagnosis of skin cancer, routine skin examination and skin surveillance is an important step in early identification of subsequent cancers. Risk of UVA and UVB damage is increased in individuals with light skin, eyes, and hair. Fitzpatrick skin type is a continuum of risk graded I to VI with the highest risk individuals (Type I—blue eyes and red hair) burning easily/never tanning, and lowest risk individuals (Type VI—dark eyes and hair) who rarely burn and are deeply pigmented.[2,3]

BASAL CELL CARCINOMA
General Principles

Definition
BCC is a neoplasm arising from basal keratinocytes of the epidermis and adnexal structures. BCCs cause damage primarily by local growth and destruction; metastasis is very rare. Exposure to UVB light damages the cellular DNA repair system, leading to atypical cells.

Epidemiology

Those at highest risk for BCC are fair skinned, with light hair/eyes and poor tanning ability. The lifetime risk for development of BCC in the Caucasian U.S. population is 30%, and is more common in men than in women. Up to 85% of BCC occur on the head and neck, although not always in areas of maximal sun exposure. Intense UVB light exposure places patients at higher risk than continuous exposure. Transplant patients are at marked increased risk of developing BCC. New BCC is common in the 3 years following an index diagnosis.[2,4]

Classification

There are five histologic subtypes of BCC and a number of clinical subtypes that vary in presentation and progression. Clinical presentation, cell type, tumor size, and location are important in planning treatment. Histologic types include nodular, superficial, micronodular, infiltrative, and morpheaform; a mixed pattern is one that includes multiple cell types. The three main clinical types are:

- **Nodular:** This is the most common type of BCC, often described as a pearly white or pink papule that ulcerates. These lesions can remain flat and can appear anywhere on the body. Nodular BCC, which is one of the less aggressive BCC clinical types, can also be pigmented or cystic in appearance.
- **Superficial:** This is the least aggressive of the BCC clinical subtypes, slow growing, round/oval, or scaling plaque, typically with a characteristic pearly border. The trunk is a common location.
- **Sclerosing/morpheaform:** Lesions are plaque-like, waxy, and often white to yellow in color, with a subtly-abnormal surface appearance allowing deep growth and extension prior to diagnosis.[2,4]

Diagnosis

History

Patients often describe a scaling or nonhealing sore, or a bleeding lesion. Typically, lesions are present for an extended period of time prior to presentation.

Physical Examination

BCCs are most easily recognized when they have a pearly border, scaling, and surface ulceration. Telangiectatic vessels are often visible throughout and surrounding the lesion. The vast majority of BCC will be found on the head and neck region and can occur in non-sun-exposed areas as well.

Differential Diagnosis

Depending on the clinical subtype at presentation, BCC can resemble dermal nevi, keratoacanthoma, irritated seborrheic keratosis, psoriasis, molluscum, and sebaceous hyperplasia. Shave, punch, or excisional biopsies are options for definitive diagnosis.[2,4]

Treatment

Medical/Surgical

In planning definitive treatment of BCC, it is important to consider histology, lesion size, clinical presentation, and location. Treatment options are determined based on level of risk. See Table 16.8-1.

Low-Risk BCC

Low-risk BCCs are clinical subtype nodular or superficial, slow growing, well-defined borders, and small (head <6 mm, neck <10 mm, trunk <20 mm). Treatment options for low-risk BCC are as follows:

- **Electrodesiccation and curettage (ED&C):** The tissue integrity of a BCC is weak and collapses with curettage in a characteristic way that is palpable at the time of removal. ED&C has a 95% cure rate when used appropriately.
- **Excision:** Use local anesthesia with sharp elliptical excision of the lesion with 2- to 3-mm margins. If pathology shows tumor extension to the borders of the specimen, re-excision is indicated.
- **Radiation:** Reserved for special cases for patients who would not tolerate other treatment, such as the elderly.[2,4]
- **Topical treatment:** Two topical treatments can be used in the treatment of BCC:
  - **Imiquimod 5%:** An immune modulator that causes a local T-cell-mediated immune response. It is applied five times per week for 6 weeks. Recurrence rate of 20% at 2 years is higher than with surgical interventions. The local skin reaction is generally well tolerated.[5]
  - **5-Fluorouracil 5%:** An antimetabolite that incorporates into DNA of rapidly dividing cells and leads to cell death. It is applied twice daily for 12 weeks. Local skin reaction occurs with erythema and flaking.[5]

High-Risk BCC

Subtypes at higher risk for recurrence and metastasis are sclerosing BCC, morpheaform, basosquamous, or micronodular, or larger lesions as described above. Special consideration must be given to lesions in the area of the nose and eyes because of possible local extension.

Mohs surgery: High-risk histologic subtypes have been associated with up to 7 mm of microscopic extension around the primary tumor. Mohs surgery is a microscopically controlled surgery to treat poorly defined tumors, large tumors, or those in challenging areas such as the nose or eyelid. It is the treatment of choice for sclerosing BCCs.[6]

SQUAMOUS CELL CARCINOMA
General Principles
Definition

SCC occurs in areas of actinic damage, thermal injury, chronic inflammation, or radiation exposure with potentially aggressive behavior depending on clinical type. SCC has significant metastatic potential. The cells affected are the epithelial keratinocytes.

Epidemiology

Those at highest risk are fair skinned with high cumulative sun exposure. Other indicators of risk include history of sunburns or evidence of sun damage (freckling, telangiectasias, wrinkling), and older age. SCC can arise from actinic keratosis (AK), cutaneous horns, Bowen disease—squamous cell carcinoma in situ (SCCIS), leukoplakia, lichen sclerosis, chronic infection, and thermal burns. SCC occurs in sun-exposed areas of the scalp, back, dorsal aspect of the hands, and pinna. Similar to BCC, transplant patients are at high risk because of immunosuppression.

Malignant potential of SCC is related to size, location, histology, immunologic status, and invasion depth. Lesions that are associated with higher metastatic potential are size >2 cm, depth >4 mm, show poorly differentiated histology, are located on lip/ear/scar, or reveal perineural involvement. Mode of spread of SCC is by direct extension, by lateral extension along tissue planes, by perineural or perivascular routes, and by local metastasis via lymphatics. If SCC has progressed, distant metastasis via hematogenous dissemination to the lungs, liver, brain, skin, and bone is possible.[2]

Classification

SCC exists as part of a continuum of disease; precursor lesions are listed below in order of progression toward SCC. Progression of disease in dysplasia and SCC itself is defined by increasing depth and invasion of the epidermis.

- **AK:** Dysplastic change ("atypia") confined to the epidermis. Progression to SCC occurs in 20% of lesions. Generally AKs are rough, red/brown, and dry in appearance often with silver-white scale. There is a higher likelihood of SCC in thicker, red, painful, ulcerated, growing or large AKs. These are commonly found in elderly patients, and may be isolated or occur as multiple lesions.
- **Bowen disease and erythroplasia of Queyrat (SCCIS):** These lesions are often slow growing, red, scaly patches that can develop into invasive SCC. Erythroplasia of Queyrat is SCCIS affecting the penis.
- **SCC:** Proliferating atypical keratinocytes penetrate the epidermal basement membrane into the dermis, resulting in induration and increased potential for local destruction and distant metastasis.[2,4]

Diagnosis
History

Patients may describe a persistent or growing lesion that has evolved over time and has grown in either size or thickness. Lesions can arise from chronically inflamed or scarred skin.

Physical Examination

SCC often appears flat, scaly, or indurated and is present in sun-exposed areas, often with other signs of sun damage surrounding lesions (except in African Americans in whom SCC commonly occurs in non-sun-exposed areas). Given the mode of extension, evaluation of regional lymph nodes is important.

Differential Diagnosis

Psoriasis, eczema, superficial BCC, seborrheic keratosis, and MM can be diagnosed. Diagnostic or excisional biopsy should be performed for uncertain diagnosis.[2]

TABLE 16.8-1 Treatment Options for Common Skin Cancers and Precursor Lesions

Lesion type	Biopsy	Cryotherapy	Topical treatment	ED&C	Excision	Specialty
Basal cell carcinoma (BCC)	Use for diagnostic uncertainty as most treatment options are destructive	• Nodular • Superficial with <3 mm depth	• Patient selection and reliability important **Superficial BCC:** • Imiquimod 5% 5–7×/wk × 6 wk • 5-Fluorouracil 5% BID × 12 wk • Lower cure rates than surgical management	• Low-risk lesions (central face <6 mm, neck, scalp <10 mm, trunk <20 mm, well-defined, low-risk histology) • 2-mm margins	• Low-risk lesions (see ED&C for definition) • 2–3-mm margins	• High-risk lesions • Moh's • Radiation used often in elderly • Larger lesions • Fast growing • Recurrent lesions
Actinic keratosis (AK)	Not needed unless recurrent or uncertain diagnosis	Preferred method of treatment	• Imiquimod 5% 2× weekly × 16 weeks • 5-Fluorouracil 5% BID × 2–4 wk • Diclofenac 3% BID × 2–3 mo • Ingenol gel 0.015% daily × 3 d or 0.05% daily 2 d • Helpful for large-field treatment	• Thicker lesions • Can reduce risk of residual atypical cells	Not indicated unless progression to SCC suspected	
Bowen disease (SCCIS) Erythroplasia of Queyrat (SCCIS of mucous membranes)	• Punch or shave • If SCC suspected full thickness biopsy indicated	Can be used for thin lesions	• Imiquimod 5% 5× weekly × 6 wk • 5-Flourouracil BID × 8 wk • Consider lidocaine ointment for pain	YES	Can be used, but may be more aggressive than needed	If distal glans and urethra involved, Mohs surgery may be indicated

(Continued)

TABLE 16.8-1   Treatment Options for Common Skin Cancers and Precursor Lesions *(continued)*

Lesion type	Biopsy	Cryotherapy	Topical treatment	ED&C	Excision	Specialty
Squamous cell carcinoma (SCC)	Punch biopsy preferred (depth of invasion important)	NO	NO	• Low-risk lesions (Central face <6 mm, neck, scalp <10 mm, trunk <20 mm, <4 mm depth, slow growing, well-defined, no signs of extension) • 4-mm margins	• Low-risk lesions (see ED&C for definition) • 4-mm margins	• High-risk lesions • Mohs • Radiation treatment often used in elderly • Large size • Poorly differentiated • Depth >4 mm • Histologic signs of spread as staging is required
Malignant melanoma (MM)	• Punch biopsy of thickest location • Excisional biopsy with 2–3-mm margins	NO	NO	NO	• Surgical excision based on Breslow depth • In situ → 5-mm margins • <1 mm Breslow depth → 1-cm margins	Surgical consultation for excision of lesions >1 mm deep, ulcerated, or Clark level 4

Treatment

Medications/Surgical

Actinic Keratosis

Preferred treatment is **cryotherapy**. Large thick lesions can be treated with curettage or excision. 5-Flourouracil is a reasonable treatment for lesions where large areas of treatment are needed ("field therapy"). Topical treatment produces significant, visible inflammation, which can be a major cosmetic concern for patients. Occasionally, treatment of superimposed infection may be needed. Topical treatment can also be painful; management with pain medications and topical lidocaine may be needed. Newer topical agents (imiquimod, diclofenac, ingenol) are expensive.

    Cryotherapy: Treatment using liquid nitrogen to destroy epithelial layer and create separation between epidermis and dermis.

Squamous Cell Carcinoma *In Situ*

Bowen disease can be treated with **ED&C**, **cryotherapy**, or **excision**. Keeping side effects and patient preference in mind, **5-flourouracil** and **imiquimod** are also options. Erythroplasia of Queyrat is most often treated with **5-flourouracil** or **imiquimod**. If urethral meatus is involved, **Mohs** is likely indicated.[5]

Squamous Cell Carcinoma

Size, location, and risk are important to consider in planning treatment of SCC.

- **Low-risk SCC** is defined as small and well-differentiated lesions with less than 4 mm depth of invasion without perineural or vascular invasion. Small lesions are face <6 mm, cheeks, forehead, neck, scalp <10 mm, trunk/extremities <20 mm. Treatment options include **ED&C** and **excision** with 4-mm margins.
- **High-risk SCC:** Larger lesions or those in high-risk locations may require **Mohs surgery** and consideration of **sentinel node biopsy**. Higher risk lesions are excised with 6-mm margins. Sentinel node mapping is required to identify node-draining lesion and region. The sentinel node is removed for histologic evaluation for SCC and treatment planning.[2,4]

MALIGNANT MELANOMA

General Principles

Definition

MM is due to the development of malignant pigment cells extending through the epidermis, into the dermis and beyond. MM can metastasize to any organ. Disordered replication of malignant melanocytes and extension leads to color, shape, and surface variation that can be distinguished from typical uniform nevi. Radial and vertical growth is possible.[2]

Epidemiology

MM is responsible for greater than 76,000 cancer diagnoses in the United States annually, and the incidence is on the rise. Males are at greater risk than females, and light-skinned individuals are at 10-fold increased risk of developing MM. Other risk factors include personal history of atypical nevi, large number of nevi (>75), previous non-melanoma skin cancer, giant congenital nevi, personal history of melanoma, family history of MM, immunosuppression, chronic tanning, UVA treatment for psoriasis, repeated blistering sunburns, and Fitzpatrick skin type I. As discussed subsequently, prognosis is based on tumor thickness (Breslow depth) at diagnosis.

    Importantly, there are precursor lesions that are associated with the development of MM. Benign acquired nevi are commonly seen in individuals and are typically uniform with little color variation. Atypical nevi are generally larger with less border regularity and confer greater risk for later development of MM. Typical progression is from benign nevus to dysplastic nevus to radial growth phase to vertical growth phase to MM.[2]

Classification

The main clinical subtypes of melanoma include:

- **Superficial spreading:** This is the most common melanoma accounting for 70% and most common in the fourth and fifth decades, often on the back and legs. This melanoma presents with irregular borders and often wide variety of colors at presentation.

- **Nodular melanoma** is the second most common melanoma, making up 15% to 20%. It occurs on the trunk and legs and is characterized by rapid growth (weeks to months) and diagnosed most commonly in the fifth and sixth decades.
- **Lentigo maligna melanoma** represents 4% to 15% of MM. These are slow growing (5 to 20 years) and occur most often in the sixth or seventh decade. They are most commonly found on the face with brown black or blue black color.
- **Acral-lentiginous melanoma** accounts for 2% to 8% of melanomas in whites and 30% to 75% of melanomas diagnosed in blacks, Asian, and Hispanic individuals. They are located on the palms and soles and have a slow radial growth phase. Periungual spread may occur as well as a new band of pigment in the nail.[2]

Diagnosis

History

Initial history often includes recent change in the color, border, surface contour, or size of a nevus. Lesions can be symptomatic with pain, itching, or ulceration.

Physical Examination

Physical examination should include careful analysis of the lesion with dermoscopy (10× magnification) if available. Given the risk of metastasis, regional lymph node examination is also indicated. Review of a worrisome lesion should involve attention to the ABCDs of melanoma: Asymmetry of lesion, Border irregularity, Color variation, Diameter enlargement, and Evolution of the lesion. If MM is diagnosed, laboratory and regional imaging may be appropriate depending on the clinical scenario and tumor stage. These may include LDH (lactate dehydrogenase), complete blood count, chemistries, CT scanning, and positron emission tomography scanning.[2,7]

Differential Diagnosis

Differential diagnosis includes hemangioma, pigmented seborrheic keratosis, benign dermal nevus, dermatofibroma, and atypical nevus. Suspicious lesions should undergo excisional biopsy where possible, with 2- to 3-mm normal margins, or punch biopsy through the thickest area if excisional biopsy is not feasible. Shave biopsy may disrupt Breslow depth, but in studies, this does not appear to affect treatment outcomes. Shave technique, even with deep shave, is not recommended for highly suspicious lesions.

Tumor Staging

Breslow depth refers to the depth in millimeters of tumor thickness and is the most important histologic feature guiding prognosis. Biopsy allows for an assessment of the depth of invasion through the epidermis, papillary dermis, reticular dermis, and into the subcutaneous fat. The Clark level is the anatomic level of extension (level 1 to 5) from epidermis→dermis→fat. Other histology seen in reports may include growth phase, lymphocytic infiltration, mitotic rates, regression, angiolymphatic invasion, and histologic subtype. Presence or absence of ulceration provides additional prognostic information.

Sentinel node involvement is the most important predictor for survival and recurrence. This is defined as melanoma cells present in the first lymph node that drains lymphatics from the lesion. Sentinel node mapping and biopsy should be done for melanoma deeper than 1 mm, if ulceration is present, or Clark level 4 or higher.

Overall, melanoma staging uses the TNM (tumor, node, metastasis) classification system. Localized (stages 1 and 2), regional metastasis (stage 3), and distant metastasis (stage 4).[2]

Treatment

Surgical

MM is treated with complete tumor resection and depending on depth of invasion, sentinel lymph node biopsy. Patients with higher risk MM and with increasing depth of invasion, or clinically enlarged regional lymph nodes, may undergo further lymph node dissection. **Recommended excision margins:** MM in situ, 5-mm margins; MM with Breslow depth <1- to 10-mm margins; and higher Breslow depth lesions increasing margins up to 20 mm.

As tumor stage increases, 10-year survival rates fall precipitously; Stage 1A has a 10-year survival rate of 95%, whereas stage IV 10-year survival rates fall to 10%. Adjuvant medical treatment with Interferon α-2b is sometimes employed for stage II and stage III lesions. Studies are ongoing to identify additional immunologically active agents that may be useful in treatment. Radiation therapy has some role, especially in palliation of systemic illness.

Frequent follow-up physical examination should be used for surveillance of additional lesions given increasing risk of recurrence as stage increases. After initial diagnosis and treatment, examinations should occur every 3 to 4 months. Spacing frequency of examinations is based on time cancer free and stage of disease.[2,7]

REFERENCES

1. The American Cancer Society. Skin Cancer Facts. http://www.cancer.org/cancer/cancercauses/sunanduv-exposure/skin-cancer-facts. Accessed January 22, 2014.
2. Habif TP. *Clinical dermatology.* 5th ed. Philadelphia, PA: Mosby Elsevier; 2010.
3. Eilers S, Bach DQ, Gaber R, et al. Accuracy of self-report in assessing Fitzpatrick skin phototypes I through VI. *JAMA Dermatol* 2013;149(11):1289–1294.
4. Firnhaber JM. Diagnosis and treatment of basal cell and squamous cell carcinoma. *Am Fam Physician* 2012;86:161–168.
5. Bahner JD, Bordeaux JS. Non-melanoma skin cancers: photodynamic therapy, cryotherapy, 5-fluorouracil, imiquimod, diclofenac, or what? Facts and controversies. *Clin Dermatol* 2013;31:792–798.
6. Morrissey M, Beachkofsky T, Ritter S. When to consider Mohs surgery. *J Fam Pract* 2013;62:558–564.
7. Sheneberger DW. Cutaneous malignant melanoma: a primary care perspective. *Am Fam Physician* 2012; 85:161–168.

CHAPTER 17

Endocrine and Metabolic Disorders

Section Editor: Kathryn K. Garner

17.1 Obesity
Matthew Barnes

OVERVIEW

Obesity remains an increasing worldwide problem. In the United States, the measured prevalence of obesity was 34.9% between 2011 and 2012.[1] Worldwide, 36.9% of men, and 38% of women are estimated to be overweight.[2] Excessive weight is noted among all age, gender, and racial/ethnic groups.[3] Although many diseases are due to either malfunctions in underlying physiology or exposure to a pathogen/toxin, most cases of obesity are due to the body's natural response to steady caloric overload and continued sedentary activity.

Obesity is associated with increased risk of death in all adult age groups for all categories of death.[4] Likewise, obesity substantially raises the risk and morbidity from metabolic syndrome (insulin resistance syndrome) related diagnoses: type 2 diabetes mellitus, coronary artery disease, hypertension (HTN), stroke, and dyslipidemia.[5] Obesity worsens symptoms of osteoarthritis,[6] obstructive sleep apnea (OSA),[7] gout,[8] dementia,[9] gallbladder disease,[10] and urinary incontinence.[11] Further, obesity has been linked to increased risk of nosocomial infection[12] and complications of flu;[13] higher rates of urolithiasis;[14] and cancers of the esophagus, colon, kidney, gallbladder, liver, pancreas, thyroid, prostate, breast, and endometrium.[15]

Clinical Assessment

The U.S. Preventive Services Task Force (USPSTF) recommends that clinicians screen all adult patients for obesity and offer intensive counseling and behavioral interventions to promote sustained weight loss for adults with a body mass index (BMI) of 30 kg per m² or higher, only intensive behavioral interventions are recommended for children aged 6 years and older (Level B recommendation).

Body Mass Index

Assessment of body fat, risk factors, and patient motivation provides the basis for development of appropriate treatment plan. The USPSTF found good evidence that BMI, an indirect measurement of body fat–based weight adjusted for height, is reliable and valid for identifying adults at increased risk for morbidity and mortality due to overweight and obesity. The following measurement scheme should not be used to evaluate growing children, frail elderly individuals, pregnant or lactating women, individuals with high muscle mass, or patients with disorders that preclude obtaining an accurate measurement of height.

$$BMI = [weight~(pounds)/height~(in.)^2] \times 704.5 ~or~ weight~(kg)/height~(m)^2$$

Underweight: BMI <18.5	Obesity Class I: BMI 30.0–34.9
Normal: BMI 18.5–24.9	Obesity Class II: BMI 35.0–39.9
Overweight: BMI 25.0–29.9	Obesity Class III: BMI ≥40

Pediatric patients are measured in the same manner, but their BMI is specifically normalized against a gender specific BMI-for-growth curve published by the Centers for Disease Control (CDC). Children are overweight when their BMI falls between the 85th and 95th percentile. Children are obese when their BMI falls above the 95th percentile.[16] Children are considered "at-risk" if they are below the 85th percentile, and cross more than 3 to 4 kg per m^2 after a year.[16]

Waist Circumference

Per the National Heart, Lung and Blood Institute, measuring waist circumference (WC) should be considered as an adjunct to BMI as an assessment of body fat in adults. WC estimates excess abdominal fat and is measured by placing a flexible tape at the height of both iliac crests, and measuring the full circumference of the abdomen.

Excess abdominal fat is a risk factor independent of obesity for development of health problems, including type 2 diabetes, HTN, and cardiovascular disease (CVD). For adults, a WC >102 cm (40 in.) in men or WC >88 cm (35 in.) in women identifies patients at additional high risk for development of obesity-associated comorbidity. However, if the patient's BMI is >35, addition of a WC measurement carries little added predictive power of disease—as their risk of obesity-associated comorbidity is already considered to be high. WC measurement is not considered standard of care in pediatric populations. Of note, for most patients, abdominal CT and MRI do not add significant predictive value beyond that of the abdominal WC.

Metabolic Syndrome

Obesity is associated with insulin resistance, particularly in the case of abdominal obesity. Insulin resistance increases the risk of developing type 2 diabetes mellitus. The resulting hyperinsulinemia, hyperglycemia, and adipocyte cytokines are thought to lead to vascular endothelial dysfunction, hyperlipidemia, HTN, and vascular inflammation promoting atherosclerotic CVD.

The World Health Organization proposed a set of criteria for defining the metabolic syndrome in 1998:

- A fasting plasma glucose >110 mg per dL, or a plasma glucose 2 hours after an oral glucose tolerance test >200 mg per dL, or hyperinsulinemia, defined as the upper quartile of a measure of insulin resistance in the nondiabetic population.

Plus at least two of the following:

- Abdominal obesity, defined as a waist-to-hip ratio of >0.90, a BMI ≥30 kg per m^2, or a waist girth ≥94 cm (37 in.).
- Dyslipidemia, defined as serum triglyceride ≥150 mg per dL or high-density lipoprotein (HDL) cholesterol <35 mg per dL.
- Blood pressure ≥140/90 mmHg or the administration of antihypertensive drugs.

The metabolic syndrome has been associated with several obesity-related disorders, including fatty liver disease, chronic renal disease, polycystic ovarian syndrome (PCOS), OSA, and increased risk of cognitive decline and dementia.

Comorbidities

Comorbidities compound the health risks associated with obesity—as obesity affects nearly every organ system (Table 17.1-1). Comorbidities are usually exacerbated by excessive weight, but also improve with weight reduction.

DIAGNOSIS

While most causes of obesity are due to a sedentary lifestyle and increased caloric intake, secondary causes of obesity should be considered in an initial evaluation.

Subjective

Evaluation of patients with a BMI >25 should include a history: ask age of onset of weight gain, events associated with weight gain, previous weight loss attempts, dietary changes, history of exercise, and history of smoking. Include behavioral interviewing, specifically factors that allow the patient to successfully enter into a weight reduction program. Ask about current motivation, previous history of weight loss, social support, capacity, and willingness to engage in physical activity.

TABLE 17.1-1   Health risks associated with obesity

Comorbidity	Impact	Study
General		
Mortality	Obesity at age 40 led to a decrease of 6–7 yr of life compared with those with normal BMI.	Framingham Study
Cardiac/vascular disease		
Ischemic heart disease	Each 5 kg/m^2 increase of BMI led to a hazard ratio increase of stroke/heart disease of 1.39.	Prospective Studies Collaboration
Diabetes	Having a BMI of >35 led to an age adjusted relative risk increase of 61.	Nurse's Health Study
Hypertension	Could account for 26% of hypertension in men, and 28% in women.	Analysis of Framingham Data
Heart failure	Obesity carries a relative risk of 2 for heart failure compared with patients with normal weight.	Analysis of Framingham Data
Coronary artery disease	Each 5 kg/m^2 increase of BMI resulted in a hazard ratio increase of coronary heart disease by 1.27.	Meta-analysis
Atrial fibrillation	Obesity led to a hazard risk of 1.52/1.46 for men and women, respectively.	Analysis of Framingham Data
Venous thromboembolism	BMI >40 led to a hazard ratio of 2.7 for risk of venous thromboembolism.	ARIC
Gastrointestinal		
Gallstones	Increases in gallstone occurrence.	Nurse's Health Study + Disease-Oriented Data
GERD	Increases in abdominal pressure, leading to increased GERD.	Disease-Oriented Data
Nonalcoholic fatty liver disease (NAFLD)	Correlated with obesity.	Retrospective Analysis
Musculoskeletal		
General osteoarthritis	Correlated with increased rates of osteoarthritis in weight-bearing and non-weight-bearing joints. Hazard ratio of 2.9 in knee, hazard ratio of 1.2.	Correlational Disease-Oriented Study
Respiratory		
Obstructive sleep apnea (OSA)	Every 10% increase in weight leads to a hazard ratio of 6 for OSA.	Correlational Study
Obesity hypoventilation syndrome	PaCO$_2$ >45 was noted in approximately 50% of those with BMI >50.	Correlational Disease-Oriented Study
Oncology		
General risk of cancer	Could contribute to 14% of all cancer deaths in men, and 20% of all cancer deaths in women.	Analysis of Prospective Cohort

(Continued)

(Continues)

Comorbidity	Impact	Study
Reproductive endocrinology		
Erectile dysfunction (ED)	If obese males lose weight, and increase physical activity, 1/3 of obese males have improvement in ED symptoms.	Randomized Controlled Trial
Polycystic ovarian syndrome (PCOS)	50% of PCOS patients are obese. Effective obesity treatment does not lessen symptoms.	Retrospective Analysis
Infertility	Decreasing spontaneous pregnancy rates, and increased time to pregnancy.	Retrospective Analysis
Psychology		
Depression	Correlated with severe obesity, most strongly with younger patients and women.	Randomized Controlled Trial
Pediatric		
Precocious puberty	Overweight and obese girls, and obese boys were correlated with earlier onset of puberty.	Retrospective Analysis
Blount disease	Obese children 13–19 yr old have a prevalence of 2.5% of Blount disease.	Retrospective Analysis
Fractures	Obese children are more prone to fractures than normal weight children.	Retrospective Analysis

Pediatric patients also have increased risk of diabetes, metabolic syndrome, hypertension, hyperlipidemia, PCOS, NAFLD, cholelithiasis, OSA, and psychological issues.

Include a medication/health reconciliation, specifically asking about medications that increase weight gain. Specifically ask about β-blockers, olanzapine (and other atypical antipsychotics), paroxetine (and other SSRIs), valproate/carbamazepine (anti-epileptics), sulfonylureas, thiazolidinediones, insulin, and steroid use. If these medications are noted, a less obesogenic regimen could be considered. Health history questions pertain specifically to the patient having a contributing depression or an obesogenic illness, such as Cushing disease, hypothyroidism, and PCOS.[17]

In children and adolescents, consider specific questions regarding caretakers who feed the child, which high-calorie foods the patient consumes, eating patterns, barriers to exercise, time spent in active play, amount of physical education, enrollment in after-school activities, and assessment of screen time. Family history should have a focus, as family history indicates the risk of the obesity's persistence into adulthood. Finally, a psychosocial assessment (HEADSS examination) should be performed.

Objective

- As noted above, BMI and WC should be obtained.
- An examination to evaluate for secondary causes should be considered, including an evaluation for Cushing disease (proximal muscle strength, striae on skin, "buffalo hump," and "moon facies"), thyroid examination (to evaluate for goiter) for hypothyroidism, and evaluation for PCOS (specifically looking for acne and hirsutism).
- Considered initial laboratory testing should include a measurement of glucose (by either fasting measures or hemoglobin A1c), thyroid-stimulating hormone (to evaluate for hypothyroidism), liver enzymes (to evaluate for nonalcoholic steatosis—"fatty liver"), and lipids (for cardiac risk assessment). Laboratory testing of children/adolescents is recommended when additional findings are present: dysmorphic features, short stature, slow growth, or delayed puberty.[18]

TREATMENT

Goals of a weight loss program are to prevent additional weight gain, reduce body weight, and maintain lower weight over time.

The USPSTF recommends that if patients are found to be obese, they should be referred to a moderate- to high-intensity comprehensive behavioral intervention for weight loss. It should be noted that a comprehensive behavioral intervention includes behavioral management activities (group sessions, individual sessions, setting weight loss goals, addressing barriers to change), improving diet/nutrition, physical activity sessions, active use of self-monitoring, and strategizing maintenance of lifestyle changes. For adults, 12 to 26 sessions per year were considered moderate to high intensity. For children, high-intensity programs were defined as having >25 hours of contact with a child and/or family over a 6-month period.[19]

As an adjunct, the USPSTF and Agency for Healthcare Research and Quality (AHRQ) developed a low-intensity counseling framework noted as the "five A's": ask, advise, assess, assist, and arrange. This method is considered an adjunctive method, as there is a lack of supporting evidence as applied to obesity. However, this method can be useful if in a setting with limited resources, or as an initial assessment.

1. Ask: Screen for obesity, and obtain a history.
2. Advise that the patient should lose weight—be clear and direct.
3. Assess if the patient is willing to lose weight at this time.
4. Assist: Set clear goals (as below). If necessary, consider pharmacotherapy and surgical options.
5. Arrange a follow-up.[17]

Attempt to initially set a 4- to 6-month goal for weight reduction of 10% or a reduction of BMI by two units. As targets are met, the patient may maintain the reduced weight or set a new goal of weight reduction. Either strategy should include permanent behavior modification, including stress reduction and self-monitoring. It is important to state that this is PERMANENT behavior modification, not temporary to avoid reengaging in unhealthy habits.

Treatment options are employed on the basis of the BMI and adjusted risk (Table 17.1-2).

Calorie Balance

- A decrease of 300 to 500 kcal per day provides a weight loss of 0.5 to 1 lb per week with a resultant 6-month 10% weight reduction for BMI 25 to 30. A decrease of 500 to 1,000 kcal per day provides weight loss of 1 to 2 lb per week, with a resultant 6-month 10% weight reduction for BMI 30 to 35.
- To calculate a 500-kcal per day deficit:
  Calculate the **resting energy expenditure (REE):**

  $(10 \times \text{weight [kg]}) + (6.25 \times \text{height [cm]}) - (5 \times \text{age [years]})^* = REE^* = +5$ for men and -161 for women

- Estimate **total caloric need** to maintain weight:total caloric need = REE × activity factor

  (activity factor = 1.6 for men and 1.5 for women)

- Calculate **adjusted caloric intake:**

  total caloric need − 500 kcal = caloric energy deficit[7]

TABLE 17.1-2	Treatment Options per BMI
BMI 18 ≤ 25, no adjusted risk	Healthy diet and physical exercise
BMI 25 ≤ 27, moderate risk	As above plus low-calorie diet
BMI 27 ≤ 30, high risk	As above
BMI 30 ≤ 35, very high risk	As above plus medication and very low–calorie diet
BMI 35 ≥ 40, extremely high risk	As above and consider surgical interventions when obesity-related comorbidities are present
BMI 40+, extremely high risk	As above plus surgical interventions

Caloric balance should first be undertaken through a diet to decrease energy intake and exercise to increase energy expenditure. Behavioral interventions such as eating breakfast, decreasing screen time, and limiting fast food have been associated with lower BMIs. Additionally, many diets have been found effective for weight loss and are summarized in Table 17.1-3.

Exercise Regimens

The USPSTF recommends that primary care clinicians selectively counsel patients to promote a healthful diet and physical activity—specifically targeting patients with increased risk of CVD who exhibit readiness to change and where there is appropriate support.[20] Exercise programs have not been shown to have large effects on initial weight loss,[21] unless rigorous (like military training).[22] However,

TABLE 17.1-3	Diet Therapy		
Diet	**Content**	**Impact**	**Evidence**
Mediterranean diet	High in fruits, vegetables, nuts, whole grains, and olive oil.	Lowers weight, improves lipid profile, insulin resistance, and lowers markers of inflammation and endothelial function.	Randomized Controlled Trial
DASH diet	Limits sodium intake to 2,400 mg and is rich in fruits, vegetables, nonfat dairy; contains whole grains, lean meats, fish/poultry, and nuts/beans.	Improve triglycerides, diastolic blood pressure, and fasting glucose in addition to leading to weight loss.	Randomized Controlled Trial
Low glycemic index diets	Replace refined grains with whole grains, fruits, vegetables. Eliminates high-glycemic beverages.	Weight loss, beneficial effects on patients with medium glycemic control (similar to non-metformin, noninsulin agents).	Randomized Controlled Trial
Portion control diets	Individually packaged foods or formula drinks as meal replacements.	Weight loss from portion-controlled diets has been maintained for 4 yr.	Retrospective Analysis
Low-fat diets	Limiting fat intake to 30% of energy intake or less. Usually needs a dietician.	Weight loss from low-fat diets has been maintained for 7.5 yr.	Retrospective Analysis
High-protein diets	Consuming 70–140 g of protein per day.	Did not lead to weight loss, could maintain weights. High intake of high protein has been linked to increased all-cause mortality.	Retrospective Analysis
Vegetarian diets	Spectrum of diets reducing animal protein intake. Vegan involves no animal protein. Lacto-ovo involves egg and milk consumption.	12% reduction in mortality risk regardless of weight loss effect. Direct correlation of amount of animal protein consumed and mortality.	Retrospective Analysis
Very low–calorie diets	Diets that contain 200–800 kcal/d.	Results in better short-term weight loss, with weight loss similar to other diets in long term.	Meta-analysis
Gluten-free diets	Diets that avoid gluten.	Associated with weight gain or stable weight, as opposed to weight loss.	Retrospective Analysis

when it comes to maintenance of weight loss, exercise consistently stands out as one of the most important factors.[23] Independent of weight loss, exercise results in a mortality benefit.[24]

The benefit of medical evaluation prior to engaging in an exercise regimen is unclear. The data are not strong enough to reach consensus on identity of which groups would benefit from exercise evaluation. However, for children and adolescence, many medical bodies have guidelines for and recommend pre-participation physicals.

An initial aerobic regimen involves an "exercise prescription" of walking >30 minutes per day, 5 to 7 days per week. This amount can lead to benefits in prevention of weight gain and mortality reduction. From that point, the patient can branch and scale their exercise regimen on the basis of personal preference, fitness level, and cardiac/musculoskeletal conditions. The emphasis should be on the patient choosing an exercise regimen that they will continue indefinitely.

Pharmacotherapy

In selected patients who have failed to achieve adequate weight loss, medication is an appropriate adjunct to a low-calorie diet, physical activity, and behavior modification. Weight loss medications create an energy deficit through reduced food consumption or reduced absorption.

In considering pharmacotherapy, a provider should base their choice of medication on positive effects beyond that for weight loss. For instance, a provider may wish to consider diet and exercise with metformin or exenatide in a patient with diabetes (as opposed to a sulfonylurea), or bupropion in a depressed patient. See Table 17.1-4 for a comparison of weight loss medications.

TABLE 17.1-4	Medications to Treat Obesity

Name (trade name—if not generic)	FDA approved for treatment of obesity	Dosage	Misc ellaneous	Impact	Contraindications/ side effects
Sympathomimetics					
Phentermine	Y	8 mg PO TID or 15–37.5 mg po QAM	Schedule IV medication; limit use to 12 wk		Obesity comorbidities, cardiovascular disease, hypertension
Lorcaserin (Belviq)	Y		Safety for valvular disease exists for only 1 yr of use	3–4 kg of weight loss	
Malabsorption agents					
Orlistat	Y (Approved for children and adolescents)	50–200 mg po with meals	Inhibits pancreatic lipases	Decreases fat absorption by 30%	
Antidepressants					
Bupropion	N		Norepinephrine modulation		Dry mouth, agitation, anxiety
Antiepileptics					
Topiramate	N		Norepinephrine + dopamine modulation	6% weight loss over 6 mo	Paresthesias, somnolence, difficulty concentrating
Zonisamide	N		Dopaminergic and serotonergic neurotransmission		Somnolence, difficulty with memory, agitation, insomnia, confusion, diplopia

(Continued)

(*Continues*)

Name (trade name—if not generic)	FDA approved for treatment of obesity	Dosage	Misc ellaneous	Impact	Contraindications/ side effects
Diabetes drugs					
Metformin	N			5% weight loss over 3 yr	Diarrhea, flatulence, indigestion
Exenatide	N				Gastrointestinal distress, pancreatitis, injection site reaction
Pramlintide	N			2+ kg weight loss	
Combination drugs					
Phentermine–topamax	Y		Approved for BMI >30, or >27 with comorbidities	8%–10% weight loss	Dry mouth and paresthesias
Bupropion–naltrexone	N			5%–6% weight loss	Nausea/headache and constipation
No longer indicated					
Sibutramine	Pulled from market				Pulled from market due to association with nonfatal myocardial infarction
Ephedrine	N (still on market for treatment of hypotension)				Adverse cardiovascular effects
Fenfluramine	Pulled from market				Heart valve destruction and pulmonary hypertension
Human chorionic gonadotropin	N			No more effective than placebo	
Testosterone	N			Decreased fat mass without weight loss	Under review due to association with nonfatal myocardial infarction
Supplements					
Chromium	N/A			1 kg weight loss over 12–16 wk	
Green Tea	N/A			Not effective	
Guar Gum	N/A			Not evidence in weight loss	Abdominal pain, flatulence, diarrhea
Hoodia Gordonii	N/A			No trial data	
B_{12}	N/A			No trial data	

Surgical Intervention

Consultation to a bariatric surgeon should be considered in patients with a BMI greater than 40, or BMI greater than 35 with serious medical comorbidities, who have not been successful with diet, exercise, and medical management. Bariatric surgery can be considered in children/adolescents if they have a BMI >35 kg per m^2 with comorbidities or BMI >40 kg per m^2, if they have reached 95% of their predicted adult stature by bone age or Tanner Stage IV, and if they have a history of failure of intensive diet/exercise programs.[25]

The three surgical procedures currently in use are:

- The Roux-en-Y gastric bypass creates a small stomach pouch and allows food to bypass some of the small intestine.
- Gastroplasty decreases the overall size of the stomach to create a feeling of fullness after eating a small amount of food leading to decreased caloric intake and weight loss.
- Lap-banding gastroplasty places a plastic band around the stomach that is connected to a subcutaneous pouch. This pouch is inflated with saline to apply a variable level of constriction to the stomach.

Bariatric surgery results in greater weight loss than conventional weight loss programs.[26] Likewise, bariatric surgery is highly effective in treating diabetes, hyperlipidemia, and HTN[27]—preventing up to 40% of disease-related mortality.[28]

Postoperative complications of bariatric surgery include infection, anemia, vitamin B deficiencies, inadequate weight loss, and gallstone formation due to rapid weight loss. The family physician should ensure that dietary changes, physical activity, and behavior modification are a part of the overall strategy for weight reduction to ensure maintenance of weight loss over time. Cold intolerance, hair loss, and fatigue are common but tend to diminish rapidly as weight loss stabilizes.

Quarterly assessment of nutritional status and supplementation needs, food intolerances, and symptoms should occur for the first year after bariatric surgery. A variety of micronutrient deficiencies have been identified because of decreased capacity for food intake. Vitamin supplementation will be required throughout the patient's lifetime, and annual metabolic and nutritional monitoring is recommended, although no standard exists. Vitamin and mineral deficiencies, such as decreased iron, B$_{12}$, vitamin D$_3$, and calcium, are common and may manifest many years following bariatric surgery.

OBESITY MANAGEMENT IN SPECIAL POPULATIONS

Absolute contraindications to weight loss are terminal illness and anorexia nervosa. Temporary contraindications include pregnancy and lactation; unstable psychiatric, medical, or surgical status; and bulimia nervosa. Patients with osteopenia or osteoporosis should undergo discussion of risk and undertake medical management to maintain bone mineral density.

Elderly persons are at increased risk of becoming overweight with loss of physical activity and decreased energy expenditure. Regular, moderate exercise and a diet low in fat and high in fiber can control weight while providing for nutritional needs. Issues of polypharmacy, drug interactions, and age-related physiologic factors should be considered before medication is prescribed for obese elderly patients.

ACKNOWLEDGMENT

The author wishes to acknowledge Meg Hayes for her work on the previous version of this chapter.

REFERENCES

1. Ogden CL, Carroll MD, Kit BK, et al. Prevalence of childhood and adult obesity in the United States, 2011–2012. *JAMA* 2014;311:806.
2. Ng M, Fleming T, Robinson M, et al. Global, regional, and national prevalence of overweight and obesity in children and adults during 1980–2013: a systematic analysis for the Global Burden of Disease Study 2013. *Lancet* 2014;384(9945):766–781.
3. Baskin ML, Ard J, Franklin F, et al. Prevalence of obesity in the United States. *Obesity Rev* 2005;6(1):5.
4. Calle EE, Thun MJ, Petrelli JM, et al. Body mass index and mortality in a prospective cohort of U.S. adults. *N Engl J Med* 1999;341:1097–1105.
5. http://www.ncbi.nlm.nih.gov/books/NBK44660/pdf/TOC.pdf. Accessed June 2014.
6. Hart DJ, Spector TD. The relationship of obesity, fat distribution and osteoarthritis in women in the general population: the Chingford Study. *J Rheumatol* 1993;20:331.
7. Young T, Skatrud J, Peppard PE. Risk factors for obstructive sleep apnea in adults. *JAMA* 2004;291:2013.
8. Choi HK, Atkinson K, Karlson EW, et al. Obesity, weight change, hypertension, diuretic use, and risk of gout in men: the health professionals follow-up study. *Arch Intern Med* 2005;165:742.

9. Singh-Manoux A, Czernichow S, Elbaz A, et al. Obesity phenotypes in midlife and cognition in early old age: the Whitehall II cohort study. *Neurology* 2012;79:755.
10. Banim PJ, Luben RN, Bulluck H, et al. The aetiology of symptomatic gallstones quantification of the effects of obesity, alcohol and serum lipids on risk. Epidemiological and biomarker data from a UK prospective cohort study (EPIC-Norfolk). *Eur J Gastroenterol Hepatol* 2011;23:733.
11. Subak LL, Richter HE, Hunskaar S. Obesity and urinary incontinence: epidemiology and clinical research update. *J Urol* 2009;182:S2.
12. Falagas ME, Kompoti M. Obesity and infection. *Lancet Infect Dis* 2006;6:438.
13. Kwong JC, Campitelli MA, Rosella LC. Obesity and respiratory hospitalizations during influenza seasons in Ontario, Canada: a cohort study. *Clin Infect Dis* 2011;53:413.
14. Taylor EN, Stampfer MJ, Curhan GC. Obesity, weight gain, and the risk of kidney stones. *JAMA* 2005;293:455.
15. Calle EE, Rodriguez C, Walker-Thurmond K, et al. Overweight, obesity, and mortality from cancer in a prospectively studied cohort of U.S. adults. *N Engl J Med* 2003;348:1625.
16. Barlow SE; Expert Committee. Expert committee recommendations regarding the prevention, assessment, and treatment of child and adolescent overweight and obesity: summary report. *Pediatrics* 2007;120 (Suppl 4):S164.
17. Rao G. Office-based strategies for the management of obesity. *Am Fam Physician* 2010; 81(12):1449–1455.
18. Allen G, Safranek S. FPIN's clinical inquiries. Secondary causes of obesity. *Am Fam Physician* 2011;83(8):972–973.
19. U.S. Preventive Services Task Force. *Guide to clinical preventive services*. 2nd ed. Washington, DC: Office of Disease Prevention and Health Promotion; 1996.
20. Moyer VA; U.S. Preventive Services Task Force. Behavioral counseling interventions to promote a healthful diet and physical activity for cardiovascular disease prevention in adults: U.S. Preventive Services Task Force recommendation statement. *Ann Intern Med* 2012;157:367.
21. Slentz CA, Duscha BD, Johnson JL, et al. Effects of the amount of exercise on body weight, body composition, and measures of central obesity: STRRIDE—a randomized controlled study. *Arch Intern Med* 2004;164:31.
22. Lee L, Kumar S, Leong LC. The impact of five-month basic military training on the body weight and body fat of 197 moderately to severely obese Singaporean males aged 17 to 19 years. *Int J Obes Relat Metab Disord* 1994;18:105.
23. Avenell A, Brown TJ, McGee MA, et al. What interventions should we add to weight reducing diets in adults with obesity? A systematic review of randomized controlled trials of adding drug therapy, exercise, behaviour therapy or combinations of these interventions. *J Hum Nutr Diet* 2004;17:293.
24. Kokkinos P. Physical Activity, Health Benefits, and Mortality Risk. *ISRN Cardiol* 2012;2012;718789.
25. Pratt JS, Lenders CM, Dionne EA, et al. Best practice updates for pediatric/adolescent weight loss surgery. *Obesity (Silver Spring)* 2009;17:901.
26. Colquitt JL, Picot J, Loveman E, et al. Surgery for obesity. *Cochrane Database Syst Rev* 2009;(2):CD003641.
27. Buchwald H, Estok R, Fahrbach K, et al. Weight and type 2 diabetes after bariatric surgery: systematic review and metaanalysis. *Am J Med* 2009;122(3):248–256.
28. Adams TD, Gress RE, Smith SC, et al. Long-term mortality after gastric bypass surgery. *N Engl J Med* 2007;357(8):753–761.

17.2 Diabetes Mellitus

John P. Sheehan, Margaret M. Ulchaker, Charles Kent Smith

CLASSIFICATION

- **Type 1 (insulin-dependent) diabetes mellitus** (DM) is characterized by insulin deficiency due to autoimmune pancreatic β-cell destruction.[1]
- **Type 2 (non–insulin-dependent) DM** is characterized by insulin resistance and variable insulin secretory defects. Abdominal obesity, hypertension, and dyslipidemia often coexist as the metabolic syndrome.[1]

- **Latent autoimmune diabetes of adulthood (LADA)**
- **Gestational DM** (see Chapter 14.6)
- **Secondary DM** (not covered in this chapter)

INITIAL APPROACH TO THE PATIENT
- **Clinical history** yields important clues to the presence and correct classification of DM.
  - Type 1 DM
    - Recent onset of polydipsia, polyuria, significant weight loss, fatigue, and ketonuria occurs in a patient generally younger than 30 years of age.
    - Clinical duration of symptoms is relatively short despite a long prodrome of autoimmune pancreatic islet destruction.
  - Type 2 DM
    - Patient may present with polydipsia, polyuria, history of weight gain or loss, fatigue, glycosuria, obesity (especially abdominal), hypertension, dyslipidemia, positive family history of DM, or previous gestational DM. Traditionally, type 2 DM presented in patients generally older than 40 years of age; however, with increasing obesity, the age of onset can be in childhood.
    - Clinical duration of mild hyperglycemia with minimal symptoms may be prolonged in such a way that patients may present with DM complications (peripheral neuropathy, retinopathy, nephropathy).
    - **LADA.** Antibody positive DM of a more indolent nature. Many individuals can be controlled for years on medications other than insulin. Eventually, patients require full insulin replacement akin to an individual with type 1 DM.
  - Gestational DM (see Chapter 14.6).
  - Secondary DM. Consider DM in the context of the primary condition such as chronic pancreatitis, post-pancreatectomy, Cushing syndrome, acromegaly, cystic fibrosis, coadministration of antipsychotic medications, etc.
- **Physical examination**
  - The presence of DM complications such as acanthosis nigricans noted on a careful initial physical examination at time of diagnosis strongly favors a diagnosis of type 2 DM.
- **Laboratory diagnosis**[1]
  - Fasting serum glucose ≥126 mg per dL on two occasions in ambulatory setting.
  - Casual serum glucose ≥200 mg per dL on two occasions in ambulatory setting.
  - An HbA1c ≥6.5% is diagnostic for DM due to better standardization of HbA1c assays.[2,3]
  - A 2-hour postload plasma glucose. (Glucose tolerance test is no longer routinely needed to diagnose DM.)
    - Indications for a 2-hour postload plasma glucose test
      - Equivocal serum glucose levels, especially in the presence of other stigmata of metabolic syndrome.
      - Presence of complications, most commonly unexplained peripheral neuropathy, suggestive of DM when casual serum glucose and fasting serum glucose are non-diagnostic.
    - Diagnostic when 2-hour postload plasma glucose ≥200 mg per dL
    - Other abnormalities of glucose tolerance testing
      - Impaired glucose tolerance (IGT)
        - Fasting plasma glucose <126 mg per dL
        - 2-Hour postload (75 g anhydrous glucose) plasma glucose of ≥140 mg per dL and ≤199 mg per dL
      - Isolated impaired fasting glucose (IFG)
        - Fasting plasma glucose ≥100 mg per dL and <126 mg per dL
      - Combined IGT and IFG
      - **Caveat:** Patients with isolated IFG are at lower risk to progress to frank DM and develop complications of DM, including increased atherosclerotic complications.
- **Laboratory classification.** Clinical history, physical examination, ambient glucose levels, and degree of ketosis usually suffice for appropriate diagnostic classification. In equivocal settings, measurement of C-peptide or insulin levels (low in type 1 patients) coupled with glutamic acid decarboxylase antibodies, insulin autoantibodies, and pancreatic islet cell antibodies (positive in new-onset type 1 DM patients and LADA patients) allows correct classification.

- **Treatment goals.** Since publication of the Diabetes Control and Complications Trial (DCCT),[4] the Epidemiology of Diabetic Complications Trial (EDIC) (the extension of the DCCT),[5] the United Kingdom Prospective Diabetes Study (UKPDS),[6] the UKPDS follow-up study,[7] and position/consensus statements from the American Diabetes Association[8] and the American Association of Clinical Endocrinologists,[9] the ultimate goal for all patients, with few exceptions, is normalization or near-normalization of blood glucose levels within the constraints of hypoglycemia. Exceptions may include extremes of age, limited life expectancy, and advanced diabetic complications, including cardiovascular and cerebrovascular disease. Intensive glucose lowering in patients with long-standing type 2 DM (median duration 10 years) and established coronary artery disease (CAD) (35% of patients) or at high risk for CAD resulted in increased mortality and no decrease in major cardiovascular events in the ACCORD trial.[10] Treatment goals will likely change on the basis of outcomes from new research; but regardless, patient training and education by a skilled team is vital to the safety and efficacy of the treatment plan.
  - Short-term goals are (a) correction of hyperglycemia and ketosis, (b) elimination of hypoglycemia, and (c) reintegration of patient into society.
  - Long-term goals include preservation of residual insulin production in type 1 DM patients through early physiologic insulin replacement, facilitating long-term optimal glycemic control, and forestalling "brittleness." The key is attainment and maintenance of normal or near-normal body weight through diet and exercise to optimize insulin sensitivity, minimize insulin requirements, and minimize cardiovascular risk. Prevention of microvascular and macrovascular complications occurs through optimal glycemic control, normotension, and avoidance of excess sodium and protein intake. Early detection and prompt intervention once complications occur is essential.
- **Patient counseling, education, and motivation.** Patient training programs in the following areas are vital for short- and long-term goal achievement: pathophysiology of DM and the prevention of complications; therapeutic options for optimal control and lifestyle flexibility; dietary instruction/counseling; exercise integration; foot care; and sick-day and minor-illness management. Patients must be well versed in integration of these principles into their daily lives.

MANAGEMENT OF TYPE 1 DIABETES MELLITUS: INSULIN CONSIDERATIONS

- **Indications for outpatient initiation of insulin** include the following: patient is not vomiting, has no evidence of clinical dehydration, has no evidence of diabetic ketoacidosis (DKA), and the necessary support staff are readily available. It is impossible to accurately predict insulin sensitivity based on weight alone. Conservative initial starting doses in an otherwise well patient are in the range of 0.25 to 0.5 units per kg of body weight.
- **Choice of insulin.** Human insulin analogues and biosynthetic human insulin are the only insulins available in the United States. See Table 17.2-1 for insulin types and kinetics. The table reflects the kinetics seen in actual clinical practice rather than those reported by the manufacturers in nondiabetic individuals. Human insulin analogues are the preferred insulins except in cases in which cost is a major issue. Human biosynthetic insulins may be the only affordable option in this situation.
- **Injection site** principles are important for insulin absorption rate.
  - Site selection
    - Buttocks are the preferred site for bedtime injections in individuals still using human Neutral Protamine Hagedorn (NPH) insulin to minimize the risk of nocturnal hypoglycemia via (a) slower absorption, (b) avoidance of the 2 A.M. counterregulatory hormonal nadir, and (c) optimization of control of dawn surge in hepatic glucose output (dawn phenomenon).
    - Upper abdomen is preferred for injections of rapid-acting insulin analogues (RAAs) due to (a) its more rapid insulin absorption and (b) better control of the early postprandial glucose level. Upper arms can be used as an alternative.
    - Avoid RAA injections into legs and buttocks before meals due to slower absorption from these sites. On the other hand, exercise can accelerate the absorption of RAA from the legs and increase risk of hypoglycemia.
  - **Site consistency.** Patients must be instructed regarding the consistent use of anatomical regions for premeal and bedtime injections with adequate site rotation within these regions to prevent lipohypertrophy from repeated insulin injections in the same anatomic site. Injecting insulin into areas of lipohypertrophy can result in erratic insulin absorption and labile glucose levels. Injection site selection is less of an issue with the long-acting analogues glargine and detemir.

TABLE 17.2-1	Insulin Kinetics as Seen in Clinical Practice				

Activity	Classification	Name	Onset (h)	Peak (h)	Duration (h)
Short-acting	Insulin	Regular	0.5–1.0	2.5–3.5	6
Rapid-acting	Insulin analogue	Aspart	0–0.25	1–1.5	3–5
		Glulisine	0–0.25	1–1.5	3–4
		Lispro	0–0.25	1–1.5	3–5
Intermediate-acting	Insulin	NPH	1–3	6–8[a]	10–19
Long-acting	Insulin analogue	Detemir	2–4	None	up to 24
		Glargine	2–4	None	24–36
Pre-mixed	Insulin	70% human NPH/30% human Regular	Kinetics reflect individual components		
	Insulin analogue	70% protaminated aspart/30% aspart	Kinetics reflect individual components		
		75% protaminated lispro/25% protaminated aspart	Kinetics reflect individual components		

[a]Considerable fluctuations in day-to-day kinetics depending on injection site and dose.

- **Insulin injection timing issues**
  - Use of the subcutaneous site versus physiologic portal insulin results in delay in insulin absorption and an unavoidable mismatch between onset and peak of the insulin action and the onset and peak of blood glucose rise after carbohydrate ingestion.
  - Injection interval
    - Inject RAA insulins (aspart, glulisine, lispro) up to 10 minutes premeal, due to their rapid onset of action. Glulisine insulin injected up to 20 minutes after the start of a meal has been reported in a clinical trial to have similar kinetics to regular insulin injected 30 minutes premeal. This may be of benefit to individuals with unpredictable carbohydrate intake such as children, the elderly, and nursing home patients.
    - For individuals still using human regular insulin, injecting 30 to 40 minutes premeal helps to optimize postprandial glycemic control.
  - A small snack (15 g carbohydrate) at the peak of the insulin action—3 hours for human regular insulin and 6 to 8 hours for human NPH—prevents hypoglycemia at this high-risk time.
- **Intensive insulin therapy programs**
  - Multiple daily insulin injections
    - Principles
      - The use of multiple injections results in (a) smaller individual insulin doses, (b) more physiologic matching of carbohydrate and insulin, and (c) reduced risk of hypoglycemia. The better postprandial control that can be achieved with intensive insulin therapy (compared with conventional therapy) may reduce microvascular and macrovascular risk even with comparable HbA1c levels.
    - Program options
      - **The qid+ program:** (a) premeal/pre-snack dose of RAA insulin titrated to carbohydrate intake and (b) bedtime insulin glargine/detemir (40% to 50% total daily dose)

- Continuous subcutaneous insulin infusion (CSII) or insulin pump therapy
  • Indications
    • Failure of multiple daily insulin injection regimens
    • Exuberant dawn phenomenon
    • Need for convenience and flexibility
    • Pregnancy
    • Preconception
  • Insulin pump setup
    • RAA insulin is programmed at set hourly basal rates to control hepatic glucose output for the entire 24-hour day (approximately 40% to 50% total daily dose).
    • Remainder of dose is premeal/snack RAA insulin titrated to carbohydrate intake.
    • RAA insulin used nearly exclusively due to superior kinetics.
  • Modern insulin pumps have algorithms that are programmed with insulin to carbohydrate ratios for carbohydrate insulin dose calculations. Additionally, there are algorithms for correction of hyperglycemia that involve target blood glucose levels, insulin sensitivity factors (the reduction in blood glucose level achieved for every additional unit of RAA administered), and insulin action time (the duration of a bolus of RAA). The patient enters into the pump his/her blood glucose level and the amount of carbohydrate to be consumed, and the pump calculates the appropriate amount of insulin to be delivered based upon the aforementioned parameters. The patient is prompted to accept/reject the calculated dosage. The hyperglycemia correction factors take into account residual insulin action from a prior bolus and reduce the risk of hypoglycemia resulting from overcorrection of hyperglycemia.
- The tid program with human NPH
  • Two thirds of total daily dose is given in the morning. One-third of dose is RAA/human regular insulin. Two thirds of dose is human NPH insulin.
  • One-third of total daily dose is given in the evening with half of the dose as RAA/human regular insulin before supper and half of the dose as human NPH given between 10 P.M. and 1 A.M.
  • Ratios must be modified pending patient's preferred mealtime carbohydrate distribution.
- **A qid program can be used:** (a) premeal dose (tid) of human regular insulin titrated to carbohydrate intake and (b) bedtime human NPH (20% of total daily dose).
- **CAVEAT:** There is NO place for pre-mixed insulin in the management of type 1 DM or pregnancy due to fixed ratios of rapid/intermediate-acting insulin and lack of flexibility.
• **Insulin adjustments**
  • Baseline dose
    ○ Doses of RAA, human regular, human NPH, glargine, or detemir insulin can be readily adjusted based on premeal, postprandial, and bedtime home blood glucose test results. Assuming a total daily dose of 0.5 unit per kg body weight, supplementing the baseline dose by 1 unit of insulin will drop an elevated blood glucose by approximately 50 mg per dL.
    ○ Algorithm
      - For the patient using supplemental RAA/human regular insulin:
        • Use before meals and at bedtime. **Example:** In a patient taking 0.5 unit of insulin per kg body weight, the following calculations apply:
          • **Premeal and bedtime dosing.** Add 1 unit of RAA/human regular insulin for every 50 mg per dL elevation in blood glucose above 100 mg per dL; that is, at 150 mg per dL, add 1 unit RAA/regular; at 200 mg per dL, add 2 units RAA/regular, etc.
          • This should be revised pending individual patient glycemic goals and hypoglycemia risk.
  • In the context of frequent follow-up, optimal control can be achieved with gradual insulin titration. Once achieved in the newly diagnosed patient, insulin requirements may gradually decline ("honeymoon phase").

MANAGEMENT OF TYPE 1 DIABETES MELLITUS: DIETARY CONSIDERATIONS

• **Basic principles.** Current emphasis is carbohydrate counting while decreasing saturated fats and trans-fats, increasing dietary fiber and moderating protein intake.[11] Most commonly, carbohydrates account for 45% to 60% of total daily calories, fat should account for less than 30%, and protein for 15% to 35% of total daily calories. Better matching of insulin to intake of total carbohydrate through gram counting of carbohydrate allows the incorporation of modest amounts of sucrose in the diet. The use of a carbohydrate counting book/smartphone apps and food scales is essential for accurate carbohydrate counting and subsequent insulin dosing.

- **Priorities for patient education**
  - Emphasize carbohydrate counting and consistency with three meals. If patients are using human regular or human NPH insulin, add 15 g carbohydrate snacks to cover insulin peaks, in the context of an appropriate total caloric intake.

MANAGEMENT OF TYPE 1 DIABETES MELLITUS

Home blood glucose monitoring (HBGM) considerations:

- **Basic principles**
  - Accuracy in HBGM is critical to safety and success of intensive therapy.
  - Frequency
    - ○ Minimum of four tests per day should be done before meals and at bedtime.
    - ○ Monitoring 2 hours after a meal is necessary to accurately determine the adequacy of the premeal RAA insulin doses and the timing of the dose. Individuals who slowly absorb insulin may need to administer their RAA doses as far as 20 to 30 minutes premeal/snack to optimize postprandial glycemic control.
    - ○ Additional testing is done when hypoglycemia or hyperglycemia is suspected.
    - ○ Periodic 2 A.M. and 4 A.M. tests
    - ○ Prior to driving if symptomatic
- Patients must follow manufacturer's instructions carefully to achieve accurate results.
- **Sources of error in HBGM:** Improper cleansing of finger; failure to wipe away first drop of blood when alcohol is used to cleanse finger; volume of blood applied to strip is too much or too little; meter is not calibrated to strip lot number; damaged strips resulting from exposure to light, heat, cold or humidity; out-of-date strips; meter not properly cleaned; and failure to use glucose control solutions to verify strip accuracy. Patient precision is vital to successful use of the insulin algorithm and sick-day management.
- Glucose sensors which measure interstitial glucose levels are an adjunct to, not a replacement for, HBGM. The sensors provide trend detection in regard to the direction of change in glucose levels via a visual display and should not be used as a substitute for HBGM. Additionally, audible alarms signal when the glucose level has reached a preprogrammed rate of fall or rise as well as when a prespecified glucose level is reached. Appropriate candidates are individuals with type 1 DM on physiologic insulin programs, are attentive to counting grams of carbohydrate, and who attend regularly for their follow-up appointments. In addition to a visual display, audible alarms signal when the interstitial glucose level reaches a prespecified rate of fall or rise in glucose as well as when a prespecified interstitial glucose level is attained. One insulin pump system, which is integrated with a glucose sensor, can be programmed to suspend basal insulin delivery for up to 2 hours in event of a hypoglycemia threshold being reached.

MANAGEMENT OF TYPE 1 DIABETES MELLITUS: EXERCISE CONSIDERATIONS

- **Physical fitness** is a goal for all individuals with DM. Safe exercise plans must be individualized based on age, cardiovascular status, foot problems, neuropathy, and retinopathy. Even increased activity, such as grocery shopping, results in a lowering of blood glucose levels. Uncompensated physical activity is a very common cause of hypoglycemia in the patient with type 1 DM.
- **Insulin adjustment for exercise or activity.** Use for planned physical activity.
  - Reduce the RAA insulin dose that is active during the exercise by 1 to 2 units or more for every 20 to 30 minutes of exercise. The amount of reduction will depend upon the intensity of the exercise.
  - Occasionally, individuals have a delayed or sustained response to physical activity such that their bedtime insulin dose may need to be reduced by 1 to 2 units or more following, for example, evening physical activity. Again, the amount of reduction will depend upon the intensity of the exercise.
  - Insulin pump patients have the option to program a temporary reduction in their basal insulin infusion rates. Temporary basal rates must be programmed 45 to 60 minutes prior to the planned physical activity due to the kinetics of subcutaneous insulin.

- **Carbohydrate adjustment for exercise or activity**
- Use for either planned or spontaneous activity.
- **Augment carbohydrate intake as follows:** Add a 15-g carbohydrate snack for every 20 to 30 minutes of physical activity, depending on the intensity of activity.

STANDARD OF CARE FOR FOLLOW-UP

Once glycemic control has been established, maintenance of glycemic control depends on the frequency of follow-up.

- Minimum visit frequency is once every 3 months.
- Review history; perform an interim physical examination; identify patient errors and omissions; adjust the patient's insulin dosage, diet, and exercise program; and do ongoing patient counseling. Laboratory evaluations should include HbA1c every 3 months and annual assessments of urine microalbumin/creatinine ratio, thyroid-stimulating hormone, blood chemistries, and a lipid panel. In addition, an electrocardiogram (EKG) and ankle–brachial indices (see following section) may be obtained annually or sooner depending on the patient symptomatology.

DAWN PHENOMENON

- **The dawn phenomenon** is a markedly elevated fasting blood glucose secondary to an exuberant rise in hepatic glucose output. This hyperglycemia results from a surge in counterregulatory hormone concentrations (growth hormone, catecholamines, and cortisol) in the absence of nocturnal hypoglycemia.
- **Treatment**
  - Delaying the timing of bedtime insulin dose until closer to midnight and titrating up the bedtime NPH, glargine, or detemir insulin usually suffices. In some instances, however, the dose increase results in hypoglycemia prior to the dawn surge. CSII is ideal in this situation, such that basal rates can be preprogrammed to coincide with the patient's individual dawn surge. Glucose sensor trends can be helpful in this regard.

AFTERNOON PHENOMENON

- **The afternoon phenomenon** is late afternoon/pre-dinner hyperglycemia in the setting of good glycemic control postlunch. In patients with insulin pumps, afternoon basal rates can be increased to accommodate this. In patients on MDI, adding a pre-breakfast or sometimes even a prelunch dose of basal insulin can help to control this.

SOMOGYI PHENOMENON

- **The Somogyi phenomenon** is post-hypoglycemia hyperglycemia due to a surge in counterregulatory hormones, rather than insulin "run-out" or overtreatment of hypoglycemia with excess carbohydrate.
- **Strategy.** Perform HBGM at 2 A.M. and 4 A.M. in addition to premeal and bedtime HBGM. If the Somogyi phenomenon is identified, a dose reduction of the evening basal insulin is indicated, coupled perhaps with a shift in the timing of the injection as late as possible (midnight or thereafter), with emphasis on the lower buttocks as the injection site of choice if human NPH insulin is being used. Glucose sensor trends can be helpful in this regard.

HYPOGLYCEMIA

Recurrent. In a well-designed, physiologic, individualized treatment program, most episodes of hypoglycemia are related to patient error.

- **Patient-related errors** include insulin–carbohydrate mismatch, delayed or missed meals, missed snacks, uncompensated exercise, erratic insulin injection site rotation, injecting into areas of lipohypertrophy, and lack of adequate HBGM (inaccurate tests or low frequency of HBGM).
- **Nonpatient-related problems** include unpredictable absorption or kinetics of basal insulin or, less frequently, insulin autoantibodies. This is best treated by utilizing a true basal-bolus insulin regimen with insulin glargine or detemir along with RAA.
- **Hypoglycemia unawareness**
  - Hypoglycemia can be a major problem in intensive therapy and a limitation to achieving glycemic targets. In most cases, it is reversible to varying degrees through program revisions designed to eliminate hypoglycemia.

- Once hypoglycemia has been eliminated for a period of 3 to 6 weeks, the patient's subjective awareness and counterregulatory hormonal response will improve, with the exception of the glucagon response. Improvement in hypoglycemia awareness facilitates safe lowering of ambient glucose levels and HbA1c.
- These patients may be very good candidates for glucose sensors assuming patient adherence to all aspects of an intensive insulin therapy regimen and pending health insurance coverage.

DIABETIC KETOACIDOSIS IN ADULTS

Prevention and management. DKA is a syndrome of hyperglycemia, ketonemia, and ketonuria of varying intensity that results in death in 10% of cases.

- **Causes.** Minor illnesses are the most common cause, such as upper respiratory and urinary tract infections. Major illnesses (such as myocardial infarction [MI] and major sepsis infarction) are a less common cause. Most cases of severe DKA can be averted through aggressive attention to the sick-day management guidelines (refer to Special Issues, below).
- Treatment
  - If intractable emesis occurs, take the following measures:
    - Administer early intravenous hydration with 1 to 2 L of normal saline fluids in emergency room.
    - Administer SC insulin bolus, not IV insulin bolus, as the half-life of an IV bolus of regular insulin is only 5 minutes.
    - Administer parenteral or rectal antiemetics.
    - Do not delay. Delay in seeking therapy is the major factor in severe DKA episodes, which result in costly hospitalizations in intensive care units and even death.
- Identify and address the underlying illness. Rule out silent MI or occult sepsis as cause of DKA.
  - Correct the volume depletion.
    - Give 1 to 2 L of normal saline in the first 1 to 2 hours to correct hypotension and establish good urine output. In children and adolescents, give 500 mL of normal saline per hour for the first 1 to 2 hours.
    - Total volume deficit is frequently 5 to 6 L. In most individuals, volume can be replaced over 12 to 24 hours, depending on the underlying cardiac and renal status.
    - Failure to adequately rehydrate and correct ketosis completely is a common cause of rapid DKA relapse despite correction of hyperglycemia. Patients need to be ketone free for 24 hours to ensure complete correction.
- **Insulin treatment.** Start a low-dose IV infusion at the rate of 0.1 unit/kg/hour to result in a 100 mg/dL/hour fall in blood glucose. Adequately dilute the insulin to allow fine titration (50 units human regular insulin in 500 mL normal saline). This dosage overcomes the common clinical problem of having 1 unit per hour be the lowest infusion rate possible. This is especially important for very insulin–sensitive patients. There is no place for RAA in IV insulin therapy. To maintain a sufficiently high insulin dose to correct ketosis without hypoglycemia, the intravenous fluids must be changed to dextrose 5% or 10% when blood glucose level falls below 250 mg per dL.
- Electrolyte replacement
  - Potassium replacement may be initiated once the serum potassium is <5.5 mEq per L and urine output is documented. Use 20 to 40 mEq per L IV fluids and monitor serum potassium values q2h.
  - Bicarbonate therapy is controversial and is rarely used unless there is severe acidosis with hemodynamic instability or severe hyperkalemia with EKG changes. Clinical trials have failed to demonstrate any benefit in the treatment of DKA. Bicarbonate should not be given by IV push because that could result in cerebral edema, especially in children, which is often fatal.
  - Phosphate repletion has more theoretical than proven practical benefits unless severe depletion is present (serum phosphorus <0.5 mg per dL).
  - **Magnesium repletion.** If deficiency is severe (serum magnesium level <1.0 mEq per L) or the patient is symptomatic (seizures, tetany, cardiac arrhythmias), then replace with magnesium chloride at a dose of 1 mEq/kg/24 hour, assuming normal renal function.
- Monitor DKA progress. Clinical and laboratory monitoring of the patient should be documented on a flow sheet. Laboratory parameters should be followed at least every 2 hours until stability emerges.

HYPERGLYCEMIC HYPEROSMOLAR NONKETOTIC COMA

- **Characteristics.** This condition occurs in type 2 DM patients, most commonly with underlying renal insufficiency or cerebrovascular disease (cerebrovascular accident or subdural hematoma). The degree of dehydration is more severe than that of DKA. Blood glucose levels range from 600 to 2,000 mg to dL, and ketosis is generally absent.
- **Treatment** is similar to that for DKA in terms of IV fluids, insulin, and electrolytes, but hydration rates must be lower.
  - The initial infusion rate of normal saline should not exceed 1 L per hour to expand the extracellular space, with the IV fluid being switched to half normal saline once blood pressure is stable and good urine output is established. Fluid should be replaced over a 24-hour period.
  - Often insulin therapy is not needed on an ongoing basis once the acute metabolic derangement has been corrected and any underlying precipitating illness treated or resolved.

INITIAL MANAGEMENT OF TYPE 2 DIABETES MELLITUS

- **Minimally decompensated presentation**
  - Clinical picture includes obesity and mild to moderate hyperglycemia with or without symptoms. Treatment strategies include patient education, training, and motivation; an individualized hypocaloric meal plan (regardless of the macronutrient distribution)[12] with dietary counseling; and an exercise plan tailored to the individual. Emphasize permanent lifestyle modification. Additionally, metformin is advocated as a component of initial therapy, assuming no contraindications.
- **Moderately decompensated presentation**
  - **Clinical picture.** Obesity, severe symptomatic hyperglycemia (fasting blood glucose >300 mg per dL), and mild dehydration or decompensation call for more urgent lowering of blood glucose levels, largely for symptomatic relief and reversal of the glucotoxic effect of the prior sustained hyperglycemia on pancreatic islet insulin secretion and peripheral insulin action.
  - Treatment strategies
    - Temporary insulin therapy with daily glargine/detemir at a starting daily dose of 0.4 units per kg of weight and an algorithm for hyperglycemia similar to that for type 1 DM patients will rapidly yield symptomatic relief and reversal of islet and peripheral/target organ glucotoxicity.
- **Severely decompensated presentation**
  - Clinical picture shows a severely symptomatic patient with blood glucose levels frequently exceeding 350 mg per dL, marked dyslipidemia (serum triglycerides >1,000 mg per dL), and hyperosmolality with absence of ketosis.
  - Treatment strategies
    - Intravenous fluids and insulin (similar to DKA) in the hospital setting are necessary for acute reversal of the metabolic derangement, followed later by a switch to daily insulin glargine/detemir.
    - Start patient training and education with an individualized meal plan,[11] dietary counseling and an exercise plan. The long-term goal may be tapering and withdrawal of insulin, pending residual insulin secretion, assuming that glycemic control can be maintained with diet, exercise, oral agent therapy and/or injectable incretin-based therapy.
- **Special situation: The nonobese type 2 diabetic patient.** Patients who are at less than 120% of IBW comprise approximately 10% of those with type 2 DM. It is important to rule out LADA in these individuals. If LADA is ruled out, these patients may benefit from modest weight loss toward IBW, with a hypocaloric meal plan (regardless of the macronutrient distribution),[12] dietary counseling, and exercise training program. Exercise is especially beneficial to these patients, many of whom are relatively insulinopenic and poor responders to oral agents. Frequently these patients will require basal insulin therapy with glargine/detemir insulin, and many will need to progress to full insulin replacement akin to an individual with type 1 DM.

DIETARY MANAGEMENT OF TYPE 2 DIABETES MELLITUS

- **Goals in overweight and obese patients**
  - Reduction in body weight
    - **Strategies.** Reduce overall caloric intake (regardless of the macronutrient distribution)[12] through carbohydrate counting and fat gram counting. Consumption of 100 kcal per day over and above caloric needs will result in a 10-pound annual weight gain. Reduction in daily caloric intake by 500 calories daily will facilitate a 1-pound weekly weight loss.

○ A reduction of even 5% to 10% in weight can have a major impact on the clinical course of a type 2 DM patient. Patients need not reduce to IBW to achieve euglycemia, but the closer they are, the better all the other markers of the metabolic syndrome will be (e.g., dyslipidemia, hypertension).

○ Weight loss results in removal of fat from the liver, pancreas, and skeletal muscle and improving insulin sensitivity.

EXERCISE THERAPY FOR TYPE 2 DIABETES MELLITUS

All of the benefits of exercise for the type 1 DM patient apply even more to the type 2 DM patient, with the added benefit of raising the frequently depressed high-density lipoprotein cholesterol (HDL-C) level. Adherence to an ongoing exercise routine is one of the most powerful predictors of maintenance of weight loss. The importance of exercise capacity and survival must be stressed. In the LOOK-AHEAD trial, intensive lifestyle modification resulted in a reduction in HbA1c of 0.7% after 1 year, equivalent to many pharmacotherapeutic agents.

PHARMACOTHERAPY OF TYPE 2 DIABETES MELLITUS

- **Introduction**
- Pharmacotherapy of type 2 DM is now directed at the specific pathophysiologic defects that have been identified as the ominous octet:[13]
  ○ Increased hepatic glucose production
  ○ Decreased insulin secretion
  ○ Decreased skeletal muscle glucose uptake
  ○ Hypersecretion of glucagon
  ○ Diminished incretin effect
  ○ Increased lipolysis
  ○ Increased renal glucose reabsorption
  ○ Neurotransmitter dysfunction in the central nervous system
  ○ All oral medications can be used as initial therapy, or as second- or third-order therapy in combination with other oral agents, injectable incretin-based therapy or insulin.
- **Insulin sensitizers**
- Metformin
  ○ **Indication.** Metformin therapy is indicated as first-line therapy for all patients with type 2 DM who are free from significant liver disease, have a serum creatinine <1.4 mg per dL in women or <1.5 mg per dL in men. Lactic acidosis is a risk if any of these underlying conditions exist. Metformin should be discontinued on the day of any iodinated dye-load procedure or surgery and should be withheld for 48 hours after the procedure. Metformin can be restarted until a normal serum creatinine is confirmed post-contrast study/surgery. Metformin should also be withheld during treatment for pneumonia or acute MI.
  ○ **Mode of action.** Metformin is an insulin sensitizer at the level of the liver with a primary mode of action of controlling excess hepatic glucose output. It is not a hypoglycemic agent; therefore, it generally cannot cause hypoglycemia when used as monotherapy.
  ○ Dosing
  - Use as monotherapy or in combination with other oral agents, injectable incretin-based therapy, and/or insulin.
  - Initial dose
    • Immediate release (IR) (500 mg bid with food) can be titrated to a maximum of 2,550 mg in an 850-mg tid dosing schedule. Maximum effective dose is generally seen at 1,000 mg bid.
  - Extended-release (ER) preparations can be used to facilitate dosing convenience and reduce the risk of diarrhea. The initial dose is 500 mg with the evening meal titrated to 2,000 mg daily.
  ○ **Other effects.** Metformin facilitates weight loss and can improve the lipid profile.
- **Adverse effects.** Gastrointestinal (GI) side effects of nausea, flatus, and diarrhea can occur but are usually self-limited (1 to 2 weeks). Side effects can be minimized by taking medication with food and using an ER preparation. Long-term discontinuation rate due to GI side effects is generally less than 4%. Vitamin B_{12} malabsorption may occur.[14]
- Thiazolidinediones (glitazones)
  ○ **Indications.** Therapy with glitazones are indicated for patients with type 2 DM who are free of significant liver disease, hepatic transaminases ≤1.5 times the upper limit of normal, and who

have good left ventricular function. Glitazones can be used as initial therapy in patients in whom metformin is contraindicated or not tolerated. Glitazone therapy is contraindicated in patients who have type 1 DM, who have New York Heart Association class III or IV CHF. They can be used safely in patients with renal disease.

- ○ **Mode of action.** Glitazones are insulin sensitizers that activate peroxisome proliferator–activated γ-receptors. Clinical effect from this activation is delayed, and the maximal effect of a given dose level may not be seen for 8 to 12 weeks. The primary mode of action of glitazones is to enhance skeletal muscle glucose uptake both directly and also indirectly via reduction in free fatty acids. At higher doses, they also reduce hepatic glucose output. They are antihyperglycemic and as such when used as monotherapy or in combination with metformin generally do not cause hypoglycemia.
- ○ Pioglitazone may have the added benefit of lowering triglyceride levels and raising HDL-C levels and may benefit patients with hepatic steatosis (fatty liver).[15]
- ○ The use of rosiglitazone was greatly reduced following a flawed meta-analysis that suggested increased cardiovascular risk. The re-review of the RECORD trial mandated by the United States Food and Drug Administration (FDA) did not show any increased cardiovascular risk.[16] Rosiglitazone has been shown also to preserve β-cell function in ADOPT (A Diabetes Outcome Progression Trial).
- ○ Dosing
  - Pioglitazone
    - Initial dose of 15 mg qd can be titrated to 45 mg qd.
  - Rosiglitazone
    - The prescribing of rosiglitazone was limited by a Risk Evaluation Mitigation Strategy (REMS) program. Although this REMS program has been lifted, rosiglitazone is no longer commonly prescribed.
    - Initial dose of 2 mg bid can be titrated to 4 mg bid. Rosiglitazone can be given qd, but better glucose-lowering effect was noted with bid dosing in clinical trials.
- ○ Adverse effects
  - **Idiosyncratic hepatic dysfunction.** The first glitazone troglitazone was voluntarily removed from the U.S. market by its manufacturer in March 2000, secondary to a small number of treated patients developing fulminant hepatic failure resulting in transplantation and/or death. The incidence of elevations in hepatic transaminases in treated patients was 2%. Rosiglitazone and pioglitazone have a lower risk of elevations in hepatic transaminases (0.35% and 0.26%). Current recommendations are for monitoring of hepatic transaminases at baseline and then periodically thereafter.
  - **Pedal edema.** Edema, varying from trace to 4+, can develop as a consequence of glitazone therapy. No predisposing factors appear to exist except concurrent insulin therapy, which may actually precipitate diastolic heart failure.
  - **Weight gain.** The weight gain seen with glitazone therapy in some patients appears to be in excess of that expected from reduction/elimination in glycosuria. Some of the weight gain may be fluid related although many patients report increased appetite with glitazones.
- **α-Glucosidase inhibitors**
  - **Indications.** Acarbose can be used as monotherapy in patients in whom metformin is contraindicated or not tolerated, is generally indicated as second- or later-line treatment for individuals with type 2 DM. They can be used in combination with oral agents, injectable incretin-based therapy or insulin. Contraindications include cirrhosis, inflammatory or other bowel disease, and malabsorption.
  - **Mode of action.** α-Glucosidase inhibitors interfere with digestion and absorption of dietary carbohydrate. Their primary effect is on postprandial blood glucose levels. They are antihyperglycemic agents and as such when used as monotherapy or in combination with metformin cannot cause hypoglycemia. However, hypoglycemia can occur when acarbose is used in combination with secretagogues or insulin. When hypoglycemia occurs, it must be managed with pure glucose because the digestion and absorption of alternative carbohydrates will be delayed.
  - **Dosing**
    - ○ Acarbose
      - Starting dose of 25 mg tid to be taken with the first bite of each meal.
      - Titration to 50 mg tid, up to a maximum dose of 100 mg tid. The need for multiple doses may hinder adherence.

- Adverse effects include flatus and nausea, which lessen over time, but have clinically limited their use. Small numbers of patients experience an elevation in transaminases (usually in individuals with a body weight of less than 60 kg).
- **Secretagogues**
  - Sulfonylureas
    - **Indications.** Although in the past sulfonylureas were considered to be first-line pharmacotherapeutic agents for type 2 DM, new treatment guidelines generally utilize these drugs as later-line agents. They can be used in combination with other non-secretagogue oral agents, injectable incretin-based therapy, or insulin. Their use is contraindicated in patients with type 1 DM, elevations in hepatic transaminases. A relative contraindication is sulfa allergy. Caution must be used in the setting of end-stage renal disease.
    - Mode of action is augmentation of non-glucose-dependent pancreatic insulin secretion via binding to sulfonylurea receptors.
    - Dosing varies with each agent.
    - Adverse effects are hypoglycemia and weight gain. Hypoglycemia frequency is reduced with the third-generation agent glimepiride versus the second-generation agents: glipizide and glyburide. The first-generation agents (chlorpropamide, tolazamide, tolbutamide, and acetohexamide) are now rarely used because they carry a poor side-effect profile.
  - Repaglinide
    - **Indications.** Although it can be used as monotherapy in patients in whom metformin is contraindicated or not tolerated, repaglinide is generally used as later-line therapy and can be used in combination with non-secretagogue oral agents, injectable incretin-based therapy, or insulin. As it has no sulfa moiety, it can be used in patients with sulfa allergy/sulfonylurea allergy. Caution should be given with coadministration with medications that are inducers or inhibitors of either the CYP3A4 pathway or CYP2C8 pathway. Caution is especially warranted when both pathways are simultaneously inhibited (CYP3A4 by such medications as ketoconazole, erythromycin, clarithromycin, itraconazole) and (CYP2C8 by medication such as gemfibrozil, trimethoprim, montelukast) as significant increases in plasma levels of repaglinide can occur.
    - **Mode of action.** Binding to a specific islet cell receptor results in more rapid secretion of insulin in response to food eaten compared with sulfonylureas. Effect is seen especially on postprandial and to a lesser extent on fasting glucose levels.
    - Dosing
      - Initial dose of 0.5 mg taken 0 to 15 minutes before a meal can be titrated to a maximum dose of 4 mg taken 1 to 15 minutes before a meal or snack for a maximal daily dose of 16 mg. The need for multiple doses may hinder adherence.
      - Must be dosed in conjunction with food to have optimum glucose-lowering effect. If a meal is skipped, the dose should be skipped.
      - **Adverse effects.** Hypoglycemia can occur, but does so less frequently than with sulfonylureas due to the rapid onset and shorter duration of action. This is pertinent especially when patients delay or miss meals. In addition, the lack of an increase in basal insulin secretion lowers the risk of hypoglycemia.
  - Nateglinide
    - **Indications.** Although it can be used as monotherapy in patients in whom metformin is contraindicated or not tolerated, nateglinide is generally used as later-line therapy and can be used in combination with non-secretagogue oral agents, injectable incretin-based therapy, or insulin. It is contraindicated in advanced hepatic disease due to lack of clinical studies. As it has no sulfa moiety, nateglinide can be used in patients with sulfa allergy/sulfonylurea allergy.
    - **Mode of action.** The phenylalanine derivative nateglinide binds to a specific islet receptor, resulting in more rapid insulin secretion from the pancreatic islets. It uniquely restores early insulin secretion, which is lost early in the course of type 2 DM. Early insulin secretion is very important in the regulation of hepatic glucose production postprandially.
    - Dosing
      - The recommended starting dose is 120 mg tid prior to meals; however, a dose of 60 mg tid prior to meals may be used in patients who are near goal HbA1c. If a meal is skipped, the dose should be skipped. The need for multiple doses may hinder adherence.
    - Adverse effects
      - Hypoglycemia is the most common side effect and is seen at a much lower rate than that with any other secretagogue.

- Dipeptidyl peptidase IV (DPP-IV) inhibitors
  - **Indications.** Although DPP-IV inhibitors can be used as monotherapy in patients in whom metformin is either contraindicated or not tolerated, DPP-IV inhibitors are most commonly used as second- or later-line agents in combination with oral agents or insulin. The currently approved DPP-IV inhibitors are sitagliptin, saxagliptin, linagliptin, and alogliptin.
  - **Mode of action.** DPP-IV inhibitors inhibit the enzyme DPP-IV, the enzyme involved in the degradation of glucagon like peptide 1 (GLP-1). As a result, GLP-1 levels return to a physiologic, not pharmacologic level, resulting in a reduction in pancreatic hypersecretion of glucagon and augmentation of glucose-dependent insulin secretion.
  - **Dosing.** Linagliptin is the only DPP-IV inhibitor with a single dose regardless of renal status, as it is excreted unmetabolized in the feces. The other DPP-IV inhibitor doses vary pending renal status. The efficacy of linagliptin is reduced when coadministered with a p-glycoprotein inducer such as rifampin.
  - **Adverse events.** The most common adverse events are upper respiratory infections, nasopharyngitis, urinary tract infections, and headaches. Postmarketing reports suggested a causal relationship with these agents and pancreatitis in addition to pancreatic cancer. Patients with type 2 DM are at increased risk for both of these conditions regardless of treatment modality. The FDA and the European Medicines Agency (EMA) have reviewed all the available data and have to date not found a causal relationship for either pancreatitis or pancreatic cancer.[17]
- Sodium-glucose co-transporter 2 (SGLT-2) inhibitors
  - **Indications.** Currently there are two FDA-approved SGLT-2 inhibitors—canagliflozin and dapagliflozin. Although SGLT-2 inhibitors can be used as monotherapy, they are most commonly used as second- or later-line therapy. Canagliflozin is contraindicated in individuals with an eGFR <45 mL per minute. It is an inducer of the UGT enzyme system; coadministration with medications, such as rifampin, phenytoin, ritonavir or phenobarbital, can result in reduced efficacy of canagliflozin. Pending eGFR, the canagliflozin dose should be increased. Canagliflozin can increase digoxin levels; monitor digoxin levels appropriately. Dapagliflozin is contraindicated in individuals with an eGFR <60 mL per minute. It should not be used in patients with active bladder cancer and should be used with caution in patients with a personal history of bladder cancer.
  - **Mode of action.** SGLT-2 transports 90% of filtered glucose from the proximal tubule into the interstitial cell for reabsorption. SGLT-2 inhibitors reduce glucose reabsorption and increase urinary glucose excretion by approximately 70 g of glucose daily. This results in improvement in glycemic control, weight loss, and blood pressure lowering.
  - Dosing
    - Canagliflozin initial dosing is 100 mg daily in the morning and can be titrated to 300 mg daily in the morning if eGFR is >60 mL per minute.
    - Dapagliflozin initial dosing is 5 mg daily in the morning, which can be titrated to 10 mg daily in the morning if eGFR remains >60 mL per minute.
  - **Adverse events.** The most common adverse events are genital mycotic infections in women and in uncircumcised males. Individuals with a history of prior genital mycotic infections are at higher risk for further genital mycotic infections. Additional adverse events include hypovolemia due to increased urinary glucose excretion and increased urine volume. It is important to ensure that individuals are volume replete before initiating therapy. Additionally, reducing diuretic dosage by 50% is prudent. SGLT-2 inhibitor therapy can result in a transient reduction in eGFR as a consequence of hypovolemia. Urinary tract infections and constipation can also occur.
- **Injectable incretin-based therapy**
  - GLP-1 receptor agonists
    - **Indications.** Three GLP-1 receptor agonists are FDA-approved and vary by half-life—exenatide, liraglutide, and exenatide LAR. Although they can be used as monotherapy in individuals in whom metformin is contraindicated or not tolerated, they are generally used as second- or later-line agents in combination with oral agents or insulin. Postmarketing reports suggested a causal relationship with these agents and pancreatitis in addition to pancreatic cancer. Patients with type 2 DM are at increased risk for both of these conditions regardless of treatment modality. The FDA and EMA have reviewed all the available data and have to date not found a causal relationship for either pancreatitis or pancreatic cancer.[17]
    - **Contraindications.** Exenatide and exenatide LAR are contraindicated in individuals with an eGFR <30 mL per minute. Liraglutide and exenatide LAR are contraindicated in individuals

with a personal or family history of medullary thyroid cancer or multiple endocrine neoplasia type 2 syndrome 2 (MEN2) due to C-cell hyperplasia being noted in rats and mice and the association of C-cell hyperplasia to medullary thyroid cancer. No sustained elevations in calcitonin levels have been seen nor have there been any cases of C-cell hyperplasia in monkeys or in humans treated with these medications. If a thyroid nodule is noted, individuals should be referred to an endocrinologist for evaluation.

- ○ **Mode of action.** GLP-1 receptor agonists bind to the GLP-1 receptor and raise GLP-1 levels to pharmacologic levels. They are resistant to degradation by the DPP-IV enzyme. Raising GLP-1 levels into the pharmacologic range results in restoration of first-phase insulin secretion, enhancement of glucose-dependent insulin secretion, suppression of glucagon hypersecretion, delayed gastric emptying, and promotion of satiety.
- ○ Dosing
  - – Exenatide with its short half-life must be administered BID and in conjunction with a meal. Exenatide is administered as a subcutaneous injection via a pen device at a dose of 5 μg within 60 minutes of the morning and evening meals. The dose can be increased after 1 month to 10 μg bid if necessary. Major effect is on postprandial glucose levels.
  - – Liraglutide with its long half-life is dosed once daily irrespective of meals. It is administered subcutaneously via a pen. The initial dose of 0.6 mg daily can be titrated week two to 1.2 mg daily and then week three to 1.8 mg daily to facilitate glycemic control. Liraglutide impacts both fasting and postprandial glucose control.
  - – Exenatide LAR with its extended half-life is administered subcutaneously at a dose of 2 mg weekly via vial and syringe or a new pen device. Steady state is achieved after 6 to 7 weeks. Exenatide LAR impacts both fasting and postprandial glucose control.
- ○ **Adverse events.** GI side effects include nausea, dyspepsia, vomiting, diarrhea, and constipation. Both liraglutide and even more so, exenatide LAR, have lower risks of GI side effects. Hypoglycemia is a potential risk with all GLP-1 agonists when administered concurrently with secretagogues and/or insulin; the dose of secretagogues/insulin should be reduced appropriately. Small subcutaneous nodules can occur at the injection site of exenatide LAR and gradually resolve spontaneously.
- • **Pramlintide.** Pramlintide is an analogue of the neuroendocrine hormone amylin that is cosecreted by the pancreatic β-cells in response to food intake. Pramlinitide delays gastric emptying, suppresses glucagon hypersecretion, and reduces food intake via central modulation of appetite. Pramlintide improves postprandial glucose and overall glycemic control and is indicated for individuals with type 1 DM as an adjunct to insulin therapy. In individuals with type 2 DM, pramlintide may be used with oral agents or insulin. In type 1 DM patients, pramlintide should be initiated at a dose of 15 μg sc immediately prior to major meals with titration in 15 μg increments to a maintenance dose of 30 to 60 μg premeal as tolerated. In patients with type 2 DM, pramlintide should be initiated at a dose of 60 μg sc immediately prior to major meals and increased to 120 μg premeal as tolerated. Concurrent insulin therapy increases the risk of insulin-induced hypoglycemia, especially in patients with type 1 DM. Reduction in premeal insulin by 50% is recommended to minimize the risk of hypoglycemia. Frequent HBGM is needed to ensure safety and efficacy. Nausea is the most common treatment-emergent adverse event that limits dose titration or ongoing use of pramlintide. No dose adjustments are needed for patients with creatinine clearance >20 mL per minute.
- • **Insulin**
  - • Long-term insulin therapy indications.
    - ○ Insulinopenic nonobese type 2 DM patients who have failed optimum diet, exercise, and oral agent therapy are best managed on insulin programs described for type 1 DM patients
    - ○ Insulin is indicated in patients in whom oral agents and/or injectable incretin-based therapies are contraindicated, are not tolerated, or have failed.
  - • **Dosing schedules.** Several dosing schedules have been advocated, and all have a tendency to cause progressive weight gain and attendant increasing insulin requirements to try to maintain glycemic control. The use of detemir insulin has been associated with less weight gain than glargine or NPH. Administration of detemir or glargine insulin at bedtime facilitates the best control of dawn hepatic glucose output, thereby minimizing islet glucotoxicity and maximizing islet insulin secretory response to daytime oral agents and/or injectable incretin-based therapy. Should this regimen fail to give adequate control, any of the regimens outlined for type 1 DM patients may be used. A rare indication for the use of CSII in type 2 DM is the lean insulinopenic patient.

- The ORIGIN Trial failed to show any increased cardiovascular risk with insulin therapy in individuals with type 2 DM.[18] Additionally, no increased risk of any cancers was documented in contradistinction to the earlier reports associating glargine prescriptions and cancer risk.[19]
- **Bariatric surgery**
  - Weight loss can result in dramatic improvement in glycemic control and other metabolic parameters. Weight loss results in removal of fat from the liver, pancreas, and skeletal muscle and greatly improves the function of these organs. Bariatric surgery is one approach to weight loss.[20] The generally accepted BMI criterion for bariatric surgery for obese type 2 DM patients is a BMI of ≥35 kg per m²; benefit has also been shown for patients with BMIs as low as 27 kg per m². The best results are seen in the first year postsurgery. Roux-en-y gastric bypass in general leads to the best weight loss but also has the most adverse metabolic derangements to include iron, vitamin B_{12}, and vitamin D malabsorption with attendant sequelae. Recidivism and regain of weight is a significant long-term issue. The use of the term "surgical cure" is thus premature at this stage. Bariatric surgery for obese type 1 DM patients has resulted in decreased insulin requirements and naturally does not cure the disease.[21]

STANDARDS OF CARE FOR FOLLOW-UP

The standard of care for follow-up for the patient with type 2 DM is the same as that for the patient with type 1 DM.

SPECIAL TESTING IN DIABETES

- **Ankle–brachial indices** are part of the standard of care because of their predictive value, not only for peripheral vascular disease (PVD) but also for CAD and cardiovascular death risk. Blood pressures are measured with a mercury sphygmomanometer and hand-held Doppler at both the dorsalis pedis and posterior tibial arteries and compared with that obtained at the brachial artery. Any reduction in the ankle–brachial index (ankle pressure divided by brachial pressure) below 0.9 is significant and warrants intensive risk factor modification.
- **Screening for asymptomatic CAD**
  - Screening for truly asymptomatic CAD is highly controversial. Silent ischemia and silent MI are more common in DM patients, especially those with cardiac autonomic neuropathy. Patients with type 2 DM are considered coronary risk equivalent to patients with established CAD and therefore deserve intensive risk factor modification. The Bari 2-D trial showed that optimization of medical treatment was non-inferior to percutaneous intervention in type 2 DM with stable CAD referred for angiography, although only 35% of stented patients received drug-eluting stents. Patients who had coronary artery bypass grafting (CABG) in the Bari 2-D trial selected on the basis of angiographic findings had an 8.1% risk reduction for the composite end point of death/non-fatal MI/stroke versus optimized medical therapy.[22] Currently, there is no consensus on finding the asymptomatic high-risk individual with type 2 DM who would benefit ultimately from CABG or a drug-eluting stent.
  - Calcium scoring (CAC) is a reasonable first test for high-risk patients with type 2 DM with subsequent imaging studies pending the results. CAC has been shown to be superior to Framingham and UKPDS risk scoring.[23]

SPECIAL ISSUES

- **Foot care**
  - The critical interplay of three pathophysiologic processes—neuropathy, ischemia, and infection—results in injury predisposition and potential amputation.
  - Patients should be instructed to inspect and wash, but not soak feet daily; to use lotion on plantar and dorsal surfaces but not on intertriginous areas; to keep nails trimmed; and to seek podiatric care if needed.
- **Sick-day guidelines**
  - Perform HBGM at a minimum qid; ideally q4h.
  - Monitor urine ketones with voiding or monitor serum ketones.
  - Maintain aggressive oral fluid intake to prevent onset of hyperglycemia or ketosis: 1 cup salted broth every hour to replace fluids and electrolytes; 2 cups hourly is needed if urine ketones are moderate or higher. Maintain aggressive oral rehydration until ketone free for 24 hours.

- Always take full basal insulin dose.
- Add more insulin per algorithm; increase algorithm (i.e., take 2 units of RAA/human regular insulin per 50 mg per dL elevation in blood glucose) if making no or slow progress.
- Replace solid carbohydrates with clear liquid carbohydrates (such as regular ginger ale, regular soda, regular gelatin) if necessary and dose with RAA accordingly.
- Obtain early medical evaluation for underlying illness.
- Obtain early emergency intervention with intravenous fluids if emesis reoccurs (more than three episodes) or diarrhea is intractable.
- The goal is prevention of DKA in patients with type 1 DM, which has up to a 10% mortality per episode.

COMPLICATIONS OF DIABETES MELLITUS

- **Hypertension in DM** (see Chapter 9.1)
  - DM type
    - **Type 1 DM patients.** Hypertension implies the presence of microalbuminuria or nephropathy until proven otherwise.
    - **Type 2 DM patients.** Blood pressure targets of a systolic blood pressure <130 mmHg and diastolic blood pressure <80 mmHg have not been shown to reduce risk of death from either cardiovascular disease or MI. There was a slight reduction in nonfatal stroke.[24]
- Treatment
  - For both type 1 DM patients and type 2 DM patients, angiotensin-converting enzyme inhibitors (ACEi) are first-line therapy. Angiotensin receptor blockers (ARBs) are useful in patients who develop an ACEi cough. Routine use of ACEis or ARBs is useful particularly in patients with type 2 DM to preserve renal function regardless of the presence of hypertension or albuminuria. There are no data to support the routine use of ACEi/ARBs in normotensive normoalbuminuric patients with type 1 DM.
  - Calcium-channel blockers are warranted in cases of intolerance of or contraindications to ACEi or inadequate blood pressure control with these agents. They may have renal protective effects. Better cardiovascular event reduction may be seen with the use of calcium-channel blockers versus hydrochlorothiazide as the second agent.
  - β-Blockers have generally been avoided by most physicians unless there are specific indications (e.g., following MI) because of hypoglycemia symptom masking and delay in recovery of hypoglycemia in type 1 DM patients and worsening dyslipidemia and PVD in type 2 DM patients. However, the combination α–β blocker carvedilol has unique properties that almost negate the potential negatives.
  - Diuretics can be used in low dose without increasing insulin resistance.
  - Combination therapy with ACEi and ARBs has been shown to increase cardiovascular risk.
  - The use of aliskerin in combination with ACEi or ARBs in patients with type 2 DM is contraindicated based on the results of a randomized clinical trial, which showed increased risk of renal impairment, hypotension, and hyperkalemia.
- **Dyslipidemia (see Chapter 17.4)**
  - In type 1 DM, in the absence of nephropathy, dyslipidemia is generally associated only with poor glycemic control or a positive family history of dyslipidemia.
  - Type 2 DM treatment priorities per current guidelines revolve around the following:
    - Low-density lipoprotein cholesterol (LDL-C) lowering with therapeutic lifestyle changes with statins as the preferred initial intervention to achieve at least a 30% reduction in LDL-C regardless of baseline LDL-C.
    - HDL-C raising with therapeutic lifestyle changes.
    - Triglyceride lowering with diet and exercise, optimization of glycemic control, the addition of high potency statins, especially for patients with LDL-C elevations.
    - In the past, niacin has been relatively contraindicated in diabetes due to its adverse effect on glucose control. However, the long-acting formulation of niacin ER tablets appears to have good clinical effect in terms of lowering triglycerides and raising HDL-C with minimal adverse effects on glucose control.
    - Routine combination therapy with statins and fibrates is not of value per the ACCORD trial with potential benefit only in patients with triglycerides >204 mg per dL or HDL-C ≤34 mg per dL.[25]

- **Microalbuminuria**
  - When elevated, urine microalbumin/creatinine ratio is a strong predictor of the progression to clinical proteinuria. Its presence is an indication for ACE inhibitor or ARB treatment. Additionally, microalbuminuria is a predictor of retinopathy, neuropathy, and cardiovascular risk.
- **Proteinuria**
  - Use of ACEi or in the case of cough ARBs is indicated in the presence of proteinuria.
  - Reduction of dietary protein intake toward 0.8 g per kg of body weight is prudent.
- **Retinopathy**
  - An annual dilated ophthalmologic examination is indicated for all, with laser therapy being well established in the preservation of vision. In the UKPDS, improved blood pressure control was positively associated with reduced microvascular complication risk. The benefits of ACE inhibitor treatment in slowing the progression of retinopathy have been documented in a clinical trial.
- **Neuropathy** (see Chapter 6.9). Symptomatic pain may be controlled with:
  - FDA-approved for diabetic peripheral neuropathic pain
    - Pregabalin, an anticonvulsant structurally related to gabapentin, has been found in clinical studies to benefit diabetic peripheral neuropathy pain as well as postherpetic neuralgia. Pregabalin can be dosed at 50 mg qhs and may be increased to 100 mg tid as necessary based on tolerability and efficacy. Many patients can achieve pain control with only an evening dose. A lower starting dose and gradual increase to a lower maximum dose should be considered in patients with renal impairment.
    - Duloxetine, a selective serotonin and norepinephrine reuptake inhibitor with antidepressant properties, has been found in clinical trials to benefit diabetic peripheral neuropathic pain. Duloxetine should be initiated at a dose of 30 mg daily irrespective of meals and can be titrated to 60 mg daily. A lower starting dose and gradual titration should be considered in patients with renal impairment.
  - Non-FDA-approved for neuropathic pain but commonly prescribed:
    - Venlafaxine XR, a selective serotonin and norepinephrine reuptake inhibitor, can be used starting at a dose of 37.5 mg daily and titrating as necessary to a dose of 150 to 225 mg daily.
    - Gabapentin, an anticonvulsant, can be used starting at a dose of 100 to 300 mg nightly and titrating to a maximum dose of 800 mg tid. Doses must be significantly reduced in the setting of reduced creatinine clearance.
    - Tricyclic antidepressants (e.g., amitriptyline), starting at low doses of 10 to 25 mg at bedtime and titrating up, pending patient tolerance.
    - Additional daytime pain relief can be obtained with topical capsaicin cream.
    - **CAVEAT:** Opiates should be avoided due to the risk of developing drug tolerance and the potential for addiction.

PREGNANCY PLANNING (SEE CHAPTER 14.6)

The congenital abnormality rate and risks of macrosomia can be reduced to almost nondiabetic levels through euglycemia at the time of conception and throughout pregnancy. This is best achieved through an intensive program of (a) RAA premeal and bedtime basal insulin, or (b) CSII. Detemir is the only basal insulin that has a pregnancy Category B rating. Individuals with type 2 DM should discontinue all oral agents and initiate intensive insulin therapy prior to conception if needed. Additionally, ACEi, ARBs, and other antihypertensives should be discontinued preconception. Methyldopa and labetalol are agents frequently used preconception and throughout pregnancy for blood pressure control.

NETWORKING TO OPTIMIZE DIABETES CARE

Physicians alone cannot provide all the care and counseling needed by patients with DM. Physicians need to identify community resources to assist in the modern multidisciplinary team-care approach: nurse educators, (especially those who are certified diabetes educators) who are hospital based or private practice based, dietitians (especially those who are certified diabetes educators), psychologists, social workers, podiatrists, and endocrinologists.

REFERENCES

1. American Diabetes Association. Diagnosis and classification of diabetes mellitus. *Diabetes Care* 2014;37:S81–S90.
2. The American Diabetes Association International Expert Committee. International expert committee report on the role of the A1c assay in the diagnosis of diabetes. *Diabetes Care* 2009;32:1327–1334.
3. American Association of Clinical Endocrinologists Board of Directors and American College of Endocrinologists Board of Trustees. American Association of Clinical Endocrinologists/American College of Endocrinology statement on the use of hemoglobin A1c for the diagnosis of diabetes. *Endocr Pract* 2010;16:155–156.
4. The Diabetes Control and Complications Trial Research Group. The effect of intensive treatment of diabetes on the development and progression of long-term complications in insulin-dependent diabetes mellitus. *N Engl J Med* 1993;329:977–986.
5. The Diabetes Control and Complications Trial/Epidemiology of Diabetes Interventions and Complications Research Group. Retinopathy and nephropathy in patients with type 1 diabetes four years after a trial of intensive therapy. *N Engl J Med* 2000;342:381–389.
6. UK Prospective Diabetes Study (UKPDS) Group. Intensive blood-glucose control with sulfonylureas or insulin compared with conventional treatment and risk of complications in patients with type 2 diabetes (UPKDS 33). *Lancet* 1998;352:837–853.
7. Holman RR, Paul SK, Bethel MA, et al. 10-year follow-up of intensive glucose control in type 2 diabetes. *N Engl J Med* 2008;359:1577–1589.
8. Iznucci SE, Bergenstal RM, Buse JB, et al. Management of hyperglycemia in type 2 diabetes: a patient-centered approach. Position statement of the American Diabetes Association (ADA) and the European Association for the Study of Diabetes (EASD). *Diabetes Care* 2012;35:1364–1379.
9. Garber AJ, Abrahmason MJ, Barzilay JI, et al. American Association of Clinical Endocrinologists' comprehensive diabetes management algorithm 2013 consensus statement. *Endocr Pract* 2013;19(Suppl 2):1–48.
10. The Action to Control Cardiovascular Risk in Diabetes (ACCORD) Study Group; Gerstein HC, Miller ME, Byington RP, et al. Effects of intensive glucose lowering in type 2 diabetes. *N Engl J Med* 2008;358:2545–2559.
11. Evert AB, Boucher JL, Cypress M, et al. Nutrition therapy recommendations for the management of adults with diabetes. *Diabetes Care* 2014;37:S120–S143.
12. Sacks FM, Bray GA, Carey VJ, et al. Comparison of weight-loss diets with different compositions of fat, protein, and carbohydrate. *N Engl J Med* 2009;360:859–873.
13. DeFronzo RA. Banting lecture. From the triumvirate to the ominous octet: a new paradigm for the treatment of type 2 diabetes mellitus. *Diabetes* 2009;58:773–795.
14. de Jager J, Kooy A, Lehert P, et al. Long term treatment with metformin in patients with type 2 diabetes and risk of vitamin B-12 deficiency: randomised placebo controlled trial. *BMJ* 2010;340:2181–2187.
15. Erdmann E, Song E, Spanheimer R, et al. Observational follow-up of the PRO-active study: a 6-year update. *Eur Heart J* 2014;16:63–74.
16. Mahaffey KW, Hafley G, Dickerson S, et al. Results of a reevaluation of cardiovascular outcomes in the RECORD trial. *Am Heart J* 2013;166:240–249.
17. Egan AG, Blind E, Dunder K, et al. Pancreatic assessment of incretin-based drugs—FDA and EMA assessment. *N Engl J Med* 2014;370:794–797.
18. The ORIGIN Trial Investigators. Basal insulin and cardiovascular outcomes in dysglycemia. *N Engl J Med* 2012;367:319–328.
19. Smith U, Gale EA. Does diabetes therapy influence the risk of cancer? *Diabetalogia* 2009;52:1699–1708.
20. Schauer PR, Kashyap SR, Wolski K, et al. Bariatric surgery vs. intensive medical therapy in obese patients with diabetes. *N Engl J Med* 2012;366:1567–1576.
21. Brethauer SA, Aminian A, Rosenthal RJ, et al. Bariatric surgery improves the metabolic profile of morbidly obese patients with type 1 diabetes. *Diabetes Care* 2014;37:e51–e52; doi:10.2337/dc13-1736.
22. The Bari 2D Study Group. A randomized trial of therapies for type 2 diabetes and coronary artery disease. *N Engl J Med* 2009;360:2503–2515.
23. Dhakshainmurthy VA, Lim E, Hopkins D, et al. Risk stratification in uncomplicated type 2 diabetes: prospective evaluation of the combined use of coronary artery calcium imaging and selective myocardial perfusion scintigraphy. *Eur Heart J* 2006;27:713–721.
24. The ACCORD Study Group. Effects of intensive blood-pressure control in type 2 diabetes mellitus. *N Engl J Med* 2010;1575–1585.
25. The ACCORD Study Group. Effects of combination lipid therapy in type 2 diabetes. *N Engl J Med* 2010;362:1563–1574.

Thyroid Disorders

Kelly Gray Koren

GENERAL PRINCIPLES

Definition

Disorders of the thyroid gland include states of hyperthyroidism, hypothyroidism, and euthyroidism. The thyroid is a common site of disease, making it imperative for the family physician to be capable of identifying systemic symptoms. The thyroid itself may be enlarged (goiter), have nodules, or have benign or malignant tumors.

Anatomy

Embryologically, the thyroid gland is derived from an evagination of the floor of the pharynx descending along the midline. The median isthmus connects the two lateral lobes. In most people, there is also a pyramidal lobe that extends superiorly from the isthmus. Oxygenated blood is supplied by the superior and inferior thyroid arteries. Venous drainage is then completed by the superior, middle, and inferior thyroid veins.

Epidemiology

Hyperthyroidism occurs 10 times more often in females than in males, with an annual incidence of 1:1,000 females. Hypothyroidism occurs in approximately 20:1,000 females and 2:1,000 males annually. Hyperthyroidism occurs most commonly between 20 and 50 years of age, while the incidence of hypothyroidism increases with age.[1,2]

HYPERTHYROIDISM

Diagnosis

Etiology

- **Graves disease** is the most common cause of hyperthyroidism in iodine-sufficient areas usually affecting women of reproductive age. It is a diffuse toxic goiter and is caused by abnormal thyroid-stimulating immunoglobulin (TSI) binding to thyroid-stimulating hormone (TSH) receptors on the follicular cells, resulting in diffuse excessive stimulation of thyroid hormone production as well as enlargement of the gland itself. Graves disease consists of the following: hyperthyroidism, ophthalmopathy (puffiness of the lids, chemosis, proptosis, extraocular muscle weakness), and dermopathy.[1]
- **Toxic multinodular goiter** is usually a mild hyperthyroidism in which there is a large, asymmetric, nodular goiter.[1]
- **Toxic thyroid adenoma** is a hyperfunctioning follicular adenoma. It is usually a firm, large, solitary nodule.[3]
- **Painless lymphocytic thyroiditis** is most common in the postpartum period and has a high recurrence rate with subsequent pregnancies. It usually presents with an initial hyperthyroid phase, a subsequent hypothyroid phase, and eventually a recovery of normal thyroid function.[1]
- **Subacute thyroiditis** (de Quervain) is often accompanied by fever, myalgia, and a history of an upper respiratory tract infection. The thyroid gland itself is painful and tender.[1]
- **Exogenous hyperthyroidism** should be suspected when there are symptoms present, yet absence of a goiter and absence of an increased serum thyroglobulin level.[4]
- **Pituitary tumors, ovarian teratomas (struma ovarii), iatrogenic (lithium therapy), and excessive ingestion of iodine-induced hyperthyroidism** are rare causes, but should be considered when more common causes are ruled out.[1]

Clinical Presentation

An increase in thyroid hormone concentration causes an increase in tissue oxygen consumption that raises heat production and also increases metabolism. This can cause excessive diaphoresis, palpitations, fatigue and weakness, heat intolerance, oligomenorrhea, frequent bowel movements, anxiety, insomnia, and irritability. Proptosis, hyperreflexia, a fine tremor, and proximal muscle weakness may also be present.[1]

Apathetic thyrotoxicosis is an atypical presentation of hyperthyroidism, usually seen in elderly patients. Patients exhibit apathy, muscle rigidity, depression, dementia, anorexia, marked weight loss, and constipation.[2] Thyrotoxic crisis, though rare, may be life-threatening. This condition is often accompanied by fever, seizures, vomiting, diarrhea, jaundice, and even coma.[1]

Physical Examination

Hyperthyroidism can cause numerous systemic effects. Cardiovascular effects often include sinus tachycardia, a widened pulse pressure (due to increased systolic blood pressure and decreased diastolic pressure), as well as arrhythmias (most commonly atrial fibrillation or premature ventricular contractions) due to increased myocardial excitability. On examination, it is also important to look for onycholysis, pretibial myxedema, tremor, lid lag, proptosis, goiter, thyroid tenderness, hyperreflexia, warm or moist skin, and gynecomastia. Thyrotoxicosis for an extended period of time may also cause osteopenia. Also, it is important to listen for a bruit over the thyroid arteries, as they are commonly present in Graves disease.

Laboratory Evaluation

Biochemical diagnosis of hyperthyroidism is made most commonly with a suppressed or undetectable TSH level and an increased serum level of free T_4 (thyroxine).[1,2] If there are normal free T_4 levels, the serum free T_3 (triiodothyronine) levels should be obtained. Occasionally, a patient may have hyperthyroid symptomatology, a suppressed TSH, normal free T_4 index, but elevated T_3—this is T_3 toxicosis.[1] A low TSH level alone is not diagnostic for hyperthyroidism as it can be found to be decreased in dopamine or glucocorticoid therapy or secondary hypothyroidism.

Serum thyroglobulin is usually used as a tumor marker to follow up on thyroid carcinomas (see below), but it is also useful when the TSH is suppressed and the radioactive iodine (I-131) uptake (RAIU) is low. The thyroglobulin level is high in lymphocytic thyroiditis and is low in exogenous hyperthyroidism.[1,3]

Graves disease is a specific form of hyperthyroidism with the TSH receptor autoantibody tests—TSI or TRab (thyroid receptor antibody)—positive in 80% of patients with the diagnosis and are diagnostic.[1,2] TSI levels can also be measured in infants born to women with Graves disease. The antibody tests are of special importance in pregnant women in whom one cannot perform an RAIU study.[2]

When subacute thyroiditis is in the differential diagnosis, an erythrocyte sedimentation rate (ESR) level may be helpful as this is usually markedly elevated in that condition.[1]

Imaging

Ultrasonography may be used to evaluate thyroid nodules and goiters. Graves disease may demonstrate an altered blood flow that can be demonstrated via ultrasound.[1]

Diagnostic Procedures

I-131 uptake study is done after thyroid function tests have been done, the thyrotropin levels are suppressed, and the diagnosis is not clear. This test evaluates hyperthyroidism by separating the high RAIU uptake disorders from the low RAIU uptake disorders. The RAIU is elevated in Graves disease, toxic adenomas, toxic multinodular goiters, TSH-secreting pituitary adenomas, metastatic follicular thyroid carcinomas, and trophoblastic tumors.[3] The RAIU is low in subacute thyroiditis, lymphocytic thyroiditis, exogenous hyperthyroidism, recent iodine load (contrast dye, diet) and struma ovarii. Low RAIU disorders comprise only 5% of all causes of hyperthyroidism.

Thyroid scanning shows a diffuse, homogeneous distribution in Graves disease, multiple areas of increased uptake in toxic multinodular goiter, and a single area of increased uptake in toxic adenoma. It can also be used to evaluate ectopic thyroid tissue (struma ovarii) or to follow up on thyroid cancer. It can be done with either pertechnetate or radioactive iodine.

Treatment

Medications

Thionamides (propylthiouracil and methimazole) are used to treat hyperthyroidism and work by blocking thyroid hormone synthesis and may also decrease the production of TSI. Propylthiouracil (PTU) at high doses also decreases the peripheral conversion of T_4 to T_3. Thionamides are used to lower thyroid hormone levels in anticipation of radioactive iodine therapy or surgery or as long-term therapy in Graves disease, with the goal of inducing a remission of the hyperthyroid condition.[1] Because the drugs only work temporarily and spontaneous remission is a possibility, treatment is given for 12 to 18 months after which a trial discontinuation is initiated. More than half of patients relapse in the first 6 months.

Monitor patients for relapse every 4 to 6 weeks for the first 3 to 6 months, and then every 3 months for the first year following cessation of the thionamides. If the patient remains euthyroid, annual monitoring is continued indefinitely. If relapse of hyperthyroidism occurs, alternative therapy is recommended.[1]

Adverse side effects include rash, urticaria, nausea, transient leukopenia (not a harbinger of agranulocytosis), and, less commonly, arthralgias, hepatic necrosis, or cholestatic jaundice. Agranulocytosis is idiosyncratic, occurring in 0.4% of patients, and is usually seen within the first 3 months of therapy. Routine monitoring of white blood cells during the initial 3 months is recommended. If agranulocytosis is detected, it is usually reversible upon discontinuation of the drug but may recur with use of another thionamide. Agranulocytosis can develop in hours and a severe sore throat is often the first symptom. Methimazole is often preferred because of its longer half-life and at doses of less than 30 mg per day may have a lower risk of agranulocytosis. It is important to perform pregnancy tests on women of reproductive potential because thionamides are contraindicated.[2] These medications cross the placenta and may disrupt thyroid hormone synthesis in the fetal thyroid.

β-Adrenergic antagonists, or β-blockers, provide rapid control of sympathetic-mediated hyperthyroid symptoms, to include tachycardia, hypertension and tremor, and are administered to those with severe symptoms and those awaiting more definitive treatment. Propranolol (nonselective β-blocker) given in doses of 20 to 40 mg by mouth every 6 hours is very effective and is prescribed most commonly.[1] Propranolol should not be used alone in the patient with hyperthyroidism as it does not prevent a potentially life-threatening thyrotoxic crisis.

Iodides are not routinely used to treat hyperthyroidism as they may cause a paradoxic increase in thyroid hormone levels. The organic iodide radiographic contrast agents iopanoic acid and ipodate sodium are used more often than the inorganic potassium iodide. All of the iodides block the peripheral conversion of T_4 to T_3 and suppress hormone. Usually they are used as adjunctive therapy before emergent surgical procedures or to decrease thyroid vascularity prior to surgery for Graves disease.

Nonoperative Treatment

I-131 is an effective thyroid gland ablating treatment. It is commonly used as initial therapy for Graves disease, toxic adenoma, or toxic multinodular goiter, or as an alternative therapy for the patient with Graves disease who fails to obtain or maintain a remission with thionamides.[1] Effective radioactive iodine therapy will leave the patient hypothyroid. Adverse effects include a painful thyroiditis that may develop within days after treatment, as well as a transient worsening of hyperthyroid symptoms. Radioactive iodine is contraindicated in women who are pregnant, plan to become pregnant within 6 months, and those who are currently breastfeeding.

Surgery

Surgical excision is recommended in patients with contraindications to radioactive iodine therapy, those with very large goiters, and for those who cannot tolerate or are not responsive to thionamides. Thionamides are the first-line treatment of thyrotoxicosis in pregnancy; however, the lowest dose should be employed. Surgery is often considered in the second or third trimester of pregnancy if reasonable doses of antithyroid drug therapy are not effective.[1] The goal of the surgery is to reduce the amount of thyroid gland, so that euthyroid levels of thyroid hormone are secreted by the tissue left behind. A "necklace" incision extends to the sternocleidomastoid muscles bilaterally to access the gland. Although there is a very low surgical risk, the rare complications are serious. If the recurrent laryngeal nerve is injured, there can be vocal cord paralysis. Permanent hypothyroidism and hypoparathyroidism can also occur.

Follow-Up

After hyperthyroidism is treated by one of the above modalities, it is critical to follow up with thyroid function tests to ensure that the patient is euthyroid. Postablation and postoperative hypo- or hyperthyroidism is common and should be treated appropriately.

HYPOTHYROIDISM
General Principles

Definition

Clinical hypothyroidism is present when characteristic physical findings are evident and laboratory analysis supports the diagnosis. Hypothyroidism can have a primary, secondary, or tertiary etiology. Subclinical hypothyroidism lacks physical characteristics, but is detected by laboratory analysis.[5]

Epidemiology

Clinical hypothyroidism is evident in up to 2% of women and 0.2% of men. Subclinical hypothyroidism has an approximate prevalence of 4% to 8.5% overall.[5] The prevalence of both clinical and subclinical hypothyroidism is higher in women. In addition, prevalence increases with age for both men and women.

Etiology

Hypothyroidism can have a primary, secondary, or tertiary etiology. Primary hypothyroidism results from a defect in the thyroid gland itself. The most common cause of primary hypothyroidism is Hashimoto thyroiditis. Other causes of primary hypothyroidism include radiation exposure, radioactive ablation therapy, iodine deficiency or excess, subacute thyroiditis, and medications. Secondary hypothyroidism results from a defect in the pituitary gland causing a deficiency in TSH production. Some causes of secondary hypothyroidism include Sheehan syndrome, a pituitary neoplasm, radiation exposure, and tuberculosis. Tertiary hypothyroidism results from a defect in the hypothalamus causing a deficiency in thyrotropin-releasing hormone (TRH) production. Tertiary hypothyroidism can be caused from a neoplasm, radiation exposure, or a granuloma.[5]

Diagnosis

Clinical Presentation

Historic findings that are suggestive of hypothyroidism include fatigue, weakness, cold intolerance, weight gain, dry skin, coarse hair, decreased sweating, constipation, muscle cramps, arthralgias, menorrhagia, and impaired cognition.[6]

Physical Examination

Physical examination findings consistent with hypothyroidism include bradycardia, dry skin, coarse hair, brittle nails, periorbital edema, carpal tunnel syndrome, slow speech, loss of the outer third of eyebrows, depression, and delayed relaxation of deep tendon reflexes.[6]

Laboratory Studies

Initial diagnostic tests of TSH and free T_4 levels should be obtained. Primary hypothyroidism can be diagnosed based on an elevation in TSH greater than twice the normal level. Subsequently, a decrease in free T_4 will also be observed. Secondary hypothyroidism presents with a decreased or normal TSH level and a decreased free T_4 level. Tertiary hypothyroidism will also present with a normal or decreased TSH level and a decreased free T_4 level; however, if the TRH level is measured, it will be normal or decreased. A TRH stimulation test may be used to differentiate secondary from tertiary hypothyroidism. Subclinical hypothyroidism presents with a normal free T_4 level, but an elevation in TSH.[6]

Other laboratory studies may be affected by a hypothyroid state. Cholesterol and triglyceride levels are often elevated. Anemia and hyponatremia can also be observed. Creatinine phosphokinase (CPK) may be elevated in addition to lactate dehydrogenase (LDH), aspartate aminotransferase (AST), and alanine aminotransferase (ALT) levels. If the hypothyroidism is due to Hashimoto thyroiditis, antithyroid peroxidase antibodies are present in the serum.[5]

Treatment

Medications

Therapy for clinical hypothyroidism is best accomplished with levothyroxine. Levothyroxine is a synthetic isomer of T_4. The use of levothyroxine precludes the need for T_3 because T_3 is produced via peripheral deiodination of T_4. Dosage requirements for levothyroxine vary according to the patient's age and weight. Elderly individuals usually require a lower dosage. If a patient has known or suspected cardiovascular disease, a low dose should initially be used to prevent angina pectoris. In general, therapy should begin at a low dose. The dosage is typically increased if necessary after re-checking thyroid levels 6 to 8 weeks after the initial dose.[6]

Subclinical hypothyroidism treatment with levothyroxine is recommended if the TSH levels are greater than 10 m per L. If TSH levels are between 4.5 and 10 μ per L, no firm guidelines direct treatment. Patients can follow thyroid hormone levels every 6 to 12 months for an elevation in TSH levels. If patients have elevated lipid levels, symptoms of hypothyroidism, or positive antithyroid peroxidase antibodies, treatment with levothyroxine should be considered.[5]

Follow-Up

Adequate replacement therapy is assured by re-measuring TSH levels 6 to 8 weeks after initiation of therapy, and 6 to 8 weeks after any change in dosage. If the TSH level remains elevated, the dose is increased. If the TSH level is suppressed, the dose is decreased. The goal of levothyroxine replacement therapy is normalization of TSH. Suppression of TSH should be avoided due to the increased risk of accelerated osteoporosis, induction of cardiac arrhythmias, and increase in left ventricular mass.

Complications

Myxedema coma occurs with severe hypothyroidism complicated by marked hypothermia, hypotension, bradycardia, hypoventilation, and unresponsiveness. Even if treated early, mortality rates are approximately 20% to 50%. Supportive measures should be started immediately and include assisted ventilation, warming devices, volume repletion for hypotension, and glucocorticoids if adrenal insufficiency is suspected. A search for precipitating causes such as infection, cardiac disease, metabolic disturbances, or drug use is critical.[6]

THYROIDITIS

- **Subacute thyroiditis**, also known as de Quervain thyroiditis, is the result of a viral infection of the thyroid gland. Women are four times more affected than men. The average age of diagnosis is 40 to 50 years. A prodromal phase characterized by pharyngitis, myalgias, fatigue, and low-grade fever precedes the development of a tender goiter with neck pain often radiating to the ear. Because of cytotoxic damage of the follicular cells, about half of individuals initially exhibit hyperthyroidism due to the release of preformed T_3 and T_4. When preformed T_3 and T_4 are depleted, transient hypothyroidism may follow. In the majority of cases, full recovery results. Laboratory studies illustrate an elevated ESR and C-reactive protein level in addition to a mild anemia and leukocytosis. Treatment consists of providing nonsteroidal anti-inflammatory drugs (NSAIDs) for pain. If no resolution of pain occurs within 1 week, prednisone can be utilized. β-Adrenergic antagonists are used for symptomatic treatment as needed.[1]
- **Acute suppurative thyroiditis** is the result of a bacterial, fungal, mycobacterial, or parasitic infection of the thyroid gland. Patients present with a warm, erythematous, tender thyroid gland as well as systemic signs of infection. Laboratory studies illustrate an ESR and elevated white blood cell count with a left shift. Treatment includes appropriate antimicrobial therapy with possible surgical drainage.[1]
- **Radiation-induced thyroiditis and trauma-induced thyroiditis** are the result of the destruction of thyroid parenchyma with subsequent release of preformed T_3 and T_4. Radiation-induced thyroiditis can occur following radioactive iodine therapy or following radiation to the head and neck area for cancer treatment. Trauma-induced thyroiditis results from physical force. Treatment includes NSAIDs or prednisone for pain and β-adrenergic antagonists for symptomatic relief.[1]
- **Hashimoto thyroiditis**, also known as chronic lymphocytic thyroiditis, is an autoimmune condition characterized by infiltration of the thyroid by lymphocytes. Women are seven times more affected than men. The average age of diagnosis is 40 to 60 years. Patients present with painless enlargement of the thyroid gland. Hypothyroidism or euthyroidism may be clinically evident at presentation. Laboratory studies illustrate the presence of antithyroid peroxidase antibodies in 90% to 95% and antithyroglobulin antibodies in 20% to 50% of affected individuals. Treatment with levothyroxine is indicated for patients with clinical hypothyroidism, subclinical hypothyroidism with a TSH greater than 10 m per L, and progressive goiter enlargement.[1]
- **Postpartum thyroiditis and silent sporadic thyroiditis** are probably the result of an autoimmune condition. About 5% to 7% of women develop postpartum thyroiditis. A firm, painless goiter is usually present 2 to 6 months after delivery. Women may experience hypothyroidism (43%), hyperthyroidism (32%), or hyperthyroidism followed by hypothyroidism (25%). The hyperthyroid variant occurs most frequently 3 months postpartum, whereas the hypothyroid variant occurs most frequently at 6 months postpartum. About 80% of patients have normal thyroid function at 1 year postpartum. Laboratory studies illustrate a normal ESR while 80% have positive antithyroid peroxidase antibodies. Treatment includes β-blockers for hyperthyroid symptom management and levothyroxine for clinical hypothyroidism. Caution should be used when prescribing β-blockers to breastfeeding mothers as it is secreted into the breast milk. Silent sporadic thyroiditis is similar to postpartum thyroiditis; however, it does not occur during pregnancy.[1,2]
- **Drug-induced thyroiditis** results from the use of amiodarone, interferon-α, interleukin-2, and lithium. This destructive thyroiditis may result in hyperthyroidism or hypothyroidism and usually resolves with discontinuation of the offending agent.[1]

THYROID NODULE

General Principles

Epidemiology

Clinically evident thyroid nodules can be found in 5% of the adult population. Solitary thyroid nodules are malignant in approximately 10% of these cases. In children younger than 13, thyroid nodules are rare, but the incidence of cancer in these children reaches approximately 20%.[3]

Diagnosis

Clinical Presentation

Historic findings that are suggestive, but not diagnostic, of malignancy include a family history of thyroid cancer, history of irradiation to the head and neck region, patient age younger than 20 or older than 60 years, rapid nodule growth, or presence of distant metastases.[7]

Physical Examination

Physical findings suspicious for malignancy include a very firm irregular nodule, fixation to adjacent structures, vocal cord paralysis, or enlarged regional lymph nodes.[7]

Laboratory Studies

A fine-needle aspiration biopsy (FNAB) and TSH levels are recommended as initial diagnostic tests in most adults presenting with a thyroid nodule. Unless the patient has signs and symptoms of thyrotoxicosis, a TSH level and FNAB should both be obtained. In the case of suspected thyrotoxicosis, a TSH level should be measured to confirm the diagnosis followed by an RAIU study. A calcitonin level should be obtained if there is a family history of medullary carcinoma. An ultrasound can be obtained to determine the presence of other nodules, nodule consistency (cystic vs. solid), and thyroid anatomic structure. In children younger than 13, the use of FNAB remains controversial. An ultrasound is recommended in this age group to further examine thyroid anatomy as well as nodule consistency and number. Because of the high incidence of malignancy in these children, further preoperative studies are not recommended, as surgical excision is currently the mainstay of treatment.[3]

The first step in diagnosis is analyzing the TSH level. If the TSH level is elevated, the thyroid nodule is hypofunctioning. Because hypofunctioning thyroid nodules represent malignancies in 10% to 20% of cases, FNAB results should be reviewed for further diagnostic information.[3] Similarly, if the TSH level is normal, the patient's FNAB results should be reviewed. If the TSH level is decreased, the thyroid nodule is most likely hyperfunctioning. Of hyperfunctioning thyroid nodules, 1% are malignant. An RAIU study is recommended in this case to determine whether the nodule is "hot" or "cold." Individuals with "cold" nodules should have a FNAB completed.

In analyzing the FNAB results, the pathologic structure of the tissue can determine whether the nodule is benign or malignant. If the FNAB results illustrate a cellular pathology, follicular adenoma and follicular carcinoma are both diagnostic possibilities. In this case, a hypofunctioning nodule as determined by TSH levels favors malignancy and surgical excision. A hyperfunctioning nodule as determined by TSH levels necessitates further studies including an RAIU study. If FNAB results are nondiagnostic, repeat FNAB testing is necessary with possible ultrasound-guided aid.[3]

Treatment

If the thyroid nodule represents a malignancy, surgical excision is necessary. Postoperative therapy is often malignancy dependent. Levothyroxine suppression therapy is recommended to decrease TSH levels and subsequent thyroid gland stimulation. Imaging studies as well as calcitonin and thyroglobulin levels, if applicable, are important for surveillance of metastasis or recurrence. If the thyroid nodule is benign, levothyroxine suppression therapy and clinical observation with or without ultrasound monitoring should be considered.[3,7]

SPECIAL CONSIDERATIONS

- Occasionally abnormal thyroid function tests can be found in patients who have a number of non-thyroidal illnesses or conditions, including caloric restriction, recent surgery, chronic liver disease, chronic renal disease, diabetes mellitus, infections, malignancy, psychiatric disorders, and with certain drugs (β-adrenergic blockers, amiodarone, phenytoin, glucocorticoids, dopamine, cholecystographic dyes, and heroin). These patients are not generally pharmacologically treated and the laboratory abnormalities typically resolve with improvement of the underlying cause.

- Whenever a patient has acute behavioral changes, consider thyrotoxicosis as a potential cause.
- If a patient presents with signs and symptoms of dementia or depression, rule out hypothyroidism as a potential etiology.
- Thyrotoxicosis symptoms may be overlooked in pregnancy as they may be mistaken for normal changes.[2]

REFERENCES

1. Bahn RS, Burch HB, Cooper DS, et al; American Thyroid Association; American Association of Clinical Endocrinologists. Hyperthyroidism and other causes of thyrotoxicosis: management guidelines of the American Thyroid Association and American Association of Clinical Endocrinologists. *Endocr Pract* 2011;17:457–520.
2. Woeber K. Update on the management of hyperthyroidism and hypothyroidism. *Arch Intern Med* 2000;160:1067–1071.
3. Gharib H, Papini E, Paschke R, et al; AACE/AME/ETA Task Force on Thyroid Nodules. American Association of Clinical Endocrinologists, Associazione Medici Endocrinologi, and European Thyroid Association Medical guidelines for the clinical practice for the diagnosis and management of thyroid nodules. *Endocr Pract* 2010;16(Suppl 1):2–43.
4. Donangelo I, Braunstein G. Update on subclinical hyperthyroidism. *Am Fam Physician* 2011;83:933–938.
5. Garber JR, Cobin RH, Gharib H, et al; American Association of Clinical Endocrinologists and American Thyroid Association Taskforce on Hypothyroidism in Adults. Clinical practice guidelines for hypothyroidism in adults: cosponsored by the American Association of Clinical Endocrinologists and the American Thyroid Association. *Endocr Pract* 2012;18:989–1028.
6. Gaitonde DY, Rowley KD, Sweeney LB. Hypothyroidism: an update. *Am Fam Physician* 2012; 86:244–251.
7. Knox M. Thyroid nodules. *Am Fam Physician* 2013;88:193–196.

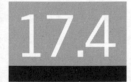

17.4 Dyslipidemias

Marvin Moe Bell

GENERAL PRINCIPLES

Hypercholesterolemia is a major risk factor for development of atherosclerotic cardiovascular disease (ASCVD). High levels of low-density lipoprotein (LDL) cholesterol have been the main target for cholesterol-lowering therapy for many years, based on the Adult Treatment Panel III (ATP3) guidelines from 2001.[1] Low levels of high-density lipoprotein (HDL) cholesterol and high levels of triglycerides (TGs) are additional risk factors for ASCVD. The benefit of statin drugs to reduce cardiovascular events has been demonstrated in both primary prevention (people without ASCVD) and secondary prevention (people with known ASCVD) trials. Updated 2013 guidelines for treatment of blood cholesterol to reduce ASCVD risk in adults[2] no longer recommend specific LDL treatment target levels. Instead, either moderate-intensity or high-intensity statin therapy is recommended for people at higher risk for developing ASCVD. Other drug classes are generally not recommended due to lack of evidence that they reduce the development of ASCVD.

DIAGNOSIS
Identify High-Risk Patients

Four major groups will benefit from statin treatment aimed to reduce ASCVD risk:

1. People with clinically established ASCVD (prior myocardial infarction, stable or unstable angina, acute coronary syndrome, revascularization procedure, stroke, transient ischemic disease, or peripheral vascular disease). Statins for secondary prevention in this risk group have the strongest medical evidence of benefit.
2. People with extremely high LDL cholesterol levels (≥190 mg per dL), likely due to familial hypercholesterolemia.

3. People who have type 2 diabetes and are between ages 40 and 75 years.
4. People between the ages of 40 and 75 who have a 10-year risk of ASCVD ≥7.5%. (This is controversial due to the arbitrary choice of the 7.5% threshold for starting statins, and concerns about the accuracy of available risk predictors.) Consider the following established ASCVD risk factors to help patients make informed decisions regarding statin use:
   - **Non-modifiable risks:** age (men older than 45, women older than 55), family history of premature coronary heart disease (first degree relative, male aged <55, female aged <65).
   - **Modifiable risks:** cigarette smoking, hypertension, obesity (BMI ≥30), low HDL (less than 40 mg per dL).
   - **Protective factor:** HDL greater than 60 mg per dL.

SCREENING

Screening with a nonfasting total cholesterol and HDL cholesterol is recommended for the following groups:[3]

- All men over age 35 (A recommendation)
- Men age 20 to 35 with one or more risk factors for ASCVD (B recommendation)
- Women over age 45 with one or more risk factors for ASCVD (A recommendation)
- Women age 20 to 45 with one or more risk factors for ASCVD (B recommendation)

Screening should identify patients with extremely high LDL levels, and will help with discussions regarding risk factor modification.

TREATMENT
Management Principles

Rule out and treat secondary causes of hyperlipidemia (especially with marked hypertriglyceridemia):

- **Endocrine:** type 2 diabetes, hypothyroidism (see Chapters 17.2 and 17.3)
- **Renal:** nephrotic syndrome, chronic renal failure (see Chapter 12.7)
- **Lifestyle:** alcoholism, anabolic steroids (see Chapters 5.3 and 5.7)

Therapeutic lifestyle changes (TLCs) such as dietary modification, weight loss, increased physical activity, and avoidance of tobacco are key components of lifelong primary and secondary prevention of ASCVD. Statins are a key component of secondary prevention for virtually all people with clinically established ASCVD.

DIETARY THERAPY

A healthy diet can improve lipids and reduce the risk of developing ASCVD. Healthy diet guidelines are available through the American Heart Association and myplate.gov, or by following a traditional Mediterranean diet. Some principles include:

- Eat mostly plant-based foods.
- Try to eat 9 to 10 servings (4.5 cups) of fruits and vegetables daily.
- Choose whole-grain and higher-fiber foods, including legumes (beans).
- Add monounsaturated fats to your diet (olive oil, canola oil, nuts, seeds, and avocados are good sources).
- Eat fish once or twice a week, especially oily fish like salmon or albacore tuna.
- Limit saturated fats and trans fats by eating lean cuts of meat with fat trimmed and removing skin from poultry; use low-fat dairy products; limit fried foods, processed meat, organ meats, butter, margarine, and highly saturated oils such as palm or coconut.
- Add water-soluble fiber in the diet or as a supplement. Sources include oat bran, beans, fruit, and psyllium (Metamucil).

DRUG THERAPY FOR RISK REDUCTION

Statins are well proven to reduce both cardiac and overall mortality rates; however, there is no evidence to support the specific LDL cholesterol targets that were in the ATP III guidelines.[1] Instead, the focus has shifted to high-risk groups on the basis of inclusion criteria for studies that found meaningful reductions in ASCVD with statin therapy.

High-intensity statins (Table 17.4-1) are indicated for the following groups:[2]

- Clinical ASCVD and age 21 to 75

TABLE 17.4-1	Statins (HMG-CoA Reductase Inhibitors) Dosing (mg)	
	Moderate intensity	**High intensity**
Atorvastatin (Lipitor)	10–20	40–80
Fluvastatin (Lescol)	40–80	
Lovastatin (Mevacor)	40	
Pitavastatin (Livalo)	2–4	
Pravastatin (Pravachol)	40–80	
Rosuvastatin (Crestor)	5–10	20–40
Simvastatin (Zocor)	20–40	

HMG-CoA, 3-hydroxy-3-methylglutaryl coenzyme A.

- Adults with LDL cholesterol ≥190 mg/dL
- Diabetics age 40 to 75 with 10-year ASCVD risk ≥7.5%[4]

Moderate-intensity statins (Table 17.4-1) are indicated for the following groups:[2]

- People in the above groups who cannot tolerate high-intensity statins
- Clinical ASCVD and age greater than 75
- Diabetics age 40 to 75 with 10-year ASCVD risk <7.5%

Moderate- or high-intensity statins should be offered to adults age 40 to 75 with a 10-year ASCVD risk ≥7.5% based on a discussion of risks versus benefits for each individual.

Unfortunately, bile acid sequestrants (resins), nicotinic acid (niacin), fibrates, omega-3 fatty acids (fish oil), and ezetimibe have not been shown to reduce major disease end points such as coronary events or stroke.

HYPERTRIGLYCERIDEMIA

Very high triglycerides (greater than 500 mg per dL [5.6 mmol per L]) warrant therapy to reduce the risk of pancreatitis. Treatment of high triglycerides to reduce ASCVD risk remains controversial. Therapy includes exercise, weight reduction, alcohol restriction, and treatment of contributing causes. Omega-3 fatty acids or fibrates can be used in resistant cases.

ISOLATED LOW HIGH-DENSITY LIPOPROTEIN (<40 MG PER DL)

The following practices may help raise HDL and reduce the risk of ASCVD:

- Smoking cessation, exercise, weight loss if obese, and avoidance of androgens and progestins.
- A low-fat, high-carbohydrate diet can lower HDL. Replacing carbohydrates with monounsaturated fats may increase HDL.

Medications to increase HDL are in clinical trials, but have not been shown to reduce ASCVD.

FORMULARY OF LIPID-LOWERING DRUGS

- **Statins** (HMG-CoA reductase inhibitors)
  - **Advantages:** These agents are extremely effective in lowering LDL and may prevent atherosclerotic plaque rupture. They are well tolerated and reduce overall mortality in primary and secondary prevention.
  - **Problems:** Elevation of liver function tests (LFTs) to three times normal occurs in 1% to 2% of patients (use caution with liver disease). Myositis or myopathy with high-serum creatinine phosphokinase (CPK) develops in 0.5% of patients, more often when statins are used with niacin or fibrates. Warn patients and check CPK if muscle soreness occurs. Statins can cause cognitive impairment (reversible) and slightly increase the risk of developing diabetes.
  - Dosing (Table 17.4-1).
- Bile acid sequestrants (resins)—limited evidence of reduction of ASCVD.
- Ezetimibe—no evidence of reduction in ASCVD.
- Omega-3 fatty acids including eicosapentaenoic acid (EPA) and docosahexaenoic acid (DHA)— mixed and inconclusive results regarding reduction of ASCVD.

- Fibric acid derivatives (fibrates) increase noncardiac mortality and risk of renal insufficiency. In the ACCORD trial, adding fenofibrate to simvastatin failed to reduce ASCVD events.
- Nicotinic acid (niacin)—both the AIM-HIGH and HPS2-THRIVE trials found that adding niacin to a statin failed to reduce ASCVD events, and actually increased stroke risk.

REFERENCES

1. Expert Panel on Detection, Evaluation, and Treatment of High Blood Cholesterol in Adults. Executive summary of the third report of the National Cholesterol Education Program (NCEP) Expert Panel on the Detection, Evaluation, and Treatment of High Blood Cholesterol in Adults (Adult Treatment Panel III). *JAMA* 2001;285:2486–2497.
2. Stone NJ, Robinson JG, Lichtenstein AH, et al. 2013 ACC/AHA Guideline on the Treatment of Blood Cholesterol to Reduce Atherosclerotic Cardiovascular Risk in Adults: a report of the American College of Cardiology/American Heart Association Task Force on Practice Guidelines. *Circulation* 2014;129 (25 Suppl 2):S1–S45.
3. United States Preventive Services Taskforce, Screening for Lipid disorders in adults, June 2008.
4. American Heart Association and American College of Cardiology 2013 Prevention Guideline Tools- CV disease risk calculator. www.myamericanheart.org.

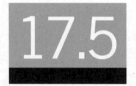

17.5 Hypercalcemia

Dawn M. Sloan

GENERAL PRINCIPLES

Definition

Hypercalcemia is defined as a serum calcium level greater than 10.5 mg per dL or 2.5 mmol per L.[1]

Epidemiology

In a retrospective study of 77,000 emergency room patients, 0.1% were found to have hypercalcemia. Of the 123 patients with identified hypercalcemia, 35% were due to malignancy; 20% were due to hyperparathyroidism (primary and secondary); 5% were due to immobilization; 3% were due to dehydration; 2% were due to Addison disease; 1% each were due to Morbus Paget, Lithium therapy, sarcoidosis, and excessive calcium intake; and 35% were due to unknown causes.[2]

Classification

Calcium is the fifth most common element in the human body; however, more than 99% of it is tied up in bones.[3] The remaining <1% is involved in numerous essential functions, including muscle contraction, intracellular communications, and transmitting nerve impulses.[3] This non-bone calcium is found as free ions, protein-bound, or in ionic complexes. In the serum, albumin and globulin are the main proteins binding calcium and phosphate. Oxalate and carbonate are the main serum anion binders. The remaining calcium found in the serum is in a free ionized form, whose levels are very tightly controlled to between 4.4 and 5.4 mg per dL (1.10 to 1.35 mM).[3]

The free ionized calcium level, approximately 50% of the serum calcium, is maintained in the short term by the pH-dependent buffering system created by the calcium-binding proteins (chiefly albumin) and in the long term by multiple hormones,[4] including parathyroid hormone (PTH), and 1,25-dihydroxyvitamin D.[3]

When any of these systems is out of balance, the calcium level can change. Conditions causing increased calcium absorption through the small intestine (usually through elevated 1,25-dihydroxyvitamin D) or a decrease in calcium excretion through the kidneys[3] will cause hypercalcemia. The other two mechanisms of hypercalcemia involve bone resorption and remodeling. If too much calcium is resorbed from the bone or too little is replaced, hypercalcemia can also result.[3] The differential diagnosis includes the following:

- **Increased dietary absorption:** vitamin D toxicity, increased 1,25-dihydroxyvitamin D levels from sarcoidosis or tuberculosis (or indirectly from elevated PTH), excessive intake of calcitriol, or similar substances.[3]
- **Decreased urinary excretion:** chronic kidney disease, familial hypocalciuric hypercalcemia;[5] also consider this as the cause of hypercalcemia in children.[3]
- **Increased bone resorption:** malignancy (solid tumors of the breast, prostate, renal cell, and non-small-cell lung carcinoma as well as multiple myeloma and lymphoma[5]), primary and secondary parathyroid hormone secretion, vitamin D toxicity,[3] hyperthyroidism.[5]
- **Decreased bone remodeling:** chronic kidney disease, elevated parathyroid hormone, immobility, weightlessness, sex hormone deficiency.[3]

Medications, such as lithium, can interfere with all of these processes.[2] Thiazide diuretics also have a reputation for causing hypercalcemia; however, in a recent study of otherwise healthy blacks taking hydrochlorothiazide, it was noted that while the calcium levels did increase slightly, hypercalcemia was very rare.[6]

DIAGNOSIS
Clinical Presentation
History
Hypercalcemia has a nonspecific set of symptoms, but should be considered in any patient with a history of malignancy. Fatigue, weakness, bone pains, nausea, vomiting, constipation, abdominal pains, weight loss, polyuria, confusion, and coma have all been reported in patients with hypercalcemia.[1] The symptoms tend to worsen as the serum calcium elevates.

Physical Examination
Physical examination findings may include any of the following:[7]

- Hypertension
- Neck mass or lymphadenopathy
- Ophthalmic band keratopathy
- Irregular heartbeat, rales, edema, third heart sound
- Flank pain, epigastric pain
- Anxiety, depression, emotional instability
- Cognitive dysfunction, dementia
- Lethargy, delirium, coma
- Muscle weakness

Laboratory Studies
Total serum calcium is the most accepted value for screening for and monitoring hypercalcemia, even though ionized calcium levels are the most physiologically relevant. Ionized calcium levels are particularly difficult to measure accurately and are very expensive.[4] Additionally, monitoring ionized calcium in the hospital setting in otherwise asymptomatic patients has been shown to increase the risk of unnecessary treatments[4] and in patients with solid tumors has been shown in at least one study not to correlate with symptoms.[1]

In patients with abnormal albumin levels, total serum calcium levels should be corrected. There are many ways to do so. The most accurate way is to use an individually validated albumin calculation that is laboratory specific, and preferably validated for the specific patient population that is being examined.[4] However, common practice is to use a formula derived from a population of healthy volunteers. One such formula is:[4]

Adjusted total calcium (mg/dL) = Total measured calcium (mg/dL) + 0.8 × [4 − measured albumin (g/dL)]

Additionally, consider obtaining a fasting glucose, creatinine, intact PTH, 25-hydroxyvitamin D levels as well as 1,25-dihydroxyvitamin D levels (the latter can be elevated in lymphomas, along with a low PTH level, demonstrating vitamin D–mediated hypercalcemia).[1]

Radiologic Imaging
No specific radiologic imaging is used to diagnose hypercalcemia. However, given the causes of hypercalcemia, consider a chest x-ray, x-rays of any areas of discrete pain, positron emission tomography scan, and/or sestamibi scan, depending on suspected causes.

Differential Diagnosis

Diabetes can cause similar none specific symptoms and polyuria. Uremia can also cause some similar symptoms.

Treatment

Initial treatment of hypercalcemia generally depends on the level of symptoms. For those patients with serum calcium >14 mg per dL, neurologic symptoms are more common and these patients require hospitalization and urgent intervention.[1]

Symptomatic patients are initially treated with intravenous fluids, as the polyuria, nausea, and vomiting usually cause significant dehydration (increased output with poor oral intake).[1] In milder cases of hypercalcemia, establishing an adequate urine output of at least 75 mL per hour can be enough to correct the calcium level.[1] Volume overload and hypernatremia are risks associated with this treatment. Use of loop diuretics has been discussed to assist on the basis of theory of increasing urine calcium excretion; however, the studies done do not support this theory, and did show increased secondary electrolyte disorders, so use of loop diuretics should be considered only in patients who develop volume overload.[1]

However, volume repletion is a transient correction to a problem that ultimately requires treatment of the underlying disease process. Work-up should be continued to identify the underlying cause.

Medications

Gallium nitrate, high-potency intravenous bisphosphonates, corticosteroids, and denosumab have been shown to be effective in malignancy-associated hypercalcemia.[1] Calcitonin works as an adjunct therapy due to modest, transient effectiveness,[1] and low-calcium hemodialysis can be considered in patients with acute kidney injury. Vitamin D supplementation works well in patients with secondary parathyroid elevation.[3]

Surgery

Particularly in those patients with primary parathyroid hormone elevations, surgery should be considered. Again, since hypercalcemia is usually secondary to another underlying disorder, identification of the underlying disorder will drive treatment.

REFERENCES

1. Rosner MH, Dalkin AC. Onco-nephrology: the pathophysiology and treatment of malignancy-associated hypercalcemia. *Clin J Am Soc Nephrol* 2012;7:1722–1729.
2. Linder G, Felber R, Schwarz C, et al. Hypercalcemia in the ED: prevalence, etiology and outcome. *Am J Emerg Med* 2013;31:657–660.
3. Peacock M. Calcium metabolism in health and disease. *Clin J Am Soc Nephrol* 2010;5:S23–S30.
4. Baird GS. Ionized calcium. *Clin Chim Acta* 2011;412:696–701.
5. Luceri PM, Haenel LC. A challenging case of hypercalcemia. *J Am Osteopath Assoc* 2013;113:490–493.
6. Chandler PD, Scott JB, Drake BF, et al. Risk of hypercalcemia in blacks taking hydrochlorothiazide and vitamin D. *Am J Med* 2014;127(8):772–778.
7. Michels TC, Kelly KM. Parathyroid disorders. *Am Fam Physician* 2013;88:249–257.

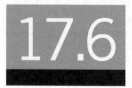

Osteoporosis

Fred E. Heidrich, Susan M. Ott

GENERAL PRINCIPLES

Definition

Osteoporosis (OP) is a syndrome in which bone strength is decreased and fractures may occur after minimal trauma.

Anatomy

Hip fractures and vertebral compression fractures are the most serious consequences. Also common fracture sites include the distal forearm and proximal humerus.

Epidemiology

Low bone density is common by age 50, especially in women. At age 65 years, only 40% of women have normal bone density and 20% have OP. Only 10% of 80-year-old women have a "normal" bone density. The lifetime risk of hip fracture for an average 50-year-old person is 17% for white women and 6% for men; risks are lower for those of African descent.[1-3]

Fractures

The fractures due to OP occur mostly in the latter half of life, but bone loss begins in the third decade. **Maximizing bone gained in childhood and adolescence and minimizing losses in the middle years** of life are key to bone health in old age.

Classification

To assess for fracture risk, obtain **dual-energy x-ray absorptiometry (DEXA)** at the hip. Other techniques include spinal DEXA and quantitative ultrasound. **Results:** T-scores indicate the number of standard deviations, SD, from the average peak bone mass (age 25 to 30). The WHO definition of OP is a bone density more than 2.5 SD below mean (T-score <-2.5) for a young Caucasian woman. A more clinically useful value is the risk of fracture, which is most commonly calculated using the FRAX algorithm.[4]

Pathophysiology

Bone is a metabolically active tissue, in which **osteoclasts resorb bone** and **osteoblasts lay down new bone.** This lets bone **remodel after injury** or in response to stressors. When bone resorption exceeds formation over a period of time, the bone loses density and strength. Bone also **serves as a reservoir** of calcium and alkali.

Etiology

The risk factors, which are part of the FRAX algorithm, include:

- **Aging** (the most common cause of OP)
- Female gender
- Low weight:height ratio
- Heredity and race (parent with hip fracture; white or Asian race)
- Personal history of low-impact fracture as an adult
- Tobacco use
- Glucocorticoid use (over 3 months of equivalent of prednisone 5 mg or more)
- Rheumatoid arthritis
- Disorders strongly associated with OP (see Differential Diagnosis)
- Alcohol intake of two or more drinks daily

Secondary OP is associated with many disease states:
Those currently mentioned in the FRAX website include:

- Type 1 (insulin-dependent) diabetes
- Osteogenesis imperfecta
- Untreated long-standing hyperthyroidism
- Hypogonadism
- Premature menopause ($<$45 years)
- Chronic malnutrition
- Malabsorption
- Chronic liver disease

    Also, secondary OP can be caused by:

- Bone-thinning drugs (anticonvulsants, antineoplastics, heparin, medications that decrease gonadal hormones, selective serotonin reuptake inhibitors, and perhaps proton pump inhibitors)
- Inactive lifestyle or immobility, especially in patients with spinal cord injury
- Chronic kidney disease
- Renal calcium wasting
- Hyperparathyroidism
- Weight loss

    Finally, a propensity for falls due to frailty is an important risk factor for fractures.

Mechanisms of Injury

Hallmark is **fracture from a degree of injury not usually expected to result in fracture,** for example, a fall from standing height.

DIAGNOSIS

Diagnosis of OP sometimes can be made based on a history of low-impact fracture and no other obvious cause (see above risks and differential dx of fracture). While not evidence-based, a 3% 10-year risk of hip fracture or a 20% 10-year risk of major osteoporotic fracture is often recommended as a threshold to initiating pharmacologic treatment.[5] A bone density T-score less than –2.5 is also often used to define OP.

Clinical Presentation

OP is usually detected by a **screening bone density and fracture risk calculation**, or after a person has a **typical fracture with minimal trauma.** Efforts to intervene early, however, depend on recognition of risks for bone loss before fractures occur.

History

Look for **risk factors and secondary causes** (see Etiology). A history of an osteoporotic fracture is a **strong** predictor of future fracture. A woman with a vertebral compression fracture is four times more likely to have a new vertebral fracture as a woman of the same age and bone density with no preexisting fracture.

Physical Examination

Look for:

- Kyphosis
- Height loss >2 to 3 in.
- Protruding abdomen
- Body mass index lower than 20

About 60% of women with spinal compression fractures are unaware of their occurrence. Height loss of up to 2 to 3 in. may be seen with disc thinning of aging, but greater loss indicates OP or scoliosis.

Laboratory Studies

- **Basic evaluation.** Complete blood count (CBC), electrolytes, creatinine, serum 25-OH-vitamin D, thyroid-stimulating hormone, liver function tests, phosphate, and calcium are normal, but alkaline phosphatase may be temporarily elevated following a fracture. Check testosterone in men, but estradiol levels are not helpful in postmenopausal women.
- **Other tests.** In otherwise unexplained cases, consider testing urinary calcium (normally 50 to 250 mg per day), parathyroid hormone, sprue panel, tryptase (in young people, for considering mastocytosis), and serum and urinary protein electrophoresis (20% of multiple myeloma is seen only in urine). Tests of bone resorption rate (such as collagen telopeptides) and formation rate (osteocalcin or bone specific alkaline phosphatase) may occasionally guide therapy, but cannot be used for screening individual patients.

Imaging

The U.S. Preventive Services Task Force (USPSTF) recommends **routine bone density screening** for all women starting at age 65, and younger women whose risk factor–based calculated risk of fracture is that of the average 65-year-old white woman without risk factors (10-year hip fracture risk of 1.7%).[6] Consensus is still pending for men, although it is reasonable to screen when the risk is similar to the 1.7% value as above. A lateral spine film or DEXA vertebral fracture assessment can screen for occult vertebral fractures.

Monitoring

DEXA scanning can be used in observation of those at risk or to monitor progress in treatment. A person must change more than 5% to be sure a change is not merely machine imprecision. Normal bone loss is slow and routine screening intervals depend on the bone density. Those with T-scores lower than −2 should be retested in 1 to 2 years; T-scores between −1.5 and −2 should be retested in 5 years.

If a woman at age 65 has T-score above −1.5, further monitoring is not necessary for 15 years unless her risk profile changes.[7]

Differential Diagnosis of Fracture

Consider metastatic lesions, multiple myeloma, osteomalacia, infections (Pott disease), pathologic fractures from Paget disease, or bone tumors. Alcoholism should always be considered, particularly when OP occurs in young people or middle-aged men and it causes more fractures than predicted by bone density. Many of these conditions can be excluded by history and physical examination.

TREATMENT

Supplements and Behavioral Interventions

Calcium is not sufficient to prevent OP, but is an important adjuvant. Recommended daily intake is 500 mg for children aged 1 to 3; 800 to 1,300 mg for ages 4 to 18; 1,000 mg for ages 19 to 50; and 1,200 mg thereafter. Quick assessment of dietary calcium intake: 300 mg for each serving of dairy product and 200 mg for the rest of the diet. Calcium carbonate is the most cost-effective supplement, and is best absorbed in chewable forms taken with food. There is controversy regarding possible coronary artery disease risk from calcium supplements, and no evidence of bone benefit from total daily intake exceeding 1,200 mg. Vitamin D is important in calcium absorption and neurologic function and the recommended daily allowance (RDA) is 600 IU per day. Persons lacking sun exposure and those older than age 70 are at risk for vitamin D deficiency and should take 800 to 1000 IU of vitamin D daily. Avoid vitamin A intake greater than the RDA.

Diets should include adequate protein, fruits, and vegetables. In underweight patients, increase caloric intake.

People at risk for **falls** should be counseled regarding footwear (laced, low heel, traction sole), vision aids, and environmental hazards (poor lighting, floor-level obstructions, slippery surfaces, lack of handrails, cool temperature). Medicines that affect alertness or cause postural syncope must be minimized in elderly people. Elderly people are more prone to postural hypotension after a large meal. Protective hip padding can reduce hip fractures, but adherence is often difficult, and many fractures occur at night when padding is often omitted.

Lifestyle

- **Weight-bearing exercise** (walking, running, dancing, aerobic exercise, sports, weight lifting, Tai Chi—as appropriate) has skeletal, cardiovascular, muscular, and emotional benefits for all age groups. Reasonable goal: 30 to 60 minutes, 4 to 6 times per week. Discourage smoking and overconsumption of alcohol. Discourage unnecessary weight loss despite cultural fashions, as women who lose weight also lose bone density. The kyphosis of established OP results in a protruding abdomen, which patients may misinterpret as excess fat.

Medications

- **Bisphosphonates** are the most commonly used therapy for OP. Fracture rates are halved in men and women with OP during the first 5 years of treatment. There are limited data about efficacy and safety after 5 years. They do, however, decrease both bone formation and resorption, with a very long half-life (over 10 years) in bone and longer-term effects remain uncertain. Alendronate (35 mg weekly for prevention/70 mg weekly for treatment), risedronate (35 mg weekly), and ibandronate (150 mg monthly) are the oral bisphosphonates currently approved for treating OP and are quite similar. They should be taken with 4 to 8 oz of water on an empty stomach, and 30 minutes should pass before any other oral intake. We prefer 4 oz of water, similar to the amount used in the pivotal study,[8] while the manufacturer recommends 6 to 8 oz. The patient should avoid reclining or bending over for at least 30 minutes after the dose to prevent esophagitis. Avoid using in pregnancy, renal failure, or hypocalcemic states, and ensure adequate intake of both calcium and vitamin D. A long-acting IV bisphosphonate (Zoledronic acid) is useful particularly in patients with dysphagia or adherence problems (such as dementia). A single dose (5 mg) will reduce bone resorption for up to 4 years. It may be given for 5 years, either every 2 years (years 0,2,4) or annually. The doses we have listed for alendronate and zoledronic acid include the FDA dose for OP prevention (the lower dose) and for OP treatment, but either is useful for fracture prevention. Osteonecrosis of the jaw has been seen with high-dose bisphosphonate use in cancer patients, but is very rare with the doses used to treat OP. Atypical femur fractures can occur with more than 5 years of continuous bisphosphonate use. Duration of treatment is controversial but many advocate a "drug holiday" after 5 years.

- **Estrogen therapy** results in about a 50% reduction in fractures, but adverse effects may limit their use. Estrogen is mainly indicated early in menopause in women with low bone mass, especially those who also want relief from hot flushes. However, after age 60, the initiation of estrogen carries a risk of myocardial infarction and thromboembolic disease, so this is not recommended. A dose of 0.625 mg conjugated estrogens daily or equivalent can promote increases in bone density, and smaller doses (0.3 mg) can be helpful in stabilizing density. Progesterone does not have additive benefits to the skeleton and it is responsible for an increased risk of breast cancer, but some form is needed to protect the uterus.[9, 10] Intrauterine progesterone is an option that may reduce cancer risk, but more studies are needed. Bone loss similar to that at natural menopause occurs on cessation of estrogen, so other management is indicated when Hormone Replacement Therapy (HRT) is stopped in women using it for OP.
- **Raloxifene,** 60 mg daily, is effective at decreasing vertebral fracture rates in postmenopausal women, although hip fracture rates are not reduced. It does not stimulate breast or uterine neoplasia, but does have prothrombotic characteristics similar to estrogen, and can worsen hot flushes. Raloxifene halves the incidence of breast cancer in studies lasting up to 8 years.
- **Teriparatide** is a potent stimulator of bone formation. It may be considered in men or women failing standard therapy. It is given by daily subQ injection, for up to 18 to 24 months. It should be avoided in pregnancy, hypercalcemia, Paget disease, active gout, and in persons with a history of bone cancer or bone irradiation. At the conclusion of therapy with teriparatide, it is important to then administer an osteoclast inhibitor (such as a bisphosphonate) for several years to avoid a rapid loss state. Currently, the FDA does not recommend a second course of this medication, and after 18 months the skeleton becomes resistant to the anabolic effects; therefore, teriparatide should not be used in mild cases or merely for prevention.
- **Denosumab**, a monoclonal antibody, decreases hip as well as vertebral and other fractures similarly to bisphosphonates,[11] but has not been as extensively studied. It is given as 60 mg subQ every 6 months. It is associated with increased risk of a variety of infections and exacerbations of eczema and can cause serious hypocalcemia. Both bone formation and resorption rates are inhibited, more than with bisphosphonates, and some cases of atypical femur fracture and osteonecrosis of the jaw have been reported.
- **Testosterone** in men can result in increased bone density but may have adverse effects on serum lipids and hematocrit, and should be avoided in men with a history of prostate cancer. Men with demonstrated low testosterone may be treated with intramuscular or transdermal testosterone.
- **Calcitonin** may reduce vertebral fractures, but bone density gains are not as great as those for other agents. It is given intranasally, 200 units daily. There is some recent controversy because some meta-analyses of clinical trials found increased cancer risk, whereas others did not.

Surgery

Percutaneous infusions of cement (vertebroplasty or kyphoplasty) have been advocated to treat acute vertebral compression fractures. These procedures carry a risk of spinal cord damage, and possibly higher risk of compression of adjacent vertebra. Long-term benefits have not been shown to be better than standard therapy, and further studies are needed.

Special Therapy

- **Thiazide diuretics** decrease renal calcium excretion and increase bicarbonate. Effects on bone density are beneficial but modest. If an antihypertensive is indicated, possible bone benefits may enter into the choice of agents. These drugs can improve bone density in patients with high urine calcium.
- **Hip pads** prevent hip fractures in elderly people if they wear the padding.
- **Strontium ranelate** is not approved by the FDA for any indication. It is used in some other countries and some trials have shown fracture benefit, but long-term effects are unclear. There is a form of strontium citrate that is sold as a food supplement; this has never been studied and use should be discouraged, especially since the strontium may be incorporated into the bone mineral and raise the bone density, making it difficult to interpret.

Referrals

Consider specialty referrals for patients with OP **prior to age 50**, with **secondary OP** where assistance is needed with the underlying cause, for cases where **fractures or density losses continue despite therapy.**

Physical Therapy

Gait and balance training may prevent falls and thus fractures. **Spinal extension exercises** and instruction in **lifting technique** may prevent vertebral crush fractures. Brief bed rest and local heat complement analgesics in managing compression fractures. In cases of severe kyphosis, back bracing may provide comfort.

Patient Education

- Calcium/vitamin D
- Exercise for bones, strength, flexibility, and balance
- Understanding DEXA
- How to take bisphosphonates

SPECIAL CONSIDERATIONS

- **Chronic steroid users:** Bone losses are greatest during first 6 months of therapy with doses of prednisone of 5 mg per day or greater. Management includes **minimizing the dose** of steroid given, maintaining **physical activity**, and aggressive implementation of **preventive and therapeutic strategies** above. Patients may suffer fractures, especially in ribs or vertebra, even with normal bone density.
- **Hypercalciuria** may be aggravated by high-dose vitamin D and helped by thiazides. In worrisome cases, measurements of vertebral or hip bone density may guide use of bisphosphonate or hormonal therapy.

REFERENCES

1. Ott SM. Osteoporosis and bone physiology. http://courses.washington.edu/bonephys/. Accessed June, 2014.
2. U.S. Department of Health and Human Services. *Bone health and osteoporosis: a report of the surgeon general.* Rockville, MD: U.S. Department of Health and Human Services, Office of the Surgeon General; 2004.
3. Marcus R, Feldman D, Dempster D, et al., eds. *Osteoporosis [the definitive textbook].* 4th ed. San Diego, CA: Academic Press, Elsevier, Amsterdam; 2013:1–2116.
4. FRAX website: http://www.shef.ac.uk/FRAX/tool.aspx. Accessed May 29, 2014.
5. Dawson-Hughes B; National Osteoporosis Foundation Guide Committee. A revised clinician's guide to the prevention and treatment of osteoporosis. *J Clin Endocrinol Metab* 2008;93:2463–2465.
6. U.S. Preventive Services Task Force. Screening for osteoporosis: U.S. preventive services task force recommendation statement. *Ann Intern Med* 2011;154:356–364.
7. Gourlay ML, Fine JP, Preisser JS, et al. Bone-density testing interval and transition to osteoporosis in older women. *New Engl J Med* 2012;366:225–233.
8. Black DM, Cummings SR, Karpf DB, et al. Randomised trial of effect of alendronate on risk of fracture in women with existing vertebral fractures. *Lancet* 1996;348:1535–1541.
9. Rossouw JE, Anderson GL, Prentice RL, et al; Writing Group for the Women's Health Initiative Investigators. Risks and benefits of estrogen plus progestin in healthy postmenopausal women: principal results from the Women's Health Initiative randomized controlled trial. *JAMA* 2002;288:321–333.
10. Anderson GL, Limacher M, Assaf AR, et al; Women's Health Initiative Steering Committee. Effects of conjugated equine estrogen in postmenopausal women with hysterectomy: the Women's Health Initiative randomized controlled trial. *JAMA* 2004;291(14):1701–7012.
11. Cummings SR, San Martin J, McClung MR. Denosumab for prevention of fractures in postmenopausal women with osteoporosis. *N Engl J Med* 2009;361:756–765.

CHAPTER 18

Disorders of the Blood

Section Editor: Jonathan Bassett

Iron-Deficiency Anemia

Josephine K. Olsen

GENERAL PRINCIPLES[1]
Definition

Anemia can be divided into three major categories: decreased number of red blood cells, low hemoglobin, and diminished volume of red blood cells. Iron-deficiency anemia (IDA) causes low hemoglobin, classically two standard deviations below normal. The current hemoglobin cutoffs vary by gender and race and decrease slightly with age. Current accepted cutoffs are as follows:

- Age 6 months to 2 years: 10.5 g per dL
- Age 2 years to 12 years: 11.5 g per dL
- Adult female: 12 g per dL (Caucasian); 11.5 g per dL (African American)
- Pregnant: 11 g per dL
- Adult male: 14 g per dL (Caucasian); 12.9 g per dL (African American)

Epidemiology[2]

Iron deficiency is the most common cause of anemia worldwide. It can also coincide with other causes of anemia. In developed countries, people at highest risk are pregnant women, dieting adolescent females, and recent immigrants. Children who tested iron deficient during infancy were later found to have lower cognitive test scores on recognition and memory.[3]

Pathophysiology

Iron is one of the main building blocks of hemoglobin. Deficiency, therefore, results in defective synthesis of hemoglobin leading to smaller red cells (microcytosis) with less hemoglobin within the cells (hypochromia).

Etiology

Etiologies for IDA include increased iron loss, inadequate iron intake, decreased iron absorption, and increased iron demand. Normal daily iron loss is 1 mg per day. Additionally, iron loss can also occur from blood loss due to menstruation (20 mg per month), frequent blood donations, and ongoing gastrointestinal (GI) bleeding. Causes of GI blood loss include use of nonsteroidal anti-inflammatory drugs, peptic ulcer disease, angiodysplasia, diverticulosis, malignancy, and, rarely, parasites such as hookworms. Inadequate iron intake can occur in individuals with eating disorders or severe malnutrition (only about 10% of dietary iron is absorbed). Malabsorption is seen with acute illness, inflammatory bowel disease, lead poisoning (which displaces iron), or surgical bowel resection. Iron demand increases in pregnancy (requiring an additional 9 mg of iron per day), lactation, and during rapid growth in infancy.

DIAGNOSIS
Clinical Presentation[4]

With an insidious onset and gradual progression of symptoms, the body can compensate and tolerate low hemoglobin levels (less than 7 g per dL). In elderly individuals, some of these signs and symptoms may be subtle or dismissed as age related. Symptoms may include weakness, leg cramping or restlessness, malaise, fatigue, dyspnea on exertion, palpitations, dizziness, chest pain, headaches, pago-phagia (ice eating), and pica. Cardiovascular signs include tachycardia, systolic murmur, and even high-output cardiac failure. Epithelial changes include pallor of the conjunctiva, lips, and palmar skin creases. Dry skin and nail changes, such as pale, brittle, or spoon-shaped nails (koilonychia), are also found. Angular stomatitis, glossitis, and, rarely, dysphagia from pharyngeal and esophageal webs may also be present.

Laboratory

Lab results vary depending on the stage of iron deficiency. Initial results may show a normocytic normochromic picture, but the ferritin, iron, or red blood cell distribution width is decreased. Once the iron stores are exhausted, the classic hypochromic microcytic picture develops with a low mean corpuscular volume. A peripheral smear may show anisocytosis, poikilocytosis, and target cells.

- A low serum ferritin level, especially below 12 µg per L (normal: 18 to 300 µg per L), indicates iron deficiency. Ferritin is also an acute phase reactant, so elevation may be a sign of inflammation and malignancy.
- Iron-binding capacity (IBC) is increased, usually to more than 375 µg per dL (normal: up to 300 µg per dL).
- Serum iron is decreased, often to less than 60 µg per dL (normal: 100 µg per dL).
- Transferrin saturation is decreased to less than 16%.
- Reticulocyte count, which is indicative of red blood cell replacement and bone marrow function, is often decreased when iron stores are exhausted.
- Other tests, such as erythropoietin level and bone marrow biopsy, can be performed but are rarely necessary.

Differential Diagnosis

Thalassemia, anemia of chronic disease, B_{12} or folate deficiency, and sideroblastic anemia.

TREATMENT

The first step in treatment is determining the underlying cause. If iron loss is determined to be the cause, iron replacement therapy can be initiated and an evaluation to rule out a GI bleed should be considered. Reticulocyte count should rise within a week and a 2-g per dL hemoglobin increase should be seen within 3 weeks. To replenish the stores, replacement should continue for 6 months. Treatment failures are due to noncompliance, malabsorption, inadequate dosing, ongoing blood loss, or incorrect diagnosis.

Iron Replacement

Oral

This is the preferred method of replacing the iron stores. Ferrous sulfate, which is inexpensive and commonly used, is better tolerated when taken with meals. GI side effects are dose related and include nausea and constipation. Ferrous sulfate 325 mg (65 mg of elemental iron) is taken one to three times daily. Target dose is 150 to 200 mg of elemental iron per day. Medications such as histamine-2 blockers and methyldopa, as well as calcium-rich foods, bran, soy, coffee, and tea all reduce iron absorption. Meat, fish, and vitamin C enhance absorption. Iron needs stomach acid in order to be absorbed, but some research suggests that proton pump inhibitors have not been shown to decrease iron absorption.[5] Ferrous fumarate 324 mg (106 mg of elemental iron) or ferrous gluconate 324 mg (38 mg of elemental iron) may be better tolerated than ferrous sulfate.

For children, iron supplements in the form of drops, elixir, and syrup are available. The regimen for management of iron deficiency in children is 3 to 6 mg per kg daily of elemental iron. Liquid preparations given by dropper or straw can help prevent staining of teeth.

Parenteral[1]

In critically ill and hemodialysis patients, iron is occasionally administered parenterally. If used, a test dose of 25 mg should be given to test for allergic reaction. Iron gluconate (125 mg of 12.5 mg per mL) or iron sucrose (100 mg of 20 mg per mL) is preferred and can be given intravenously daily, if needed, over 5 to 10 minutes. Arthralgias, myalgias, or phlebitis may occur as a delayed reaction, and severe reactions have been noted in patients with collagen vascular disease.

Prevention[6]

Infants over the age of 4 to 6 months require iron supplementation through oral drops or fortified formula. This recommendation is derived from the weight-based iron needs of infants. Their requirements eventually exceed the amount of iron that can be obtained in a practical volume of breast milk. Cow's milk is not only a poor source of iron, but also inhibits its absorption. Current recommendations are to screen all infants for IDA at the age of 1. During pregnancy, women are screened twice for iron deficiency and all are encouraged to take an iron-containing prenatal vitamin.

REFERENCES

1. Causey MW, Miller S, Foster A, et al. Validation of noninvasive hemoglobin measurements using the Masimo Radical-7 SpHb Station. *Am J Surg* 2011;201:592.
2. Price EA, Mehra R, Holmes TH, et al. Anemia in older persons: etiology and evaluation. *Blood Cells Mol Dis* 2011;46:159.
3. Congdon EL, Westerlund A, Algarin CR, et al. Iron deficiency in infancy is associated with altered neural correlates of recognition memory at 10 years. *J Pediatr* 2012;160(6):1027.
4. Allen RP, Auerbach S, Bahrain H, et al. The prevalence and impact of restless legs syndrome on patients with iron deficiency anemia. *Am J Hematol* 2013;88:261.
5. Annibale B, Capurso G, Chistolini A, et al. Gastrointestinal causes of refractory iron deficiency anemia in patients without gastrointestinal symptoms. *Am J Med* 2001;111:439.
6. Baker RD, Greer FR. Diagnosis and prevention of iron deficiency and iron-deficiency anemia in infants and young children (0–3 years of age). *Pediatrics* 2010;126(5):1040–1050.

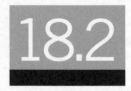

18.2 Megaloblastic Anemia

Sarah M. Balloga

GENERAL OVERVIEW

Macrocytosis is the general term for anemia, with a mean corpuscular volume (MCV) greater than 100 fL. Macrocytosis can be further delineated as megaloblastic and nonmegaloblastic anemia. Common nonmegaloblastic anemia causes include alcoholism, medications, hypothyroidism, liver disease, and myelodysplastic syndromes.

Megaloblastic anemia specifically refers to anemia that is caused by a disruption in RNA and DNA synthesis. This is manifest by the characteristic findings on peripheral smear of macro-ovalocytes and hypersegmented neutrophils. Typically this is caused by vitamin B_{12} and folate deficiencies.

VITAMIN B_{12} (COBALAMIN) DEFICIENCY

General Principles

Vitamin B_{12} plays a vital role in neurologic function, red blood cell production, and DNA synthesis. Humans cannot synthesize B_{12} and rely solely on dietary sources. Main dietary sources include animal proteins and fortified cereal products. Daily recommended intake is 2.4 mcg per day. Older adults and strict vegetarians often have difficulties obtaining the required B_{12} from dietary sources.

Digestion begins in the stomach, where gastric acid separates B_{12} from the food products. B_{12} is then bound to intrinsic factor that is produced by the gastric parietal cells. Final absorption occurs in the terminal ileum and is stored in the liver. Liver stores can last for up to 5 to 10 years.

Causes of B_{12} Deficiency

Pernicious anemia is the most common cause of B_{12} deficiency worldwide. This is an autoimmune atrophic gastritis characterized by the destruction of parietal cells and subsequent reduction in intrinsic factor. Nonimmune-mediated gastritis causes include

- *Helicobacter pylori* infection and Zollinger–Ellison syndrome
- Dietary deficiencies (elderly, alcoholics, strict vegetarians, breastfed infants of B_{12}-deficient mothers)

- Gastrointestinal malabsorption
  - Surgical, that is, ileal resection, gastrectomy, gastric bypass
  - Medical, that is, Crohn disease, tapeworm *Diphyllobothrium latum*
- Prolonged medication use
  - **Common:** histamine H_2 blockers, proton pump inhibitors, and metformin
  - Reverse transcriptase inhibitors typically cause macrocytosis and may lead to megaloblastic changes. This known side effect is an effective monitoring tool of patient compliance and no treatment is necessary.

Manifestations of B_{12} Deficiency

Diagnostically, B_{12} deficiency can be a challenge as clinical symptoms can lag 5 to 10 years after the onset of dietary deficiencies. Hematologic manifestations include fatigue, weakness, palpitations, tachycardia, and pallor—less commonly, thrombosis. Neurological signs and symptoms include paresthesias, weakness, ataxia, decreased proprioception, and cognitive and behavioral changes.

Other clinical manifestations include dermatological findings (hyperpigmentation, vitiligo), gastrointestinal findings (glossitis, jaundice), and reproductive implications (infertility).

Laboratory Findings

- Anemia (WHO definition: Hgb <13 for men, <12 for women; up to 28% of affected patients may have normal Hgb)
- MVC >100 (up to 17% may have normal MVC)
- Low normal to low B_{12} levels
  - True deficiency is defined as level <200 pg per mL, with low normal levels 200 to 400 pg per mL. Variation depends on local laboratory values.
- Elevated homocysteine *and* methylmalonic acid levels (substrates that are produced in the process of RNA and DNA synthesis). These become elevated when lacking B_{12} to complete necessary metabolic steps.
  - Methylmalonic acid is considered more sensitive and is the recommended confirmatory test of choice when B_{12} or folate levels are equivocal.
- Pernicious anemia
  - Schilling test is no longer available in the United States
  - Elevated levels of anti-intrinsic factor antibodies or antiparietal cell antibodies
  - Elevated serum gastrin or pepsinogen.

Treatment

- Treat underlying disorder
- **Replacement:** Oral supplementation and intramuscular injections are equally efficacious.
- **Oral:** 1 to 2 mg daily
- **Intramuscular:** 1 mg daily for 1 week, weekly for 8 weeks, then 1 mg monthly for life.

Follow-Up

- **Pernicious anemia:** Perform at least one endoscopic evaluation at the time of diagnosis to screen for gastric cancer, monitor for other autoimmune disorders.
- Monitor for other causes of anemia, including iron-deficiency anemia, anemia of chronic disease.
- Perform complete blood count (CBC) every 6 to 12 months to ensure resolution of anemia.

FOLIC ACID DEFICIENCY
General Principles

Similar to B_{12}, folate is a necessary cofactor in DNA synthesis. Daily total intake requirement is 400 to 1,000 mcg. Dietary sources include leafy vegetables, beans, fruits, and fortified cereal grains. The body does not have a large reservoir for folate storage and thus can become depleted rapidly. Clinical symptoms typically begin 6 months after onset of deficiency. Deficiency is becoming uncommon in the United States as federal law mandates cereal grains to be supplemented with folate.

Causes

- Inadequate intake (alcoholics, fad diets, institutionalized individuals, elderly)
- Increased requirements (pregnancy, prematurity)

- **Malabsorption:** inflammatory bowel disease, gastric bypass, tropical sprue, rare enzyme deficiencies
- Drugs (methotrexate, sulfasalazine, triamterene, trimethoprim–sulfamethoxazole, metformin, phenytoin)

Manifestations

Similar to B_{12} deficiency with the notable exception of neuropsychiatric findings.

Laboratory Findings

- Anemia
- Macrocytosis
- Hypersegmented neutrophils
- Low folate levels (<4 ng per mL)
- Elevated homocysteine with *normal* methylmalonic acid levels

Treatment

Treatment includes oral replacement 1 to 5 mg per day. This is continued indefinitely unless the underlying cause of deficiency can be corrected.

Follow-Up

- CBC every 6 to 12 months to ensure resolution of anemia

REFERENCES

1. Antony AC. Megaloblastic anemias. In: Hoffman R, Benz EJ Jr, Silberstein LE, et al., eds. *Hematology: basic principles and practice*. Philadelphia, PA: Elsevier Saunders; 2013:473–504.
2. Langan RC, Zawistoski KJ. Update on vitamin B_{12} deficiency. *Am Fam Physician* 2011;83(12):1425–1430.
3. Kaferle J, Strzoda CE. Evaluation of macrocytosis. *Am Fam Physician* 2009;79(3):203–208.
4. Stabler SP. Vitamin B_{12} deficiency. *N Engl J Med* 2013;368:149–160.

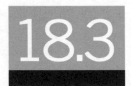

18.3 Bleeding Disorders
Matthew G. Balderston

GENERAL PRINCIPLES

Bleeding disorders are caused by abnormalities in coagulation factors, platelets, or blood vessels and result in bleeding anywhere in the body. Such disorders may be inherited or acquired. Occasionally, an asymptomatic patient is found to have an abnormal platelet or coagulation study that generates concern.

DIAGNOSIS

History

- A **bleeding score system** can be utilized when taking the history.
- **Bleeding episodes** should be characterized.
- Not all easy bruising is abnormal. **Spontaneous bruising** on the trunk or bruising of areas greater than 3 cm in diameter on the extremities is more likely pathologic.
- Childhood onset of symptoms or a family history of bleeding problems suggests an inherited disorder. Family history should prompt historical screening. When an inherited disorder is mild, it may not be evident until adulthood or until significant trauma or surgery occurs.
- **Important aspects of the history** are prior transfusion need, iron responsive anemia, surgery or dental procedures complicated by bleeding, epistaxis, oral cavity bleeds, hematomas, hemarthroses, gastrointestinal (GI) bleeds, central nervous system (CNS) bleeds, postpartum hemorrhage, and menstruation.

- **Underlying diseases** such as infection and liver dysfunction can lead to acquired bleeding problems. **Poor nutrition** can lead to vitamin K deficiency.
- A thorough **review of medications**, including antiplatelet agents—aspirin, nonsteroidal anti-inflammatory drugs (NSAIDs), clopidogrel, and ticlopidine—and anticoagulants is essential.
- **Symptoms of significant blood loss**, such as lightheadedness, dyspnea, and chest pain, may trigger more urgent inpatient evaluation.

Physical Examination

- The **CNS, GI tract, joints, deep tissue, skin, and mucous membranes** should be evaluated for bleeding.
- **Petechiae, purpura, mucocutaneous bleeding, or slow oozing after trauma** suggests deficient platelet number or function.
- On the other hand, **deep or visceral bleeding** (hemarthroses, deep hematomas), **large hematomas,** and **delayed bleeding** following injury are indicative of a problem with coagulation factors.
- There may be evidence of **accompanying medical problems**, such as infections, malignancy, and liver/renal disease.

Laboratory Studies

- A **complete blood count (CBC)** assesses platelet number.
- The **peripheral smear** confirms CBC abnormalities and may provide additional diagnostic clues (e.g., schistocytes in disseminated intravascular coagulation (DIC), large platelets in idiopathic thrombocytopenic purpura).
- **Prothrombin time (PT)** and **activated partial thromboplastin time (aPTT)** evaluate coagulation factors. **PT** evaluates the extrinsic and common pathways, including vitamin K–dependent factors II, VII, and X. **PTT** evaluates the intrinsic and common pathways, including factors VIII (deficient in hemophilia A) and IX (deficient in hemophilia B). Factor VIII inhibitors can also prolong PTT.
- **Bleeding time** will be prolonged (more than 7 minutes) in qualitative platelet dysfunction, thrombocytopenia, and von Willebrand disease (vWD). The **Platelet Function Analyzer 100 (PFA-100)** test analyzes the clotting of the patient's blood on a collagen- or epinephrine-coated surface and a collagen- or adenosine diphosphate–coated surface. The PFA-100 may be more useful than bleeding time in detecting vWD.
- **Mixing studies** evaluate for factor deficiencies or presence of clotting factor inhibitors.

TREATMENT

- The choice of **outpatient versus inpatient** management depends on the severity and location of bleeding.
- **Hemodynamic compromise** or **marked anemia** requires supportive therapy.
- **Management of underlying etiologies** or concurrent medical problems is often imperative in improving the bleeding disorder.
- Patients should **avoid aspirin-containing products and NSAIDs** in bleeding disorders.
- **Contact sports** should be avoided in significant bleeding disorders.
- Patients requiring frequent blood product transfusions should have their **HIV and hepatitis B and C status** checked. If nonimmune, hepatitis B vaccination should be performed.
- A **hematology consult** should be considered for severe, chronic, or familial bleeding problems.

COAGULATION DISORDERS

Hemophilia A

Definition

Hemophilia A is an X-linked disease due to **deficiency of coagulation factor VIII.** As a general rule, only men and boys are affected, but occasionally female carriers are clinically affected.

Clinical Presentation

The **bleeding tendency varies** with factor VIII levels. Patients with mild hemophilia (5% to 50% of normal concentrations) bleed only in response to major trauma or surgery. Patients with moderate hemophilia (1% to 5%) bleed in response to mild trauma or surgery, and those with severe hemophilia (less than 1%) bleed spontaneously.

Laboratory Studies

Laboratory findings are prolonged aPTT and decreased factor VIII assay.

Treatment

Selection and dosing of therapy depend on severity of bleeding and levels of factor VIII and factor VIII inhibitor. Hematology consultation can guide treatment. For patients with severe hemophilia, chronic prophylactic treatment may be desired.

- **Desmopressin acetate (DDAVP)** may raise factor VIII levels prior to minor surgery in mild hemophiliacs and can be re-administered in 8 hours.
- **Cryoprecipitate** can raise factor VIII levels.
- Purified IV human and porcine **factor VIII concentrates** may be given, although effectiveness may be limited when significant factor VIII inhibitors are present. Recombinant DNA-derived clotting factors are available, eliminating the risks of viral transmission.
- For patients with significant inhibitor levels, **recombinant activated factor VIIa (rFVIIa)** or **activated prothrombin complex concentrates (APCCs)** may be used to bypass the inhibitor. Plasmapheresis or immunoadsorption can temporarily lower inhibitor levels.
- **ε-Aminocaproic acid** is an inhibitor of fibrinolysis that can be used as an adjunct to factor VIII concentrate or DDAVP.
- **Gene therapies** are being developed for chronic management of hemophilias.

Hemophilia B

Definition

Hemophilia B is an X-linked bleeding disorder due to **deficiency of coagulation factor IX**. It is clinically identical to hemophilia A but less common. Acquired factor IX deficiency may occur concomitantly with deficiencies of factors II, VII, and X and in patients with **vitamin K** deficiency.

Laboratory Studies

Laboratory findings are prolonged aPTT and decreased factor IX assay.

Treatment

- **Factor IX concentrates**, available as recombinant preparations to eliminate risks of viral transmission, are administered.
- **Fresh frozen plasma** (FFP) contains low levels of factor IX activity and may be used in patients with mild disease.
- DDAVP is ineffective in management of hemophilia B.

Factor XI Deficiency

Definition

Factor XI deficiency is an autosomal recessive bleeding disorder common in Ashkenazi Jews. Spontaneous hemorrhage and hemarthrosis are rare.

Laboratory Studies

The **aPTT** is prolonged. **Factor XI assay** is usually decreased to less than 10% in homozygotes and to 20% to 60% in heterozygotes.

Treatment

Give **FFP** 10 to 20 mL per kg body weight initially, and 5 to 10 mL/kg/day maintenance. Factor XI activity level of 30% is usually sufficient for hemostasis.

Prothrombin (Factor II) and Factors V, VII, X, and XIII and Fibrinogen Deficiencies

These are exceedingly rare coagulation disorders that may sometimes present with spontaneous hemorrhage. The treatment mainstay is FFP, although factor concentrates are available for deficiencies of factors II, VII, and X.

Circulating Anticoagulants

Antibodies may inhibit specific coagulation factors, prolonging the aPTT or PT. **Factor VIII inhibitor** is the most common inhibitor that causes bleeding. Lupus anticoagulant prolongs aPTT but causes excessive thrombosis rather than bleeding. Inhibitors may be detected when adding normal plasma to patient plasma fails to correct prolonged coagulation times (1:1 dilution test). Management of bleeding may involve massive plasma or concentrate infusion, use of APCCs, plasmapheresis, and immunosuppression.

Vitamin K Deficiency

Vitamin K has an important role in hemostasis as a cofactor in the carboxylation of glutamic acid residues for coagulation factors II, VII, IX, X, protein C, and protein S. Vitamin K deficiency may develop within a week if both intake and endogenous production of vitamin K are eliminated. Vitamin K deficiencies may occur with warfarin use, postsurgical states, antibiotic therapy, biliary obstruction, liver disease, nutritional deficiencies, and malabsorption syndromes, such as inflammatory bowel diseases and ingestion of nonabsorbed fat substitutes in diet foods. Newborns are deficient in vitamin K until approximately 1 week of life.

Laboratory Studies
The PT is prolonged. The aPTT may be prolonged if the deficiency is severe. Assays for factors II, VII, IX, and X are typically low if measured.

Treatment
- Mild deficiencies may be corrected with **vitamin K**. It may be given PO, SC, IM, or IV.
- Severe bleeding should be managed by transfusion of **FFP** along with vitamin K administration.
- Hospitalized patients at risk for vitamin K deficiency should receive prophylactic vitamin K.

Liver Disease

Many patients with acute or chronic liver disease develop hemostatic abnormalities. The bleeding disorder may range from asymptomatic to significant hemorrhage.

Laboratory Studies
The PT and aPTT are prolonged from decreased clotting factor synthesis. Thrombocytopenia, decreased fibrinogen concentration, and prolonged bleeding time may be seen. Platelet dysfunction may also occur.

Treatment
- **Vitamin K** administration may be attempted, although it may be ineffective.
- **FFP** may transiently improve hemostatic function for the actively bleeding patient.
- **Platelet transfusions** may be required if the patient is thrombocytopenic, actively bleeding, or about to undergo surgery.
- Certain causes of bleeding may require **targeted therapy**, such as sclerotherapy for esophageal varices.

Disseminated Intravascular Coagulation

DIC is the consequence of activation of both the coagulation and fibrinolytic systems and may be a life-threatening condition. Usually a predominance of bleeding or thrombosis exists. DIC occurs secondarily to an initiating event, such as malignant neoplasm, infection, leukemia, obstetric complications, liver disease, shock, connective tissue diseases, massive trauma, snake bite, or extensive tissue damage, such as burns or frostbite.

Laboratory Studies
Laboratory findings include decreased **fibrinogen** (often the cardinal manifestation of DIC that correlates closely with bleeding), elevated **fibrin degradation products, thrombocytopenia**, prolonged **PT** and **aPTT**, and **schistocytes** (fragmented red blood cells) on blood smear.

Treatment
Treatment of the underlying condition is paramount. Use of cryoprecipitate, FFP, and platelet transfusions is considered in the event of major bleeding. Heparin is indicated if there are thrombotic complications.

PLATELET DISORDERS

Platelet disorders can be quantitative or qualitative. Thrombocytopenia is defined as a platelet count less than 150,000 per μL. It can be the result of decreased platelet production, increased consumption, or sequestration. In general, platelet counts greater than 50,000 per μL are not associated with significant bleeding. Severe spontaneous bleeding usually does not occur with platelet counts exceeding 20,000 per μL. A platelet count less than 5,000 per μL is considered a hematologic emergency. Bleeding may occur despite normal platelet counts if there is a qualitative defect in platelet function.

Von Willebrand Disease

vWD is a family of predominantly autosomal dominant disorders characterized by **deficient or defective von Willebrand factor (vWF)**. vWF facilitates platelet adhesion by linking platelet membrane receptors to vascular subendothelium, and it serves as the plasma carrier for factor VIII. The severity of bleeding is highly variable even within an individual patient over time. There are three subtypes of vWD: type 1—partial quantitative vWF deficiency, type 2—qualitative vWF deficiency, and type 3—virtually complete vWF deficiency.

Laboratory Studies

Bleeding time may be prolonged but correlates poorly with bleeding risk. Prolonged **aPTT** may occur. Prolonged or normal aPTT and normal PT, platelet count, and fibrinogen in the presence of bleeding symptoms should prompt vWD specific testing. Reduced **ristocetin cofactor activity (vWF activity)** is the most sensitive and specific test. Measurements of **vWF antigen, vWF multimers**, and **ristocetin-induced platelet agglutination** are useful for the subclassification of vWD.

Treatment

- Regular prophylaxis is **not** typically indicated, and treatment is given prior to scheduled procedures or in response to bleeding.
- **Oral contraceptives** may be given to women who currently do not desire to become pregnant. They mimic the hormonal changes of pregnancy, increasing vWF and factor VIII levels. A **levonorgestrel** IUD may also be used in appropriate patients.
- **DDAVP** increases vWF concentrations two- to fivefold. A nasal spray is now available, making administration easier. DDAVP is contraindicated in patients with type IIB or severe type III vWD because of the potential for exacerbating thrombocytopenia. DDAVP functions by releasing endogenous vWF stores from the endothelium.
- **Certain plasma-derived factor VIII concentrates** that contain vWF in high-molecular-weight form have been used successfully.
- **Cryoprecipitate** is no longer a recommended treatment for factor VIII or vWF deficiency.
- Factor replacement may need to be continued for 5 to 10 days following major surgery or trauma.
- **Antifibrinolytics**, including ε-aminocaproic acid and tranexamic acid, may help stabilize clots once they have formed, and are useful for mucous membrane bleeding.
- **Topical agents** such as animal or human thrombin and fibrin products are useful in minor bleeding.

Qualitative Platelet Disorders

Abnormal platelet function with normal platelet counts may occur with uremia, liver disease, cardiopulmonary bypass surgery, paraproteinemia, Glanzmann thrombasthenia, and myeloproliferative disorders. It may also occur with the use of drugs such as NSAIDs, aspirin, ticlopidine, clopidogrel, β-lactam antibiotics, alcohol, antihistamines, calcium-channel blockers, dipyridamole, and quinidine. Therapy is directed at the underlying disease or at removing the offending agent. Treatments that have been of use in some of the above conditions include DDAVP, corticosteroids, conjugated estrogen, cryoprecipitate, and platelet transfusions.

Drug-Induced Thrombocytopenia

Drug-induced thrombocytopenia is one of the most common platelet disorders encountered in the outpatient setting. Thrombocytopenia has been associated with the use of heparin, quinidine, thiazide diuretics, alcohol, H_2 antagonists, estrogens, quinine, gold salts, phenytoin, carbamazepine, rifampin, vancomycin, ticlopidine, cephalosporins, and chemotherapeutic agents. Thrombocytopenia usually resolves within days of discontinuation of the offending drug unless there is slow excretion of the drug. Prednisone may decrease the duration of thrombocytopenia in some cases. Plasma exchange or platelet transfusions may be considered if hemorrhage is severe. Platelet count should be repeated 1 week after discontinuing causative medication.

Autoimmune ("Idiopathic") Thrombocytopenia

Idiopathic thrombocytopenia (ITP) is a disorder of antibody-mediated platelet destruction. This syndrome occurs primarily in otherwise healthy patients. Less commonly, autoimmune platelet destruction occurs with other diseases, including thyroid disease, pregnancy, HIV infection, malignancies, granulomatous disorders, systemic lupus erythematosus, and other rheumatologic disorders. The presence of lymphadenopathy or splenomegaly should trigger a search for secondary causes of thrombocytopenia.

Acute ITP

- **Acute ITP** usually occurs in **children** and often follows a viral infection of the preceding 3 weeks.
- Most cases **resolve spontaneously** within 6 months.
- **Platelet count is often less than 20,000 per μL.** Peripheral smear shows large platelets.
- Prednisone is the mainstay of treatment, and intravenous immunoglobulin (IVIg) may be used as well. Platelet transfusions are usually reserved for severe hemorrhage.

Chronic ITP

- **Chronic ITP** is usually seen in adults, and spontaneous remissions are rare.
- **Platelet count usually is greater than 20,000 per μL** but may drop lower.
- **Initial treatment** is traditionally with **prednisone.** Immunoglobulin, splenectomy, danazol, immunosuppressive therapy, and anti-Rh(D) antibodies may be considered, depending on the severity of the disease.

Thrombotic Thrombocytopenic Purpura

Thrombotic thrombocytopenic purpura (TTP) is a life-threatening disorder characterized by thrombocytopenia, microangiopathic hemolytic anemia, neurologic abnormalities, fever, and renal dysfunction. Most patients have only part of this classic pentad of abnormalities. Peripheral smear shows fragmentation of red blood cells (RBCs). High lactate dehydrogenase and reticulocyte count result from hemolysis. Hemolytic uremic syndrome (HUS) is closely related to TTP, but renal failure is the predominant manifestation and there are no neurologic disturbances. It is usually preceded by diarrhea. Dialysis for renal failure may be required.

Treatment

- Initial therapy **must** include **plasmapheresis** if available or **FFP infusion** until plasmapheresis is available.
- Treat renal failure, seizures, and hypertension with **supportive measures**.
- Platelet transfusions are avoided and severe anemia is treated with platelet-depleted RBCs.
- Glucocorticoids are sometimes used.

Other Causes of Thrombocytopenia

Other causes of thrombocytopenia include hypersplenism; transfusions; DIC; nutritional deficiencies of folic acid or vitamin B_{12}; bone marrow infiltration due to myelophthisic disease (e.g., tuberculosis, metastatic carcinoma, myelofibrosis); primary hematopoietic disorders (e.g., leukemia, aplastic anemia, myelodysplasia, multiple myeloma); radiotherapy; Wiskott–Aldrich syndrome; Bernard–Soulier syndrome; congenital amegakaryocytic thrombocytopenia; and various viral, bacterial, and rickettsial infections. Therapy is directed at the underlying disorder.

ABNORMALITIES OF VASCULAR STRENGTH OR STRUCTURE

Bleeding in the absence of a hematologic defect may occur when vascular strength or structure is abnormal. For example, **senile purpura** presents with dark purple, irregularly shaped areas of skin bleeding on sun-exposed areas in elderly people. **Purpura simplex** presents with ecchymoses of the legs in healthy females, especially during menses. Management of these conditions consists of reassurance and avoidance of antiplatelet medications. **Cushing syndrome** and **scurvy (vitamin C deficiency)** also may present with abnormal skin bleeding, and treatment is directed at the underlying condition. **Osler–Weber–Rendu disease** (hereditary hemorrhagic telangiectasia) is an autosomal dominant disorder associated with bleeding from abnormal capillaries in the GI tract and nasal mucosa. Patients with **Marfan and Ehlers–Danlos syndromes** have fragile skin vessels, bruise easily, and have a tendency to form aneurysms of large arteries with potential rupture.

REFERENCES

1. Ballas M, Kraut EH. Bleeding and bruising: a diagnostic work-up. *Am Fam Physician* 2008;77:1117–1124.
2. Tosetto A, Castaman G, Plug I, et al. Prospective evaluation of the clinical utility of quantitative bleeding severity assessment in patients referred for hemostatic evaluation. *J Thromb Haemost* 2011;9:1143.
3. Yawn BP, Nichols WL, Rick ME. Diagnosis and management of von Willebrand disease: guidelines for primary care. *Am Fam Physician* 2009;80:1261–1268.
4. Gauer RL, Braun MM. Thrombocytopenia. *Am Fam Physician* 2012;85:612–622.
5. Lambert MP. What to do when you suspect an inherited platelet disorder. *Hematology* 2011;377–383.

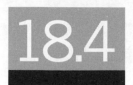

18.4 The Leukemias
Philip T. Dooley, Kevin L. Gray

The leukemias are a group of illnesses characterized by malignant infiltration of bone marrow by abnormal cell lines that produce high numbers of leukocytes, which are often nonfunctional. These disorders are categorized according to the type of cell produced and the chronic or acute clinical course of the disease. Any cell line can be affected. The following is an overview of the most common leukemias found in children and adults.

ACUTE LEUKEMIAS
Acute Lymphoblastic Leukemia

Acute lymphoblastic leukemia (ALL) is characterized by replacement of bone marrow with neoplastic lymphoid cells. ALL is the most common pediatric malignancy, with a peak incidence in early childhood (ages 1 to 4).

- **Presentation:** Symptoms include fatigue, shortness of breath, pallor, bleeding, fever, frequent minor infections, bone pain, arthralgias, adenopathy, and hepatosplenomegaly.
- **Diagnosis:** Bone marrow aspiration and biopsy generally show the presence of leukemic blast cells. Subtypes of ALL can be further classified by immunophenotyping.
- **Management:** Multiple factors contribute to the choice of treatment for ALL. In general, treatment begins with induction therapy to remove leukemic blast cells. Consolidation therapy typically continues for months, whereas maintenance therapy may continue for years. Central nervous system treatment may also help to eliminate ALL cells deposited in the meninges.
- **Prognosis:** There is increased mortality in children less than 1 year of age and children more than 10 years of age. In adults, increased mortality occurs for those over age 35. Higher WBC counts at the time of presentation and certain ALL subtypes also correlate with higher mortality.[1] Up to 89% of children achieve 5-year event-free survival.[2] Adult 3-year survival rates for those less than 30, 30 to 59, and greater than 60 years of age are 58%, 38%, and 12%, respectively.[3]
- **Complications:** Blood-related complications include anemia, thrombocytopenia, neutropenia, and monocytopenia. Increased rates of infection (bacterial, viral and fungal) are also common. Treatment side effects include diarrhea, hair loss, rashes, nausea, vomiting, and fatigue.

Acute Myeloid Leukemia

Acute myeloid leukemia (AML) is a heterogeneous group of disorders characterized by replacement of bone marrow with neoplastic hematopoietic cells. AML's peak incidence occurs later in life (ages 80 to 84). Although only 15% to 20% of leukemia in children is classified as AML, it accounts for 80% of acute leukemia in adults.[4]

- **Presentation:** Common findings include pallor, bleeding (ecchymosis, petechiae, prolonged bleeding from minor cuts), fatigue, dizziness, palpitations, dyspnea, infections, fever, lymphadenopathy, hepatosplenomegaly, weight loss, and anorexia.
- **Diagnosis:** Bone marrow aspirate includes greater than 20% leukemic blast cells and the presence of Auer rods. Subtype classification can be completed by immunophenotyping.
- **Management:** The choice of treatment depends on age, subtype, and potential for stem cell match. Induction therapy requires multiple chemotherapy agents in an ordered sequence, whereas subsequent treatment is guided by the response to induction. Remission is defined as the removal of blast cells from blood and bone marrow. Consolidation therapy is chosen based on the risk of relapse, which is a function of AML subtype and WBC count at presentation. Allogeneic stem cell transplantations can also be included when the risk of relapse following remission is high.
- **Prognosis:** Survival rates vary drastically depending on age and AML subtype. A patient less than 60 years old with a favorable cytogenetic profile may have a 5-year survival as high as 76%, whereas patients over age 60 experience 3-year relapse rates around 90%.[5]

- **Complications:** Blood-related complications include myelosuppression, pancytopenia, and leukostasis related to the initial high WBC counts. Opportunistic infections and tumor lysis syndrome can occur with treatment. Other treatment-related side effects include diarrhea, hair loss, rash, nausea, vomiting, and fatigue.

CHRONIC LEUKEMIAS

Chronic Lymphocytic Leukemia

Chronic lymphocytic leukemia (CLL) arises from acquired mutations in the DNA of a bone marrow cell; 95% of these cases occur in B cells. Mutations are possible in T lymphocytes and natural killer cells as well (5% of cases). Proliferation of these cells can spread to organs and lymphatic tissue. Increased incidence occurs with age. CLL is rarely seen in patients under the age of 25 and the median age at diagnosis is around 61.

- **Presentation:** Clinical symptoms may be absent and elevations in WBC count may be found incidentally. Symptoms at diagnosis may include fatigue, shortness of breath, weight loss, anorexia, lymphadenopathy, and hepatosplenomegaly.
- **Diagnosis:** WBC count will be elevated with a monoclonal lymphocytosis. Smudge cells may be present on the smear as well. Bone marrow aspirate and immunophenotyping can be used to confirm the diagnosis.
- **Management:** Treatment of CLL is based on a number of factors. These include absolute lymphocyte count, symptoms, age, lymph node enlargement, spleen enlargement, and thrombocytopenia. Treatment guidelines are constantly changing on the basis of research and new clinical trials. CLL treatments range from surveillance of asymptomatic patients to single- and multiple-agent chemotherapy or allogeneic stem cell transplantation with high-dose chemotherapy.
- **Prognosis:** Outcomes vary greatly depending on stage of the disease and age of the patient. Low-risk individuals can have a median survival in excess of 25 years. Higher risk patients with certain genetic abnormalities have an average survival of only 2 to 3 years.
- **Complications:** CLL may be complicated by opportunistic infections, Richter transformation (development of an aggressive lymphoma), autoimmune hemolytic anemia, and secondary malignancies. Chemotherapy complications include anemia, neutropenic fever, and tumor lysis syndrome.

Chronic Myeloid Leukemia

Chronic myeloid leukemia (CML) is characterized by increases in myeloid cells within the bone marrow. It is typically an indolent disease, called the chronic stable phase, which progresses to an accelerated phase and eventually blast crisis (greater than 20% blasts) over a period of weeks to years. Approximately 90% of patients test positive for the Philadelphia chromosome, a reciprocal translocation between the long arms of chromosomes 9 and 22. CML is rare before 40 years of age, with an incidence of less than 1 per 100,000. The median age at diagnosis is 53.[6]

- **Presentation:** Elevated WBC counts are often found incidentally as clinical symptoms may be absent. Otherwise, patients may present with fatigue, shortness of breath, pallor, splenomegaly, weight loss, or night sweats.
- **Diagnosis:** Bone marrow aspirate shows a decrease in RBCs and an increase in WBCs. Identification of the Philadelphia chromosome (using fluorescent in situ hybridization or real-time polymerase chain reaction) is diagnostic.
- **Management:** Chronic phase treatment uses tyrosine kinase inhibitors (TKIs) to remove as many CML cells as possible while maintaining quality of life. Allogeneic hematopoietic stem cell transplant (AHSCT) with high-dose induction chemotherapy can be curative but is rarely considered in patients who have never experienced the accelerated phase or blast crisis due to increased early mortality. TKIs are also the primary treatment for accelerated phase CML, with the goal of eliminating malignant cells or at least returning the patient to chronic phase disease. A different TKI or combination chemotherapy may be used in patients who have previously been treated with one TKI. AHSCT is utilized more frequently in these advanced stages if the disease can be returned to the chronic phase.
- **Prognosis:** Indicators of poor outcome include advanced stage at time of diagnosis, splenomegaly, increased number of blasts, and older age. Five-year survival rates vary drastically based on these indicators.
- **Complications:** Blood-related complications include anemia and thrombocytopenia, whereas pancytopenia occurs with blast crisis. Common TKI side effects include myelosuppression, edema, cramping, rash, and nausea.

Hairy Cell Leukemia

Hairy cell leukemia (HCL) is caused by the accumulation of B lymphocytes with hair-like projections in the blood, bone marrow, and spleen. The etiology of the disease is unproven. It represents only 2% of leukemia cases, with 600 to 800 cases per year in the United States. The median age at diagnosis is 52, with an approximately 5:1 male-to-female ratio.[7]

- **Presentation:** The most common presenting complaint is abdominal discomfort from splenomegaly. Other possible signs and symptoms include fatigue or shortness of breath from anemia, bleeding from thrombocytopenia, or infections from leukopenia. Cytopenia may also be discovered incidentally.
- **Diagnosis:** The diagnosis can usually be made by visualization of hairy cells in peripheral blood smears or bone marrow aspirate. Immunophenotyping can also be used to help confirm the diagnosis.
- **Management:** HCL treatment aims to remove malignant cells from the blood and marrow while returning the spleen and lymph nodes to normal size. Although many patients remain asymptomatic for years, most patients eventually receive treatment. First-line treatment uses a purine analogue called cladribine. Pentostatin is another purine analogue that can be used. Indications for treatment include any of the symptoms described above.
- **Prognosis:** 85% of patients treated with a single cycle of cladribine will achieve complete remission. Life expectancy exceeds 10 years for most HCL patients.
- **Complications:** The side effects of treatment include infection from immunosuppression and secondary malignancies.

ADDITIONAL RESOURCES

Updated treatment guidelines are available at the National Comprehensive Cancer Network Web site (http://www.nccn.org). In addition, the National Cancer Institute (http://www.cancer.gov) and the European Society for Medical Oncology (http://www.esmo.org) are excellent sources of information.

REFERENCES

1. Rowe JM, Buck G, Burnett AK, et al. Induction therapy for adults with acute lymphoblastic leukemia: results of more than 1500 patients from the international ALL trial: MRC UKALL XII/ECOG E2993. *Blood* 2005;106:3760–3767.
2. Surveillance, Epidemiology and End Results (SEER) Program. *Cancer Statistics Review, 1975–2007.* Bethesda, MD: National Cancer Institute; 2010.
3. Larson RA. Acute lymphoblastic leukemia: older patient and newer drugs. *Hematology Am Soc Hematol Educ Program* 2005(1):131–136.
4. Howlader N, Noone AM, Krapcho M, et al., eds. *SEER Cancer Statistics Review, 1975–2010.* Bethesda, MD: National Cancer Institute. http://seer.cancer.gov/csr/1975_2010/. Based on November 2012 SEER data submission, posted to the SEER Web site, April 2013.
5. British Committee for Standards in Haematology, Milligan DW, Grimwade D, Cullis JO, et al. Guidelines on the management of acute myeloid leukaemia in adults. *Br J Haematol* 2006;135(4):450–474.
6. Jemal A, Siegel R, Ward E, et al. Cancer statistics, 2006. *CA Cancer J Clin* 2006;56:106–130.
7. Besa EC. Hairy Cell Leukemia. Medscape. http://emedicine.medscape.com/article/200580-overview. Accessed March 18, 2014.

CHAPTER 19

Infectious Diseases

Section Editor: Laeth Nasir

Viral Upper Respiratory Infections, Influenza, and Flu

Stella C. Major

INFLUENZA VIRUS
General Principles

- An Orthomyxovirus (enveloped virus) with segmented RNA genome and two surface glycoproteins HA (hemagglutinin) and NA (neuraminidase).
- Three types exist: A, B, and C.
- A and B are responsible for seasonal illness (commonly winter months).
- Account for 10% to 15% of "common cold" illnesses.
- Infection is by droplet spread.

Epidemiology

- The CDC surveys determine the respiratory illness incidence and virus etiologies, and provide weekly updates to practitioners (http://www.cdc.gov/mmwr/mmwr_wk/wk_cvol.html).
- During 2013 to 2014 season, severe illness was reported among young and middle aged adults who were infected with 2009 H1N1 virus.

Diagnosis

Clinical Presentation

"Flu"—Sudden Onset
- Fever, cough, sore throat, runny or stuffy nose, myalgia, headaches, and fatigue lasting from few days to 2 weeks. Children may present with associated vomiting and diarrhea. Complications include pneumonia, bronchitis, and ear or sinus infections.

Bronchiolitis
- Typically in children below 2 years of age.
- Coryza, decreased appetite, coughing, sneezing, and fever. There may be associated wheezing. Very young infants may show irritability, dyspnea, and tachypnea.

Pneumonia
- Typically more gradual in onset than bacterial pneumonia.
- Productive cough, fever, breathlessness, pleuritic chest pain, generalized weakness, and fatigue.

Laboratory Studies

- A variety of diagnostic tests exist from the conventional viral culture to rapid influenza diagnostic tests, with test times ranging from 3 to 10 days for culture to less than 30 minutes for the rapid tests. Specificity and sensitivity vary for the individual tests, often very expensive. Typically used only if the results will influence clinical decision making.

Treatment

- Antiviral drugs are important adjuncts to the influenza vaccine, in controlling influenza illnesses.
- In the 2013 to 2014 season, FDA approved two neuraminidase inhibitors with low resistance levels to influenza: oseltamivir (oral) and zanamivir (inhaled).
- Standard treatment regimen for antiviral agents is one administration twice daily for 5 days.

Prevention

- Seasonal flu vaccines are designed to protect against the strains of viruses, which have been identified on surveillance to date.
- Different vaccines exist (trivalent, quadrivalent) with different virus strain contents, live or attenuated, with different modes of administration (intramuscular, intradermal, intranasal, etc.) in order to provide coverage to patients in all recommended age groups, including those with egg allergies.

Prophylaxis

- Influenza vaccine administration before influenza season should provide safe and effective immunity. Antiviral agents act as adjuvant.
- CDC does not recommend pre-exposure use of antiviral agents for prophylaxis except in very high-risk vaccinated individuals. Some groups recommend chemoprophylaxis regardless of vaccination status in outbreaks in long-term care facilities.
- If indicated (high-risk individuals with exposure to infected persons), antiviral agents (oseltamivir and zanamivir) are most effective if commenced <48 hours from exposure.

RESPIRATORY SYNCYTIAL VIRUS
General Principles
Infants

- Commonest cause of bronchiolitis in <1 years in United States
- Causes upper and lower respiratory illnesses, such as bronchitis, croup, bronchiolitis, and pneumonia. Very young and severe cases in infants will need hospitalization.

Adults

- A common cause of "cold-like" illness lasting <5 days
- Typically effects health care workers, child care workers, and elderly
- In immunosuppressed adults, may lead to pneumonia

Epidemiology

- Respiratory syncytial virus (RSV) infections are most common in the winter. Most infants will have been infected by the age of 2 years.

Diagnosis
Clinical Presentation
Bronchiolitis (as in Influenza)

- Acute bronchitis is typically a combination of cough (productive), chest pain, fatigue, fever, shortness of breath on exertion, and wheezing.

Laboratory Studies

- Highly sensitive reverse transcriptase polymerase chain reaction (RT-PCR) diagnostic kits are commercially available.
- Many laboratories offer Antigen (Ag) detection tests and Cell Culture.
- Ag detection tests are 80% to 90% sensitive (especially in young children).
- Although done rarely, paired acute and convalescent serological tests can be done.

Treatment

- No specific treatment exists for RSV illnesses in children. Treatment is supportive. Inhaled β-agonists may be effective in individual cases.
- In severe cases oxygen, suctioning and/or mechanical ventilation may be required. Ribavirin use in children with severe illness may be considered. In subgroups of immunocompromised adults, ribavirin may be helpful.

Prevention

- Palivizumab prophylaxis should be considered in high-risk subgroups of children. Updated guidance is available from the American Academy of Pediatrics (http://pediatrics.aappublications.org/content/134/2/415.full).

HUMAN PARAINFLUENZA VIRUSES

General Principles

- These are single-stranded RNA viruses of the paramyxovirus family.
- Cause a variety of different types of upper and lower respiratory illnesses.
- Most commonly human parainfluenza viruses (HPIVs) cause self-limiting "cold-like" illness in adults.
- However, they can cause serious illnesses in elderly and are a known cause of morbidity in immunosuppressed persons.

Epidemiology

- HPIV infections are more common in the spring, summer, and fall seasons.
- Like RSV, the HPIV can cause repeated infections throughout life.
- The viruses exist in four types (1, 2, 3, and 4) and two subtypes 4A and 4B.
- Each type has a different clinical manifestation and epidemiology.
- HPIV-1 and -2 (less commonly) cause croup.
- HPIV-3 causes bronchiolitis, bronchitis, and pneumonia.
- HPIV-4 is rarely isolated and may cause mild to severe infections.

Diagnosis

Clinical Presentation

- Croup typically appears in a febrile child, without coryzal symptoms, who presents with hoarseness, seal-like barking cough, acute inspiratory stridor, and varying degrees of respiratory distress.
- Pharyngitis presents with sore throat and pain on swallowing.
- Laryngitis presents with hoarseness or loss of voice.
- Asthma and bronchiolitis (see above).

Imaging

- An anteroposterior x-ray view of the neck shows the classic "pencil" or "steeple sign" in the subglottic area.

Laboratory Studies

- Identification tests are not routinely recommended.
- Direct detection of the viral genome by polymerase chain reaction.
- Direct viral antigen (Ag) detection in respiratory fluids.
- Isolation of the virus in culture.
- Serological tests—paired IgG or IgM.

Treatment

- **Mild croup:** Observation and hydration are initiated, and if treatment is desired, a single dose of oral dexamethasone 0.6 mg per kg is recommended.
- In moderate or severe cases, in addition to a single dose of parenteral steroids as above, humidified oxygen, nebulized racemic epinephrine, and close observation should be initiated to assess for the need for airway management.

Prevention

- Droplet and surface transmission.
- Strict adherence to infection control protocols, including hand washing and protective equipment, is recommended.

RHINOVIRUSES

General Principles

- These are small single-stranded RNA viruses of the Picornaviridae family. There are >100 different subtypes, which are subdivided into three major groups. Rhinovirus (RV) is the most common cause (25% to 80%) of the self-limiting "common cold" illness, which may occur all year round, but most commonly in spring and autumn.

Clinical Presentation

- With a short incubation period of 12 to 72 hours, the symptoms are a combination of dry irritated nostrils, throat soreness, followed by nasal congestion and discharge, headaches, ear and facial pain, loss of sense of taste and smell, possible cough, and possibly low-grade fever. The illness may last up to 2 weeks.

Laboratory Studies

- Viral cultures and PCR of respiratory fluids are available, though rarely used in the clinical setting.

Treatment

- Symptomatic relief.

Prevention

- Recommend effective patient education regarding hand hygiene.

CORONAVIRUS
General Principles

- Enveloped RNA viruses characterized by "crown-like" spikes on the surface.
- Exist worldwide and can infect humans and animals.
- Known subgroups exist: alpha, beta, gamma, and delta.
- Five types of coronavirus are known to infect humans. These include alpha coronavirus 229E and NL63, beta coronaviruses OC43 and HKU1, and the SARS Co-V, which caused the severe acute respiratory syndrome, first diagnosed in 2003 and not isolated anywhere since 2004.
- MERS-CoV (Middle East Respiratory Syndrome) is a new coronavirus, which has led to more severe respiratory illnesses and deaths. It was first isolated in 2012 in the Arabian Gulf region and continues to be isolated to date.
- Spread is mostly occurring in healthcare settings and the CDC continues to monitor its spread globally and provides guidance to the public and professionals worldwide.

Epidemiology

- Commonly these viruses cause mild–moderate upper respiratory tract infections all year round and especially in fall and winter in United States accounting for 10% to 20% of "common cold" infections.

Diagnosis

- The clinical presentation ranges from symptoms of a common cold to severe acute respiratory distress syndrome.

Laboratory Studies

- Viral serology tests and viral cultures, and respiratory sample PCR testing exist to confirm the organism.

Treatment

- Supportive with strict isolation guidance that CDC regularly updates.

Prevention

- Health care workers must follow CDC recommendations in case of contact with MERS Co-V patients. At all times, contact and airborne precautions and monitoring of own health are advised.

ADENOVIRUSES
General Principles

Epidemiology
- Adenoviruses are typically associated with viral illness all year round and may cause a variety of different illnesses. They account for 5% of common cold illnesses.

Diagnosis

Clinical Presentation
- Acute respiratory disease, diarrhea, bronchiolitis, pharyngoconjunctivitis, conjunctivitis (pinkeye), and epidemic keratoconjunctivitis.

Laboratory Studies
- Adenovirus can be isolated by virus isolation, Ag-detecting PCR assays, and serum serology testing.
- Asymptomatic shedding is frequent.

Treatment

- Treatment with selected antivirals in life-threatening illness may be considered. Vaccines against types 4 and 7 are administered to military recruits in the United States to prevent acute respiratory diseases.

Prevention

- Infection control practices (contact and airborne precautions).

HUMAN METAPNEUMOVIRUS
General Principles

Epidemiology
- First isolated in 2001 in Netherlands.
- Are associated with upper and lower respiratory infections in all ages.
- Infections typically occur in the fall and winter.

Diagnosis

- RT-PCR is the most efficient method for diagnosis, but is rarely available, and not well standardized.

Clinical Presentation

- Presentations might be mild or severe.
- Mild upper respiratory symptoms include cough, coryzal, sore throat, and fever.
- Severe respiratory symptoms include high fever, severe cough and shortness of breath, wheezing, vomiting, and diarrhea.

Laboratory Studies

- Currently, human metapneumovirus is isolated only in research laboratories.

Treatment and Prevention

- Symptomatic treatment plus contact and airborne precautions.

REFERENCES

1. Shi L, Loveless M, Spagnuolo P, et al. Antiviral treatment of influenza in children: a retrospective cohort study. *Adv Ther* 2014;31(7):735–750.
2. Plint AC, Grenon R, Klassen TP, et al. Bronchodilator and steroid use for the management of bronchiolitis in Canadian pediatric emergency departments. *CJEM* 2014;16:1–8.
3. Gao HN, Lu HZ, Cao B, et al. Clinical findings in 111 cases of influenza A (H7N9) virus infection. *N Engl J Med* 2013;368(24):2277–2285.
4. Bresee J, Hayden FG. Epidemic influenza—responding to the expected but unpredictable. *N Engl J Med* 2013;368(7):589–592.
5. Milési C, Baleine J, Matecki S, et al. Is treatment with a high flow nasal cannula effective in acute viral bronchiolitis? A physiologic study. *Intensive Care Med* 2013;39(6):1088–1094.
6. Raj VS, Osterhaus AD, Fouchier RA, et al. MERS: emergence of a novel human coronavirus. *Curr Opin Virol* 2014;5:58–62.
7. Skjerven HO, Hunderi JO, Brügmann-Pieper SK, et al. Racemic adrenaline and inhalation strategies in acute bronchiolitis. *N Engl J Med* 2013;368(24):2286–2293.
8. Center for Disease Control and Prevention. MMWR. http://www.cdc.gov/mmwr/mmwr_wk/wk_cvol .html. Accessed May 8, 2014.
9. Center for Disease Control and Prevention. Flu symptoms. http://www.cdc.gov/flu/about/disease/symptoms.htm. Accessed May 8, 2014.
10. Center for Disease Control and Prevention. Bronchiolitis symptoms. http://www.cdc.gov/rsv/about/ symptoms.html. Accessed May 8, 2014.
11. Center for Disease Control and Prevention. RSV. http://www.cdc.gov/rsv/about/infection.html. Accessed May 8, 2014.

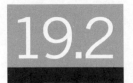

Gastroenteritis
Charles E. Henley

GENERAL PRINCIPLES
Diarrhea due to gastroenteritis is one of the leading causes of infant mortality worldwide and results in the hospitalization of approximately 55,000 children each year in the United States, affecting over 600,000 children annually worldwide. Most gastroenteritis in the United States is viral, with the main causative agent being rotavirus, which causes sporadic viral gastroenteritis, mainly in infants and young children. Norovirus is the most common form of gastroenteritis worldwide, and can affect both adults and children. It tends to occur in family, school, or community outbreaks.

DIAGNOSIS
Clinical Presentation
Viral gastroenteritis usually presents with symptoms of nausea, vomiting, and crampy abdominal pain of varying intensity due to excessive fluid in the upper gastrointestinal tract and increased peristalsis. Blood and fecal leukocytes are usually not present in the stool. In this way it can be differentiated from most of the bacterial pathogens that are inflammatory and invade the mucosa of the colon, producing a bloody diarrhea. Other physical signs besides the voluminous non-bloody stools are those associated with dehydration, such as decreased urination, mental status changes, dry mucosal membranes, and lethargy. A history of daycare exposure, foods eaten, and recent exposure to antibiotic use is also important. Patients with bloody diarrhea, abdominal tenderness, and fever or severe dehydration should be hospitalized.

    Diagnostic testing should be focused rather than all-inclusive. If the history and examination of the stool do not confirm the presence of blood and leukocytes, then the conclusion should be that the diarrhea is noninflammatory. If that is the case, then routine stool cultures may be an expensive waste of time.

- **Laboratory tests**, in general, are not helpful in differentiating between inflammatory and noninflammatory diarrhea, although lactoferrin is commonly used as a marker for leukocytes, with a sensitivity of 90% and a specificity of 70%. The plasma glucose; creatinine; and electrolytes of sodium, potassium, and HCO_3 may be useful in assessing volume and acid–base status.
- **Viral detection** is expensive and may be unnecessary, but the best test for rotavirus is the enzyme-linked immunosorbent assay, which detects viral antigens.

TREATMENT
Because the course of viral gastroenteritis is self-limiting, the goals of therapy are to replace fluids and electrolytes lost secondary to the diarrhea. Most patients can be treated at home with oral rehydration therapy (ORT).

- **Mild to moderate dehydration** can be managed with ORT, even in the face of continued vomiting. It is rapid, safe, and inexpensive. Several ORT solutions, such as Pedialyte and Rice-Lyte, are commercially available, with 45 and 50 mEq per L of sodium, respectively. ORT has also been used successfully in more severe dehydration, but if there are signs of altered mental status, shock, uremia, and ileus, then treatment with intravenous fluids is indicated. In addition, patients with short gut syndrome or carbohydrate malabsorption are not good candidates for ORS.
- **Refeeding:** The question of when and how to initiate feedings again can be simplified by following certain guidelines. ORT can be continued during the diarrhea, even if there is nausea and vomiting. Breastfeeding should continue uninterrupted, in addition to ORT. Formula-fed infants should have a lactose-free, full-strength formula reintroduced after 6 hours of ORT. The American Academy of Pediatrics recommends starting with a 1:1 dilution and gradually progressing to full strength. If the diarrhea worsens, return to ORT and gradually refeed with dilute formula, up to full strength over 6 to 72 hours. In weaned children, foods such as rice, wheat noodles, and bananas are good initially, but lactose-containing foods, caffeine, and raw fruits should be avoided for 24 to 48 hours.

• **Antidiarrheal agents** should be used with caution. Anticholinergic agents are generally ineffective and are contraindicated in children. Absorbents, such as kaolin and pectin (Kaopectate), may create more formed stools but may not actually cause a reduction in fluid loss or duration of the diarrhea. Antisecretory agents, such as bismuth subsalicylate (Pepto-Bismol), can increase intestinal sodium and water reabsorption and block the effects of enterotoxins. Antimotility agents, such as loperamide (Imodium) and diphenoxylate plus atropine (Lomotil), work by decreasing intestinal motility and reducing the distention that causes cramping and pain associated with gastroenteritis. Side effects include drowsiness, tachycardia, and ileus. Antimotility agents should be avoided in infants and used cautiously, if at all, in older children or adults because they can increase the morbidity associated with certain bacterial diseases, such as shigellosis.

VACCINES

Two vaccines for rotavirus are currently approved by the FDA. Rota Teq (RV5), a pentavalent vaccine, is dosed orally at 2, 4, and 6 months of age. A monovalent vaccine, Rotarix (RV1), is given orally in two doses 1 to 2 months apart.

SPECIAL CONSIDERATIONS
Food-Borne Gastroenteritis

• The etiology of food-borne gastroenteritis includes viruses, such as Norovirus; bacteria, such as *Salmonella typhi*, Campylobacter, *Staphylococcus aureus*, and their enterotoxins; as well as some parasites, such as *Giardia lamblia*. These illnesses are usually associated with ingestion of undercooked meats, contaminated seafood or water, or foods left unrefrigerated. Because most cases of food-borne gastroenteritis resolve with supportive care alone, an extensive workup may be unnecessary except for public health concerns; if one suspects botulism, which requires therapy with a specific antibody to the neurotoxin; or for patients who exhibit signs of extreme toxicity. Prophylaxis for travelers' diarrhea can be accomplished in limited clinical circumstances using some quinolones, rifaximin, or bismuth subsalicylate.

• **Patients with AIDS** commonly have gastrointestinal symptoms that may be caused by an array of agents such as *Salmonella, Mycobacterium avium, Cytomegalovirus, Cryptosporidium, Isospora belli,* and *Campylobacter jejuni.* They are also at risk for *Clostridium difficile* infection as a result of frequent antibiotic use. Therapy should be focused on the treatable causes of the diarrhea and the therapeutic measures that alleviate morbidity, such as the previously discussed antidiarrheal agents. Attention should also be paid to prevention of the spread of gastrointestinal infection, especially in hospitalized patients where there is potential for fecal–oral transmission of enteric pathogens.

BIBLIOGRAPHY

1. Centers for Disease Control and Prevention. CDC-INFO. Atlanta, GA: Centers for Disease Control and Prevention. http://www.cdc.gov/rotavirus/index.html
2. Wendy B, Andrew S. Acute Diarrhea. *Am Fam Physician.* 2014;89(3):181
3. American Academy of Pediatrics. Rotavirus Infections. In: Peter G, ed. *Red Book: Report of the Committee on Infectious Disease.* 24th ed. Elk Grove Village, IL: American Academy of Pediatrics; 1997:626-628.
4. Glass R, Parashar UD. The promise of new rotavirus vaccines. *N Engl J Med* 2006:354(1):75–77
5. Rotavirus/Vaccines.Gov. http://vaccines.gov/diseases/rotavirus.%202013.
6. Smith PD. Infectious diarrheas in patients with AIDS. *Gastroenterol Clin North Am* 1993;22:535.

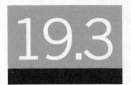

19.3 Epstein–Barr Virus Infections

Arwa Nasir

GENERAL PRINCIPLES

Definition

The Epstein–Barr virus (EBV) is a double-stranded DNA virus from the herpes virus family (also known as herpes virus 4). The major target tissue for EBV is the lymphatic system, specifically the B lymphocytes and epithelial cells.

The most common clinical syndrome associated with EBV is infectious mononucleosis (IM).

EBV is also associated with several other clinical conditions that include lymphomas (most notably Burkitt lymphoma and Hodgkin and non-Hodgkin lymphomas) and various epithelial malignancies (most commonly nasopharyngeal and gastric carcinoma). In the immune compromised host, EBV can cause various complex immunoproliferative syndromes.

Epidemiology

Humans are the only natural hosts of EBV. Like all herpes viruses, EBV has a latency phase, and often remains in the body after the acute infection. It is transmitted during acute infection via body fluids, most commonly saliva. It can also be transmitted through blood transfusion or organ transplantation. Transmission is common in families and in group settings such as dormitories where close personal contact is common. The incubation period following natural infection is 4 to 7 weeks. EBV is excreted intermittently in the saliva for long periods after infection.

In developing countries, and among lower socioeconomic groups, 90% of children have positive antibody titers by age 6. In higher socioeconomic conditions, only 40% to 50% of adolescents show evidence of prior infection.

Diagnosis

Clinical findings of IM result from the viral invasion of epithelial and lymphatic tissues and the resulting immune response.

Among younger children, infections are often asymptomatic, or produce mild nonspecific symptoms. Adolescents and adults often display more typical and severe symptoms.

Physical findings include fever, exudative pharyngitis, tonsillar enlargement, cervical or generalized lymphadenopathy, and splenomegaly. Hepatomegaly is less common, but laboratory evidence of hepatitis is present in the majority of patients. Skin rashes are observed in some patients. A characteristic morbilliform rash commonly occurs if a patient with IM is treated with penicillin or penicillin derivatives.

In more severe cases, patients present with clinical manifestations such as meningitis, encephalitis, hemolytic anemia, agranulocytosis, pneumonia, or myocarditis.

Complications

1. Splenic rupture is an uncommon but potentially fatal complication of IM. It is more common in adolescents than in younger children, and occurs without traumatic injury in half of patients with IM who suffer this complication.
2. Airway obstruction secondary to Waldeyer ring hypertrophy and surrounding tissue edema is more common in younger children, and can potentially lead to airway compromise.
3. Dehydration due to decreased oral intake.
4. Chronic fatigue syndrome occurs in fewer than 10% of patients.
5. Neurologic complications occur in about 5% of patients and include Guillain–Barre syndrome, transverse myelitis, cranial nerve palsy, peripheral neuropathy, and cerebellar ataxia.
6. Disseminated infections and lymphomas are rare complications, and may occur in both immune compromised and apparently immune competent patients.
7. "Alice in Wonderland" syndrome has been described in younger children and consists of distortion of perception of sizes and shapes and spatial relations of objects. It is usually transient.

Laboratory Findings

Serum from patients with IM contains IgM "the heterophile antigen," which causes the agglutination of horse RBCs. This phenomenon is the basis for the "Monospot" test, which has a high specificity for detecting infection. The Monospot test is often negative in young children less than 4 years of age. In early infection, or among patients with a negative Monospot test, when clinical suspicion persists, serum testing for IgM and IgG against EBV viral capsid antigen is sensitive and specific for confirmation of infection. While IgM levels wane about 3 months after infection, IgG typically persists for life.

Total WBC counts may be increased or decreased in the first week of infection. Atypical lymphocytes or Downey cells are characteristic of IM. Atypical lymphocytes are seen less commonly in younger children.

Differential Diagnosis

• Other viral infections, such as cytomegalovirus.
• Streptococcal pharyngitis.
• Lymphoma or hematologic disorders (especially with abnormal WBC counts).

Treatment

• **Supportive care:** pain control, hydration, rest, and avoidance of contact sports.
• Although evidence is lacking to support the use of systemic steroids in IM, they are occasionally used in severe cases, especially in hospitalized patients with significant airway narrowing. Corticosteroids are not necessary in mild uncomplicated cases and should not be administered to all patients with IM.
• Antiviral therapy is not recommended.

Counseling and Patient Education

1. The disease is self-limited.
2. Hydration, fever management, rest, and avoidance of contact sports are the mainstays of treatment.
3. Avoid sharing secretions to prevent spreading the virus.
4. Follow up to ensure splenomegaly is resolving before resuming vigorous activity and contact sports.

REFERENCES

1. Katz B. Epstein-Barr virus infections mononucleosis and lymphoproliferative disorders. In: Long S, Pickering L, Prober C, eds. *Principles and practice of pediatric infectious diseases.* Philadelphia, PA: Churchill Livingstone-Elsevier; 2008:1036–1044.
2. Jenson HB. Acute complications of Epstein-Barr virus infectious mononucleosis. *Curr Opin Pediatr* 2000;12(3):263–268.
3. Rinderknecht AS, Pomerantz WJ. Spontaneous splenic rupture in infectious mononucleosis: case report and review of the literature. *Pediatr Emerg Care* 2012;28(12):1377–1379.
4. Connelly KP, DeWitt LD. Neurologic complications of infectious mononucleosis. *Pediatr Neurol* 1994;10(3):181–184.
5. Jenson H. Epstein-Barr virus. In: Kleigman RM, Stanton BF, St Geme J, et al., eds. *Nelson textbook of pediatrics.* Philadelphia, PA: Elsevier; 2011.

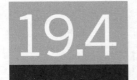

19.4 Human Immunodeficiency Virus Infections and the Acquired Immunodeficiency Syndrome

Paul E. Lyons

GENERAL PRINCIPLES

Human immunodeficiency virus (HIV) is a retrovirus that infects human lymphocytes and other cells, causing progressive immune dysfunction resulting in acquired immunodeficiency syndrome (AIDS). AIDS is characterized by opportunistic infections, malignancies, and other clinical manifestations. Without treatment, the latency period from initial HIV infection to the development of AIDS may be as long as a decade. Within 1 year of HIV diagnosis, one-third of patients will be diagnosed with AIDS, suggesting a significant lag between infection and diagnosis.

Epidemiology

According to the CDC, over 1 million persons in the United States are living with HIV. There are approximately 50,000 new infections and 30,000 deaths per year. Approximately 20% of HIV-infected individuals are unaware they are infected. Risk factors associated with an increased risk for HIV include intravenous drug use, unprotected/at-risk sexual activity, occupational exposures, and maternal HIV status (for newborns). Physician-initiated discussion of safe sex and drug use are appropriate at well-adolescent and health care maintenance visits, and may influence patient behavior. The United States Preventive Services Task Force (USPSTF) recommends that all pregnant patients (and those considering pregnancy) should be encouraged to undergo screening as a routine part of preconception/prenatal care or at the time of labor if not previously tested. USPSTF also recommends routine screening for all individuals 15 to 65 years old.

DIAGNOSIS

HIV Testing

HIV testing should be offered to all patients, especially those with a history of injection drug use or high-risk sexual activity. A positive screening (immunoassay) test result is confirmed by Western blot or other specific test. Immunoassay tests of blood samples can be positive as soon as 3 weeks following infection. HIV infection is generally considered to have been ruled out with a final negative test at 6 months. Direct viral detection may be indicated in some circumstances, especially in patients with suspected acute HIV infection.

- **Initial history** should be comprehensive, highlighting concomitant infections—sexually transmitted diseases, tuberculosis (TB), hepatitis, and opportunistic infections—travel, drug allergies, illicit drug use, and psychiatric illness, and, for women, Pap smears, and past pregnancies. Social history should assess the impact of infection on support systems, work history, etc. Review of systems for fever, night sweats, recurrent oral or vaginal candidiasis, diarrhea, lymphadenopathy, and dermatitis may help in disease staging, as may physical examination of the mouth, skin, lymph nodes, and abdomen. Particular attention should be paid to history of AIDS-related conditions, including recurrent/diffuse zoster, esophageal candidiasis, invasive cervical cancer, Kaposi sarcoma (KS), or chronic herpes simplex.
- **Laboratory screening.** A complete blood cell count and platelet count, renal and liver chemistries, fasting glucose and lipid panel, albumin, as well as syphilis and hepatitis B and C serologies should be obtained. Baseline CD4 lymphocyte count and viral load (VL) should be determined with two measurements. Genotypic resistance testing should be obtained at baseline. Skin testing for TB should be performed annually. Cervical Pap smears should be performed every 6 months for the first year, then annually if normal.

MANAGEMENT

Management of HIV-infected patients. With the advent of potent combination antiretroviral therapy (ART), HIV is becoming a chronic disease necessitating long-term care for many patients. There are currently over two dozen distinct HIV drugs with the FDA identifying 36 uniquely branded medications or combination pills. Expert consultation is encouraged for clinicians with limited experience in managing HIV disease.

Antiretroviral Therapy

According to the National Institute of Allergy and Infectious Disease (NIAID), antiretroviral agents can be identified in six distinct drug types based on where in the HIV replication cycle they act: (a) entry inhibitors, (b) fusion inhibitors, (c) nucleoside reverse transcriptase inhibitors (NRTIs), (d) nonnucleoside reverse transcriptase inhibitors (NNRTIs), (e) integrase inhibitors, and (f) protease inhibitors (PIs). There are also a number of multiclass combination products. Potent regimens have been shown to suppress viral replication, elevate CD4 cells, decrease transmission, and reconstitute the immune system. Historically, treatment initiation was dependent on three factors: HIV-related symptoms, CD4 count, and VL. With increasing evidence of the benefit of early treatment in modifying disease course and reducing transmission, guidelines are evolving toward less reliance on CD4 counts as a key indicator for initiation of therapy. The 2013 World Health Organization (WHO) consolidated guidelines suggest the use of combination ART for all patients with CD4 ≤500. Regardless of CD4 count, these guidelines recommend ART for all children up to 5 years old, patients with active TB or hepatitis B, and any patient in a serodiscordant partnership. Combination therapy with three agents from two classes of drugs is the standard of care for initial therapy. Second- and third-line regimens, typically chosen in the case of viral resistance, are increasingly difficult to tolerate. Optimal regimens balance potency with tolerability in order to promote maximum adherence. Complex drug interactions with and among antiretroviral agents should be recognized and addressed. Genotypic and phenotypic resistance testing may also be helpful in designing an optimal antiretroviral regimen.[1,2]

- **NRTIs.** These drugs inhibit reverse transcriptase by competing with host nucleotides. The agents in this class are zidovudine (azidothymidine, AZT; 300 mg bid), lamivudine (3TC; 150 mg bid), didanosine (ddI; 400 mg qd), abacavir (ABC; 300 mg bid), emtricitabine (FTC), and tenofovir (TDF). The WHO has recommended phasing out the use of d4T (stavudine) where possible due to toxicity associated with its use. Lactic acidosis has been identified as a rare but potentially fatal side effect of all drugs in this class. All drugs in this class have also been associated with lipodystrophy. Common side effects include gastrointestinal (GI) intolerance with AZT and ddI; peripheral neuropathy with ddI, ddC, and d4T; pancreatitis with ddI; and bone marrow suppression with AZT. ABC can cause a potentially fatal hypersensitivity reaction characterized by fever, rash, nausea, and malaise. Patients who have discontinued ABC should not be rechallenged with this agent.
- **NNRTIs.** These drugs inhibit reverse transcriptase by binding to it and changing its shape. The agents in this class are nevirapine [NVP] (Viramune; 200 mg bid), efavirenz [EFV] (Sustiva; 600 mg qd), delavirdine [DLV] (Rescriptor; 400 mg tid), rilpivirine (Edurant; 25 mg po qd), and etravirine (Intelence; 200 mg po bid). Rash (including occasional Stevens–Johnson syndrome) and increased transaminase levels are common class side effects. EFV can cause central nervous system (CNS) side effects. These drugs all affect the P450 system, so drug interactions must be considered.
- **PIs.** These drugs inhibit protease, thereby preventing formation of new virus. The agents in this class are saquinavir (Invirase, not recommended as a single protease inhibitor), indinavir (Crixivan 800 mg q8h), ritonavir (Norvir, 600 mg bid), and nelfinavir (1,250 mg bid). Lopinavir (Norvir) is a second-generation protease inhibitor formulated as Kaletra in combination with ritonavir and dosed at 400/100 mg bid. Additional agents in this class include tipranavir (Aptivus; 500 mg bid with ritonavir 200 mg bid), fosamprenavir (Lexiva; 700 to 1,400 mg bid), darunavir (Prezista; 800 mg po qd with ritonavir 100 mg po qd), and atazanavir (Reyataz; 300 mg po qd with ritonavir 100 mg po qd). Class side effects include GI intolerance, hyperglycemia/diabetes mellitus, fat redistribution, hyperlipidemia, and liver function test abnormalities. Drug-specific side effects include diarrhea with nelfinavir and lopinavir, paresthesias with ritonavir and amprenavir, rash with amprenavir, and nephrolithiasis with indinavir. These drugs, especially ritonavir, can inhibit enzymes in the P450 system, so drug interactions need to be carefully considered. Sometimes these drug interactions can be employed to therapeutic advantage when using a combination of PIs.

- **Fusion inhibitors.** These drugs act to block HIV-1 entry into CD4 cells. Currently, the only medication in this class is enfuvirtide (Fuzeon; 90 mg subcutaneous bid). It is not considered first-line therapy for HIV infection.
- **Integrase inhibitors.** This class of medications inhibits HIV-1 integrase. This enzyme is required for HIV-1 replication. Medications in this class include dolutegravir (Tivicay; 50 mg po qd) and raltegravir (Isentress; 400 mg po bid).
- **Entry inhibitors** are also known as CCR5 antagonists. This class of medications blocks CCR5—a protein necessary for HIV-1 entry into CD4 cells. One medication is currently marketed in this class, maraviroc (Selzentry; 300 mg po bid).

Immunizations

Influenza and pneumococcal vaccines are recommended. Hepatitis B vaccine is indicated for hepatitis B–seronegative patients. Live virus vaccines are generally contraindicated in patients with AIDS but should not be withheld when indicated in less immunocompromised patients. The use of measles–mumps–rubella (MMR) vaccine is not contraindicated in patients who are not severely immunocompromised.

Prophylaxis Against Opportunistic Infections

Prophylaxis against *Pneumocystis carinii* pneumonia (PCP) is indicated when the CD4 count falls to less than 200 cells per mL, or following an episode of PCP.[3] Trimethoprim–sulfamethoxazole (TMP–SMX), one double-strength (DS) tablet daily, is the drug of choice; alternatives include single-strength (SS) TMP–SMX, TMP–SMX DS three times weekly, dapsone—check for glucose-6-phosphate dehydrogenase (G6PD) deficiency before administering—with or without pyrimethamine, or inhaled pentamidine if no other options are available. Toxoplasmosis prophylaxis is indicated for patients with positive *Toxoplasma* titers who have a CD4 count less than 100. TMP–SMX is an effective prophylactic agent against *Toxoplasma gondii*; alternative prophylaxis is usually with dapsone plus pyrimethamine and folinic acid (Leucovorin). Prophylaxis against *Mycobacterium avium complex* (MAC) disease is indicated for a CD4 count less than 50; clarithromycin and azithromycin are the preferred agents. Increasing evidence suggests that prophylaxis against these illnesses can be safely discontinued in individuals who respond to combination ART, with a sustained rise in their CD4 count greater than the CD4 thresholds noted above.

COMPLICATIONS OF HIV DISEASE
Systemic

- **Fungal infections** with *Cryptococcus neoformans*, *Histoplasma capsulatum*, *Blastomyces dermatitidis*, and *Coccidioides immitis*, often with disseminated disease in blood, bone marrow, liver, spleen, and CNS, require management with amphotericin B and/or oral azole drugs (itraconazole, fluconazole).
- **MAC disseminated infection** typically presents with progressively worsening constitutional symptoms such as fevers, night sweats, and weight loss in patients with CD4 counts less than 50. Bone marrow involvement is common. MAC is generally managed with ethambutol plus either clarithromycin or azithromycin; rifabutin, ciprofloxacin, or amikacin can be added for severe infections.
- ***Mycobacterium tuberculosis* infection** (TB) can occur early or late in the course of HIV disease. With advanced HIV disease, disseminated TB is more common than the localized pulmonary form. TB involving the bone marrow, GI tract, pericardium, CNS, or lungs is most common. Initial treatment with a four-drug regimen, including isoniazid, pyrazinamide, ethambutol, and rifampin or rifabutin for the first 2 months, is generally recommended, followed by an additional 7 months of therapy based on sensitivity results.[1,4] Directly observed therapy should be considered if compliance is a concern. Potentially dangerous drug interactions between rifampin and some antiretroviral agents often require substitution of rifabutin for rifampin. Guidelines regarding the treatment of tuberculosis, especially HIV-related tuberculosis, change frequently; updated CDC guidelines on the management of comorbid tuberculosis and HIV disease can be found at http://www.cdc.gov (also see Chapter 10.4).
- **Weight loss and wasting** are common in AIDS. Opportunistic infections and malignancies, inadequate oral intake, chronic diarrhea, and depression can accelerate the wasting process. Consultation with a nutritionist can be helpful. Megestrol and tetrahydrocannabinol can promote increase in weight by improving appetite; resistance exercise training has shown benefit in increasing lean body mass. Growth hormone can also increase lean body mass, but it is expensive and the safety of its long-term use is unclear.[5]

- **KS**, although typically confined to the dermis, can involve the viscera as well (see below).
- **Hematologic** complications of HIV infection commonly include leukopenia, anemia, and, less commonly, thrombocytopenia. Destruction of CD4 cells; HIV-mediated disruption of the hematopoietic system; low erythropoietin levels; anemia of chronic disease; and bone marrow suppression by HIV-related medications, opportunistic infections (such as MAC or B19 parvovirus), or malignancies should all be considered in the differential diagnosis of hematologic abnormalities. Treatment is generally directed at the underlying cause; granulocyte colony-stimulating factor can be used for significant neutropenia (absolute neutrophil count less than 500).
- **Skin disease.** KS typically presents as raised or flat violaceous lesions on the skin and/or hard palate (see below). Sometimes a biopsy is needed to distinguish KS from bacillary angiomatosis, which results from *Bartonella henselae* infection. Perioral and anogenital recurrent herpes simplex virus (HSV) infections are treated with oral acyclovir; intravenous acyclovir or foscarnet can be used for refractory or resistant infections. Herpes zoster infection confined to one or two dermatomes is treated with oral acyclovir, but disseminated infections or those involving the eye should be treated with IV acyclovir. Staphylococcal folliculitis and seborrheic dermatitis are more common in HIV infection. Cutaneous reactions to medications are also common, including maculopapular or urticarial rashes, erythema multiforme, fixed drug eruptions, or more severe reactions such as the Stevens–Johnson syndrome or toxic epidermal necrolysis.
- **Oral cavity diseases** include candidiasis (thrush), KS, hairy leukoplakia, aphthous ulcers, and periodontal disease. Thrush can appear as erythematous patches or white plaques. Treatment with topical clotrimazole is usually effective, but systemic treatment with ketoconazole or fluconazole is sometimes required. Oral and esophageal aphthous ulcers often respond to prednisone; thalidomide has shown benefit for these conditions as well.
- **Eye disease.** Cytomegalovirus (CMV) retinitis occurs in persons with advanced HIV disease (CD4 <50). Patients may note floaters, visual defects, or frank peripheral or central vision loss. Induction therapy with IV ganciclovir or foscarnet, followed by maintenance therapy with IV or oral ganciclovir or IV foscarnet, can be effective in halting or slowing disease progression. Current guidelines recommend oral valganciclovir, oral or IV ganciclovir, or IV foscarnet. Ganciclovir intraocular implants are no longer marketed as of May 2013. For specific indications, intraocular ganciclovir may be indicated. *Treponema pallidum*, *Toxoplasma gondii*, and fungi may also be associated with symptomatic disease and ophthalmologic findings.
- **Pulmonary disease**
  - **PCP** most commonly occurs in patients with a CD4 count less than 200. Patients usually present with nonproductive cough, fever, and progressive dyspnea. Chest radiograph shows infiltrates or diffuse interstitial involvement but can be normal. Diagnosis is confirmed with induced sputum, bronchoalveolar lavage, or biopsy specimens. The treatment of choice is TMP–SMX; adjuvant prednisone therapy improves survival in patients with a PaO_2 of less than 70 mmHg. Second-line therapies for PCP include intravenous pentamidine, dapsone and trimethoprim, dapsone and trimetrexate, or clindamycin and primaquine.
  - **Bacterial pneumonia.** *Mycobacterium tuberculosis* (TB) can occur at any stage in the course of HIV disease. Pulmonary infiltrates should be carefully evaluated for TB because of the severity of its course in HIV-infected persons, and significant public health implications. Typical bacterial pneumonias, especially those caused by *Streptococcus pneumoniae*, *Haemophilus influenzae*, and *Staphylococcus aureus*, are common in HIV disease. Standard antibiotic therapy is usually effective.
  - **Fungal infections.** Pulmonary involvement with *Cryptococcus*, *Histoplasmosis*, *Aspergillus*, *Blastomyces*, or *Coccidioides*, while not as common as PCP or bacterial pneumonias, should be considered in patients with low CD4 counts.
  - **KS** can cause pulmonary disease, occasionally without dermal lesions. Radiographs characteristically show reticulonodular interstitial disease with pleural effusions.

GI Disease

- **Candidal esophagitis** causes dysphagia, odynophagia, and retrosternal pain. Response to empirical therapy with fluconazole or ketoconazole establishes the diagnosis and avoids endoscopic evaluation. Treatable HSV and CMV infections, which can cause painful ulcerations, are identified by endoscopic biopsy. Aphthous ulcers have a similar presentation and can be treated with prednisone and/or thalidomide.
- **Diarrhea**, often with severe weight loss, occurs in more than half of AIDS patients. Bacterial stool cultures can identify *Salmonella*, *Campylobacter*, and *Shigella* species. In patients with fever, blood

cultures should also be obtained. *Clostridium difficile* enteritis, identified by *C. difficile* antigen in stool, is managed with oral metronidazole. Stool tests for ova and parasites can reveal *Entamoeba histolytica, Giardia lamblia*, and other infectious agents that respond to usual therapies. *Cryptosporidium* infection produces watery diarrhea, abdominal pain, nausea, and vomiting; treatment with paromomycin or azithromycin might help, but the most effective intervention appears to be potent ART. Symptomatic control of diarrhea with diphenoxylate hydrochloride with atropine, loperamide, tincture of opium, or octreotide can be helpful. Sigmoidoscopy with biopsy and culture is indicated when results of initial stool studies are negative. CMV enterocolitis is often accompanied by diarrhea, weight loss, abdominal pain, fever, and anorexia, and can lead to severe complications such as perforation. Ganciclovir and foscarnet provide limited benefit.

Neurologic Disease

- *Cryptococcus neoformans* causes meningoencephalitis in 6% to 10% of AIDS patients, usually in patients with a CD4 count less than 100. The most common symptoms are fever, headache, and altered mental status. Meningeal signs and symptoms are uncommon. Serum and cerebrospinal fluid cryptococcal antigen is positive in 95% and 90% of patients, respectively. Acute treatment with amphotericin B for at least 2 weeks, usually in combination with flucytosine, and followed by fluconazole for 8 to 10 weeks is recommended. Patients with mild disease, low cerebrospinal fluid titers, and normal mental status can be treated initially with fluconazole alone. Lifetime maintenance therapy with fluconazole is currently recommended to prevent reoccurrence of disease; the safety of discontinuing lifelong suppressive therapy against cryptococcosis in patients who enjoy a sustained immunologic response to combination ART is under investigation.
- *Toxoplasma gondii* encephalitis usually presents in patients with a CD4 count less than 100. Symptoms and signs include altered sensorium, seizures, focal motor or sensory abnormalities, cerebellar dysfunction, or neuropsychiatric manifestations. Empirical therapy is recommended for patients with multiple ring-enhancing lesions on computed tomography (CT) scans or magnetic resonance images; CNS lymphoma presents similarly and should be considered if empirical antitoxoplasmosis therapy is not effective. Treatment with pyrimethamine and folinic acid (Leukovorin) plus either clindamycin or sulfadiazine is continued for 6 to 8 weeks. Clinical or radiographic improvement can be expected within 2 to 3 weeks. Failure to respond usually indicates an evaluation for lymphoma. Maintenance therapy with pyrimethamine and clindamycin or sulfadiazine is required to prevent relapse.
- **AIDS–dementia complex** is a common condition in advanced AIDS. It is characterized by cognitive, motor, and behavioral dysfunction. Early manifestations include difficulties with concentration and memory. Eventually, performance of complex tasks becomes more difficult; slowing of thought processes and verbal response is typical. As the disease progresses, motor impairment and behavioral disturbances can become severe. The condition may respond to potent combination ART, ideally including at least two antiretroviral agents that cross the blood–brain barrier.
- **Distal symmetric polyneuropathy (DSPN)** presents as painful or burning paresthesias in a stocking-glove distribution on the extremities. It usually begins in the lower extremities but can include the upper extremities as well. DSPN is a common adverse effect of combination ART, especially to regimens including d4T and ddI, but can also be caused by HIV itself. The most effective therapeutic options include tricyclic antidepressants and gabapentin.
- **Progressive multifocal leukoencephalopathy (PML)**, caused by infection by JC virus, occurs late in the course of HIV disease. PML usually develops insidiously with a single focus (e.g., limb weakness, ataxia, visual defects) but can progress to multiple foci, delirium, seizures, and death. Prolonged survival and remission has been reported with effective combination ART.

Gynecologic Disease

Chronic vaginal candidiasis, recurrent HSV infection, and condyloma acuminatum are common. Cervical dysplasia can progress rapidly in HIV-infected women, resulting in cervical neoplasia. Pelvic inflammatory disease can be difficult to diagnose because leukocytosis is uncommon (see also Chapters 13.1 and 13.5).

Malignancies

KS is the most common AIDS-associated malignancy. Treatment modalities include radiation therapy, cryotherapy, intralesional chemotherapeutic drug injections, systemic chemotherapy, and α-interferon therapy. Non-Hodgkin lymphoma often presents at an advanced stage, behaves aggressively, and responds poorly to treatment. Primary CNS lymphoma is usually managed with radiation but can be difficult to distinguish from *T. gondii* encephalitis.

SPECIAL CONSIDERATIONS
Pregnancy and HIV

Women with advanced HIV disease are at risk for having low-birth-weight infants, prematurity, chorio-amnionitis, and fetal demise. Perinatal transmission occurs in about 25% of births unless ART is given. ART during pregnancy, labor, and delivery and for the newborn during the first weeks of life can decrease the risk of perinatal transmission. Combination ART may decrease transmission, promote maternal health, and may clear infection in newborns.[1,6] An appropriate regimen can be chosen with the help of an expert consultant. Invasive procedures that might promote transmission, such as fetal scalp monitoring, scalp sampling, and episiotomy, should be utilized only when clearly indicated. Cesarean section should be offered to all HIV-infected women with a VL greater than 1,000 but has increased morbidity in HIV-positive women. Breastfeeding is contraindicated because it promotes transmission of HIV.

HIV in Children

Because neonates acquire maternal HIV antibody that is transplacentally transmitted, an HIV DNA polymerase chain reaction test, repeated at designated intervals, is necessary to diagnose HIV in most infants by 4 months of age.[7] Common early manifestations of HIV infection in children include oral candidiasis, lymphadenopathy, hepatosplenomegaly, fever, diarrhea, recurrent bacterial infections, failure to thrive, and developmental delay.

REFERENCES

1. Guidelines for the use of antiretroviral agents in HIV-1 infected adolescents and adults. http://aidsinfo.nih.gov. Accessed March 28, 2014.
2. Hirsch MS, Brun-Vezinet F, D'Aquila RT, et al. Antiretroviral drug resistance testing in adult HIV-1 infection. *JAMA* 2000;283:2417–2444.
3. U.S. Centers for Disease Control and Prevention. 2002 USPHS/IDSA guidelines for the prevention of opportunistic infections in HIV-infected adults and adolescents. http://aidsinfo.nih.gov. Accessed July 8, 2013.
4. U.S. Centers for Disease Control and Prevention. Prevention and treatment of tuberculosis among patients infected with human immunodeficiency virus: principles of therapy and revised recommendations. *MMWR* 1998;47(No. RR-20):1–58.
5. Goldschmidt RH, Dong BJ. Treatment of AIDS and HIV-related conditions: 2000. *J Am Board Fam Pract* 2000;13:274–298.
6. Public Health Service Task Force recommendations for the use of antiretroviral drugs in pregnant HIV-1 infected women for maternal health and interventions to reduce perinatal HIV-1 transmission in the United States. http://aidsinfo.nih.gov. Accessed November 17, 2005.
7. Guidelines for the use of antiretroviral agents in pediatric HIV infection. http://aidsinfo.nih.gov. Accessed November 6, 2013.

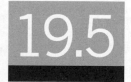

19.5 Syphilis
Mark Duane Goodman

GENERAL PRINCIPLES
Definition

Brought from the New World to Europe in 1495 by Columbus's sailors, syphilis has influenced human misery, morality and medical policy to this very day. The name "Syphilis" is given to a shepherd who defied Apollo in a poem by Girolamo Fracastoro in 1530. The spirochete *Treponema pallidum* is finally discovered as the causative organism in 1905. In 1908, arsenic is touted as the first therapy, and in 1927 the Nobel Prize for medicine is granted to Julius Wagner for developing therapeutic fever for neurosyphilis by inducing malaria. In the 1940s, penicillin becomes the primary treatment for syphilis, which remains true to this day. Along the way, syphilis modifies fashion (in high society, makeup and beauty spots concealed syphilitic skin lesions), physician–patient relationships (confidentiality in modern medicine has its roots in the treatment of syphilis), art, literature, and war.

Epidemiology

The Centers for Disease Control and Prevention (CDC) have reported a steady increase in the incidence of syphilis since 2000, largely among men who have sex with men. In the United States, nearly 50,000 new cases are discovered annually.

Etiology

T. pallidum is a thin, motile spirochete bacterium. Impossible to culture outside of the host (as of yet), infection is determined by visualization of host material, or by a variety of antibody tests.

Classification and Physical Findings

Incubation period can range from 10 to 90 days, typically 3 weeks.

Primary Syphilis

An average incubation period of 3 weeks is followed by the appearance of a painless skin lesion known as a *chancre* (papules that ulcerate), which lasts 3 to 90 days at the site of inoculation, which can be on the external genitals, vagina, anus, rectum, lips, and in the mouth.

Secondary Syphilis

A secondary bacteremia develops 2 weeks to 2 months after the appearance of the chancre. It is usually associated with systemic signs, such as generalized skin rash, mucocutaneous lesions, and lymphadenopathy. Relapses of secondary syphilis in untreated patients are not uncommon. The rash usually does not cause itching, and may appear as red or red-brown spots often on the palms and soles (salmon-colored patches). Large raised gray-white lesions may also develop in warm moist areas of the mouth, skin folds, and groin. Other symptoms include fever, lymphadenopathy, pharyngitis, patchy hair loss, weight loss, myalgias, and fatigue.

Latent Syphilis

- **Early:** Subclinical infection is believed to have begun within 1 year. Infection is reported if seroconversion or fourfold increase in non-treponemal titer, seroconversion on a treponemal test, and history consistent with primary or secondary syphilis or sexual contact only within the last 12 months are documented.
- **Late:** Subclinical infection is believed to have been more than 1 year ago.

Tertiary Syphilis

Tertiary syphilis can include:

- **Cardiovascular syphilis:** aortitis, aortic aneurysms.
- **Gummas:** local destruction of skin and bones and neurologic involvement.
- **Neurosyphilis:** Neurosyphilis is syphilis infection of the nervous system: it can occur at ANY stage of infection, and should be reported by stage of infection "with neurologic manifestations." Appearing 10 to 30 years after infection, 15% of untreated patients can develop symptoms of incoordination, paralysis, numbness, blindness, and dementia. Signs can include Argyll-Robertson pupils (react to accommodation, but not to light), tabes dorsalis (destruction of the dorsal roots of the spinal column) with a characteristic steppage gait, seizures, incontinence, and early death.
- **Congenital syphilis:** A pregnant woman with syphilis can pass the disease to her unborn baby. Babies born with syphilis can have profound health problems, which may include pregnancy complications (low birth weight, premature delivery, and stillbirth) and postnatal health problems (cataracts; deafness; seizures; and physical manifestations such as Hutchinson teeth, nasal bridge deformities, and frontal bossing).

DIAGNOSIS

Laboratory Studies

Direct visualization of *T. pallidum* by darkfield examination or direct fluorescent antibody tests of biopsied lesions is the gold standard of diagnosis. However, interpretation requires considerable expertise, and most often indirect methods of diagnosis, such as serologic tests, are employed.

Non-Treponemal Tests

- Venereal disease research laboratory (VDRL) and rapid plasma reagin (RPR)
- VDRL and RPR tests have sensitivities of 78% and 86%, respectively, and are used for screening. They become positive 4 to 6 weeks after infection and 1 to 3 weeks after the appearance of the

primary lesion. The titers correlate well with the disease activity, and can be used to measure response to treatment, but can be falsely negative at the very early or late stage, initially due to developing antibody response and later due to waning antibody response. Common causes of false positives are viral infections (hepatitis), pregnancy, malignancy, immunizations, connective tissue disorders (rheumatoid and lupus), and intravenous drug use.

Treponemal Tests
- PCR (polymerase chain reaction)
- TPPA (*T. pallidum* particle agglutination)
- CIA (chemiluminescence immunoassay)
- FTA-ABS (fluorescent antibody)
- MHA-TP (micro-hemagglutination assay-*T. pallidum*)
- Confirm a positive VDRL or RPR. MHA-TP is positive in 76% of patients with primary syphilis, and the FTA-ABS is positive in 84%. Compared with non-treponemal tests, treponemal tests may become positive earlier in the course of the infection. These tests do not correlate well with disease activity and should not be used to monitor treatment response. The FTA-ABS remains positive for life in most people despite treatment.

For the diagnosis of **neurosyphilis**, cerebrospinal fluid (CSF) evaluation is required.

- CSF examination is indicated for any patients with neurologic or ophthalmic symptoms or signs potentially attributable to syphilis. Other indications for CSF evaluation include tertiary syphilis without neurologic symptoms, treatment failure, and HIV coinfection, according to some experts. All children with syphilis should have a CSF examination to exclude neurosyphilis, with a review of birth and maternal medical records to determine whether syphilis was acquired perinatally.
- When CSF evaluation is performed, it should include determination of protein and glucose levels, cell count, and VDRL.
- An elevated CSF leukocyte count (more than five white blood cells per mm^2), a CSF protein measurement greater than 40 mg per dL (40 mg per L), and low CSF glucose levels are consistent with neurosyphilis. The CSF should not be tested routinely for RPR nor treponema-specific antibodies (MHA-TP or FTA-ABS), because false-positive tests occur frequently.

The workup for **congenital syphilis** should include a complete blood count with differential, CSF analysis for VDRL, cell count and protein, and other tests as indicated, such as long bone radiography, chest radiography, liver function testing, cranial ultrasonography, ophthalmologic examination, and auditory brainstem response.

A diagnosis can be confirmed when *T. pallidum* has been identified from darkfield microscopy or fluorescent antibody test of lesions, placenta, umbilical cord, or any other tissue from the infant.

A presumptive diagnosis can be made in any infant whose mother had untreated or inadequately treated syphilis at delivery, regardless of symptoms or signs in the infant, or in any infant or child who has a reactive specific treponemal test for syphilis *and* any of the following: evidence of congenital syphilis on physical examination; evidence of congenital syphilis on long bone radiographs; reactive CSF VDRL; elevated CSF cell count or protein (without other cause); or reactive test for FTA-ABS-IgM using fractional serum.

Differential Diagnosis

For primary syphilis, the differential diagnosis for a genital ulcer includes genital herpes (usually painful with a red base), chancroid (typically painful), and trauma. The presentation of secondary and tertiary syphilis can be similar to a wide array of inflammatory and infectious syndromes. Neurosyphilis must be considered in the workup of any neurologic condition.

TREATMENT
Medications

Parenteral penicillin G (Bicillin L-A) is the drug of choice for management of all stages of syphilis. The **Jarisch–Herxheimer** reaction (fever, hypotension, headache, and myalgias) can occur within 24 hours after appropriate therapy, particularly in patients with early syphilis. This reaction is thought to be the result of an inflammatory response to the destruction of *Treponema*. It can be treated symptomatically with antipyretics, but there is no known preventive treatment. Patients should be advised that this is not a manifestation of penicillin allergy.

Treatment for **primary, secondary**, and **early latent syphilis**:

- **Adults:** benzathine penicillin G, 2.4 million units IM in a single dose.
- **Children:** benzathine penicillin G, 50,000 units per kg (up to the adult dose) IM in a single dose.[1]

Treatment for **late latent syphilis**:

- **Adults:** benzathine penicillin G, 2.4 million units IM every week for 3 weeks.
  - For penicillin-allergic nonpregnant adults, doxycycline 100 mg twice daily for 2 weeks or tetracycline 500 mg four times day for 4 weeks.
- Children are given benzathine penicillin G, 50,000 units per kg (up to the adult dose) IM every week for 3 weeks.

Treatment for **tertiary syphilis**:

- **Adults:** benzathine penicillin G, 2.4 million units IM every week for 3 weeks.
  - For penicillin-allergic nonpregnant adults, doxycycline 100 mg twice daily for 2 weeks or tetracycline 500 mg four times day for 2 weeks.

For **neurosyphilis,** the treatment regimen is as follows:

- Aqueous crystalline penicillin G, 18 to 24 million units daily (2 to 4 million units every 4 hours) for 10 to 14 days, followed by benzathine penicillin G, 2.4 million units IM weekly for 3 weeks.

For **congenital syphilis,** the treatment regimen is as follows:

- Aqueous crystalline penicillin G, 50,000 units/kg/dose IV every 8 to 12 hours for 10 to 14 days; *or* procaine penicillin G 50,000 units/kg/dose IM per day in a single dose for 10 days.
- Treatment for congenital syphilis is recommended in the absence of confirmatory serologic testing when the mother has untreated syphilis; when the mother has a fourfold or greater increase in non-treponemal titer; when she was treated with erythromycin or other non-penicillin regimen during pregnancy; or if she was treated for syphilis within the month prior to delivery.

For **penicillin-allergic patients,** the treatment regimen is as follows:

- For penicillin-allergic nonpregnant adults, doxycycline 100 mg twice daily for 2 weeks or tetracycline 500 mg four times day for 2 weeks for primary, secondary, and early latent syphilis. Extend treatment to 4 weeks total if treating tertiary syphilis.
- Penicillin-allergic pregnant women, patients with neurosyphilis, and HIV-infected patients and children, should undergo penicillin desensitization orally or intravenously, and be treated with penicillin. The procedure should be treated as a potential medical emergency, and be carried out in a supervised medical setting.

Patient Education and Counseling

Health education and prevention services are imperative to combat the spread of syphilis. Patients should be advised that the highest risk of syphilis transmission is unprotected sex with one who has multiple partners. Other risk factors include sexual activity that occurs in exchange for drugs, high-risk sexual activity among adolescents, men who have sex with men, and sexual behavior in correctional facilities. Intimacy decisions made with under the influence of alcohol or drugs can increase the likelihood of transmission of sexually transmitted infections, including syphilis. HIV infection is two to five times higher in the presence of mucosal lesions, including syphilitic chancres.

Follow-Up and Monitoring

No studies have established the absolute laboratory criteria for successful therapy. However, evidence from large epidemiologic studies suggests obtaining serum VDRL or RPR titers at 6, 12, and 24 months after treatment. The titers are both qualitative and quantitative and can be ensued to monitor response to treatment. The tests are not interchangeable. The test that is used initially must be used for subsequent testing. It is expected that patients will become nonreactive following treatment; however, some patients demonstrate a **serofast** reaction, maintaining persistently low titers for life (usually 1:8 or less). Other causes of reactive tests post treatment include reinfection, HIV coinfection, and undiagnosed neurosyphilis.

In patients treated for **primary** and **secondary syphilis,** a fourfold decrease in antibody titers should be seen by 6 months, and those with **early latent syphilis** should have a fourfold decrease by 1 year posttreatment. In the absence of a fourfold change in titers, which is equivalent to a change of two dilutions (from 1:16 to 1:4), retreatment should be considered.

Successful treatment of **late latent** and **tertiary syphilis** should lead to a fourfold decrease by 12 to 24 months. If titers increase fourfold, fail to drop at least fourfold within 12 to 24 months, or syphilitic signs and symptoms develop, treatment should be considered a failure and retreatment considered.

For **neurosyphilis,** predicting the response to treatment is somewhat more complicated. The purpose of treatment is to arrest further disease progression, and attempt to reverse the ongoing symptoms. Patients should be monitored with CSF examination every 6 months for decreasing cell count if CSF pleocytosis was initially present. If there is no decrease in 6 months or failure to return to normal in 2 years, retreatment should be considered.

Because of the enormous public health implications, all partners of syphilis patients should be aggressively sought and offered testing and treatment. In addition, every pregnant woman should be tested for syphilis during pregnancy and at delivery, if indicated.

REFERENCES

1. Krigger KW. *Manual of family medicine*. Philadelphia, PA: Lippincott Williams & Wilkins; 2002.
2. Mandell GL, Bennett JE, Dolin R. *Bennett's principles and practice of infectious disease*. 6th ed. Philadelphia, PA: Elsevier; 2005:2773–2781.
3. Centers for Disease Control and Prevention. *STDFact-Syphilis 2-1-2014*.
4. Myint M, Bashiri H, Harrington RD, et al. Relapse of secondary syphilis after benzathine penicillin G: molecular analysis. *Sex Transm Dis* 2004;31(3):196–199.
5. Birnbaum NR, Goldschmidt RH, Buffett WO. Resolving the common dilemmas of syphilis. *Am Fam Physician* 1999;59:2233–2240.
6. Cohen J, Powderly WC. *Infectious diseases*. 2nd ed. London, England: Mosby; 2004:720.
7. Brown DL, Frank JE. Diagnosis and management of syphilis. *Am Fam Physician* 2003;68:286.
8. Dunant S. Syphilis, Sex and Fear: How the French disease conquered the world. The Guardian http://www.theguardian.com/books/2013/may/17/syphilis-sex-fear-borgias. Published May 17, 2013. Accessed March 10, 2014.

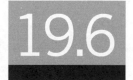

19.6 Gonorrhea
Amy E. Lacroix

GENERAL PRINCIPLES

Gonorrhea (gonococcus or "GC") continues to have both a national and worldwide burden as a well-recognized sexually transmitted infection (STI). It is the second most commonly reported notifiable disease in the United States. Efforts to identify, treat, and eliminate the infection resulted in its prevalence reaching its nadir in the United States in 1998. In recent years, however, its prevalence has increased. The U.S. prevalence as of 2012 based on CDC data was 107 cases per 100,000 people. There were over 330,000 cases reported in the United States that year. Prevalence is highest in adolescents and young adults (ages 15 to 24, with the highest rates being among 20 to 24 year olds); however, the section of the population in which the rates are increasing most rapidly are the older adult population. Rates are similar among men and women. The disease burden is borne disproportionately by the black population in the United States (20 times the prevalence of the white population). Gonococcus is a bacterium with an impressive ability to adapt, and has become resistant to many of the drugs used to treat it in the past 60 years. As resistance is increasing, treatment recommendations continue to change. Co-occurrence of Chlamydia infection continues to be common, and should always be considered.

ETIOLOGY

Neisseria gonorrhea is a fastidious, aerobic, Gram-negative, oxidase-positive coccus that occurs in pairs (diplococcus). It adheres to mucosal surfaces by means of tenacious pili. It is differentiated from *Neisseria meningitidis* by its absence of a polysaccharide capsule. Testing for GC has traditionally been done on Thayer-Martin (sheep blood) agar plates by culture, but in the last 10 years, this has largely been replaced by very sensitive and rapid nucleic acid amplification tests (NAATs). It can be recovered from many mucosal surfaces, including conjunctivae, pharynx, urethra, vagina, and rectum. It is strongly associated with the presence of white blood cells (purulent discharge), and its presence in white cells on Gram stain is also diagnostic.

CLINICAL PRESENTATION

Presenting symptoms relate to the site of infection. Dysuria or penile discharge in a sexually active male should be presumed to be an STI until proven otherwise. Asymptomatic infections occur as well, and are more common in women than in men. Clinical presentation may include exudative pharyngitis, purulent urethritis (in either men or women, though more commonly in men), vaginal discharge, pelvic pain (in women), purulent conjunctivitis, and rectal pain or discharge. Local adenopathy is common. Disseminated infections, including bacteremia, endocarditis, dermatitis, infectious arthritis, and teno-synovitis, are less common. Meningitis is rare but can occur. Arthritis tends to be mono-articular and often involve large joints. Arthritis can also be reactive.

Conjunctivitis most commonly occurs as a result of vertical maternal to infant transmission at birth. Topical application of 0.5% erythromycin ointment (neither silver nitrate nor tetracycline ophthalmic solutions are available in the United States at this time) to the eyes of newborns immediately after birth is commonly used as a prophylaxis. It may be delayed for up to 1 hour to allow for maternal infant bonding. Conjunctivitis may also be seen in adults.

The presence of any GC in prepubertal children outside of the newborn period is strongly associated with sexual abuse and should be thoroughly investigated.

TESTING

At this time, routine testing of asymptomatic men is not recommended by the U.S. Preventive Services Task Force (USPSTF). Screening is recommended in women who are at high risk (adolescents and young adults who are sexually active) and in pregnancy. Testing should be done on symptomatic patients or when patients are at high risk by virtue of exposure or known positivity for other STIs. A Gram stain performed on discharge will show intracellular Gram-negative diplococci. Urinalysis may be positive for leukocyte esterase, but is not diagnostic. Cultures will grow organisms usually within 24 to 48 hours. NAATs have become routine in diagnosis. They are rapid and very sensitive. Specificity depends on the local prevalence in the population. They are approved for use on specimens that include cervical swabs (obtained from the os), vaginal swabs, urine specimens (should NOT be clean catch), and urethral swabs. There is not a significant difference in sensitivity/specificity depending on the site from which they are obtained, so the least invasive site should be used. Self-obtained vaginal swabs from females are perfectly acceptable. NAATs have not been approved by the FDA for use in diagnosis of rectal, pharyngeal, eye infections, or pediatric infections. Locally run validation studies may facilitate their use from specimens such as these. In cases of suspected child abuse, traditional cultures should always be obtained. All positive tests must be reported to the local health department. Many local health departments have Disease Information Specialists who can follow up on positive tests and assist patients in making sure they are treated and that partners are notified and treated.

Positive testing for GC is a risk factor for acquisition of other STIs. Patients who are positive should be encouraged to obtain testing for concurrent infections, including Chlamydia (10% to 30% concurrent infection rates), Trichomonas, HIV, and syphilis. Routine vaccination to prevent Hepatitis B and Human Papilloma Virus at appropriate ages is the best prevention for those STIs and their oncologic sequelae.

Reinfection with GC is common in adolescents and young adults, and a repeat test after 3 months should be strongly considered. Anyone who is treated suboptimally (perhaps due to medication allergy) should be subsequently cultured to assure efficacy. Treatment failures should be cultured also; however, account must be taken of whether a second positive test is a failure or repeat infection.

TREATMENT

Treatment of GC should be based on a positive NAAT or culture, or positive symptoms with a known exposure to disease. Because of increasing bacterial resistance, recommended primary treatment of uncomplicated GC (pharyngitis, urethritis, cervicitis, and proctitis) in adults now includes only IM ceftriaxone 250 mg PLUS concurrent administration of either oral azithromycin 1,000 mg once or oral doxycycline 100 mg BID for 1 week. It is recommended by the CDC to treat all patients with

GC for Chlamydia, this regimen covers both infections. Pregnant patients should not be treated with tetracyclines. Quinolones and oral cephalosporins are not recommended. Test of cure is not currently recommended. Exposed partners should be tested and treated as well. Many states now have explicit laws which allow for partner treatment without establishment of care (expedited partner therapy), which is approved by the CDC and has been demonstrated to decrease disease STI prevalence.

Complicated infections should be hospitalized and treated with IV or IM ceftriaxone as per CDC guidelines. Infants born to mothers known to be infected should get a single dose of 25 to 50 mg per kg of ceftriaxone (up to a maximum of 125 mg).

REFERENCES

1. Centers for Disease Control. Gonorrhea. http://www.cdc.gov/std/stats12/gonorrhea.htm. Accessed April 10, 2014.
2. Elias J, Frosch M, Vogel U. Neisseria. In: Versalovic J, ed. *Manual of clinical microbiology*. 10th ed. Washington, DC: ASM Press; 2011:106–233.
3. United States Preventive Services Task Force. Screening for Gonorrhea: Recommendation Statement. http://www.uspreventiveservicestaskforce.org/uspstf05/gonorrhea/gonrs.htm. Accessed April 14, 2014.
4. Centers for Disease Control. Sexually Transmitted Diseases (STDs) Legal Status of Expedited Partner Therapy. http://www.cdc.gov/sTd/ept/legal/default.htm. Accessed April 14, 2014.
5. Centers for Disease Control. Sexually Transmitted Diseases (STDs) Treatment Guidelines 2010. Includes updates http://www.cdc.gov/std/treatment/2010/gonococcal-infections.htm. Accessed April 14, 2014.

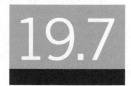

19.7 Chlamydia Infection

Kent Jian Zhao

GENERAL PRINCIPLES

Chlamydia and *Chlamydophila* species include *Chlamydia trachomatis*, *Chlamydophila* (formerly Chlamydia) *pneumonia* and *Chlamydophila* (formerly Chlamydia) *psittaci*. *C. trachomatis* is the cause of the **most commonly** reported notifiable disease in the United States. Direct medical costs of *C. trachomatis* infections were estimated at $516.7 million in 2008 ($2012). Sexually active **females 25 years old and younger, older women who have new or multiple sex partners,** and **men who have sex with men (MSM)** need **annual screening** because most infected people are **asymptomatic.** Although it is easy to cure, serious complications such as pelvic inflammatory disease (PID), tubal factor infertility, and ectopic pregnancy can happen if untreated. *C. pneumonia* and *C. psittaci* caused pneumonia are being reported more recently.

Epidemiology

- *C. trachomatis* urogenital infection is the **most common notifiable disease** in the United States. It is a reportable disease in every state.
- In 2012, **1,422,976 cases** of *Chlamydia* were reported to CDC, but an estimated 2.86 million infections occur annually. The **highest prevalence** is among 15- to 24-year-old women. Although *Chlamydia* screening is expanding, many women who are at risk are still not being tested—reflecting, in part, the lack of awareness among some health care providers and the limited resources available to support these screenings.
- *Chlamydia* **screening and treatment may reduce PID** incidence dramatically. Posttreatment **repeat infections usually result from reinfection** and are associated with an elevated risk of PID and other complications. Men most commonly have urethral infections. **Nongonococcal urethritis** in men is often (15% to 55%) caused by *Chlamydia*. Women and men can develop acute or chronic conjunctivitis when exposed to infectious genital secretions during oral–genital sexual contact or autoinoculation. Women and men who practice receptive **anal intercourse** can develop **proctitis** or proctocolitis. *Chlamydia* serovars L1, L2, and L3 cause **lymphogranuloma venereum**

(LGV), which is rare in the United States. **Infected infants** develop **conjunctivitis** 5 to 12 days after exposure and chlamydial **pneumonia** presents as early as 2 weeks or as late as 4 months after delivery. Although perinatally transmitted *Chlamydia* infections may persist for >1 year, **sexual abuse** must also be **considered in preadolescent children** infected with *C. trachomatis*.

- *C. pneumoniae* causes **lower respiratory tract infection** most commonly in school-age children and adults.
- **Psittacosis** is caused by *Chlamydophila psittaci*, a **zoonotic infection** acquired from infected birds.

DIAGNOSIS
Clinical Presentation

- Exposure to *C. trachomatis* usually occurs through sexual intercourse. The cervix is the most common site for women; urethra and rectum are other initial sites; but majority of women are asymptomatic. The urethra is the most common site for men, but majority of men are asymptomatic also; other anatomical sites include epididymis and prostate.

History

- Women are asymptomatic or can have nonspecific symptoms such as dysuria, abnormal vaginal discharge, abdominal pain, intermenstrual vaginal bleeding, or postcoital bleeding. **Men** are often asymptomatic or can have mild to severe symptoms of **dysuria** and penile discharge. Symptoms of **proctitis** or proctocolitis include anorectal pain, discharge, tenesmus, rectal bleeding, and constipation and are almost exclusively seen in MSM.
- Physical examination in women is normal or can show cervical friability, green or yellow endocervical mucopus (from **mucopurulent cervicitis**), abdominal tenderness, or cervical motion and adnexal tenderness consistent with PID. Testicular and/or epididymal pain, which is typically unilateral, is present with **epididymitis**. Physical examination may be normal or can show white, gray, or clear urethral discharge; meatal edema and erythema; and pyuria. Tenderness and swelling of the epididymis are present with epididymitis.
- *Chlamydia* **conjunctivitis** shows unilateral or bilateral conjunctival erythema, mucopurulent discharge, cobblestone appearance of conjunctiva, and preauricular adenopathy on physical examination.
- **LGV** causes a self-limited **genital ulcer** followed by tender inguinal adenopathy located above and below the inguinal ligament. The adenopathy frequently becomes suppurative. LGV also can cause anorectal disease such as proctitis or proctocolitis usually seen in MSM or women practice anal sexual activity.
- *C. trachomatis* is the most common pathogen of the rare **reactive arthritis** and **reactive arthritis triad (RAT)**, formerly known as Reiter syndrome (urethritis, uveitis, and arthritis).
- Infected **infants** who present with *Chlamydia* **conjunctivitis** may have tearing, erythematous conjunctiva, purulent discharge, and eyelid swelling. Infants with chlamydial **pneumonia** present with paroxysmal cough and tachypnea without fever. Physical findings include rales and sometimes wheezing. Approximately 50% of infants with chlamydial pneumonia also have conjunctivitis.
- *C. pneumoniae* symptoms include pharyngitis, hoarseness, and headache. Cough is prominent and can persist for weeks to months if the infection is not managed effectively. Pneumonia and bronchitis can also be present.
- **Psittacosis** symptoms include fever, chills, headache, nonproductive cough, malaise, and myalgias. Complications include confusion, abdominal pain, hepatitis, endocarditis, and Stevens–Johnson syndrome.

Laboratory Studies

- **Nucleic acid amplification tests (NAATs)** that are cleared by the Food and Drug Administration (FDA) are recommended for detection of genital tract infections caused by *C. trachomatis* infections in men and women with and without symptoms.
- For detecting these infections of the genital tract, optimal specimen types for NAATs are **vaginal swabs** from women and **first catch urine** from men.
- Older nonculture tests and non-NAATs have inferior sensitivity and specificity characteristics and no longer are recommended.
- NAATs have not been cleared by FDA for the detection of rectal and oropharyngeal infections caused by C. trachomatis.

- CDC is recommending NAATs to test for these extragenital infections based on increased sensitivity, ease of specimen transport, and processing. Because these specimen types have not been cleared by FDA for use with NAATs, laboratories must establish performance specifications when using these specimens to meet Clinical Laboratory Improvement Amendments (CLIAs) regulatory requirements and local or state regulations as applicable prior to reporting results for patient management.
- *C. trachomatis* and culture capacity might still be needed in instances of child sexual assault and extragenital infections.
- A self- or clinician-collected vaginal swab is the recommended sample type. Self-collected vaginal swab specimens are an option for screening women when a pelvic examination is not otherwise indicated.
- An endocervical swab is acceptable when a pelvic examination is indicated.
- A first catch urine is the recommended sample type for men and is equivalent to a urethral swab in detecting infection.
- NAATs for *C. trachomatis* and *N. gonorrhoeae* are preferred for the diagnostic evaluation of adult sexual assault victims, from any sites of penetration or attempted penetration.
- Culture remains the preferred method for urethral specimens from boys and extragenital specimens (pharynx and rectum) in boys and girls.
- Genital and lymph node specimens (i.e., lesion swab or bubo aspirate) can be tested for *C. trachomatis* by culture, direct immunofluorescence, or nucleic acid detection. Commercially available NAATs for *C. trachomatis* detect both LGV and non-LGV *C. trachomatis* but cannot distinguish between them.
- For patients presenting with proctitis, *C. trachomatis* NAAT testing of a rectal specimen is recommended. Although a positive result is not a definitive diagnosis of LGV, the result might aid in a presumptive clinical diagnosis of LGV proctitis.
- Routine additional testing following a positive NAAT screening test for *C. trachomatis* is no longer recommended by CDC unless otherwise indicated in the product insert.
- Certain NAATs have been FDA-cleared for use on liquid-based cytology specimens.
- All pregnant women should be routinely screened for *C. trachomatis* during the first prenatal visit.
- Pregnant women aged ≤25 years and those at increased risk for *Chlamydia* (e.g., women who have a new or more than one sex partner) should also be retested during the third trimester to prevent maternal postnatal complications and chlamydial infection in the infant.
- Women found to have chlamydial infection during the first trimester should be retested within approximately 3 to 6 months, preferably in the third trimester.

TREATMENT
- **Behavioral—Prevention**
  - Primary prevention of sexually transmitted diseases (STDs) begins with changing the sexual behaviors that place persons at risk for infection. Health care providers have a unique opportunity to provide education and counseling to their patients.
  - A reliable way to avoid transmission of STDs is to abstain from oral, vaginal, and anal sex or to be in a long-term, mutually monogamous relationship with an uninfected partner.
  - For persons who are being treated for an STD (or whose partners are undergoing treatment), counseling that encourages abstinence from sexual intercourse until completion of the entire course of medication is crucial.
  - **Male condoms**, when used consistently and correctly, are effective for reducing the transmission of *Chlamydia*.
- Except in pregnant women, test-of-cure (i.e., repeat testing 3 to 4 weeks after completing therapy) is not advised for persons treated with the recommended or alterative regimens, unless therapeutic compliance is in question, symptoms persist, or reinfection is suspected.
- Coinfection with *C. trachomatis* frequently occurs among patients who have gonococcal infection; therefore, dual therapy for gonococcal and chlamydial infections is appropriate.
- Patients who have chlamydial infection and also HIV infection should receive the same treatment regimen as those who are HIV negative.

Medications
Table 19.7-1 presents medications.

TABLE 19.7-1	Medications	

Infection	Primary antibiotic treatment	Alternative regimens
C. trachomatis urethral, endocervical, rectal infections	Azithromycin (Zithromax), 1 g PO single dose, or Doxycycline (Vibramycin), 100 mg PO bid for 7 d (These have equal efficacy, but azithromycin should always be available to give patients when there is a question of compliance.)[1]	Erythromycin[a] base (E-Mycin, Eryc) 500 mg PO qid for 7 d, or erythromycin[a] ethylsuccinate (EES) 800 mg PO qid for 7 d, or ofloxacin[b] (Floxin) 300 mg PO bid for 7 d, or levofloxacin[b] (Levaquin) 500 mg/d for 7 d
C. trachomatis during pregnancy[c]	Azithromycin 1 g PO in a single dose or amoxicillin (Amoxil) 500 mg PO tid for 7 d	Erythromycin base 500 mg PO qid for 7 d (or 250 mg PO four times a day for 14 d), or EES 800 mg PO qid for 7 d (or 400 mg qid for 14 d)
LGV	Doxycycline, 100 mg PO bid for 21 d	Erythromycin base 500 mg PO qid for 21 d
Chlamydia conjunctivitis[d] or pneumonia in infants/children	Erythromycin base or ethylsuccinate 50 mg/kg/d PO divided into four doses daily for 14 d (weight <45 kg) Azithromycin 1 g PO in a single dose (weight ≥45 kg but age <8 yr) Azithromycin 1 g PO in a single dose or doxycycline 100 mg PO twice a day for 7 d (aged ≥8 yr)	
C. pneumoniae	Doxycycline 100 mg PO bid for 7 d or erythromycin base 500 mg PO qid for 7 d, or EES 800 mg PO qid for 7 d	Fluoroquinolones taken for 7–14 d have also been shown to be effective
C. psittaci[e]	Doxycycline 100 mg PO bid	Tetracycline 500 mg qid

[a]Consider retesting 3 weeks after completion of treatment with erythromycin because side effects can lead to decreased patient compliance. False positives on retesting can occur if tests are conducted <3 weeks after completion of therapy due to excretion of dead organisms.
[b]Ofloxacin and levofloxacin are not recommended for adolescents <18 years or in pregnant or lactating women.
[c]CDC recommends retesting 3 weeks after completion of treatment.
[d]Ocular prophylaxis does not prevent transmission of *Chlamydia* from infected mother to her infant.
[e]Erythromycin is the best alternative for patients in whom tetracyclines are contraindicated, although its in vivo efficacy has not been determined. Continue treatment for 10 to 14 days after defervescence.

REFERENCES

1. Centers for Disease Control and Prevention. Sexually Transmitted Diseases Treatment Guidelines, 2010. *MMWR* 59(RR-12):1–49.
2. Centers for Disease Control and Prevention. Recommendations for the Laboratory-Based Detection of Chlamydia trachomatis and Neisseria gonorrhoeae—2014. *MMWR* 2014;63(RR-02):1–9.
3. U.S. National Library of Medicine—Chlamydia.
4. File TM Jr, Tan JS, Plouffe JF. The role of atypical pathogens: *Mycoplasma pneumoniae, Chlamydia pneumoniae,* and *Legionella pneumophila* in respiratory infection. *Infect Dis Clin North Am* 1998;12:569.
5. Latham-Sadler BA, Morell VW. Community-acquired respiratory infections in children. *Primary Care Clin Office Pract* 1996;23:837.
6. Smith KA, Bradley KK, Stobierski MG, et al. Compendium of measures to control Chlamydophila psittaci (formerly *Chlamydia psittaci*) infection among humans (psittacosis) and pet birds. *J Am Vet Med Assoc* 2005;226(4):532–539.

Herpes Virus Infections

Sanjeev K. Sharma

GENERAL PRINCIPLES

Definition

Herpes virus infections are the third leading cause of viral diseases in humans. These infections can be silent or lead to overt disease. The name *herpes* is from the Greek Herpein meaning "to creep," and is reminiscent of the spreading nature of characteristic skin lesions. There are about 25 herpes viruses, but only 7 are known to cause disease in humans (Table 19.8-1). The herpes viruses primarily infect epithelial mucosal cells or lymphocytes and subsequently travel up peripheral nerves. These viruses then live in the nucleated neurons for the life of the host, and may be reactivated in the future. Infection or reactivation is manifested by vesicular skin lesions filled with fluid; these lesions heal usually without scarring. Some of the common infections are described subsequently.

Herpes Simplex Virus—Types 1 and 2

In general, herpes simplex virus 1 (HSV-1) tends to cause disease above the waist and HSV-2 causes disease below the waist. The initial lesion "dewdrop on a rose petal" is a clear vesicle with erythematous base, which may subsequently become pustular, encrusted or an ulcerated lesion.

- **Oral herpes** can be caused by HSV-1 or -2 in adults, whereas HSV-1 is the main cause in children. It usually starts in the lips and can spread to mouth and pharynx (gingivostomatitis). Reactivation from the trigeminal ganglion can lead to recurrent cold sores. A prodrome of tingling and itching precedes the appearance of vesicles on the lip. The lesions are typically blisters, which become a whitish ulcer. This heals without scarring (cold sore). The disease is more severe in immunocompromised people. Lesions may be brought on by stress, fever, ultraviolet light, or trauma. Gingivostomatitis may be associated with fever, and cervical lymphadenopathy (LAP).
- **Herpes keratitis.** HSV-1 is the leading cause of corneal blindness in the United States. It presents as a unilateral keratoconjunctivitis with pain, photophobia, chemosis, blurred vision, and tearing. Fluorescein staining may reveal the characteristic dendritic ulcer.
- **Herpetic whitlow** is a paronychia caused by HSV-1 or -2 via small wounds on hands or wrist either by autoinoculation or by direct contact with infected persons.

TABLE 19.8-1	Diseases caused by herpes virus infections in humans
Herpes simplex virus 1 (HSV-1)	Oral herpes, cold sores, herpes keratitis, herpes whitlow, herpes gladiatorum, eczema herpeticum, genital herpes, proctitis, encephalitis
Herpes simplex virus 2 (HSV-2)	Oral herpes, cold sores, herpes whitlow, herpes gladiatorum, eczema herpeticum, genital herpes, proctitis, meningitis, HSV infection of neonates
Epstein–Barr virus (EBV)	Infectious mononucleosis, Burkitt lymphoma, nasopharyngeal cancer, hairy leukoplakia
Cytomegalovirus (CMV)	Glandular fever, congenital CMV infections, infections in immunosuppressed patients (retinitis, esophagitis, pneumonitis, encephalitis, and colitis)
Varicella zoster virus (VZV)	Chickenpox, shingles (zoster)
Human herpes virus 6 (HHV-6)	Exanthum subitum or roseola infantum
Human herpes virus 8 (HHV-8)	Kaposi sarcoma–associated herpes virus

- **Herpes gladiatorum** is transmitted by close physical contact in sports such as wrestling and rugby. Lesions are usually in the head and neck region and often on the right side of the body. In rugby, it is also called scrum pox.
- **Eczema herpeticum** is usually seen in children at site of active eczema or preexisting atopic dermatitis.
- **Genital herpes** is usually caused by HSV-2, but 10% of cases are caused by HSV-1. These lesions are transmitted genital-to-genital or oral-to-genital contact. Asymptomatic shedding of virus frequently occurs. The primary infection can be asymptomatic or present as painful vesicular lesions on the glans or shaft of penis, vulva, vagina, cervix, or urethra. The patient may present with itching, dysuria, and vaginal or urethral discharge. Primary infection may also cause systemic symptoms of fever, headache, malaise, myalgia, and tender inguinal LAP (80%). Typically, lesions of primary infections last 2 weeks with full re-epithelialization in 3 weeks. Recurrent lesions begin with a prodrome of itching and tingling 12 to 24 hours before lesions appear. The duration of recurrent lesions tends to be shorter, with an average of 4 to 6 days. Symptoms in recurrent disease typically are much less severe and lesions are less extensive.
- **HSV proctitis** is more common in male homosexuals with receptive anal intercourse. It may presents as signs of anal inflammation, including anal ulcers, tenesmus, and diarrhea.
- **HSV encephalitis** is the most common cause of sporadic viral encephalitis and usually the result of HSV-1 infection. It presents as a nonspecific febrile illness with headache. Patients may develop seizures and focal neurological deficits later in the course of disease.
- **HSV meningitis** is often due to HSV-2 infection and presents typically with fever, vomiting, headache, and meningismus. It is often seen in patients with active genital herpes.
- **Neonatal HSV infection** is usually acquired during delivery (mother shedding viruses in the genital tract) or less commonly, postpartum contact. With a primary genital infection, 30% to 60% of neonates may be infected, compared with only 1% to 3% if the infection is recurrent. Since the neonate has an underdeveloped immune system, the infection spreads rapidly to lungs, liver, and the central nervous system. Only one-third of neonates with HSV have typical skin lesions; consider HSV in an infant showing signs of sepsis. If the mother has active genital lesions at the time of delivery, a cesarean section is the recommended mode of delivery.

Diagnosis

The diagnosis is suspected on the basis of the patient's medical history and physical examination. HSV cultures, polymerase chain reaction (PCR) testing, direct fluorescence antibody, and serologic testing for type-specific HSV antibodies are available to confirm the diagnosis. Scrapings from the base of the lesions and histochemistry performed (Tzank smear) for viral inclusions or multinucleated giant cells are rapid but have low sensitivity (60%) and specificity. Viral culture and PCR-based testing are preferred tests in patients with active lesions. Despite isolation of virus from vesicular fluid, cerebrospinal fluid (CSF) or tissue culture remains the gold standard, sensitivity of viral culture is only 50%, and results take 2 to 7 days to obtain. PCR-based HSV DNA probe essays have emerged as the most sensitive method to confirm diagnosis of HSV infections in most patients. The sensitivity and specificity of PCR-based testing in the diagnosis of HSV infection in CSF approach 100%. Serological testing is available to diagnose genital HSV infections and can differentiate past from active disease. This can be useful in pregnant women at risk of shedding the virus at the time of delivery.

Treatment

Nucleoside analogs are the drugs of choice for the treatment of HSV infections. These agents are active against only replicating viruses and have no effect on latent viruses. These drugs are activated in HSV-infected cells only and hence are relatively nontoxic to the host. Treatment options are shown in Table 19.8-2.

EPSTEIN–BARR VIRUS INFECTIONS

Epstein–Barr virus (EBV) causes infectious mononucleosis (IM) in the western world, Burkitt lymphoma in Africa, and nasopharyngeal cancer in oriental countries. It is also associated with oral hairy leukoplakia in human immunodeficiency virus (HIV) patients. (See Chapter 19.3 for further details.)

The majority of patients with EBV infections are asymptomatic. The infection is transmitted by close contact (kissing disease), also may be spread by blood transfusion.

TABLE 19.8-2 Treatment for Herpes virus Infections

Viral infection	Drug of choice	Dosage	Duration (d)
Herpes simplex virus (HSV)			
Orolabial herpes in immunocompetent recurrence	Penciclovir (Denavir) Docosanol (Abreva)	1% cream applied q2h w/a apply 5 times a day until healed	4
Genital			
First episode	Acyclovir (Zovirax)	400 mg PO tid or 200 mg PO 5 times a day[a]	7–10
	or Famciclovir[b] (Famvir)	250 mg PO tid	7–10
	or Valacyclovir (Valtrex)	1 g PO bid	7–10
Recurrence	Acyclovir	400 mg PO tid or 200 mg 5 times a day or 800 mg bid	5
	or Famciclovir	125 mg PO bid	5
	or Valacyclovir	500 mg PO bid or 1 g/d	5
Chronic suppression	Acyclovir	400 mg PO bid	—
	or Famciclovir or Valacyclovir	250 mg PO bid 500 mg to 1 g PO daily	—
Mucocutaneous disease in immunocompromised	Acyclovir	5 mg/kg IV q8h[b]	7–14
		or 400 mg PO 5 times a day	7–14
Encephalitis	Acyclovir	20 mg/kg IV q8h	14–21
Neonatal	Acyclovir[b]	20 mg/kg IV q8h	10–21
Acyclovir resistant	Foscarnet (Foscavir)	40 mg/kg IV q8h	14–21
		5 mg/kg IV once weekly	14
Acyclovir and foscarnet-resistant HSV	Cidofovir (Vistide)		
Keratoconjunctivitis	Trifluridine (Viroptic) Vidarabine	1 drop of 1% solution topically q2h, up to 9 drops per day ½ in. q3h with a maximum of 5 times per day until healed	10
Varicella zoster virus (VSV)			
Varicella	Acyclovir	20 mg/kg (800 mg max. qid)	5
Herpes zoster	Valacyclovir	1 g PO tid	7
	or Famciclovir	750 mg once daily or 500 mg PO bid, or 250 mg tid	7
	or Acyclovir	800 mg PO 5 times a day	7–10
Varicella zoster in immunocompromised	Acyclovir	10 g/kg IV q8h[c]	7
Acyclovir resistant	Foscarnet	40 mg/kg IV q8h	10

[a]For severe initial genital herpes, intravenous acyclovir (5 mg/kg q8h for 5–7 days) can be used. Dosage reduction is recommended for creatinine clearance less than 50 mL/min.
[b]For children <12. 10 mg/kg IV every 8 hours × 7 days.
[c]Pediatric dosage is 500 mg/m^2 q8h for 7–10 days.

Infectious Mononucleosis

A usually benign disease characterized by fever, malaise, LAP, and tonsillitis. Patients may have hepatosplenomegaly and generalized maculopapular rash. The illness usually resolves in 1 to 4 weeks, but complications such as secondary infection, meningitis, encephalitis, myelitis, and Guillain–Barre syndrome can occur.

Burkitt Lymphoma

Burkitt lymphoma is endemic in Africa. It often presents as a tumor of the jaw and face in children. For unknown reasons, it is rarely seen in other parts of the world.

Nasopharyngeal Cancer

This disease occurs in Alaska, South China, and East Africa. It may present as a neck mass due to cervical nodal metastasis, nasal obstruction with epistaxis, or headache caused by cranial nerve involvement.

Oral Hairy Leukoplakia

It is an opportunistic infection in HIV patients. It presents as white corrugated painless plaques that cannot be scraped off, mainly on lateral sides of tongue. Other parts of the oral cavity may be involved such as soft palate and buccal mucosa. It is specific to HIV, and is not seen in patients with other kinds of immunodeficiency.

Diagnosis

The most common laboratory finding in IM is lymphocytosis with absolute count >4,500 per μL or differential count of more than 50%, and it is also associated with atypical lymphocytes >10%. A latex agglutination test (monospot test) is readily available and detects heterophile antibodies.

Treatment

Primary treatment of most EBV infections is supportive. Acetaminophen or nonsteroidal anti-inflammatory agents are recommended for fever or pain.

CYTOMEGALOVIRUS

Cytomegalovirus (CMV) infection has affected nearly 50% of the U.S. population by age 35. It is transmitted sexually, or via saliva, urine, or by blood transfusion.

It is usually asymptomatic, but in patients with organ transplant or other immunosuppressive diseases such as AIDS it can cause retinitis, esophagitis, pneumonitis, encephalitis, or colitis.

CMV Mononucleosis

It is a syndrome closely resembling IM in immunocompetent individuals. Systemic symptoms such as fever are more prominent than cervical LAP or splenomegaly compared with IM.

Diagnosis

Diagnosis includes enzyme-linked immunosorbent assay (ELISA) testing or characteristic inclusion bodies in biopsy specimens. Detection of CMV specific IgM antibodies suggests recent seroconversion. PCR testing for quantifying CMV DNA is widely available for diagnosis or monitoring of these patients.

Treatment

Treatment is symptomatic in immunocompetent patients. Ganciclovir is used especially in treatment of retinitis. Foscarnet can also be used. Acyclovir is not recommended.

VARICELLA (CHICKENPOX)

This virus is highly infectious and 90% of susceptible household contacts with the patient will become infected. Spread is primarily by respiratory secretions (cough and sneeze) or through direct contact with skin lesions.

Chicken pox has an incubation period of 14 to 16 days after contact with a varicella or herpes zoster patient. This is followed by a prodrome of fever and malaise for 1 to 2 days, and then appearance of the characteristic rash. The disease is more severe in older children and adults, especially if they are immunocompromised. Fifteen percent of adolescent or adult patients with varicella may develop pneumonia. Other complications are fulminant encephalitis, cerebellar ataxia, and, rarely, transverse myelitis and aseptic meningitis. Recovery from infection provides immunity for life.

Congenital varicella syndrome occurs in 2% of affected pregnancies, with limb hypoplasia, ocular atrophy, and psychomotor retardation. It may be caused by an infection in utero during first trimester of pregnancy. Neonatal varicella occurs when the mother develops varicella around the time of delivery; it has mortality up to 30%.

Diagnosis

Diagnosis is primarily by history of exposure and presence of characteristic rash. Rash is generalized and pruritic and starts from head and face and spread to chest and back and then spread to rest of the body. It starts as maculopapular rash and rapidly changes to vesicles that subsequently crust. The rash is concentrated mainly on chest and back and is in different stages of evolution simultaneously.

Treatment

Symptomatic treatment with antihistamines and acetaminophen is recommended. Aspirin should be avoided as it may lead to Reyes syndrome. Acyclovir is recommended within 24 hours of appearance of rash in patients 12 years of age or older, those with chronic pulmonary disorders, or patients receiving immunosuppressive treatment such as steroids. Acyclovir may be considered for prophylaxis of secondary household contacts within 24 hours without preexisting immunity. Intravenous acyclovir should be used in immunocompromised hosts. Passive immunization with varicella zoster immune globulin (VZIG, 1 vial 5 = 125 units = 1.25 mL, 125 units per 10 kg up to 625 units, with minimum of 1 vial, IM), administered within 96 hours of a significant exposure, is indicated for neonates, pregnant women, and immunocompromised patients.

HERPES ZOSTER (SHINGLES)

Reactivation of varicella zoster virus occurs, often unpredictably, or among those with immunosuppressive conditions. Zoster usually manifests as radicular pain in the affected nerve segment, followed by vesicular lesions after few days in the discrete areas of that dermatomal nerve segment. New lesions may appear in adjacent dermatomes. Involvement of the ophthalmic branch of cranial nerve V may cause visual impairment or blindness, uveitis, keratitis, or conjunctivitis, whereas involvement of CN 7 and 8 can lead to Bell palsy or Ramsay–Hunt syndrome (facial palsy, tinnitus, vertigo, and impairment of taste and hearing), respectively. The presence of the Hutchinson sign (vesicles on the side and tip of the nose) is an indication that ocular involvement is likely, and slit-lamp examination is mandatory. Postherpetic neuralgia (PHN) is characterized by pain persisting 4 to 6 weeks beyond crusting of lesions. It is more common in older patients, occurring in more than 50% of persons older than 60 years.

Diagnosis

History of chickenpox, herpes zoster, or lack of varicella immunization in the past with the appearance of characteristic rash helps make the diagnosis. The lesions are vesicular with an erythematous base. Definitive diagnosis can be made by culture of the virus from the lesion.

Treatment

Supportive care includes analgesics and wet compresses with water or a 5% Burlow solution may be helpful. The use of nucleoside analog (acyclovir and valacyclovir) within 72 hours of appearance of the rash is recommended (see Table 19.8-2). Systemic steroids have demonstrated no additional benefit in reduction of PHN. Studies examining amitriptyline, narcotics, capsaicin, anticonvulsants, and percutaneous nerve stimulation for PHN have been inconclusive.

Patients with eye involvement should be referred to an ophthalmologist.

REFERENCES

1. Hunt R. Virology, Chapter 11. Herpes Virus. http://pathmicro.med.sc.edu/virol/herpes.htm.
2. CDC.gov
3. Wenner C, Nashelsky J. Antiviral agents for pregnant women with genital herpes. *Am Fam Physician* 2005;72:1807.
4. Holten KB, Britigan DH. Treatment of herpes zoster. *Am Fam Physician* 2006;73:882.
5. Patel R. Antiviral agents for the prevention of the sexual transmission of herpes simplex in discordant couples. *Curr Opin Infect Dis* 2004;17:45–48.
6. Brady RC, Bernstein DI. Treatment of herpes simplex virus infections. *Antiviral Res* 61:73–81.

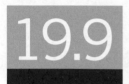

Lyme Disease
Jennifer Parker

GENERAL PRINCIPLES

Lyme disease is a tick-borne illness transmitted by the bite of certain Ixodes ticks. It is caused by the bacterial spirochete *Borrelia burgdorferi* in the United States, whereas other species of *Borrelia* cause the disease in Europe. Lyme disease is a multisystem illness manifesting initially as a systemic and dermatologic condition. If not treated, the infection can lead to rheumatologic, neurologic, or cardiac sequelae.

Definition

Any infection with *B. burgdorferi* can be considered Lyme disease. Infection can range from asymptomatic seroconversion to severe neurologic sequelae.

Pathophysiology (Epidemiology)

Lyme disease was first discovered in the 1970s, with standardized case definitions developed in 1991. In the United States, most cases occur in New England, the mid-Atlantic states, and in Minnesota and Wisconsin, with less frequent cases along the Pacific coast in Oregon and Northern California.[1,2] The incidence has been increasing over the past decade. Mice, chipmunks, and birds are natural reservoirs for the spirochete, and ticks acquire the bacteria by feeding on infected animals. Deer are not competent hosts, but they do play a role in sustaining the life cycle of the ticks.[2]

DIAGNOSIS

Clinical Manifestations

Early disease is characterized by the erythema migrans (EM) rash, which occurs 3 to 30 days after the tick bite. The rash occurs at the site of the bite and classically expands with a ring of central clearing,[2] hence the description target lesion. However, the lesion can be uniformly erythematous or have enhanced central erythema. Systemic flu-like symptoms including fever, fatigue, and myalgia often accompany the rash.

If untreated, the organism can spread hematogenously, leading to early disseminated disease. This stage presents with multiple, smaller EM lesions and/or central nervous system (CNS) involvement, Lyme neuroborreliosis. Common CNS manifestations are cranial nerve palsy or lymphocytic meningitis. Systemic symptoms of myalgias, arthralgias, headache, and fatigue may also occur in this phase with cardiac complications such as atrioventricular node block or carditis being less common.

Late Lyme disease occurs weeks to months after initial infection and presents as a monoarticular arthritis, most often of the knee. This is seen less commonly because most affected people are treated prior to this stage.[2,3]

History

History should focus on potential exposure, including geographic location and possibility of tick bite. If this is present, timing of clinical symptoms, including rash, systemic, neurologic, cardiac, and rheumatologic symptoms, should be explored.

Physical Examination

Physical examination should focus on the systems involved in the disease process as well. A thorough skin examination, neurologic examination including cranial nerve testing, and musculoskeletal examination are important. Vital signs (pulse and blood pressure) and cardiac auscultation are necessary to determine whether there is cardiac involvement.

Laboratory Studies

Serologic testing in a two-tiered approach with screening enzyme immunoassay or immunofluorescent assay and confirmatory Western immunoblot is recommended. However, the testing lacks sensitivity in early Lyme as IgM antibodies can take 3 to 4 weeks to develop.[2,3] Thus, history of potential exposure and presence of EM rash is sufficient for diagnosis and initiating treatment. Serologic testing is helpful when illness has been present for several weeks and/or the diagnosis is in question.

If there is CNS involvement, antibody testing should be done on cerebrospinal fluid (CSF).[1,3] PCR is available for detection in the CSF or in synovial fluid, but it lacks sensitivity and is not currently recommended.[4,5]

Mildly elevated erythrocyte sedimentation rate and liver enzyme testing may be seen. In neuroborreliosis, CSF may show a lymphocytic pleocytosis and mildly elevated protein.

Genetics

There is currently no evidence that there is a genetic predisposition to Lyme disease or its sequelae.

Differential Diagnosis

The disease that most closely mimics cutaneous Lyme disease is Southern Tick Associated Rash Illness (STARI), which occurs in southern and south central United States. STARI does not have any of the other features of Lyme such as neurologic or rheumatologic manifestations. The differential diagnosis for EM includes nummular eczema, cellulitis, insect or spider bite, granuloma annulare, tinea corporis, erythema multiforme, and urticaria. When symptoms are more systemic, Rocky Mountain Spotted Fever, relapsing fever, Colorado tick fever, babesiosis, tularemia, ehrlichiosis, and syphilis should be considered. Differential diagnosis of Lyme arthritis includes septic arthritis, reactive arthritis, and inflammatory arthritis. Coinfection with *Babesia*, *Anaplasma*, *Ehrlichia*, deer tick virus, or other species of *Borrelia* can occur.[2]

TREATMENT
Medications

For early disease including localized or disseminated, uncomplicated arthritis or cranial nerve palsy, doxycycline 100 mg orally twice daily is recommended for adults and children 8 years of age and over. For children under 8 years old, amoxicillin 50 mg/kg/day orally divided three times daily up to 1,500 mg is recommended; if penicillin allergic, cefuroxime 30/mg/kg/day orally divided twice daily up to 1,000 mg is recommended. Recommended length of therapy is 14 to 21 days.[3] For meningitis, IV therapy with either ceftriaxone 2 g IV daily (50 to 75 mg/kg/day pediatric dose) or cefotaxime 2 g IV every 8 hours (150 to 200 mg/kg/day pediatric dosing) is the recommended treatment for a total of 14 to 28 days. For complicated arthritis or carditis, either oral or IV therapy is recommended. One-time treatment with doxycycline within 72 hours of removal of deer tick has been studied and can be effective, but there are currently no recommendations to treat empirically as such.[2]

Complications

There is a debate about whether chronic Lyme or post-Lyme syndrome is a true clinical phenomenon. Chronic Lyme implies continued infection with *B. borgdorferi* despite antibiotic treatment, which has not been demonstrated in studies. Thus, the term post-Lyme syndrome has been used to describe the symptoms of arthralgia, myalgia, sleep disorders, and difficulty with concentration that some patients describe. Some studies suggest that there may be an autoimmune or other immunogenic mechanism causing this syndrome, whereas others indicate that incidence of this nonspecific constellation of symptoms is no higher in patients treated for Lyme than it is in the general population or following other infections and thus may not be an actual clinical entity. There is currently no evidence for prolonged antibiotic treatment for these late symptoms.[6]

Patient Education

Avoiding tick bites in endemic areas by wearing long pants and shirts, using at least 20% N,N-diethyl-meta-toluamide (DEET) and frequent checking for ticks is important for prevention. Educating patients about signs and symptoms of Lyme disease can lead to earlier presentation and treatment. A previous vaccination, LYMErix was on the market from 1998 to 2002 but was withdrawn by the manufacturer. The vaccine was directed against the outer surface protein A (Osp A) and there are currently new Osp A vaccines being studied.[7,8]

REFERENCES

1. Graham J, Stockley K, Goldman R. Tick-borne illnesses: a CME update. *Pediatr Emerg Care* 2011;27:141–7.
2. Shapiro ED. Clinical practice. Lyme disease. *N Engl J Med* 2014;370:1724–31.

3. American Academy of Pediatrics. Lyme disease (Lyme borreliosis, *Borrelia burgdorferi* infection). In: Pickering LK, ed. *Red book: 2012 report of the Committee on infectious diseases.* 29th ed. Elk Grove Village, IL: American Academy of Pediatrics; 2012:474–479.
4. Nelson CA. CDC Expert Commentary. PCR for Diagnosis of Lyme Disease: Is It Useful? Medscape website. http://www.medscape.com/partners/cdc/public/cdc-commentary. Accessed on June 11, 2012.
5. CDC. Notice to readers: Caution regarding testing for Lyme disease. *MMWR. Morb Mortal Wkly Rsp* 205; 54: 125. http://www.medscape.com/viewarticle/764501.
6. Sordet C. Chronic Lyme disease: fact or fiction? *Joint Bone Spine* 2014;81:110–1.
7. Lantos PM. Lyme disease vaccination: are we ready to try again? *Lancet Infect Dis* 2013;13:643–4.
8. Stricker RB, Johnson L. Lyme disease vaccination: safety first. *Lancet Infect Dis* 2014;14:12.

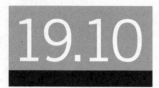

19.10 Rocky Mountain Spotted Fever

Ashley J. Falk, Nathan P. Falk

GENERAL PRINCIPLES

Definition

Rocky Mountain spotted fever (RMSF) is a potentially fatal, tick-borne illness caused by *Rickettsia rickettsii*.

Epidemiology

- Most prevalent in the southeastern and south central states
- 2,221 cases of RMSF reported to the Centers for Disease Control and Prevention in 2010[1]
- Incidence is highest among persons aged 40 to 64 years[2]
- Most common between the months of April and September
- Two principal vectors for bacterial transmission within the United States
  - The wood tick (*Dermacentor andersoni*) in the western United States
  - The dog tick (*Dermacentor variabilis*) in the eastern and southern United States

Etiology

RMSF is caused by the Gram-negative obligate intracellular bacterium *R. rickettsii*.

DIAGNOSIS

Clinical Presentation

- Based on clinical signs and symptoms after an incubation period of 4 to 12 days (mean 7 days).
- Classic presentation is rapid onset of headache and fever followed in 2 to 3 days by rash.
- Other symptoms are nonspecific and may include myalgias, nausea, vomiting, abdominal pain (especially in children) malaise, sore throat, nonproductive cough, and pleuritic chest pain.
- Classic triad of fever, headache, and rash present in less than 50% of cases at initial presentation.[3,4]

History

A tick bite is recalled by 50% to 70% of patients.

Physical Examination

- Rash initially appears on the distal extremities (palms, soles, wrists, ankles, and forearms) and consists of small, pink, blanchable macules.
- Rash later spreads centripetally to the trunk, neck, and face.
- Lesions become maculopapular and petechial and may then coalesce and form large ecchymotic areas and ulcerations.
- From 5% to 15% of patients may never develop a rash.[5]

Laboratory Studies

Laboratory studies include primarily a clinical diagnosis as there are no completely reliable tests in the early phase of illness when therapy should be initiated.

- Skin biopsy
  - May be used if rash is present, however, very few laboratories have the ability to perform, so often of little or no use in initial patient management
  - 100% specific and 60% sensitive (very low sensitivity once treatment has been initiated)[6]
- Serologic testing
  - Confirmation may be done using indirect fluorescent antibody testing.[7]
  - Overall sensitivity is 95% and is available through most state health departments.
  - False negatives may occur during the first 5 days of symptoms as antibody response is not yet detectable, or if treatment is initiated within 48 hours of symptom onset as these patients may never develop an antibody response.
- General laboratory testing is nonspecific but may reveal thrombocytopenia, hyponatremia; elevated liver transaminases; azotemia; and an increased, decreased, or normal white blood cell count.

Differential Diagnosis

Measles, meningococcemia, streptococcal infection, parvovirus infection (Fifth disease), roseola, enteroviral infection, viral meningitis, ehrlichiosis, drug reaction, infectious mononucleosis, leptospirosis, immune thrombocytopenic purpura, immune complex vasculitis, or bacterial sepsis.

TREATMENT

Medications

- Antibiotics should be initiated immediately when there is suspicion of RMSF rather than waiting for confirmatory testing, especially in patients from endemic areas with fever and rash during the summer months.[5]
- Delay in initiating therapy may increase mortality, especially in children.[7]
- **Adults** (and children weighing >45 kg): doxycycline 100 mg bid for at least 7 days or 3 days after fever is gone.[8]
  - **Pregnancy:** chloramphenicol 500 mg qid (or 50 mg/kg/day divided qid).
- **Children:** doxycycline 2.2 mg per kg IV/PO bid (maximum dose 200 mg daily).[9]

Complications

Multisystem illness may occur, including renal failure, pneumonitis, adult respiratory distress syndrome, myocarditis, hepatitis, gastrointestinal bleeding, diarrhea, skin necrosis, coagulopathy, hemolysis, encephalitis, and seizure.

SPECIAL CONSIDERATIONS

- **Prevention.** No vaccine exists and routine prophylaxis following tick exposure is not recommended as less than 1% of ticks in endemic areas are infected with *Rickettsia*.
- Patients reporting tick bites should inform their physician if they develop fever, headache, or rash within 14 days of exposure.

REFERENCES

1. CDC. Summary Notifiable Diseases United States June 30th, 2011. *MMWR Morb Mortal Wkly Rep* 2012;53:1–111.
2. Hopkins RS, Jajosky RA, Hall PA, et al. Summary of notifiable diseases—United States, 2003. *MMWR Morb Mortal Wkly Rep* 2005;52:1.
3. Abramson JS, Givner LB. Rocky Mountain spotted fever. *Pediatr Infect Dis J* 1999;18:539.
4. Ustaine RP. Dermatologic emergencies. *Am Fam Physician* 2010;82:773.
5. Thorner AR, Walker DH, Petri WA. Rocky Mountain spotted fever: state of the art clinical review. *Clin Infect Dis* 1998;27:1353.
6. Bratton RL, Corey GR. Tick-borne disease. *Am Fam Physician* 2005;71:2323.
7. Kirkland KB, Wilkinson WE, Sexton DJ. Therapeutic delay and mortality in cases of Rocky Mountain spotted fever. *Clin Infect Dis* 1995;20:1118.
8. Consequences of delayed diagnosis of Rocky Mountain spotted fever in children—West Virginia, Michigan, Tennessee, and Oklahoma, May–June 2000. *MMWR Morb Mortal Wkly Rep* 2000;49:885.
9. American Academy of Pediatrics. Rocky Mountain spotted fever. In: Pickering LK, ed. *Red Book: 2012 Committee on infectious diseases.* 29th ed. Elk Grove Village, IL: American Academy of Pediatrics; 2012

19.11 Parasitic Diseases

Matthew R. Anderson, Manel Silva

GENERAL PRINCIPLES

Definition

A parasite is an organism that lives on or in another living organism (the host) from which it derives nutrition. Medically important parasites include the single-celled protozoans, ectopods (e.g., lice and scabies), and helminths (roundworms or flatworms). Although commonly thought of as intestinal pathogens, parasites produce clinical syndromes as diverse as seizures and heart failure.

A few parasitic infections are common in primary care; these include infections caused by bed bugs, lice, *Giardia*, pinworms, scabies, and Trichomonas.. However, with an increasingly mobile population, doctors may also encounter less common parasitic diseases. The CDC's Division of Parasitic Diseases and Malaria has identified five neglected parasitic diseases in the United States: Chagas disease, cysticercosis, toxocariasis, toxoplasmosis, and trichomoniasis. The Division's Web site is an excellent resource for both providers and patients: www.cdc.gov/parasites.

Anatomy

During the course of their lifecycle, parasitic infections can involve multiple organs. Parasitic infection and symptomatology are listed here by organ system:

- **Skin.** Dermatitis (*Ascaris*, *Capillaria hepatica*, hookworms, *Strongyloides*, chigoe flea, cutaneous and visceral larva migrans, *Dracunculus*, lice, *Mansonella*, scabies, mites); migratory pruritic swellings (*Loa loa*); subcutaneous nodules, skin ulcers, and scars (cutaneous leishmaniasis, *Dracunculus*, *Dirofilaria*, *Onchocerca*, sparganum, *Taenia*, *Trypanosoma brucei gambiense*); swimmer's itch (schistosomiasis); pruritus and skin depigmentation (onchoceriasis); temporal and periorbital swelling with conjunctivitis (acute *Trypanosoma cruzi* infection); facial and periorbital edema during acute infection (*Trichinella*); and ulcers (cutaneous and mucocutaneous leishmaniasis, *T. gambiense*, *Dracunculus*, *Tungiasis*)
- **Central nervous system.** Meningoencephalitis (African trypanosomiasis, *Acanthamoeba*, *Angiostrongylus*, *Naegleria*, cerebral malaria, schistosomiasis), new-onset seizures, or focal neurologic signs consistent with a space-occupying lesion (cysticercosis, malaria, toxoplasmosis, trichinosis, hydatid and coenurus cysts, *Sparganosis*)
- **Eyes.** Vitreous infestation (onchocercosis, ascariasis, ocular toxocariasis), conjunctivitis (*Loa loa*), keratoconjunctivitis and corneal ulcers (caused by free-living amebas), uveitis, choroiditis and choroidoretinitis (toxoplasmosis), anterior uveitis (*Wuchereria bancrofti*) periorbital swelling, and conjunctivitis (*Trypanosoma cruzi*)
- **Hematologic.** Microcytic anemia (malaria, *Babesia*, hookworm, *Trichuris*, trypanosomes), macrocytic anemia (fish tapeworms), leukopenia (malaria, visceral leishmaniasis), eosinophilia (invasive helminths, especially *Schistosoma* and *Trichinella*, *Dientamoeba fragilis*, and *Cystoisospora belli*)
- **Lymphatic.** Elephantiasis (lymphatic filariasis), lymphadenopathy (African trypanosomiasis, *Mansonella ozzardi*, toxoplasmosis, visceral leishmaniasis)
- **Respiratory.** Loeffler syndrome (*Ascaris lumbricoides*, *Strongyloides*), pneumonitis (hookworms, *Pneumocystis*, *Strongyloides*), chest pain and hemoptysis (paragonimiasis), pulmonary mass lesion (*Dirofilaria*, echinococcosis, paragonimiasis), tropical pulmonary eosinophilia (filariasis)
- **Cardiovascular.** Heart block, congestive heart failure (*Trypanosoma cruzi*)
- **Intestinal.** Appendicitis (*Ascaris*, *Trichuris*, pinworms); colic, diarrhea, and vomiting (*Capillaria philippinensis*, *Cryptosporidium*, intestinal flukes, *Isospora belli*, *Strongyloides*, *Cyclospora*, *Giardia*); mucoid and bloody diarrhea (amebiasis), bloody stool (schistosomiasis), obstruction (*Ascaris*, *Hymenolepis nana*, *Taenia saginata*); colitis (*Trichuris*); pruritus ani (*Enterobius*)
- **Hepatobiliary.** Liver abscess or cyst (*Entamoeba histolytica*, cysticercosis, hydatid disease), biliary obstruction (*Ascaris lumbricoides*), portal hypertension (schistosomes), hepatosplenomegaly (malaria, babesiosis, *Capillaria hepatica*, visceral leishmania, visceral larva migrans, Katayama fever in acute schistosomiasis)

- **Genitourinary.** *Chyluria* (lymphatic filariasis), hematuria (schistosomes), prostatitis, urethritis, and vaginitis (trichomonads)
- **Musculoskeletal.** Myositis (trichinosis, toxoplasmosis, Chagas disease), cysts (*Echinococcus, cysticercosis*)

Transmission

Transmission of parasites may occur via the fecal–oral route, through the skin, by blood transfusion or organ transplant, or by a suitable local vector such as a mosquito.

Epidemiology

- **Populations at risk.** International travelers (especially those traveling outside of industrialized countries and major cities), missionaries, and immigrants are at particular risk. Backpackers who drink untreated groundwater are at risk for acquiring *Giardia*, amebiasis, guinea worm, and *Cryptosporidium* as well as bacterial pathogens.
- Residents of institutions, including daycare centers, group homes, and nursing homes, are at risk for acquiring *Giardia*, amebiasis, as well as bacterial pathogens spread by fecal contamination. People who engage in oral–anal sex are at risk for acquiring *E. histolytica* and *Giardia lamblia* as well as viral pathogens such as hepatitis A virus, and bacteria such as *Shigella*.
- **Risk by geographic area.** For continuously-updated information about specific risks in various geographic regions, consult the U.S. Centers for Disease Control and Prevention (CDC) web page (http://www.cdc.gov/travel/). The World Health Organization (WHO) also provides information for travelers (http://www.who.int/ith/en/).
- **Immunosuppressed patients** show increased susceptibility to some parasites. This group includes malnourished individuals, patients with cancer, patients on steroids, and patients with AIDS (discussed later in the chapter).

Screening and Prevention

- Routine testing for asymptomatic parasite carriage in travelers or food handlers is not recommended because of the low yield.
- Individuals with a high likelihood of exposure to parasites (missionaries, refugees, and immigrants arriving from endemic regions) can be treated empirically for intestinal helminths.[1] Although not Food and Drug Administration (FDA)-approved for this indication, a single dose of albendazole (400 mg taken orally for both children and adults) may be superior to treating only those with positive ova and parasite examinations; testing is more expensive and results in fewer carriers receiving treatment.
- Individuals with suspected exposure to *Giardia*, amebiasis, or platyhelminths may need repeated stool examinations for ova and parasites (three is recommended) because of intermittent excretion. Giardia and amebiasis can also be diagnosed based on stool antigen tests.

Prevention Advice

- Travelers should avoid inhaling water mist while swimming, or swimming with open cuts or abrasions. They should not swim in freshwater areas where schistosomiasis is endemic (see http://wwwnc.cdc.gov/travel/yellowbook/2014/chapter-3-infectious-diseases-related-to-travel/schistosomiasis#4116).
- In areas where chlorinated or filtered tap water is not available, and hygiene and sanitation are poor, people should drink canned or bottled beverages, or beverages made with boiled water such as tea or coffee. Decontamination options include
  - Boiling water for 1 minute at low altitudes, or for three minutes if above 6,500 feet. Water should be filtered through a cloth or allowed to settle prior to boiling.
  - Disinfecting water can be done with chlorine bleach or iodine. Water should be filtered first. For each gallon, add 1/8 teaspoon (eight drops) of chlorine. Iodine dosing will depend upon formulation.
  - Filters should be small enough to remove bacteria and *Cryptosporidium*.
- To prevent fecal–oral transmission of diseases, strict hand washing should be practiced.
- For mosquito-borne diseases, the best strategy is to avoid getting bitten. Travelers should use clothing that covers extremities and sleep under bed nets; ideally these items should be pretreated with Permethrin. DEET-containing repellants are probably the best agents for use on the skin. Mosquito activity is highest at dawn and dusk.
- Travelers should avoid foods that may harbor parasites, especially raw or undercooked foods. The general advice is: *Boil it, Cook it, Peel it or Forget it!* Salads and cut fruits are potentially a source of infections. Travelers should avoid consuming foods from street vendors, as well as unconventional foods or animal products.

- Infants under 6 months benefit from exclusive breastfeeding to prevent parasitic infections.
- Travelers should obtain prophylactic vaccines and medicines if traveling to endemic areas and consult with a travel clinic if they have any predisposing illnesses that increases their risks. The CDC maintains a list of travel clinics at http://wwwnc.cdc.gov/travel/page/find-clinic

DIAGNOSIS
History

The most important step in assessing risk is a careful history, including the patient's social and physical environment (including past exposures to immigrants from endemic areas), travel history including duration of potential exposure, and personal habits. It is unnecessary to rule out parasitic infection in asymptomatic individuals who were never in environments where they might have been infected. Because parasitic infections can affect diverse systems, a thorough review of systems may be necessary to obtain the appropriate differential (see Clinical Presentations mentioned previously). If this history suggests a risk for parasitic disease, the clinician must then determine which parasites are potential pathogens.

- **Parasites seen in stool.** Roundworms or flatworm segments can be passed in stool. Specimens brought in by patients should be preserved in 70% alcohol and sent to a diagnostic laboratory. Objects such as earthworms or mucus plugs can be mistaken for parasites.
- **HIV infection** with certain parasites has been associated with either increased susceptibility or more severe diseases. The major parasitic infections include visceral leishmaniasis and those caused by *Toxoplasma gondii*, *Cryptosporidium* spp., *Cyclospora* spp., *C. belli*, *Trypanosoma cruzi*, *Microsporum* spp., *Strongyloides stercoralis*, and *Plasmodium* species.

Laboratory Studies

Diagnosis of Symptomatic Infection
- The CDC Division of Parasitic Diseases maintains an excellent Web site on the diagnostic evaluation of parasites (http://www.cdc.gov/dpdx/).
- Appropriate laboratory work should be obtained for symptomatic patients with risk factors for parasitic disease. In U.S. laboratories, only about 1% of ova and parasite tests indicate the presence of some form of parasite and most of these are nonpathogenic protozoans.
- Clinically useful diagnoses come almost exclusively from outpatients or hospitalized patients within the first 3 days of their admission. Testing asymptomatic patients is not recommended.

Office Examination
- **Stool examination (ova and parasites).** Three separate stool samples taken every other day increase the likelihood of finding pathogens. Examination of a fresh stool specimen permits visualization of short-lived motile forms that cannot be found in preserved or refrigerated specimens. Purged stools that are examined immediately are superior to preserved specimens, especially when one is looking for ameba; magnesium citrate can be used as a purgative. Ideally a thin, fresh slide of feces should be examined within an hour of collection, looking for trophozoites and amebas. Then, a drop of Gram iodine or Lugol solution is added to provide better visualization of cysts. Part of the sample should be placed in separate preservative containing vials according to supplied directions and sent to a reference laboratory. Care should be taken to avoid contamination with urine or water. Testing for *Cryptosporidium* and *Cyclospora* cysts requires special staining.
- **The cellophane tape test** is used to detect *Enterobius* (pinworm) and *Taenia saginata* eggs. Clear cellophane (Scotch) tape is placed with the sticky side down on the unwashed perianal area, preferably in the early morning before bathing or after defecation. The tape is placed (again sticky side down) on a microscope slide, which is examined for eggs. Adult pinworms can be seen with this technique. Sensitivity is improved by repeating the examination on subsequent days.
- **Clinical Laboratory Improvement Amendment (CLIA):** Offices performing these tests should be CLIA-certified.

Clinical Laboratory Examination
- **Stool examination (ova and parasites).** Various techniques exist for concentrating and staining stool specimens. When looking for helminth eggs, one or two concentrated preserved specimens are usually sufficient. Table 19.11-1 provides a guide to the interpretation of findings in the ova and parasite examination.

TABLE 19.11-1	Interpreting Stool Ova and Parasite Results		
Definite pathogens	**Pathogens primarily in immunosuppressed hosts**	**Pathogenicity disputed**	**Nonpathogens**
Cryptosporidium parvum	*Balantidium coli*	*Blastocystis hominis*	*Chilomastix mesnili*
Cyclospora spp.	*Microsporidia* spp.		*Endolimax nana*[a]
Dientamoeba fragilis			*Entamoeba coli*
Entamoeba histolytica			*Entamoeba dispar*
Enterobius vermicularis			*Entamoeba hartmanni*
Giardia lamblia			*Iodamoeba buetschlii*
Cystoisospora belli			

Note: The presence of a "nonpathogenic" organism implies fecal contamination of the food or water supply and therefore may be clinically significant.
[a]Morphologically similar to *E. histolytica* by light microscopy.

- **Antigen tests** for amebiasis (*E. histolytica*), cryptosporidiosis, giardiasis, and trichomoniasis are now available in many clinical laboratories. Antigen tests often have better sensitivity than microscopy and are considered the test of choice for giardiasis.
- **Blood smear.** Blood smear is indicated for malaria (thick and thin film done at time of fever), filariasis (blood drawn during hours of periodic release, usually midnight), trypanosomiasis, and babesiosis. For periodic fevers, blood drawing must be timed appropriately for the clinical syndrome.
- **Directed biopsy** is often necessary for diagnosis of parasites that do not colonize the intestinal tract.
- **Serology:** Serologic tests are available for a variety of parasitic infections, including leishmaniasis and toxoplasmosis.
- **Sputum samples** can be useful in identifying *Pneumocystis jiroveci* pneumonia, *Paragonimus westermani* eggs, *Strongyloides* larvae, hookworm larvae, and rarely *E. histolytica*. Bronchoscopic samples obtained early in the morning have a higher yield.
- **Urine specimens** can be examined to look for *Schistosoma haematobium* eggs (collected near noontime) or *Trichomonas vaginalis*.
- **Vaginal swab** is indicated in female patients to assess for *Trichomonas vaginalis* infections; antigen tests are also available.
- **Endoscopy** may reveal *Giardia* and *Strongyloides* in patients where the ova and parasite examination is negative.
- **Other testing modalities.** Antibody, antigen, as well as molecular diagnostic techniques are available for a variety of parasitic infections. For details, consult the CDC Division of Parasitic Diseases (http://www.dpd.cdc.gov/dpdx/HTML/DiagnosticProcedures.htm).
- **Eosinophilia.** Helminths that invade tissue can produce eosinophilia. Among these are *Ancylostoma duodenale* (hookworm), *Dientamoeba fragilis*, *C. belli*, *Sarcocystis*, and those causing *filariasis*, *scabies*, *schistosomiasis*, *strongyloidiasis*, *toxocariasis*, and *trichinellosis*.

Imaging

Imaging can be useful for diagnosis and for localization for biopsies. A chest radiograph or computed tomography (CT) scan of the chest may suggest parasites that cause respiratory and cardiovascular findings. Abdominal ultrasound or CT of abdomen may be useful for those parasites causing hepatobiliary and spleen findings. A head CT may suggest parasites causing central nervous system pathologies.

TREATMENT

The CDC Web site offers open-access, authoritative recommendations for the treatment of parasitic infections.

SPECIAL CONSIDERATIONS
Common Parasitoses

Giardia lamblia
In about 60% of patients, *Giardia* produces no symptoms (asymptomatic cyst passer) and infection resolves spontaneously. Acute giardiasis (1 to 3 weeks after infection) presents with watery diarrhea and other abdominal symptoms. These symptoms may last for months. Chronic giardiasis presents with symptoms of malabsorption and lactose intolerance.

Diagnosis
Fecal examination may reveal trophozoites or cysts and should be done in all patients. Examination of three stool samples is only 85% sensitive in chronic giardiasis, so that enzyme immunoassay (EIA) testing for *Giardia* antigen is now considered the test of choice. If stool tests are negative, but clinical suspicion is high, more invasive testing may be necessary and referral to a gastroenterologist should be considered.

Treatment
Metronidazole (Flagyl), 500 mg bid for 5 days (pediatric dose is 15 mg/kg/day in three doses for 5 days), or Nitazoxanide 500 mg bid for 3 days (pediatric dose varies by age). Treatment is generally not indicated for persons who are asymptomatic.

Enterobius vermicularis
Pinworms cause intense anal pruritus, usually at night. They can occasionally be visualized as thread-like worms that migrate outside the anus at night. Diagnosis is generally via visualization of pin-worm eggs using the cellophane tape test (see above). Treat both adults and children with albendazole 400 mg once, repeated in 2 weeks. It is recommended to treat the entire family if one individual is infected. Clothes and bedding should be cleaned and fingernails kept short.

Ascaris lumbricoides
Ascaris is the world's most common intestinal worm. Infections are usually asymptomatic, but large infestations can cause intestinal obstruction. Worms occasionally migrate into the biliary tree, causing cholangitis. Diagnosis is by stool ova and parasite examination. Treatment is with albendazole 400 mg once. Pediatric and adult doses are the same. Treatment should be deferred in patients with Ascaris-associated pulmonary infections.

Entamoeba histolytica
Amebiasis usually results in asymptomatic colonic infection. When *E. histolytica* invades the intestinal wall, it produces colitis with clinical presentations ranging from dysentery to perforation. Amebas can spread hematogenously to any organ in the body; liver abscesses are the most common extraintestinal manifestation.

Diagnosis
Stool for ova and parasite examination can be obtained from aspirates obtained during colonoscopy. The mucus portion is more likely to contain amebas than the other parts of the stool. For abscesses, ultrasound-directed needle aspiration or serology, or both, may be necessary. *Entamoeba dispar*, which is morphologically indistinguishable from *E. histolytica*, is nonpathogenic; the two species can be distinguished by antigen testing.

Treatment
All patients require treatment. Asymptomatic intraluminal infection is usually treated with iodoquinol (Yodoxin) 650 mg tid × 20 days or paromomycin (Humatin) 25 to 35 mg/kg/day (adults) or 30 to 40 mg/kg/day (children) divided tid and given over 7 days. Symptomatic disease is treated with metronidazole (Flagyl), 750 mg tid for 7 to 10 days (pediatric dose 35 to 50 mg/kg/day in three doses for 10 days). This is followed by paromomycin or iodoquinol for an additional 7 days to eliminate intraluminal cysts.

Cystoisospora belli, cyclospora cayetanensis, and blastocystis spp.
These are protozoans that can cause diarrhea and intestinal cramping. Whether *Blastocystis* is truly a pathogen remains in dispute.

Diagnosis
Diagnosis is done by ova and parasite stool examination.

Treatment

Diseases caused by both *Cystoisospora* and *Cyclospora* are treated with co-trimoxazole (Bactrim, Septra), 160/800 mg PO bid for 10 days. If there are symptoms, blastocystosis can be treated with metronidazole 750 tid × 5 to 10 days).

Delusional parasitosis

This is an uncommon psychiatric condition in which patients insist that there are bugs or insects crawling on their bodies or into body openings. Patients may bring samples of what they believe to be such insects inside matchboxes or envelopes (the "matchbox" sign). Treatment is difficult; antipsychotics are generally recommended.

REFERENCE

1. Muennig P, Pallin D, Challah C, et al. The cost-effectiveness of ivermectin vs. albendazole in the presumptive treatment of strongyloidiasis in immigrants to the United States. *Epidemiol Infect* 2004;132:1055–1063. doi:10.1017/S0950268804003000.

CHAPTER 20

Injuries and Violence

Section Editor: Courtney Ann Dawley

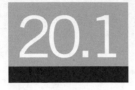

Bites of Humans and Animals

Richard W. Pretorius

Approximately half of all Americans are bitten by an animal during their lives, with 3 million animal bites per year in the United States. The vast majority (80% to 90%) of these bites are from dogs, usually the family pet or an animal known to the victim.[1] The remainder are inflicted by various wild and domestic animals, including farm animals, foxes, coyotes, skunks, rodents, and reptiles. Snakes account for approximately 45,000 bites annually in the United States, but less than 20% of these bites are inflicted by poisonous snakes. Dog and cat bites specifically represent 1% of all emergency room visits, with 1% of dog bites and 6% of cat bites requiring hospitalization.

Prophylactic antibiotics for cat or dog bites have not been shown to be effective in controlled trials.[2] However, antibiotics may prevent hand infection, particularly if there is a delay in obtaining medical attention. Human bites, other than the hand, do not appear to have any higher risk of infection than animal bites.[2] Deeper wounds can carry increased risk of infection,[3] which is usually polymicrobial involving several genera of bacteria, fungi, viruses, spirochetes, and rickettsia. Other potential complications include tenosynovitis, cellulitis, sepsis, arthritis, osteomyelitis, and fractures of underlying bony structures. Peritonitis and meningitis have also occurred in patients as a result of bites that have penetrated the abdominal cavity or the thin cranial bone of children.

HUMAN BITES

Epidemiology

The majority (80%) of human bites result from closed-fist injuries sustained during fist fights. The resulting lacerations are typically 3 to 8 mm in length, overlie the third metacarpophalangeal joint of the dominant hand, and can have a poor prognosis as they are frequently infected by the time the patient seeks medical care. Bacteria are often introduced into the joint when the joint capsule is broken and may spread into the deeper spaces of the hand when the digits are extended. Swelling and edema may decrease mobility of the involved digit. The majority of the remaining bites (15%) are accidental, occlusional bites from "love nips," which are most commonly seen on the genitalia, breasts, shoulders, arms, and hands. Occlusional bites found on children are usually inflicted by other children, although an intercanine distance of 3 cm or greater are likely from an adult and require an evaluation for abuse.

Treatment

The mainstay of treatment is cleansing with povidone–iodine and thorough irrigation with a large volume of sterile saline, 500 mL for small wounds and a liter or more for larger wounds. Although the culture of uninfected wounds is not recommended, infected wounds should be cultured prior to irrigation.[4] Human bites left open to close by secondary intention have the least incidence of infection, although they are accompanied by the greatest scar formation and can require several weeks to close completely. Delayed primary closure, which is often done, has a slightly higher risk of infection. Primary closure which poses a significant risk for infection is not advised in the treatment of hand bites, although it may be used in areas with excellent blood supply such as the face.[5] After dressing the wound, splint the hand in the position of function to minimize the tension on the tendons and muscles. Elevate all hand bites, especially when swelling is present, as the lack of elevation frequently leads to treatment failures. Reevaluate the injury within 24 hours. Obtain radiographs of the bite site to rule out underlying fractures and the presence of foreign bodies, joint space air, and osteomyelitis.

α-Hemolytic streptococci are the most common organisms cultured from infected hand injuries. Other bacteria commonly cultured from these injuries include *Staphylococcus aureus, Eikenella corrodens, Haemophilus influenzae,* and β-lactamase-producing oral, anaerobic bacteria.

Outpatient Antibiotic Therapy

Antibiotic prophylaxis for a minimum of 5 to 7 days should be considered for all patients with closed-fist injuries and occlusional bites to the hand or fingers, even when presenting within 8 hours of the injury, or prior to overt signs of infection. This is best accomplished with amoxicillin–clavulanate potassium (Augmentin, 875/125 mg) 1 pill orally twice daily for 10 days for adults and (600/42.9 mg/5 mL) 45 mg per kg orally bid for children. Alternatively, a second-generation cephalosporin, such as cefuroxime axetil (Ceftin), may be used at a dosage of 250 to 500 mg every 12 hours in adults and 20 to 30 mg/kg/day in divided doses in children.

Hospitalization

Intravenous antibiotics are necessary for all patients with clinically infected hand wounds. A surgeon should be consulted for bites over joints, especially the metacarpophalangeal joint, due to the frequent need for early surgical intervention with intrasynovial irrigation and drain placement. Aerobic and anaerobic cultures must be obtained before starting antibiotics. Intravenous antibiotic options include ampicillin sodium/sulbactam sodium (Unasyn) 1.5 to 3.0 g every 6 hours, cefoxitin (Mefoxin) 1 to 2 g every 6 to 8 hours, cefotetan disodium (Cefotan) 1 to 2 g every 6 to 12 hours, and imipenem–cilastatin (Primaxin) 500 mg every 6 hours.[6] Patients with diabetes who do not respond to initial treatment with oral antibiotics should be considered for coverage with gentamicin (Garamycin) 2 g per kg load, then 1.7 mg per kg every 8 hours, or similar aminoglycoside antibiotic, because these patients frequently have Gram-negative infections.

DOG BITES

Epidemiology

Dog bites cause 10 to 20 deaths annually with the majority of deaths from exsanguination associated with bites to the head and neck in children younger than 4 years.[7] Elderly patients are also at increased risk. Tears, avulsions, punctures, scratches, and crush injuries may also be present. The overall risk of infection is about 8%.[8] Primary suturing is recommended as leaving the wound to heal by secondary intention does not reduce the infection rate and diminishes the cosmetic appearance.[8]

Treatment

All wounds should be thoroughly cleaned and irrigated. Devitalized tissue should be debrided and the wound thoroughly examined for foreign bodies. Dog bites to the hand, wrist, and foot should be left open to close by secondary intention. Bites to the face and other areas with excellent blood supply that appear clinically uninfected may undergo primary closure. Children with severe facial or neck injuries from dog bites should be considered for primary closure under general anesthesia. In children with dog bites to the head by a moderate- to large-sized dog, evaluation with radiographs or computed tomography (CT) scan should be considered to evaluate for a potential open skull fracture. Positive cultures have been obtained in 90% of clinically infected wounds.[9] One study found that *Pasteurella multocida* was isolated in 53% of cases, whereas *Streptococcus* was cultured in 29%, and *Staphylococcus* in about 24%.[9] Another study[10] found that α-hemolytic streptococci were the most frequently isolated organisms. Patients with poorly functioning immune systems are at risk for the development of *Capnocytophagia canimorsus* sepsis (examine peripheral smear for bacilli) and disseminated intravascular coagulation and should be immediately hospitalized at their initial presentation for treatment of the bite. Anaerobic bacteria, including *Bacteroides, Fusobacterium, Peptostreptococcus,* and *Eubacterium,* have also been cultured from infected dog bite wounds.

Outpatient Antibiotic Therapy

Antibiotic therapy should be administered to patients with moderate to severe bites; bites on the hands, neck, or face; bites that appear clinically infected; and immunocompromised patients. The routine culturing of uninfected wounds is not recommended as they often grow multiple organisms and will not assist in guiding the treatment of an infection if one occurs. Facial bites have a relatively low risk of infection (7%); consequently, some authors feel that these wounds should be managed with reconstructive surgery without prophylactic antibiotics.[11] Amoxicillin–clavulanate potassium (Augmentin), 250 to 500 mg every 8 hours, is the drug of choice for outpatient therapy. Children are dosed at 20 mg/kg/day in divided doses. Penicillin V potassium (Pen-Vee K), 250 to 500 mg for every 6 hours, and ampicillin (Omnipen), 250 to 500 mg every 8 hours (in children, 50 to 100 mg/kg/day), are other possible choices. In the absence of overt infection, a 3- to 5-day prophylaxis regimen is prudent for crush injuries or injuries that involve the hand or a joint.

Hospitalization

Hospitalization is indicated for patients with systemic manifestations of infection and in patients with severe cellulitis or in whom the infection has spread rapidly and has not responded to outpatient therapy. Intravenous antibiotic therapy can be accomplished with ampicillin sodium/sulbactam sodium, 1.5 to 3.0 g every 6 hours. Alternative intravenous antibiotics include ceftriaxone sodium (Rocephin), given 1 to 2 g once daily or administered in divided doses. Children may be administered 50 to 75 mg per kg once daily or in divided doses.

CAT BITES

Epidemiology

Cats bite approximately 400,000 humans annually. The majority occur on the arms, forearms, and hands. Feline canine teeth are sharp and pointed, which facilitates the penetration of bones and joints. The resulting puncture wounds are difficult to clean and irrigate adequately, and 50% of these bites become infected. Patients may develop septic arthritis and osteomyelitis following a cat bite.[12] Other patients have developed *Pasteurella* meningitis, pneumonia, and prosthetic joint infections after a cat bite.

Treatment

Puncture wounds should be carefully irrigated, with care given to prevent extravasation of fluid and bacteria into surrounding tissues. Puncture wounds should be left open to heal by secondary intention. *P. multocida* is the most common bacterium isolated from the oral cavity and teeth of cats.[13] This organism can cause an intense inflammation with a rapidly expanding cellulitis. A purulent drainage is noted in approximately 40% of patients. Cultures frequently show growth of *Pasteurella* within 24 hours of the bite.[2] Wounds that become infected 24 hours post-bite usually culture *Staphylococcus* or *Streptococcus*.[14] Other isolates cultured from cat bite wounds include *Eikenella* and various Gram-negative enteric bacteria and anaerobic bacteria, including *Bacteroides* and *Actinomyces*. *Bartonella henselae*, the etiologic agent of cat-scratch disease, may be inoculated in both cat scratches and bites.[15] Infection with this agent may also result in a reactive arthritis with polyarthralgia of the knees and elbows.[16]

Outpatient Antibiotic Therapy

The drug of choice for the outpatient treatment of cat bites is amoxicillin–clavulanate potassium, 250 to 500 mg every 8 hours. Children are dosed at 20 mg/kg/day in divided doses based on the amoxicillin component.

Hospitalization

Severely infected bites requiring hospitalization may be treated with ceftriaxone sodium (Rocephin), 1 to 2 g in adults and 50 to 75 mg/kg/day in children. Tularemia has also been shown to be transmitted by cat bites and scratches[17] and should be considered where bites have failed to improve with appropriate treatment. This kind of infection is most appropriately managed with streptomycin, 1 g per kg every 12 hours IM or IV for 7 to 14 days. Children should be dosed at 15 mg/kg/day IM in two divided doses for 10 days. In adults, *Bartonella henselae* infections should be managed with erythromycin 500 mg qid or doxycycline 100 mg bid. Children may be treated with erythromycin 30 to 50 mg/kg/day in divided doses.

EXOTIC PETS

Epidemiology

The ownership of exotic pets in the United States is rapidly increasing with 3% of U.S. homes keeping exotic pets.[18] The most common exotic pets are reptiles such as iguanas, monitor lizards, anoles, and chameleons. Some unusual mammals are kept as pets as well, including rats, chinchillas, hedgehogs, and simians.

Treatment

As with all other bites, the mainstay of treatment is copious irrigation with sterile saline and debridement if necessary. Because exotic pets are far less common than cats and dogs, their bites are not seen very often, and the treatment of these bites has not been well studied. It is generally recommended that the bites of simians be treated the same as a human bite because their oral flora is very similar. Lizards, on the other hand, harbor unusual subtypes of *Salmonella*. Routine prophylaxis of these bites is not necessary. If a lizard bite does become infected, the antibiotic treatment should provide coverage for *Salmonella*.[18] Clindamycin 450 mg four times a day for adults or 20 to 30 mg per kg in divided doses four times a day is one option.

SNAKE BITES

Epidemiology

Poisonous snakes, found in every state except for Maine, Alaska, and Hawaii, inflict approximately 7,000 to 8,000 bites yearly in the United States, resulting in 9 to 15 deaths. Up to 50% of poisonous snake bites are "dry bites" and do not result in envenomation. Snake venoms are complex mixtures of enzymes that result in the disruption of cell membranes, precipitation of free hemoglobin, muscle and local tissue necrosis, thrombocytopenia, abnormal clotting times, and—in severe cases—death. Patients may experience breathing difficulties; perioral tingling; weakness; diplopia; nausea; vomiting; and muscle fasciculations of the tongue, face, and upper chest and arms after pit viper envenomation. Patients may also experience a metallic taste in the mouth. Patients will commonly experience severe pain and marked swelling at the bite site.

Treatment

A poisonous snake bite is a medical emergency. Field treatment includes having the victim stop physical exertion and resting, calmly reassuring, splinting of the bitten extremity below heart level, considering loose application only for coral snake bites of a wide lymphatic constriction band (that easily allows two fingers between the skin and the band), and transporting to the nearest emergency facility. Cryotherapy, restricting arterial or venous blood flow, and incision and suction are contraindicated.

- Emergency treatment includes an assessment of envenomation, cleansing of the wound, and administration of antivenom where indicated. Bites from pit vipers (rattlesnakes, cottonmouths, copperheads) are primarily hemotoxic in nature. Hallmark findings of pit viper envenomation are pain and swelling. If pain and swelling are not present within 30 minutes of a pit viper bite, the patient was probably not envenomated. Patients thought to have received a dry bite can be observed for an additional 2 to 4 hours and be treated as outpatients if no signs of envenomation occur with 8 hours of the bite.[19] Patients remaining asymptomatic may be safely discharged home after routine wound care has been accomplished. However, coral snake bites are primarily neurotoxic, and patients envenomated by coral snakes may show minimal signs and symptoms for several hours. Hospitalization (24-hour observation) is indicated for patients of coral snake bites even when it is suspected that the patient received a dry bite. Serial measurements of the bitten extremity should be made and recorded at 15- to 30-minute intervals. Envenomation may be graded as follows: grade 1, no envenomation; grade 2, mild envenomation with pain and edema extending up to 6 inches from the bite site during the first 12 hours; grade 3, moderate envenomation with edema extending up to 12 inches from the bite site accompanied by nausea, vomiting, prolonged bleeding times, and decreases in platelet counts and hematocrit; and grade 4, severe envenomation with marked swelling and extensive systemic involvement.

- **Antivenom administration.** Not all venomous bites require the administration of antivenom. The major indications are rapid progression of swelling, coagulation defect, neuromuscular paralysis, and cardiovascular collapse. A polyvalent Fab crotalid antivenom (CroFab) quickly reverses the local effects of the venom and has the unique capacity to completely reverse the neurotoxicity associated with bites of the potent Mojave rattlesnake.[19] Prior to starting the antivenom, a complete blood count, prothrombin time, partial thromboplastin time, electrolytes, blood urea nitrogen, urinalysis, and arterial blood gases should be done. Blood should also be typed and cross-matched. Two large-bore intravenous lines of normal saline or lactated Ringer solution are typically started, and a Foley catheter should be inserted for accurate urine measurements. A syringe of 0.3 to 0.5 mL of a 1:1,000 solution of epinephrine must be available for management of anaphylaxis. Grade 2 envenomations may require up to six vials of antivenom, whereas grade 3 and 4 envenomations may require up to 15 and 30 vials, respectively. Antivenom is only effective when administered intravenously and should not be injected intramuscularly, subcutaneously, or directly into the bite site. There is no maximal dose of antivenom. The patient's condition must be continuously reevaluated after each antivenom dosing. A small vial of venous blood (5 to 10 mL) may be collected after each dose of antivenom dosing. If this blood clots after 20 minutes, no additional antivenom is needed.[20] In cases where the patient develops an allergy to the antivenom and has sustained a severe poisoning, the antivenom can be temporarily stopped while the patient is treated with intravenous diphenhydramine (Benadryl), 10 to 50 mg in adults and 5 mg/kg/day in children. The antivenom may then be restarted at a lower rate.

- **Antibiotics.** Antibiotics should be reserved for actual infections as prophylaxis with intramuscular ceftriaxone, 1 to 2 g per day in adults and 50 to 75 mg/kg/day in children, does not decrease the 5% risk of local abscess from crotalid's bites.

VACCINATION PROPHYLAXIS

Tetanus

The patient's tetanus vaccination status must be determined.[21] Patients who have completed the primary three-shot regimen will need a booster shot if it has been 10 or more years since their last shot. A wound that is large and dirty needs a booster if it has been longer than 5 years since their last one. If the patient has not completed the primary three-shot series, that series should be started when the patient presents for treatment. If the wound is small and clean, beginning the vaccination series is adequate. If the wound is large and/or dirty, the patient should be given human tetanus immune globulin (250 units for adults and children). The vaccine and immune globulin should be administered at separate sites that are distant from the other, so that they do not interfere with each other.

Rabies

Rabies prophylaxis includes both vaccination and human rabies immune globulin (RIG).[22,23] If a patient has been previously immunized against rabies, the vaccine is given on days 0 and 3. If there is no history of vaccination and the patient has a high-risk bite, the vaccine is given on days 0, 3, 7, and 14 (with an additional dose on day 28 for the immunocompromised). Additionally, the unvaccinated patient should be given RIG as a single dose of 20 IU per kg. As much of the RIG as possible is infiltrated around the wound, and the rest injected IM at a site distant from the vaccine. The difficult part is determining which bites need rabies prophylaxis. The best source for an answer to this is the local public health department. Some basic guidelines include bites from any dog, wild animal, or bat that is not available for observation. If the animal is available, prophylaxis can be held for up to 10 days to allow for observation and examination to determine whether the animal was carrying rabies. One absolute indication is for people who have been in a room with a bat, and it cannot be determined whether a bite, scratch, or mucous membrane exposure has occurred (Advisory Committee on Immunization Practices recommendation). This includes small children, the disabled, intoxicated persons, and anyone who awakens to find a bat in the room. Bats have very small sharp teeth and it can be very difficult to determine whether a bite occurred.

REFERENCES

1. Gandhi RR, Liebman MA, Stafford BL, et al. Dog bite injuries in children: a preliminary survey. *Am Surg* 1999;65(9):863–864.
2. Medeiros I, Saconato H. Antibiotic prophylaxis for mammalian bites. *Cochrane Database Syst Rev* 2001; (2):CD001738.
3. Abrahamian FM, Goldstein EJ. Microbiology of animal bite wound infections. *Clin Microbiol Rev* 2011; 24(2):231–246.
4. Hagen M, Goldstein E, Sanford JP. Bites from pet animals. *Hosp Pract* 1993;28(9):79–86.
5. Donkor P, Bankas DO. A study of primary closure of human bite injuries to the face. *J Oral Maxillofac Surg* 1997;55(5):479–481.
6. Kahn RM, Goldstein EJ. Common bacterial skin infections: diagnostic clues and therapeutic options. *Postgrad Med* 1993;93(6):175–182.
7. Weis HB, Friedman DI, Coben JH. Incidence of dog bite injuries treated in emergency departments. *JAMA* 1988;279(1):51–53.
8. Paschos NK, Makris EA, Gantsos A, et al. Primary closure versus non-closure of dog bite wounds. a randomised controlled trial. *Injury* 2014;45:237–240.
9. Dire DJ, Hogan DE, Riggs MW. A prospective evaluation of risk factors from dog-bite infections. *Acad Emerg Med* 1994;1(3):258–266.
10. Goldstein EJ. Bite wounds and infection. *Clin Infect Dis* 1992;14(3):633–638.

11. Wolff KD. Management of animal bite injuries of the face: experience with 94 patients. *J Oral Maxillofac Surg* 1998;56(7):838–843.
12. Chodakewitz J, Bia FJ. Septic arthritis and osteomyelitis from a cat bite. *Yale J Biol Med* 1988;61(6): 513–518.
13. Dendle C, Looke D. Management of mammalian bites. *Aust Fam Physician* 2009;38(11):868–874.
14. Aghababian RV, Conte JE. Mammalian bite wounds. *Ann Emerg Med* 1980;9(2):79–83.
15. Piemont Y, Heller R. Bartonellosis: I. Bartonella henselae [in French]. *Ann Biol Clin (Paris)* 1998;56(6): 681–692.
16. Jendro MC, Weber G, Brabant T, et al. Reactive arthritis after cat bite: a rare manifestation of cat scratch disease-case report and overview. *Z Rheumatol* 1998;57(3):159–163.
17. Capellan J, Fong IW. Tularemia from a cat bite: case report and review of feline associated tularemia. *Clin Infect Dis* 1993;16(4):472–475.
18. Warwick C, Steedman C. Injuries, envenomations and stings from exotic pets. *J R Soc Med* 2012; 105(7):296–299.
19. Singletary EM, Rochman AS, Bodmer JCA, et al. Envenomations. *Med Clin North Am* 2005;89(6): 1195–1224.
20. Warrell DA, Fenner PJ. Venomous bites and stings. *Br Med Bull* 1993;49(2):423–439.
21. Centers for Disease Control and Prevention (CDC). Updated recommendations for use of tetanus toxoid, reduced diphtheria toxoid and acellular pertussis (Tdap) vaccine from the Advisory Committee on Immunization Practices, 2010. *MMWR Morb Mortal Wkly Rep* 2011;60(1):13–15.
22. Rupprecht CE, Briggs D, Brown CM, et al; Centers for Disease Control and Prevention (CDC). Use of a reduced (4-dose) vaccine schedule for postexposure prophylaxis to prevent human rabies: recommendations of the Advisory Committee on Immunization Practices. *MMWR Recomm Rep* 2010;59(RR-2):1–9.
33. Rabies Vaccine. www.cdc.gov/rabies/medical_care/vaccine.html. Accessed March 31, 2014.

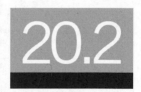

20.2

Burns
Chantell R. Hemsley

GENERAL PRINCIPLES
Epidemiology
Each year in the United States, 2.5 million people seek medical care for burns. Although 95% of burn victims do not require hospitalization, burns can be devastating.[1] They are the third leading cause of accidental death and can cause lifelong scarring and disfigurement. Major risks of death consist of smoke inhalation injuries, shock due to inadequate fluid resuscitation, and infection.

Severity Classification
The severity of the burn should be categorized as minor, moderate, or major. This is based on the burn depth and size, burn location, patient age, patient comorbidities, and the presence of trauma or inhalation injury.

- **Minor burns** can be treated on an outpatient basis:
  - ≤10% total body surface area (TBSA) partial-thickness burn in a patient 10 to 40 years of age
  - ≤15% TBSA partial-thickness burn in an adult
  - ≤2% full-thickness burn in a child or adult, not involving eyes, ears, face, or genitalia
  - Cannot cross a major joint and cannot be circumferential
- **Moderate burns** should be admitted to the hospital:[2]
  - 10% to 20% TBSA partial-thickness burn in children <10 and adults >40 years of age with <10% full-thickness burn
  - 15% to 25% TBSA in adults with <10% full-thickness burn
  - ≤10% TBSA full-thickness burn in children or adults without cosmetic or functional risk to eyes, ears, face, hands, feet, or perineum[2]
- **Major burns** should be referred to a burn center:

- Coinciding major trauma or inhalation injury
- Medical comorbidities predisposing to infection (e.g., diabetes, sickle cell disease)
- ≥20% TBSA partial-thickness burn in a child <10 or in an adult >40 years of age
- ≥25% TBSA
- ≥10% full-thickness burn in a child or adult
- All burns involving eyes, ears, face, hands, feet, or genitalia
- High-voltage electrical burns[2]

Pathophysiology

The depth of the burn determines the need for medical interventions as well as the risk for complications. Burn depth can be viewed as **superficial** (epidermal involvement only), **superficial partial-** and **deep partial-thickness** (involving the superficial or deep dermal layers), and **full-thickness** (destroys the entire dermis). Burn depth estimation revisions are often necessary in the first 24 to 72 hours, especially if involving thin-skinned areas.[2]

Burns to **thin-skinned areas** should always be treated initially as at least partial-thickness. Thin-skin areas include volar forearm surfaces, medial thighs, perineum, ears, and burns in children less than age of 5 and adults over the age of 55.

Mechanisms of Injury

Most burns are due to thermal injuries, such as scalding water or fires. Electrical burns due to high voltage can cause significant damage to muscles, including the heart. **High-voltage burns** are characterized by entry and exit burn sites; if none is present, then the patient has a high-voltage injury that places the patient at risk for occult muscle damage.[2]

DIAGNOSIS

Clinical Presentation

Remove any hot or burned clothing. Immediately begin cooling using room temperature or cool tap water. Cool with caution in people with >10% TBSA involvement and avoid ice and freezing to prevent frostbite.[3]

History

Burn victims from enclosed spaces are at greater risk for smoke inhalation. The time of injury is important for determining fluid resuscitation during the first 8 hours following injury.

Physical Examination

Minor, moderate, or major burns should be categorized by classifying injuries as superficial, superficial partial-thickness, deep partial-thickness, and full-thickness (see "classification," below). It is important to estimate the burn size of all partial-thickness and full-thickness burns. Examination is necessary for signs of smoke inhalation (persistent coughing, wheezing, dyspnea, hoarseness, facial burns, sooty mucus, and laryngeal edema).

Burn size is expressed as a percentage of TBSA. Superficial burns can be ignored. **The rule of nines** method is an appropriate way to estimate TBSA in adults; each leg represents 18% TBSA, each arm 9%, the anterior and posterior trunk each 18%, and the head 9%. For small burns, the surface of the patient's palm represents 0.4% of the TBSA. With electrical burns, all tissue in between the entry and exit wounds should be considered; it should be treated as a full-thickness burn.

Laboratory Studies

In an electrical injury, evaluate for occult rhabdomyolysis by checking blood creatinine kinase (CK) levels. Arterial blood gas (ABG) can access for carbon monoxide poisoning and further elucidate pulmonary status in the case of a suspected smoke inhalation.

Imaging

Electrocardiogram (ECG) should be done if an electrical injury has occurred.

Monitoring

- A total of 12 to 24 hours of cardiac monitoring is warranted after an electrical injury if there are any ECG abnormalities.
- Observe patients with suspected inhalation injury for 12 to 24 hours if unable to directly visualize the airway (see below).

Surgical Diagnostic Procedures

Fiberoptic laryngoscopy and bronchoscopy can assess the extent of airway injury and assist with intubation with suspected smoke inhalation victims. If unavailable, monitor for declining pulmonary function using serial peak expiratory flow rates and repeat ABGs.[4,5]

Depth Classification

Burns are classified according to the depth of the burn. Hallmarks distinguishing burn depth are as follows:

- **Superficial burns** result from UV exposure and are painful, dry, red, and blanch with pressure. They usually take 3 to 6 days to heal without scarring.
- **Superficial partial-thickness burns** result from splash or spill scalds and are painful to temperature and air. Blisters are present. Wounds are moist, red, weeping, and blanch with pressure. They heal in 7 to 20 days; scarring is unusual although pigment changes may occur.
- **Deep partial-thickness burns** result from prolonged spill scalds, flame, or hot oil or grease and are painful to pressure only. Blisters are apparent and are easily unroofed. The wound is wet or waxy and dry. Color varies from cheesy white to red to patchy, and they do not blanch with pressure. They take more than 21 days to heal, and scarring may be severe.
- **Full-thickness burns** result from immersion scalds, flame, steam, hot oil or grease, or chemical or electrical sources. They are usually painless. The skin is waxy white to leathery gray to charred and black, is dry and inelastic, and does not blanch with pressure. Healing is very slow, if at all, and may require skin grafting if >2% of the TBSA is involved. Scarring is very severe with contractures.[2]

TREATMENT

Initial treatment of minor burns consists of cooling, cleansing, appropriate dressing, and pain management. Moderate and severe burns require intravenous (IV) fluid resuscitation. All patients should be assessed for smoke inhalation with aggressive airway management.

Medications

Superficial burns do not require infection prophylaxis. All other burns benefit from applying a topical antibiotic.

- **1% silver sulfadiazine** (SSD) is a good first-line agent, but avoid using near eyes or mouth; in persons with sulfonamide hypersensitivity; and in pregnant women, newborns, and nursing mothers.
- **Bacitracin** is an effective alternative topical antibiotic when SSD cannot be used. Other therapies, which have not been extensively studied, include honey or aloe vera.
  Administer a **tetanus booster** to all burn victims who are not with current tetanus immunization.[2] Pain control should focus on both an around-the-clock regimen, as well as a rescue medication before dressing changes and during increased physical activity.[2]
- **Pregabalin** or **Gabapentin** have been shown to be equivalent or superior to **antihistamines** for post-burn pruritis in preliminary studies.[6–8]

Surgery

Full-thickness burns >2 cm usually require skin grafting. Timing of the procedure is crucial: Skin grafting begun within 72 hours is beneficial for non-scald burns in children and adults younger than 30 years old. Observe all other non-scald full-thickness burns for 8 to 10 days. Wait 2 weeks before performing surgery in children with hot water scald burns; earlier interventions in this group have resulted in worse outcomes.[9,10]

Nonoperative

Airway management is critical in patients with major burns. Intubation should not be delayed if severe inhalation injury or respiratory distress is present or anticipated.

Prevention of shock using aggressive **fluid resuscitation** is crucial in those with ≥15% TBSA or in major burns. However, over resuscitation can also result in significant morbidity and mortality.

- In adults, initially give IV crystalloid solution, standard of care being lactated Ringer's. Major burns should be treated with two large bore IVs preferably placed in nonburned skin. The Parkland formula estimates the rate of fluids for the first 24 hours at 4 mL per kg body weight for each % TBSA effected. One half of this total amount should be given over the first 8 hours, with the remainder given over the next 16 hours.

- Maintenance fluids can continue after the first 24 hours with additional boluses titrated to maintain urinary output of at least 5 mL per kg (1 mL per kg for electrical injuries). Poor urinary output is correlated with higher mortality. After the first 24 hours, the crystalloid solution can be changed to 5% dextrose in 0.45% normal saline with 20 mEq of potassium chloride.
- In children weighing <25 kg, maintain hourly urine output at 1 mL per kg.
- The use of colloids (e.g., albumin) appears to offer no advantage over the use of crystalloids.[5,11,12]

Remove ruptured blisters. Intact blisters should be left undisturbed unless there are signs of infection. If blisters persist without resorption past 2 weeks, refer to a surgeon as there could be an underlying deep partial burn warranting grafting. Avoid needle aspiration of blisters.[13]

Special Therapy

Dressings. Superficial burns do not require wound dressings. Simple skin lubricants (e.g., aloe vera cream) are sufficient. All partial- and full-thickness burns should have dressings.

- First, gently clean the burn with mild soap and water. Skin disinfectants (Hibiclens, Betadine) can actually inhibit the healing process and are discouraged. Apply a thin layer of topical 1% silver sulfadine or other antimicrobial. Then, cover with fine-mesh gauze (e.g., Telfa) and secure in place with a moderate degree of pressure.
- Change dressings whenever they become soaked with excessive exudates or other fluids. Wound should be cleansed before each redressing.
- Deep wounds may require biologic dressings or skin grafts.[14,15]

After epithelialization occurs, use an unscented moisturizing cream such as Cetaphil or Eucerin until natural lubricating mechanisms return. Avoid the use of preparations high in lanolin. Evidence for the efficacy of vitamin E lotions is limited.[16]

Referrals

Refer minor burn patients to a surgeon with burn care expertise if a full-thickness burn >2 cm is discovered or at 2 weeks if wound epithelialization has not begun. Wound complications can also be the grounds for referral. Full-thickness burns <2 cm in diameter can be allowed to heal by contracture when it is in a nonfunctional, noncosmetic area and the skin is not thin.

Follow-Up

See patients the day after injury to adjust pain medications and assess dressing change competence. In the right patient, visits can then be weekly until wound epithelialization occurs. More frequent follow-up is required if there is insufficient pain control, any concern about the patient or family's ability to provide care, or if synthetic or biologic dressings have been used.

Complications

- All suspected **burn infections** warrant aggressive management to include admission and parenteral antibiotics. Burn infections are prone to sepsis and will extend the depth and extent of the burn. Diagnosing infection in burn patients is challenging. It should be suspected whenever increasing erythema, edema, pain, or tenderness is associated with lymphangitis, fever, malaise, or anorexia.
- **Necrotic tissue** in deep burn wounds may cause progressive tissue injury as well as increasing the risk for infection. Wound excision and grafting is usually beneficial.
- **Hypertrophic scarring** is usually inevitable whenever epithelialization takes longer than 2 weeks in African Americans and in young children, and 3 weeks in all others. Early application of pressure is recommended. Refer patients promptly if the wound misses its epithelialization milestone or if hypertrophic scarring appears.[17]
- Increased mortality is associated with age >60 years, nonsuperficial burns covering >40% TBSA, coexisting trauma, pneumonia, and, in one study, female sex.[18,19]

REFERENCES

1. Deitch EA. The management of burns. *N Engl J Med* 1990;323:1249–1253.
2. Waitzman AA, Neligan PC. How to manage burns in primary care. *Can Fam Physician* 1993;39: 2394–2400.
3. Pushkar NS, Sandorminsky BP. Cold treatment of burns. *Burns Incl Therm Inj* 1982;9:101–110.
4. Miller K, Chang A. Acute inhalation injury. *Emerg Med Clin North Am* 2003;21:533–537.
5. Monafo WW. Current concepts: initial management of burns. *N Engl J Med* 1996;335:1581–1586.
6. Ahuja RB, Gupta GK. A four arm, double blind, randomized and placebo controlled study of pregabalin in the management of post-burn pruritus. *Burns* 2013;39(1):24–29.

7. Ahuja RB, Gupta R, Gupta G, et al. A comparative analysis of cetirizine, gabapentin and their combination in the relief of post-burn pruritis. *Burns* 2011;37(2):203–207.
8. Gray P, Kirby J, Smith MT, et al. Pregabalin in severe burn injury pain: a double-blind, randomised placebo-controlled trial. *Pain* 2011;152(6):1279–1288.
9. Baxter CR. Management of burn wounds. *Dermatol Clin* 1993;11:709–714.
10. Desai MH, Rutan RL, Herndon DN. Conservative treatment of scald burns is superior to early excision. *J Burn Care Rehabil* 1991;12:482–484.
11. Alderson P, Schierhout G, Roberts I, et al. Colloids versus crystalloids for fluid resuscitation in critically ill patients. *Cochrane Database Syst Rev* 2000;2:CD000567.
12. Muller MJ, Herndon DN. The challenge of burns. *Lancet* 1994;343:216–220.
13. Rockwell WB, Ehrlich HP. Should burn blister fluid be evacuated? *J Burn Care Rehabil* 1990;11:93–95.
14. Hartford CE. Care of outpatient burns. In: Herndon D, ed. *Total burn care*. Philadelphia, PA: WB Saunders; 1996:71–80.
15. Mertens DM, Jenkins ME, Warden GD. Outpatient burn management. *Nurs Clin North Am* 1997; 32:343.
16. Barbosa E, Faintuch J, Machado Moreira EA, et al. Supplementation of vitamin E, vitamin C, and zinc attenuates oxidative stress in burned children: a randomized, double-blind, placebo-controlled pilot study. *J Burn Care Res* 2009;30(5):859–866.
17. Deitch EA, Wheelahan TM, Rose MP, et al. Hypertrophic burn scars: analysis of variables. *J Trauma* 1983; 23:895–898.
18. McGwin G Jr, George RL, Cross JM, et al. Improving the ability to predict mortality among burn patients. *Burns* 2008;34(3):320–327.
19. Moore EC, Pilcher DV, Bailey MJ, et al. The Burns Evaluation and Mortality Study (BEAMS): predicting deaths in Australian and New Zealand burn patients admitted to intensive care with burns. *J Trauma Acute Care Surg* 2013;75(2):298–303.

BIBLIOGRAPHY

1. Ulmer JF. Burn pain management: a guideline-based approach. *J Burn Care Rehabil* 1998;19:151–159.

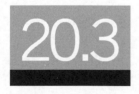

20.3 Smoke Inhalation and Carbon Monoxide Poisoning

Richard W. Pretorius

SMOKE INHALATION
General Principles

The inhalation of heated gas and the products of combustion can cause serious respiratory injury and is responsible for the majority of fire deaths, more so than surface burns and their complications. Any patient with carbon deposits in the mouth, singeing of nasal hair, or other findings suspicious for significant smoke inhalation should be admitted to the hospital for observation, treatment, and possible intubation. Approximately one-third of patients admitted to burn units have smoke inhalation as a compounding complication. Hypoxia, heat, and chemicals can all injure lung parenchyma.

Pathophysiology/Etiology
- **Impaired tissue oxygenation** results from the carbon monoxide and—with increased frequency—cyanide found in smoke. It can be immediately life-threatening.
  - Carbon monoxide (CO) accounts for over half of the fatalities in smoke inhalation (see "Carbon Monoxide Poisoning").
  - Suspect cyanide, which impairs cellular oxidative metabolism, when plastics or organic chemicals are fuels,[1] especially with high-temperature and low-oxygen settings.
- **Thermal injury** results from the inhalation of heated gases.

- The supraglottic mucosa, which has little protection from heated gases, often develops edema and subsequent airway obstruction within 18 to 24 hours after exposure.
- The subglottic tissues are generally protected from thermal injury because smoke is dry with a low specific heat and the upper airway has excellent heat exchange properties, although steam inhalation can result in tracheobronchial burns.
- Elective intubation needs to be considered early in all patients with suspected thermal injury.
- **Chemical injury** is primarily caused by insoluble irritant gases that affect the lower airways.
  - Insoluble irritant gases include aldehydes, amines, chlorine, hydrochloric acid, and sulfur dioxide.
  - As with thermal injury, there may be a delay between exposure and clinical manifestation.

Diagnosis of Smoke Inhalation

History
- Positive predictive factors for significant smoke inhalation include unconsciousness, entrapment in an enclosed space, and exposure to known toxins.[2]

Physical Examination
- Facial burns, singeing of eyebrows and nasal vibrissae, carbonaceous sputum, and oropharyngeal carbon deposits are suggestive of inhalation injury.
- Cyanosis, tachypnea, stridor, wheezing, and crackles are suggestive of the need for aggressive treatment; however, these signs are infrequently found despite the presence of significant injury.

Laboratory Studies
- Carboxyhemoglobin testing should be carried out on all patients. Elevated levels (>2%) should raise suspicion regarding the presence of other toxins (e.g., CO and cyanide).
- **Arterial blood gases.** Hypoxemia and elevated alveolar–arterial (P_AO_2–P_aO_2 >15 mm) gradient are frequently seen in inhalation injury, although they are insensitive indicators of injury and do not predict clinical outcome.
- Pulse oximetry can also be used as a noninvasive measure of oxygenation,[1] but may be normal despite the presence of carboxyhemoglobin as CO displaces oxygen from hemoglobin but does not change the concentration of oxygen dissolved in the blood.

Imaging
- Chest radiography generally is an insensitive initial test and should be reserved for hospitalized patients and those with suspected thoracic injury.

Diagnostic Procedures
- Bronchoscopy with direct fiberoptic visualization of the upper and lower airway provides an assessment of the extent of injury. Since the appearance of the subglottic tissues is an unreliable predictor of the need for ventilation, laryngoscopy may suffice for management decisions.[3]

Treatment

Protocol
- **Immediate.** Early mortality occurs from asphyxiation due to CO and cyanide.
- Remove patient from offending environment.
  - Provide 100% oxygen via a non-rebreathing mask until carboxyhemoglobin level is in the normal range. Maintain a partial pressure of oxygen (PO_2) greater than 75.
  - If cyanide poisoning is present, induce methemoglobinemia. This can be expedited by contacting the local poison control center.
- **Early.** Upper airway obstruction causing fatal injury occurs in the first 8 to 48 hours after exposure.
  - Endotracheal intubation should be strongly considered on initial assessment if physical findings are suggestive of inhalation injury.[2]
  - If direct visualization of the upper airway with laryngoscopy or bronchoscopy reveals even minimal early swelling or obstruction, endotracheal intubation should be performed because swelling will continue for the first 24 hours.
  - Bronchoscopy within the first 24 hours can remove foreign particles that may worsen the inflammatory reaction and may decrease time spent in the intensive care unit.[1]
  - Humidified oxygen or air should be given to thin the viscous bronchorrhea that is produced by injured airways.
  - Bronchodilators (albuterol 5% solution, 0.5 mL) may have variable effects, depending on whether obstruction is due to edema or bronchospasm. There is no contraindication to its use in smoke inhalation.

- Steroids and prophylactic antibiotics are contraindicated.
- Antibiotics are indicated for proven infection, which tends to occur with the onset of bronchorrhea 2 to 3 days after the injury.
- **Late.** Adult respiratory distress syndrome is a late complication.

CARBON MONOXIDE POISONING

General Principles

CO, which causes up to 80% of fatalities from smoke inhalation, is a colorless, odorless, tasteless, non-irritating gas produced by incomplete combustion of carbonaceous materials. It is responsible for 500 accidental and 5,000 suicidal deaths in the United States every year. The CO molecule has 240 times the affinity of oxygen for hemoglobin. Toxic effects are due to tissue hypoxia as carboxyhemoglobin is incapable of carrying oxygen and interferes with oxygen release.

Diagnosis

Clinical Presentation

Although exposure levels do not consistently correlate with carboxyhemoglobin levels and symptoms, the following associations are commonly seen:

- Mild exposure (1% to 15% carboxyhemoglobin) causes headache, dizziness, and nausea.
- Moderate exposure (16% to 40% carboxyhemoglobin) causes severe headache, nausea, vomiting, loss of coordination, and unconsciousness.
- Severe exposure (40% to 60% or greater carboxyhemoglobin) causes seizures, coma, and death.[3]

History

History may include suicidal or accidental exposure to auto exhaust, smoke inhalation, or exposure to a poorly vented heater or appliance.

Laboratory Findings

- Increased carboxyhemoglobin level. Normal levels are 1% to 3%; levels in smokers are 5% to 6%.
- Patients may have a normal arterial partial pressure of oxygen (PaO_2).
- Pulse oximetry should be considered unreliable; it cannot differentiate oxyhemoglobin from carboxyhemoglobin.

Management

Medications

- Remove the patient from exposure, maintain vital functions, and support ventilation artificially if necessary. Patient should remain quiet so as to decrease oxygen consumption.
- Administer 100% oxygen until carboxyhemoglobin is less than 5%; 40% to 50% of the body's CO can be eliminated in 1 hour with high-dose oxygen.

Special Therapy

- Hyperbaric oxygen can reduce the half-life of CO to 22 minutes, although it cannot be routinely recommended due to equivocal trials.[1,4] Despite unproven benefit, it can be considered for severe cases, including CO >40%, loss of consciousness, severe metabolic acidosis (pH <7.1), and end-organ ischemia. Because of the increased binding of CO to fetal hemoglobin, consider hyperbaric oxygen for CO >20% in the pregnant patient.
- Consider transfusion of blood or packed cells to increase the oxygen-carrying capacity of the blood.
- Cerebral edema should be managed with diuretics and steroids.

Follow-Up

Monitor the patient after severe exposure for the following neurologic symptoms: tremors, mental deterioration, and psychotic behavior.

REFERENCES

2. Dries DJ, Endorf FW. Inhalation injury: epidemiology, pathology, treatment strategies. *Scand J Trauma Resusc Emerg Med* 2013;21:31.
3. Committee on Trauma. Thermal injuries. In: *ATLS manual,* 9th ed. Chicago, IL: American College of Surgeons; 2012:230–235.
4. American Burn Association. Inhalation injury: diagnosis. *J Am Coll Surg* 2003;196:307–312.
5. Buckley NA, Juurlink DN, Isbister G, et al. Hyperbaric oxygen for carbon monoxide poisoning. *Cochrane Database Syst Rev* 2011;4:CD002041.

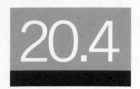

20.4 Intimate Partner Violence

Jessica-Renee Gamboa

GENERAL PRINCIPLES

Domestic violence or intimate partner violence (IPV) is defined as "a pattern of behavior used to establish power and control over another person through fear and intimidation, often including the threat or use of violence."[1] It is described as assaultive and coercive behavior to include physical injury, psychological abuse, sexual assault, enforced social isolation, stalking, deprivation, intimidation, and threats. A woman's lifetime risk for abuse is 23%.[2] Nearly 5.3 million incidents occur each year among women 18 years of age and older and 3.2 million occur among men.[3] Thirty-one percent of women and 26% of men report some form of IPV in their life. These numbers are likely lower than the actual rates due to underreporting of such actions.[2] IPV occurs in same-sex relationships as well with 22% to 46% of all gays and lesbians reporting having been in a physically violent same-sex relationship.[4]

Domestic violence is not a disease present in the body; rather it is a health-related risk factor.[5] It leads to adverse health outcomes such as sexually transmitted infections, pelvic inflammatory disease, unintended pregnancy, chronic pain, neurological disorders, gastrointestinal disorders, migraines, as well as other disabilities. Abuse is a common and complex public health issue. Costs of IPV from direct medical and mental health services are estimated to be around $4.1 billion, with total costs exceeding $5.8 billion annually.[6] A public health approach seeks to identify a combination of individual, relational, community, and societal factors that contribute to the risk of being a victim or perpetrator of domestic violence.[5] Awareness of the prevalence and effects of IPV in all sectors will assist family physicians in addressing this important health issue effectively.

DIAGNOSIS

The CDC has identified several risk factors and signs and symptoms for IPV, and they are outlined in Table 20.4-1. Many risk factors for both victimization and perpetration are the same. Physicians should be aware that those who are identified as at risk may not be involved in IPV.[7]

As of 2013, the U.S. Preventive Services Task Force (USPSTF) recommends clinicians screen all women of childbearing age for IPV, to include those that have no signs or symptoms of domestic violence. Those that screen positive should be provided or referred for intervention. The American Congress of Obstetricians and Gynecologists (ACOG) as well as the American Medical Association (AMA) recommend routine inquiry about IPV with all patients.[2] The American Academy of Family Physicians (AAFP) notes it is imperative family physicians be aware of the prevalence of violence in all sectors of society, be alert for its effects in their encounters with virtually every patient, and be capable of providing an appropriate response when these issues are identified. With this awareness, physicians are able to work to prevent violence for patients who are at risk within their practices and communities.[4]

Several screening tools are adequate for identifying IPV in the primary care setting. The Hurt, Insult, Threat, Scream (HITS); Ongoing Abuse Screen/Ongoing Violence Assessment Tool (OAS/OVAT); Slapped, Threatened and Throw (STaT); Humiliation, Afraid, Rape, Kick (HARK); and Woman Abuse Screen Tool (WAST) have the highest sensitivity and specificity and many can be self-administered.

TREATMENT

For patients exposed to IPV, the SOS-DoC framework can aid physicians in responding to these situations.[6]

- S—offer **S**upport and assess **S**afety: Keep the discussion private and confidential. Ask questions regarding severity and frequency of violence and safety of others in the household.
- O—discuss **O**ptions: safety plans, legal options and community resources.
- S—validate the patient's **S**trength.
- Do—**Do**cument observations, assessment and plans including safety plans.

TABLE 20.4-1	Domestic Violence Risk Factors

Risk type	Victimization	Perpetration
Individual	Prior history	Victim of physical/psychologic
	Being female	abuse (strongest predictor)
	Young age	Low self-esteem
	Heavy alcohol/drug use	Low income
	High-risk sexual behavior	Low academic achievement
	Being less educated	Heavy alcohol/drug use
	Unemployment	Depression
	For men: different ethnicity from	Anger/hostility
	partners	Personality disorders
	For women: greater education	Few friends/social isolation
	than their partners	Economic stress
	Verbally abusive, jealous, or	Belief in strict gender roles
	possessive partner	Desire for power/control
		Involvement in aggressive
		behavior
Relational	Couples with income,	Marital conflict
	educational, or job status	Marital instability
	disparities	Dominance and control of the
	Dominance and control of the	relationship by one partner
	relationship by one partner	over the other
	over the other	Economic stress
		Unhealthy family relationships
		and interactions
Community	Poverty	Poverty
	Low social capital	Low social capital
	Weak community sanctions	Weak community sanctions
	against domestic violence	against domestic violence
Societal	Traditional gender norms	Traditional gender norms

Associated signs and symptoms with intimate partner violence

Acute injuries	Psychologic	Nonspecific
Multiple bruises/anatomical	Acute/chronic anxiety	Abdominal/chest/pelvic pain
sites involved	Depression	Headaches
Mechanism inconsistent with	Posttraumatic stress disorder	Insomnia/fatigue
findings	Suicidal ideation	Sexual dysfunction
Firearm wounds	Sleep disturbance	Chronic pain
Knife wounds	Substance abuse	Missed appointments
Fractures	Social isolation	
Delay in seeking care		

- C—offer Continuity, follow-up appointments and identify barriers to access.
  - **In the case of an injury.** Suspect domestic abuse if unexplained injuries are present or if the patient's explanation seems implausible. Ask direct questions, talk with the patient privately, and provide enough space to answer questions. If a patient discloses abuse, be explicit that physical and sexual violence are never acceptable. Offer assurance and unconditional positive regard. Skill in establishing rapport and communication are critical to help a patient feel comfortable and safe. Accept the answers given, reaffirming your desire to understand and help when you can. Remember, abuse and violence are never easy to talk about.
  - **Complete documentation.** A physician's notation in the medical record should include an objective report of the abuse history as reported by the patient, detailed drawings of physical findings, laboratory and radiologic findings, and any photographs of abuse injuries. Document in the chart that the symptoms or injuries treated are abuse related and request a follow-up appointment.

SPECIAL CONSIDERATIONS

- **Know your state's legal requirements.** Every state has legislation designed to protect victims of domestic violence because spouse and partner abuse has been defined as a criminal act. Physicians must be aware of the specific laws and support services for abused persons available in their practice community. Remember to obtain informed consent from an abused person before disclosing the abuse diagnosis to a third party or the police. Elder and child abuse carries mandated reporting in all 50 states, including the District of Columbia.
- **Assess the safety of children in the home.** Ask directly whether or not children are safe in the home. If the children have been mistreated or are at risk for abuse, refer them to an emergency shelter or child protection services.
- **Assess psychologic needs.** Determine whether an abused person is using drugs or alcohol or is suicidal. Each requires urgent and appropriate intervention.
- **Pregnancy and reproductive coercion.** IPV contributes to unintended pregnancies and delayed prenatal care; however, becoming pregnant may also increase the frequency and severity of IPV. Poor outcomes also associated with IPV during pregnancy include preterm birth, low birth weight, and perinatal death. Reproductive coercion is defined by coercion from male partners to make their female partners pregnant or discontinue a current pregnancy.[8] It also includes birth control sabotage, which is when a partner interferes with contraception, such as discarding birth control methods (pills/patches/rings, etc.), refusing to use barrier methods, and denying partner access to medical care to obtain birth control.
- **Knowledge of community service providers.** In caring for an abused patient, the physician's primary role is to provide that person with good medical care and safe, reliable information about support services. These community services include counseling, home visits, mentoring support, and other community services and providers who have been specifically trained to help survivors of domestic violence. Respect an abused person's ability to make appropriate choices and decide if and when he or she will leave a violent partner.
- **Work to make the office a safe place to discuss domestic abuse.** Work with local service providers to obtain sensitive posters and educational materials. Provide patients with educational materials about family violence and community resources. Ensure that these materials are offered in ways that allow patients privacy to access them. Placing them in bathrooms as well as waiting rooms is important. Local agencies may help you with this educational outreach. There are excellent online resources such as "The Family Violence Prevention Fund" (www.endabuse.org) or "The National Coalition Against Domestic Violence" (www.ncadv.org). Toll-free numbers such as the National Domestic Violence Hotline, 1-800-799-SAFE (1-800-799-7233) are also valuable resources for victims. These can be useful tools for working with women and men who experience interpersonal violence in their intimate relationships.

Domestic violence is a common problem and a complex public health issue that must be recognized and treated with sensitivity. In addition to recognizing abuse-related injuries and symptoms, family physicians can provide patients with life-saving information on community resources available to address domestic violence.

REFERENCES

1. National Coalition against Domestic Violence. www.ncadv.org. Accessed March 12, 2014.
2. U.S. Preventative Service Task Force. Screening for Intimate Partner Violence and Abuse of Elderly and Vulnerable Adults, U.S. Preventive Services Task Force Recommendation Statement. http://www.uspreventiveservicestaskforce.org/uspstf12/ipvelder/ipvelderfinalrs.htm. Accessed March 12, 2014.
3. National Center for Injury Prevention and Control. Intimate partner violence; fact sheet. www.cdc.gov/ncipc/factsheets/ipvfacts.htm. Accessed March 26, 2014.
4. AAFP. Violence (Position Paper) (1994) (2011). http://www.aafp.org/about/policies/all/violence.html. Accessed March 18, 2014.
5. Tacket A, Wathen CN, MacMillan H. Should health professionals screen all women for domestic violence? *Plos Med* 2004;1:1–4.
6. Cornholm PF, Fogarty CT, Ambuel B, et al. Intimate partner violence. *Am Fam Physician* 2011;83(10): 1165–1172.
7. Center for Disease Control and Prevention. Intimate partner violence. 2013. http://www.cdc.gov/violenceprevention/intimatepartnerviolence/. Accessed March 26, 2014.
8. Modi MN, Palmer S, Armstrong A. The role of Violence Against Women Act in addressing intimate partner violence: a public health issue. *J Womens Health* 2014;23(3):253–259.

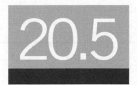

20.5 Child Maltreatment

Sara Shelton Kerley

GENERAL PRINCIPLES

Child maltreatment is an issue that ought to be in the forefront of a family physician's mind any time they are evaluating and treating a child. Moreover, family physicians have a uniquely advantageous position for identifying possible abuse, given their relationship to the entire family unit as well as the pediatric patient.

It is important to remember that child abuse has not only immediate, but also long-term health consequences for the victims. As adults, they are more likely to suffer from cardiovascular disease, liver disease, hypertension, diabetes, and obesity. Childhood trauma is a risk factor for borderline personality disorder, depression, anxiety, and other mental health disorders. Victims are more likely to engage in sexual risk-taking as they reach adolescence, and they are nine times as likely to become involved in criminal activities. There is an increased likelihood that victims will smoke cigarettes, abuse alcohol, or take illicit drugs during their lifetime, and they are more likely to themselves become perpetrators of interpersonal violence.[1,2]

Definition and Classification

The Child Abuse Prevention and Treatment Act (CAPTA) of 2010 defines child abuse as "at a minimum, any recent act or failure to act on the part of a parent or caretaker, which results in death, serious physical or emotional harm, sexual abuse or exploitation, or an act or failure to act which presents an imminent risk of serious harm."[3] This federal definition is a minimum, and definitions may vary from state to state.[4] From a clinical perspective, child maltreatment can include neglect, physical abuse, emotional abuse, and sexual abuse. Neglect, or the failure of a parent or caregiver to provide for a child's basic needs, may be in the form of physical, medical, educational, or emotional neglect. Physical abuse, that is, nonaccidental trauma inflicted by a parent or caregiver, may include shaking, hitting, choking, burning, or any number of other acts of harm. Emotional abuse, also known as psychological abuse, can include withholding affection, excessive criticism, threats of harm, and other behaviors that can ultimately damage a child's emotional development and well-being. Finally, sexual abuse is defined by CAPTA as "the employment, use, persuasion, inducement, enticement, or coercion of any child to engage in, or assist in any other person to engage in, any sexually explicit conduct for the purpose of producing a visual depiction of such conduct; or the rape, and in cases or caretaker or interfamilial relationships, statutory rape, molestation, prostitution, or other form of sexual exploitation of children, or incest with children."[3]

Prevalence

According to the U.S. Department of Health and Human Services, in 2012 there were 3.4 million referrals made to CPS agencies nationwide involving concerns of maltreatment of 6.3 million children. Of these, 2.1 million reports were investigated, and as a result one-fifth of these found at least one child victim of abuse or neglect—a total of 686,000 children. The vast majority of these cases were neglect (>75%), followed by physical abuse (>15%), sexual abuse (<10%), and finally psychological maltreatment (<10%).[1] Per the National Incidence Study of Child Abuse and Neglect (NIS-4), which looked at the years 2005 to 2006, one child in every 25 is a victim of abuse each year.

Fatalities occurred at a rate of 2.2 deaths per 100,000 children. Of these, 70% were attributed to neglect or a combination of neglect and another form of abuse, and 44.3% were attributed to physical abuse or a combination of physical abuse and another form of abuse. 70% of those that died were under the age of 3.[5]

A significant amount of data amassed over the last several decades gives insight into victim, perpetrator, and family characteristics. Children are most vulnerable from birth to 1 year of age, and girls are abused at just slightly higher rates than boys. Caucasian children are at highest risk, followed by Hispanic and African American children.[5] Children with disabilities have been found to have lower rates of physical abuse but significantly higher rates of emotional neglect, and those who are physically abused have higher rates of serious injury or harm.[6]

Greater than 80% of perpetrators are parents, followed by other relatives and unmarried partners of parents, and a greater number of perpetrators are women than men. The incidence of maltreatment is higher for children with no parent in the labor force and those with an unemployed parent and lowest for those with employed parents. According to the NIS-4, children in low socioeconomic households experienced abuse at a rate five times higher than other children—they are three times more likely to be abused and seven times more likely to be neglected. Children whose single-parent had a live-in partner had more than 10 times the rate of abuse and 8 times the rate of neglect compared with children living with married biological parents.[7]

DIAGNOSIS

Clinical Presentation

Abuse or neglect may come to the attention of a clinician through any number of presentations. Physical injuries are often not detected or reported, particularly if they are minor and do not require medical attention, and sexual abuse rarely results in abnormal physical examination findings. Rather, children are reported as suspected victims of abuse when an individual reports a suspicious injury or witnesses an abusive event, a caregiver notices symptoms and brings the child for medical attention without recognizing that the child has been injured, the abuser is concerned that the injury is severe enough to warrant medical care, or the child discloses the abuse.[8,9]

History

As with any medical problem, a thorough and detailed medical history is of vital importance in the evaluation of suspected child abuse. In addition to a standard general medical, developmental, and social history, caregivers should also be asked about pregnancy history, child behavior (do they consider the child to be difficult?), home life stressors, substance abuse by people living in the home with the child, and the overall discipline philosophy of the caregiver(s). It is important to maintain a nonjudgmental tone throughout the interview, and use open-ended questions whenever possible. If the child is able to give a history, they should be questioned separately from the caregiver. Statements made by the caregiver and the child concerning the mechanism of injury and the accompanying circumstances should be documented verbatim. The following should raise suspicion for nonaccidental trauma: vague or incomplete explanations for significant injuries, changing explanations, explanations that are inconsistent with a child's developmental stage or with the severity of injury, or inconsistent explanations from one witness to another.[8]

If sexual abuse is suspected, it is essential to interview the caregiver and the child separately in order to avoid any biasing of the child. Explain that this interview is for medical purposes and that a more detailed, forensic interview may be required at a later time. To establish rapport, the clinician should start by talking to the child about nonthreatening topics, letting the child know that it is okay to talk to doctors about embarrassing or uncomfortable things. Leading questions should be avoided, and developmentally appropriate language should be used. Again, any descriptions of abuse should be recorded verbatim.[9]

Physicians must be aware of their local resources, and if a child advocacy center or specialized clinic is available and acuity allows, it is often most appropriate to refer the child for comprehensive interviewing, examination, and treatment in order to minimize the number of interviews required.[9]

Physical Examination

Minor accidental trauma is a common occurrence in childhood, and it is important to consider the stated mechanism of injury in addition to the injury pattern before concluding that abuse has occurred. While injuries in various stages of healing; injuries to multiple body parts; bruising on the torso, ear, or neck in a child younger than 4; or bruising of any body part in a child younger than 4 months are all concerning for abuse, no pattern of injury indicates abuse with absolute certainty. A thorough physical examination is crucial, particularly because the history is often incomplete or falsified.[10]

Children should be observed for level of consciousness, responsiveness, and overall demeanor, and their height, weight, and head circumference should be obtained. Findings concerning for neglect may be noted during the general assessment, including failure to thrive, dental caries, patchy hair loss (secondary to malnutrition), and severe diaper dermatitis. Information gained via nonverbal cues may be helpful in safety planning, particularly if the child displays fear of the abuser.[8]

All injuries should be carefully described and documented as well as photographed. Some bruising may take some days to appear, so reexamination in 1 to 2 days can be useful. Bruising from accidental trauma tends to occur overlying bony prominences where bruising secondary to abuse tends to involve the buttocks, trunk, neck, and head. Additionally bruising from nonaccidental trauma may have a pattern consistent with an object used to inflict injury, that is, linear bruising inflicted by a belt or cord, hand-shaped bruises. Inflicted burns are typically well demarcated, and splash marks are notably absent.[8]

The neck, torso, and extremities should be palpated to detect occult fracture, and a neurologic examination should be performed to check for spinal cord injury. If possible, a fundoscopic examination should be performed looking for retinal hemorrhages. Finally, the mouth and teeth should be evaluated looking for caries or inflicted injury.[10]

When sexual abuse is suspected, if there is not an injury that demands emergent examination, physicians should consider referring the child to a center specializing in abuse. Forensic evidence can be collected if the abuse has occurred within the past 72 hours, and some states recommend collecting evidence even up to 96 hours after the abuse. The examination should be explained to the child, and a chaperone should be present for support. Instrumentation is rarely required—female genitalia can typically be examined with labial traction and separation. If instrumentation is required, consider sedating the child for comfort. Finally, it is important to explain to the parents and the child (if appropriate) that sexual abuse rarely results in examination abnormalities and that a normal examination does not rule in or rule out the possibility of abuse.[9]

Laboratory Studies

The type and severity of injury will dictate appropriate laboratory tests for each case. A coagulopathy workup may be indicated if abuse is suspected on the basis of significant bruising. Liver enzymes and an electrolyte panel may be indicated to look for occult renal and abdominal injuries. Additionally, a complete metabolic panel, albumin, alkaline phosphatase, and a parathyroid hormone levels can be obtained to evaluate for malnutrition and bone mineralization disorders.[10]

Because the transmission of STIs is uncommon in sexual abuse cases, universal screening is not recommended. Rather, consider screening for STIs under the following circumstances: child has experienced penetration of the genitalia or anus, the abuser is a stranger, the abuser is known to be infected or suspected to be infected with STIs, the child has another household contact with an STI, the child lives in a community with high rates of STIs, and of course, if the child has signs or symptoms of an STI.[9]

Imaging

When abuse is suspected and a child has a known fracture or is under the age of 2, a complete skeletal survey is recommended. A so-called "babygram" is not adequate to fully evaluate for skeletal injuries in an infant. If intracranial injury is suspected, an MRI of the head and neck is recommended. This may be more sensitive than CT in finding subtle intracranial injury patterns and is more sensitive than CT and plain films in detecting cervical spine injuries.[8]

Certain radiographic findings are more concerning for abuse than others. Rib fractures; sternal, scapular, and spinous process fractures; and metaphyseal fractures are considered highly specific for nonaccidental trauma. Multiple fractures and fractures in different stages of healing also raise concerns for child abuse.[10]

Differential Diagnosis

As discussed previously, no injury pattern or radiographic finding is absolutely pathognomonic for child abuse. It may be important to rule out coagulopathies, osteogenesis imperfecta, and other genetic disorders whose signs may mimic those of abuse. Certainly accidental trauma must be ruled out, although it is important to keep in mind that accidental and nonaccidental trauma can coincide.

TREATMENT

Treatment of immediate injuries is the physician's top priority, and ensuring the child's continuing safety follows closely behind. It may be appropriate to admit the child to the hospital throughout the evaluation and treatment process to provide that safety.[11] Beyond immediate concerns, the treatment of child abuse requires a multidisciplinary approach and should involve the entire family. Physicians should be aware of local resources available for not only the abused child but also the abusive caregiver and the rest of the family.[12]

Reporting

Physicians are mandated by law to report any suspected child abuse to local child protective services or law enforcement. Child protective services will then determine whether the case warrants an investigation and proceed accordingly. The Childhelp National Child Abuse Hotline at 800-4-A-CHILD (800-422-4453) is an excellent resource and can assist physicians in contacting the appropriate agencies.[10]

Referrals

Once again, the evaluation and treatment of child maltreatment is a complex endeavor and requires a multidisciplinary approach. If the local area has a child advocacy center or other practice that specializes in child abuse, it is in the best interest of the child to engage with this center early in the process, so that they can benefit from the medical and psychological resources that are available.

REFERENCES

1. Child Welfare Information Gateway. *Long-term consequences of child abuse and neglect.* Washington, DC: U.S. Department of Health and Human Services, Children's Bureau; 2013. https://www.childwelfare.gov/pubs/factsheets/long_term_consequences.cfm. Accessed July 17, 2014.
2. Felitti VJ, Anda RF, Nordenberg D, et al. Relationship of childhood abuse and household dysfunction to many of the leading causes of death in adults: the adverse childhood experiences (ACE) study. *Am J Prev Med* 1998;14:245–258.
3. U.S. Department of Health and Human Services Administration for Children and Families Administration on children, Youth and Families Children's Bureau. *The Child Abuse Prevention and Treatment Act of 2010.* Washington, DC: U.S. Department of Health and Human Services, Children's Bureau; 2010. http://www.acf.hhs.gov/programs/cb/resource/capta. Accessed July 17, 2014.
4. Child Welfare Information Gateway. Definitions of Child Abuse and Neglect in Federal Law. https://www.childwelfare.gov/can/defining/federal.cfm. Accessed July 17, 2014.
5. Child Welfare Information Gateway. *What is child abuse and neglect? Recognizing the signs and symptoms.* Washington, DC: U.S. Department of Health and Human Services, Children's Bureau; 2013. https://www.childwelfare.gov/pubs/factsheets/whatiscan.cfm. Accessed July 17, 2014.
6. Sedlak AJ, Mettenburg J, Basena M, et al. *Fourth National Incidence Study of Child Abuse and Neglect (NIS–4): Report to Congress, executive summary.* Washington, DC: U.S. Department of Health and Human Services, Administration for Children and Families; 2010 http://www.acf.hhs.gov/sites/default/files/opre/nis4_report_congress_full_pdf_jan2010.pdf. Accessed July 17, 2014.
7. Child Welfare Information Gateway. *Child maltreatment 2012: summary of key findings.* Washington, DC: U.S. Department of Health and Human Services, Children's Bureau; 2014. https://www.childwelfare.gov/pubs/factsheets/canstats.cfm. Accessed July 17, 2014.
8. Kellogg ND; American Academy of Pediatrics Committee on Child Abuse and Neglect. Evaluation of suspected child physical abuse. *Pediatrics* 2007;119:1232.
9. Jenny C, Crawford-Jakubiak JE, Committee on Child Abuse and Neglect. The evaluation of children in the primary care setting when sexual abuse is suspected. *Pediatrics* 2013;132:e558.
10. Kodner C, Wetherton A. Diagnosis and management of physical abuse in children. *Am Fam Physician* 2013;88:669–675.
11. American Academy of Family Physicians Policy. Child Abuse. 2013. http://www.aafp.org/about/policies/all/child-abuse.html. Accessed July 17, 2014.
12. American Academy of Family Physicians Policy. Medical Necessity for the Hospitalization of the Abused and Neglected Child. 2013. http://www.aafp.org/about/policies/all/medical-necessity.html. Accessed July 17, 2014.

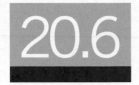

20.6

Evaluation and Management Sexual Assault Victim

Michael Ryan Odom

GENERAL PRINCIPLES

According to the U.S. Department of Justice, sexual assault is a crime of violence against a person's body and will. Sex offenders use physical and/or psychological aggression or coercion to victimize, in the process often threatening a victim's sense of privacy, safety, autonomy, and well-being. Sexual assault is the most underreported violent crime secondary to multiple pressures on the victim.[1]

Many misconceptions are perpetuated about sexual assault. The most common is the assumption that rape is motivated by sexual desire. Rape is a violent crime, motivated by anger or the need for power and control.[2] Another is that sexual assault is limited to a specific gender; rather, no gender or sexual preference is immune from assault.[3]

Epidemiology

National Intimate Partner and Sexual Violence 2010 Survey underscored the pervasiveness of this violence, the immediate impacts of victimization, and the lifelong health consequences related to sexual violence. There was a significantly disproportionate impact on women compared with men. Nearly 1 in 5 women (17%) and 1 in 71 men (1%) have been raped in their lifetime. Most female victims of completed rape (80%) experienced their first rape before the age of 25 and almost half (42%) experienced their first rape before the age of 18 (30% between 11 and 17 years old and 12% at or before the age of 10). More than a quarter of male victims of completed rape (28%) were first raped when they were 10 years old or younger.

The survey was also one of the first to attempt to survey sexual preference minorities in order to evaluate the impact on the lesbian, gay, bisexual, and transgender (LGBT) community as well. The survey found lifetime prevalence of rape in women to be approximately 1 in 8 lesbian women (13%), nearly 1 in 2 of bisexual women (46%), and 1 in 6 heterosexual women (17%). In contrast, while underpowered to report completed rape except for heterosexual men (0.7%), gay and bisexual men had similar rates of sexual violence compared with women. Four in 10 gay men (40%), nearly 1 in 2 bisexual men (47%), and 1 in 5 heterosexual men (21%) have experienced sexual violence other than rape in their lifetime,[3] and approximately 50% of rape victims have some acquaintance with their attackers.[4]

A 2012 Swedish study in the *Journal of Interpersonal Violence* reported extragenital injuries were almost three times as common as genital injuries, 58% (263/465) compared with 20% (90/450).[5] Genital injuries are not an inevitable consequence of rape, and lack of genital injuries does not imply consensual intercourse.[4] Only 1% to 2% of sexual assault victims require hospitalization.[2,4]

DIAGNOSIS[6,7]

Evidence beyond 48 to 72 hours after an assault often is difficult to recover or may be invalid; however, with advances in technology, evidence should be collected and submitted regardless if it is beyond the cutoff point. It is imperative to document the time frame (from time of assault to medical examination) and to encourage victims to proceed with evidence collection as soon as possible, regardless if the victim plans to report the sexual assault at the time of presentation. Multidisciplinary sexual assault teams are encouraged by the U.S. Department of Justice and the American College of Emergency Physicians and may be available in some medical centers.

Consent[6]

Informed consent or refusal in a language the patient understands should be obtained for each of the following components of the sexual assault evaluation. Follow facility policy for seeking patients' consent for medical evaluation and treatment. Informed consent of patients for medical evaluation and treatment typically is needed for the following:

General medical care	Evidence collection
• Notification to law enforcement or other authority	• Pregnancy testing and care
• Evidence collection and release	• Testing and prophylaxis for sexually transmitted infection (STIs)
• Toxicology screening	• HIV prophylaxis
• Release of information and evidence to criminal justice system personnel, SART/ SARRT members, and partnering service providers	• Photographs, including colposcopic images
• Contact with patients for reasons related to their criminal sexual assault case	• Permission to contact the patient for medical purposes
• Patient notification in case of a DNA match or additional victims	• Release of medical information
• Transferal of evidence to law enforcement personnel	

History of Present Illness[6,7]

The history should focus on explicit details of the sexual assault for forensic purposes. Avoid legal terms such as "rape" or "abuse." Provide a quiet, secure, and private environment. Allow 30 to 60 minutes for the history and the physical examination. Victims should be offered a chaperone for any interaction.

The following details of the history should be obtained:

• Was there drug or alcohol use by the patient before, during, or after the assault?
• Where and when did the assault take place?
• Was there touching or penetration of any part of the patient's body with a penis, finger, or any object?
• Was a condom used?
• Was there use of any kind of spermicidal foam or gel?
• Is the patient using any other form of birth control (intrauterine device, oral, etc.)?
• Is the patient undergoing fertility treatment?
• Was the patient kissed, licked, or bitten by the assailant? If so where?
• Did the patient clean up in any way after the assault?
  • Specifically, did the patient:
    • Void
    • Insert or remove a tampon
    • Change a sanitary pad
    • Shower, bathe, douche, wipe
    • Change clothes
    • Brush their teeth, gargle, chew gum, smoke, eat, drink OR
    • Take medications before coming to the emergency department (ED)? If so, when?
• Where are the original clothes, sanitary pads, or cleaning accessories?
• Who brought the patient to the ED?
  • What are the names and agencies of the emergency medical services (EMS) providers OR the name and contact information of any stranger, friend, or family member who accompanied the patient?

Physical Examination

Most hospitals have a standard rape kit with instructions to help guide the clinician through the collection and preservation of evidence for forensic evaluation.[3] Once the kit is opened, the "chain of evidence" must be maintained; evidence cannot be left unattended.[4,8]

The examiner should prevent cross-contamination of evidence by changing gloves whenever cross-contamination could occur. Clearly document all findings.

• Before the patient undresses, place a clean hospital sheet on the floor to be a barrier for the collection paper.

- Allow the patient to remove and place each piece of clothing being collected in a separate paper bag. Handle all clothing with gloved hands to prevent contamination of evidence, and it should be handled primarily by the patient.[7] A female chaperone should be present for a male physician.
  - Clothing can be collected up to 1 month after the assault, provided the items have not been laundered. Clothing should be placed in paper bags.[8]
- Photograph and recover any trace evidence, including sand, soil, leaves, grass, and biological secretions. Note the body location of the collection.
- Note all injuries by documenting the location, size, and complete description of any trauma, including bite marks, strangulation injuries, or areas of point tenderness, especially those occurring around the mouth, breasts, thighs, wrists, upper arms, legs, back, and anogenital region. A body map may be useful to aid in documentation. Genital trauma occurs more commonly in postmenopausal women.[7,9]
- Identify and recover moist secretions with a dry swab. Dry secretions should be moistened with a damp swab and then recovered with a dry swab. Debris should be scraped onto a bindle.
  - Use a Wood's lamp to examine the patient's thighs for fluorescing semen and urine stains. Swab any highlighted areas.
- On the basis of the history obtained, follow the instructions for the pertinent portions of the sexual assault evidence collection kit.
  - Toluidine blue dye may be used to identify minor external genital and anal injuries, but it may cause discomfort (burning). Lacerations expose the deeper dermis containing nuclei that absorb this stain.
  - A wet mount should be done to check for the presence of bacterial vaginosis, trichomonads, yeast, and sperm. Motile sperm may be seen up to 8 hours postcoitus and nonmotile sperm can be detected beyond 72 hours. Vaginal swabbing should also be collected during pelvic examination for *Chlamydia* and *Neisseria gonorrhoeae*.
  - The absence of sperm may indicate that the assailant had undergone a vasectomy.
  - If blood is present at the rectum, anoscopy or sigmoidoscopy and rectal digital examination should be performed on the basis of patient's history.[4,10]
  - The patient should pluck approximately 15 to 20 pubic hairs to serve as samples for reference.[10]
  - Obtain rectal aspiration in case of anal assault by injecting sterile saline into the rectum and then aspirating.
  - Swabs from the victim's penis should be collected and may be examined for saliva if there is a history of oral copulation.[4]

Laboratory Studies[1,2,7,8,11]

In cases where the laboratories are going to be processed by a crime laboratory, following the appropriate local procedure at initial presentation is critical for proper evidence collection. This may require duplicate laboratory collection if laboratories are required to treat the patient. Consider tests that may be appropriate for a given patient:

- Serum or urine pregnancy test
  - Rule out an established pregnancy; 1% to 5% of sexual assaults result in pregnancy.
- Gonorrhea, *Chlamydia*, and syphilis testing
  - In cases where prophylaxis will be given and chronic abuse is not suspected, cultures and syphilis testing are not necessary.
  - Test at initial presentation and repeat at 6 weeks, 3 and 6 months.
- Hepatitis B surface antibody
  - Check for the immune status in the previously immunized patient. Hepatitis B testing is not indicated in the nonimmunized patient.
- **HIV risk assessment and screening:** Patients should be assessed for risk of HIV transmission following assault. (See HIV prophylaxis for additional information.)
  - Initial visit and repeated at 3, 6, and 12 months from the date of exposure.
  - There is a risk of less than 1% of infection after a one-time sexual encounter.
- Drugs of abuse and alcohol level in serum, urine, and toxicology.
- Gamma-hydroxybutyrate (GHB), flunitrazepam ("date rape drug") serum, and/or urine level are often screened in the Rape Kits but may be performed at the primary hospital as well if medically indicated.

- Laboratory and radiographic studies as indicated.
- Additional testing may be performed with the Rape Kit and a contracted forensic lab.

TREATMENT
Medications

- **Pregnancy prophylaxis:** Regardless of a victim's menstrual cycle, postcoital emergency contraception should be offered. In the United States, some of the available regimens for emergency contraception include levonorgestrel (Plan B) alone, the Yuzpe regimen (combination of oral contraceptive pills given in two doses 12 hours apart), and the progestin antagonist/agonist, ulipristal. Levonorgestrel is highly effective up to 72 hours postcoitus, and moderately effective up to 120 hours. Ulipristal, where available, is effective up to 120 hours after intercourse and is the preferred drug beyond 72 hours after unprotected intercourse.[12]
- **Sexually transmitted disease (STD) prophylaxis:**[12,13] The CDC recommends empiric therapy for common STIs. The recommendations are given below.

Empiric Therapy, per Centers for Disease Control 2010 Guidelines

Gonorrhea	Ceftriaxone 125 mg IM or Cefixime 400 mg PO
Chlamydial infection	Azithromycin 1 g PO (single dose) or Doxycycline 100 mg PO twice daily for 7 d
Trichomoniasis	Metronidazole 2 g PO (single dose)
Hepatitis B	Hepatitis B vaccine without HBIG at the time of visit, then repeated at 1–2 and 4–6 mo[a]

[a]The CDC recommends Hepatitis B vaccine as adequate protection. If there is known exposure to Hepatitis B, provider may consider HBIG within 14 days of exposure.

- **HIV prophylaxis.** HIV prophylaxis is controversial because of presumed low risk of transmission and the efficacy of antiretroviral drugs after sexual assault is extrapolated from a study of healthcare workers who had percutaneous exposures to HIV-infected blood.[12–14]
  - Postexposure prophylaxis (PEP) should be based on risk factors of HIV exposure (penetration, ejaculation occurred on mucous membranes, multiple assailants, mucosal lesions present on the assailant or survivor, or any other suspicious characteristics).
  - PEP consists of zidovudine, and it should be prescribed with the consultation of an Infectious Disease Provider. The CDC recommends that patients be given an initial prescription for PEP for only 3 to 7 days with short-term follow-up for further counseling, medication, and HIV antibody monitoring.[1,6,13]

Referral

Provide patients with oral and written medical discharge instructions. Include a summary of the examination (e.g., evidence collected, tests conducted, medication prescribed or provided, information provided, and treatment received), medication doses to be taken, follow-up appointments needed or scheduled, and referrals. The discharge form could also include contact information and hours of operation for local advocacy programs.[15,16]

Follow-Up

An optimal time for a first medical follow-up contact is 24 to 48 hours following discharge. A medical visit should occur within 2 weeks of the acute evaluation; ongoing psychological and counseling support should be provided. A male victim should be referred to an urologist or proctologist. A child should be referred to a pediatrician.[15,16]

Follow-up appointment should include:[14,16]

- Pregnancy testing
- STD testing for patients who develop interim symptoms or who declined initial evaluation
- HIV testing
- Continuing Hepatitis B vaccine

Complications

Many victims can experience rape trauma syndrome. In the first phase, days to weeks, symptoms may include anger, fear, anxiety, physical pain, sleep disturbance, anorexia, shame, guilt, and intrusive thoughts. The second phase, "reorganization," which may last for months, includes physical and emotional symptoms. Patients may experience musculoskeletal, genital, pelvic and or abdominal pain, anorexia, and insomnia. Dreams and nightmares are common and phobias may develop. Patients may develop chronic pain (pelvis, back), fibromyalgia, headaches, irritable bowel syndrome, poor overall health status, sexual dysfunction, somatoform disorders, alcohol and drug abuse, anxiety, depression, eating disorders, sleep disorders, and posttraumatic stress disorder.[14] Children who are sexually assaulted or abused may display variable nonspecific symptoms and/or physical findings.[17]

REFERENCES

1. U.S. Department of Justice, Office on Violence against Women; Kristin L. *A national protocol for sexual assault medical forensic examinations: adults/adolescents*. 2nd ed. Washington, DC: U.S. Department of Justice, Office on Violence Against Women; 2013.
2. Geist RF. Sexually related trauma. *Emerg Med Clin North Am* 1988;6:439.
3. Basile KC, Black MC, Breiding MJ, et al. *National Intimate Partner and Sexual Violence Survey 2010 Summary Report*. Atlanta GA: Centers for Disease Control and Prevention, National Center for Injury Prevention and Control, Division of Violence Prevention; 2011.
4. Fled Haus KM. Female and male sexual assault. In: Tintinalli JE, Kelen GD, Stapczynski JS, eds. *Emergency medicine—a comprehensive study guide*. 5th ed. New York, NY: McGraw-Hill; 2000:1952–1955.
5. Moller AS, Backstrom T, Sondergaard HP, et al. Patterns of injury and reported violence depending on relationship to assailant in female Swedish sexual assault victims. *J Interpers Violence* 2012;27(16):3131–3148.
6. Workowski KA, Berman SM. *Sexually transmitted diseases treatment guidelines, 2010*. Atlanta GA: Department of Health and Human Services, Centers for Disease Control and Prevention; 2010.
7. Asher S, Award SH, Blackburn C, et al. *Evaluation and management of the sexually assaulted or sexually abused patient*. 2nd ed. Dallas, TX: American College of Emergency Physicians; 2013.
8. Hochbaum SR. The evaluation and treatment of the sexually assaulted patient. *Emerg Med Clin North Am* 1987;5:601.
9. Ramim SM, Stain AJ, Stone IC, et al. Sexual assault in postmenopausal women. *Obstet Gynecol* 1992; 80:860.
10. Dupre AR, Hampton HL, Morrison H, et al. Sexual assault. *Obstet Gynecol Surv* 1993;48:640–648.
11. The California medical protocol for examination of sexual assault and child sexual abuse victims; 2001:98. www.calema.ca.gov
12. Bates CK. Evaluation and Management of Adult Sexual Assault Victims. In: Moreira ME, ed. Uptodate. UpToDate.com. Published November 5, 2012. Accessed March 18, 2014.
13. Workowski KA, Berman S. Sexually transmitted diseases treatment guidelines, 2010. *MMWR Recomm Rep* 2010;59:1–110.
14. Luce H, Schrager S. Sexual assault of women. *Am Fam Physicians* 2010;81(4):489–495.
15. Burgess AW, Holmstrom LL. *Rape: crisis and recovery*. Bowie, MD: Robert J. Brady; 1979.
16. Support services: the Rape Abuse and Incest National Network (RAINN at 1-800-656-HOPE). https://www.rainn.org/get-help/national-sexual-assault-hotline. Accessed June 2014.
17. Berkowitz CD. Abuse and neglect of children. In: Tintinalli JE, Kelen GD, Stapczynski JS, et al., eds. *Emergency medicine—a comprehensive study guide*. 5th ed. New York, NY: McGraw-Hill; 2000:115–117.

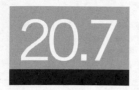

Acute Musculoskeletal Injury

Rebecca L. Peebles, Sabrina L. Silver

GENERAL PRINCIPLES

Definition

Acute musculoskeletal injuries are insults to bone, muscle, ligament, or tendon, resulting in a disruption of the normal anatomy. There is no consensus as to when an acute injury is considered chronic. The "acute phase" varies from 6 weeks to 6 months.

Epidemiology

- Ankle sprains account for 2 million injuries per year and 20% of all sports injuries.[1]
- Knee injuries account for around 1 million emergency department (ER) visits a year.[2]
- Low back pain has an estimated prevalence of 20% in the U.S. population and acute low back pain is the fifth most common complaint in a primary care setting.[3]

Etiology

Underlying conditions such as deconditioning, poor biomechanics, or osteoporosis can decrease tolerance of outside stressors and often contribute to acute symptoms, with or without trauma.

General Treatment Approach

Initial treatment involves stabilizing surrounding tissue to protect the injury, decreasing inflammation, and pain control. More specifically this includes:

- **Imaging.** Choice varies, but can include x-ray, ultrasound (US), computed tomography (CT), and magnetic resonance imaging (MRI).
- **Reductions** for joint dislocations.
- **Splints or casts** for fractures, ligament, and some tendon tears.
- **Immobilization** for sprains, strains, and fractures.
- **Rest, ice, compression, and elevation (RICE)** to reduce inflammation.
- **Nonsteroidal anti-inflammatory drugs (NSAIDs)** can be used but are controversial. A short course (5 to 7 days) can be beneficial for reducing inflammation and controlling pain, but in the long run may slow inflammatory-mediated healing.
- **Opioids** for pain control in fractures and dislocations.
- **Muscle relaxants** for pain control; this is most commonly used for acute back pain.

After initial treatment allows for healing and regeneration of affected tissue, most patients do well with physical therapy for strengthening and rehabilitation of the injured area. Some injuries require surgery for definitive treatment.

FRACTURES

Diagnosis

History

History should be obtained with attention to mechanism of injury and risk factors that render the patient susceptible for fracture or impaired healing. The type, direction, and speed of the force applied to the bone can help predict the injury before imaging is obtained. Fractures result from compressive, tensile, and/or sheer stress that overcomes the intrinsic strength of the normal bone. This may happen acutely or over time with repetitive loading, resultant microdamage of cortical bone, and subsequent failure of bone integrity. Acutely, the speed at which this force is loaded will determine the extent of the fracture. Rapid loading diminishes the bone's ability to absorb force causing fragmentation, whereas slow loading causes a single fragment.

Physical Examination

For a suspected fracture, inspect the affected area for swelling, ecchymosis, asymmetry, and gross deformity; palpate for tenderness; and assess strength, range of motion (ROM), and neurovascular compromise. Key findings that favor fracture include point tenderness over bone, loss of function, and apprehension with movement. Examine the joints distal and proximal to the suspected fracture to evaluate for associated injuries.

Imaging

X-rays are the diagnostic imaging of choice. Multiple views should be obtained as a fracture must be visualized in two or more views to make the diagnosis. Fractures should be described in terms of location, open or closed, direction of fracture line, fragments, displacement, and angulation. If the radiograph does not reveal evidence of a fracture, CT or MRI may be indicated. Imaging of the joint above and below the fracture should be considered.

Treatment

Understanding the three stages of bone healing provides insight into the treatment process. The inflammatory stage begins within the first few hours of injury with hematoma formation and recruitment of inflammatory cells. Soft callus is laid around week 2 at the transition into the repair stage. By week 6, a hard callus replaces the soft, marking clinical union. During the final stage, remodeling, immature bone is replaced with mature bone and strength is regained by 3 to 6 months.

Bone healing is inhibited by smoking, malnutrition, diabetes, rheumatoid arthritis, osteoporosis, and use of steroid, cytotoxic, or NSAID medications.[4] Furthermore, other comorbidities such as bone density, nutrition, endocrine abnormalities, and the female athlete triad should be considered for patients having recurrent stress or low-impact fractures.

Immobilization via splinting or casting throughout the inflammatory and repair stages of bone healing is crucial. Any fracture that has significant displacement should be reduced prior to immobilization. Reduction can often be achieved in the office or emergency department, but more complicated fractures may require general anesthesia and/or surgery for definitive care. Always perform postreduction imaging and neurovascular examination. Surgery is indicated if misalignment or neurovascular complications are present or if reduction cannot be maintained. If clinical suspicion for fracture is high but radiographs are negative, immobilize as if a fracture is visualized. Specific management of common fractures is reviewed in Table 20.7-1.

TABLE 20.7-1	Common Fractures and Treatments[a]			
Fracture name	**Bone involved**	**Mechanism**	**Clinical notes**	**Treatment**
Clavicle	Most commonly middle third of clavicle	Fall onto shoulder	Present with arm adducted across chest and supporting injured arm; may have tenting of the skin at proximal end of fracture	Immobilization with sling for 4–6 wk
Humerus	Most commonly middle third with proximal third being second	Trauma	May have shortening of affected arm; check radial nerve for integrity	Reduction followed by hanging cast for 1–2 wk and finally bracing for another 6–7 wk
Colles'	Distal radius	Fall onto outstretched arm with hyperextended and radial deviated wrist	Fracture has dorsal displacement and angulation, resulting in the "dinner fork" deformity on x-ray	Reduction followed by either splint- or short-arm cast for 6 wk

TABLE 20.7-1 | **Common Fractures and Treatments** *(continued)*

Fracture name	Bone involved	Mechanism	Clinical notes	Treatment
Scaphoid	Scaphoid	Fall onto outstretched arm with dorsiflexed and ulnar deviated wrist	Present with wrist swelling and tenderness over anatomical snuff box; if not seen on x-ray but high clinical suspicion repeat x-ray in 1–2 wk	Long-arm thumb spica cast for 6 wk followed by short-arm thumb spica for 6 wk
Boxer's	Neck of fifth metacarpal	Direct force to 5th metacarpal (i.e., punching a hard surface)	Obtain less than 40 degrees of angulation with reduction	Ulnar gutter splint for 4 wk
Metacarpal shaft	Metacarpal	Direct force	Must have less than 10 degrees of rotation otherwise need surgery	Cast or splint for 4 wk
Jersey Finger	Avulsion of FDP	Hyperextension of DIP	Inability to flex affected joint	Surgery
Mallet finger	Disruption of extensor tendon at DIP	Hyperflexion of DIP	Inability to extend affected joint	Splint in full extension for 6–8 wk
Fibula	Distal fibula	Trauma to ankle	Weber classification based on location relative to ankle mortise: A = below, B = at mortise, C = above mortise; have low suspicion for syndesmosis involvement	If no syndesmosis involvement (most commonly Weber A), then short-leg cast or removable boot for 6 wk; otherwise, surgery
Fibula avulsion	Distal fibula where ATFL attaches	Supination and external rotation of foot	Associated with ankle sprains	Rest, ice, elevation, aircast if needed for pain control
Lisfranc	Tarsometatarsal	Forceful abduction of forefoot	Can be easily overlooked, so need high suspicion; Look for plantar bruising; If <2 mm of displacement and <15 degrees of angulation can do conservative management	Conservative management is 6–8 wk in cast or boot. Initially non–weight bearing then advance as tolerated
Jones	Base of fifth metatarsal	Trauma	High rate of nonunion	Can do cast with non–weight bearing for 6–8 wk; in active patient consider going straight to surgery
Phalangeal	Phalanges	Direct blow	Nonunion is uncommon; the great toe is the most likely be unstable	Hard sole shoe for patient comfort

FDP, flexor digitorum profundus; DIP, distal interphalangeal joint; ATFL, anterior talofibular ligament.

[a]Information compiled from Egol et al. (2010)[5] and Monteleone (2006).[6]

Pain should be controlled with ice, acetaminophen, or judicious use of opiates. Anti-inflammatory medications should be avoided during the first week of injury as they inhibit the necessary inflammatory process and can lead to prolonged healing. Once clinical union is achieved, mobilization and physical therapy should be initiated.

MUSCLE STRAIN
Diagnosis
History
Strains occur when overexertion causes injury to the tendons or muscle. Lifting heavy objects, rapid pivoting and turning, or direct blows are mechanisms that may cause a strain. The patient may complain of pain in the muscle or at the insertion site that worsens with movement requiring that muscle.

Physical Examination
Swelling or bruising may be appreciated, as well as tenderness to palpation or a palpable muscle spasm. ROM may be limited due to weakness secondary to pain.

Imaging
Imaging is not indicated initially, but with worsening pain, ultrasound may be indicated to rule out hematoma or complete rupture of a tendon.

Treatment
Advise NSAIDs and RICE. Encourage use of the affected muscle limited only by activities that cause excessive pain. Patients should be educated that some strains can take 6 to 8 weeks to heal.

TENDON AND LIGAMENT INJURY
Diagnosis
History
Tendon and ligament injuries can result from direct laceration, but more commonly occur with tensile overload. Tendons can withstand significant load; hence, disruption usually occurs at the musculotendon junction or bony avulsion.[4]

Physical Examination
Palpation directly over the tendon or ligament often reveals tenderness. Special tests have been developed for most of the major tendons and ligaments to help isolate the affected segment and will be covered in the sections to follow.

Ligamentous injuries are graded on the basis of the extent of laxity with manual testing.

- **Grade I (minor tear):** minimal laxity
- **Grade II (partial tear without complete disruption):** 5 to 10 mm of translation with a firm endpoint
- **Grade III (complete tear):** greater than 10 mm of translation with soft or no endpoint.

Imaging
Imaging is often not necessary. When indicated, modality will vary on the basis of the clinical suspicion and location, and is generally accomplished through US and MRI.

Treatment
Grade I and II ligament and most tendon injuries are managed conservatively. A period of relative rest (usually 72 hours or less) and modified activity are necessary immediately after insult. Immobilization will vary by injury, but in general, prolonged immobilization will result in stiffness and decreased strength of the structure. Load should be decreased to allow pain-free activity and will vary from non–weight bearing to modified activity.

Use of NSAIDs and corticosteroid injections are controversial. NSAIDs can be used to decrease pain and swelling with the initial injury but may result in decreased recruitment of repair mechanisms and prolonged healing. Corticosteroid injections decrease inflammation around injured tendons, which reduces adhesion formation. Care must be taken to avoid injecting directly into the tendon as elevated tissue pressure will result in further damage. Case reports have associated rupture of weight-bearing tendons such as the Achilles tendon with corticosteroid injection; however, no studies have been completed to further assess this correlation.

Surgical repair should be considered for Grade III ligament tears and tendon injuries refractory to conservative treatment after 4 to 6 months.

SPINE
Acute Back Pain
Diagnosis
History
Acute back pain is defined by pain that has been present for less than 12 weeks. Typically there is a history of overexertion that correlates with the onset of pain. It is important to check for 'red flag symptoms' which include age >50, fevers and chills, trauma, saddle anesthesia, abnormal bowel or bladder function, and new motor or sensory deficits.

Physical Examination
Red flag findings must be assessed. Ensure intact sensory and motor function of both lower extremities. A negative straight leg raise helps rule out radicular pain, whereas a positive one can point toward sciatica or degenerative disc disease. Palpate bony landmarks for suspicious fractures, and paraspinal muscles for muscle spasms. Tenderness to palpation over paraspinals will often be the only physical finding.

Imaging
In the absence of any red flag findings, no imaging is indicated. If other signs or symptoms of fracture are present, then x-ray is the imaging of choice.

Treatment
Conservative treatment with NSAIDS or acetaminophen (up to 4 g per day in patients without liver disease) is recommended for pain determined to be of musculoskeletal etiology.[3] In patients with palpable muscle spasm, a short course of muscle relaxants (i.e., cyclobenzaprine 10 mg TID) can help improve back pain.[7] Patients should be encouraged to keep active and educated on the natural history of the disease, which can take up to 3 months to fully recover. Other alternative treatments such as manipulation, massage, and acupuncture may be of benefit to some patients.

UPPER EXTREMITY
Shoulder Dislocation
Diagnosis
History
Shoulder dislocations occur in the anterior direction 95% of the time as a result of a force on the shoulder when the arm is abducted and externally rotated. Nontraumatic shoulder dislocations occur secondary to intrinsic laxity or repetitive microtraumas such as in swimmers and gymnasts. Posterior shoulder dislocations are rarer and occur in setting of seizures or electrocution. In general, the patient will report a popping sensation with pain and obvious deformity. Dislocations can result from trauma, with complications including fractures and labral tears.

Physical Examination
With an anterior dislocation, the arm is typically in slight abduction and external rotation with a flexed elbow. Patients typically have obvious deformity of the shoulder joint and will experience pain and apprehension with any addition of abduction or external rotation. Patients with a posterior dislocation will hold their arm in adduction and internal rotation, and also have obvious deformity of the shoulder joint. It is important to assess integrity of the axillary nerve. They should be able to at initiate abduction or at least have contraction of the deltoid if the axillary nerve is intact.

Imaging
Radiographs of the affected shoulder in the anteroposterior and axillary scapular view should be ordered. An orthogonal view should be used if a posterior fracture is suspected.[8] Radiographs allow visualization of the direction of dislocation as well as diagnosis of any associated fractures such as a Hill–Sachs or Bankhart lesion.

Treatment
Reduction of the joint should be obtained as soon as possible. For an anterior dislocation, Stimson's method is a good technique as it is the least traumatic. The patient should lie prone on an examination table, with

the arm of the dislocated shoulder hanging off the table at 90 degrees of forward flexion. Gentle downward traction by a weight should be applied to facilitate the relaxation of muscles and spontaneous reduction. Other techniques include Rockwood traction–countertraction and Milch techniques. Relocation of a posterior dislocation is done with patient supine and application of lateral traction with external rotation. After reduction, the patient should then be immobilized in a sling for 2 to 4 weeks with early physical therapy.[8]

Biceps Tendon Rupture

Diagnosis

History

Biceps tendon ruptures occur at the insertion of the long head on the labrum about 90% of the time.[9] Rupture of the short head insertion on the acromion and the distal insertion on the radius are far less common. Most commonly a proximal rupture occurs with an eccentric force on a flexed elbow in a patient with a history of chronic shoulder problems.[9] Patients will often present with a story of sharp, tearing pain, of anterior shoulder that radiates down the anterior arm along the route of the bicep muscle. Distal ruptures occur in a similar population due to the wear and tear on the distal insertion. With either rupture, the patient may be able to describe an audible popping noise in conjunction with the formation of a muscle deformity in the anterior arm.

Physical Examination

In a complete rupture, there will be an obvious mass near the elbow as a result of the muscle bundles bunching after rupture, frequently referred to as a "popeye" deformity. With a proximal rupture, patients will have point tenderness over the biceps tendon groove along with a positive Speed test and Yergason test. The hook test is good for diagnosing distal biceps tendon rupture.

Imaging

Shoulder films should be ordered but are commonly negative. With a convincing examination, there is no need for further initial images. However, with a skilled user, US of the bicipital groove can show the ruptured tendon. Furthermore, if diagnosis of a proximal rupture is not certain or a distal rupture is suspected, then MRI will show the ruptured anatomy. A proximal biceps tendon rupture can often result in a labral tear secondary to the anatomy of the tendon anchoring in the labrum. If this is suspected, an MRI with contrast should be obtained.

Treatment

For a proximal biceps tendon rupture, physical therapy should be initiated. If the tendon rupture has an associated labral tear, the patient should be referred to a surgeon to discuss surgical management. A distal biceps tendon rupture should be referred to a surgeon for definitive treatment in order to maintain ability to supinate the elbow.[9]

KNEE

Patellar Dislocation

Diagnosis

History

Patellar dislocations occur as a result of direct trauma to the knee or from twisting with the knee extended. Dislocations almost always occur laterally. Typically the patella reduces spontaneously with knee extension and many patients will be unsure if dislocation occurred. If the patient presents remote from injury, the chief compliant might be recurrent sensation of patellar subluxation.

Physical Examination

Knee effusion will often be present. If relocation has not occurred, obvious deformity will be noted. The medial retinaculum and lateral femoral condyle will be tender to palpation. Patellar apprehension test will be positive and laxity may be observed.

Imaging

X-rays of the knee, including sunrise views, should be obtained to assess for fractures. MRI should be reserved for ruling out associated ligamentous or meniscal tears.

Treatment

Flexing the hip and applying medial force on the patella while extending the knee can achieve relocation of the patella. The patient should be immobilized in full extension for 1 to 2 weeks. Early isometric quadriceps strengthening exercises and ROM exercises should be initiated once pain and swelling have decreased. After the first dislocation, patients have a 50% chance of recurrence. Patients with recurrent dislocations necessitate orthopedic evaluation.

Ligament Tears

See Table 20.7-2 for discussion of anterior cruciate ligament (ACL), medial collateral ligament (MCL), lateral collateral ligament (LCL), and posterior cruciate ligament (PCL) tears.

Meniscus Tear

Diagnosis

History

Traumatic meniscus tears frequently result from forceful twisting or hyperflexion. Patients often report locking sensation, inability to fully extend the knee, or pain with excessive knee flexion. Swelling may develop over time, but is not typically present immediately after injury. Anatomic variants in the lateral meniscus predispose patients to meniscal injury.

Physical Examination

Posterior joint line tenderness and effusion are often noted on palpation. McMurray, Apley compression, and Thessaly tests are positive only when reproduction of the patient's reported symptoms is achieved.

Imaging

X-rays should be obtained to assess for associated fracture or osteochondral loose body. If surgical intervention is being considered, MRI is recommended as it is 93% sensitive and 95% specific for evaluation of meniscal tears.[8]

Treatment

Acute meniscus tears should be treated conservatively with use of crutches, ice, and NSAIDs. ROM and isometric quadriceps strengthening can be started immediately and progressed as tolerated. Orthopedic consult is indicated for symptoms persisting more than 3 months, frequent locking, or expedited return to sport. Patients presenting with locked knee or inability to achieve full extension warrant orthopedic evaluation within 24 hours.

ANKLE

Achilles Tendon Rupture

Diagnosis

History

Achilles tendon ruptures occur predominantly in males with a bimodal distribution, with the majority occurring in middle age and a small second peak in 70- to 79-year olds.[10] Patients will frequently report a "pop" or "snap" sensation followed by immediate intense pain in the posterior distal leg. The initial pain and swelling resolves quickly but patients often present with complaint of lingering weakness, poor balance, or abnormal gait. Predisposing biomechanical factors include pronation, lower extremity varus, tight heel cord, weak dorsiflexion, weak plantar flexion, ankle instability,[4] or use of fluoroquinolones or corticosteroid medications (systemic or locally injected).

Physical Examination

Within the first 3 days of injury, a gap will be palpable 2 to 7 cm proximal to the insertion of the Achilles at the calcaneal enthesis. After 48 to 72 hours, hematoma and fibrous tissue formation fill this gap, making diagnosis more difficult. The Thompson test distinguishes between partial and complete tears.

Imaging

The diagnosis is usually made clinically. However, if the injury is longstanding or partial tear is suspected, diagnosis can be confirmed with ultrasound or MRI.

Treatment

Nonsurgical

Conservative approach should be considered for patient who are elderly, inactive, or have poor wound healing. The lower leg should be immobilized in gravity equines position for 4 weeks and then neutral position for an additional 4 weeks. Evaluation by an orthopedic surgeon is warranted even if conservative approach is taken.

TABLE 20.7-2 Ligamentous Knee Injuries

Ligament	Mechanism	Clinical notes	Imaging	Treatment
ACL	Typically noncontact; forced anterior movement of the tibia with sudden pivot, hyperflexion, or landing a jump	C/C: instability of knee Sx: pop, swelling F: ligament laxity AI: meniscal tear (90%) ST: Lachmans (most sensitive) Anterior drawer	X-ray MRI	Rest, ice, and compression to decrease initial swelling. Crutches and knee brace until able to bear weight without significant pain. ROM and quadriceps strengthening exercises as soon as tolerated. **Surgery:** Indicated for recurrent instability or athletes in sports requiring cutting and pivoting. Urgent referrals unnecessary as surgery is delayed 3–6 wk to minimize fibrosis from initial hemarthrosis. PT prior to surgery improves post-op outcomes.
MCL	Lateral/valgus force	C/C: pain at joint line Sx: less instability, swelling F: joint line TTP, ligament laxity AI: ACL tear ST: valgus stress	X-ray MRI	Rest, ice, and compression to decrease initial swelling. **MCL/LCL Grade I and II:** Crutches only if unable to initially bear weight. ROM and strengthening exercises of the quadriceps and hamstrings should initiated immediately after Grade I sprain and after 1 wk of rest for Grade II sprains. **MCL/LCL Grade III sprains:** Orthopedic evaluation necessary.
LCL	Anteromedial/varus force while knee in extension or excessive internal rotation on tibia, uncommon to occur without PCL injury	C/C: lateral knee pain Sx: if CPN injury— lateral leg numbness/tingling or weakness with dorsiflexion F: joint line TTP, ligament laxity AI: PCL and/or CPN injury ST: varus stress		
PCL	Hyperextension, posterior trauma, hyperflexion while in plantarflexion	C/C: instability Sx: posterior knee pain F: posterior knee effusion, TTP AI: LCL tear ST: Posterior drawer test, Godfrey test	X-ray MRI	Rest, ice, and compression to decrease initial swelling. **Grade I and II injuries:** ROM and quadriceps strengthening exercises using a hinged knee brace. **Grade III injuries:** 2–4 wk of immobilization. Non–weight bearing until patient can ambulate with normal gait. ROM and quadriceps strengthening after the initial immobilization period and continued for up to 3 mo. **Surgery:** Indicated if injuries necessitating operative repair are present.

ACL, anterior cruciate ligament; MCL, medial collateral ligament; LCL, lateral collateral ligament; PCL, posterior cruciate ligament; C/C, chief complaint; Sx, common symptoms; F, examination findings; AI, commonly associated injuries; ST, special tests; TTP, tenderness to palpation; CPN, common peroneal nerve; ROM, range of motion; PT, physical therapy.

X-rays should be obtained to assess for fractures. MRI is indicated to confirm ligament tear and evaluate for associated meniscal or osteochondral injuries.

Surgical

Surgical management should be considered for young, healthy, or active patients. Compared with those managed with conservative treatment, postsurgical patients have increased strength, greater rate of return to play, and lower re-rupture rate (0% to 5% vs. 40%).

Rehabilitation

Accelerated rehabilitation with no increased risk of re-rupture is seen in both groups with early ROM, eccentric strength training, and flexibility drills of the gastrocnemius and soleus muscles.[4,11]

Ankle Sprain

See Table 20.7-3 for discussion of ankle sprains.

Imaging

On initial examination, it is important to determine the need for imaging by using the five Ottawa ankle rules. X-rays are indicated if any of the following five physical examination findings are present:

- Inability to bear weight for four steps immediately after the injury or in the examination room,
- Bony tenderness over posterior aspect of the medial malleolus,
- Bony tenderness over posterior aspect of the lateral malleolus,
- Bony tenderness over base of the fifth metatarsal head,
- Bony tenderness over the navicular.

By using these rules appropriately, the number of unnecessary x-rays can be reduced by 30% to 40%.[12] Stress radiographs can help diagnose lateral ligament injury, but are not required.

OTHER

Rhabdomyolysis

Diagnosis

History

Rhabdomyolysis occurs with excessive breakdown of muscle tissue, resulting in the release of muscle fibers and breakdown products into the blood stream. These by-products can damage the kidney causing acute kidney injury and electrolyte abnormalities. Most often this is a result of a crush injury causing muscle damage. Other historical causes include substance abuse, history of inflammatory muscle disease, lengthy exertion, trauma, prolonged immobility, and seizures. Rhabdomyolysis can also be induced by medications, with antipsychotics, statins, selective serotonin reuptake inhibitors, and colchicine being the most common.[13] The patient may have complaints of muscle or joint pain. They also can present with dark urine due to the filtering of these breakdown products by the kidney.

Physical Examination

The physical examination is nonspecific and may only reveal muscle tenderness. In crush injuries, it is important to assess neurovascular integrity. Urine output should be assessed to determine the extent of kidney injury.

Laboratory

No imaging is indicated. Laboratory work should include electrolytes, creatine kinase, urinalysis, and urine and serum myoglobin. Calcium and potassium may be elevated. The creatine kinase may be significantly elevated—often up to five times normal.[13] Urine may test positive for blood and be negative for red blood cells due to the presence of myoglobin.

Treatment

Once rhabdomyolysis is diagnosed, the inciting factor should be determined in order to prevent further damage. Otherwise, treatment is supportive of kidneys and electrolyte abnormalities. Aggressive fluid resuscitation is first-line treatment, with a recommendation to alternate normal saline with 5% glucose solution every 500 mL at a rate of 500 mL per hour.[14] Cardiac monitoring is important as the patients can develop cardiac arrhythmias secondary to hyperkalemia. Monitoring of renal function and urine output should be done to determine the extent of kidney injury. In the acute phase, the target urine output is 200 mL per hour until patients' creatine kinase starts to drop and electrolytes stabilize.[14]

TABLE 20.7-3 Ankle Sprains

Type	Ligaments involved	Mechanism	Clinical notes	Treatment
Lateral	Anterior talofibular Posterior talofibular Calcaneofibular	Excess lateral force on an inverted, plantarflexed ankle	Most common ankle sprain F: ligament laxity, TTP over injured ligament AI: high ankle sprains, Maisonneuve fractures ST: anterior drawer (often falsely negative in first 48 h); talar tilt to assess the ATFL or, if performed in neutral flexion, CFL	*Grade I and II* I: Ice, NSAIDS, and relative rest. PT: Initiated within 48 h with focus of ROM, muscle strengthening, and proprioception. Grade I and II sprains typically heal in 1–3 and 2–4 wk, respectively. *Grade III* I: 5–7 d in boot or short-leg cast and use of crutches until full weight bearing is tolerated. Semirigid or lace-up brace should be worn throughout rehabilitation period. PT: Initiate after the first week. Lateral and medial Grade III injuries typically heal in about 5–8 and 6 mo, respectively.
Medial	Deltoid	Eversion	F: TTP at Deltoid ligament AI: injury to surrounding structures common due to significant force required to tear Deltoid ligament ST: reverse talar tilt	Same as lateral ankle injuries.
High	Syndesmotic ligaments	Synchronous ankle external rotation and hyperdorsiflexion	F: TTP along proximal fibula or interosseous region AI: medial or lateral ankle sprains, fibular fracture ST: Squeeze test	*Grade I and II* Immobilization, protected weight bearing for up to 3 and 6 wk, respectively, followed by functional rehabilitation *Grade III* Surgical intervention.

F, examination findings; AI, commonly associated injuries; ST, special tests; TTP, tenderness to palpation; ATFL, anterior talofibular ligament; CFL, calcaneofibular ligament; I, Initial treatment; ROM, range of motion; PT, physical therapy.

Decision to obtain x-rays should be based on the Ottawa ankle rules: inability to bear weight for more than four steps, or bony tenderness over one of the following structures: the posterior aspect of the medial or lateral malleoli, base of the fifth metatarsal, navicular. Stress radiographs can help diagnose lateral ligament injury, but are not required.

Compartment Syndrome

Diagnosis

History

Acute compartment syndrome occurs when the blood flow and circulation within a fascia compartment is compromised. Most frequently, there is trauma to a limb resulting in increased fluid or blood within the compartment. Fractures, crush injuries, or casts placed too tightly are all possible sources. The ischemia causes severe pain in the affected limb. This pain typically starts within a few hours of the injury but can present as far out as 48 hours. This pressure can also cause nerve damage, and the patient may complain of paresthesia in the distribution of the damaged nerve.

Physical Examination

Traditionally, the five Ps (pain, paresthesia, pallor, pulselessness, and poikilothermia) have been taught as the diagnostic findings, but quite frequently the patient presents sooner than the development of these symptoms. Often a pulse is still present and palpable. Pain that worsens with movement and an appropriate history should raise the clinical suspicion of compartment syndrome.

Imaging

No imaging is necessary, but an intracompartmental pressure should be obtained. Pressures higher than 30 mmHg are considered significant. Another measurement—diastolic blood pressure minus the intracompartmental pressure—can be used for diagnosis when the value is ≤20 mmHg.[15] This delta pressure has been shown to be a more accurate diagnostic value for determining treatment and avoiding unnecessary surgeries.[15]

Treatment

In true compartment syndromes, fasciotomy is the treatment of choice. This allows the muscle to expand and relieves the pressure on the tissues. Nerves start to experience damage within 2 hours of elevated pressures, and irreversible damage can occur after 8 hours of elevated pressures, so it is important to have a low suspicion for diagnosis and treatment.[15]

REFERENCES

1. Tiemstra JD. Update on acute ankle sprains. *Am Fam Physician* 2012;85(12):1170–1176.
2. Jackson JL, O'Malley PG, Kroenke K. Evaluation of acute knee pain in primary care. *Ann Intern Med* 2003;139(7):575–588.
3. Roelofs PDDM, Deyo RA, Koes BW, et al. Non-steroidal anti-inflammatory drugs for low back pain. *Cochrane Database Syst Rev.* 2008;(1):CD000396. doi:10.1002/14651858.CD000396.pub3
4. O'Connor FG, Casa DJ, St. Pierre P, et al. *ACSM's Sports Medicine: A Comprehensive Review*. Philadelphia, PA: Wolters Kluwer/Lippincott Williams & Wilkins Health; 2010:chaps 7, 9, 18, 45, 48, 49, 60, 63, 64.
5. Egol KA, Koval KJ, Zuckerman JD, et al. *Handbook of fractures*. Philadelphia, PA: Wolters Kluwer/Lippincott Williams & Wilkins Health; 2010.
6. Monteleone GP. Common Fractures: Recognition and Management. AAFP Board Review 2006. PDF file. http://medicine.hsc.wvu.edu/Fammed-Sports-Med/MediaLibraries/Fammed-Sports-Med/Media/Documents/PDFs/Common-Fractures.pdf. Accessed February 15, 2014.
7. Browning R, Jackson JL, O'Malley PG. Cyclobenzaprine and back pain: a meta-analysis. *Arch Intern Med* 2001;161:1613–1620.
8. Luke A, Benjamin C. Sports medicine and outpatient orthopedics. In: Papadakis MA, McPhee SJ, Rabow MW, eds. *Current medical diagnosis and treatment 2014*. 53rd ed. New York, NY: McGraw-Hill Global Education Holdings, LLC; 2014:chap 41.
9. Quach T, Jazayeri R, Sherman OH, et al. Distal biceps tendon injuries—current treatment options. *Bull NYU Hosp Jt Dis* 2010;68(2):103–111.
10. Seidenberg PH, Beutler AI. *The sports medicine resource manual*. Philadelphia, PA: Saunders; 2008: chaps 6, 9, 12.
11. Willits K, Amendola A, Bryant D, et al. Operative versus nonoperative treatment of acute achilles tendon ruptures: a multicenter randomized trial using accelerated functional rehabilitation. *J Bone Joint Surg Am* 2010;92(17):2767–2775.
12. Bachmann LM, Kolb E, Koller MT, et al. Accuracy of Ottawa ankle rules to exclude fractures of the ankle and mid-foot: systematic review. *BMJ* 2003;326:417.
13. Melli G, Chaudhry V, Cornblath DR. Rhabdomyolysis: an evaluation of 475 hospitalized patients. *Medicine (Baltimore)* 2005;84:377.
14. Cervellin G, Comelli I, Lippi G. Rhabdomyolysis: Historical background, clinical, diagnostic and therapeutic features. *Clin Chem Lab Med* 2010;48:749–756.
15. Konstantakos EK, Dalstrom DJ, Nelles ME, et al. Diagnosis and management of extremity compartment syndromes: an orthopedic perspective. *Am Surg* 2007;73(12):1199–1209.

CHAPTER 21

Occupational and Environmental Problems

Section Editor: Timothy J. Coker

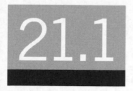

Disability Determination

Timothy J. Coker

GENERAL PRINCIPLES

Disability evaluation and determination is an important medical function because it impacts both the patient and the economy. Although it is important, it can be quite challenging for clinicians to accomplish. Clinicians must synthesize clinical and nonclinical information to make a medical decision and communicate it to multiple administrative and legal entities. Primary care clinicians will continue to perform evaluations because as the treating provider, they can provide the best medical evidence to make an appropriate disability determination.[1]

Definition

Disability is often confused with impairment. It is important for clinicians to know the difference between the two to provide appropriate evaluation. There are several definitions for each of these terms from different organizations and the most common definitions have been included at the end of this chapter (Table 21.1-1). The following are general definitions of the term.

TABLE 21.1-1	Disability Definitions

Definitions of impairment

A significant deviation, loss, or loss of use of any body structure or body function in an individual with a health condition, disorder or disease.[2]

A loss, loss of use or derangement of any body part, organ system or organ function.[3]

Results from anatomical, physiological, or psychological abnormalities, which can be shown by medically acceptable clinical and laboratory diagnostic techniques. A physical or mental impairment must be established by medical evidence consisting of signs, symptoms, and laboratory findings—not only by the individual's statement of symptoms.[4]

Definitions of disability

Activity limitations and/or participation restrictions in an individual with a health condition disorder or disease.[2]

An alteration of an individual's capacity to meet personal, social, or occupational demands or statutory or regulatory requirements because of an impairment.[3]

The inability to engage in any substantial, gainful activity (SGA) by reason of a medically determinable physical or mental impairment(s), which can be expected to result in death or which has lasted or can be expected to last for a continuous period of not less than 12 months.[4]

Impairment is typically defined as "a significant deviation, loss, or loss of use of any body structure or body function in an individual with a health condition, disorder or disease."[2] It can be defined as permanent or temporary or partial or total depending on the issue. It does not vary based on environment.

Disability is typically defined as a limitation due to impairment in the ability to perform activities of daily living or complex activities, like work.[4] It is determined by environmental factors. A person with an impairment may be disabled only in certain situations or jobs.

Epidemiology

In 2005, the United States Census Bureau found that 54.4 million people in the noninstitutional population had some level of disability, with 35 million of them reporting severe disability.[5] In that population, African Americans and Hispanics had higher rates of disability than whites.[5]

Arthritis, back or spinal problems, and heart conditions are the top three conditions that cause disability.[6-8] In addition, disability also increases with age. The United States Census Bureau found that 41.9% of those over 65 years old had a disability compared with 18.6% of younger people.[6,7]

Classification

There are several guides available that can be used to classify impairment and disability. One of the most popular ones, The American Medical Association (AMA) "Guides to the Evaluation of Permanent Impairment," has standardized the approach to impairment assessment. There are several editions of the guides and each state has mandated specific editions or portions of them as the standard for impairment determination. Provider should check with their respective states to determine which one they should use.

The predominant guides for disability determination, the Blue Book and the Green Book, were created by the Social Security Administration (SSA). The Blue Book describes the disability process and contains a listing of impairments for treating clinicians to determine disability. The Green Book is for consulting clinicians. If a patient meets criteria for a medical diagnosis, the condition is on the list of impairments, and it has lasted or is expected to last at least 12 months or death, he or she will meet the medical criteria for disability.

History and Physical Examination

Clinicians should gather information about the individual's medical problems and their functional limitations, which may involve performing diagnostic testing and imaging, completing a detailed physical examination, and collecting consultant reports. The clinician needs to then determine whether the patient has an impairment based on the medical issues. Once impairment has identified, additional factors can be evaluated to determine whether there are situations where the individual has disability.

Documenting the medical and limitation information is as important as collecting it. Clinicians need to create a coherent picture in their documentation to assist disability agencies, such as the SSA, which can make an appropriate decision.

TREATMENT

Treatment is determined by the underlying medical problem and does not change based on disability status. All therapy should be directed to minimizing or eliminating impairment. Treatment may include medications, surgeries, physical and occupational therapy, and behavioral and mental health care.

Referrals

Depending on the nature of the patient's impairment, referrals may be necessary for additional recommendations or treatment. There should be ongoing communication between the referring and primary physician.

Patient Education

Patients should be educated about the difference between impairment and disability. They should also be directed to resources that can educate them about the disability process.

Follow-Up

Follow-up with the primary physician and consultants will be based on the patient's medical problems.

HELPFUL INTERNET SITES

- http://www.nhchc.org/wp-content/uploads/2012/02/DocumentingDisability2007.pdf
- www.geriatric.theclinics.com
- www.acoem.org
- www.who.int/classifications/icf/en/
- http://www.socialsecurity.gov/disability/professionals/bluebook/

REFERENCES

1. O'Connell JJ, Zevin BD, Quick PD. Documenting Disability: Simple Strategies for Medical Providers. The National Health Care for the Homeless Council. September 2007. http://www.nhchc.org/wp-content/uploads/2012/02/DocumentingDisability2007.pdf. Accessed June 1, 2014.
2. Rondinelli R. *Guides to the evaluation of permanent impairment.* 6th ed. Washington, DC: American Medical Association; 2007.
3. Cocchiarella L, Anderson GB. *Guides to the evaluation of permanent impairment.* 5th ed. Washington, DC: American Medical Association; 2001.
4. Social Security Administration. Disability Evaluation Under Social Security (Blue Book). http://www.socialsecurity.gov/disability/professionals/bluebook/. Accessed June 1, 2014.
5. National Council on Disability (NCD). The Current State of Health Care for People with Disabilities. http://www.ncd.gov/publications/2009/Sept302009/. Accessed June 16, 2014.
6. Brault M. *Americans with disabilities: 2005.* Washington, DC: U.S. Census Bureau; 2008.
7. Altman B, Bernstein A. *Disability and health in the United States, 2001–2005.* Hyattsville, MD: National Center for Health Statistics; 2008.
8. Centers for Disease Control and Prevention (CDC). Public Health and aging: projected prevalence of self-reported arthritis or chronic joint symptoms among persons aged >65 years—United States, 2005–2030. *MMWR Morb Mortal Wkly Rep* 2003;52:489.

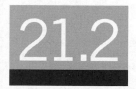

21.2 Pesticide and Related Poisoning

Scott W. Hughes

GENERAL PRINCIPLES

Pesticides represent hundreds of chemicals mixed into thousands of formulations targeted at a specific pest, crop, or structure. They are used throughout the world in home, office, industrial, agricultural, and military applications. These chemicals are used in gaseous, liquid, and in solid forms. The range of chemicals includes organophosphates, organochlorides, carbamates, dipyridyls, chlorophenoxy compounds, anticoagulants, hydrocarbons, organic and inorganic compounds, and many more.[1]

Epidemiology

A person's presence in an area where pesticides are used does not necessarily mean that there will be exposure. Exposure does not necessarily mean there will be adequate contact to produce the physiologic changes of poisoning. Poisoning may not automatically lead to impairment or disability. There is accumulating evidence to support that pesticide self-poisoning is one of the most commonly used methods of suicide worldwide, with approximately 250,000 deaths annually.[2]

Pathophysiology

As in all poisonings, time since exposure, dosage, and route of exposure (inhalation, ingestion, or absorption) will influence the effects on the patient's systems. Organophosphates and carbamates are acetylcholinesterase inhibitors used in insecticides and nerve agents. This class of pesticides accounts for the majority of severe exposures due to its mechanism of action.[1] Organophosphates immediately penetrate the central nervous system (CNS) and inactivate acetylcholinesterase, producing acute cholinergic symptoms from the accumulation of acetylcholine in the body. Inactivation is initially reversible, but becomes irreversible with time.[3] The duration of the reversible period is based primarily on the agent of exposure. Treatment during this reversible phase greatly reduces systemic effects.[4] Although organophosphates enter the CNS immediately, carbamates do not and their action on the enzyme is reversible leading to limited toxicity.

Symptoms

The effects of the increased acetylcholine are felt by the muscarinic and nicotinic receptors producing miosis and mydriasis, bradycardia or tachycardia, salivation, lacrimation, urination, nausea, vomiting, bronchorrhea, bronchospasm, weakness, hypertension, and diaphragmatic failure. The most life-threatening concerns are the bronchorrhea, bronchospasm, and respiratory insufficiency. Persons affected can also develop severe pancreatitis, which can be painless and fatal.[5,6] Effects on the CNS include headache, confusion, delirium, seizures, and coma. Exercise caution as some pesticides may exhibit delayed onset of symptoms and signs. Organophosphates, for example, have a well-documented intermediate syndrome that can begin 2 to 4 days after initial symptoms have resolved and results in rapidly developing respiratory distress and failure often requiring ventilator support for up to 21 days after onset.[7] The signs and symptoms of other pesticide and related poisonings vary and the diagnosis is many times made upon history alone.

DIAGNOSIS

Mild poisonings are associated with few symptoms and normal vital signs. Moderate poisonings are associated with more severe symptoms, objective signs, and normal vital signs. Severe poisonings are associated with multiple complaints, objective signs, and unstable vital signs. Whenever possible, physicians should learn the name of the chemical and its properties before embarking on nonemergency treatment. Sources include the safety data sheet (SDS), reference texts, poison control centers, telephone numbers on the pesticide container, TOXLINE, and MEDLINE. In suspected poisonings where the substance is not known and the clinical picture is confusing, consulting the poison control center and local toxicologists is highly recommended. In any poisoning, early communication with the poison control center is advisable as it will have the latest information on diagnosis and treatment.

History

- Contact the employer or applicator for the name of the formulation and the material SDS.
- Question how the exposure occurred, with emphasis on the exact mechanism of exposure, cause and effect relationship of exposure and symptoms, previous exposures and poisonings, and drug- or alcohol-related problems.
- Symptoms (and signs) may vary by the type of formulation to which the person was exposed, the length and concentration of exposure, and decontamination. Nausea, vomiting, and fatigue are common to most poisonings but may also represent other diseases as well as psychogenic illness. Symptoms may also be attributable to solvents used as the carriers for the pesticides, such as xylene, benzene, carbon tetrachloride, and several others.

Physical Examination

- **Skin.** Rashes should be carefully described and secondary changes caused by scratching and treatment documented. Halogenated hydrocarbons can produce chloracne, often confused with acne vulgaris.
- **Respiratory.** Inhalation of dusts, mists, and gases may cause instantaneous or delayed bronchospasm with only minimal reversibility.[6]
- **Gastrointestinal (GI).** Nausea, vomiting, diarrhea, and abdominal pain occur as a result of eating contaminated food or by direct ingestion of poison in attempted suicides and homicides.
- **Neurologic.** Acute or delayed polyneuropathy and chronic lapses in concentration and memory can result from exposure to organophosphates and halogenated hydrocarbons. Electroencephalogram abnormalities can be noted without frank seizure activity at even low levels of exposure to organophosphates and may require benzodiazepine administration for normalization.[3]
- **Ocular.** Sprays or mists to the eyes can cause problems ranging from simple conjunctivitis to corneal opacities.

Laboratory Tests

Laboratory tests are of limited usefulness and care should not be delayed waiting for them. Blood, liver, and kidney test results may be clouded by the presence of other diseases and may be abnormal only in the most severe poisonings. Cholinesterase (ChE) activity tests are useful only in organophosphate and carbamate poisoning and are most effective when used in a monitoring program for applicators where baselines have been established.[4] These tests do have usefulness in tracking a return to normal function of ChE activity, and may guide longer term clinical treatment.[8] Many military facilities are able to detect weaponized agents from samples and may represent a useful confirmatory tool for suspected exposures.

DIFFERENTIAL DIAGNOSIS

Until a specific agent is identified and confirmed as the cause of the exposure, a wide differential should be maintained. These can include many of the following general categories:

- Medication toxicity
- Viral syndromes
- Idiopathic epilepsy
- Non-pesticide toxin ingestion

TREATMENT

As previously stated, the cornerstone of pesticide treatment is decontamination, stabilization, and supportive care. In more severe cases, this may include airway and circulation support. Decontamination should not be ignored in the hospital setting. Many pesticides and nerve agents are formulated for persistence, placing medical workers at risk for contamination. Decontamination, both at the site and again upon arriving at a medical facility, should be considered a high priority to protect others from harm, especially if the exposure was during a terrorist or other malicious act, as these are more likely to involve weapon-grade chemicals. Inadvertent exposures from agricultural pesticides do not represent the same level of risk, and emergency medical treatment should not be delayed for extensive decontamination.[4] Gastric elimination of the substance, if ingested, may be performed, but studies have shown no evidence of benefit, likely due to the rapid absorption of the agents involved.[4] Mild poisonings may be able to be evaluated and followed on an outpatient basis, depending on the poison. Individuals may require only decontamination, reassurance, antiemetics for nausea and vomiting, and steroids for rash. Contact with the poison control centers will help determine whether this is an option, as many pesticides have delayed action and an initially stable patient may not remain so. Moderate symptoms (to include eye irritation without intense blepharospasms, minor skin erythema, and small blisters less than 2 cm in size) should be hospitalized and monitored for any deterioration in clinical condition.

Severe poisonings (from early eye irritation worsening to severe blepharospasm, obvious skin blister, weakness, neurologic involvement, and respiratory difficulty) require hospitalization and intensive physiologic support. Forced diuresis, exchange transfusion, and chelation are replete with complications and should be considered only when the patient's condition is severe, on an inpatient basis, when the specific agent has been identified, and after consulting toxicology experts. Atropine is the hallmark of initial treatment in organophosphate and carbamate poisoning. Goal-directed therapy with atropine is aimed at increasing heart rate to over 80, systolic blood pressure to over 80, and minimizing bronchospasm and bronchorrhea.[4] The initial dosage is 2 to 4 mg IV every 2 to 5 minutes as needed for control of airway secretions. Dosages as high as 70 mg in the first 30 minutes of therapy may be required.[4] Nerve agent poisonings generally require less atropine than agricultural pesticides. More lipid-soluble poisons may require large doses of atropine (up to a total of 40 to 100 mg per day). Continuous IV infusion of atropine, starting at 0.05 mg/kg/hour and titrated, can also be used in severe cases.[4]

Pralidoxime (2-PAM) or obidoxime should be given to all symptomatic patients who require atropine. Oxime therapy allows for the reactivation of ChEs if it is given before irreversible binding of the toxin occurs (24 to 48 hours depending on the specific agent). Initial dosing is a 2-g loading dose given IV, then 1 g every 1 to 4 hours for 48 hours, then another 1 g every 4 hours until recovery.[4]

Benzodiazepines, specifically diazepam, should be used in cases of agitated delirium or in the event of seizure activity.[4]

Complications

As discussed earlier, organophosphate-induced intermediate syndrome may present 2 to 4 days after exposure and affects approximately 20% of patients with an oral exposure to organophosphates. Respiratory distress and failure may develop rapidly requiring ventilator support for as long as 21 days.[7]

Follow-Up

Serial examinations to follow chronic problems may be necessary, especially with neurologic and respiratory involvement. Work impairments and disability status must be documented.

SPECIAL CONSIDERATION

In jurisdictions where required, reports must be made to the appropriate agencies in accidental poisonings. Intentional poisoning and any suspected terrorist or malicious poisoning should be immediately reported to the appropriate authorities. Long-term exposure to organophosphates has the potential to cause adverse reproductive outcomes, certain malignancies, and cause neurodevelopmental issues. Women, especially those in agricultural settings, should receive counsel to avoid exposure during routine prenatal counseling.[9-12]

REFERENCES

1. Roberts JR, Karr CJ. Pesticide exposure in children. *Pediatrics* 2012;130(6):e1757–e1763.
2. Gunnell D, Eddleston M, Phillips M, et al. The global distribution of fatal pesticide self-poisoning: systematic review. *BMC Public Health* 2007;7:357.
3. Barthold CL, Schier JG. Organic phosphorus compounds—nerve agents. *Crit Care Clin* 2005;21(4): 673–689.
4. Eddleston M, Buckley N, Eyer P, et al. Management of acute organophosphorus pesticide poisoning. *Lancet* 2008;371:597–607.
5. Jett D. Neurotoxic pesticides and neurologic effects. *Neurol Clin* 2011;29:667–677.
6. Hernandez A, Parron T, Alarcon R. Pesticides and asthma. *Curr Opin Allergy Clin Immunol* 2011; 11:90–96.
7. Karalliedde L, Baker D, Marrs TC. Organophosphate-induced intermediate syndrome: aetiology and relationships with myopathy. *Toxicol Rev* 2006;25(1):1–14.
8. Black RM, Read RW. Biological markers of exposure to organophosphate nerve agents. *Arch Toxicol* 2013;87:421–437.
9. Shirangi A, Nieuwenhuijsen M, Vienneau D, et al. Living near agricultural pesticide applications and the risk of adverse reproductive outcomes: a review of the literature. *Paediatr Perinat Epidemiol* 2010; 25:172–191.
10. Rosas LG, Eskenazi B. Pesticides and child neurodevelopment. *Curr Opin Pediatr* 2008;20:191–197.
11. Sankpal UT, Pius H, Khan M, et al. Environmental factors in causing human cancers: emphasis on tumorigenesis. *Tumor Biol* 2012;33:1265–1274.
12. Sathyanarayana S, Focareta J, Dailey T, et al. Environmental exposures: how to counsel preconception and prenatal patients in the clinical setting. *Am J Obstet Gynecol* 2012;207(6):463–470.

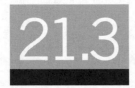

21.3 Occupational Lung Diseases

Brian N. Julich

The most common occupational lung diseases are occupational asthma, hypersensitivity pneumonitis (HP), toxic pneumonitis, pneumoconiosis (asbestosis, coal worker's pneumoconiosis, and silicosis), work-related pulmonary infections, and lung cancer.[1] Because patients may present with nonspecific or undifferentiated pulmonary symptoms, documentation of the nature and duration of exposure is essential. As these illnesses may present years after the occupational exposure, a detailed past medical and occupational history is required.[2-4] Since work products may contain multiple chemicals, the Material Safety Data Sheet (MSDS) should be obtained from the company's safety officer and reviewed for possible causes for symptoms. In addition, timing of symptoms should be identified to better determine etiology.

Differential diagnosis of patients with nonspecific pulmonary symptoms that appear to be related to work exposures includes asthma, allergy to indoor allergens, HP, bronchiolitis obliterans, byssinosis, organic toxic dust syndrome, metal fume fever, organic dust toxic syndrome, sarcoidosis, tuberculosis (TB), miliary TB, *Pneumocystis carinii* pneumonia, bronchiolitis obliterans with organizing pneumonitis, berylliosis, viral syndrome, pneumonia, allergic alveolitis, connective tissue disorders, idiopathic pulmonary fibrosis, sarcoidosis, histoplasmosis, pneumoconiosis, and chronic fungal diseases.

OCCUPATIONAL ASTHMA
General Principles
Definition

Occupational asthma is characterized by variable airflow limitation, bronchial hyperresponsiveness, and airway inflammation caused by conditions attributable to a particular work environment not otherwise found outside of the work place. The variable airflow obstruction can be reversed spontaneously or with treatment. Pre-existing asthma made worse by the workplace exposure is not considered occupational asthma and is referred to as work-exacerbated asthma.

Epidemiology

This condition accounts for approximately 25% to 50% of all occupational lung diseases, 10% to 25% of cases of adult onset asthma, and is responsible for approximately 5% to 15% of all asthma cases.

Etiology

More than 350 plausible causes have been associated with occupational asthma.[5] Occupational asthma is caused by either large-molecular-weight or low-molecular-weight sensitizers. Large-molecular-weight agents include latex, animal proteins, plant proteins, and flour. Low-molecular-weight agents include isocyanates, anhydrides, metals, drugs, dyes, bleaches, amines, glues, resins, and formaldehyde.

Diagnosis
Clinical Presentation

The most common symptoms of occupational asthma are cough (to include nocturnal cough), wheezing, chest tightness, and shortness of breath. Respiratory symptoms typically occur while at work or within 1 to 8 hours after work. Symptoms that worsen during the workweek but improve during weekends or vacations are also suggestive of occupational asthma. Extrapulmonary symptoms such as itchy eyes, tearing, sneezing, nasal congestion, and rhinorrhea often precede occupational asthma.[6–8] Potential exposures should be documented as well as their duration and intensity. A personal history of asthma, atopy, hay fever, pulmonary disorders, a family history of asthma, medication use, the home environment, tobacco use, and personal habits are additional important historical information that should be gathered.

Physical Examination

The physical examination for occupational asthma is generally nonspecific and may be normal during office visits away from the occupational exposure. However, the following findings may be suggestive of occupational asthma: expiratory wheezing, shortness of breath, atopic dermatitis, nasal polyps, rhinoconjunctivitis, and/or sinusitis.

Diagnostic Testing

Pulmonary function tests can assist in the diagnosis of occupational asthma. Office spirometry can demonstrate a reversible obstructive pattern but may be normal in those who develop symptoms only in work settings.

Because of the setting specific reactions, serial measurements of peak expiratory flow rates (PEFRs) have been useful in the assessment of occupational asthma.[9,10] Patients are properly instructed on the use of the peak flow meter and are asked to record their PEFR, at a minimum, four times a day for at least 2 weeks. This should be performed for equal time periods at work and away from work. Serial PEFRs are limited by patient compliance, self-reporting, reproducibility, sensitivity, and specificity. A 20% change in peak expiratory flow measured while at work for 2 weeks and while off work for 2 weeks is indicative of a positive result and should be further evaluated with spirometry if not already completed.[11]

If unable to confirm with serial PEFRs or spirometry, inhalation provocation test can be completed. A specific inhalation challenge, one using a suspected trigger, is the gold standard for confirmation of occupational asthma. The challenge can be accomplished by exposing subjects to occupational agents in a hospital laboratory or at the workplace, and comparing their spirometry results pre- and postexposure. Nonspecific inhalation challenge testing with methacholine or histamine can also be beneficial and is accomplished by the patient breathing a sequence of nebulized mists containing progressively increased concentrations of bronchoconstricting agents. See section on asthma diagnosis for results indicating a positive test.

Immunologic studies, such as a skin prick test, a radioallergosorbent test (RAST), or a basophil histamine release test may assist in determining the trigger but is limited by the type of allergen and whether the allergen is well characterized in the testing panels.

A chest radiograph is useful only to exclude other pulmonary conditions or complications of asthma. Additional imaging is rarely beneficial.

Treatment

Treatment of occupational asthma is similar to asthma treatment, which includes inhaled agents such as β-agonists, corticosteroids, and mast cell membrane stabilizers. Noninhaled agents include leukotriene antagonists, theophylline, and systemic corticosteroids.

Prevention

Early detection of reversible airway disease may facilitate a plan to prevent development of chronic symptoms. Complete avoidance of the offending substance is the primary means of preventing recurrence of symptoms. This may be accomplished by transferring the worker from the specific area of causation. Alternatively, the work area may be changed, such as by making an open system into a closed system or by improving or redirecting the ventilation. Personal protective equipment and high-efficiency particulate air (HEPA) filters may be used in certain circumstances.

Prognosis

Usually good, provided exposure to causative agent can be controlled or the patient's reaction to the agent can be reduced.

HYPERSENSITIVITY PNEUMONITIS (EXTRINSIC ALLERGIC ALVEOLITIS)
General Principles
Definition

HP is a form of interstitial lung disease characterized by diffuse lung inflammation due to exposure to airborne organic antigens and it encompasses a group of occupational lung diseases that include farmers' lung, bird fanciers' disease, Japanese summer-type HP, humidifier lung, bagassosis, and mushroom workers' lung.

Epidemiology

Not well characterized due to few population-based studies. It is thought that the prevalence and incidence are low. Agricultural workers and bird handlers are at particularly increased risk.

Etiology

There have been over 300 etiologies of HP reported.[12] The most common exposures are the following: agricultural work (farming, vegetable, and dairy/cattle workers), bird and poultry handling, exposure to contaminated ventilation and water, veterinarian work and animal handling, grain processing, wood working (lumber mills, construction, paper mills, etc.), plastic manufacturing, and textile workers.

Diagnosis
Clinical Presentation

HP can be categorized as acute, subacute, and chronic. Acute HP consists of flulike symptoms and signs, to include cough, fever, chills, myalgias, malaise, dyspnea without wheezing, nausea, and tachycardia, within 3 to 8 hours after exposure to an environmental antigen.[13] Removal from exposure will result in subsiding symptoms within 12 hours, but these reoccur upon reexposure. Patients with subacute HP show gradual development of productive cough, dyspnea, fatigue, anorexia, and weight loss. Chronic HP can include insidious onset of progressive shortness of breath, chronic cough, fatigue, and weight loss.

Physical Examination

During acute phase, auscultation usually reveals bilateral inspiratory crackles with fever. Wheezing is rarely noted. During the subacute phase, auscultation reveals diffuse crackles and tachypnea. In the chronic phase, digital clubbing and respiratory findings consistent with pulmonary fibrosis are typically noted.

Diagnostic Testing

Testing not only confirms the diagnosis of HP but determines severity. Laboratory testing is of limited benefit but may show a positive rheumatoid factor (RF), an elevated C-reactive protein, an elevated erythrocyte sedimentation rate, and increased circulating immune complexes.

Pulmonary function tests may demonstrate a restrictive or a mixed obstructive–restrictive pattern. Diffusion capacity (DLCO) testing will be decreased in both subacute and chronic HP. Mild arterial hypoxemia is present in subacute HP, whereas more severe resting and exertional hypoxia are seen with chronic HP.

Chest x-rays are often normal but may reveal a fleeting micronodular interstitial pattern in the lower and middle lung zones. The radiographic findings of chronic HP usually show progressive fibrotic changes with decrease in lung volumes, especially in the upper lobes.

High-resolution computed tomography (HRCT) is usually necessary to confirm the diagnosis and will show ground-glass attenuation and parenchymal micronodules with honeycombing and/or emphysematous changes.

When the diagnosis is still unclear, bronchoscopy with lavage or lung biopsy may be necessary. Bronchoalveolar lavage (BAL) demonstrates lymphocytosis and CD4+/CD8+ ratio less than 1. As HP progresses, lavage may show neutrophilia or eosinophilia. Lung biopsy can be accomplished by open technique or video-assisted technique. Acute HP biopsies demonstrate poorly formed noncaseating interstitial granulomas or mononuclear cell infiltrates in a peribronchial distribution with giant cells. Subacute HP demonstrates more well-formed noncaseating granulomas located in the interstitium as well as bronchiolitis, and interstitial fibrosis.

Treatment

Corticosteroids, oxygen, and bronchodilators are the mainstay of treatment. Workers who have severe symptoms or hypoxemia require hospitalization for more aggressive treatment.

Prevention

Avoidance of exposure to the precipitating antigen is best. Use of respirators may reduce exposure to relatively safe levels.

Prognosis

The prognosis for HP is good as long as the patient can avoid exposure to the offending agent and allow his or her lungs to recover. However, chronic HP can lead to debilitating pulmonary fibrosis and emphysematous changes that may not be able to be reversed.

TOXIC PNEUMONITIS
General Principles

Definition

Acute inflammation of the lungs caused by inhalation of metal fumes, toxic gases/vapors, or organic agents.

Epidemiology

Toxic pneumonitis accounts for less than 2% of interstitial lung disease diagnoses in a year in the United States.

Etiology

Toxic pneumonitis is caused by two types of agents: inorganic agents and organic agents. Inorganic agents include ammonia, chlorine, nitrogen oxides, sulfur dioxide, cadmium, trimellitic anhydrides, and vanadium pentoxide. Organic agents include bacteria, fungi, grain dust, and animal particles. It usually requires a high level of exposure. Workers in welding, refrigeration, oil refining, alkali/bleach, paper, cadmium smelter and processor, boilermaker, textile, grain, livestock, and horticulture industries are at risk. Most of the inorganic agents that cause toxic pneumonitis can also cause chemical burns.

Diagnosis

Clinical Presentation

Patients present with flulike symptoms (fever, myalgias, chest tightness, cough, headache, and/or nausea) that normally start 4 to 24 hours after the initial exposure. Depending on the agent and its concentration, chemical burns may also be seen. With certain organic agent exposures, symptoms may occur on the first day of returning to work from some period of time off (sometimes called Monday morning fever), especially in environments with very high amounts of moldy dust seen by workers.

Physical Examination
Examination may show fever, increased respiratory rate, bibasilar crackles, wheezing, cyanosis, lacrimation, and rhinitis.

Diagnostic Testing
Spirometry shows a mild restrictive pattern with a decrease in total lung capacity and diffusion capacity. Chest radiographs may show patchy infiltrates and are necessary to rule out pulmonary edema. BAL may be helpful.

Treatment
Supportive measures until symptoms resolve. Corticosteroids are *not* recommended.

Prevention
Once causal agent has been identified, recurrences should be prevented by avoiding that agent by modifying job tasks and using respiratory protection.

Prognosis
The course is usually benign with no long-term sequelae. However, there is the potential with high concentration exposures to develop life-threatening pulmonary edema.

INHALATION FEVERS (METAL FUME FEVER AND POLYMER FUME FEVER)
General Principles
Definition
Acute chemical pneumonitis caused by exposure to inhaled chemical fumes.

Etiology
Chemical fumes that may trigger symptoms include ammonia, chlorine, nitrogen oxides, sulfur dioxide, cadmium, trimellitic anhydride, and vanadium pentoxide. Metal fume fever is due to direct inhalation of heated zinc (zinc oxide) Polymer fume fever is due to inhalation of heated Teflon, plastics, polymers, and polyurethane.

Epidemiology
There have been no recent studies documenting the prevalence and incidence of this condition. Although approximately 30% of workers reported symptoms of metal fume fever in the early 1900, rates have thought to have decreased since then.[14]

Diagnosis
Clinical Presentation
Typically present with flulike symptoms (fever, chills, headaches, malaise, cough, myalgias, sore throat, and nausea) and ocular and or respiratory irritant symptoms that occur 4 to 8 hours after exposure.

Physical Examination
Auscultation of the lungs is often normal. Crackles may be heard in severe cases.

Diagnostic Testing
Chest radiographs may show transient infiltrates or even pulmonary edema with severe exposures. Spirometry test can be normal.

Treatment
Supportive measures to include anti-inflammatory medication as needed and removal from environment containing the offending agent.

Prevention
Metal fumes should be kept below the occupational threshold limit value and decreasing exposure times to offending agent.

Prognosis
Usually follow a self-limited, benign course.

Acute Chemical Pneumonitis

General Principles

Definition
Acute inflammation of the lungs caused by inhalation of irritant gases.

Etiology
Acute chemical pneumonitis can be caused by irritant gases (NH_3, SO_2, HCl, Cl_2, H_2S, O_3, NO_2), organic chemicals (acetic acids, aldehydes, isocyanates, amines, tear gas, organic solvents, and agrichemicals), metallic compounds (mercury, metallic oxides, halides, hydrides), and complex mixtures (fire smoke, pyrolysis products, solvent mixtures).

Diagnosis

Clinical Presentation
Includes irritation of eyes, nose, and throat. Patient may have cough, hoarseness, wheezing, and/or chest pain.

Physical Examination
Auscultation of the lungs is usually normal, but wheezing and rhonchi can be heard.

Diagnostic Testing
Chest radiographs may demonstrate patchy infiltrates or pulmonary edema in severe exposures. Spirometry is usually consistent with obstructive or mixed patterns.

Treatment
Removal of patient from environment containing the offending agent or decreasing the patient's exposure time to offending agent in the workplace are the mainstays of treatment. Nonsteroidal anti-inflammatory drugs may be used for mild cases with steroids being used for severe cases.

Prognosis
Most patients recover quickly after being removed from the offending exposure. However, those with a history of asthma or other chronic lung diseases may take longer to recover.

PNEUMOCONIOSIS

General Principles
Describes the group of pulmonary diseases caused by the deposition of dust in the lungs that results in diffuse fibrosis. The dusts that cause pneumoconiosis are asbestos, coal dust, silica, beryllium, graphite, aluminum, and others. Asbestos, coal dust, and silica have affected the largest number of workers. The International Labour Office (ILO) has standardized procedures for radiologic evaluation of pneumoconiosis, and the National Institute for Occupational Safety and Health (NIOSH) and the National Coal Workers' Health Surveillance Program has adopted these standards along with specific certification requirements for radiologists.[1]

Asbestosis

Definition
Asbestosis is a type of pneumoconiosis caused by inhalation of the naturally occurring fibrous mineral silicate, resulting in a slowly progressive diffuse fibrotic condition of the lung. Other diseases associated with asbestos exposure are carcinoma of the lung, malignant mesothelioma, and benign pleural lung disease (pleural plaques, pleural thickening, and pleural effusion).[1]

Epidemiology
The prevalence of asbestosis is variable and depends on the type of asbestos fiber, the type of industry, dose of exposure, and age. The main occupational exposures have been asbestos mining, asbestos removal, building demolition, textile and tile manufacturing, shipbuilding, pipefitting, and application of asbestos fireproofing and insulation. The highest prevalence of asbestosis has been found among insulation workers.[1] The latency period for the disease is generally 15 to 20 years.

Etiology
Asbestos fibers irritate and scar lung tissue overtime causing the tissue to become stiff and making breathing difficult. The two most common forms of asbestos fibers are chrysotile and amphibole, with the latter being more toxic than the former.[15] Smoking increases the attack and progression rate of asbestosis, likely by decreasing ciliary motility, thus decreasing clearance of inhaled fibers.[16]

Diagnosis

Specific diagnostic criteria have been set for asbestosis. The following criteria need to be fulfilled: (a) a reliable history of asbestos exposure, (b) appropriate duration from time of exposure to time of disease detection, (c) end expiratory crackles on auscultation of lungs, (d) restrictive pattern on lung function test with forced vital capacity (FVC) less than normal limit, (e) DLCO less than normal limit, (f) chest radiographs or HRCT with findings consistent with interstitial lung disease, (g) histologic evidence of interstitial fibrosis, and (h) absence of other causes of diffuse parenchymal lung disease.

Clinical Presentation

The earliest symptom is usually the insidious onset of breathlessness with exertion that is slowly progressive even in the absence of exposure. Cough, sputum production, and wheezing are uncommon and if present tend to be caused by cigarette smoking.

Physical Examination

Findings include inspiratory crackles in the lower lung fields. Clubbing of the fingers may be seen occasionally. Cor pulmonale may occur in advanced cases resulting in peripheral edema, jugular venous distention, hepatojugular reflux, and/or right ventricular heave or gallop.

Diagnostic Testing

- Laboratory studies are generally nonspecific and not clinically useful.
- Pulmonary function tests show decreased lung volumes as well as decreased DLCO. Pulmonary compliance is decreased and there is an absence of airflow obstruction.
- Chest x-ray will show small, irregular opacities in the lower lung fields. Honeycombing may be seen in severe cases and in end-stage disease. However, posteroanterior chest x-rays have poor sensitivity and specificity. HRCT with 1-mm sections is more accurate at detecting asbestosis in asymptomatic subjects.

Treatment

Only supportive care, as there is no effective treatment. Smoking cessation is strongly encouraged. Pneumococcal and influenza vaccines should be administered. Supplemental oxygen should be used when resting hypoxemia is present.

Prevention

Controlling asbestos dust as well as avoiding direct contact with asbestos particles can reduce development of asbestosis. This usually requires workers to wear protective suits and respirators when performing tasks such as removal of insulation. The 1995 Occupational Safety and Health Administration asbestos standard requires employers to provide medical surveillance for employees who work with or around asbestos for more than 30 days in a year.

Prognosis

Progression of disease is usually slow and is dependent on the total dose of exposure, fiber type, and susceptibility of the individual. The severity of parenchymal opacities with a multinodular or reticular pattern on chest x-ray has been shown to correlate positively with probability disease progression. The two main complications of asbestosis exposure are respiratory failure and malignancy.

Coal Worker's Pneumoconiosis

General Principles

Definition

An interstitial lung disease due to chronic exposure to coal dusts. Black lung is the term used in the Federal Coal Mine Health and Safety Act, which defines the coal miners' benefits program. Coal dust can result in a spectrum of conditions, including simple or complicated pneumoconiosis, progressive massive fibrosis (PMF), chronic bronchitis, and emphysema.

Epidemiology

The prevalence in the United States is approximately 9% in those with about 25 years of potential coal dust exposure. Occupations including underground mining, face working, roof bolting, and tunnel drilling are at increased risk for exposure.[1]

Etiology

Repeated exposure to coal or graphite dust from either coal mining or work with graphite.

Diagnosis

Clinical Presentation

Patients present with productive cough and shortness of breath with exertion. Coal worker's pneumoconiosis (CWP) has been associated with rheumatoid disease (Caplan syndrome; see section of rheumatic diseases for further discussion), TB, bronchitis, and emphysema.

Physical Examination

No specific findings may be noted. In advanced stages of complicated CWP, findings of emphysematous changes can be present.

Diagnostic Testing

Chest radiograph may show round, small densities in the upper lung zones initially with middle and lower zones involvement at later stages. PMF is associated with increased radiologic nodularity, sometimes coupled with bullous emphysematous changes. Computed tomography (CT) of the chest has higher sensitivity than chest radiography in simple CWP. Advanced disease is associated with both obstructive and restrictive impairment of lung function with decreases in FEV_1 and FVC, and decreased diffusion capacity (DLCO).

Treatment

Treatment of persons with CWP, PMF, and emphysema caused by coal dust is largely supportive with bronchodilator therapy being used for symptom reduction.

Prevention

Prevention is accomplished by dust control primarily by ventilation and respiratory protection. Periodic medical examinations are required for all coal mine workers. Workers who have early radiologic evidence of CWP should be removed from exposure.

Prognosis

Simple CWP usually has a good prognosis. However, complicated CWP may lead to progressive shortness of breath and emphysematous changes.

Silicosis

General Principles

Definition

Silicosis is a chronic fibrotic (fibronodular) disease of the lungs caused by exposure to free crystalline silica. Industrial sources of free silica include mining, stonework, sandblasting, foundry work, and glass manufacturing.[1]

Epidemiology

Accurate assessment of the incidence and prevalence in the United States is difficult as the exact number of people who are at risk and affected by the disease is unknown due to poor record-keeping practices, time delays in exposure to diagnosis, and poor understanding of the disease. The disease is usually seen after 10 to 30 years of exposure (chronic silicosis), but can occur as soon as 10 years after exposure (accelerated silicosis) or even a few weeks to a few years after heavy exposure (acute silicosis).

Etiology

Exposure to silica dust with enough frequency or in a high enough single dose to cause inflammation of the lungs. Silica is found in sand, quartz, and certain mining products. Industrial sources include mining, stonework, sandblasting, foundry work, and glass manufacturing.[1]

Diagnosis

Clinical Presentation

Different phases of silicosis are only differentiated by their time to development of symptoms. Patients may be asymptomatic and only have chest radiograph findings. Symptomatic patients will have chronic cough and dyspnea on exertion. Patients with acute silicosis can have rapid onset of symptoms, including cough, weight loss, fatigue, and occasionally pleuritic pain.

Physical Examination

Findings on auscultation may include crackles and wheezes. In advanced stages, emphysematous changes and digital clubbing may develop.

Diagnostic Testing

Spirometry is usually normal in early disease. In more advanced stages, restrictive pattern can be expected but a mixed obstructive and restrictive pattern is also common.

Chest radiographs can show several distinct patterns. Simple silicosis is characterized by small, round opacities in the upper lung zones with hilar enlargement. The radiographic appearance of simple silicosis can be confused with the presentation of military distribution of mycobacterial or fungal respiratory disease. PMF (conglomerate silicosis) is characterized by small opacities gradually enlarging and coalescing to form larger opacities in the upper and mid-lung zones greater than 10 mm in diameter.[17] As the opacities enlarge, the hila may retract upward in association with upper lobe fibrosis and lower lobe hyperinflation. Eggshell calcification of the hilar nodes is also characteristic. Silicoproteinosis is a radiographic hallmark of acute silicosis and demonstrates basilar alveolar filling pattern without rounded opacities or lymph node calcifications.[18]

Treatment

Treatment is supportive, including treatment of air flow limitation with bronchodilators, corticosteroids for acute exposures, aggressive treatment of respiratory tract infections, and supplemental oxygen for chronic hypoxemia. Patients with silicosis should be immunized against pneumococcal pneumonia and undergo yearly TB skin tests with treatment of any positive tests.

Prevention

Workers with any degree of silicosis should be prevented from working in areas of silica dust, although the disease may progress despite this measure. Controlling exposure to silica dust through the use of strict environmental control techniques (masks, filters, and/or avoidance) is essential to decreasing risk.

Prognosis

Prognosis varies based on exposure and phase at presentation. Acute silicosis often worsens quickly with death coming in months, but progressive pulmonary fibrosis shows a more gradual decrease in lung function. Those with simple silicosis may be asymptomatic and remain stable for years.

OCCUPATIONAL NONTUBERCULOUS LUNG INFECTIONS

General Principles

Etiologic agent can come from a myriad of different infectious sources. Infections from humans include influenza, *Streptococcus* infection, pneumococcus infection, and *Chlamydia* pneumonia. Animal infections include anthrax, *Coxiella burnetii*, brucellosis, psittacosis, tularemia, and plague. Environment infections include sporotrichosis, coccidioidomycosis, and legionellosis.

Clinical Presentation

Usual presentations include fever, chills, malaise, weight loss, cough, chest pain, and shortness of breath.

Diagnosis

Diagnosis of occupational lung infections involves a detailed history of exposure, physical examination, chest radiograph, appropriate cultures, and serologic testing.

Treatment

Treatment requires precise diagnosis based on cultures and is directed toward the agent.

Prevention

Prevention of occupational lung infections may require respiratory protection in the presence of potential exposure. Consider vaccine availability and safety. Monitor and control potential for pathogen transmission by removing infected workers and sterilizing the workplace as necessary.

REFERENCES

1. Hendrick DJ, Sherwood B, eds. *Occupational disorders of the lung, recognition, management, and prevention*. Philadelphia, PA: WB Saunders; 2002.
2. U.S. Centers for Disease Control and Prevention. *Work related lung disease surveillance report*. Washington, DC: U.S. Department of Health and Human Services; 1999.
3. Levin SM, Kahn PE, Lax MB. Medical examination for asbestos-related disease. *Am J Ind Med* 2000;37:6.
4. Beckett WS, Bascom R. Occupational lung disease. *Occup Med State Art Rev* 1992;7:2.

5. Maestrelli P, Boschetto P, Fabbri LM, et al. Mechanisms of occupational asthma. *J Allergy Clin Immunol* 2009;123(3):531.
6. Malo JL, Lemière C, Desjardins A, et al. Prevalence and intensity of rhinoconjunctivitis in subjects with occupational asthma. *Eur Respir J* 1997;10(7):1513.
7. Castano R, Gautrin D, Thériault G, et al. Occupational rhinitis in workers investigated for occupational asthma. *Thorax* 2009;64(1):50.
8. Vandenplas O, Ghezzo H, Munoz X, et al. What are the questionnaire items most useful in identifying subjects with occupational asthma? *Eur Respir J* 2005;26(6):1056.
9. Moscato G, Godnic-Cvar J, Maestrelli P. Statement on self-monitoring of peak expiratory flows in the investigation of occupational asthma. Subcommittee on Occupational Allergy of European Academy of Allergy and Clinical Immunology. *J Allergy Clin Immunol* 1995;96(3):295.
10. Park D, Moore VC, Burge CB, et al. Serial PEF measurement is superior to cross-shift change in diagnosing occupational asthma. *Eur Respir J* 2009;34(3):574.
11. Tarlo SM, Balmes J, Balkissoon R, et al. Diagnosis and management of work-related asthma: American College of Chest Physicians Consensus Statement. *Chest* 2008;134(3 Suppl):1S.
12. Salvaggio JE. The identification of hypersensitivity pneumonitis. *Hosp Pract* 1995;30(5):57.
13. Richerson HB, Bernstein IL, Fink JN, et al. Guidelines for the clinical evaluation of hypersensitivity pneumonitis. Report of the Subcommittee on Hypersensitivity Pneumonitis. *J Allergy Clin Immunol* 1989;84(5, pt 2):839.
14. Antonini JM, Lewis AB, Roberts JR, et al. Pulmonary effects of welding fumes: review of worker and experimental animal studies. *Am J Ind Med* 2003;43(4):350.
15. Mossman BT, Gee JB. Asbestos-related diseases. *N Engl J Med* 1989;320(26):1721.
16. Churg A, Stevens B. Enhanced retention of asbestos fibers in the airways of human smokers. *Am J Respir Crit Care Med* 1995;151(5):1409.
17. Wade WA, Petsonk EL, Young B, et al. Severe occupational pneumoconiosis among West Virginian coal miners: one hundred thirty-eight cases of progressive massive fibrosis compensated between 2000 and 2009. *Chest* 2011;139(6):1458.
18. Marchiori E, Ferreira A, Müller NL. Silicoproteinosis: high-resolution CT and histologic findings. *J Thorac Imaging* 2001;16(2):127.

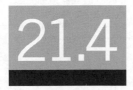

21.4

Heat-Related Illnesses
Richard E. Gray

GENERAL PRINCIPLES

Heat-related illnesses occur when the effects of environmental and metabolic heat production overwhelm the body's ability to dissipate heat.[1] This risk is elevated when ambient temperatures exceed 90°F. Risk factors include dehydration, lack of acclimatization, decreased fitness levels, exertion activities that exceed fitness, excessive alcohol use, sleep deprivation, excess body fat, sunburn, heart and lung disease, age less than 15 years or greater than 65 years, chronic disease, and medications that limit sweating.[2,3] Lack of proper clothing that allows heat dissipation, inadequate medical triage/support, and noncompliance with organization recommendations for rest and participation also place patients at risk for heat-related illness.[2,3]

MINOR HEAT-RELATED ILLNESSES

• **Heat cramps.** Patients complain of brief, intense cramps that last approximately 1 to 3 minutes in severely stressed muscles. In addition, patients may experience diffuse muscle twitches and tenderness. Workers and athletes are typically affected after profuse sweating from vigorous physical activity, which causes fluid and electrolyte depletion including dilutional hyponatremia related to dehydration and additional consumption of free water.[1] Physical examination may reveal cool and moist skin, but body temperature will be within the normal range. Heat cramps generally resolve with rest, oral electrolyte and fluid replacement, and prolonged stretching of affected muscles.[3]

- **Heat edema** is a benign condition that responds well to rest in a cool environment and elevation of the lower extremities.[1] Diuretics should be **avoided** in patients with edema secondary to heat exposure. Diagnostic workup for more serious conditions (congestive heart failure, liver failure, kidney failure, etc.) is warranted if additional physical signs and symptoms are present that support these diagnoses.
- **Heat syncope** involves transient loss of consciousness that is associated with heat exposure.[1] Ultimately, dilation of the vascular space leads to compromised venous return and loss of consciousness. Advanced age, dehydration, prolonged standing, orthostatic hypotension, and medical conditions that reduce cardiac output are common precipitating factors.[1] In addition, medications such as anticholinergics and diuretics may contribute to heat syncope and should be adjusted as needed. Management consists of rest and rehydration with close observation of the patient while resting in the recumbent position in a cool environment.[1] Rapid recovery and return to baseline is expected.[1]

MAJOR HEAT-RELATED ILLNESSES

Heat exhaustion results from water and salt depletion during strenuous activity or high heat exposure that results in the inability to continue activity.[3] Heat exhaustion can progress to heat stroke if diagnosis and proper treatment are delayed.[1,3]

Clinical Presentation

Heat exhaustion typically presents with profuse sweating, cutaneous flushing, nausea, vomiting, diarrhea, headache, muscle weakness, loss of coordination, and normal mentation.[3]

Diagnosis

A patient with heat exhaustion will present with a clear sensorium and without focal neurologic findings. Core body temperature will be less than 40°C (104°F).[1,3] Tachycardia, hyperventilation, and hypotension occur in serious cases of heat exhaustion.[3]

Management

The patient must be immediately taken to a shaded, cool environment with excess clothing removed and placed in a supine position with their legs elevated. Oral rehydration should be initiated and vital signs monitored. Patients should be transported to a medical facility if not improving after 30 minutes.[3]

    Heatstroke is generally divided into two categories: classic heatstroke due to passive exposure to high ambient temperatures and exertional heatstroke related to strenuous activity.[1-4] Mortality rate ranges as high as 20% to 50%, but early recognition and appropriate treatment can reduce the mortality risk to near 0%.[1-4]

Background Information

Heatstroke most often affects those with chronic diseases, limited mobility, obesity, and the elderly. Other risk factors include limited access to air conditioning, alcohol use, dehydration, illicit drug abuse, prior history of heat exhaustion or heat stroke, and use of certain medications (e.g., sedatives, diuretics, anticholinergics, antipsychotics).[1,3] During periods of extreme heat, individuals become progressively dehydrated until their body's cooling mechanisms fail. Exertional heatstroke occurs in unacclimatized individuals who overexert themselves in conditions of extreme heat.[1,3]

Clinical Presentation and Diagnosis

Physical examination will reveal a core body temperature of greater than 40°C (104°F) and central nervous system signs/symptoms ranging from irritability and confusion to a deep coma or seizures.[1-3] The presence of neurological deficits and a normal core body temperature should prompt investigation for other causes of the neurological symptoms.[3]

    Classic heatstroke occurs slowly over a number of days due to exposure to excessive ambient temperatures and most often occurs in the debilitated individual (chronic disease, elderly). Exertional heatstroke onset is generally more rapid and is associated with high levels of physical activity in high ambient temperatures by individuals without proper acclimatization or with other risk factors.[3] Heatstroke patients may present with hypotension, tachycardia, and tachypnea.[2]

Management

Heatstroke victims must be treated by protection of airway, breathing, and circulation immediately followed by cooling techniques.[1-3] First-line treatment includes removal of clothing and equipment and submersing the patient into cold water to take advantage of the quick conduction of heat into cold water while protecting the patient's airway.[1-3] Second-line treatment involves removing unnecessary clothing, spraying the body with tepid (~32°C) water, and enhancing airflow across the patient during transport to an emergency facility.[5] Other options include placing ice packs on the neck, groin, and axilla after removing the patient's clothing. Reducing core body temperature to less than 40°C (104°F) in less than 30 minutes seems to improve outcomes and limit complications. Lack of cooling in the field (pre-hospital environment) increases the risk of death and other moderate to severe complications.[2,3]

Respiratory assistance with intubation is often required for critically ill patients. Continuous cardiac monitoring and oxygen therapy should be initiated as soon as possible. Core temperature is continuously measured with a flexible rectal probe. Baseline laboratory tests should include a complete blood count, complete metabolic profile, arterial blood gases, chest radiography, electrocardiography, cardiac isoenzymes, prothrombin time, partial thromboplastin time, fibrin degradation products, creatine kinase, urinalysis, and urine myoglobin.

Complications

Systemic inflammatory response syndrome is the most common complication associated with heat stroke.[2-4] The duration of body temperature exceeding less than 40°C (104°F) appears to be more predictive of severe complications than the absolute maximum core body temperature reached during heatstroke.[2,4] Other complications include cardiac arrhythmias, hypotension, acute kidney injury, elevated liver enzymes, respiratory failure requiring mechanical ventilation, and multisystem organ dysfunction.[4] Rhabdomyolysis is also a common complication and appropriate laboratories should be ordered for evaluation once hospital care is available.[4] Ideally, intravenous fluid resuscitation to help maintain blood pressure and minimize acute kidney injury should be started before transport to the hospital.[4] Obtaining intravenous access should not delay cooling efforts.[1]

Prevention

A National Weather Service heat index of over 90°F should be considered hazardous. Exposure to direct sunlight can raise the "real feel" temperature an additional 15°F. Patients with any physical impairment or limitation and those taking medications that decrease their ability to sweat should avoid heat and drink plenty of liquids. More active individuals can minimize their risk of heat-related illness by gradually acclimating themselves to the heat over a period of 10 to 14 days, drink plenty of water before and during exposure to the heat, and wear vapor-permeable, light clothing.[1-3] Athletes and workers at risk for heat-related illness should replenish fluid losses with frequent and small quantities of fluid, but should not exceed 0.5 to 1 L per hour. A commercially available carbohydrate electrolyte beverage may be beneficial in the case of prolonged physical exertion.

REFERENCES

1. Lipman GS, Eifling KP, Ellis MA, et al. Wilderness medical society practice guidelines for the prevention and treatment of heat-related illness. *Wilderness Environ Med* 2013;24(4):351–361. doi:10.1016/j.wem.2013.07.004.
2. Casa DJ, Armstrong LE, Kenny GP, et al. Exertional heat stroke: new concepts regarding cause and care. *Curr Sports Med Rep* 2012;11(3):115–123.
3. Becker JA, Stewart LK. Heat-related illness. *Am Fam Physician* 2011;83(11):1325–1330.
4. Zeller L, Novack V, Barski L, et al. Exertional heatstroke: clinical characteristics, diagnostic and therapeutic considerations. *Eur J Intern Med* 2011;22:296–299.
5. Sinclair WH, Rudzki SJ, Leicht AS, et al. Efficacy of field treatments to reduce body core temperature in hyperthermic subjects. *Med Sci Sports Exerc* 2009;41(11):1984–1990.

CHAPTER 22

Therapeutic Choices

Section Editor: Rick Kellerman

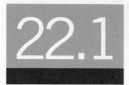

Bacterial Endocarditis Prophylaxis

Bruce M. Bushwick

GENERAL PRINCIPLES

Definition

Bacterial endocarditis is an infection of the endocardium. The infection develops on heart valves, septal defects, or mural endocardium. Individuals at risk for the infection have a damaged or altered endothelial surface that becomes colonized and infected by bacteria. The subsequent inflammation causes vegetations composed of platelets, fibrin, and bacteria to develop on the endocardial surface. The vegetations cause structural damage to valves and can embolize throughout the body, resulting in systemic disease.[1]

There are no definitive controlled clinical trials of prevention strategies in humans, so recommendations are inferred from animal models, *in vitro* studies, and clinical experience. Most cases of bacterial endocarditis are believed to be caused by random bacteria and are not preventable, but a small number of cases may be prevented by prophylaxis strategies. Bacterial endocarditis is hypothesized to result from transient (less than 30 minutes) low-grade bacteremia. Prevention strategies are directed toward reducing bacteremia following oral mucosal trauma.[2] In endocarditis cases implicated from oral mucosal trauma, the most common blood culture isolates are oral (viridans) streptococci and Group D streptococci (enterococci). These isolates remain sensitive to penicillin.[3]

Epidemiology

Between 10,000 and 20,000 patients develop endocarditis each year in the United States.[1] The incidence of infectious endocarditis has shifted from young adults with rheumatic valvular disease to older adults with prosthetic valves or no previously known valve disease. The male-to-female ratio is over 2 to 1 for reasons not well understood. Women, however, do worse with the disease and undergo fewer surgical procedures. The incidence of infectious endocarditis peaks at 14.5 episodes per 100,000 person-years for patients 70 to 80 years old.[3]

PREVENTION STRATEGIES[2]

New recommendations follow two steps—identify your high-risk patients and use antibiotic prophylaxis only on those undergoing dental or oral procedures that traumatize oral mucosa. This strategy is greatly simplified from the past recommendations. For individuals undergoing gastrointestinal or genital urinary procedures, prophylaxis is no longer recommended (transesophageal echocardiogram, esophagogastroduodenoscopy, or colonoscopy). It may be necessary to communicate with the patient's dentist in order to understand the dental diagnosis and procedure that is planned.

Identify your high-risk patients with:

- Prosthetic heart valves or prosthetic material used for cardiac valve repair.
- A prior history of infective endocarditis.
- Unrepaired congenital cyanotic heart disease.

- Repaired congenital heart defect with prosthetic material or device for the first 6 months after the procedure.
- Repaired congenital heart disease with residual defects at or adjacent to the site of the prosthetic patch or device.
- Cardiac transplant patients with valve regurgitation due to a structurally abnormal valve.

Identify high-risk dental or oral procedures:

- Procedures that involve manipulation of either gingival tissue or the periapical region of teeth.
- Procedures that perforate the oral or throat mucosa (this can include tonsillectomy and adenoidectomies).
- Procedures on actively infected tissue.

Prophylaxis is not recommended for dental procedures not considered high risk:

- Anesthetic injections through uninfected tissue.
- Radiographs of teeth.
- Adjustment, placement, or removal of prosthodontic/orthodontic appliances.
- Placement of orthodontic brackets.
- Shedding of deciduous teeth.
- Bleeding from trauma to the lips or oral mucosa.

TREATMENT WITH PROPHYLACTIC ANTIBIOTICS[2]

Administer antibiotics, once, 30 to 60 minutes in advance of procedure. Avoid cephalosporins for those with a history of anaphylaxis, angioedema, or urticaria with penicillins or ampicillin.

- Oral administration
  - Amoxicillin 2 g
- Oral administration for those allergic to penicillins or ampicillin
  - Cephalexin 2 g or
  - Clindamycin 600 mg or
  - Azithromycin 500 mg or
  - Clarithromycin 500 mg
- For those unable to take oral medications
  - Ampicillin 2.0 g IM or IV or
  - Cefazolin 1 g IM or IV or
  - Ceftriaxone 1 g IM or IV
- For those unable to take oral medications and allergic to penicillins or ampicillin
  - Cefazolin 1 g IM or IV or
  - Ceftriaxone 1 g IM or
  - Clindamycin 600 mg IM or IV
- Dose adjustments for children (total dose should not exceed adult dose):
  - Amoxicillin or ampicillin 50 mg per kg
  - Azithromycin or clarithromycin 15 mg per kg
  - Cefazolin or ceftriaxone 50 mg per kg
  - Clindamycin 20 mg per kg
  - Cephalexin 50 mg per kg

Patient Education

When endocarditis prophylaxis is given, the rationale for treatment, including risks and benefits, should be explained to the patient. Early signs and symptoms of endocarditis should be reviewed, such as unexpected fevers, night sweats, chills, weakness, myalgias, arthralgias, or malaise, so that emergent infections can be rapidly identified and treated.

The American Heart Association offers a wallet card that patients can carry—Prevention of Infective (Bacterial) Endocarditis. It is available at www.americanheart.org. It outlines antibiotic choices and indications for prophylaxis.

There are patient-dependent risks of antibiotic adverse reactions. No prevention strategy is perfect. Only a small number of infective endocarditis cases will be prevented with prophylaxis for dental procedures.[2] For all patients at risk, an effective oral health program, including regular dental care, should be promoted to minimize bacterial seeding from chronically inflamed tissues.[3]

REFERENCES

1. Fowler VG Jr, Scheld WM, Bayer AS. Endocarditis and intravascular infections. In: Mandell G, Bennett J, Dolin R, eds. *Principles and practice of infectious diseases*. 7th ed. Philadelphia, PA: Churchill-Livingstone/Elsevier; 2009:chap 77.
2. Nishimura RA, Carabello BA, Faxon DP, et al; American College of Cardiology/American Heart Association Task Force. ACC/AHA 2008 guideline update on valvular heart disease: focused update on infective endocarditis: a report of the American College of Cardiology/American Heart Association Task Force on Practice Guidelines: endorsed by the Society of Cardiovascular Anesthesiologists, Society for Cardiovascular Angiography and Interventions, and Society of Thoracic Surgeons. *Circulation* 2008;118:887–896.
3. Habib G, Hoen B, Tornos P, et al. Guidelines on the prevention, diagnosis, and treatment of infective endocarditis (new version 2009): the Task Force on the Prevention, Diagnosis, and Treatment of Infective Endocarditis of the European Society of Cardiology (ESC). Endorsed by the European Society of Clinical Microbiology and Infectious Diseases (ESCMID) and the International Society of Chemotherapy (ISC) for Infection and Cancer. *Eur Heart J* 2009;30(19):2369–2413.

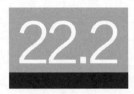

22.2 Medication Use During Pregnancy

Jacintha S. Cauffield, Marilyn S. Darr

In general, common sense suggests that medication use during pregnancy should be limited. Nevertheless, pregnant women sometimes present with clinical syndromes that may warrant drug therapy.

The U.S. Food and Drug Administration (FDA) has established five categories for drugs based on their potential for causing birth defects in infants born to women who use the drugs during pregnancy. The categories are as follows:[1]

- **A** Controlled studies in women fail to demonstrate a risk to the fetus in the first trimester, and fetal harm appears remote (e.g., folic acid, levothyroxine).
- **B** Animal studies have not demonstrated a fetal risk, but there are no human studies in pregnant women, or animal studies have shown an adverse effect that was not confirmed in human studies (e.g., amoxicillin, ceftriaxone, cetirizine, and loratadine).
- **C** Animal studies are either lacking or showing adverse effects, and there are no controlled studies in women. Drugs should be given only if benefit outweighs the potential risk to the fetus (e.g., budesonide, lamotrigine, and propranolol).
- **D** Positive evidence of human fetal risk exists, but benefits may outweigh risks in certain situations (e.g., angiotensin-converting enzyme [ACE] inhibitors, carbamazepine, lithium, phenytoin, propylthiouracil, and valproic acid [for all indications except migraine headaches]).
- **X** Studies or experience have shown fetal risk that clearly outweighs any possible benefits (e.g., isotretinoin, methotrexate, misoprostol, thalidomide, and warfarin [for all indications except mechanical heart valves between 12 and 36 weeks gestation]).

Drugs used during pregnancy and others that should be avoided are discussed here by system category. Commonly used herbal agents considered safe and those to avoid are listed at the end of the chapter. Most medications are followed by the FDA category in parentheses if available. Clinicians who prescribe medications during pregnancy should observe the following guidelines: Try to avoid any medication during the first trimester. Use single, non-combination agents. Choose topical treatments (if available) over oral. Use the lowest effective dose. Remember, use medication only if the benefit appears to outweigh the risk.

INFECTIOUS DISEASES

Colds (Upper Respiratory Tract Infection)

The best treatment is symptomatic management with fluids, humidity, and rest for 10 days. For sore throat, acetaminophen and topical lidocaine (B) may be used. For severe rhinorrhea, ipratropium bromide nasal spray (B) is an option. If absolutely necessary, first-generation antihistamines, particularly chlorpheniramine (B) appear safest, but cetirizine (B) (Zyrtec) and loratidine (B) (Claritin) are reasonable alternatives. If a decongestant is indicated, use a topical agent first. Preparations containing guaifenesin (C) or dextromethorphan (C) may be used for the management of cough. In general, no data are available on the teratogenic risk of most other over the counter agents for relief of cold symptoms. *Avoid* iodine-containing expectorants (e.g., potassium iodide) (D) because of the potential for thyroid toxicity in the newborn, and also *avoid* alcohol-containing products.[2,3]

Pneumonia (Community Acquired)

Pneumonia during pregnancy can become very severe. Always consider admission for close monitoring and treatment. *Streptococcus pneumoniae*, *Mycoplasma pneumoniae*, and *Chlamydia pneumoniae* are the most common bacterial organisms. *Haemophilus influenzae* is commonly found in patients who smoke. For empirical outpatient treatment, use azithromycin (B) (Zithromax), 500 mg followed by 250 mg per day PO for 4 days. Alternative treatment includes azithromycin plus a β-lactam. Preferred agents include amoxicillin 1 g tid, amoxicillin/clavulanate 2 g bid, cefpodoxime 200 mg bid, and cefuroxime 500 mg bid. The β-lactams are *not* active against *M. pneumoniae* or *C. pneumoniae*. *Avoid* clarithromycin (C), doxycycline (D), and fluoroquinolones (C)[4] (see also Chapter 10.2).

Sexually Transmitted Diseases[5]

- **Chlamydial infection.** Manage with azithromycin (B) (Zithromax), 1 g orally × 1 or amoxicillin (B), 500 mg PO tid for 7 days. Alternative regimens are erythromycin base (B) (Eryc, E-Mycin), 500 mg PO qid for 7 days or erythromycin ethylsuccinate 800 mg qid × 7 days. If gastrointestinal symptoms are problematic with the erythromycin regimens, the dose can be reduced to 250 mg base or 400 mg ethylsuccinate and given for 14 days. Repeat culture 3 to 4 weeks after completion of antibiotic course. *Avoid* erythromycin estolate (Ilosone), doxycycline (D), and fluoroquinolones (C).
- **Genital warts, external (*Condyloma acuminata*).** Safe treatments during pregnancy include topical bi- or trichloroacetic acid weekly, cryotherapy, or liquid nitrogen. *Avoid* podophyllin (D-), podofilox (C) (Condylox), sinecatechins (C) (Veregen), and imiquimod (C) (Aldara) until further data are available.
- **Gonorrhea (GC) (uncomplicated).** Treat for both GC and *Chlamydia* with ceftriaxone (Rocephin) (B), 250 mg IM or cefixime (Suprax) (B), 400 mg PO single dose plus azithromycin (B), 1 g orally. Women who cannot tolerate a cephalosporin should be administered a single 2-g dose of azithromycin (B) orally. Re-culture in 7 days after treatment only in those patients who received azithromycin alone or cefixime regimen. *Avoid* fluoroquinolones and tetracyclines.
- **Herpes genitalis.** For severe first episodes, late-onset disease in the second or third trimester, or disseminated herpes simplex virus infections, use of acyclovir (B) (Zovirax) appears justified. Famciclovir (B) (Famvir) and valacyclovir (B) (Valtrex) are newer agents with better absorption, but have limited information for use in pregnant women. Doses vary with indication. For daily suppressive therapy at 36 weeks until delivery, use acyclovir, 400 mg PO three times daily due to increased glomerular filtration in pregnancy.
- **Pediculosis (*Phthirus humanus capitis* or "*head lice*" and *Phthirus pubis* or "*crabs*").** Treat with topical, poorly absorbed permethrin (B) 5% (Elimite) cream or pyrethrins with piperonyl butoxide (C) (Nix) 1% liquid. Wash hair, apply lotion for 10 minutes, and then rinse off. *Avoid* lindane (C) (Kwell) due to the potential for neurotoxicity and aplastic anemia. *Avoid* ivermectin (C).
- **Scabies (*Sarcoptes scabei*).** Treat with topical permethrin (B) (Elimite) 5% cream. Apply to entire skin from chin to toes. Leave on for 8 to 10 hours. Avoid crotamiton (C) (Eurax), lindane (C) (Kwell), and ivermectin (C) Sklice.
- **Syphilis.** Manage primary, secondary, and latent infection of less than 1-year duration with benzathine penicillin (B) (Bicillin LA), 2.4 million units IM (1.2 MU in each buttocks). Higher doses are used in late latent or when the duration of disease is unknown. There is no alternative to penicillin in pregnancy. If there is a penicillin allergy, skin test and desensitize if necessary. Follow treated patients at 1, 3, 6, 12, and 24 months with non-treponemal antibody tests (venereal disease research laboratory or rapid plasma reagin). Retreatment is indicated if there is a fourfold increase in titer or the titer does not decrease appropriately after the appropriate time period (see also Chapter 19.5).

Urinary Tract Infection (Uncomplicated)[6]

Empirical treatment includes Nitrofurantoin (B) (Macrobid) 100 mg orally twice daily for 5 days or 3 to 7 days of cefpodoxime (B) 100 mg twice daily, Amoxicillin–clavulanate (B) (Augmentin) 500 mg twice daily. Nitrofurantoin should be avoided near-term due to risk of hemolytic anemia in the neonate. Trimethoprim–sulfamethoxazole (D) (Bactrim, Septra) can also be used in the second and third trimesters, but *avoid* near-term due to risk of kernicterus. Obtain a repeat urine culture after treatment. *Avoid* fluoroquinolones (C), which are associated with fetal cartilage damage, and doxycycline (D) due to offspring teeth staining and maternal hepatotoxicity (see also Chapters 12.1 and 12.2).

Vaginitis
(see also Chapter 13.1)[5]

- **Bacterial vaginosis.** Manage with metronidazole (B) (Flagyl), 250 mg PO bid for 7 days or clindamycin (B) (Cleocin), 300 mg PO bid for 7 days. Although providers may avoid use of metronidazole during the first trimester, the CDC no longer discourages use in early pregnancy. Use oral metronidazole and clindamycin rather than topical therapy during pregnancy.
- **Candidiasis.** Treat with topical agents, such as clotrimazole (B) (Mycelex, Gyne-Lotrimin), miconazole (Monistat) (C), and terconazole (Terazol) (C) vaginal cream. Use vaginally every night for 7 days. Avoid oral fluconazole (Diflucan) (C) until more safety data are available.
- ***Trichomonas vaginalis* infection.** If symptomatic, Metronidazole (B), as a single 2-g dose or 500 mg PO bid for 7 days, is the treatment of choice.

RESPIRATORY DISORDERS[7]
Allergic Rhinitis

Allergic rhinitis can worsen in predisposed women, particularly in the presence of concomitant asthma. First-line therapy includes intranasal cromolyn (B) (Nasalcrom) or budesonide (B) (Rhinocort, Rhinocort AQ). If symptoms are not controlled, then antihistamines, such as chlorpheniramine (B), loratadine (B), and cetirizine (B), can be used. Pseudoephedrine (C) (Sudafed), 30 to 60 mg PO qid has the best safety record if an oral decongestant is required.

Asthma

It is safer for pregnant women with asthma to be treated than to have symptoms. Like nonpregnant patients, management is stepwise. Whenever possible, treatment should be by inhalation rather than oral. Preferred agents include short-acting β-agonist albuterol (C) (Ventolin, Proventil), and inhaled corticosteroids, particularly budesonide (B) (Pulmicort). Long-acting β-agonists salmeterol (C) or formoterol (C) are preferred add-on therapy. Leukotriene receptor antagonists zafirlukast (Accolate) (B) or montelukast (Singulair) (B) are also options, and should not be discontinued if the patient is already taking them. Although not preferred therapy, cromolyn (B) (Intal) or theophylline (C) can be used. During exacerbations, IV and oral glucocorticoids may be used in the usual manner. Zileuton (C) (Zyflo) should be *avoided* during pregnancy (see also Chapter 10.1).

GASTROINTESTINAL DISORDERS
Nausea and Vomiting[8]

Attempt conservative measures, including small frequent meals, a bland diet, and acupressure wristbands or acupressure on the volar surface of the forearm. Ginger tea up to 1 g per day (about four cups) may help. Initial medications include pyridoxine (A), 10 to 25 mg PO q8h. If monotherapy is ineffective, an antihistamine such as doxylamine (A) can be used either as an individual agent (12.5 to 25 mg PO q6h prn) or in combination (Declegis extended release pyridoxine 10 mg/pyridoxine 10 mg tablets, up to four doses per day). Other antihistamines such as meclizine (B) (Antivert) 25 mg PO q6h prn can be used. Other safe antiemetics include promethazine (C) (Phenergan), 25 mg PO/IM/PR every 4 to 6 hours prn and ondansetron (B) (Zofran) 8 mg q12h. Metoclopramide (B) (Reglan), 10 mg PO qid and prochlorperazine (C) (Compazine) are commonly used, but the patient should monitored for extrapyramidal symptoms.[8]

Gastroesophageal Reflux (GERD)[9]

GERD can affect 40% to 80% of pregnant women. Treatment includes routine antireflux measures. Antacids, alginic acid (Gaviscon), and sucralfate are first-line agents. Avoid antacids containing sodium bicarbonate or magnesium trisilicate. Antacids may interfere with iron absorption. H_2 receptor antagonists cimetidine (B) (Tagamet), 400 mg PO at bedtime, and ranitidine (B) (Zantac) 150 mg PO bid, have the most published human data, but famotidine (B) and nizatidine (B) may also be used. In refractory cases, the proton pump inhibitors lansoprazole (B) (Prevacid), pantoprazole (B) (Protonix), esomeprazole (B) (Nexium), and omeprazole (C) (Prilosec) can be used (see also Chapter 11.2).

Constipation

Nonpharmacologic management, including physical activity, increased fiber and fluid intake, and education, is preferred. A supplemental fiber, preferably calcium polycarbophil, and docusate (C) are the preferred first-line agents. For refractory symptoms, lactulose (B), polyethylene glycol, sorbitol, bisacodyl, and senna (C) may be used.[9]

Diarrhea

Attempt conservative measures, such as fluid replacement and bland diet, first. If medication is needed, loperamide (B) (Imodium) is the preferred agent. *Avoid* bismuth salicylate (C) (Pepto Bismol) and atropine/diphenoxylate (C) (Lomotil).[9]

Inflammatory Bowel Disease

Active Crohn's disease and ulcerative colitis can have an adverse impact on pregnancy. First-line treatment in active disease is sulfasalazine (B) (Azulfidine), 500 mg PO qid, or mesalamine (B) (Asacol), 800 mg PO tid, and rectal or systemic glucocorticoids. Like other sulfonamides, sulfasalazine is considered category D near-term because of the theoretical risk of kernicterus. Folic acid 1 mg PO bid is advised in women receiving sulfasalazine. Adverse fetal effects have been documented with the use of 6-mercaptopurine (D) and azathioprine (D). They should be considered only in patients with refractory, steroid-dependent disease. *Avoid* cyclosporine. Methotrexate (X) is *contraindicated*. Consultation with a gastroenterologist is warranted in active disease (see also Chapter 11.9).[9]

ENDOCRINE DISORDERS

Diabetes

Diet is the cornerstone of management. All patients should receive nutritional counseling with a registered dietician. If medication is needed, insulin (B) is the drug of choice. Metformin (B) may be considered in women with impaired fasting glucose or impaired glucose tolerance (IGT). Glyburide (B/C depending on manufacturer) has also been used. Efficacy appears similar to insulin, but safety data are limited for both metformin and glyburide. Avoid other oral agents (see also Chapter 17.2).[10]

Thyroid disorders

(see also Chapter 17.3)

- **Hypothyroidism.** Untreated hypothyroidism adversely affects pregnancy outcomes. Oral levothyroxine (A) is the thyroid preparation of choice. Desiccated thyroid and levothyroxine/L-triiodothyronine combinations should not be used, and women taking them should be switched over to levothyroxine. Levothyroxine requirements may increase during pregnancy.[11]
- **Hyperthyroidism.** Medication management is preferred. Propylthiouracil (PTU) (D) is preferred over methimazole (MMI; Tapazole) (D) in the first trimester, due to a possible lower incidence of major malformations and slower placental transfer. MMI is preferred in the second and third trimesters due to risk for hepatotoxicity with PTU. Adjust to the lowest dose effective to maintain thyroid hormone levels slightly above normal range for total T4 and T3 pregnancy values and to keep the thyroid-stimulating hormone suppressed. Free T4 should be kept at or slightly above the nonpregnancy levels. Assess thyroid function monthly. *Avoid* β-blockers, such as propranolol (C) (Inderal). Monitor for intrauterine growth retardation. The use of radioactive iodine (X) is *contraindicated*. Endocrinology consultation for management issues is recommended.[12]

NEUROLOGIC AND PSYCHIATRIC DISORDERS

Headaches, Migraine

Nondrug therapies, such as relaxation, sleep, massage, ice packs, and biofeedback, should be tried first. If drug therapy is needed, the most acceptable analgesic is acetaminophen (B) (Tylenol), 1,000 mg at first sign of headache. An antiemetic may also be required, such as promethazine (C) (Phenergan) or metoclopramide (B) (Reglan). Nonsteroidal anti-inflammatory drugs are considered safe until the third trimester (category D), due to risk of premature closure of ductus arteriosus. In severe cases, hydrocodone (C) may be given for short-term use only. *Avoid* use of serotonin 5-HT$_1$ receptor agonists such as sumatriptan (C) until more data are available. Prophylactic treatment is rarely indicated. Valproic acid and divalproex sodium (X for migraines) (Depakene, Depakote) are *contraindicated*. Ergotamine (X) is an abortifacient and is *contraindicated* during pregnancy[13] (see also Chapter 6.1).

Depression

Psychotherapy is considered first-line treatment for depression during pregnancy. Fluoxetine (Prozac) (C) and sertraline (C) (Zoloft) are agents of choice. Alternatives include citalopram (C), bupropion (C), duloxetine (C), mirtazapine (C), and venlafaxine (C), but data are limited. Tricyclic antidepressants, including nortriptyline (C), desipramine (C), amitriptyline (D), and imipramine (D) should be used *very* judiciously, due to unsubstantiated teratogenic activity. *Avoid* paroxetine (D) due to an FDA advisory of possible fetal ventricular septal defects and monoamine oxidase (MAO) inhibitors (see also Chapter 5.2).[14]

Seizure Disorders

Benefits of specific agents must be weighed against adverse pregnancy outcomes from uncontrolled seizures. Treat with as few agents and at the lowest dose possible to maintain control. Evidence for congenital malformations with older agents, including phenytoin, carbamazepine, and phenobarbital, is inconclusive but reassuring. Lamotrigine and levetiracetam may have minimal risk for congenital malformations, but more data are needed. Valproic acid and its derivatives (D) should be avoided if possible due to increased risk for neural tube defects. If valproate must be taken, minimize the dose. Supplementation with folic acid (0.4 to 4 mg per day) may or may not decrease risk.[15]

CARDIOVASCULAR DISEASES

Hypertension

Methyldopa (B) (250 mg bid–tid, titrated to max 3 g per day) has the most data supporting efficacy and use, but may be limited by side effects, including sedation. Labetalol (C) (usually 200 to 800 mg per day in two divided doses) is increasingly prescribed for its low incidence of side effects and strong evidence for efficacy. Nifedipine (C), hydralazine (C), and hydrochlorothiazide (B) can also be used. ACE inhibitors (D) and angiotensin receptor blockers (ARBs) (D) are *contraindicated*.[16]

VACCINES

Women who are pregnant should receive the inactivated influenza vaccine. Tdap is also indicated for each pregnancy, preferably between weeks 27 and 36 regardless of the interval of the previous Tdap or Td vaccine. Live vaccines, including varicella, zoster, the intranasal live, attenuated, influenza vaccine (LAIV), and measles, mumps, and rubella (MMR) are contraindicated during pregnancy.[17]

HERBAL AGENTS

Herbal agents generally recognized as safe for use as a food supplement by the FDA include chamomile, garlic, ginger, and mints. Raspberry leaf is also likely safe in amounts found in food, but not is larger quantities (see also Chapter 22.3).

Herbal agents to avoid during pregnancy include but are not limited to bitter orange, black and blue cohosh, cascara, castor oil, chasteberry, chondroitin, dihydroepiandrosterone, dong quai, feverfew, ginkgo, ginseng (*Panax* species), goldenseal, guarana, horse chestnut, kava kava, passionflower, pau d'arco, pennyroyal, St. John's wort, soy isoflavones, and valerian.[18]

REFERENCES

1. FDA labeling requirements for prescription drugs and/or insulin. 21 C.F.R. § 201.57. Subpart B. (b) (9) (i)(A) (2013).
2. Erebara A, Bozzo P, Einarson A, et al. Treating the common cold during pregnancy. *Can Fam Physician* 2008;54:687–689.
3. Briggs GG, Freeman RK, Yaffe SJ. *Drugs in pregnancy and lactation.* 9th ed. Baltimore, MD: Lippincott Williams & Wilkins; 2011.
4. Mandell LA, Wunderink RG, Anzueto A, et al. Infectious Diseases Society of America/American Thoracic Society consensus guidelines on the management of community-acquired pneumonia in adults. *Clin Infect Dis* 2007;44:S27–S72.
5. U.S. Centers for Disease Control and Prevention. Sexually transmitted diseases treatment guidelines 2010. *MMWR Recomm Rep* 2010;59(RR-12):1–110.
6. Macejko AM, Schaeffer AJ. Asymptomatic bacteriuria and symptomatic urinary tract infections during pregnancy. *Urol Clin North Am* 2007;34:35–42.
7. Yawn B, Knudtson M. Treating asthma and comorbid allergic rhinitis in pregnancy. *J Am Board Fam Med* 2007;20:289–298.

8. Niebyl JR. Nausea and vomiting in pregnancy. *N Engl J Med* 2010;363:1544–1550.
9. Tukral C, Wolf JL. Therapy insight: drugs for gastrointestinal disorders in pregnant women. *Nat Clin Pract Gastroenterol Hepatol* 2006;3:256–266.
10. Committee on Practice Bulletins—Obstetrics. Practice Bulletin No. 137: gestational diabetes mellitus. *Obstet Gynecol* 2013;122(2, pt 1):406–416.
11. Garber JR, Cobin RH, Gharib H, et al. Clinical practice guidelines for hypothyroidism in adults: co-sponsored by the American Association of Clinical Endocrinologists and the American Thyroid Association. *Endocr Pract* 2012;18:988–1028.
12. Bahn RS, Burch HB, Cooper DS, et al. Hyperthyroidism and other causes of thyrotoxicosis: management guidelines of the American Thyroid Association and American Association of Clinical Endocrinologists. *Endocr Pract* 2011;17:456–520.
13. Gilmore B, Michael M. Treatment of acute igraine headache. *Am Fam Physician* 2011;83:271–280.
14. Yonkers KA, Wisner KL, Stewart DE, et al. The management of depression during pregnancy: a report from the American Psychiatric Association and the American College of Obstetricians and Gynecologists. *Gen Hosp Psychiatry* 2009;31:403–413.
15. Battino D, Tomson T. Management of epilepsy during pregnancy. *Drugs* 2007;67:2727–2746.
16. American College of Obstetricians and Gynecologists. ACOG Practice Bulletin No. 125: chronic hypertension in pregnancy. *Obstet Gynecol* 2012;119(2, pt 1):396–407.
17. Centers for Disease Control. Adult Immunization Schedule-2014. http://www.cdc.gov/vaccines/schedules/downloads/adult/adult-schedule.pdf. Accessed March 17, 2014.
18. The Pharmacist's Letter/Physician's Letter Natural Medicines Comprehensive Database. http://www.naturaldatabase.com. Accessed March 18, 2014.

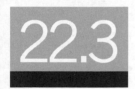

22.3 Herbal Medicine

Mari A. Ricker, David K. Solondz

GENERAL PRINCIPLES

- **Variety.** Herbs come in many different forms: whole fresh, whole dried, encapsulated powder, extract tablets, teas, tinctures, juice, essential oils, decoctions, lyophilized herb, standardized extract, cold and hot infusions, and topical preparations.
- **Standardization.** In an attempt to ensure consistency of herbal dosing, herbs are standardized to a constituent marker within the herb. For example, St. John wort is often standardized to an active component known as hypercin. Standardized products will reflect that they contain 0.3% hypercin in their St. John wort.

DOSING AND ADMINISTRATION

- **Normal dosage.** Unless noted differently on the packaging, a dosage is given for oral intake for an adult weighing approximately 150 pounds (70 kg).
- **Dosing for children/elderly.** There are several rules that can be used for determining the appropriate dose:
  - **Young's rule.** *Children*: The fraction of the adult dose is the child's age divided by the child's age plus 12. For example, 500 mg tid is the adult dose. For a 7-year-old child, the fraction is 7/(7 + 12) = 7/19. So the appropriate dose would be approximately 180 mg tid for a 7-year-old child.
  - **Cowling's rule.** *Children 12 to 18*: Take the age of the child at the child's next birthday and divide by 24 to determine the fraction. For example, 500 mg tid for a 14-year-old (at next birthday) child would be 14/24 or 300 mg tid approximately.
  - **Clark's rule.** *Elderly or weight adjustment:* Using the patient's weight in pounds, you can divide the weight by 150 to calculate the fraction. For example, 500 mg tid, a 94-pound woman would have a fraction of 94/150 and a dose of approximately 300 mg tid (See Table 22.3-1).

TABLE 22.3-1 Common Herbal Medications

Herb (taken orally)	Common uses	Dosing	Standardization	Contraindications	Side effects	Medicine interactions
Black Cohosh *Cimicifuga racemosa*	Menopause, PMS, dysmenorrhea	20–80 mg bid	1 mg triterpene glycosides per dose	• Estrogen-dependent tumors • Endometrial cancer • Pregnancy • Breastfeeding	• Nausea/vomiting • Headache • Hypotension	• Theoretical interaction with antihypertensive medications, due to increased hypotensive effect • Contains trace amounts of salicylic acid, theoretical interaction with antiplatelet agents
Butterbur *Petasites hybridus*	Migraine headaches, allergic rhinitis	• **Migraine:** 50–100 mg bid with meals (hepatotoxic pyrrolizidine alkaloids free) • **Allergies:** butterbur, one tablet 3–4 times daily	• **Migraine:** 15% petasin and isopetasin • **Allergies:** leaf extract standardized to 8 mg of petasin per dose	Caution if allergy to ragweed, chrysanthemums, marigolds, daisies	• Highest concern with preparations that are not pyrrolizidine alkaloid-free; this can cause hepatotoxicity with cumulative use • Mild drowsiness • Stomach upset	• Use with caution with drugs that induce CYP3A4, such as carbamazepine (Tegretol), phenobarbital, phenytoin (Dilantin), rifampin
Chamomile *Matricaria recutita*	Insomnia, diarrhea, colic, anxiety, gastrointestinal spasm	• **Tea:** 3 g (1 tsp)/cup water, 1–4 cups/d • **Tincture:** 3–10 mL tid (1:5 g/mL in 45% alcohol)	Oral: 1.2% apigenin and 0.5% essential oil per dose	• Known allergy to chamomile • Some cross over with mugwort or birch pollen allergy	• Drowsiness	• Caution with use of other sedative medications • Theoretical interaction with CYP3A4 isoenzyme (causes inhibition per in vitro data) though no herb–drug interactions in the literature
Cranberry *Vaccinium macrocarpon*	Urinary tract infection prevention	• **Oral:** 400–500 mg bid • **Juice:** 1–2 glasses/ daily of 100% juice (need higher volume if less than 100% cranberry juice)	11%–12% quinic acid per dose	• Limit to <1 L/d with history kidney stones • Contains small amounts of salicylic acid, avoid large amounts in patients with aspirin allergy	• Large doses can cause gastrointestinal upset and diarrhea	• In vitro studies suggest that flavonoids in cranberry inhibit CYP2C9 enzymes; however, no clinical studies have shown impact in humans
Cinnamon *Cinnamomum aromaticum*	Type 2 diabetes	• 1–6 g (1 tsp = 4.75 g) daily	None	Advanced liver disease (contains small amounts of coumarin)	None	• Hypoglycemic agents • Hepatotoxic medications

Herb	Uses	Dose	Standardization	Cautions	Side Effects	Drug Interactions
Echinacea *Echinacea angustifolia* or *E. purpurea*	Upper respiratory infections, otitis media, arthritis, (some antiviral, antibacterial, and antifungal effects)	• **Capsule:** 500 mg tid × 1 d then 250 mg qid • **Juice:** freshly expressed (*E. purpurea*) 60 gtt tid × 1 d then 40 gtt tid for up to 10 d	• **Capsule:** 4% echinacosides or 4% sesquiterpene esters per dose • **Juice:** 2.4% soluble β-1,2-D5-fructofuranosides per dose	• Caution in patients with renal insufficiency • Avoid in patients allergic to Asteraceae/Compositae family (ragweed, chrysanthemums, marigolds, daisies, etc.) or ragweed pollens. Anaphylactic reactions have occurred	Mild gastrointestinal symptoms	• Theoretical interactions with immunosuppressant medications, corticosteroids, and CYP3A3 isoenzyme (causes inhibition per in vitro data)
Fever Few *Tanacetum parthenium*	Migraines (used as prophylaxis)	• **Migraines:** 50–250 mg 0.2% parthenolide daily		• Pregnancy due to uterine stimulation • Avoid in patients allergic to Asteraceae/Compositae family (ragweed, chrysanthemums, marigolds, daisies, etc.) or ragweed pollens • Discontinue 14 d prior to surgery	• Gastrointestinal upset • Mild irritation of mucosa • Withdrawal symptoms in abrupt discontinuation of use	• Anticoagulant medications (aspirin, warfarin, NSAIDS, antiplatelet medication)
Garlic *Allium sativum*	HTN, hypercholesterolemia, (antioxidant and antimicrobial effects)	• **Dried:** 500–1,000 mg/d • **Fresh:** 4,000 mg daily	Allicin: approximately 4,000 mcg of Allicin	• Must be stopped 7–10 d prior to surgery because of interaction with platelet aggregation	• GI distress, irritation • Hypoglycemia	• Anticoagulant medications (aspirin, warfarin, NSAIDS, antiplatelet medication) • Hypoglycemic agents • Antihypertensive agents • Theoretical CYP2D6 or CYP3A4 though no reports of interactions
Ginger *Zingiber officinale Roscoe*	Nausea and vomiting, especially during pregnancy	• 2–4 g/d • 1 g/d in pregnancy	None	• Caution in patients with gallstones, ginger increases flow of bile • Must be stopped 14 d prior to surgery because of interaction with platelet aggregation • German commission E contraindicate use in pregnancy, but no studies have shown embryonic loss or toxic effects	• **Large doses:** reflux symptoms	• Anticoagulant medications (aspirin, warfarin, NSAIDS, antiplatelet medication)

(continued)

TABLE 22.3-1 Common Herbal Medications *(Continued)*

Herb (taken orally)	Common uses	Dosing	Standardization	Contraindications	Side effects	Medicine interactions
Ginkgo *Ginkgo biloba*	Alzheimer dementia, cognition, memory, claudication	40–80 mg tid	24%–27% ginkgo flavone glycosides and 5%–7% triterpenes per dose	• Bleeding disorders, discontinue 14 d prior to surgery	• Restlessness • Diarrhea • Headache • Nausea/vomiting • Lack of muscle tone • Weakness	• Anticoagulant medications (aspirin, warfarin, NSAIDS, antiplatelet medication) • May increase clearance of insulin and hypoglycemic agents causing increase in blood glucose
Ginseng, panax *Panax ginseng* (NOT American ginseng)	General tonic and immune system booster, cognition, COPD, erectile dysfunction	• 100–600 mg daily in divided doses • Regimen of 4 weeks on, 2 weeks off is recommended	4%–5% ginsenosides per dose	• Hypertension • Renal failure • Autoimmune diseases (MS, SLE, RA) • Hormone-sensitive conditions (i.e., cancers, endometriosis, fibroids) • Possible QT prolongation on initiation of use • Pregnancy/lactation • Discontinue 14 d prior to surgery	• Insomnia • Mastalgia, • Metrorrhagia • Palpitations/ tachycardia • **Ginseng abuse syndrome:** from prolonged use at high dosage (diarrhea, hypertension, nervousness, insomnia, and skin eruptions)	• MAOIs • Stimulants/caffeine • Hormonal therapies • Antihypertensive medications and hypoglycemic agents • Anticoagulant medications (aspirin, warfarin, NSAIDS, antiplatelet medication)
Ginseng, Siberian *Eleutherococcus senticosus*	Adaptogen and tonic, increase in energy and well-being, common cold, HSV	• 400 mg qd to tid or 400 mg daily • Regimen of 4 wk on, 2 wk off is recommended	0.8% eleutherosides B and E per dose	• Hypertension • Atherosclerotic and rheumatic heart disease • MI • Mental illness • Hormone-sensitive conditions (i.e., cancers, endometriosis, fibroids) • Discontinue 14 d prior to surgery	• Anxiety/irritability • Mastalgia • Uterine bleeding	• Stimulants/caffeine • Barbiturates • Digoxin • Antihypertensive medications and hypoglycemic agents • Anticoagulant medications (aspirin, warfarin, NSAIDS, antiplatelet medication)

Herb	Uses	Dose	Standardization	Contraindications	Adverse effects	Drug interactions
Golden Seal *Hydrastis canadensis*	Immune booster, URI, dyspepsia, GU inflammation, UTI, infectious diarrhea	250 mg bid-qid	• 10% alkaloids or 2.5% berberine and 1.5%–5% hydrastine per dose	• Newborn • Pregnancy	• Gastrointestinal distress • Hypotension • Bradycardia • Hypertension • Can displace albumin • Kernicterus	• Theoretical interaction with CYP3A3 isoenzyme (causes inhibition per in vitro data) • May increase digoxin level
Hawthorn *Crataegus oxyacantha*	Congestive heart failure, angina, hypotension, hypertension, anxiolytic	250 mg qd to tid	• 2% vitexin or 20% procyanidins per dose or 30–168 mg procyandins or 3.5–19 mg flavonoids	• None	• Dizziness • Headache • Hypotension	• Caution with digoxin, vasodilators (β-blockers/CCB, nitrates) ARB/ACE-I
Licorice *Glycyrrhiza glabra*	Dyspepsia, ulcers, oral irritation, hepatitis, muscle cramps	300 mg tid or 7 mL tid	Use deglycrrhizinated (DGL) forms to reduce mineralocorticoid activity	• Hypertension/CHF • Hormone-sensitive cancers • CKD • Pregnancy • Discontinue 14 d prior to surgery	• Hypertension • Risk for hypokalemia	• Potassium wasting medications • Coumadin • Digoxin
Milk thistle *Silybum marianum*	Acute or chronic liver conditions (hepatoprotective), digestive tonic, lactation stimulant, increases bile flow Diabetes	80–200 mg qd-tid	70%–80% silymarin extract per dose	• Ragweed allergy • Avoid plant extracts in hormone-sensitive cancer due to estrogenic effect (seed extract ok)	• Mild laxative, bloating, anorexia	• None
Saw Palmetto *Serenoa repens*	Benign prostatic hyperplasia	160 mg bid	80%–90% fatty acids and sterols per dose	• Discontinue 14 d prior to surgery	• Mild gastrointestinal symptoms	• Not recommended for use with α-blockers • Theoretical interaction with hormonal therapies (i.e., OCPs)

(continued)

TABLE 22.3-1 Common Herbal Medications (*Continued*)

Herb (taken orally)	Common uses	Dosing	Standardization	Contraindications	Side effects	Medicine interactions
Stinging Nettles *Urtica dioica*	Allergies, urinary symptoms (i.e., IC, nocturia, frequency)	**Freeze dried leaf:** 300–1,200 mg bid–qid	None	• Renal insufficiency (mild diuretic) • Pregnancy	• GI upset • Skin reaction	• MAOIs • Has high vitamin K content; theoretical interaction with anticoagulant medications (aspirin, warfarin, NSAIDS, antiplatelet medication) • Antihypertensive medications and hypoglycemic agents
St. John wort *Hypericum perforatum*	Mild to moderate depression	300 mg tid Up to 1,800 mg/d	• 0.1%–0.3% hypericin or • 0.3%–0.5% hypericum or • 3%–5% hyperforin per dose	• Severe depression • Alzheimer's • Caution with anesthesia (may cause severe hypotension)	• Photosensitivity • Transaminase elevation • Drowsiness • Elevated TSH • May be associated with hypertension crisis (serotonin syndrome)	• May decrease serum concentrations of cyclosporine, digoxin, theophylline, amitriptyline, protease inhibitors, chemotherapeutic agents, warfarin, oral contraceptives • Caution with SSRIs, MAOIs, reserpine, and narcotics
Tumeric *Curcima longa*	Joint inflammation (RA, OA), anti-inflammatory, antioxidant, dyspepsia	• 300 mg tid to 500 mg qid with meals	95% curcuminoids per dose	• Biliary obstruction • Caution with PUD, IBD • Bleeding disorders • Discontinue 14 d prior to surgery	• GI upset (diarrhea, nausea)	• Anticoagulant medications (aspirin, warfarin, NSAIDS, antiplatelet medication)
Valerian *Valeriana officinalis*	Insomnia, anxiety, PMS, menopause	• 200 mg daily qid **Sedative dose:** 200–400 mg qhs	0.3%–1% valerenic acids per dose	• Caution in children, never in <3 yr old • Discontinue 14 d prior to surgery	• Sedation or drowsiness • Headache • Restlessness	• CNS depressants—sedatives, hypnotics, benzodiazepines, alcohol

NSAIDS, nonsteroidal antiinflammatories; MAOIs, monoamine oxidase inhibitors; MS, multiple sclerosis; SLE, systemic lupis erythematosus; RA, rheumatoid arthritis; CCB, calcium channel blocker; CKD, chronic kidney disease; MI, myocardial infarction; URI, upper respiratory infection; GU, genitourinary; UTI, urinary tract infection; HSV = herpes simplex virus; SSRI, selective seratonin reuptake inhibitor; CNS, central nervous system; GI, gastrointestinal; PUD, peptic ulcer disease; IBD, inflammatory bowel disease; IC, interstitial cystitis; OA, osteoarthritis; PMS, premenstrual syndrome.

WEB ADDRESSES

- American Botanical Council: http://www.herbs.org/
- U.S. Pharmacopeia: http://www.usp.org
- Food and Drug Administration (FDA): http://vm.cfsan.fda.gov

REFERENCES

1. *German Commission E Monographs*. Austin, TX: American Botanical Council; 1998.
2. Natural medicines comprehensive database. Stockton, CA: Prescriber's letter; 2014. http://www.naturaldatabase.com. Accessed March 8, 2014.
3. DerMarderosian A. *The review of natural products by facts and comparisons*. St. Louis, MO: Wolters Kluwer; 1999.
4. Rotblatt M, Ziment I. *Evidence-based herbal medicine*. Philadelphia, PA: Hanley and Belfus; 2002.
5. Krinsky DL, LaValle JB, Hawkins EB, et al. *Natural therapeutics pocket guide*. 2nd ed. Hudson, OH: Lexi-Comp; 2003.
6. Brown DJ. *Herbal prescriptions for health and healing*. Roseville, CA: Prima Health; 2003.

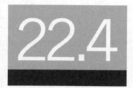

22.4 Management of Acute and Chronic Nonmalignant Pain

Amy E. Curry

GENERAL PRINCIPLES

"The aim of the wise is not to secure pleasure, but to avoid pain." Aristotle

Definitions

Pain is a frequent reality in the human condition and is one of the most common reasons people seek out medical attention. Chronic pain affects up to one-third of all Americans at some point in their lives. It is the leading cause of disability and has caused the loss of more than $100 billion to the U.S. economy in direct costs and lost productivity.

Pain is defined as an "unpleasant sensory and emotional experience associated with actual or potential tissue damage."[1] It is also, "whatever the experiencing person says it is, existing whenever s/he says it does."[1] These definitions convey the complex human response to pain, hint at the suffering that often accompanies it, and acknowledge the reality that some patients feel pain, yet have no objective findings or identifiable cause.

Nociception is the process by which pain from tissue or nerve damage is communicated to the central nervous system. Nociceptive pain is caused by a noxious stimulus within the context of an intact healthy nervous system, whereas neuropathic pain is caused by nervous system malfunction or damage. Often, both nociceptive and neuropathic pain coexist.

Injured tissues undergo cell breakdown and release various products and mediators of inflammation: prostaglandins, substance P, bradykinin, histamine, serotonin, and cytokines. These substances activate sensory nociceptors to generate nerve impulses and also sensitize them to increase their excitability and frequency discharge.

Nerve impulses travel from the periphery into the dorsal horn of the spinal cord, and are propagated by the release of excitatory amino acids, such as glutamate and aspartate, and neuropeptides, such as substance P. Repeated stimulation activates the N-methyl d-aspartate (NMDA) receptors in a process known as "wind up." Impulses within the dorsal horn are then projected to various parts of the brain in ascending tract bundles. Pain impulses are not simply related to the brain unrestricted, however. Pain traffic is inhibited inside the dorsal horn by spinal interneurons as well as descending inhibitory input from the brain. Inhibition in both pathways occurs via the release of inhibitory amino acids such as γ-aminobutyric acid (GABA), endogenous opioids, serotonin, and norepinephrine.

Pain impulses are transmitted to many areas of the brain, including the cortex and the limbic system. This perception of pain involves not only the neurochemical impulse at the molecular level, but also the patient's emotions, memories, cultural values, ethics, mental state, and previous pain experiences, making pain perception unique and individualized to each patient.

Prolonged exposure to noxious pain generating stimulation or inflammatory mediators, can lead to sensitization of the pain pathway in both the peripheral and the central nervous system. Sensitization can trigger changes in the nervous system that can persist indefinitely. This sensitization can lead to clinical pain states such as (a) hyperalgesia—an increased response to painful stimuli that can even extend beyond the region of injury, (b) allodynia—a painful response to a normally innocuous stimulus, (c) persistent pain—a prolonged pain, from minutes to hours, after a transient stimulus, and (d) referred pain—the spread of pain to uninjured tissues.

Understanding the pain pathway and sensitization has many clinical implications and allows for the direct targeting of various places in the treatment of pain.

ACUTE PAIN

Acute pain by definition is a new onset of pain, usually from an identifiable cause and with a predictable course and time of resolution. It is a "complex, unpleasant experience with emotional and cognitive, as well as, sensory features that occur in response to tissue trauma."[1] Even brief exposure to painful stimuli can cause intense suffering, neuronal remodeling, and the development of chronic pain. Therefore, aggressive treatment of acute pain may decrease the risk of these complications.

Assessment of acute pain involves taking a detailed history with attention to the mechanism of injury, if known, and the characteristics of the pain, followed by a full physical examination of the painful area. The patient should be provided analgesia as soon as possible after initial assessments have been made and relief of the pain should not be delayed while work-up is completed.

Pharmacologic treatment of acute pain can be guided by the patient's reported numeric pain score (see Figure 22.4-1) and the World Health Organization Analgesic Ladder (see Figure 22.4-2). For mild to moderate pain scores, non-opioids and weak opioids are indicated. These include acetaminophen, nonsteroidal anti-inflammatory medications (NSAIDs), tramadol, hydrocodone, and oxycodone. Combination therapy with acetaminophen, NSAIDs, and one of the weak opioids is safe and may provide significant analgesia by targeting many areas along the pain pathway. For more severe pain, strong opioids, such as morphine, hydromorphone, and intravenous (IV) fentanyl can be used, along with the non-opioid medications. There is little use of methadone in the setting of acute pain and the potential of significant harm exists.

If clinically feasible, use oral or mucosal forms of analgesia, followed by parenteral forms, preferably IV. Intramuscular analgesia should be limited due to its inconsistent absorption, painful administration, and risk of tissue fibrosis. Those topical analgesics designed to only affect surrounding tissue, such as lidocaine, capsaicin, and EMLA cream, may be of benefit. Fentanyl patches, however, have limited use in the treatment of acute pain as they are contraindicated in the opiate-naïve patient and take up to 72 hours to achieve full analgesic dosing.

Useful adjuvants in the treatment of acute pain include muscle relaxants, heat, transcutaneous electrical nerve stimulation (TENS), and PRINCE, which refers to protection, rest, immobilization, ice, compression, and elevation. If the patient is experiencing significant neuropathic pain, usually described as a burning, stinging, "pins and needles" sensation, the addition of antiseizure medications as well as the above-mentioned topical medications may be of benefit.

If opioids are needed beyond the first few days to weeks, short-acting forms should be used initially, but can be transitioned to long-acting formulations. Patients should be counseled on the side effects of opioid therapy to include nausea, vomiting, constipation, pruritus, urinary retention, and respiratory depression, as well as the risks of driving or operating heavy machinery.

Although the benefit of aggressively treating acute pain does exist, the growing problem of opioid addiction in America, especially among the adolescent population, makes both judicious prescribing

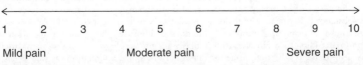

| 1 | 2 | 3 | 4 | 5 | 6 | 7 | 8 | 9 | 10 |

Mild pain   Moderate pain   Severe pain

Figure 22.4-1. A numeric pain scale can assist the patient in communicating pain level in an objective manner.

Step 1: Mild pain (1–4 on pain assessment scale)
Non-opioid +/– adjuvant

Step 2: Moderate pain (5–6 on pain assessment scale)
Weak opioid +/– non-opioid +/– adjuvant

Step 3: Severe pain (7–10 on pain assessment scale)
Strong opioid +/– non-opioid +/– adjuvant

Figure 22.4-2. World Health Organization Analgesic Ladder can help guide appropriate selection of pain treatment based on numeric pain assessment scores.

of opioids necessary as well as careful consideration to the realistic quantity of medication that needs to be dispensed. Patients should be advised to keep all medications in a safe and preferably locked area and to safely dispose of any unused medications. Patients may dispose of opioids by returning them to the pharmacy, taking them to a law enforcement facility or placing them in an inedible substance inside a sealed container in the trash. The Food and Drug Administration does allow the following opioids to be flushed down the toilet: fentanyl (including the patches), hydromorphone, methadone, morphine, oxycodone, and oxymorphone.

Finally, the depth of emotional, mental, and psychological pain that the patient may also be experiencing beyond that of the physical, needs to be identified, fully validated, and treated, if present. A multidisciplinary team approach involving law enforcement, social work, and mental health workers may be required to ensure that all aspects of the patient's pain are addressed.

CHRONIC NONMALIGNANT PAIN

Chronic nonmalignant pain (CNMP) is pain that extends beyond the expected period of healing, usually 3 to 6 months, and is not caused by cancer. It may develop de novo with no apparent cause or there may be an identifiable level of tissue pathology, progress from an acute injury, or be caused by a chronic condition such as rheumatoid arthritis. Regardless of its etiology, CNMP often disrupts sleep and normal living; ceases to serve a protective function; and may cause vocational, social, and psychological problems.

Assessment

Assessment of CNMP requires considerable time and attention and may require longer appointments dedicated to addressing the patient's CNMP complaints. A detailed pain history should be taken, in addition to the patient's past medical history, and should include characteristics of the pain, all previous testing or consultations, past and present pain management treatments, and their outcomes. This may surprisingly reveal areas in the work-up and treatment of the patient's pain complaint that are incomplete or have been neglected. All past medical records should also be reviewed and a full physical examination should be performed with careful attention to the painful area.

Additional time should be given to screening the patient for mental illness, specifically depression and anxiety, which is overrepresented in patients with CNMP compared with the general population. Measureable, objective treatment goals should be agreed upon in addition to that of eliminating the patient's pain.

Treatment

A multidisciplinary approach should be employed in the treatment of CNMP, involving both nonpharmacologic and pharmacologic treatments.

Nonpharmacologic Treatment of CNMP

Psychological methods in the treatment of CNMP include

1. Patient education concerning CNMP
2. Contingency management to decrease "sick role" behavior
3. Cognitive-behavioral therapy to include both cognitive restructuring and coping skills training to alter patient's responses to pain
4. Relaxation techniques
5. Hypnosis
6. Distraction to draw attention away from the pain and to include social and recreational activities
7. Biofeedback
8. Psychotherapy

Physical methods in the treatment of CNMP include

1. Stretching
2. Exercise/reconditioning
3. Gait and posture training
4. Applied heat or cold
5. Immobilization
6. TENS
7. Nerve stimulation via implantable devices
8. Massage
9. Acupuncture
10. Chiropractic or osteopathic manipulation

Pharmacologic Treatment of CNMP

Non-opioid analgesics, as mentioned above, include acetaminophen and NSAIDs. Although acetaminophen has no anti-inflammatory effects, it is well tolerated and can be used in the elderly, but can be hepatotoxic at doses greater than 4,000 mgs per day and 2,000 mg per day in patients with liver diseases. NSAIDs should be used cautiously in elders due to their significant side effect profile to include renal toxicity, bleeding risk, increase in blood pressure, and fluid retention; however, they can be very helpful in inflammatory conditions.

Adjuvant or coanalgesics are useful drugs that can be used to disrupt the pain pathway, treat comorbid conditions associated with CNMP, such as insomnia and mental illness, and are particularly useful in the treatment of neuropathic pain. These include the antiseizure medications, the tricyclic antidepressants, the selective serotonin and norepinephrine reuptake inhibitors, muscle relaxants, lidocaine patches, and capsaicin cream. Additionally, injectable glucocorticoid steroids are an important adjuvant therapy and can be safely administered via an intra-articular or intraspinal route as well as in limited amounts via oral, IV, or IM routes.

The use of opioid analgesics in the treatment of CNMP has increased dramatically in the past decade; however, an increase in prescription opioid abuse, addiction, diversion, and overdose deaths has also occurred. In response to this, the American Pain Society and the American Academy of Pain Medicine released evidence-based guidelines on the use of opioids in CNMP in 2009.[2] These guidelines recently received the highest ratings for evidence-based guidelines in a systematic review and critical appraisal study of 13 pain guidelines.[3] It is recommended that a clinician considering the use of opioids in a patient's treatment of CNMP follow these guidelines.[4]

A summary of the guidelines is as follows:

1. A trial of opioid therapy should be considered only after a complete work-up of the pain complaint has been performed, if the pain is severe to moderate, if other modalities have failed, and the benefits outweigh the potential harms. The patient should be assessed for risk of substance abuse, misuse, or addiction. Several validated tools that stratify this risk include the Screener and Opioid Assessment for Patients with Pain (SOAPP) version 1, and the revised version (SOAPP-R), the Opioid Risk Tool (ORT), and the Diagnosis, Intractability, Risk, Efficacy (DIRE) instrument.

2. Before starting opioid therapy, informed consent should be obtained from the patient. The risks of long-term use of opioid therapy, to include hyperalgesia, endocrine and immune dysfunction, should be reviewed. Consideration should be given to the creation of a written management plan agreed upon by both the provider and the patient. The plan would include objective treatment goals, the need for compliance monitoring, the use of one pharmacist and one physician

to provide opioid medications, and the behaviors that might lead to discontinuation of opioid treatment.

3. The initiation of opioid treatment should be on a trial basis and discontinued if the patient's goals are not being met. There is insufficient evidence to support the use of short-acting versus long-acting opioids and whether long-acting opioids decrease the risk of addiction or abuse. It is also unknown whether as-needed dosing or scheduled around the clock dosing is better. The opioid selection and dosing should be individualized to the patient's goals, health problems, prior exposure to opioids, and risk of opioid abuse.

4. Methadone should be used only by clinicians familiar with its risks and variable pharmacokinetics. Methadone can cause QTc prolongation in a dose-dependent fashion or if used with other drugs known to prolong the QTc as well. Its metabolism is highly variable between individuals and can be enhanced or inhibited by other medications competing for the same enzymatic pathways. The very long half-life, as high as 120 hours in some patients, exceeds that of its analgesic effects; therefore, it should be started at no more than 1 to 2.5 mg every 8 to 12 hours, and not increased for 5 to 7 days. Lower amounts and daily dosing may also be indicated. Accordingly, methadone is not recommended for use in breakthrough pain or as an as-needed medication. When converting patients to methadone, several equianalgesic algorithms exist and insufficient evidence exists to support one over another; however, starting doses should not exceed 30 to 40 mg per day, regardless of the calculated conversion dose.

5. Monitoring of patients on opioid treatment should occur at a frequency and to the degree warranted by their risk for opioid abuse, misuse, or diversion. Monitoring should include an assessment of pain severity, progress toward treatment goals, evidence of medication compliance in the form of urine drug screens and pill counts, and the presence of adverse effects. Use of tools such as the Pain Assessment and Documentation Tool (PADT) and the Current Opioid Misuse Measure (COMM), as well as reports from state prescription drug-monitoring programs may be helpful.

6. Opioid treatment may be used in patients with a history of drug abuse, psychiatric problems, or serious aberrant drug-related behaviors, only if the clinician can implement stringent and frequent monitoring measures. If patients are unable to comply or develop opioid addiction, referral to a structured opioid agonist treatment program with methadone or buprenorphine or to mental health and addiction specialists may be warranted.

7. Caution should be used in patients requiring repeated dose escalations and reevaluation of potential causes, to include misuse and abuse, should be performed. The benefit of exceeding >200 mg daily of morphine equivalents may not exceed the risks of adverse effects. Opioid rotation can be considered and equianalgesic dosing can be calculated. Because of incomplete cross tolerance and individual variation, the calculated initial equianalgesic dose should be reduced by 25% to 50%. Clinicians should taper or wean patients off of opioids who show no benefit from therapy, develop adverse effects, or display behaviors of misuse or abuse. In order to avoid the unpleasant, although not life-threatening symptoms of withdrawal, a slow taper of 10% dose reduction per week can be used. In some circumstances, a faster reduction of 25% to 50% every few days or referral to a structured detoxification program may be beneficial.

8. Clinicians should anticipate and treat opioid-induced adverse effects. Most side effects will resolve with time, except for constipation; thus, a bowel regimen should be instituted. Long-term use of sustained-release opioids has been associated with hypogonadism.[5] Patients reporting fatigue, decreased libido, sexual dysfunction, menstrual irregularities or who are found to have osteoporosis, should be tested and treated for hormonal deficiencies. Respiratory depression can occur in patients with sleep apnea, pulmonary disorders, excessive doses of or rapid titration of initial opioid therapy or the concurrent use of opioids and other depressive substances, such as alcohol or benzodiazepines.

9. Opioid therapy should not be used as the sole means of analgesia in CNMP, but is likely to be most effective if used in conjunction with psychotherapeutic interventions, such as cognitive–behavioral therapy, functional restoration, interdisciplinary therapy, and other adjunctive non-opioid therapies.

10. Opioids can impair driving and work safety and patients should be counseled not to drive or engage in dangerous activities if they are demonstrating signs of impairment, starting opioid therapy, increasing the dose or rotating to a new opioid, taking other sedating medications, drinking alcohol, or using illegal substances.

11. Patients on opioid therapy should have a medical home and should be referred to pain specialists if additional skills or procedures are needed.

12. All patients on around the clock opioid therapy should have a plan in place for the treatment of breakthrough pain. There is insufficient evidence to suggest the optimum method for the treatment of breakthrough pain. Options include nonpharmacologic and non-opioid therapies or the addition of a short- or rapid-acting opioid, dosed at 10% to 20% of the patient's total daily opioid dose. The risks and benefits of the addition of an opioid for breakthrough pain should be considered in light of the patient's risk of opioid misuse or abuse.

13. Opioids should not be used in pregnancy, unless substantial benefit outweighs the risks, due to the potential adverse effects to the newborn found to be associated with maternal opioid use. These include neonatal abstinence syndrome, low birth weight, premature birth, hypoxic–ischemic brain injury, and neonatal death.

14. Clinicians should understand the federal and state guidelines, policies, and laws concerning their responsibilities when prescribing opioids in CNMP.

REFERENCES

1. Berry PH, Chapman CR, Covington EC, et al., eds. *Pain: current understanding of assessment, management, and treatments.* National Pharmaceutical Council, Inc. and Joint Commission on Accreditation of Healthcare Organizations. Monograph. December, 2001. http://www.npcnow.org/publication/pain-current-understanding-assessment-management-and-treatments. Accessed March 30, 2014.
2. Chou R, Fanciullo G, Fine P, et al. Clinical guidelines for the use of chronic opioid therapy in chronic noncancer pain. *J Pain* 2009;10(2):113–130.
3. Nuckols TK, Anderson L, Popescu I, et al. Opioid prescribing: a systematic review and critical appraisal of guidelines for chronic pain. *Ann Intern Med* 2014;160:38–47.
4. Huntzinger A. Guidelines for the use of opioid therapy in patients with chronic noncancer pain. *Am Fam Physician* 2009;80(11):1315–1318.
5. Katz N, Mazer NA. The impact of opioids on the endocrine system. *Clin J Pain* 2009;25(20):170–175.

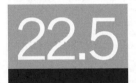

22.5 End-of-Life Care

James J. Helmer Jr., Marc Tunzi, Wendell M. Harry

GENERAL PRINCIPLES

Everybody dies. The aim of end-of-life care is to make life's last transition as comfortable and meaningful as possible for dying patients and their families. Death is not failure; not caring properly for dying patients is failure. Many aspects of end-of-life care planning apply to everyone, but especially to geriatric patients and to patients with life-limiting diseases. Similarly, certain aspects of end-of-life symptom and problem management apply to patients who are severely ill but are not yet considered terminally ill.

COMMUNICATION AND PLANNING ISSUES

- **Break bad news in a quiet, unhurried, comfortable setting.** Find out what patients know, and how much they want to know, before delivering information in a sensitive but straightforward manner, using clear language. Check for patient's understanding and emotional response. Schedule follow-up.
- **The goals of care** for end-of-life patients and their families are to maximize comfort and function and to minimize pain and suffering. Achieving these goals relies on effective communication and planning.
  - After assessing patient's understanding of their clinical situation, discuss expectations and the goals of care directly with those who have decision-making capacity (see below). When possible, patients should be empowered to control their own treatment and to resolve conflicts among competing goals of care (see below). *Ask* patients if and how they might wish to share decision making for difficult and complex issues.
  - After obtaining the patient's permission, assess the family's understanding of the clinical situation and discuss expectations and treatment goals with them as well. *Ask* patients if they need help

talking to their family about their condition and clinical decisions. When meeting with families—unless otherwise directed by the patient (or by a legally appointed surrogate; see below)—try to involve all those present, probe for questions, clarify misunderstandings gently, and plan for follow-up.

- Be sensitive to cultural differences in end-of-life care values and practices. Encourage patients and families to consider community resources and pastoral care. Be aware of how your own social, moral, and religious values influence life-and-death decision making with your patients.
- "Be there." All patients and families experience a wide range of emotions during the dying process. Anger, denial, depression, and bargaining are typical reactions. In addition, personal psychosocial problems, interpersonal family relationships, and the time line of the death (whether chronic or acute) all influence how patients and families react. The family physician's continued presence and validation of these reactions—even when other medical specialists are involved in patient management—may be therapeutic for everyone.

- **Ethical planning issues.** Addressing patients' desires about end-of-life care and life-sustaining treatment should be part of health care maintenance performed during regular office visits. Normalize this "informed consent" for the future by making such statements as, "I discuss life-sustaining treatments and advance directives, such as the living will and the power of attorney for health care, with all my patients; do you have any questions about them?" or "I discuss medical values with all my patients; have you ever discussed them with your family?"
  - Personal values ultimately guide patient decision making. Patients must be asked whether they want to live at all costs or whether they might compromise some life expectancy for a better quality of life. Patients must also be asked about a variety of other potentially competing values, such as maintaining mobility and physical independence, maintaining the ability to think clearly and communicate with others, being treated in accordance with their cultural and religious/spiritual beliefs, not becoming a burden on family, and avoiding unnecessary pain and suffering.
  - Advance directives are written or oral instructions that enable patients to guide their future health care decisions in the event that they cannot do so themselves.
  - Living wills are documents that allow patients to choose one of two or three scenarios for their end-of-life care (choices vary by state): Do everything medically possible to maintain life; do no extraordinary intervention but maintain comfort and allow death to occur "naturally"; or do no extraordinary intervention but continue nutrition and hydration in addition to other comfort care. In most states, laws require a patient to be diagnosed as terminal (prognosis less than 6 to 12 months) by two physicians for a living will to be legally binding.
  - Durable powers of attorney for health care (DPAHC) are legal documents that enable patients to appoint another specific individual (known as a proxy, agent, or surrogate) to make decisions for them, should they be unable to do so for themselves. These documents are most effective when patients and their surrogates have thoroughly discussed treatment options, so that the standard of substituted judgment may be applied (see below). Many DPAHC documents include a "living will" section within them. Patients do not need a lawyer to complete a DPAHC.
  - Many states now have POLST (Physician Orders for Life-Sustaining Treatment) documents. Signed by the patient (or surrogate) and physician, the POLST is a set of orders that travels with patients to all sites of care—home, hospital, skilled nursing facility, etc. Most POLST documents have three sections:
    - **a. Cardiopulmonary Resuscitation**—Attempt *or* Do Not Attempt CPR if a patient has no pulse and is not breathing;
    - **b. Medical Interventions**—Comfort Only; Limited Interventions (such as intubation, antibiotics, dialysis, blood products, etc., while the patient is not in "arrest"); or Full Treatment;
    - **c. Artificially Administered Nutrition**—*no* artificial nutrition (including feeding tubes); allow a *trial* of artificial nutrition; or accept *long-term* artificial nutrition.
  - Oral directives are the most common kind of advance directives and are often sufficient in guiding terminal care decisions. Unfortunately, the legal benefits of oral directives to family and friends vary by state and may not be upheld in cases of a family dispute or family physician disagreement. Oral directives to physicians, on the other hand, when clearly documented in the medical record, are usually honored by the courts.
- Medical decision-making capacity refers to the ability to make a rational decision about medical treatment options. Capacity should be viewed on a sliding scale: a patient may have the ability to understand and make decisions about some treatment options but not others, and this ability should be re-evaluated for each pending decision. Determining capacity requires assessment of a patient's

ability to accept responsibility for making the treatment decision; to understand the medical situation and prognosis; to understand the alternatives for care; to decide on an alternative based on reasoning that fits his or her general goals and values; and to communicate that decision clearly. Appropriate questions include, "What can you tell me about your condition?" "What is your understanding of this treatment and why do you think it is right for you?" "What can you tell me about the alternatives we've discussed?" Medical decision-making capacity should not be confused with *competency*, which is a legal status determined by a court of law.

- **Surrogacy.** When an individual does not have medical decision-making capacity, surrogate decisions must be made. When possible, a legal surrogate, appointed by the patient in a DPAHC, should make decisions. A POLST or living will may also guide care. When these are not available, surrogate decision makers should generally follow the traditional family hierarchy: spouse, adult children, parents, siblings, other relatives, and friends. The two standards most often used for making surrogate decisions are *substituted judgment* ("If the patient were still able to make decisions for herself, what would she want in this situation?") and *best interests* ("What do you think is the best thing to do for the patient, all things considered?").

Surrogate decision making is very stressful for most people. Ideally, patients and surrogates should discuss choices and values beforehand, with patients directing surrogates to follow previously-expressed preferences. Alternatively, patients should empower surrogates to simply use their own judgment and make decisions for the patients they are representing the same way they would for themselves.

MEDICAL CARE ISSUES

Palliative Care is a team approach to caring for the "whole person," and focuses on improving quality of life for patients and their families who are experiencing a life-threatening or life-limiting illness or injury. It facilitates comprehensive care for patients who are at any stage in the continuum of their illness, which may include curative, chronic management, and end of life. Palliative Care takes place in any care setting, and does not preclude interventions and therapies (such as hospitalization, IV antibiotics, IV fluids, High-Flow Therapy [Vapotherm], BiPAP, intubation, thoracentesis, paracentesis, surgery, chemotherapy, radiation, and CPR) that are consistent with the patient's goals of care.

In contrast, Hospice is intended for patients who are at the end stage on the continuum of their illness. Hospice should be strongly considered if the patient has 6 months or less to live based on the expected natural course of their illness. Instead of using doctors' offices, clinics, urgent cares, or ERs, patient care is provided at the patient's home, nursing home, or "hospice house" and typically does not involve invasive therapies. The goal of Hospice is to allow a patient a natural death while minimizing suffering, so that patients may carry out those goals that are most important to them. If symptoms cannot be controlled at the home, patients may be admitted to the hospital under the General Inpatient Hospice Coverage for several days without having to revoke their Medicare Hospice benefit. Additionally, hospice provides bereavement follow-up for 13 months after the patient's death. Hospice may be viewed as a subset of Palliative care.

DOMAINS OF PAIN

The domains of care for both Hospice and Palliative Care relate to the **domains of pain** as described by Cicely Saunders SW, RN, MD (considered the founder of the modern hospice movement), who focused on treating a patient's "Total Pain." Total Pain refers to Physical Pain, Emotional Pain, Social Pain, and Spiritual Pain.

- **Physical pain** (discussed in greater detail below and elsewhere in this manual) includes nociceptive, neuropathic, and mixed pain syndromes. Other aspects of physical suffering within this domain include dyspnea, nausea, dysphagia, fatigue, anorexia–cachexia, and delirium.
- **Emotional pain** includes symptoms such as anxiety and depression. Patients with a terminal illness often experience a predictable and normal grief reaction. Grief usually follows a typical progression: shock/disbelief, denial, anger, bargaining, guilt, depression, and finally, acceptance/hope. Some aspects of emotional pain should be normalized, and do not require "medical" treatment. For example, it is normal for a person to feel angry and sad when they have an incurable disease. However, when emotional pain interferes with meaningful activities, goals, spiritual discovery, and relationships medical intervention is warranted (see below).
- **Social pain** refers to barriers in a patient's support network and infrastructure. Social pain can arise from damaged relationships, loss of cultural identity, language barriers, homelessness, loss of work,

poverty, and loss of medical insurance are essential in maximizing therapeutic gain. Strategic use of family meetings, with involvement from clinical social workers and medical interpreters, can be very instrumental in recognizing and addressing social pain.

- **Spiritual pain** includes the disruption in one's ability to find sources of strength, hope, joy, and sense of purpose. Spirituality does not necessarily equate with a belief in God or a specific religion. Spirituality can be any connection a patient experiences that brings peace, hope, joy, and sense of purpose. For example, a patient may define their spirituality through a love of nature, cooking, gardening, or being with family and friends. It is important to begin with taking a spiritual history taken from EPERC Fast Fact #019 (Table 22.5-1).

- The premise for diagnosing Total Pain is that each domain of pain: Physical, Emotional, Social, and Spiritual, impacts the other domains creating a harmful synergy. By the same token,

TABLE 22.5-1	Taking a Spiritual History

S—spiritual belief system
- Do you have a formal religious affiliation? Can you describe this?
- Do you have a spiritual life that is important to you?
- What is your clearest sense of the meaning of your life at this time?

P—personal spirituality
- Describe the beliefs and practices of your religion that you personally accept.
- Describe those beliefs and practices that you do not accept or follow.
- In what ways is your spirituality/religion meaningful for you?
- How is your spirituality/religion important to you in daily life?

I—integration with a spiritual community
- Do you belong to any religious or spiritual groups or communities?
- How do you participate in this group/community? What is your role?
- What importance does this group have for you?
- In what ways is this group a source of support for you?
- What types of support and help does or could this group provide for you in dealing with health issues?

R—ritualized practices and restrictions
- What specific practices do you carry out as part of your religious and spiritual life (e.g. prayer, meditation, services, etc.)
- What lifestyle activities or practices do your religion encourage, discourage or forbid?
- What meaning do these practices and restrictions have for you? To what extent have you followed these guidelines?

I—implications for medical care
- Are there specific elements of medical care that your religion discourages or forbids? To what extent have you followed these guidelines?
- What aspects of your religion/spirituality would you like to keep in mind as I care for you?
- What knowledge or understanding would strengthen our relationship as physician and patient?
- Are there barriers to our relationship based upon religious or spiritual issues?
- Would you like to discuss religious or spiritual implications of health care?

T—terminal events planning
- Are there particular aspects of medical care that you wish to forgo or have withheld because of your religion/spirituality?
- Are there religious or spiritual practices or rituals that you would like to have available in the hospital or at home?
- Are there religious or spiritual practices that you wish to plan for at the time of death, or following death?
- From what sources do you draw strength in order to cope with this illness?
- For what in your life do you still feel gratitude even though ill?
- When you are afraid or in pain, how do you find comfort?
- As we plan for your medical care near the end of life, in what ways will your religion and spirituality influence your decisions?

improving pain symptoms in one domain has the potential to improve symptoms found in the other domains, thereby creating a beneficial synergy. For example, a patient dying of ovarian cancer who is estranged from her adult son (social pain) may experience a lower threshold of her physical, emotional, and spiritual pain. Assisting in healing the relationship with her son will relieve her social pain and allow her to experience a higher threshold for her physical, emotional, and spiritual pain symptoms.

FUNCTIONAL ASSESSMENT

Tools that describe a patient's level of function are helpful in identifying ways to improve quality of life, for communication between healthcare providers, and for prognostication. Useful tools include the Palliative Performance Scale (PPS), the Karnofsky Performance Status (KPS) scale, and the Eastern Cooperative Oncology Group (ECOG). The PPS, KPS, and ECOG address the patient's ability to carry out normal activities and work. The PPS also addresses oral intake and level of consciousness. PPS and KPS scales use percentages of maximum capacity (e.g., 100% indicates no deficits, 0% indicates death). The ECOG uses a grade from 0 (fully active, able to carry on all pre-disease activities) to a grade of 4 (completely disabled, cannot carry out any self-care, totally confined to bed or chair). A PPS score of less than 60% to 70% roughly correlates with a short (6 weeks) prognosis, depending on the life-limiting diagnosis. Most oncologists will not pursue chemotherapy if a patient has an ECOG greater than 2.

PAIN AND SYMPTOM MANAGEMENT

Under-treatment of pain during end-of-life care remains a widespread problem that increases suffering for patients, families, and caregivers. Pain should be anticipated and prevented when possible (e.g., pre-medicate for re-positioning or wound care; prevent bedsores; avoid futile tests/treatments). When treating pain, however, other symptoms should be carefully assessed as well; sometimes "pain" is really fatigue, dyspnea, nausea, constipation, loneliness (i.e., social/spiritual pain), anxiety (i.e., emotional pain), or other condition.

The most effective agents for initial and adjunctive treatment of pain are specific to the *type* of pain, and often to the *site* of pain as well. Some classic examples are the use of gabapentin and/or nortriptyline for neuropathic pain, NSAIDS and/or bisphosphonates for pain from bony metastases, and corticosteroids for pain from tumor-related compression/swelling. Opiates are appropriate for all types of pain at the end of life, and should be used early in the course of pain treatment.

When initiating pain medications, low-potency agents should be used first (e.g., morphine 2.5 mg to 10 mg PO q2–4h, oxycodone 2.5 to 5 mg PO q3–4h, or hydrocodone/APAP 5/325-10/325, 1–2 PO q4h) and titrated quickly to obtain the desired relief, increasing the dose by 25% to 50% per increment. Combination analgesics such as hydrocodone/APAP and oxycodone/APAP have the obvious limitation of a "ceiling dose" due to potential APAP toxicity. In the opiate-tolerant patient or during a pain crisis, opiate titration must be carefully calculated and appropriately aggressive, increasing the dose by 50% to 100% per increment, and using a shorter dosing interval (e.g., time to Cmax or 1 to 2 hours for most oral opiates). Once the effective dose and interval is determined, the use of scheduled/routine pain medication is more effective and thus preferred over "as-needed" (i.e., prn) use. As-needed pain medication should be used for "breakthrough" pain, at a dose proportional to the scheduled opiate dose (typically 10% to 25% of the total daily opiate usage). In general for end-of-life care, opiates need not be delayed or withheld for fear of respiratory depression, as the dose required for analgesia is generally well below the dose likely to suppress respiratory drive.

Both pharmacokinetics (duration of onset/action) and the delivery system should be carefully considered (i.e., pill vs. liquid; IV vs. SQ vs. transdermal; oral vs. rectal, etc.), and tailored to individual patient. Effective end-of-life care requires some facility with alternate delivery routes (transdermal, subcutaneous, sublingual, nasal), as the oral, rectal, or IV routes may not be appropriate for a given patient. Side effects (nausea, constipation, unwanted sedation, delirium, and neurotoxicity) should be anticipated, monitored closely, and treated promptly. Some analgesics used for end-of-life care require special expertise and caution (e.g., methadone, fentanyl, buprenorphine).

The goal of complete pain relief is sometimes elusive, and must be weighed against the competing goals of function and alertness. Generally, drug dependency is not a concern. Chronic nonmalignant pain is a disease in its own right, and is not addressed in this section/chapter.

Non-Pain Suffering/Symptoms

Symptom management should focus on minimizing suffering and maximizing function (e.g., control of nausea or anxiety while preserving alertness). This balance between relief of suffering and improvement in function may change during the progression of illness as the patient's goals of care change. Symptom assessment may be challenging; patients may be too afraid, proud, weak, or tired to divulge symptoms on their own, but will usually discuss them if asked. When a patient is cognitively impaired, the particulars of pain, fatigue, nausea, etc. must be solicited from caregivers, family, and staff as well as the patient, using culturally appropriate tools and language. A formal Palliative Care consult should be considered when symptoms are difficult to control and an unacceptable level of suffering persists. Some very common causes of suffering for dying patients are not addressed here due to space limitations (constipation, urinary problems, fatigue, end-of-life emergencies, etc.). *Note*: all medications recommended below are for "typical" adults and adolescents, and may not apply to children or to the very elderly.

Dyspnea is the "sensation of breathlessness." Dyspnea is present in a majority of patients near the end of life. Treating the underlying cause(s), when appropriate and possible, may provide adequate relief (e.g., oxygen for hypoxia, bronchodilators for bronchospasm, anxiolytics for anxiety, etc.). Much relief can be provided by simple interventions such as a bedside fan or relaxation and breathing techniques. The mainstay medications for relief of dyspnea are opiates. Morphine sulfate is the drug of choice to decrease the sensation of air hunger, though any opiate should provide relief of dyspnea. Low doses of concentrated liquid morphine (20 mg per mL) given PO or SL will be effective for most patients. Opiates should not be withheld for fear of respiratory depression in the context of end-of-life care. The effective dose of an opiate for treatment of dyspnea is typically well below the dose that will suppress respiratory drive; a low starting dose with fairly rapid titration is safe and effective for dyspnea as well as pain. Audible, excessive respiratory secretions shortly before death (i.e., the "death rattle") are often treated by administration of potent anticholinergics, such as atropine drops (1% ophthalmic solution) one to four drops SL q4h, or scopolamine transdermal patch, though evidence for efficacy is lacking. Consider stopping any unnecessary hydration or gastric tube feeding that may contribute to pulmonary congestion or aspiration.

Treatment of **nausea and vomiting** depends on its cause(s) (e.g., peptic ulcer disease, constipation, offending odors, medications, etc.), and may include behavioral, environmental, medical, and pharmacologic interventions. The *vomiting center* (in the medulla) receives stimuli from various sites, so choosing medication(s) that targets the appropriate receptor/mechanism improves the likelihood of relief with the least number of medications. For example, nausea caused by anxiety (higher cortical stimulus) may not be relieved by an agent that primarily targets the GI tract (e.g., metoclopramide) or the chemoreceptor trigger zone (CTZ) (e.g., ondansetron). When uncertain about the causes of nausea, start empiric therapy using an agent with action at multiple receptor sites and with the lowest risk of toxicity for your patient (e.g., metoclopramide, prochlorperazine). For persistent nausea, scheduled/routine as well as "prn" dosing is recommended, analogous to treatment of persistent pain. A combination of agents is often needed. Some common agents include: **dopamine agonists,** effective at the CTZ for nausea caused by chemotherapy, metabolic derangements, etc. (prochlorperazine 5 to 20 mg PO/PR/IV Q4–8h [*also anti-histamine], haloperidol 0.5 to 1 mg PO/SQ/IV Q6–12h); **H1 antagonists (anti-histamines),** effective for GI and vestibular-related nausea (promethazine 25 mg PO/IV Q4–6h [Not SQ], meclizine 25 mg PO Q6–12h); **5-HT3 (serotonin) antagonists,** effective for GI and CTZ-related nausea (ondansetron 4 to 8 mg BID–TID PO/SQ/IV); **pro-motility agents** (metoclopramide 5 to 20 mg PO/IV/SQ/PR Q4–8h [max 60 mg per day; *also has dopamine and 5HT3 antagonist effects at higher doses]); **corticosteroids,** effective for GI- and tumor-related nausea (dexamethasone 2 to 4 mg PO/SQ/IV daily-QID, prednisone 10 to 40 mg* PO daily-QID); **anxiolytics,** for the "higher cortical" stimuli, such as anticipatory or anxiety-related nausea (lorazepam 0.5 to 2 mg PO/SL/SQ/IV q4–6h); **cannabinoids** (dronabinol 2.5 mg PO BID, titrated up; medical cannabis in various forms; **substance P antagonists,** i.e., NK1 antagonists, for chemotherapy-related nausea (aprepitant, variable dosing, usually given with a corticosteroid and 5-HT3 antagonist).

Anorexia–cachexia. Food is often seen as a sign of life and hope, and compromised intake may be seen as a sign of despair or abandonment. End-of-life patients often have decreased hunger and thirst, however, and should control their own dietary intake. Trial of an appetite stimulant may result in weight gain and improved quality of life for some patients but does not decrease mortality. Agents include megestrol 800 mg daily, dexamethasone 1 to 2 mg PO BID, and dronabinol 2.5 to 5 mg PO BID for a trial of 8 to 12 weeks. Forced feedings do not prolong life. Tube feeding in demented patients does not increase longevity or improve quality of life for the patient. And for some cancers, increased feeding may speed the rate of cancer growth. Potential benefits of artificial (assisted) nutrition and hydration (ANH) in terminally ill patients may include improvement in strength and function, and reduction of fatigue. Potential burdens include increasing patient pain or anxiety with forced oral intake, gastric distention and aspiration, worsening CHF or ascites, and the surgical risks of tube placement. Families may need repeated education and support to avoid confusing anorexia and cachexia (a normal part of the disease/dying process) with starvation (suffering or death caused by hunger).

When anorexia occurs in a patient for whom oral intake is desired and appropriate, he/she should be evaluated for pain control, depression, constipation, oral candidiasis/mucositis, and dysphagia. **Dysphagia** (difficulty swallowing) is a common issue with very ill patients and has many possible causes. **Painful swallowing** (odynophagia) caused by chemotherapy-induced mucositis is managed by providing softer, colder, nonacidic foods, by offering lidocaine 2% swish/spit q4–8h, by using compounded analgesic mouthwashes (e.g., "magic mouthwash" containing Maalox/Benadryl/lidocaine, or morphine-containing mouthwash), or by using doxepin oral rinse (5 mg per 5 mL) every 4 to 6 hours. **Dry mouth** can significantly impair swallowing, and is caused by medications, radiation, mouth-breathing, and systemic dehydration. In addition to minimizing anticholinergic medication use, consider providing humidified air, saliva substitutes, sugar-free gum, sips of water, ice chips, a moist sponge stick, pilocarpine 5 to 10 mg PO BID or TID, or systemic hydration if appropriate (via IV, SQ, or enteral route). Oropharyngeal **infections** are treated according to suspected cause. Candidiasis, gingivitis (best prevented with attentive oral hygiene), and herpetic infections are addressed elsewhere in this text.

Anxiety may be due to dyspnea, pain, or a specific patient fear (fear of dying, suffering, abandonment, etc.). Treatment, when needed, will depend in part on the patient's other symptoms: some pain and nausea medications, for example, may also be anxiolytic. Treatment may also depend on how much sedation is acceptable to the patient/caregiver. The mainstay for treating anxiety is the short-acting benzodiazepines, such as lorazepam, 0.5 to 2 mg PO, SL or SQ BID–QID, or alprazolam, 0.25 to 1 mg PO BID–QID. If the prognosis is greater than 6 to 8 weeks, a trial of a selective serotonin re-uptake inhibitor (e.g., citalopram, sertraline, etc.) is reasonable. When **insomnia** is present, use of a sedating antidepressant such as nortriptyline 10 to 100 mg PO at bedtime, or trazodone, 50 to 100 mg PO BID–TID is reasonable. However, especially in elderly, the well-known risks of sedation, falls, confusion, and delirium with benzodiazepines and anticholinergics must be measured against their benefits and against the patient's goals of care.

Agitation should always be approached as a sign of another underlying problem, though it may be a sign/symptom in its own right, especially among patients with dementia or other cognitive impairment (tumor, stroke, encephalopathy, etc.). Common causes include anxiety, constipation, bladder distention, pain, and medication side effects. For patients who cannot communicate their needs (e.g., with advanced dementia), a trial of analgesics is indicated as evaluation for other causes is under way. **Delirium,** often manifesting as agitation, is a distinct clinical entity defined by the following: acute onset; waxing/waning course; altered level of consciousness; cognitive deficits; and inattentiveness. Delirium may be hyperactive, hypoactive, or a mixed type. Delirium is known to cause suffering, and the signs of agitation and confusion are distressing to family and caregivers. After addressing the underlying "organic" causes of delirium (see section on Delirium for more info), the most effective medications for relief of symptoms are the antipsychotics, such as haloperidol, 0.5 to 2 mg PO/SL/SQ/IV q2–4h (titrated up to effect), risperidone (Risperdal), 0.25 to 2 mg PO BID or TID (ODT available), quetiapine (Seroquel) 12.5 to 200 mg PO QHS or BID, or olanzapine (Zyprexa), 1.25 to 5 mg PO QD (ODT available). Irreversible or "terminal" delirium is a diagnosis made in retrospect, and refers to delirium in the patient with signs of impending death: mottled skin; cool extremities; Cheyne–Stokes breathing; deepening somnolence; talking to/about dead family/friends, or about taking a trip, packing up, leaving. The key difference in managing terminal delirium is permissive use of sedating medications (benzodiazepines, barbiturates) that are normally contraindicated in "reversible" delirium.

- **Ethical treatment issues**
  - **Do not attempt resuscitate (DNAR) orders** refer to the withholding of CPR in the event of a cardiac or pulmonary arrest. Before writing a DNAR order, the patient's clinical condition and prognosis, a description of what CPR entails, and an estimate of the patient's likely chance for survival should be discussed with the patient and family and documented in the medical record. Advance directives and POLSTs should be reviewed and/or considered. Studies suggest that when CPR is attempted in hospital, approximately 17% of patients survive to discharge and 83% die

acutely. Survival rates for patients over 75 years old and for patients with metastatic cancer are 1% to 2%.[1] Patients who choose not to be resuscitated should be reassured that other treatments will not be affected by this decision. Patients who are still at home should be advised that if an ambulance is called and emergency medical services personnel respond, CPR may be automatically initiated. Depending on the clinical situation, these patients and families should be instructed to call their physician or hospice or home health nurse first.

- **Withholding versus withdrawing care.** There is no ethical difference between withholding and withdrawing care that cannot or has not achieved its desired effect. Psychologically, however, it usually *feels* different to withdraw care. Clear communication about expectations is critical. The judicious use of treatment time trials may also be helpful. If a particular treatment is tried over a predetermined, fixed period of time and if at the end of that time the desired outcomes are not achieved, the treatment may be discontinued without guilt. In general, the concept of "benefits versus burdens" should guide decisions on the appropriateness of care. This involves engaging the patient, family, and health care team in listing the benefits and burdens of an intervention and weighing them against each other to determine use.
- **Determination of futility** depends on who decides what is futile: the patient, the family, or the physician. A treatment may be physiologically futile but may be extremely important to a patient's sense of hope or may give a family enough time to gather together. On the other hand, a patient or a family who strongly values life at all costs might insist on an intervention that clearly has no benefit but does have great burdens (e.g., administering chemotherapy to a patient with metastatic cancer who is now failing medical therapy for sepsis). If clear communication with the patient and family does not resolve disagreements regarding futile care, an ethics consultation should be obtained in order to address persistent disagreements or conflicts in patient care. Alternatively, care may be transferred to another physician who feels able to meet the patient's or family's treatment requests. A few states have specific laws and procedures governing futility decision making.
- **Euthanasia and physician-assisted suicide** are beyond the scope of this manual. However, if a patient inquires about them, the opportunity should be used to explore the reasons behind the request. Often, these patients have great fears about pain, isolation, or becoming a physical or financial burden to their families. Some may have treatable depression. Others may simply need a clarification of their medical problems and a discussion of their medical care plans.
- **Determination of death**
  - Traditionally, death has been clinically defined as the absence of spontaneous pulse and blood pressure (no circulatory function) and the absence of spontaneous breathing (no respiratory function). Often, the absence of pupillary responses (no brain function) is added.
  - Brain death criteria have been established in most states because intensive care life support systems may physiologically sustain certain organs even after a patient's cerebral functions have been permanently lost. These clinical criteria generally include coma that is documented to be irreversible (i.e., not due to drugs or hypothermia), absence of motor function and reflexes (though spinal cord reflexes may still be intact), and absence of brainstem function, established by apnea and the lack of pupillary and oculovestibular reflexes.[2]
    - Electroencephalograms and other studies may be confirmatory but are not usually required. However, some hospitals do require formal neurologic consultation before allowing a patient to be declared brain dead. Organ donation is sometimes an issue with brain-dead patients whose other organs remain viable. In these cases, death should first be declared by a physician clearly unassociated with the transplant team, and the discussion of organ donation should follow.

BEREAVEMENT AND FOLLOW-UP ISSUES

- **Autopsy** should be considered when the physician or the patient's family wants certainty about the cause of death, to confirm the clinical diagnosis, to evaluate the level of response to a particular treatment, or to be reassured that care was appropriate and death unavoidable. Legally, the local coroner's office must be notified when an individual dies without medical attendance, when the attending physician is unable to state the cause of death, or when death follows an accident or injury, including suicide or homicide. Asking about autopsies should be simple and direct, emphasizing the considerations outlined previously. The discussion should follow family notification of the death and preferably occur in person (though, in most states, consent for autopsy may be obtained over the phone). If an autopsy is performed, a family conference should be arranged afterward to discuss the findings. The costs of an autopsy are usually not covered by health insurance plans. However, many hospitals provide autopsies as a quality control measure at no charge.

- **Family follow-up issues** focus on promoting the tasks of bereavement, which include feeling sadness and pain, accepting the reality of the loss, and redirecting time and energy from caring for the deceased to other activities. Reassuring family members that they will not be abandoned, normalizing their reactions, and encouraging open communication are all helpful. Appropriate comments include "It's OK to feel both sad and angry" and "Death is hard to understand; have you talked with your family or minister about how you're handling things?"
- **Physician follow-up issues.** The death of a patient who has had a very complicated course of disease or with whom the physician has developed a close relationship is often a great personal loss. Complicating this loss may be a sense of guilt or personal failure. Just as family and friends must grieve to recover, physicians too should be allowed to grieve by discussing a patient's death with staff, colleagues, or their own families, if appropriate. Attending a patient's funeral service should be considered a means of both assisting the physician's own grief work and showing support for the patient's family.

Conclusion

End-of-life care requires a thoughtful blend of the "art and science" of medicine delivered to a "whole person" (patient, family, caregivers). To provide effective and compassionate care at the end of life, physicians must be facile in the areas of palliative medicine and prognostication, communication and culture, bioethics, and a team approach to patient care. By clarifying the goals of care, by remaining flexible and nonjudgmental, and by facilitating excellent communication, the care team can maintain hope and support meaning for a "whole person," and provide a dignified and comfortable death for most patients.

REFERENCES

1. Tunzi M. A new standard for incapacitated patient decision making: the clinical standard of surrogate empowerment. *J Clin Ethics* 2012;23:316–330.
2. Elsayem A, Driver L, Bruera E. *The M.D. Anderson supportive and palliative care handbook*. 3rd ed. Houston, TX: The University of Texas; 2008.
3. Geoffrey H, Cherny NI, Christakis NA, et al. *Oxford textbook of palliative medicine*. 4th ed. New York, NY: Oxford University Press; 2011.
4. *Hospice and palliative care training for physicians: self-study program (AAHPM, UNIPAC Book Series)*. 4th ed. Glenview, IL: American Academy of Hospice and Palliative Medicine; 2012.
5. Buckman R. *How to break bad news: a guide for health care professionals*. Baltimore, MD: Johns Hopkins University Press; 1992.
6. Kubler-Ross E. *On death and dying*. New York, NY: Macmillan; 1969.
7. Lo B. *Resolving ethical dilemmas*. 5th ed. Baltimore, MD: Lippincott Williams & Wilkins; 2013.
8. Doyle D, Hanks G, Cherny N, et al. *Oxford textbook of palliative medicine*. 3rd ed. New York, NY: Oxford University Press; 2003.
9. Wijdicks EFM. The diagnosis of brain death. *N Engl J Med* 2001;344:1215–1221.
10. Wade DT, Johnston C. The permanent vegetative state: practical guidance on diagnosis and management. *BMJ* 1999;319:841–844.

Index

Note: Page numbers followed by "f" refer to illustrations; page numbers followed by "t" refer to tables.